Medications *and* Mothers' Milk

A Manual of Lactational Pharmacology

2012

Medications *and* Mothers' Milk

Fifteenth Edition

Thomas W. Hale, R.PH., Ph.D.

Professor

Department of Pediatrics

Texas Tech University

School of Medicine

Amarillo, TX 79106

Medications and Mothers' Milk

Fifteenth Edition

Hale Publishing, L.P.

1712 N. Forest

Amarillo, TX 79106-7017

Cover photograph by Paola Paschetto

DISCLAIMER

The information contained in this publication is intended to supplement the knowledge of healthcare professionals regarding drug use during lactation. This information is advisory only and is not intended to replace sound clinical judgment or individualized patient care. The author disclaims all warranties, whether expressed or implied, of this information for any particular purpose.

Printed in the United States of America

Printed by Edwards Brothers Malloy

ISBN: 978-0-9847746-3-0

Library of Congress Number: 2012932138

Foreward

New Changes In This Edition:

This edition has the largest number of changes I have ever placed in this book. It contains hundreds of new drugs, diseases, herbals, and many other additions.

Because of this mass of new data, I have changed the size of the book in order to place this new data. We simply ran out of space with the smaller formatted book.

In addition, in May of 2010, the American Academy of Pediatrics withdrew and retired (redacted) their old policy statement on the transfer of drugs and other chemicals into human milk. Since this publication was both retired and withdrawn, I decided it was only proper to remove all safety recommendations by the AAP.

Other Changes include:

- We transferred all the radiocontrast agents, and anti-cancer drugs out of the appendix into the body of the book, and added many more.

- We placed a new set of radiation tables into Appendix A, which now includes much new data, including close contact restrictions, which suggest how long mothers should be away from their infant to preclude irradiating their infant from close contact.

- We have included more over-the-counter drugs this year, although it is not as complete as the *Nonprescription Drugs for the Breastfeeding Mother* by Frank Nice.

- We have added numerous diseases, vaccines, and many new immune-modulating drugs.

Lastly, I would also like to thank all the pharmacy students who worked diligently to help in this edition. Most specially, I would like to thank two wonderful colleagues, Dr. Almas Zane and Dr. Maria Milla, who helped so much in the production of this work.

TWH

Preface

INTRODUCTION

Everyone now agrees that human milk is best for human infants. The benefits to growth and development are obvious and confirmed by many studies. However, the use of medications in breastfeeding mothers is often controversial and steeped in misconception by the medical field. This book is dedicated to reducing some of these misconceptions. The truth is most drugs don't enter milk in levels that are hazardous to a breastfed infant. The problem is which drugs are safe and which are hazardous?

Because so few clinicians understand lactational pharmacology, the number of women who discontinue breastfeeding in order to take a medication is still far too high. Fortunately, many mothers are now becoming aware of the enormous benefits of breastfeeding and simply refuse to follow some of the advice given by their healthcare professionals. They seek out the information on their own and invariably find this book.

Because so many women ingest medications during the early neonatal period, it is not surprising that one of the most common questions encountered in pediatrics concerns the use of various drugs during lactation. Unfortunately, most healthcare professionals simply review the package insert or advise the mother not to breastfeed without having done a thorough study of the literature to find the true answer. Discontinuing breastfeeding is often the wrong decision, and most mothers could easily continue to breastfeed and take the medication without risk to the infant.

In the last 25 years we have collected a lot of data on many current medications and their use in breastfeeding. This book contains most of this knowledge.

It is generally accepted that all medications transfer into human milk to some degree, although it is almost always quite low. Only rarely does the amount transferred into milk produce clinical doses in the infant. Ultimately, it is the clinician's responsibility to review the research we have on the drugs in this book and make a clear decision as to whether the mother should continue to breastfeed.

Since the PDR basically lists only the pharmaceutical manufacturer's package insert, the standard recommendation is to not take the medication while breastfeeding. Therefore, the PDR is the poorest source for obtaining accurate breastfeeding information.

Drugs may transfer into human milk if they:

Attain high concentrations in maternal plasma

Are low in molecular weight (< 500)

Are low in protein binding

Pass into the brain easily

However, once medications transfer into human milk, other kinetic factors are involved. One of the most important is the oral bioavailability of the medication to the infant. Numerous medications are either destroyed in the infant's gut, fail to be absorbed through the gut wall, or are rapidly picked up by the liver. Once in the liver, they are either metabolized or stored, but often never reach the mother's plasma.

Drugs normally enter milk by passive diffusion, driven by equilibrium forces between the maternal plasma compartment and the maternal milk compartment. They pass from the maternal plasma through capillaries into the lactocytes lining the alveolus. Medications must generally pass through both bilayer lipid membranes of the alveolar cell to penetrate milk; although early on, they may pass between the alveolar cells (first 72 hours postpartum). During the first three days of life, large gaps between the alveolar cells exist. These gaps permit enhanced access into the milk for most drugs, many immunoglobulins, maternal living cells (lymphocytes, leukocytes, macrophages), and other maternal proteins. By the end of the first week, the alveolar cells swell under the influence of prolactin, subsequently closing the intracellular gaps and reducing the transcellular entry of most maternal drugs, proteins, and other substances into the milk compartment. It is generally agreed that medications penetrate into milk more during the colostrum period than in mature milk. However, the absolute dose transferred during the colostrum period is still low as the total volume of milk is generally less than 30-100 mL total volume/day for the first few days postpartum.

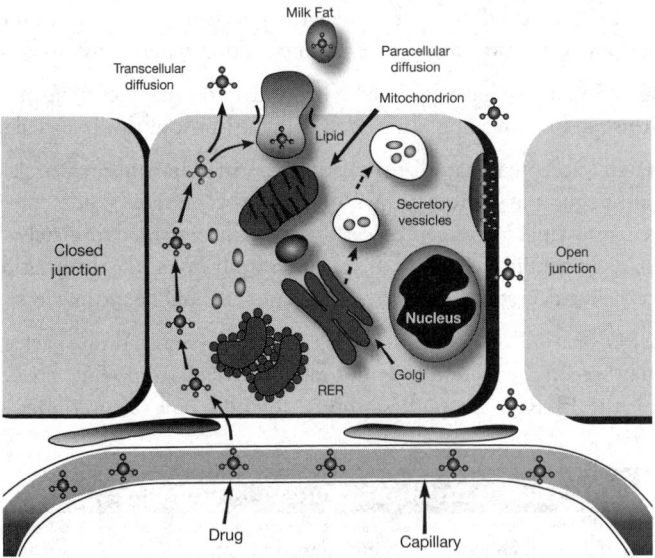

In most instances, the most important determinant of drug penetration into milk is the mother's plasma level. Almost without exception, as the level of the medication in the mother's plasma rises, the concentration in milk increases as well. Drugs enter and exit milk as a function of the mother's plasma level. As soon as the maternal plasma level of a medication begins to fall, equilibrium forces drive the medication out of the milk compartment back into the maternal plasma for elimination. In some instances, drugs are trapped in milk (ion trapping) due to the lower pH of human milk (7.0-7.2). With drugs with a high pKa, the ionic state of the drug changes and stops its exit back into the maternal circulation. This is important in weakly basic drugs, such as the barbiturates (drugs with high pKa). There are a few known cellular pumping systems that actively pump drugs into milk. The most important is iodine. The iodine pump is the same as found in everyone's thyroid gland. Its purpose is to make sure the infant receives iodine to maintain thyroxine production.

The iodides, such as ^{131}I or any "ionic" form of iodine, concentrate in milk due to this pump. Thus iodides, particularly radioactive ones, should be avoided as their milk concentrations are exceedingly high. Two other physicochemical factors are important in evaluating drugs in breastfeeding mothers—the degree of protein binding and lipid solubility. Drugs that are very lipid soluble penetrate into milk in higher concentrations almost without exception. Of particular interest are the drugs that are active in the central nervous system (CNS). CNS-active drugs invariably have the unique characteristics required to enter milk. Therefore, if a drug is active in the central nervous system, higher levels in milk can be expected; although, the amounts still are often subclinical. Many of the neuroactive drugs produce Relative Infant Doses of >5%. Protein binding also plays an important role. Drugs circulate in the maternal plasma, either bound to albumin or freely soluble in the plasma. It is the free component (unbound fraction) that transfers into milk, while the bound fraction stays in the maternal circulation. Therefore, drugs that have high maternal protein binding (warfarin, many NSAIDs) have reduced milk levels simply because they are excluded from the milk compartment.

Once a drug has entered the mother's milk and has been ingested by the infant, it must traverse through the infant's GI tract prior to absorption. Some drugs are poorly stable in this environment due to the proteolytic enzymes and acids present in the infant's stomach. This includes the aminoglycoside family, Omeprazole, and large peptide drugs, such as Heparin or Insulin. Other drugs are poorly absorbed by the infant's gastrointestinal tract and do not enter the infant's blood stream. Thus, oral bioavailability is a useful tool to estimate just how much of the drug will be absorbed by the infant. Many drugs are sequestered in the liver (first pass) and may never actually reach the plasma compartment where they are active. Absorption characteristics such as these ultimately tend to reduce the overall effect of many drugs in breastfed infants. There are certainly exceptions to this rule, and one must always be aware that the action of a drug in the GI tract can be profound, producing diarrhea, constipation, and occasionally syndromes such as pseudomembranous colitis. One of the more popular methods for estimating risk is to determine the Relative Infant Dose (RID). The RID is calculated by dividing the infant's dose via milk (mg/kg/day) by the mothers dose in mg/kg/day. The RID gives the clinician a feeling for just how much medication the infant is exposed to on a weight-normalized basis. However, many authors calculate the infant dose without normalizing for maternal and infant weight, so be cautious.

Relative Infant Dose

$$RID = \frac{Dose.infant\ \frac{mg/kg}{d}}{Dose.mother\ \frac{mg/kg}{d}}$$

Dose.infant = dose in infant

Dose.mother = dose in mother

Key Points About Breastfeeding and Medications

- Avoid using medications that are not necessary. Herbal drugs, high dose vitamins, unusual supplements, etc. that are simply not necessary should be avoided

- If the Relative Infant Dose is less than 10%, most medications are quite safe to use. The RID of vast majority of drugs is <1%.

- Choose drugs for which we have published data, rather than those recently introduced.

- Evaluate the infant for risks. Be slightly more cautious with premature infants or neonates.

- Medication used in the first three to four days generally produce subclinical levels in the infant due to the limited volume of milk

- Recommend that mothers with symptoms of depression or other mental disorders seek treatment. Most of the medications used to treat these syndromes are safe.

- Most drugs are quite safe in breastfeeding mothers. The hazards of using formula are well known and documented.

- Discontinuing breastfeeding for some hours/days may be required, particularly with radioactive compounds. Follow the guidelines in the appendices of this book.

- Choose drugs with short half-lives, high protein binding, low oral bioavailability, or high molecular weight.

Lastly, it is terribly important to always evaluate the infant's ability to handle small amounts of medications. Some infants, such as premature or unstable infants, may not be suitable candidates for certain medications. But remember that early postpartum (and in late stage lactation), the amount of milk produced (30-100 cc/day) is so low that the clinical dose of drug transferred is often low, so even premature neonates would receive only a limited amount from the milk.

Evaluation of the Infant

- Inquire about the infant—always inquire as to the infant's age, size, and stability. This is perhaps the most important criterion to be evaluated prior to using the medication.

- Infant age—premature and newborn infants are at somewhat greater risk. Older infant are at somewhat lower risk due to high metabolic capacity.

- Infant stability—unstable infants with poor GI stability may increase the risk of using medications.

- Pediatric Approved Drugs—generally are less hazardous if long-term history of safety is recognized.

- Dose vs Age—the age of an infant is critical. Use medications cautiously in premature infants. Older, mature infants can metabolize and clear medications much easier. Remember the dose of the drug is dependent on milk supply. In mothers in late-stage lactation (>1 year), milk production is often low, so is the dose of drug delivered.

- Drugs that alter milk production—avoid medications that may alter the mother's milk production. See the appendices for lists of such drugs.

GENERAL SUGGESTIONS FOR THE CLINICIAN

Determine if the drug is absorbed from the GI tract. Many drugs, such as the aminoglycosides, vancomycin, cephalosporin antibiotics (third generation), morphine, magnesium salts, and large protein drugs (heparin), are so poorly absorbed that it is unlikely the infant will absorb significant quantities. At the same time, observe for GI side effects from the medication trapped in the GI compartment of the infant (e.g., diarrhea).

Review the Relative Infant Dose (RID) and compare that to the pediatric dose if known. Most of the RID were derived from the C_{max} (highest milk concentration of the drug) that were published. In this edition, I've added 'ranges' of RID, so the reader can see the various dose estimates from different studies. The milk/plasma ratio is virtually worthless unless you know the maternal plasma level. It does not provide the user with information as to the absolute amount of drug transferred to the infant via milk. Even if the drug has a high milk/plasma ratio, if the maternal plasma level of the medication is very small (such as with propranolol), then the absolute amount (dose) of a drug entering milk will still be quite small and often subclinical.

Try to use medications with shorter half-lives as they are generally eliminated from the maternal plasma rapidly, thus exposing the milk compartment (and the infant) to reduced levels of medication. This is particularly true with anti-cancer drugs.

Be cautious of drugs (or their active metabolites) that have long pediatric half-lives as they can continually build up in the infant's plasma over time. The barbiturates, benzodiazepines, and meperidine are classic examples where higher levels in the infant can and do occasionally occur.

If you are provided a choice, choose drugs that have higher protein binding because they are generally sequestered in the maternal circulation and do not transfer readily into the milk compartment or the infant. Remember, it's the free drug that transfers into the milk compartment. Without doubt, the most important parameter that determines drug penetration into milk is plasma protein binding. Choose drugs with high protein binding.

Although not always true, I have generally found centrally active drugs (anticonvulsants, antidepressants, antipsychotic) frequently penetrate milk in higher (not necessarily 'high') levels simply due to their physicochemistry. If the drug in question produces sedation, depression, or other neuroleptic effects in the mother, it is likely to penetrate the milk and may produce similar effects in the infant. Thus, with CNS-active drugs, one should always check the data in this book closely and monitor the infant routinely.

Be cautious of herbal drugs as many contain chemical substances that may be dangerous to the infant. Numerous poisonings have been reported. Prior to using, advise the mother to contact a lactation consultant or herbalist who is knowledgeable about their use in breastfeeding mothers. Do not exceed standard recommended doses. Try to use pure forms, not large mixtures of unknown herbals. Do not overdose, use only minimal amounts.

For radioactive compounds, I have gathered much of the published data in this field into several new tables. The Nuclear Regulatory Commission recommendations are quite good, but they differ from some published data. They can be copied and provided to your radiologist. They are available from the Nuclear Regulatory Commission's web page address in the appendix.

Use the Relative Infant Dose. The box below shows the calculation. In general, a Relative Infant Dose of < 10% is considered safe, and its use is becoming increasingly popular by numerous investigators.

Most importantly, it is seldom required that a breastfeeding mother discontinue breastfeeding just to take a medication. It is simply not acceptable for the clinician to stop lactation merely because of heightened anxiety or ignorance on their part. The risks of formula feeding are significant and should not be trivialized. Few drugs have documented side effects in breastfed infants, and we know most of these.

The following review of drugs, and even diseases, is a thorough review of what has been published and what we presently know about the use of medications in breastfeeding mothers.

THE AUTHOR MAKES NO RECOMMENDATIONS AS TO THE SAFETY OF THESE MEDICATIONS DURING LACTATION, BUT ONLY REVIEWS WHAT IS CURRENTLY PUBLISHED IN THE SCIENTIFIC LITERATURE. INDIVIDUAL USE OF MEDICATIONS MUST BE LEFT UP TO THE JUDGEMENT OF THE PHYSICIAN, THE PATIENT, AND OTHER HEALTHCARE CONSULTANTS.

Thomas W. Hale

How To Use This Book

This section of the book is designed to aid the reader in determining risk to an infant from maternal medications and in using the pharmacokinetic parameters throughout this reference.

Drug Name and Generic Name:

Each monograph begins with the generic name of the drug. Several of the most common USA trade names are provided under the Trade section.

Other Trades:

This book is used all over the world. Thus many other trade names from other countries are now included in this section.

Category:

This lists the class or 'family of drugs' that the medication belongs to and gives a general idea of the pharmacology, mechanism of action and probable use of the drug.

Drug Monograph:

The drug monograph lists what we currently understand about the drug, its ability to enter milk, the concentration in milk at set time intervals, and other parameters that are important to a clinical consultant. I have attempted at great length to report only what the references have documented.

PREGNANCY RISK CATEGORY:

Pregnancy risk categories have been assigned to almost all medications by their manufacturers and are based on the level of risk the drug poses to the fetus during gestation. They are not useful in assigning risk via breastfeeding. The FDA has provided these five categories to indicate the risk associated with the induction of birth defects. Unfortunately, they do not indicate the importance of when during gestation the medication is used. For this reason, I have added small comments to indicate that some drugs are more dangerous during certain trimesters of pregnancy. The definitions provided below are, however, a useful tool in determining the possible risks associated with using the medication during pregnancy. Some of the herbal supplements, infectious agents and newer medications may not have pregnancy classifications and are therefore not provided herein. Instead, for such drugs, based on published data, I have given a pregnancy rating. Note that this rating is only to give the patient and the healthcare professional an idea of what the probable consequence of the drug during pregnancy might be.

Category A:

Controlled studies in women fail to demonstrate a risk to the fetus in the first trimester (and there is no evidence of a risk in later trimesters) and the possibility of fetal harm appears remote.

Category B:

Either animal-reproduction studies have not demonstrated a fetal risk, but there are no controlled studies in pregnant women, or animal reproduction studies have shown an adverse effect (other than a decrease in fertility) that was not confirmed in controlled studies in women in the first trimester (and there is no evidence of a risk in later trimesters).

Category C:

Either studies in animals have revealed adverse effects on the fetus (teratogenic or embryocidal, or other) and there are no controlled studies in women, or studies in women and animals are not available. Drugs should be given only if the potential benefit justifies the potential risk to the fetus.

Category D:

There is positive evidence of human fetal risk, but the benefits from use in pregnant women may be acceptable despite the risk (e.g., if the drug is needed in a life-threatening situation or for a serious disease for which safer drugs cannot be used or are ineffective).

Category X:

Studies in animals or human beings have demonstrated fetal abnormalities, or there is evidence of fetal risk based on human experience, or both, and the risk of the use of the drug in pregnant women clearly outweighs any possible benefit. The drug is contraindicated in women who are or may become pregnant.

DR. HALE'S LACTATION RISK CATEGORY:

L1 Safest:

Drug which has been taken by a large number of breastfeeding mothers without any observed increase in adverse effects in the infant. Controlled studies in breastfeeding women fail to demonstrate a risk to the infant and the possibility of harm to the breastfeeding infant is remote; or the product is not orally bioavailable in an infant.

L2 Safer:

Drug which has been studied in a limited number of breastfeeding women without an increase in adverse effects in the infant. And/or, the evidence of a demonstrated risk which is likely to follow use of this medication in a breastfeeding woman is remote.

L3 Probably Safe:

There are no controlled studies in breastfeeding women; however, the risk of untoward effects to a breastfed infant is possible, or controlled studies show only minimal non-threatening adverse effects. Drugs should be given only if the potential benefit justifies the potential risk to the infant. (New medications that have absolutely no published data are automatically categorized in this category, regardless of how safe they may be.)

L4 Possibly Hazardous:

There is positive evidence of risk to a breastfed infant or to breastmilk production, but the benefits from use in breastfeeding mothers may be acceptable despite the risk to the infant (e.g., if the drug is needed in a life-threatening situation or for a serious disease for which safer drugs cannot be used or are ineffective.)

L5 Hazardous:

Studies in breastfeeding mothers have demonstrated that there is significant and documented risk to the infant based on human experience, or it is a medication that has a high risk of causing significant damage to an infant. The risk of using the drug in breastfeeding women clearly outweighs any possible benefit from breastfeeding. The drug is contraindicated in women who are breastfeeding an infant.

Relative Infant Dose:

The Relative Infant Dose (RID) is calculated by dividing the infant's dose via milk in "mg/kg/day" by the maternal dose in "mg/kg/day" (see page 9). This weight-normalizing method indicates approximately how much of the "maternal dose" the infant is receiving. Many authors now use this preferred method because it gives a better indication of the relative dose transferred to the infant. In this edition, I now report RID ranges, which is the RID published by various authors. This gives the reader an estimate of all the Relative Infant Doses published by the various authors.

Please understand, however, that many authors use different methods for calculating RID. Some are not weight-normalized. In these cases, their estimates may differ slightly from this book. While I often place the 'authors' estimates of Relative Infant Dose, the RID range that I calculate is based on a 70 Kg mother and is weight-normalized in all instances. So RID may be slightly different according to how it is calculated.

Many researchers now suggest that anything less than 10% of the maternal dose is probably safe. This is usually correct. However, some drugs (metronidazole, fluconazole) actually have much higher Relative Infant Doses, but because they are quite non-toxic, they do not often bother an infant. To calculate this dose, I chose the data I felt was best, and this often included larger studies with AUC calculations of mean concentrations in milk. I also chose an average body weight of 70 kg for an adult. Thus, the RIDs herein are calculated assuming a maternal average weight of 70 kg and a daily milk intake of 150 mL/kg/day in the infant. Please note, many authors fail to normalize their data for weight. Others provide a

RID for 'each' feeding, not a daily average. Therefore, my values may vary slightly from others simply due to differences in the method of calculation.

Adult Concerns:

This section lists the most prevalent undesired or bothersome side effects listed for adults. As with most medications, the occurrence of these is often quite rare, generally less than 1-10% of the time. Side effects vary from one patient to another and should not be overemphasized, since most patients do not experience untoward effects.

Pediatric Concerns:

This section lists the side effects noted in the published literature as associated with medications transferred via human milk. Pediatric concerns are those effects that were noted by investigators as being associated with drug transfer via milk. In some sections, I have added comments that may not have been reported in the literature, but are well known attributes of this medication and are useful information to provide the mother so that she can better care for her infant ("Observe for weakness, apnea").

Drug Interactions:

Drug interactions generally indicate which medications, when taken together, may produce higher or lower plasma levels of other medications, or they may decrease or increase the effect of another medication. These effects may vary widely from minimal to dangerous. Because some medications have hundreds of interactions and because I had limited room to provide this information, I have listed only those that may be significant. Therefore, please be advised that this section may not be complete. In several references, I have suggested that due to the large number of interactions the reader consult a more complete drug interaction reference. Please remember that the drugs administered to a mother could interact with those being administered concurrently to an infant.

Alternatives:

Drugs listed in this section may be suitable alternate choices for the medication listed above. In many instances, if the patient cannot take the medication or it is a poor choice due to high milk concentrations, these alternates may be suitable candidates. WARNING: The alternates listed are only suggestions and may not be at all proper for the syndrome in question. Only the clinician can make this judgment. For instance, nifedipine is a calcium channel blocker with good antihypertensive qualities, but poor antiarrhythmic qualities. In this case, verapamil would be a better choice.

Adult Dosage:

This is the usual adult oral dose provided in the package insert. While these are highly variable, I chose the dose for the most common use of the medication.

T½ =

This lists the most commonly recorded adult half-life of the medication. It is very important to remember that short half-life drugs are preferred. Use this parameter to determine if the mother can successfully breastfeed around the medication by nursing the infant, then taking the medication. If the half-life is short enough (1-3 hours), then the drug level in the maternal plasma will be declining when the infant feeds again. This is ideal. If the half-life is significantly long (12-24 hours) and if your physician is open to suggestions, then find a similar medication with a shorter half-life (compare ibuprofen with naproxen).

M/P=

This lists the milk/plasma ratio. This is the ratio of the concentration of drug in the mother's milk divided by the concentration in the mother's plasma. If high (> 1-5), it is useful as an indicator of drugs that may sequester in milk in high levels. If low (< 1), it is a good indicator that only minimal levels of the drug are transferred into milk (this is preferred). While it is best to try to choose drugs with LOW milk/plasma ratios, the amount of drug which transfers into human milk is largely determined by the level of drug in the mother's plasma compartment. Even with high M/P ratios and LOW maternal plasma levels, the amount of drug that transfers is still low. Therefore, the higher M/P ratios often provide an erroneous impression that large amounts of drug are going to transfer into milk. This simply may not be true.

T_{max} =

This lists the time interval from administration of the drug until it reaches the highest level in the mother's plasma (C_{max}), which we call the peak or "time to max", hence T_{max}. Occasionally, you may be able to avoid nursing the baby when the medication is at the peak. Rather, wait until the peak is subsiding or has at least dropped significantly. Remember, drugs enter breastmilk as a function of the maternal plasma concentration. In general, the higher the mother's plasma level, the greater the entry of the drug into her milk. If possible, choose drugs that have short peak intervals, and suggest mom not breastfeed when the drug is at C_{max}.

PB=

This lists the percentage of maternal protein binding. Most drugs circulate in the blood bound to plasma albumin and other proteins. If a drug is highly protein bound, it cannot enter the milk compartment as easily. The higher the percentage of binding, the less likely the drug is to enter the maternal milk. Try to choose drugs that have high protein binding in order to reduce the infant's exposure to the medication. Good protein binding is typically greater than 90%.

Oral=

Oral bioavailability refers to the ability of a drug to reach the systemic circulation after oral administration. It is generally a good indication of the amount of medication that is absorbed into the blood stream of the patient. Drugs with low oral bioavailability are generally either poorly absorbed in the gastrointestinal tract, are destroyed in the gut, or are sequestered by the liver prior to entering the plasma compartment. The oral bioavailability listed in this text is the adult value; almost none have been published for children or neonates. Recognizing this, these values are still useful in estimating if a mother or perhaps an infant will actually absorb enough drug to provide clinically significant levels in the plasma compartment of the individual. The value listed estimates the percent of an oral dose that would be found in the plasma compartment of the individual after oral administration. In many cases, the oral bioavailability of some medications is not listed by manufacturers, but instead terms such as "Complete", "Nil", or "Poor" are used. For lack of better data, I have included these terms when no data are available on the exact amount (percentage) absorbed.

Vd=

The volume of distribution is a useful kinetic term that describes how widely the medication is distributed in the body. Drugs with high volumes of distribution (Vd) are distributed in higher concentrations in remote compartments of the body and may not stay in the blood.

For instance, digoxin enters the blood compartment and then rapidly leaves to enter the heart and skeletal muscles. Most of the drug is sequestered in these remote compartments (100 fold). Therefore, drugs with high volumes of distribution (1-20 liter/kg) generally require much longer to clear from the body than drugs with smaller volumes (0.1 liter/kg). For instance, whereas it may only require a few hours to totally clear gentamycin (Vd=0.28 l/kg), it may require weeks to clear amitriptyline (Vd=10 l/kg), which has a huge volume of distribution. In addition, some drugs may have one half-life for the plasma compartment, but may have a totally different half-life for the peripheral compartment, as half-life is a function of volume of distribution. I have found that drugs with high Vd also produce lower milk levels. For a complete description of Vd, please consult a good pharmacology reference. In this text, the units of measure for Vd are liters/kg.

pKa=

The pKa of a drug is the pH at which the drug is equally ionic and nonionic. The more ionic a drug is, the less capable it is of transferring from the milk compartment to the maternal plasma compartment. Hence, the drug becomes trapped in milk (ion-trapping). This term is useful because drugs that have a pKa higher than 7.2 may be sequestered to a slightly higher degree than one with a lower pKa. Drugs with higher pKa generally have higher milk/plasma ratios. Hence, choose drugs with a lower pKa.

MW=

The molecular weight of a medication is a significant determinant as to the entry of that medication into human milk. Medications with small molecular weights (< 200) can easily pass into milk by traversing small pores in the cell walls of the mammary epithelium (see ethanol). Drugs with higher molecular weights must traverse the membrane by dissolving in the cells' lipid membranes, which may significantly reduce milk levels. As such, the smaller the molecular weight, the higher the relative transfer of that drug into milk. Protein medications (e.g., Heparin, Insulin), which have enormous molecular weights, transfer at much lower concentrations and are virtually excluded from human breastmilk. Therefore, when possible, choose drugs with higher molecular weights to reduce their entry into milk.

Common Abbreviations

$T\frac{1}{2}$	Adult elimination half-life
T_{max}	Time to peak plasma level (PK)
M/P	Milk/Plasma Ratio
RID	Relative Infant Dose
C_{max}	Plasma or milk concentration at peak
Vd	Volume of Distribution
PB	Percent of protein binding in maternal circulation
PHL	Pediatric elimination half-life
Oral	Oral bioavailability (adult)
µg/L	Microgram per liter
ng/L	Nanogram per liter
mg/L	Milligram per liter
mL	Milliliter. One cc
NSAIDs	Non-steroidal anti-inflammatory
ACEI	Angiotensin converting enzyme inhibitor
MAOI	Monoamine oxidase inhibitors
MW	Molecular Weight
µCi	Microcurie of Radioactivity
mmol	Millimole of weight
µmol	Micromole of weight
X	Times
AUC	Area under the Curve
BID	Twice daily
TID	Three times daily
QID	Four times daily
PRN	As needed
QD	Daily
d	Day
SSRIs	Selective serotonin reuptake inhibitors
SNRIs	Serotonin norepinephrine reuptake inhibitors
TCAs	Tricyclic antidepressants
GI	Gastrointestinal
NR	Not rated
et. al	"and others"

¹¹¹INDIUM OCTREOTIDE   L4

Trade: Indium Octreotide
Other Trades:
Category: Radiopharmaceutical agent

Octreotide (Sandostatin LAR) is a long acting form consisting of microspheres containing octreotide. Octreotide is a close analog of and provides activity similar to the natural hormone somatostatin. Like somatostatin, it also suppresses LH response to GnRH, decreases splanchnic blood flow, and inhibits release of serotonin, gastrin, vasoactive intestinal peptide, secretin, motilin, and pancreatic polypeptide. It is used to treat acromegaly and carcinoid tumors. This product, if present in milk, would not likely be absorbed to any degree.

The radioactive form (^{111}Indium) leaves the plasma rapidly; one-third of the radioactive injected dose remains in the blood pool at 10 minutes after administration. Plasma levels continue to decline so that by 20 hours post-injection, about 1% of the radioactive dose is found in the blood pool. The "biological" half-life of indium In^{111} pentetreotide is only 6 hours while the radioactive half-life is 2.8 days. Half of the injected dose is recoverable in urine within six hours after injection, 85% is recovered in the first 24 hours, and over 90% is recovered in urine by two days. Hepatobiliary excretion represents a minor route of elimination, and less than 2% of the injected dose is recovered in feces within three days after injection. The return to breastfeeding is largely dependent on the dose, but a waiting period of 3 days would largely eliminate any risks at the lower dose, but this is largely dependent on the dose.

Radioactive ^{111}Indium Octreotide: This is an imaging agent that can help find primary and metastatic neuroendocrine tumors. The concentration of radioactive octreotide in breastmilk in a 10 weeks postpartum woman was measured at daily intervals for three days after injection of 5.3 mCi (196 MBq) of ^{111}Indium-octreotide.[1] The disappearance of radiolabeled octreotide from the breastmilk exhibited a bi-exponential pattern with a maximum concentration of 14.2 nCi (0.54 kBq) per 125 mL feeding at 4 hours. The maximum reading was 8.3 mrem x h(-1) (0.83 mSv x h(-1)) immediately after administration. This decreased rapidly (85%) due to rapid urinary clearance by 24 hours. Breastmilk content of radioactive octreotide and external surveys at the breast surface were determined at 3 hour intervals for up to 10 days. Assuming an infant is breastfed for the first 10 days following therapy, the internal and external dose equivalents would be 22.97 mrem (0.23 mSv) and 27.86 mrem (0.28 mSv) respectively, for a total of 50.83 mrem (0.5 mSv). In this paper, the patient resumed breastfeeding on day 10, when the newborn received a total dose equivalent of 1.55 mrem (0.016 mSv). The 10 day waiting period used in this study was based on very conservative assumptions and assumed 100% of the ingested ^{111}In is orally bioavailable. However, oral indium has been shown to be poorly absorbed from the gastrointestinal tract (approximately 0.15%), which suggests the infant's dose could be considerably less. The authors suggest that a briefer interruption deserves attention although they provide no numbers.

Breastfeeding restrictions: ^{111}In-Octreotide (CSF-imaging neuroendocrine tumors): 5.3 mCi dose: <10 days interruption.

Close contact restrictions (6 feet separation from infant): Avoid close contact for the first 4 hours, limit close contact to 35 min per hour with maximum 9 hours per day.[2] Restricting close contact to 35 minutes every 4 hours for 3 days reduces radiation exposure by 30%.[2]

Note: These recommendations still permit a minimal amount of <1 mSv of radiation transfer to the infant. Exposure of 1 mSv has a cancer incidence risk of 1 in 10,000 people. This amount of exposure is less than the amount an average American is exposed to from the environment (6.2 mSv/year). The only way to avoid any radiation exposure is to wait for 5–10 half-lives, until all of the radioisotope decays (14–28 days).

Pregnancy Risk	Possibly Hazardous	Lactation Risk	L4
T ½	= 2.8 days	M/P	=
Vd	=	PB	=
Tmax	=	Oral	=
MW	=	pKa	=

Adult Concerns: May inhibit gallbladder contractility and decrease bile secretion. Hypoglycemia or hyperglycemia, hypothyroidism may result. Bradycardia, arrhythmias in acromegalic patients. Numerous other adverse effects, consult package insert.

Pediatric Concerns:

Drug Interactions: Not compatible with Total Parenteral Nutrition solutions.

Relative Infant Dose:

Adult Dose: 3–6 mCi intravenously.

Alternatives:

References:
1. Castronovo FP, Jr., Stone H, Ulanski J. Radioactivity in breast milk following 111In-octreotide. Nucl Med Commun 2000; 21(7): 695–699.
2. Mountford PJ, O'Doherty MJ, Forge NI, Jeffries A, Coakley AJ. Radiation dose rates from adult patients undergoing nuclear medicine investigations. Nucl Med Commun. 1991 Sep; 12(9): 767–77

[11]C-WAY 100635 or ^{11}C-RACLOPRIDE | L2

Trade: C-Way 100635, C-Raclopride

Other Trades:

Category: Diagnostic Agent, Radiopharmaceutical Imaging

[11]C-WAY 100635 and ^{11}C-raclopride (sequentially) are used to measure brain serotonin-1A and dopamine-2 receptor binding, respectively, in depressed and non-depressed postpartum research subjects. In a study of 5 lactating women the ^{11}C-WAY 100635 injection was followed by 90 min of scanning.[1] Sixty minutes later, ^{11}C-raclopride injection was followed by 60 min of scanning. Approximately

15 min after the conclusion of each scan, study participants expressed their milk for the study. The mean infant age was 9.4 ±3.4 week; the range was 4–13 week. The mean activity of ^{11}C in breast milk (455 ± 107 Bq/mL) was similar to that in plasma (355 ± 99 Bq/mL) 60 minutes after 526 ± 61 MBq of ^{11}C-WAY 100635 had been injected. For ^{11}C-raclopride, the mean activity concentration of ^{11}C in breast milk (105 ±32 Bq/mL) was significantly less than that in plasma (913± 361 Bq/mL) 60 min after radiopharmaceutical injection (384 ± 24 MBq). Using worst-case scenario, the mean radioactive dose to the nursing infant at 1 h was 2.7 ± 0.6 μSv after ^{11}C-WAY 100635 and 0.6 ± 0.2 μSv after ^{11}C-raclopride injection.

The authors concluded that interruption of breastfeeding was not warranted. A brief interruption of breastfeeding for only 100 minutes would remove all risk to the infant.

Pregnancy Risk	Possibly Hazardous	Lactation Risk	L2
T ½	= 20.3 minutes	M/P	=
Vd	=	PB	=
Tmax	=	Oral	=
MW	= 346.2	pKa	=

Adult Concerns: Possible akathisia and extrapyramidal effects if given in therapeutic doses. No side effects likely in diagnostic dosages.

Pediatric Concerns: Milk levels were equal to or less than maternal plasma levels. However, the half-life of this radioisotope is brief (20.3 min), so only limited exposure would result.

Drug Interactions:

Relative Infant Dose:

Adult Dose:

Alternatives:

References:
1. Moses-Kolko EL, Meltzer CC, Helsel JC, Sheetz M, Mathis C, Ruszkiewicz J, et al. No interruption of lactation is needed after (11)C-WAY 100635 or (11)C-raclopride PET. J Nucl Med 2005 Oct; 46(10): 1765.

5-HYDROXYTRYPTOPHAN   L3

Trade:

Other Trades:

Category: Precursor of serotonin

5–Hydroxytryptophan (5–HTP) is a natural aromatic amino acid which is the immediate precursor of the neurotransmitter serotonin. L-Tryptophan is another amino acid formerly used to treat depression.

L-Tryptophan: L-tryptophan (LTP), once absorbed, is rapidly transported to the liver where some of it is incorporated into proteins, and some passes unchanged into the general circulation. It is a precursor of serotonin. One of the major problems with the use of LTP is that when used at higher doses, metabolism to kynurenine is highly induced, and the majority of LTP is subsequently metabolized rather than converted into serotonin. Even under the best of circumstances, less than 3% of the LTP is likely to be converted to serotonin in the brain. L-Tryptophan crosses the blood-brain barrier only poorly. As the doses increase, the creation of the metabolite kynurenine tends to block entry of LTP into the brain. As the doses of LTP used are extraordinarily high, 2000–6000 mg/day cost and adverse effects are significant.[1] Older formulations created with contaminates were responsible for the eosinophilia-myalgia syndrome.

5–HTTP: 5–HTP is rapidly absorbed, and approximately 70% of the dose is bioavailable. The remaining 30% is converted to serotonin by intestinal cells which may lead to some nausea. 5–HTP readily crosses the blood-brain barrier (24% in CSF) and is one step closer to serotonin production. The dose of 5–HTP is much lower, averaging 100–300 mg/day, and some studies have found it equivalent to tricyclic antidepressants[2] and fluvoxamine (an SSRI) in treating depression.[3] Although several cases of eosinophilia-myalgia syndrome have been reported with the use of 5–HTP[4,5], both of these patients had defective metabolic mechanisms for converting 5–HTP.

Unfortunately, there are no data on the transfer of exogenously supplied LTP or 5–HTP into human milk. For instance, it is not apparently known if high maternal plasma levels would produce high milk levels. While it is true human milk contains higher levels of LTP, presumably to stimulate serotonin levels in the infant's CNS, it is not known if high maternal doses would likewise produce high milk levels. Because the infant's neurologic development is incredibly sensitive to serotonin levels, and because we do not know if supplementation with LTP or 5–HTP could produce high milk levels leading to overdose in the infant, this author does not recommend the use of L-tryptophan or 5–HTP supplementation in breastfeeding mothers until we know corresponding milk levels.

Pregnancy Risk	C	Lactation Risk	L3
T ½	= 4.3 hours	M/P	=
Vd	= 0.6 l/kg	PB	= 19%
Tmax	= 3–6 hours	Oral	= <70%
MW	= 393	pKa	= 6.96

Adult Concerns: Adverse anorexia, diarrhea, nausea, and vomiting have been reported.

Pediatric Concerns: None reported via milk.

Drug Interactions: Carbidopa may increase absorption of 5-HT. Use with MAOI is potentially dangerous. 5-HT may potentiate the serotonergic effect of selective serotonin reuptake inhibitors (SSRIs).

Relative Infant Dose:

Adult Dose:

Alternatives: Selective serotonin reuptake inhibitors, Tricyclic antidepressants.

References:

1. Murray MT, Pizzorno JE. 5-Hydroxytryptophan. In: Murray MT, Pizzorno JE, editors. Textbook of Natural Medicine. Churchill Livingstone, 1999: 783–796.
2. van Praag HM. Management of depression with serotonin precursors. Biol Psychiatry 1981; 16(3): 291–310.
3. Poldinger W, Calanchini B, Schwarz W. A functional-dimensional approach to depression: serotonin deficiency as a target syndrome in a comparison of 5-hydroxytryptophan and fluvoxamine. Psychopathology 1991; 24(2): 53–81.
4. Sternberg EM, Van Woert MH, Young SN, Magnussen I, Baker H, Gauthier S, Osterland CK. Development of a scleroderma-like illness during therapy with L-5-hydroxytryptophan and carbidopa. N Engl J Med 1980; 303(14): 782–787
5. Michelson D, Page SW, Casey R, Trucksess MW, Love LA, Milstien S, Wilson C, Massaquoi SG, Crofford LJ, Hallett M, An eosinophilia-myalgia syndrome related disorder associated with exposure to L-5-hydroxytryptophan. J Rheumatol 1994; 21(12): 2261–2265

ABACAVIR   L3

Trade: Ziagen

Other Trades: Ziagen

Category: Antiretroviral agent for HIV

Abacavir is an antiretroviral agent used in the treatment of HIV infections. It is typically used in combination with two or more antiretroviral agents. Breastfeeding is not recommended for women who have HIV due to possibility of transmission of the virus. Due to its large molecular weight and structure, levels in milk when determined will probably be low. Data suggests that the HIV virus is not usually transmitted until the viral load exceeds 1500 copies/mL.

Pregnancy Risk	C	Lactation Risk	L3
T ½	= 1.54 hours	M/P	=
Vd	= 0.86 l/kg	PB	= 50%
Tmax	= 0.7–1.7 hours	Oral	= 83%
MW	= 671	pKa	= 5.01

Adult Concerns: Nausea, headache, malaise and fatigue, nausea/vomiting/diarrhea, depression, and dreams/sleep disorders.

Pediatric Concerns: In pediatric HIV-1 clinical studies the most common side effects were fever and/or chills, nausea/vomiting/diarrhea, skin rashes, and ear/nose/throat infections. But these were reported with the clinical administration of the drug to infants, not via milk.

Drug Interactions: In humans, abacavir does not appear to inhibit cytochrome P450 isoforms (2C9, 2D6, 3A4). Thus, it is unlikely that major drug interactions will occur between abacavir and other drugs metabolized through these pathways.

Relative Infant Dose:

Adult Dose: 300 BID or 600 mg daily

Alternatives:

References:

1. Pharmaceutical manufacturer prescribing information, 2010.

ABATACEPT   L3

Trade: Orencia

Other Trades: Orencia

Category: Antirheumatic

Abatacept is a soluble fusion protein that is linked to the A modified portion of human immunoglobulin G1(IgG1).[1] The apparent molecular weight of abatacept is 92 kilodaltons. Abatacept inhibits T cell activation by binding to CD80 and CD86 receptors which down regulates the T cells which are implicated in inflammation of rheumatic disorders. *In vitro*, abatacept decreases T cell proliferation and inhibits the production of the cytokines TNF alpha (TNFα), interferon-γ, and interleukin-2. There are no data on the transfer of this antibody into human milk. Due to its large molecular weight and unusual structure, it is not likely to enter milk in clinically relevant amounts. But as yet we have no studies to confirm this.

Pregnancy Risk	C	Lactation Risk	L3
T ½	= 13.1 days	M/P	=
Vd	= 0.02–0.13 l/kg	PB	=
Tmax	=	Oral	= Nil
MW	= 92,000	pKa	= 15.12

Adult Concerns: The adverse events most frequently resulting in clinical intervention were infections. The most frequent infection listed is upper respiratory tract infections, bronchitis, and herpes zoster. Other side effects include: headache, nasopharyngitis, dizziness, COPD exacerbation, cough, rhonchi, and dyspnea.

Pediatric Concerns: None yet reported in breastfeeding infants.

Drug Interactions: Do not use with other anti TNF products such as adalimumab, etanercept, and infliximab because such combination therapy may increase their risk for infections.

Relative Infant Dose:

Adult Dose: 750 mg (for 60–100 Kg weight) Intravenous

Alternatives: Infliximab, etanercept

References:
1. Pharmaceutical manufacturer prescribing information, 2011.

ACAMPROSATE   L3

Trade: Campral

Other Trades: Campral

Category: GABA Agonist / Glutamate Antagonist

Acamprosate is a medication used for ethanol dependency. Its mechanism of action is not fully known, however it does increase levels of GABA and decrease levels of glutamate. During use, it reduces alcohol intake with out the disulfiram-like effects.[1] There are no data available on the transfer of acamprosate to human milk. It is not a sedative and is not additive, and its oral absorption is minimal. Due to the relatively low molecular weight and the lack of protein binding, transfer could be possible. In addition, alcohol-dependent mothers may not be a good risk for breastfeeding. However, this drug poses a minimal risk to infants.

Pregnancy Risk	C	Lactation Risk	L3
T ½	= 20–33 hours	M/P	=
Vd	= 1 l/kg	PB	= Nil
Tmax	=	Oral	= 11%
MW	= 400	pKa	= 15.12

Adult Concerns: Adverse effects seen include diarrhea, insomnia, anxiety, anorexia, weakness, and nausea.

Pediatric Concerns:

Drug Interactions: None reported.

Relative Infant Dose:

Adult Dose: 666 mg TID

Alternatives:

References:
1. Pharmaceutical manufacturer prescribing information, 2005.

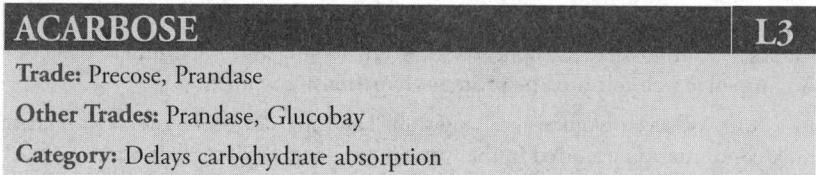

ACARBOSE   L3

Trade: Precose, Prandase

Other Trades: Prandase, Glucobay

Category: Delays carbohydrate absorption

Acarbose is an oral alpha-glucosidase inhibitor used to reduce the absorption of carbohydrates in the management of Type II (NIDDM) diabetics.[1] The reduction of carbohydrate absorption reduces the rapid rise in glucose following a meal; hence, glycosylated hemoglobin (Hemoglobin A1C) levels are reduced. Acarbose is less than 2% bioavailable as an intact molecule.[2] No data are available on the transfer of acarbose into human milk but with a bioavailability of less than 2%, it is very unlikely any would reach the milk compartment or be orally absorbed by the infant.

Pregnancy Risk	B	Lactation Risk	L3
T ½	= ~2 hours	M/P	=
Vd	= 0.32 l/kg	PB	=
Tmax	= ~1 hour	Oral	= 0.7– 2%
MW	= 645	pKa	= 12.01

Adult Concerns: Adverse effects include flatulence, abdominal pain and distention, diarrhea, and borborygmi. Isolated cases of elevated liver enzymes have been reported. Elevated liver enzymes occurred in approximately 15% of acarbose-treated patients and is apparently dose related with doses >300 mg daily.

Pediatric Concerns: None reported via milk.

Drug Interactions: May increase hypoglycemia when used with other antidiabetic medications such as the sulfonylureas.

Relative Infant Dose:

Adult Dose: Initial Dose: 25 mg TID Maintenance Dose: 50–100 mg TID

Alternatives:

References:
1. Pharmaceutical manufacturer prescribing information, 1999.
2. Balfour JA, McTavish D. Acarbose. An update of its pharmacology and therapeutic use in diabetes mellitus. Drugs 1993; 46(6): 1025–1054.

ACEBUTOLOL   L3

Trade: Sectral

Other Trades: Monitan, Sectral

Category: Antihypertensive, beta blocker

Acebutolol is predominately a beta-1 blocker, but can block beta-2 receptors at high doses. It is low in lipid solubility, and contains some intrinsic sympathetic activity (partial beta agonist activity). It increases cold sensitivity. Studies indicate that on a weight basis, Acebutolol is approximately 10–30% as effective as propranolol. It is 35–50% bioavailable orally.[1] After relatively high doses in animal studies, acebutolol does not appear to be overly teratogenic or harmful to the fetus. Acebutolol is well tolerated by pregnant hypertensive women.

In a study of seven women receiving 200–1200 mg/day acebutolol, the highest milk concentration occurred in the women receiving 1200 mg/day and was 4123 µg/L.[2] In women receiving 200, 400, or 600 mg/day of acebutolol, milk levels were 286 µg/L, 666 µg/L and 539 µg/L respectively. Acebutolol and diacetolol (its major metabolite) appear in breast milk with a milk/plasma ratio of 1.9 to 9.2 (Acebutolol) and 2.3 to 24.7 for the metabolite (diacetolol). These levels are considered relatively high and occurred following maternal doses of 400–1200 mg/day. When the metabolite is added, the dose may approach 10% of maternal dose. Neonates appear much more sensitive to acebutolol.

Pregnancy Risk	B/D in 2nd and 3rd trimester	Lactation Risk	L3
T ½	= 3–4 hours	M/P	= 7.1–12.2
Vd	= 1.2 l/kg	PB	= 26%
Tmax	= 2–4 hours	Oral	= 35–50%
MW	= 336	pKa	= 14.56

Adult Concerns: Hypotension, bradycardia, and transient tachypnea have been reported. Drowsiness has been reported.

Pediatric Concerns: Hypotension, bradycardia, hypoxemia and transient tachypnea have been reported.

Drug Interactions: Decreased effect when used with aluminum salts, barbiturates, calcium salts, cholestyramine, NSAIDs, ampicillin, rifampin, and salicylates. Beta blockers may reduce the effect of oral sulfonylureas (hypoglycemic agents). Increased toxicity/effect when used with other antihypertensives, contraceptives, MAO inhibitors, cimetidine, and numerous other products. See drug interaction reference for complete listing.

Relative Infant Dose: 0.9%–3.6%

Adult Dose: 200–400 mg BID

Alternatives: Propranolol, Metoprolol

References:
1. Facts and Comparisons. St. Louis: 2010..
2. Boutroy MJ, Bianchetti G, Dubruc C, Vert P, Morselli PL. To nurse when receiving acebutolol: is it dangerous for the neonate? Eur J Clin Pharmacol 1986; 30(6): 737–739.

ACETAMINOPHEN   L1

Trade: Tylenol, Genapap, Feverall, Actamin Maximum Strength, Altenol, Aminofen, Anacin aspirin free, Apra, Aceta

Other Trades: 222 Af Extra Strength, Abenol

Category: Analgesic

Acetaminophen is an analgesic/antipyretic used in the treatment of fever and pain. When taken orally, only minimal amounts are secreted into breast milk and are considered too small to be hazardous. In a study of 11 mothers who received 650 mg of acetaminophen orally, the highest milk levels reported were from 10–15 mg/L.[1] The milk/plasma ratio was 1.08. In another study of three patients who received a single 500 mg oral dose, the reported milk and plasma concentrations of acetaminophen was 4.2 mg/L and 5.6 mg/L respectively.[2] The milk/plasma ratio was 0.76. The maximum observed concentration in milk was 4.4 mg/L. In another study of women who ingested 1000 mg acetaminophen, milk levels averaged 6.1 mg/L and provided an average dose of 0.92 mg/kg/day according to the authors.[3] There seems to be wide variation in the milk concentrations in these studies, but the relative infant dose is probably less than 8.8% of the maternal dose. This is significantly less than the pediatric therapeutic dose.

Acetaminophen is increasingly being used intravenously for the relief of moderate to severe pain conditions. Some reports have suggested that the analgesic efficacy of intravenous acetaminophen is equivalent to that of intravenous morphine, and is probably preferred due to its minimal side-effects.[4,5] Following 1 gram IV dose of acetaminophen, the peak plasma concentrations attained are in the order of 28 mg/L at the end of 15 min. According to one report, following a 2 gm IV dose of acetaminophen in postpartum mothers, the plasma levels decreased from 22.5 mg/L to 3.9 mg/L within 1–6 hours post-dose.[6] Following a single IV dose, a maternal peak plasma concentration of 28 mg/L suggests that a breastfed infant would receive a dose of 19.6–28 mg/day (M/P ratio = 1) or about 4–6 mg/kg/day. This is far lower than the clinical doses for infants (15 mg/kg/dose). The dose ingested could be higher in premature infants or younger infants, but would probably still be lower than the clinically used pediatric doses. Nevertheless, some caution is advised. IV acetaminophen has been successfully used in premature infants born at 25–32 weeks of gestation, without any reported side-effects.[7] The serum concentrations at the end of 8–12 doses ranged between 8–64 mg/L. The authors reported that the infants tolerated the drug well. Based on these studies it may be said that infants seem to tolerate IV acetaminophen well. The dose ingested by an infant following IV acetaminophen in a lactating mother would most probably not be clinically relevant.

There is growing evidence that acetaminophen use may be linked to an increased prevalence of asthma among children and adults. In one published paper, it has been recommended, "any child with asthma or a family history of asthma avoid using acetaminophen."[8] Prenatal exposure and exposure to acetaminophen in the first year of life has also been linked to development of asthma later in life.[9,10,11,12,13] Subsequently, the issue of lactational exposure to acetaminophen and its association with development of asthma has also been addressed. In one such short-term study, out of 11 wheezing, exclusively breastfed infants, mothers of 7 of the infants had admitted intake of acetaminophen at the time of onset of wheezing symptoms in the infants.[14] However, these claims have been refuted by a few other authorities, based on various grounds. Nevertheless, due to the immaturity of metabolic pathways in the infant, a customary recommendation of judicious use of medications (including acetaminophen), during lactation has been advocated.

Pregnancy Risk	B	Lactation Risk	L1
T ½	= 2 hours	M/P	= 0.91–1.42
Vd	= 0.8–1.0 l/kg	PB	= 10–25%
Tmax	= 10–60 minutes	Oral	= >85%
MW	= 151	pKa	= 9.5

Adult Concerns: Few when taken in normal doses. Diarrhea, gastric upset sweating in overdose. Note: numerous cases of liver toxicity have been reported following 'chronic' abuse of acetaminophen at >200 mg/kg/day. Do not exceed 3000 mg in a 24 hour period or 1000 mg/dose. Exceedingly high doses can cause severe hepatic toxicity and death.

Pediatric Concerns: None reported via milk. Probably safe.

Drug Interactions: Rifampin can interact to reduce the analgesic effect of acetaminophen. Increased acetaminophen hepatotoxicity when used with barbiturates, carbamazepine, hydantoins, sulfinpyrazone, and chronic alcohol abuse.

Relative Infant Dose: 8.8%–24.2%

Adult Dose: 325–650 mg every 4–6 hours PRN

Alternatives:

References:
1. Berlin CM, Jr., Yaffe SJ, Ragni M. Disposition of acetaminophen in milk, saliva, and plasma of lactating women. Pediatr Pharmacol (New York) 1980; 1(2): 135–141.
2. Bitzen PO, Gustafsson B, Jostell KG, Melander A, Wahlin-Boll E. Excretion of paracetamol in human breast milk. Eur J Clin Pharmacol 1981; 20(2): 123–125.

3. Notarianni LJ, Oldham HG, Bennett PN. Passage of paracetamol into breast milk and its subsequent metabolism by the neonate. Br J Clin Pharmacol 1987; 24(1): 63–67.

4. Serinken M, Eken C, Turkcuer I, Elicabuk H, Uyanik E, Schultz CH. Intravenous paracetamol versus morphine for renal colic in the emergency department: a randomised double-blind controlled trial. Emerg Med J. 2011 Dec 20.

5. Craig M, Jeavons R, Probert J, Benger J. Randomised comparison of intravenous paracetamol and intravenous morphine for acute traumatic limb pain in theemergency department. Emerg Med J. 2012 Jan; 29(1): 37–9. Epub 2011 Mar 1.

6. Kulo A, van de Velde M, de Hoon J, Verbesselt R, Devlieger R, Deprest J,Allegaert K. Pharmacokinetics of a loading dose of intravenous paracetamol post caesarean delivery. Int J Obstet Anesth. 2012 Feb 14.

7. van Ganzewinkel CJ, Mohns T, van Lingen RA, Derijks LJ, Andriessen P. Paracetamol serum concentrations in preterm infants treated with paracetamol intravenously: a case series. J Med Case Reports. 2012 Jan 4; 6(1): 1.

8. McBride JT. The association of acetaminophen and asthma prevalence and severity. Pediatrics. 2011 Dec; 128(6): 1181–5. Epub 2011 Nov 7.

9. Eyers S, Weatherall M, Jefferies S, Beasley R. Paracetamol in pregnancy and the risk of wheezing in offspring: a systematic review and meta-analysis. ClinExp Allergy. 2011 Apr; 41(4): 482–9. doi: 10.1111/j. 1365–2222.2010.03691. x. Epub2011 Feb 22. Review.

10. Etminan M, Sadatsafavi M, Jafari S, Doyle-Waters M, Aminzadeh K, Fitzgerald JM. Acetaminophen use and the risk of asthma in children and adults: a systematic review and metaanalysis. Chest. 2009 Nov; 136(5): 1316–23. Epub 2009 Aug 20. Review.

11. Rebordosa C, Kogevinas M, S√∏rensen HT, Olsen J. Pre-natal exposure to paracetamol and risk of wheezing and asthma in children: a birth cohort study. Int J Epidemiol. 2008 Jun; 37(3): 583–90. Epub 2008 Apr 9.

12. Shaheen SO, Newson RB, Henderson AJ, Headley JE, Stratton FD, Jones RW,Strachan DP; ALSPAC Study Team. Prenatal paracetamol exposure and risk of asthma and elevated immunoglobulin E in childhood. Clin Exp Allergy. 2005Jan; 35(1): 18–25.

13. Shaheen SO, Newson RB, Sherriff A, Henderson AJ, Heron JE, Burney PG, Golding J; ALSPAC Study Team. Paracetamol use in pregnancy and wheezing in earlychildhood. Thorax. 2002 Nov; 57(11): 958–63.

14. Verd S, Nadal-Amat J. Paracetamol and asthma and lactation. Acta Paediatr. 2011 Jul; 100(7): e2–3; author reply e3. doi: 10.1111/j. 1651–2227.2011.02163. x. Epub 2011 Feb 25.

ACETAMINOPHEN + HYDROCODONE | L3

Trade: Lorcet, Lortab, Vicodin, Anexsia, Maxidone, Norco, Zydone, Ceta Plus
Other Trades:
Category: Analgesic

Acetaminophen and Hydrocodone bitartrate is a drug combination product indicated for alleviation of moderate to moderately-severe pain. This combination has been found to be very effective in the relief of postpartum and post-operative pain. It has also been found to very effective for the alleviation of pain associated with mastitis.[1]

Only small amounts of acetaminophen are secreted into breast milk and are considered too small to be hazardous. There seems to be wide variation in the milk concentrations of acetaminophen in studies, but the relative infant dose is probably less than 8.8% of the maternal dose. This is significantly less than the pediatric therapeutic dose. Acetaminophen is compatible with breastfeeding.[2–4]

Hydrocodone is a narcotic analgesic and antitussive structurally related to codeine although somewhat more potent. Its active metabolite is hydromorphone. Hydrocodone is commonly used in breastfeeding mothers throughout the USA.

Its relative infant dose is 2.4–3.7%. While standard clinical doses of 5–10 mg every 4–6 hours appear to be compatible with breastfeeding, higher doses of hydrocodone, especially when used in breastfeeding mothers of premature or newborn infants, may be concerning.[5] It is recommended that for treatment of postpartum pain, hydrocodone dosages should be limited to no more than 30 mg per day. If higher doses are required, then the infant should be closely monitored for possible untoward effects such as sedation and apnea. Doses more than 40 mg/day should be avoided.[6]

Mothers should be advised to watch for sedation and appropriate weight gain in their infants.

Pregnancy Risk	C		Lactation Risk	L3
$T\frac{1}{2}$	= acetaminophen/ hydrocodone: 2 hours/5.6–14.8 hours		M/P	= acetaminophen/ hydrocodone: 0.91–1.42/0.25
Vd	= acetaminophen/ hydrocodone: 0.8–1/3 l/kg		PB	= acetaminophen/ hydrocodone: 25%/58%
Tmax	= acetaminophen/ hydrocodone: 0.5–2 hours/2 hours		Oral	= acetaminophen/ hydrocodone: >85%/72%
MW	= acetaminophen/ hydrocodone: 151/297		pKa	= acetaminophen/ hydrocodone: 9.5/7.9,9.2

Adult Concerns: Common side-effects include nausea, vomiting, dizziness, light-headedness and sedation. Serious side-effects are Stevens-Johnson syndrome, agranulocytosis thrombocytopenia, hepatotoxicity and respiratory depression.

Pediatric Concerns: Sedation observed in one infant whose mother consumed 20 mg hydrocodone + 1300 mg acetaminophen every 4 hours.[4] Neonatal sedation and apnea possible, especially with doses more than 30 mg/day.

Drug Interactions: Use with caution when being used concomitantly with other CNS depressants such as other narcotic analgesics, antihistamines, antipsychotics, antianxiety agents, or other CNS depressants (including alcohol) due to additive effect. Also use with caution in those on tricyclic antidepressants and Monoamine oxidase inhibitors.

Relative Infant Dose:

Adult Dose: hydrocodone/acetaminophen: 5 mg/500 mg:1–2 tabs every 4–6 hours or as needed. Do not exceed more than 8 tabs in a 24 hr period.

Alternatives: Acetaminophen + oxycodone

References:
1. Bodley V, Powers D. Long-term treatment of a breastfeeding mother with fluconazole-resolved nipple pain caused by yeast: a case study. J Hum Lact. 1997 Dec; 13(4): 307–11.
2. Berlin CM, Jr., Yaffe SJ, Ragni M. Disposition of acetaminophen in milk, saliva, and plasma of lactating women. Pediatr Pharmacol (New York) 1980; 1(2): 135–141.
3. Bitzen PO, Gustafsson B, Jostell KG, Melander A, Wahlin-Boll E. Excretion of paracetamol in human breast milk. Eur J Clin Pharmacol 1981; 20(2): 123–125.
4. Notarianni LJ, Oldham HG, Bennett PN. Passage of paracetamol into breast milk and its subsequent metabolism by the neonate. Br J Clin Pharmacol 1987; 24(1): 63–67.

5. Anderson PO et al. Hydrocodone Excretion into Breast Milk: The First Two Reported Cases. Breastfeeding Medicine Vol 2 (1) 2007; 10–14.

6. Sauberan JB, Anderson PO, Lane JR, Rafie S, Nguyen N, Rossi SS, Stellwagen LM. Breast milk hydrocodone and hydromorphone levels in mothers using hydrocodone forpostpartum pain. Obstet Gynecol. 2011 Mar; 117(3): 611–7. PubMed PMID: 21343764.

ACETAMINOPHEN + OXYCODONE | L3

Trade: Endocet, Percocet, Roxicet, Roxilox, Tylox, Narvox, Magnacet, Perloxx, Primalev

Other Trades: Oxycocet

Category: Analgesic

Acetaminophen and Oxycodone hydrochloride is a combination drug used for alleviation of moderate to moderately-severe pain.

Only small amounts of acetaminophen are secreted into breast milk and are considered too small to be hazardous. There seems to be wide variation in the milk concentrations in these studies, but the relative infant dose is probably less than 8.8% of the maternal dose. This is significantly less than the pediatric therapeutic dose. Acetaminophen is compatible with breastfeeding.[1-3]

Oxycodone is similar to hydrocodone and is a mild analgesic somewhat stronger than codeine. Small amounts are secreted in breastmilk. Following a dose of 5–10 mg every 4–7 hours, maternal levels peaked at 1–2 hours, and analgesia persisted for up to 4 hours.[4] Reported milk levels range from <5 to 226 µg/L. Maternal plasma levels were 14–35 µg/L. The authors suggest a milk/plasma ratio of approximately 3.4. Although active metabolites were not measured, the authors suggest that an exclusively breastfed infant would receive a maximum 8% of the maternal dosage of oxycodone. No reports of untoward effects in infants have been found although sedation is a possibility in some infants. In another study, 50 post-cesarean women received 30 mg oxycodone rectally, and 10 mg orally up to every 2 hours as needed. The average maternal plasma levels at 0–24 hours and 24–48 hours were 18 (range 0–42) ng/mL and 12 (range 0–40) ng/mL, respectively. Average milk concentrations in samples taken during 0–24 hours and 24–48 hours were 58 (range 7–130) ng/mL and 49 (range 0–168) ng/mL, respectively. Milk/Plasma ratios were therefore calculated to be 3.2–3.4. Only one infant had a detectable level of oxycodone in their plasma, with a concentration of 6.6–7.4 ng/mL.[5] These plasma and milk levels suggest that oxycodone concentrates in the milk compartment, however, the authors suggest that at doses less than 90 mg/day for up to 3 days, maternal use of oxycodone poses only a minimal threat to breastfeeding infants. This study did not measure plasma or milk concentrations at steady state or during peak plasma concentrations, therefore, levels may have been higher at times. In a recent retrospective study, the rate of CNS depression in breastfeeding infants was compared between 3 cohorts of breastfeeding women receiving oxycodone, codeine and acetaminophen, respectively, for alleviation of postpartum pain.[6] The mothers were receiving doses which were within the recommended adult dosages. The rates of infant CNS depression in the three groups was as follows: oxycodone group–20.1%; codeine group–16.7%; acetaminophen group–0.5%. While in the oxycodone group, symptoms appeared in mothers receiving median doses of

0.4 mg/kg/day (28 mg for a 70 kg individual), symptoms in the codeine group appeared at a median dose of 1.4 mg/kg/day (98 mg/day for a 70 kg individual). Although CNS depression seemed to appear over a wide range of doses, it was found that higher doses were more likely to cause symptoms in the breastfed infant. This pattern held true for both the oxycodone as well as the codeine group. Further, maternal sedation was more likely with the use of oxycodone than with the use of codeine. Based on these findings, the authors conclude that oxycodone should not be considered a safer alternative to codeine in breastfed infants.

The data suggests that oxycodone is somewhat more risky and that the risks are dose-related. The use of doses greater than 40 mg/day should be avoided in breastfeeding mothers.

Pregnancy Risk	C		Lactation Risk	L3
T ½	= Acetaminophen/oxycodone: 2 hours/3–6 hours		M/P	= Acetaminophen/oxycodone: 0.91–1.42/3.4
Vd	= Acetaminophen/oxycodone: 0.8–1.0/3.7 l/kg		PB	= Acetaminophen/oxycodone: 25%/
Tmax	= Acetaminophen/oxycodone: 0.5–2 hours/1–2 hours		Oral	= Acetaminophen/oxycodone: >85%/50%
MW	= Acetaminophen/oxycodone: 151/315		pKa	= Acetaminophen/oxycodone: 9.5/8.5

Adult Concerns: Common side-effects are nausea, vomiting, dizziness, sedation. Some of the serious side-effects include hypotension, shock, liver toxicity, agranulocytosis, apnea and respiratory depression. Also refer individual agents.

Pediatric Concerns: Sedation has been reported in some infants (20.1%) at doses higher than 30 mg/day (median = 0.4 mg/kg/day).

Drug Interactions: Oxycodone may enhance the effect of skeletal muscle relaxants and cause respiratory depression. Use with caution while using with other CNS depressants such as other opioid analgesics, general anesthetics, sedatives, alcohol etc. due to additive effect. When used in high doses, increased risk of hepatotoxicity due to the acetaminophen component.

Relative Infant Dose:

Adult Dose: Acetaminophen/oxycodone: 325–650 mg/2.5–10 mg every 6 hours or as needed.

Alternatives: Acetaminophen + hydrocodone

References:
1. Berlin CM, Jr., Yaffe SJ, Ragni M. Disposition of acetaminophen in milk, saliva, and plasma of lactating women. Pediatr Pharmacol (New York) 1980; 1(2): 135–141.
2. Bitzen PO, Gustafsson B, Jostell KG, Melander A, Wahlin-Boll E. Excretion of paracetamol in human breast milk. Eur J Clin Pharmacol 1981; 20(2): 123–125.
3. Notarianni LJ, Oldham HG, Bennett PN. Passage of paracetamol into breast milk and its subsequent metabolism by the neonate. Br J Clin Pharmacol 1987; 24(1): 63–67.
4. Marx CM, Pucin F, Carlson JD. et. al. Oxycodone excretion in human milk in the puerperium. Drug Intel Clin 1986; 20: 474.

5. Seaton S, Reeves M, McLean S. Oxycodone as a component of multimodal analgesia for lactating mothers after Caesarean section: Relationships between maternal plasma, breast milk and neonatal plasma levels. Aust NZ J Obstet Gyn 2007; 47: 181–85.
6. Lam J, Kelly L, Ciszkowski C, Landsmeer ML, Nauta M, Carleton BC, Hayden MR, Madadi P, Koren G. Central nervous system depression of neonates breastfed by mothers receiving oxycodone for postpartum analgesia. J Pediatr. 2012Jan; 160(1): 33–37. e2. Epub 2011 Aug 31.

ACETAMINOPHEN + TRAMADOL   L2

Trade: Ultracet

Other Trades:

Category: Analgesic

Acetaminophen and Tramadol hydrochloride drug combination is indicated for alleviation of acute pain. Only small amounts of acetaminophen are secreted into breast milk and are considered too small to be hazardous. There seems to be wide variation in the milk concentrations in these studies, but the relative infant dose is probably less than 8.8% of the maternal dose. This is significantly less than the pediatric therapeutic dose. Acetaminophen is compatible with breastfeeding.[1–3]

Following a single IV 100 mg dose of tramadol, the cumulative excretion in breastmilk within 16 hours was 100 µg of tramadol (1.05% of the maternal dose) and 27 µg of the M1 metabolite.[4] In a recent study of 75 mothers who received 100 mg of tramadol every 6 hours after caesarian section, milk samples were taken on days 2–4 postpartum in transitional milk.[5] At steady state, the milk/plasma ratio averaged 2.4 for rac-tramadol and 2.8 for rac-O-desmethyltramadol. The estimated absolute and relative infant doses were 112 µg/kg/day and 30 µg/kg/day for rac-tramadol and its desmethyl metabolite. The relative infant dose was 2.24% and 0.64% for rac-tramadol and its desmethyl metabolite, respectively. No significant neurobehavioral adverse effects were noted between controls and exposed infants. Based on these studies, tramadol appears to be compatible with breastfeeding.

Pregnancy Risk	C		Lactation Risk	L2	
T½	= Acetaminophen/tramadol: 2 hours/7 hours		M/P	= Acetaminophen/tramadol: 0.91–1.42/2.4	
Vd	= Acetaminophen/tramadol: 0.8–1.0/ l/kg		PB	= Acetaminophen/tramadol: 10.25%/20%	
Tmax	= Acetaminophen/tramadol: 10–60 min/2 hours		Oral	= Acetaminophen/tramadol: > 85%/60%	
MW	= Acetaminophen/tramadol: 151/263		pKa	= Acetaminophen/tramadol: 9.5/9.4	

Adult Concerns: Somnolence, dizziness, pruritus, hot flashes, constipation, diarrhea, nausea, loss of appetite, dry mouth, prostatic disorder, diaphoresis, weakness.

Pediatric Concerns:

Drug Interactions: Concomitant administration with agents such as quinidine, fluoxetine, paroxetine, amitriptyline, ketoconazole and erythromycin may decrease its clearance and cause serious side-effects such as seizures. Caution to be exercised when used with other serotoninergic agents such as selective serotonin reuptake inhibitors, monoamine oxidase inhibitors, lithium and St. John's Wort.

Relative Infant Dose:

Adult Dose: Acetaminophen/tramadol: 325 mg/37.5 mg, 1–2 tablets every 4 -6 hours or as needed. Do not exceed 8 tablets in a 24 hour period.

Alternatives:

References:

1. Berlin CM, Jr., Yaffe SJ, Ragni M. Disposition of acetaminophen in milk, saliva, and plasma of lactating women. Pediatr Pharmacol (New York) 1980; 1(2): 135–141.
2. Bitzen PO, Gustafsson B, Jostell KG, Melander A, Wahlin-Boll E. Excretion of paracetamol in human breast milk. Eur J Clin Pharmacol 1981; 20(2): 123–125.
3. Notarianni LJ, Oldham HG, Bennett PN. Passage of paracetamol into breast milk and its subsequent metabolism by the neonate. Br J Clin Pharmacol 1987; 24(1): 63–67.
4. Pharmaceutical manufacturer prescribing information, 1996.
5. Ilett KF, Paech MJ, Page-Sharp M, et. al. Use of a sparse sampling study design to assess transfer of tramadol and its O-desmethyl metabolite into transitional breast milk. Br J Clin Pharmacol 65(5): 661–666, 2008

ACETAZOLAMIDE   L2

Trade: Dazamide, Diamox, Sequels

Other Trades: Acetazolam, Apo-Acetazolamide, Diamox,

Category: Diuretic

Acetazolamide is a carbonic anhydrase inhibitor dissimilar to other thiazide diuretics. In general, diuretics have in the past been suggested to decrease the volume of breast milk although this is totally undocumented. In a patient receiving 500 mg of acetazolamide twice daily, acetazolamide concentrations in milk were 1.3 to 2.1 mg/L while the maternal plasma levels ranged from 5.2–6.4 mg/L.[1] Plasma concentrations in exposed infants were 0.2 to 0.6 µg/mL two to 12 hours after breastfeeding. These amounts are unlikely to cause adverse effects in the infant.

Pregnancy Risk	C	Lactation Risk	L2
T ½	= 2.4–5.8 hours	M/P	= 0.25
Vd	= 0.2 l/kg	PB	= 70–95%
Tmax	= 1–3 hours	Oral	= Complete
MW	= 222	pKa	= 10.35

Adult Concerns: Anorexia, diarrhea, metallic taste, polyuria, muscular weakness, potassium loss. Malaise, fatigue, depression, renal failure have been reported.

Pediatric Concerns: None reported via milk.

Drug Interactions: Increases lithium excretion, reducing plasma levels. May increase toxicity of cyclosporine. Digitalis toxicity may occur if hypokalemia results from acetazolamide therapy.

Relative Infant Dose: 2.2%

Adult Dose: 500 mg BID

Alternatives:

References:
1. Soderman P, Hartvig P, Fagerlund C. Acetazolamide excretion into human breast milk. Br J Clin Pharmacol 1984; 17(5): 599–600.

ACETOHEXAMIDE   L3

Trade: Dymelor

Other Trades: Dimelor

Category: Hypoglycemic agent

Acetohexamide is an intermediate-acting hypoglycemic sulfonylurea anti-diabetic agent.[1] Its structure is similar to tolbutamide, chlorpropamide, and tolazamide. No data are available on its transfer to human milk, but other sulfonylureas transfer to milk in minimal levels (see tolbutamide). The use of sulfonylureas in breastfeeding mothers is somewhat controversial due to limited studies but has not been noted in the literature to produce any problems. Observe infant closely for hypoglycemia if used.

Pregnancy Risk	C	Lactation Risk	L3
T ½	= 1.3–6 (metabolite) hours	M/P	=
Vd	= 0.2 l/kg	PB	= 65–90%
Tmax	= 3–5 hours	Oral	= Good
MW	= 324	pKa	= 15.77

Adult Concerns: The most common adverse effects include hypoglycemia, nausea, epigastric fullness, heartburn, and rashes.

Pediatric Concerns: None reported via milk, but observe for hypoglycemia.

Drug Interactions: Numerous drugs interact with sulfonylureas, please consult further references. Increased hypoglycemic effects occur when used with salicylates, beta blockers, MAO inhibitors, oral anticoagulants, NSAIDs, sulfonamides, insulin, etc. Reduced hypoglycemic effects may occur when used with cholestyramine, diazoxide, hydantoins, rifampin, and thiazides.

Relative Infant Dose:

Adult Dose: 250–1000 mg daily

Alternatives: Metformin

References:
1. Pharmaceutical manufacturer prescribing information, 1999.

ACITRETIN   L5

Trade: Soriatane
Other Trades: Soriatane
Category: Retinoid-like compound

Acitretin is used in the treatment of severe psoriasis. It should only be used in non-pregnant patients who are unresponsive to other treatment options. Its exact mechanism of action is unknown, but it helps to normalize cell differentiation and thin the cornified layer of the skin by reducing the rate of proliferation.[1] This product produces major human fetal abnormalities, and is retained in the body for long periods of time. Chronic use in breastfeeding mothers is probably not recommended. In the only study conducted on the transfer of acitretin into human milk, a 31-year-old mother was taking 40 mg once daily and had milk concentrations of 30–40 µg/L. This indicated that an infant would receive only 1.8% of the maternal dose; however, due to the toxic potential of this medication, the authors concluded that acitretin should be avoided during breastfeeding.[2]

Pregnancy Risk	X	Lactation Risk	L5
T ½	= 49 hours	M/P	=
Vd	=	PB	= >99.9%
Tmax	= 2–5 hours	Oral	= 72%
MW	= 326	pKa	=

Adult Concerns: Adverse effects include cheilitis, alopecia, skin peeling, hypercholesterolemia, hypertriglyceridemia, increased liver function tests, and rhinitis. It is significantly teratogenic and should never be used in pregnant or women who intend to become pregnant during therapy or anytime for at least three years after discontinuation of treatment. It must not be used by females who do not use reliable contraception.

Pediatric Concerns: No data are available.

Drug Interactions: Ethanol, methotrexate, progestins, sulfonylureas, tetracycline, and vitamin A.

Relative Infant Dose: 1.8%

Adult Dose: 25–50 mg/day

Alternatives:

References:
1. Pharmaceutical manufacturer prescribing information, 2004.
2. Rollman O, Pihl-Lundin I. Acitretin Excretion into Human Breast Milk. Acta Derm Venereol 1990; 70: 487–90.

ACORUS CALAMUS   L4

Trade: Sweet Flag Root

Other Trades:

Category: Antispasmotic, antisecretory

Acorus Calamus, also known as Sweet Flag Root is an antispasmodic and antisecretory herbal. It is also believed to have a nematocidal effect. It is primarily used for dyspepsia and as an appetite stimulant in anorexia. Because of its potential mutagenic properties, it is considered unsafe for use by humans.

Pregnancy Risk	Possibly Hazardous	Lactation Risk	L4
T ½	=	M/P	=
Vd	=	PB	=
Tmax	=	Oral	=
MW	=	pKa	=

Adult Concerns: Antisecretory, antispasmotic effects. Some common side effects include breathing problems, chest pain, hives, itchiness, or vomiting.

Pediatric Concerns:

Drug Interactions:

Relative Infant Dose:

Adult Dose:

Alternatives:

References:

ACYCLOVIR   L2

Trade: Zovirax, Lipsovir

Other Trades: Acyclo-V, Zyclir, Aciclover, Apo-Acyclovir, Aviraz, Zovirax

Category: Antiviral

Acyclovir is converted by herpes simplex and varicella zoster virus to acyclovir triphosphate which interferes with viral HSV DNA polymerase. It is currently cleared for use in HSV infections, Varicella-Zoster, and under certain instances such as Cytomegalovirus and Epstein-Barr infections. There is virtually no percutaneous absorption following topical application and plasma levels are undetectable. The pharmacokinetics in children is similar to adults. In neonates, the half-life is 3.8–4.1 hours, and in children one year and older it is 1.9–3.6 hours.

Acyclovir levels in breastmilk are reported to be 0.6 to 4.1 times the maternal plasma levels.[1] Maximum ingested dose was calculated to be 1500 µg/day assuming 750 mL milk intake. This level produced no overt side effects in one infant. In a study by Meyer,[2] a patient receiving 200 mg five times daily produced breast milk concentrations averaging 1.06 mg/L. Using this data, an infant would ingest less than 1 mg acyclovir daily. In another study, doses of 800 mg five times daily produced milk levels that ranged from 4.16 to 5.81 mg/L (total estimated infant ingestion per day = 0.73 mg/kg/day).[3] Topical therapy on lesions other than nipple is probably safe. But mothers with lesions on or close to the nipple should not breastfeed on that side. Toxicities associated with acyclovir are few and usually minor. Acyclovir therapy in neonatal units is common and produces few toxicities. Calculated intake by infant would be less than 0.87 mg/kg/day.

Pregnancy Risk	B	Lactation Risk	L2
T ½	= 2.4 hours	M/P	= 0.6–4.1
Vd	= 0.8 l/kg	PB	= 9–33%
Tmax	= 1.5–2 hours	Oral	= 15–30%
MW	= 225	pKa	= 15.12

Adult Concerns: Nausea, vomiting, diarrhea, sore throat, edema, and skin rashes.

Pediatric Concerns: None reported via milk in several studies.

Drug Interactions: Increased CNS side effects when used with zidovudine and probenecid.

Relative Infant Dose: 1.1%–1.5%

Adult Dose: 200–800 mg every 4–6 hours

Alternatives: Valacyclovir

References:
1. Lau RJ, Emery MG, Galinsky RE. Unexpected accumulation of acyclovir in breast milk with estimation of infant exposure. Obstet Gynecol 1987; 69(3 Pt2): 468–471.
2. Meyer LJ, de Miranda P, Sheth N, Spruance S. Acyclovir in human breastmilk. Am J Obstet Gynecol 1988; 158(3Pt1): 586–588.
3. Taddio A, Klein J, Koren G. Acyclovir excretion in human breastmilk. Ann Pharmacother 1994; 28(5): 585–587.

ADALIMUMAB   L3

Trade: Humira

Other Trades: Humira

Category: Anti-rheumatic, anti-tumor necrosis antibody

Adalimumab is a recombinant humanized IgG1 monoclonal antibody specific for human tumor necrosis factor (TNF). TNF is implicated in the pain and destructive component of arthritis and other autoimmune syndromes. This product would be similar to others such as etanercept (Enbrel) and infliximab (Remicade). IgG transfer into human milk is significant the first 4 days postpartum, then is minimal afterwards. The primary immunoglobulin in mature human milk is IgA. Immunoglobulins are transferred into human milk by a very specific carrier protein which inhibits the transfer of IgG-like products. It is not known if these unusual immunoglobulins are transferred into milk, but it is unlikely. Specific data from my laboratories suggests that no infliximab transfers into human milk in mothers receiving IV doses.[1] It is not likely that adalimumab would transfer in clinically relevant amounts after the first week postpartum, but no data are available at this time.

Pregnancy Risk	B	Lactation Risk	L3
T ½	= 2 weeks	M/P	=
Vd	= 4.7 l/kg	PB	= Nil
Tmax	= 131 hours	Oral	= Low
MW	= 148,000	pKa	=

Adult Concerns: May induce tuberculosis reactivations. May induce immunosuppression and reduce host defenses against infections. Serious infections, neurologic events, and malignancies have been reported.

Pediatric Concerns: None reported via milk. Unlikely to enter milk in clinically relevant amounts.

Drug Interactions: None reported.

Relative Infant Dose:

Adult Dose: 40 mg every other week subcutaneously

Alternatives: Infliximab

References:
1. Hale TW, Fasanmade A. Unpublished data. 2002.

ADAPALENE   L3

Trade: Differin
Other Trades: Differin
Category: Topical acne remedy

Adapalene is a retinoid-like compound(similar to Tretinoin) used topically for treatment of acne. No data are available on its transfer into human milk. However, adapalene is virtually unabsorbed when applied topically to the skin.[1] Plasma levels are almost undetectable (<0.25 mg/mL plasma), so milk levels would be infinitesimally low and probably undetectable.[2]

Pregnancy Risk	C	Lactation Risk	L3
T ½	=	M/P	=
Vd	=	PB	=
Tmax	=	Oral	= Very low
MW	= 412.52	pKa	=

Adult Concerns: Exacerbation of sunburn, irritation of skin, erythema, dryness, scaling, burning, itching.

Pediatric Concerns: None reported via milk. Very unlikely due to minimal maternal absorption.

Drug Interactions: Avoid sunlight.

Relative Infant Dose:

Adult Dose: Apply topical daily.

Alternatives: Tretinoin

References:
1. Pharmaceutical manufacturer prescribing information, 2005.
2. Drug Facts and Comparisons 1999 ed. St. Louis: 1999.

ADEFOVIR   L4

Trade: Hepsera

Other Trades: Hepsera

Category: Anti-Hepatitis B Virus agent

Adefovir inhibits hepatitis B virus replication.[1] No data are available on the transfer of adefovir into in human milk, yet based on the kinetic profile (low protein binding and moderate oral bioavailability, it is possible that the drug would cross into the milk compartment to some degree. Because this drug is potentially toxic to a rapidly growing infant, and because it is used over long periods of time, it is not recommended for use in lactating mothers at this time.

Pregnancy Risk	C	Lactation Risk	L4
T ½	= 7.5 hours	M/P	=
Vd	= 0.4 l/kg	PB	= <4%
Tmax	= 1.75 hours	Oral	= 59%
MW	= 501	pKa	=

Adult Concerns: Adverse reactions include nephrotoxicity, or kidney dysfunction, lactic acidosis, severe hepatomegaly, feeling of weakness, headache, and abdominal pain.

Pediatric Concerns: No data are available. Milk levels are likely to be low.

Drug Interactions: Ibuprofen increases the oral bioavailability of adefovir. When used in combination with tenofovir, serum concentrations of both may be elevated.

Relative Infant Dose:

Adult Dose: 10 mg daily

Alternatives: Lamivudine, if not resistant

References:
1. Pharmaceutical manufacturer prescribing information, 2009.

ADENOSINE   L2

Trade: Adenocard, Adenoscan

Other Trades: Adenocard, Adenoscan

Category: Adenosine Receptor Agonist

Adenosine produces a direct negative chronotropic, dromotropic and inotropic effect on the heart, presumably due to A1-receptor stimulation, and produces peripheral vasodilation, presumably due to A2-receptor stimulation. The net effect of Adenoscan in humans is typically a mild to moderate reduction in systolic, diastolic and mean arterial blood pressure associated with a reflex increase in heart rate. Rarely, significant hypotension and tachycardia have been observed. There are no adequate well controlled studies in breastfeeding.[1] However, adenosine has a half-life <10 seconds and is not likely bioavailable long enough to enter the milk. Based on this information, it is probably safe to use in breastfeeding.

Pregnancy Risk	C	Lactation Risk	L2
T ½	= <10 secs	M/P	=
Vd	=	PB	=
Tmax	=	Oral	= Nil
MW	= 267.2	pKa	= 13.89

Adult Concerns: Flushing, chest discomfort, dyspnea or urge to breathe deeply, headache, throat, neck or jaw discomfort, gastrointestinal discomfort, lightheadedness/dizziness.

Pediatric Concerns:

Drug Interactions:

Relative Infant Dose:

Adult Dose: 6–12 mg

Alternatives:

References:
1. Pharmaceutical Manufacturing Information. 2011.

AIRBORNE   L4

Trade: Airborne
Other Trades:
Category: HERBAL

Airborne contains Vitamins: A, C, E, K plus riboflavin, selenium, zinc sulfate, magnesium, glutamine, lysine, mineral oil, sucralose, sorbitol, citric acid, NaHCO3, KHCO3, echinacea, schizonepeta ginger, chinese vitex, magnesium, zinc, Na, K, maltodextrin, Lonicera, Forsythia. The dose of vitamin A is 100% USDA (5,000 IU/tablet) recommended dose and directions on the bottle say to take up to three times daily, so the vitamin A dose would be excessive. The presence of various herbal drugs is problematic, as none of them have been studied in breastfeeding or pregnant women.

Pregnancy Risk	Hazardous	Lactation Risk	L4
T ½	=	M/P	=
Vd	=	PB	=
Tmax	=	Oral	=
MW	=	pKa	=

Adult Concerns: None listed except for sensitivity to any of the components. Large doses of certain vitamins and minerals can cause symptoms of toxicity such as anorexia, nausea and vomiting, diarrhea, irritability, drowsiness, altered mental status, blurred vision, low blood pressure, irregular heartbeat, headache, muscle pain and weakness.

Pediatric Concerns:

Drug Interactions:

Relative Infant Dose:

Adult Dose:

Alternatives: oxymetazoline

References:

ALBENDAZOLE   L3

Trade: Albenza

Other Trades: Eskazole

Category: Anthelminic for treatment of numerous varieties of worms

Albendazole is a broad-spectrum anthelmintic used for treating intestinal parasite infections. It is virtually unabsorbed (<5%) orally and would be unlikely to harm an infant even if present in milk. It is often used to treat common parasitic infections in pediatric patients all over the world.

Pregnancy Risk	C	Lactation Risk	L3
T ½	= 8–12 hours	M/P	=
Vd	=	PB	= 70%
Tmax	= 2–5 hours	Oral	= <5%
MW	= 265	pKa	= 13.94

Adult Concerns: Abdominal pain, nausea, vomiting, headache, dizziness, and fever have been reported.

Pediatric Concerns: No data are available in breastfeeding mothers. Milk levels are unlikely to be clinically relevant. Commonly used in infants and children.

Drug Interactions: Avoid use with corticosteroids including dexamethasone due to increased side effect profile. Avoid concomitant use with ginseng. Do not use with theophylline.

Relative Infant Dose:

Adult Dose: Highly variable and due to individual parasite. Check other source.

Alternatives: Mebendazole

References:
1. Pharmaceutical manufacturer prescribing information, 2005.

ALBUTEROL   L1

Trade: Proventil, Ventolin

Other Trades: Respax, Respolin, Ventolin, Asmol, Novo-Salmol, Ventolin, Asmavent, Salbulin, Salbuvent, Salamol

Category: Bronchodilator for asthma

Albuterol is a very popular beta-2 adrenergic agonist that is typically used to dilate constricted bronchi in asthmatics.[1] It is active orally but is most commonly used via inhalation. When used orally, significant plasma levels are attained and transfer to breastmilk is possible. When used via inhalation, less than 10% is absorbed into maternal plasma. Small amounts are probably secreted into milk although no reports exist. It is very unlikely that pharmacologic doses will be transferred to the infant via milk following inhaler use. However, when used orally, breastmilk levels could be sufficient to produce tremors and agitation in infants. Commonly used via inhalation in treating pediatric asthma. This product is safe to use in breastfeeding mothers.

Pregnancy Risk	C	Lactation Risk	L1
T ½	= 3.8 hours	M/P	=
Vd	= 2.2 l/kg	PB	= 36–93%
Tmax	= 5–30 minutes	Oral	= 100%
MW	= 239	pKa	= 10.3

Adult Concerns: Hypersensitivity reaction, angina, atrial fibrillation, diabetic ketoacidosis.

Pediatric Concerns: None reported via milk. Observe infant for tremors and excitement.

Drug Interactions: Albuterol effects are reduced when used with beta blockers. Cardiovascular effects are potentiated when used with MAO inhibitors, tricyclic antidepressants, amphetamines, and inhaled anesthetics (enflurane).

Relative Infant Dose:

Adult Dose: 2–4 mg TID or QID

Alternatives:

References:
1. Pharmaceutical manufacturer prescribing information, 1997.

ALBUTEROL + IPRATROPIUM BROMIDE   L1

Trade: DuoNeb, Combivent

Other Trades:

Category: Bronchodilators

Albuterol Sulfate and Ipratropium Bromide is a combination drug product indicated for use in chronic obstructive pulmonary disease in patients requiring a second bronchodilator.

When used via inhalation, less than 10% is absorbed into maternal plasma. Small amounts are probably secreted into milk although no reports exist. It is very unlikely that pharmacologic doses will be transferred to the infant via milk following inhaler use. However, when used orally, breastmilk levels could be sufficient to produce tremors and agitation in infants. Commonly used via inhalation in treating pediatric asthma. This product is safe to use in breastfeeding mothers.

Ipratropium is a quaternary ammonium compound, and although no data exists, it probably penetrates into breastmilk in exceedingly small levels due to its structure. It is unlikely that the infant would absorb any, due to the poor tissue distribution and oral absorption of this family of drugs.

Pregnancy Risk	C	Lactation Risk	L1
$T\frac{1}{2}$	= Albuterol/ipratropium bromide: 3.8 hours/2 hours	M/P	= Albuterol/ipratropium bromide:
Vd	= Albuterol/ipratropium bromide: 2.2/ l/kg	PB	= Albuterol/ipratropium bromide: 39–93%/
Tmax	= Albuterol/ipratropium bromide: 5–30 min/1–2 hours	Oral	= Albuterol/ipratropium bromide: 100%/0–2%
MW	= Albuterol/ipratropium bromide: 239/412	pKa	= Albuterol/ipratropium bromide: 10.3/

Adult Concerns: Bronchitis, upper respiratory tract infection, chest pain.

Pediatric Concerns:

Drug Interactions: Due to the Albuterol component, there is an increased risk of tachycardia and increased blood pressure when used concomitantly with Monoamine oxidase inhibitors. Albuterol when combined with beta-blockers have antagonistic action on each other.

Relative Infant Dose:

Adult Dose: 2 metered dose inhalations 4 times a day

Alternatives:

References:

ALCAFTADINE OPHTHALMIC SOLUTION | L3

Trade: Lastacaft
Other Trades:
Category: Topical H_1 histamine receptor

Alcaftadine is an H_1 histamine receptor antagonist used for allergic conjunctivitis. Following bilateral topical ocular administration of alcaftadine ophthalmic solution, 0.25%, the mean plasma C_{max} of alcaftadine was approximately 60 pg/mL and the median T_{max} occurred at 15 minutes. Plasma concentrations of alcaftadine were below the lower limit of quantification (10 pg/mL) by 3 hours after dosing. The mean C_{max} of the active carboxylic acid metabolite was approximately 3 ng/mL and occurred at 1 hour after dosing. Plasma concentrations of the carboxylic acid metabolite were below the lower limit of quantification (100 pg/mL) by 12 hours after dosing. There was no indication of systemic accumulation or changes in plasma exposure of alcaftadine or the active metabolite following daily topical ocular administration.

While no breastfeeding studies are available the levels in plasma are so low that milk levels would be far subclinical.

Pregnancy Risk	B		Lactation Risk	L3
T ½	= 2 hours (metabolite)		M/P	=
Vd	=		PB	= 40–60%
Tmax	= 15 minutes		Oral	=
MW	= 307		pKa	=

Adult Concerns: Eye irritation, burning and/or stinging upon instillation, eye redness and eye pruritus.

Pediatric Concerns: Levels in maternal plasma too low to produce clinical effects in breastfed infant.

Drug Interactions: None reported.

Relative Infant Dose:

Adult Dose: One drop twice daily

Alternatives:

References:
1. Pharmaceutical manufacturer prescribing information, 2010.

ALEFACEPT   L3

Trade: Amevive
Other Trades:
Category: Immunosuppresant

Alefacept is an immunosuppressant used in the treatment of chronic plaque psoriasis. It binds to the lymphocyte antigen CD2, thus inhibiting the LFA-3/CD2 interaction.[1] Although levels in milk have not been determined, its transfer into the milk compartment is highly unlikely due to its enormous molecular size (94 kilodaltons). Furthermore, due to low oral bioavailability, even if present in milk, it would be unabsorbed in an infant.

Pregnancy Risk	B		Lactation Risk	L3
T ½	= 270 hours		M/P	=
Vd	= 0.094 l/kg		PB	=
Tmax	=		Oral	= 63%
MW	= 91,400		pKa	=

Adult Concerns: Adverse reactions include lymphopenia, malignancies, infections and hypersensitivity.

Pediatric Concerns: No data are available, but it is unlikely to transfer into milk.

Drug Interactions: No data available.

Relative Infant Dose:

Adult Dose: 7.5 mg IV weekly

Alternatives:

References:
1. Pharmaceutical manufacturer prescribing information, 2005.

ALEMTUZUMAB   L4

Trade: Campath
Other Trades: MabCampath
Category: anticancer drug

Alemtuzumab is a recombinant DNA-derived humanized monoclonal antibody that is directed against specific cell receptors on leukemic cells. It is indicated for treatment of chronic B-cell lymphocytic leukemia. It is a large IgG1 antibody.[1] No data are available on its transfer to human milk, but it is very unlikely to enter milk, due to its large molecular weight. However, the first 72 hours postpartum, IgG levels in milk are higher, and this should be considered with this agent. While some IgG is still transferred into human milk, it is done so by a very specialized transporter. It is unlikely this transporter would transport this unusual monoclonal antibody.

Mothers should avoid breastfeeding, if this product is used within 2 weeks of delivery. Otherwise, the amount present in milk is likely quite low. This is a large molecular weight antibody that is unlikely to enter milk in significant quantities.

Pregnancy Risk	C	Lactation Risk	L4
T ½	= 12 days	M/P	=
Vd	= 0.1–0.4 l/kg	PB	= 0.18
Tmax	=	Oral	= Nil
MW	= 150 kD	pKa	=

Adult Concerns: Adverse events include rigors post-infusion, fever, nausea, vomiting, hypotension, rash, fatigue, urticaria, dyspnea, pruritus, headache, and diarrhea. An elevated risk of infection is reported.

Pediatric Concerns: None reported via milk. Unlikely to penetrate milk after first 2 weeks postpartum.

Drug Interactions:

Relative Infant Dose:

Adult Dose: Maintenance dose is 30 mg/day three times weekly on alternate days.

Alternatives:

References:
1. Pharmaceutical manufacturer prescribing information, 2003.

ALENDRONATE SODIUM   L3

Trade: Fosamax
Other Trades: Fosamax
Category: Inhibits bone resorption

Alendronate is a specific inhibitor of osteoclast-mediated bone resorption, thus reducing bone loss and bone turnover.[1] It is indicated for use in osteoporosis and paget's disease of the bone. While incorporated in bone matrix, it is not pharmacologically active. Because concentrations in plasma are too low to be detected (<5 ng/mL), it is very unlikely that it would be secreted into human milk in clinically relevant concentrations. Concentrations in human milk have not been reported. Because this product has exceedingly poor oral bioavailability, particularly when ingested with milk, it is very unlikely that alendronate would be orally absorbed by a breastfeeding infant. In one case of an unknown pregnancy, the mother was taking alendronate 0.12 mg/kg/day orally. Her baby was born with no physical abnormalities, and the baby's growth was normal.[2] No data was collected on the concentrations of alendronate in the mother's milk.

Pregnancy Risk	C	Lactation Risk	L3
T ½	= <3 hours (plasma)	M/P	=
Vd	= 0.4 l/kg	PB	= 78%
Tmax	=	Oral	= <0.7%
MW	= 325	pKa	= 1.45

Adult Concerns: Abdominal pain, nausea, dyspepsia, constipation, muscle cramps, headache, taste perversion. There are a number of case reports of esophagitis and esophageal ulceration in patients taking Fosamax.

Pediatric Concerns: None reported via milk.

Drug Interactions: Ranitidine will double the absorption of alendronate. Calcium, milk, and other multivalent cation containing foods reduce the bioavailability of alendronate.

Relative Infant Dose:

Adult Dose: 10 mg daily.

Alternatives:

References:
1. Pharmaceutical manufacturer prescribing information, 1997.
2. Rutgers-Verhage AR, DeVries TW, Torringa MJL. No Effects of Bisphosphonates on the Human Fetus. Birth Defects Res., Part A 2003; 67: 203–204.

ALFENTANIL   L2

Trade: Alfenta
Other Trades: Rapifen, Alfenta
Category: Narcotic analgesic

Alfentanil is an opiate that is used for pain relief during labor and delivery and given prior to induction of anesthesia for surgery. Alfentanil is secreted into breastmilk. Following a dose of 50 µg/kg IV (plus several additional 10 µg/kg doses), the mean levels of alfentanil in colostrum at 4 hours varied from 0.21 to 1.56 µg/L of colostrum, levels probably too small to produce overt toxicity in breastfeeding infants.[1] Mean levels 28 hours post-alfentanil were 0.05 µg/L.

Pregnancy Risk	C	Lactation Risk	L2
T ½	= 1–2 hours	M/P	=
Vd	= 0.3–1.0 l/kg	PB	= 92%
Tmax	= Immediate	Oral	= 43%
MW	= 417	pKa	= 6.5

Adult Concerns: Observe for bradycardia, shivering, constipation and sedation. In neonates observe for severe hypotension.

Pediatric Concerns: None reported via milk.

Drug Interactions: Phenothiazines may antagonize the analgesic effects of opiates. Dextromethorphan may increase the analgesia of opiate agonists. Other CNS depressants such as benzodiazepines, barbiturates, tricyclic antidepressants, erythromycin, reserpine and beta blockers may increase the toxicity of this opiate.

Relative Infant Dose: 0.4%

Adult Dose: 8–40 µg/kg total

Alternatives: Remifentanil

References:
1. Giesecke A, Rice L, Lipton J. Alfentaril in colostrum. Anesthesiology 63: A284 1985.
2. Spigset O. Anaesthetic agents and excretion in breast milk. Acta Anaesthesiol Scand 1994; 38(2): 94–103.

ALFUZOSIN   L4

Trade: Uroxatral
Other Trades:
Category: Alpha1 adrenergic antagonist

Alfuzosin is not approved for use in women, but is used in men for benign prostatic hyperplasia. It is occasionally used in women to assist in the passage of a kidney stone or for bladder motility problems. It works by antagonizing the alpha1 adrenoreceptors, thus reducing ureter contractility. There are no data regarding alfuzosin transfer into breastmilk. However, due to possibility of hypotension in infant, breastfeeding while taking alfuzosin is not recommended.

Pregnancy Risk	B	Lactation Risk	L4
T ½	= 10 hours	M/P	=
Vd	= 3.2 l/kg	PB	= 82–90%
Tmax	= 8 hours	Oral	= 49%
MW	= 389	pKa	=

Adult Concerns: Postular hypotension, syncope, dizziness, fatigue, constipation, abdominal pain, nausea, bronchitis, upper respiratory track infection.

Pediatric Concerns:

Drug Interactions:

Relative Infant Dose:

Adult Dose: 10 mg once daily.

Alternatives:

References:
1. Alfuzosin packge insert. Bridgewater, NJ. Sanofi-Adventis U. S. LLC; 2010.

ALISKIREN   L3

Trade: Tekturna, Valturna, Tekturna HCT
Other Trades:
Category: Renin inhibitor

Aliskiren is a direct renin inhibitor, blocking the formation of angiotensin II and thus decreasing blood pressure. It works directly on renin, and therefore may be more clinically advantageous than a typical ACE inhibitor.[1] No data are available on its transfer into human milk. However, due to its high molecular weight and low oral absorption (3%), it is unlikely that an infant would absorb enough to receive a therapeutic dose from breastmilk. Aliskiren should be avoided while breastfeeding premature infants, as the nephrons of the kidney are undeveloped. A risk versus benefit analysis should be conducted in each individual.

Pregnancy Risk	C/D in 2nd and 3rd trimester	Lactation Risk	L3
T ½	= 24 hours	M/P	=
Vd	= 135 l/kg	PB	= 47–51%
Tmax	= 1–3 hours	Oral	= 3%
MW	= 609	pKa	= 15.90

Adult Concerns: Adverse reactions include dizziness, rash, diarrhea, increased serum creatinine and BUN.

Pediatric Concerns: No data are available.

Drug Interactions: Atorvastatin and ketoconazole may increase the effect of aliskiren, while furosemide may decrease the effect.

Relative Infant Dose:

Adult Dose: 150–300 mg/day

Alternatives: Methyldopa, metoprolol, hydrochlorothiazide, captopril, enalapril

References:
1. Pharmaceutical manufacturer prescribing information, 2011.

ALLANTOIN   L3

Trade:

Other Trades:

Category: Astringent

Allantoin is an astringent, keratolytic and also has anti-inflammatory properties and has been used to promote wound healing.[1] It is frequently present in mouthwashes, toothpaste, and other oral hygiene products. It is also present in shampoos, lipsticks, anti-acne products, sun care products, and other cosmetic and pharmaceutical products. There are no adequate and well-controlled studies or case reports in breastfeeding women, although its topical use is probably not a contraindication to breastfeeding.

Pregnancy Risk	Probably Safe	Lactation Risk	L3
T ½	=	M/P	=
Vd	=	PB	=
Tmax	=	Oral	=
MW	= 158.1	pKa	=

Adult Concerns: Rash, skin irritation at application site.

Pediatric Concerns:

Drug Interactions:

Relative Infant Dose:

Adult Dose:

Alternatives:

References:
1. Pharmaceutical manufacturer prescribing information, 2010.

ALLERGY INJECTIONS   L3

Trade:

Other Trades:

Category: Desensitizing injections

Allergy injections consist of protein and carbohydrate substances from plants, animals, and other species. There are no reported untoward effects. They are unlikely to enter milk. Observe for allergic reactions, although adverse effects are unlikely in the breastfed infant.

Pregnancy Risk	Probably Safe	Lactation Risk	L3
T ½	=	M/P	=
Vd	=	PB	=
Tmax	=	Oral	=
MW	=	pKa	=

Adult Concerns: Allergic pruritus, anaphylaxis, other immune reactions.

Pediatric Concerns: None reported in breastfeeding mothers.

Drug Interactions:

Relative Infant Dose:

Adult Dose: N/A

Alternatives:

References:

ALLOPURINOL   L2

Trade: Zyloprim, Lopurin

Other Trades: Allorin, Capurate, Zygout, Zyloprim, Alloprin, Apo-Allopurinol, Novo-Purol, Zyloprim, Aluline, Caplenal, Cosuric, Hamarin, Zyloric

Category: Reduces uric acid levels

Allopurinol is a potent antagonist of xanthine oxidase, an enzyme involved in the production of uric acid. It is used to reduce uric acid levels in gouty individuals. In a nursing mother receiving 300 mg/day allopurinol, the breastmilk concentration at 2 and 4 hours was 0.9 and 1.4 μg/mL respectively.[1] The concentration of the metabolite, oxypurinol, was 53.7 and 48.0 μg/mL at 2 and 4 hours respectively. The milk/plasma ratio ranged from 0.9 to 1.4 for allopurinol and 3.9 for its metabolite, oxypurinol. The average daily dose that an infant would receive from milk would be approximately 0.14–0.20 mg/kg of allopurinol and 7.2–8.0 mg/kg of oxypurinol. No adverse effects were noted in the infant after 6 weeks of therapy. Pediatric dosages for ages 6 years and under is generally 10 mg/kg/24 hours.

Pregnancy Risk	C	Lactation Risk	L2
T ½	= 1–3 hours (allopurinol)	M/P	= 0.9–1.4
Vd	= 1.6 l/kg	PB	=
Tmax	= 2–6 hours	Oral	= 90%
MW	= 136	pKa	= 9.4

Adult Concerns: Itching skin rash. Fever, chills, nausea and vomiting, diarrhea, gastritis

Pediatric Concerns: No adverse effects were noted in one infant after 6 weeks of therapy.

Drug Interactions: Alcohol decreases allopurinol efficacy. Inhibits metabolism of azathioprine and mercaptopurine. Increased incidence of skin rash when used with amoxicillin and ampicillin. Increased risk of kidney stones when used with high doses of vitamin C. Allopurinol prolongs half-life of oral anticoagulants, theophylline, chlorpropamide.

Relative Infant Dose: 4.9%

Adult Dose: 100–400 mg BID

Alternatives:

References:
1. Kamilli I, Gresser U. Allopurinol and oxypurinol in human breast milk. Clin Investig 1993; 71(2): 161–164.

ALMOTRIPTAN | L3

Trade: Axert

Other Trades: Almogran

Category: Acute migraine treatment

Almotriptan is a selective serotonin receptor antagonist similar to sumatriptan although it is slightly more bioavailable orally. No data are available on its transfer to human milk. Clinically, it is not much better than oral sumatriptan[1], which has been well studied in breastfeeding women. See sumatriptan for alternative.

Pregnancy Risk	C	Lactation Risk	L3
T ½	= 3–4 hours	M/P	=
Vd	= 2.85 l/kg	PB	= 35%
Tmax	= 2–4 hours	Oral	= 80%
MW	= 469.65	pKa	= 8.77

Adult Concerns: Nausea, somnolence, headache, dry mouth, tachycardia, myocardial ischemia.

Pediatric Concerns: None reported.

Drug Interactions: Higher plasma level of almotriptan could result from use with ketoconazole, amiodarone, cimetidine, clarithromycin, erythromycin, nefazodone, and other inhibitors of CYP3A4. Do not use with ergot alkaloids, MAO inhibitors, verapamil, SSRIs such as fluoxetine, sertraline, etc.

Relative Infant Dose:

Adult Dose: 6.25–12.5 mg

Alternatives: Sumatriptan

References:
1. Spierings EL, Gomez-Mancilla B, Grosz DE, Rowland CR, Whaley FS, Jirgens KJ. Oral almotriptan vs. oral sumatriptan in the abortive treatment of migraine: a double-blind, randomized, parallel-group, optimum-dose comparison. Arch Neurol 2001; 58(6): 944–950.

ALOE VERA | L3

Trade:

Other Trades:

Category: Extract from A. Vera

There are over 500 species of aloes. The aloe plant yields two important products: Aloe latex derived from the outer skin and Aloe gel, a clear, gelatinous material derived from the inner tissue of the leaf. The aloe gel is the most commonly used product in cosmetic and health food products. The gel contains a polysaccharide glucomannan, similar to guar gum, which is responsible for its emollient effect. Aloe also contains tannins, polysaccharides, organic acids, enzymes, and other products. Bradykininase, a protease inhibitor, is believed to relieve pain and decrease swelling and pruritus. Other components such as an anti-prostaglandin compound is believed to reduce inflammation.[1] Aloe latex, a bitter yellow product derived from the outer skin, is a drastic cathartic and produces a strong purgative effect on the large intestine due to its anthraquinone barbaloin content. Do not use the latex orally in children.[2] The most common use of the aloe gel is in burn therapy for minor burns and skin irritation. Thus far, well controlled studies do not provide evidence of a clear advantage over aggressive wound care. Two FDA advisory panels failed to find sufficient evidence to show Aloe Vera is useful in treatment of minor burns, cuts, or vaginal irritation. Recent evidence suggests that Aloe vera may accelerate wound healing such as in frostbite and in patients undergoing dermabrasion although another study suggests a delay in healing.[3,4] Numerous studies have suggested accelerated wound healing, reduction in arthritic inflammation, and other inflammatory diseases although these are, in many cases, poorly controlled. The toxicity of Aloe vera gel when applied topically is minimal. Oral use of the latex derived from the outer skin of Aloe vera is strongly discouraged as they are drastic cathartics. Aloe emodin and other anthraquinones present in Aloe vera latex may cause severe gastric cramping and should never be used in pregnant women and children.

Aloe vera is probably okay to use during breastfeeding if used acutely and topically. Caution is advised when used orally. No adverse effects have been reported in breastfed infants. Avoid oral use in breastfeeding mothers.

Pregnancy Risk	Possibly Hazardous	Lactation Risk	L3
T ½	=	M/P	=
Vd	=	PB	=
Tmax	=	Oral	=
MW	=	pKa	=

Adult Concerns: Severe gastric irritation, strong purgative effect and diarrhea when gel used orally.

Pediatric Concerns: No reports of untoward effects following maternal use or via milk ingestion.

Drug Interactions:

Relative Infant Dose:

Adult Dose: N/A

Alternatives:

References:

1. Review of Natural Products Ed: Facts and Comparisons 1997.
2. Leung AY. Encyclopedia of Common Natural Ingredients used in Food, Drugs and Cosmetics. J Wiley and Sons, 1980.
3. Fulton JE, Jr. The stimulation of postdermabrasion wound healing with stabilized aloe vera gel-polyethylene oxide dressing. J Dermatol Surg Oncol 1990; 16(5): 460–467.
4. Schmidt JM, Greenspoon JS. Aloe vera dermal wound gel is associated with a delay in wound healing. Obstet Gynecol 1991; 78(1): 115–117.

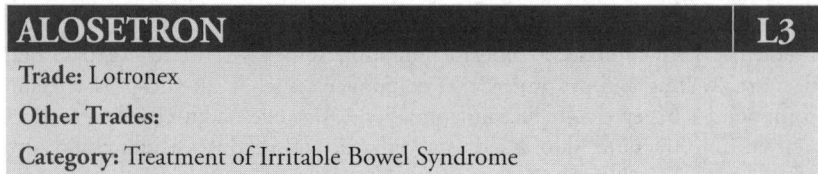

ALOSETRON   L3

Trade: Lotronex

Other Trades:

Category: Treatment of Irritable Bowel Syndrome

Alosetron is a new 5–HT3 receptor antagonist which is used to control the symptoms of irritable bowel syndrome. No data are available on the transfer of this medication into human milk. While the manufacturer suggests it is present in animal milk, no data are provided.[1] The peak plasma levels (in young women) of this product are quite small, only averaging 9 ng/mL following a 1 mg dose. Although the half-life of the parent alosetron is short (1.5 hours), its metabolites have much longer half-lives although their importance is unknown. Bioavailability is lessened (<25%) when mixed with food. With this data it is unlikely milk levels will be extraordinarily high, or that the levels transferred to the infant will be clinically relevant to the infant. However, its use in breastfeeding patients should be approached with caution until we have more clinical experience with this new product.

Pregnancy Risk	B	Lactation Risk	L3
T ½	= 1.5 hours	M/P	=
Vd	= 1.36 l/kg	PB	= 82%
Tmax	= 1 hour	Oral	= 50–60%
MW	= 294.351	pKa	=

Adult Concerns: Constipation is very common, hypertension, nausea less so.

Pediatric Concerns: None reported via milk, but no studies exist.

Drug Interactions: It is unlikely alosetron will inhibit the metabolism of drugs metabolized by the major CYP 450 enzymes.

Relative Infant Dose:

Adult Dose: 1 mg twice daily.

Alternatives:

References:
1.   Pharmaceutical manufacturer prescribing information, 200..

ALPHA–GALACTOSIDASE ENZYME | L3

Trade:

Other Trades:

Category:

Alpha galactosidase is an enzyme that systemically hydrolyses the terminal alpha-galactosyl moieties from glycolipids and glycoproteins.[1] Used orally, it is used to reduce gas production in the gastrointestinal tract by breaking down complex carbohydrates and oligosaccharides such as raffinose. There are no adequate and well-controlled studies or case reports in breastfeeding women, however used orally, this product is probably safe for breastfeeding mothers.

Pregnancy Risk	Probably Safe	Lactation Risk	L3
T ½	=	M/P	=
Vd	=	PB	=
Tmax	=	Oral	=
MW	= 101,000	pKa	=

Adult Concerns: Observe for gastric side effects. Few are listed in these products.

Pediatric Concerns:

Drug Interactions:

Relative Infant Dose:

Adult Dose:

Alternatives:

References:
1.   Pharmaceutical manufacturer prescribing information, 2010.

ALPRAZOLAM | L3

Trade: Xanax

Other Trades: Kalma, Ralozam, Apo-Alpraz, Novo-Alprazol, Xanax

Category: Benzodiazepine antianxiety agent

Alprazolam is a prototypic benzodiazepine drug similar to valium but is now preferred in many instances because of its shorter half-life. In a study of 8 women who received a single oral dose of 0.5 mg, the peak alprazolam level in milk was 3.7 µg/L which occurred at 1.1 hours; the observed milk/serum ratio (using AUC method) was 0.36.[1] The neonatal dose of alprazolam in breastmilk is low. The author estimates the average between 0.3 to 5 µg/kg per day. While the infants in this study did not breastfeed, these doses would probably be too low to induce a clinical effect. In a brief letter, Anderson reports that the manufacturer is aware of withdrawal symptoms in infants following exposure in utero and via breastmilk.[2] In a mother who received 0.5 mg 2–3 times daily orally during pregnancy, neonatal withdrawal syndrome was evident in the breastfed infant the first week postpartum. This data suggests that the amount of alprazolam in breastmilk is insufficient to prevent a withdrawal syndrome following prenatal exposure. In another case of infant exposure solely via breastmilk, the mother took alprazolam (dosage unspecified) for nine months while breastfeeding and withdrew herself from the medication over a 3 week period. The mother reported withdrawal symptoms in the infant including irritability, crying, and sleep disturbances. The benzodiazepine family, as a rule, are not ideal for breastfeeding mothers due to relatively long half-lives and the development of dependence. However, it is apparent that the shorter-acting benzodiazepines are safest during lactation provided their use is short-term or intermittent, and at a low dose.[3]

Pregnancy Risk	D	Lactation Risk	L3
T ½	= 12–15 hours	M/P	= 0.36
Vd	= 0.9–1.3 l/kg	PB	= 80%
Tmax	= 1–2 hours	Oral	= Complete
MW	= 309	pKa	= 2.8

Adult Concerns: Drowsiness, fatigue, insomnia, confusion, dry mouth, constipation, nausea, vomiting.

Pediatric Concerns: Rarely, withdrawal syndrome reported in one breastfed infant. Observe for sedation, poor feeding, irritability, crying, insomnia on withdrawal. Use on an acute or short term basis is not contraindicated.

Drug Interactions: Decreased therapeutic effect when used with carbamazepine, disulfiram. Increased toxicity when used with oral contraceptives, CNS depressants, cimetidine and lithium.

Relative Infant Dose: 8.5%

Adult Dose: 0.5–1 mg TID

Alternatives: Lorazepam

References:
1. Oo CY, Kuhn RJ, Desai N, Wright CE, McNamara PJ. Pharmacokinetics in lactating women: prediction of alprazolam transfer into milk. Br J Clin Pharmacol 1995; 40(3): 231–236.
2. Anderson PO, McGuire GG. Neonatal alprazolam withdrawal--possible effects of breast feeding. DICP 1989; 23(7–8): 614.
3. Maitra R, Menkes DB. Psychotropic drugs and lactation. N Z Med J 1996; 109(1024): 217–218.

ALTEPLASE | L3

Trade: Activase
Other Trades: Actilyse
Category: Thrombolytic agent

Alteplase is a thrombolytic agent commonly known as tissue-type plasminogen activator (tPA). Alteplase is a large protein with 527 amino acids and with a large molecular weight. It binds to fibrin in a thrombus and converts the plasminogen to plasmin which subsequently leads to a breakdown of the clot. Alteplase is rapidly cleared from the plasma, with an initial half-life of 5 minutes following rapid IV therapy and a somewhat longer half-life of 26–46 minutes following prolonged infusion.[1,2] Its transfer into mature milk would be negligible, but it could potentially pass in small amounts in colostrum. Whether it would be bioavailable in the gut of a newborn infant is questionable, but it would almost certainly not be bioavailable in an older infant. It is very unlikely it would produce adverse effects in breastfed infants.

Pregnancy Risk	C	Lactation Risk	L3
T ½	= 26–46 minutes	M/P	=
Vd	= 8.1 l/kg	PB	=
Tmax	= 20–40 minutes	Oral	= Nil
MW	= Large	pKa	=

Adult Concerns: Hemorrhage, reperfusion arrhythmias, bradycardia and possibly seizures.

Pediatric Concerns: None reported.

Drug Interactions: May potentiate hemorrhage when used with other anticoagulants such as dicoumarol, warfarin, anisindione, acenocoumarol, phenindione, heparin and etc. Nitroglycerin may increase clearance of TPA.

Relative Infant Dose:

Adult Dose: 100 mg

Alternatives:

References:
1. Pharmaceutical manufacturer prescribing information, 2001.
2. Verstraete M, Su CA, Tanswell P, Feuerer W, Collen D. Pharmacokinetics and effects on fibrinolytic and coagulation parameters of two doses of recombinant tissue-type plasminogen activator in healthy volunteers. Thromb Haemost 1986; 56(1): 1–5.

ALTRETAMINE   L4

Trade: Hexalen
Other Trades: Hexalen
Category: Anticancer drug

Used to treat ovarian, breast, cervix, pancreatic, and other cancers, altretamine requires metabolism to the cytotoxic derivative. While it is well absorbed orally, its oral bioavailability is low, due to first pass metabolism and uptake by the liver. Its usefulness is limited by its toxicity. Following oral administration of radiolabeled altretamine, urinary recovery of radioactivity was 61% at 24 hours and 90% at 72 hours.[1] Human urinary metabolites were N-demethylated homologues of altretamine with <1% unmetabolized altretamine excreted at 24 hours. No data on entry into human milk are available. Withhold breastfeeding for at least 72 hours.

Pregnancy Risk	D	Lactation Risk	L4
T ½	= (beta) 4.7–10.5 hours	M/P	=
Vd	=	PB	= 94%
Tmax	= 0.5–3 hours	Oral	=
MW	= 210.3	pKa	=

Adult Concerns: Anxiety, clumsiness, confusion, seizures, dizziness, mental depression, numbness in arms or legs, weakness, nausea, vomiting

Pediatric Concerns:

Drug Interactions:

Relative Infant Dose:

Adult Dose: 260 mg/m²/day in 4 divided doses

Alternatives:

References:
1. Pharmaceutical manufacturer prescribing information, 2005.

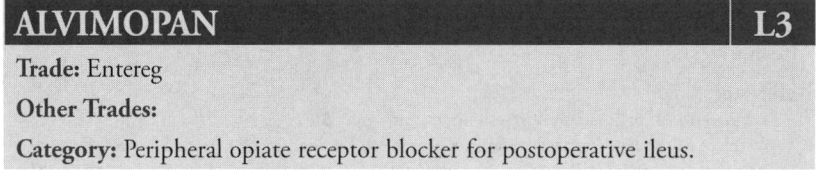

ALVIMOPAN   L3

Trade: Entereg
Other Trades:
Category: Peripheral opiate receptor blocker for postoperative ileus.

Alvimopan is a peripherally acting μ-opioid receptor antagonist indicated to accelerate the time to upper and lower gastrointestinal recovery following partial large or small bowel resection surgery with primary anastomosis.[1] No data are available on its transfer into human milk. However, adult plasma levels are incredibly low, the oral bioavailability is low, and the molecular weight is slightly high, so milk levels are estimated to be quite low.

Pregnancy Risk	B	Lactation Risk	L3
T ½	= 10–17 hours	M/P	=
Vd	= 0.42 l/kg	PB	= 80–94%
Tmax	= 2 hours	Oral	= 6%
MW	= 460	pKa	= 9.75

Adult Concerns: Side effects appear minimal but include: anemia, constipation, dyspepsia, flatulence, hypokalemia, back pain and urinary retention.

Pediatric Concerns: None yet reported via milk. Observe for constipation.

Drug Interactions: No data yet.

Relative Infant Dose:

Adult Dose: 12 mg BID

Alternatives:

References:
1. Pharmaceutical manufacturer prescribing information, 2010.

AMANTADINE   L3

Trade: Symmetrel, Symadine

Other Trades: Symmetrel, Endantanine, Gen-Amantadine, Mantadine

Category: Anti-viral and antiparkinsonian

Amantadine is a unique compound that has both antiviral activity against influenza A and is effective in treating Parkinsonian symptoms.[1] Pediatric indications for prevention of influenza for ages 1–10 are available. Only trace amounts are believed to be secreted in milk although no reports are found. Adult plasma levels following doses of 200 mg daily are 400–900 nanograms/mL.[2] Even assuming a theoretical milk/plasma ratio of 1.0, the average daily dose to a breastfeeding infant would be far less than 0.9 mg, a dose that would be clinically irrelevant compared to the 4–8 mg/kg dose used in 1-year-old infants. However, amantadine is known to suppress prolactin production and should not be used in breastfeeding mothers or at least should be used with caution while observing for milk suppression.[3,4]

Pregnancy Risk	C	Lactation Risk	L3
T ½	= 1–28 hours	M/P	=
Vd	= 4.4 l/kg	PB	= 67%
Tmax	= 1–4 hours	Oral	= 86–94%
MW	= 151	pKa	= 10.1

Adult Concerns: Urinary retention, vomiting, skin rash in infants. Insomnia, depression, confusion, disorientation, nausea, anorexia, constipation, vomiting.

Pediatric Concerns: None reported via milk but a major reduction in prolactin levels has been reported. Avoid.

Drug Interactions: May increase anticholinergic effects when used with anticholinergic or CNS active drugs. Increased toxicity/levels when used with hydrochlorothiazide plus triamterene, or amiloride.

Relative Infant Dose:

Adult Dose: 100 mg BID

Alternatives:

References:
1. Pharmaceutical manufacturer prescribing information, 1997.
2. Cedarbaum JM. Clinical pharmacokinetics of anti-parkinsonian drugs. Clin Pharmacokinet 1987; 13(3): 141–178.
3. Correa N, Opler LA, Kay SR, Birmaher B. Amantadine in the treatment of neuroendocrine side effects of neuroleptics. J Clin Psychopharmacol 1987; 7(2): 91–95.
4. Siever LJ. The effect of amantadine on prolactin levels and galactorrhea on neuroleptic-treated patients. J Clin Psychopharmacol 1981; 1(1): 2–7.

AMIKACIN   L2

Trade: Amikin

Other Trades: Amikin

Category: Aminoglycoside antibiotic

Amikacin is a typical aminoglycoside antibiotic used for gram negative infections. Other aminoglycoside antibiotics are poorly absorbed from the gastrointestinal tract in infants although they could produce changes in the gastrointestinal flora. Only very small amounts are secreted into breastmilk. Following 100 and 200 mg IM doses, only trace amounts have been found in breastmilk and then in only 2 of 4 patients studied.[1] In another study of 2–3 patients who received 100 mg IM, none to trace amounts were found in milk.[2]

Pregnancy Risk	D	Lactation Risk	L2
T ½	= 2.3 hours	M/P	=
Vd	= 0.28 l/kg	PB	= 4%
Tmax	= 0.75–2.0 hours	Oral	= Poor
MW	= 586	pKa	= 12.71

Adult Concerns: Diarrhea, changes in gastrointestinal flora.

Pediatric Concerns: None reported via milk. Commonly used in neonates.

Drug Interactions: Increased aminoglycoside toxicity when used with indomethacin, amphotericin, loop diuretics, vancomycin, enflurane, methoxyflurane, depolarizing neuromuscular blocking agents.

Relative Infant Dose:

Adult Dose: 5–7.5 mg/kg/dose TID

Alternatives:

References:
1. Matsuda C. A study of amikacin in the obstetrics field. Jpn J Antibiot 1974; 27: 633–636.
2. Matsuda S. Transfer of antibiotics into maternal milk. Biol Res Pregnancy Perinatol 1984; 5(2): 57–60.

AMILORIDE | L3

Trade: Midamor
Other Trades:
Category: Diuretic

Amiloride is a potassium-sparing diuretic agent used in the management of hypertension and congestive heart failure.[1] It is usually administered along with thiazide diuretics. Studies in rats have shown that the concentrations of amiloride in milk are higher than those in the plasma. It is not known if amiloride is transferred into human milk, but a review of the drug's pharmacokinetic profile suggests that transfer into milk is likely. Due to the potential of untoward effects in the breastfed infant with its use, this drug is best avoided in breastfeeding mothers. Use in lactating mothers only if the potential benefit to the mother outweighs the potential risks to the infant.

Pregnancy Risk	B	Lactation Risk	L3
T ½	= 6–9 hours	M/P	=
Vd	= 350–380 L l/kg	PB	= Not significant
Tmax	= 3–4 hours	Oral	= 30–90%
MW	= 302.12	pKa	= 8.7

Adult Concerns: Nausea, vomiting, headache, dizziness, diarrhea, hyperkalemia, postural hypotension. Do not use in those with hyperkalemia, those on potassium supplements and in those with impaired renal function.

Pediatric Concerns:

Drug Interactions: Concomitant use with ACE inhibitors, angiotensin receptor blockers, cyclosporine or tacrolimus will increase the risk of hyperkalemia. Concurrent use with lithium may cause lithium toxicity. Efficacy is reduced when administered concomitantly with NSAIDs.

Relative Infant Dose:

Adult Dose: 5–20 mg once daily.

Alternatives: Spironolactone

References:
1.   Pharmaceutical manufacturer prescribing information, 2010.

AMINOCAPROIC ACID | L4

Trade: Amicar
Other Trades:
Category: Hemostatic agent

Aminocaproic acid is an antifibrinolytic agent used in prevention of bleeding with cardiac surgery, bleeding disorders, or in patients who are currently on anticoagulant therapies.[1,2] It also prevents spontaneous fibrinolysis. There are no data on its transfer into human milk. If we were to assume a 1 to 1 milk/plasma ratio (which is probably high), and a normal maternal therapeutic plasma range of 130 µg/mL, then milk levels would be 130 µg/mL and with a relative infant dose of 19%. While high, this is very unlikely. Use caution. Observe the infant closely during therapy.

Pregnancy Risk	C	Lactation Risk	L4
T ½	= 2 hours	M/P	=
Vd	= Oral: 0.328 ; IV: 0.42 l/kg	PB	=
Tmax	= 2 hours	Oral	= Complete
MW	= 131	pKa	= 4.4

Adult Concerns: Arrhythmia, bradycardia, edema, hypotension, confusion, dizziness, fatigue, headache, abdominal pain, diarrhea, nausea, vomiting, agranulocytosis, leukopenia, thrombocytopenia, myalgia, vision decreased, watery eyes, nasal congestion.

Pediatric Concerns: Observe for abdominal pain nausea, vomiting. None yet reported in breastfeeding mothers.

Drug Interactions: Hemostatic agents can increase the effects of anti-inhibitor coagulant complexes. Hemostatic agents may also increase the adverse effect of Factor IX and fibrinogen concentrate in humans. Tretinoin may increase the effect of hemostatic agents.

Relative Infant Dose:

Adult Dose: 50–100 mg/kg but variable

Alternatives:

References:
1. Lexi-Comp Online, Lexi-Drugs Online, Hudson, Ohio: Lexi-Comp, Inc. ; July 11, 2011.
2. McAuley, David F. The Clinician's Ultimate Reference. Last updated July 25, 2010. Accessed July 12, 2009. http: //www. globalrph. com/aminocaproic_acid_dilution. htm.

AMINOPTERIN   L5

Trade:

Other Trades:

Category: Antineoplastic

Aminopterin is a 4-amino analog of folic acid that is used as an antineoplastic immunosuppressive agent in cancer chemotherapy. It results in the reduction and depletion of nucleotide precursors used in the synthesis of DNA, RNA, and proteins. Its use is not supplanted by the more effective methotrexate. While there are no studies of the use of this product in breastfeeding mothers, it is extraordinarily dangerous and should never be used in breastfeeding mothers.

Pregnancy Risk	X	Lactation Risk	L5
T ½	= 3.64 Hours	M/P	=
Vd	=	PB	=
Tmax	=	Oral	=
MW	= 440	pKa	= 6.5–8.5

Adult Concerns: Strong abortifacient. Nausea, vomiting, anorexia, weight loss, fever, chills, mucositis, GI hemorrhage.

Pediatric Concerns: Extremely dangerous. Do not use in breastfeeding mothers. If used, supplement infant with folic acid or leucovorin.

Drug Interactions: Blocks effect of folic acid. Use leucovorin as antidote.

Relative Infant Dose:

Adult Dose:

Alternatives:

References:

AMINOSALICYLIC ACID (ASA)   L3

Trade: Paser, PAS

Other Trades: Tubasal, Nemasol

Category: Antitubercular

Paraminosalicylic acid (P-ASA) inhibits folic acid synthesis and is selective only for tuberculosis bacteria. Following a maternal dose of 4.0 gm/day, the peak maternal plasma level was 70.1 mg/L and occurred at 2 hours. The breastmilk concentration of 5–ASA at 3 hours was 1.1 mg/L.[1] In another study, the concentration in milk ranged from 0.13 to 0.53 µmol/liter.[2] In a 29-year-old mother who received 3 gm/day of 5– ASA for ulcerative colitis, the estimated intake for an infant receiving 120–200 mL of milk was 0.02 to 0.012 mg of 5–ASA.[3] The concentrations of 5–ASA and its metabolite Acetyl-5–ASA present in milk appear too low to produce overt toxicity in most infants. Only one report of slight diarrhea in one infant has been reported.

Pregnancy Risk	C	Lactation Risk	L3
T ½	= 1 hour	M/P	= 0.09–0.17
Vd	=	PB	= 50–73%
Tmax	= 2 hours	Oral	= >90%
MW	= 153	pKa	= 13.23

Adult Concerns: Nausea, vomiting, diarrhea.

Pediatric Concerns: Only one report of slight diarrhea in one infant has been reported.

Drug Interactions: Reduces levels of digoxin and vitamin B_{12}.

Relative Infant Dose: 0.3%

Adult Dose: 150 mg/kg/day BID or TID

Alternatives:

References:
1. Holiness MR. Antituberculosis drugs and breast-feeding. Arch Intern Med 1984; 144(9): 1888.
2. Christensen LA, Rasmussen SN, Hansen SH. Disposition of 5-aminosalicylic acid and N-acetyl-5-aminosalicylic acid in fetal and maternal body fluids during treatment with different 5-aminosalicylic acid preparations. Acta Obstet Gynecol Scand 1994; 73(5): 399–402.
3. Klotz U, Harings-Kaim A. Negligible excretion of 5-aminosalicylic acid in breast milk. Lancet 1993; 342(8871): 618–619.

AMIODARONE   L4/L5

Trade: Cordarone

Other Trades: Aratac

Category: Strong antiarrhythmic agent

Amiodarone is a potent and sometimes dangerous antiarrhythmic drug and requires close supervision by clinicians. Although poorly absorbed by the mother (<50%), maximum serum levels are attained after 3–7 hours. This drug has a very large volume of distribution, resulting in accumulation in adipose, liver, spleen, and lungs and has a high rate of fetal toxicity (10–17%). It should not be given to pregnant mothers unless critically required.

Significant amounts are secreted into breastmilk at levels higher than the plasma level. Breastmilk samples obtained at birth and at 2 and 3 weeks postpartum in 2 patients, contained levels of amiodarone and desethylamiodarone varying from 1.7 to 3.0 mg/L (mean=2.3 mg/L) and 0.8 to 1.8 mg/L (mean=1.1 mg/L), respectively.[1] Despite the concentrations of amiodarone in milk, the amounts were apparently not high enough to produce plasma levels of both drugs higher than about 0.1 µg/mL, which are minimal compared to the maternal plasma levels of 1.2 µg/mL or higher.

McKenna reported amiodarone milk levels in a mother treated with 400 mg daily.[2] In this study, at 6 weeks postpartum, breastmilk levels of amiodarone and desethylamiodarone varied during the day from 2.8–16.4 mg/L and 1.1–6.5 mg/L respectively. Reported infant plasma levels of amiodarone and desethylamiodarone were 0.4 mg/L and 0.25 mg/L respectively. The dose ingested by the infant was approximately 1.5 µg/kg/day. The authors suggest that the amount of amiodarone ingested was moderate and could expose the developing infant to a significant dose of the drug and should be avoided.

Because amiodarone inhibits extrathyroidal de-iodinases, conversion of T4 to T3 is reduced. One case of hypothyroidism has been reported in an infant following therapy in the mother. Because of the long half-life and high concentrations in various organs, amiodarone could continuously build up to higher levels in the infant although it was not reported in the above studies. This product should be used only under the most extraordinary conditions, and the infant should be closely monitored for cardiovascular and thyroid function. Thus, breastfeeding should be avoided if this product is used chronically. Brief, 3–7 days use is probably not contraindicated if a 24–48 hour interruption is used before re-instating breastfeeding. One case reported a mother who took 200 mg amiodarone three times daily to treat fetal ascites and tachycardia. Upon delivery, the mother stopped taking amiodarone. Breastmilk was tested to determine the levels of amiodarone, which were found to be 0.6 mg/L, 2.1 mg/L, and undetectable on days 5, 11, and 25, respectively. The baby was monitored closely during this period. The authors suggest that in some instances, with close monitoring, breastfeeding can occur during amiodarone therapy.[3]

Pregnancy Risk	D		Lactation Risk	L4 acute / L5 Chronic
T ½	= 26–107 days		M/P	= 4.6–13
Vd	= 18–148 l/kg		PB	= 99.98%
Tmax	= 3–7 hours		Oral	= 22–86%
MW	= 643		pKa	= 6.6

Adult Concerns: Hypothyroidism, myocardial arrhythmias, pulmonary toxicity, serious liver injury, congestive heart failure.

Pediatric Concerns: Hypothyroidism has been reported. Extreme caution is urged.

Drug Interactions: Amiodarone interferes with the metabolism of a number of drugs including: oral anticoagulants, beta blockers, calcium channel blockers, digoxin, flecainide, phenytoin, procainamide, quinidine. Plasma levels of these drugs tend to be increased to hazardous levels.

Relative Infant Dose: 43.1%

Adult Dose: 200–800 mg BID

Alternatives: Disopyramide, Mexiletine

References:
1. Plomp TA, Vulsma T, de Vijlder JJ. Use of amiodarone during pregnancy. Eur J Obstet Gynecol Reprod Biol 1992; 43(3): 201–207.
2. McKenna WJ, Harris L, Rowland E, Whitelaw A, Storey G, Holt D. Amiodarone therapy during pregnancy. Am J Cardiol 1983; 51(7): 1231–1233.
3. Hall CM, McCormick KPB. Amiodarone and breast feeding. Arch Dis Child Fetal Neonatal Ed 2003 May; 88(3): F255–F254.

AMITRIPTYLINE   L2

Trade: Elavil, Endep, Limbitrol

Other Trades: Endep, Mutabon D, Tryptanol, Apo-Amitriptyline, Novo-
Tryptin, Domical, Lentizol

Category: Tricyclic antidepressant

Amitriptyline and its active metabolite, nortriptyline, are secreted into breastmilk in small amounts. In one report of a mother taking 100 mg/day of amitriptyline, milk levels of amitriptyline and nortriptyline (active metabolite) averaged 143 µg/L and 55.5 µg/L respectively; maternal serum levels averaged 112 µg/L and 72.5 µg/L respectively.[1] No drug was detected in the infants serum. From this data, an infant would consume approximately 21.5 µg/kg/day, a dose that is unlikely to be clinically relevant. In another study following a maternal dose of 25 mg/day, the amitriptyline and nortriptyline (active metabolite) levels in milk were 30 µg/L and <30 µg/L respectively.[2,3] In the same study when the dosage was 75 mg/day, milk levels of amitriptyline and nortriptyline averaged 88 µg/L and 69 µg/L respectively. Both drugs were essentially undetectable in the infant's serum. Therefore, the authors estimated that a nursing infant would receive less than 0.1 mg/day. In another mother taking 175 mg/day, amitriptyline levels in the mother's milk were the same as in her serum on day one (24–27 µg/mL), but milk levels decreased to 54% of the serum concentration on days 2 to 26. Milk concentrations of nortriptyline were 74 percent of that in the mother's serum (87 ng/mL). Thus, the authors reported the absolute infant dose as 35 µg/kg, 80 times lower than the mother's dose. Neither compound could be detected in the infant's serum on day 26, nor were there any signs of sedation or other adverse effects.[4]

Pregnancy Risk	C	Lactation Risk	L2
T ½	= 31–46 hours	M/P	= 1.0
Vd	= 6–10 l/kg	PB	= 94.8%
Tmax	= 2–4 hours	Oral	= Complete
MW	= 277	pKa	= 9.4

Adult Concerns: Anticholinergic side effects, such as drying of secretions, dilated pupil, sedation.

Pediatric Concerns: No untoward effects have been noted in several studies. In studies of neurobehavioral development in at least 23 infants, no untoward effects or changes were noted from normal.[2,5,6,7]

Drug Interactions: Phenobarbital may reduce effect of amitriptyline. Amitriptyline blocks the hypotensive effect of guanethidine. May increase toxicity of amitriptyline when used with clonidine. Dangerous when used with MAO inhibitors, other CNS depressants. May increase anticoagulant effect of coumadin, warfarin. SSRIs (Prozac, Zoloft,etc) should not be used with or soon after amitriptyline or other TCAs due to serotonergic crisis.

Relative Infant Dose: 1.9%–2.8%

Adult Dose: 15–150 mg BID

Alternatives: Amoxapine, Imipramine

References:

1. Bader TF, Newman K. Amitriptyline in human breast milk and the nursing infant's serum. Am J Psychiatry 1980; 137(7): 855–856.
2. Brixen-Rasmussen L, Halgrener J, Jorgensen A. Amitriptyline and nortriptyline excretion in human breast milk. Psychopharmacology (Berl) 1982; 76(1): 94–95.
3. Matheson I, Skjaeraasen J. Milk concentrations of flupenthixol, nortriptyline and zuclopenthixol and between-breast differences in two patients. Eur J Clin Pharmacol 1988; 35(2): 217–220.
4. Breyer-Pfaff U, Nill K, Entenmann A, Gaertner HJ. Secretion of Amitriptyline and Metabolites Into Breast Milk. Am J Psychiatry 1995; 152(5): 812–813.
5. Misri S, Sivertz K. Tricyclic drugs in pregnancy and lactation: a preliminary report. Int J Psychiatry Med. 1991; 21: 157–71.
6. Yoshida K, Smith B, Kumar R. Psychotropic drugs in mothers' milk: a comprehensive review of assay methods, pharmacokinetics and safety of breast-feeding. J Psychopharmacol. 1999; 13: 64–80.
7. Nulman I, Rovet J, Stewart DE et al. Child development following exposure to tricyclic antidepressants or fluoxetine throughout fetal life: a prospective, controlled study. Am J Psychiatry. 2002; 159: 1889–95.

AMITRIPTYLINE + PERPHENAZINE | L3

Trade: Triavil, Etrafon, Etrafon 2–10, Etrafon A

Other Trades: Mutabon DElavil Plus, Entrafon

Category: Phenothiazine antipsychotic and antidepressant

Amitriptyline and Perphenazine is a combination drug product indicated for use in mixed depression and anxiety disorders.

Amitriptyline and its active metabolite, nortriptyline, are secreted into breastmilk in small amounts. In one report of a mother taking 100 mg/day of amitriptyline, milk levels of amitriptyline and nortriptyline (active metabolite) averaged 143 µg/L and 55.5 µg/L respectively; maternal serum levels averaged 112 µg/L and 72.5 µg/L respectively.[1] No drug was detected in the infants serum. From this data, an infant would consume approximately 21.5 µg/kg/day, a dose that is unlikely to be clinically relevant. In another study following a maternal dose of 25 mg/day, the amitriptyline and nortriptyline (active metabolite) levels in milk were 30 µg/L and <30 µg/L respectively.[2] In the same study when the dosage was 75 mg/day, milk levels of amitriptyline and nortriptyline averaged 88 µg/L and 69 µg/L respectively. Both drugs were essentially undetectable in the infant's serum. Therefore, the authors estimated that a nursing infant would receive less than 0.1 mg/day. In another mother taking 175 mg/day, amitriptyline levels in the mother's milk were the same as in her serum on day one (24–27 µg/mL), but milk levels decreased to 54% of the serum concentration on days 2 to 26. Milk concentrations of nortriptyline were 74 percent of that in the mother's serum (87 ng/mL). Thus, the authors reported the absolute infant dose as 35 µg/kg, 80 times lower than the mother's dose. Neither compound could be detected in the infant's serum on day 26, nor were there any signs of sedation or other adverse effects.[3]

Perphenazine is a phenothiazine derivative used as an antipsychotic or sedative. In a study of one patient receiving either 16 or 24 mg/day of perphenazine divided in two doses at 12 hour intervals, milk levels were 2.1 µg/L and 3.2 µg/L respectively.[4] The authors estimated the dose to the infant at 1.06 µg (0.3 µg/kg) or 1.59 µg

(0.45 µg/kg) respective of dose. Serum perphenazine levels in the mother drawn 12 hours after doses of 16 or 24 mg/day were 2.0 and 4.9 ng/mL respectively. Hence milk/plasma ratios were approximately 1.1 and 0.7 respective of the dose. The authors estimate the dose to be approximately 0.1% of the weight-adjusted maternal dose. The authors report that during a 3 month exposure, the infant thrived and had no adverse response to the medication.

Relative Infant Dose: - Amitriptyline/perphenazine: 1.9–2.8%/0.13–0.15%

Pregnancy Risk	C	Lactation Risk	L3
T ½	= Amitriptyline/perphenazine: 31–46 hours/8–20 hours	M/P	= Amitriptyline/perphenazine: 1.0/0.7–1.1
Vd	= Amitriptyline/perphenazine: 6–10/ l/kg	PB	= Amitriptyline/perphenazine: 94.8%/
Tmax	= Amitriptyline/perphenazine: 2–4 hours/	Oral	= Amitriptyline/perphenazine: complete/40%
MW	= Amitriptyline/perphenazine: 277/904	pKa	= Amitriptyline/perphenazine: 9.4/7.94

Adult Concerns: Sedation, extrapyramidal symptoms, tardive dyskinesia, anticholinergic symptoms, postural hypotension, obstructive jaundice.

Pediatric Concerns: None reported via milk. Observe for sedation. Rate of SIDS may be increased in infants exposed to phenothiazines.

Drug Interactions: Anticholinergics used to control extrapyramidal side effects may reduce oral absorption of perphenazine, and antagonize the behavioral and antipsychotic effects of the drug. They may also enhance the anticholinergic side effects. Enhanced cardiotoxicity with cisapride. Check drug reference for numerous others.

Relative Infant Dose: 0.1%

Adult Dose: 12–64 mg daily

Alternatives:

References:
1. Bader TF, Newman K. Amitriptyline in human breast milk and the nursing infant's serum. Am J Psychiatry 1980; 137(7): 855–856.
2. Brixen-Rasmussen L, Halgrener J, Jorgensen A. Amitriptyline and nortriptyline excretion in human breast milk. Psychopharmacology (Berl) 1982; 76(1): 94–95.
3. Breyer-Pfaff U, Nill K, Entenmann A, Gaertner HJ. Secretion of Amitriptyline and Metabolites Into Breast Milk. Am J Psychiatry 1995; 152(5): 812–813.
4. Olesen OV, Bartels U, Poulsen JH. Perphenazine in breast milk and serum. Am J Psychiatry 1990; 147(10): 1378–1379.

AMLODIPINE + BENAZEPRIL   L3

Trade: Lotrel

Other Trades:

Category: Calcium channel blocker/ ACE inhibitor

Amlodipine besylate and Benazepril hydrochloride is a combination drug product of a calcium channel blocker (amlodipine) combined with an ACE inhibitor (benazepril). It is indicated in the treatment of hypertension.[1]

Amlodipine is a typical calcium channel blocker, antihypertensive agent which has greater bioavailability and a longer duration of action.[2] No data are currently available on transfer of amlodipine into breastmilk. Because most calcium channel blockers (CCB) readily transfer into milk, we should assume the same for this drug. Use caution if administering to lactating women.

Benazepril belongs to the ACE inhibitor family. Oral absorption is rather poor (37%). The active component (benazeprilat) reaches a peak at approximately 2 hours after ingestion.[3] In a patient receiving 20 mg daily for 3 days, milk levels averaged 0.15 ng/L. Peak benazepril levels (C_{max}) were 0.92 ng/L. Thus, the levels in milk are almost unmeasurable. The manufacturer suggests a newborn infant ingesting only breast milk would receive less than 0.1% of the mg/kg maternal dose of benazepril and benazeprilat.[4,5] My calculations suggest much less, or a maximum of 0.00005% of the weight-adjusted maternal dose.

Pregnancy Risk	D	Lactation Risk	L3
T ½	= Amlodipine/benazepril: 30–50 hours/10–11 hours	M/P	= Amlodipine/benazepril:
Vd	= Amlodipine/benazepril: 21/0.124 l/kg	PB	= Amlodipine/benazepril: 93%/96.7%
Tmax	= Amlodipine/benazepril: 6–9 hours/0.5–1 hour	Oral	= Amlodipine/benazepril: 64–65%/37%
MW	= Amlodipine/benazepril: 408/424	pKa	= Amlodipine/benazepril: 8.7/18.01

Adult Concerns: Edema, cough, angioedema, jaundice, hyperkalemia. Use with caution in those with renal disease.

Pediatric Concerns:

Drug Interactions: Hypotension when used concomitantly with diuretics. Hyperkalemia may occur when used concomitantly with potassium supplements or potassium sparing diuretics such as spironolactone, amiloride or triamterene. May increase plasma levels of lithium and cause lithium toxicity.

Relative Infant Dose:

Adult Dose: Amlodipine/benazepril: 2.5 -10 mg/10–80 mg once daily

Alternatives:

References:
1.   Pharmaceutical manufacturer prescribing information,2011.

2. Pharmaceutical manufacturer prescribing information, Amlodipine 2002.
3. Pharmaceutical manufacturer prescribing information, Benazepril 2005.
4. Product Information: LOTENSIN(R) oral tablets, benazepril hcl oral tablets. Novartis Pharmaceuticals Corporation, East Hanover, NJ, 2006.
5. Kaiser G: Benazepril: Pharmacokinetic Profile in Specific Subpopulations. In: Brunner HR, Salvetti A, Sever PS, eds. Benazepril: Profile of a New ACE Inhibitor, Royal Society of Medicine Press, London, UK, 1990, pp 29–39.

AMLODIPINE + HYDROCHLOROTHIAZIDE + OLMESARTAN — L3

Trade: Tribenzor

Other Trades:

Category: Antihypertensive

Amlodipine besylate + hydrochlorothiazide + olmesartan medoxomil is a combined drug product used to treat hypertension which is not responsive to initial therapy.[1]

Amlodipine is a typical calcium channel blocker, antihypertensive agent which has greater bioavailability and a longer duration of action.[2] No data are currently available on transfer of amlodipine into breastmilk. Because most calcium channel blockers (CCB) readily transfer into milk, we should assume the same for this drug. Use caution if administering to lactating women. Hydrochlorothiazide (HCTZ) is a typical thiazide diuretic. In one study of a mother receiving a 50 mg dose each morning, milk levels were almost 25% of maternal plasma levels.[3] The dose ingested (assuming milk intake of 600 mL) would be approximately 50 µg/day, a clinically insignificant amount. The concentration of HCTZ in the infant's serum was undetectable (<20 ng/mL). Some authors suggest that HCTZ can produce thrombocytopenia in nursing infant, although this is remote and unsubstantiated. Thiazide diuretics could potentially reduce milk production by depleting maternal blood volume although it is seldom observed. Most thiazide diuretics are considered compatible with breastfeeding if doses are kept low. Olmesartan is an angiotensin II receptor antagonist.[4] While it is different from the ACE inhibitors, it effectively produces the same end result, hypotension. Use in pregnancy is contraindicated. No data are available on its transfer to human milk, but its use in mothers with premature infants could be risky.

Use the combined drug product of amlodipine + hydrochlorothiazide + olmesartan with caution in mothers with premature infants.

Pregnancy Risk	D	Lactation Risk	L3
T ½	= Amlodipine/hctz/ olmesartan: 30–50 hours/5.6–14.8 hours/13 hours	M/P	= Amlodipine/hctz/ olmesartan: /0.25/
Vd	= Amlodipine/hctz/ olmesartan: 21/3/0.24 l/kg	PB	= Amlodipine/hctz/ olmesartan: 935/58%/
Tmax	= Amlodipine/hctz/ olmesartan: 6–9 hours/2 hours/1–2 hours	Oral	= Amlodipine/hctz/ olmesartan: 65%/72%/26%
MW	= Amlodipine/hctz/ olmesartan: 408/297/558	pKa	= Amlodipine/hctz/ olmesartan: 8.7/7.9,9.2/

Adult Concerns: Nausea, vomiting, headache, dizziness, edema, upper respiratory tract infections, diarrhea, joint swelling, gout.

Pediatric Concerns:

Drug Interactions: Amlodipine interactions: Cyclosporine levels may be increased when used with calcium channel blockers. Use with azole antifungals (fluconazole, itraconazole, ketoconazole, etc) may lead to enhanced amlodipine levels. Use with rifampin may significantly reduce plasma levels of calcium channel blockers. HCTZ interactions: May increase hypoglycemia with antidiabetic drugs. May increase hypotension associated with other antihypertensives. May increase digoxin associated arrhythmias. May increase lithium levels. No major drug-drug interactions are noted with the use of olmesartan.

Relative Infant Dose:

Adult Dose: Amlodipine/hydrochlorothiazide/olmesartan: 5–10 mg/12.5–50 mg/20–40 mg once daily.

Alternatives: Nifedipine, nimodipine, captopril, enalapril

References:
1. Pharmaceutical manufacturer prescribing information for Azor, 2012.
2. Pharmaceutical manufacturer prescribing information, Amlodipine 2002.
3. Miller ME, Cohn RD, Burghart PH. Hydrochlorothiazide disposition in a mother and her breast-fed infant. J Pediatr 1982; 101(5): 789–791.
4. Pharmaceutical manufacturer prescribing information, 2003.

AMLODIPINE + OLMESARTAN   L3

Trade: Azor
Other Trades:
Category: Antihypertensive

Amlodipine besylate + olmesartan medoxomil is a combined drug product used to treat hypertension.[1]

Amlodipine is a typical calcium channel blocker, antihypertensive agent which has greater bioavailability and a longer duration of action. No data are currently available on transfer of amlodipine into breastmilk. Because most calcium channel blockers (CCB) readily transfer into milk, we should assume the same for this drug. Use caution if administering to lactating women. Olmesartan is an angiotensin II receptor antagonist. While it is different from the ACE inhibitors, it effectively produces the same end result, hypotension. Use in pregnancy is contraindicated. No data are available on its transfer to human milk, but its use in mothers with premature infants could be risky.

Use the combined drug product of amlodipine + olmesartan with caution in mothers with premature infants.

Pregnancy Risk	C/D in 2nd and 3rd trimester	Lactation Risk	L3
T ½	= Amlodipine/olmesartan: 30–50 hours/13 hours	M/P	= Amlodipine/olmesartan:
Vd	= Amlodipine/olmesartan: 21/0.24 l/kg	PB	= Amlodipine/olmesartan: 93%/
Tmax	= Amlodipine/olmesartan: 6–9 hours/1–2 hours	Oral	= Amlodipine/olmesartan: 65%/26%
MW	= Amlodipine/olmesartan: 408/558	pKa	= Amlodipine/olmesartan: 8.7/

Adult Concerns: Nausea, vomiting, dizziness, headache, edema, liver impairment, renal failure, hypersensitivity reactions.

Pediatric Concerns:

Drug Interactions: Amlodipine interactions: Cyclosporine levels may be increased when used with calcium channel blockers. Use with azole antifungals (fluconazole, itraconazole, ketoconazole, etc) may lead to enhanced amlodipine levels. Use with rifampin may significantly reduce plasma levels of calcium channel blockers. No major drug-drug interactions are noted with the use of olmesartan.

Relative Infant Dose:

Adult Dose: Amlodipine/olmesartan: 5–10 mg/20–40 mg once daily.

Alternatives: Nifedipine, nimodipine, captopril, enalapril

References:
1. Pharmaceutical manufacturer prescribing information for Azor, 2012.

AMLODIPINE BESYLATE | L3

Trade: Norvasc

Other Trades: Norvasc, Istin

Category: Antihypertensive, calcium channel blocker

Amlodipine is a typical calcium channel blocker, antihypertensive agent which has greater bioavailability and a longer duration of action.[1] No data are currently available on transfer of amlodipine into breastmilk. Because most calcium channel blockers (CCB) readily transfer into milk, we should assume the same for this drug. Use caution if administering to lactating women.

Pregnancy Risk	C	Lactation Risk	L3
T ½	= 30–50 hours	M/P	=
Vd	= 21 l/kg	PB	= 93%
Tmax	= 6–9 hours	Oral	= 64–65%
MW	= 408	pKa	= 8.7

Adult Concerns: Hypotension, bradycardia, edema, headache, or nausea.

Pediatric Concerns: None reported but observe for bradycardia, hypotension upon prolonged use.

Drug Interactions: Cyclosporine levels may be increased when used with calcium channel blockers. Use with azole antifungals (fluconazole, itraconazole, ketoconazole, etc) may lead to enhanced amlodipine levels. Use with rifampin may significantly reduce plasma levels of calcium channel blockers.

Relative Infant Dose:

Adult Dose: 5–10 mg daily.

Alternatives: Nifedipine, Nimodipine

References:
1. Pharmaceutical manufacturer prescribing information, 2002.

AMOXAPINE | L2

Trade: Asendin

Other Trades: Asendin, Asendis

Category: Tricyclic antidepressant

Amoxapine and its metabolite are both secreted into breastmilk at relatively low levels. Following a dose of 250 mg/day, milk levels of amoxapine were less than 20 µg/L and 113 µg/L of the active metabolite.[1] Milk levels of the active metabolite varied from 113 to 168 µg/L in two other milk samples. Maternal serum levels of amoxapine and metabolite at steady state were 97 µg/L and 375 µg/L respectively.

Pregnancy Risk	C	Lactation Risk	L2
T ½	= 8 hours (parent)	M/P	= 0.21
Vd	= 65.7 l/kg	PB	= 15–25%
Tmax	= 2 hours	Oral	= 18–54%
MW	= 314	pKa	=

Adult Concerns: Dry mouth, constipation, urine retention, drowsiness or sedation, anxiety, emotional disturbances, parkinsonism, tardive dyskinesia, seizures.

Pediatric Concerns: None reported via milk.

Drug Interactions: Decreased effect of clonidine, guanethidine. Amoxapine may increase effect of CNS depressants, adrenergic agents, anticholinergic agents. Increased toxicity with MAO inhibitors.

Relative Infant Dose: 0.6%

Adult Dose: 25 mg BID or TID

Alternatives:

References:
1. Gelenberg AJ. Single case study. Amoxapine, a new antidepressant, appears in human milk. J Nerv Ment Dis 1979; 167(10): 635–636.

AMOXICILLIN   L1

Trade: Larotid, Amoxil

Other Trades: Alphamox, Moxacin, Cilamox, Amoxil, Apo-Amoxi, Novamoxin, Betamox

Category: Penicillin antibiotic

Amoxicillin is a popular oral penicillin used for otitis media and many other pediatric/adult infections. In one group of 6 mothers who received 1 gm oral dose, the concentration of amoxicillin in breastmilk ranged from 0.68 to 1.3 mg/L of milk (average= 0.9 mg/L).[1] Peak levels occurred at 4–5 hours. Milk/plasma ratios at 1, 2, and 3 hours were 0.014, 0.013, and 0.043. Less than 0.95% of the maternal dose is secreted into milk. This amounts to less than 0.5% of a typical infant dose of amoxicillin. No harmful effects have been reported.

Pregnancy Risk	B	Lactation Risk	L1
T ½	= 1.7 hours	M/P	= 0.014–0.043
Vd	= 0.3 l/kg	PB	= 18%
Tmax	= 1.5 hours	Oral	= 89%
MW	= 365	pKa	= 9.48

Adult Concerns: Diarrhea, rashes, and changes in GI flora. Pancytopenia, rarely pseudomembranous colitis.

Pediatric Concerns: None reported. Commonly used in neonates and children.

Drug Interactions: Efficacy of oral contraceptives may be reduced. Disulfiram and probenecid may increase plasma levels of amoxicillin. Allopurinol may increase the risk of amoxicillin skin rash.

Relative Infant Dose: 1%

Adult Dose: 500–875 mg BID

Alternatives:

References:
1. Kafetzis DA, Siafas CA, Georgakopoulos PA, Papadatos CJ. Passage of cephalosporins and amoxicillin into the breast milk. Acta Paediatr Scand 1981; 70(3): 285–288.

AMOXICILLIN + CLARITHROMYCIN + LANSOPRAZOLE   L3

Trade: Prevpac

Other Trades:

Category: Antibiotic/ proton pump inhibitor

Amoxicillin + clarithromycin + lansoprazole is a combined drug product indicated for treatment of H. pylori infections which cause stomach ulcers.[1]

Amoxicillin is a popular oral penicillin. In one group of 6 mothers who received 1 gm oral dose, the concentration of amoxicillin in breastmilk ranged from 0.68 to 1.3 mg/L of milk (average= 0.9 mg/L).[2] Peak levels occurred at 4–5 hours. Milk/plasma ratios at 1, 2, and 3 hours were 0.014, 0.013, and 0.043. Less than 0.95% of the maternal dose is secreted into milk. This amounts to less than 0.5% of a typical infant dose of amoxicillin. No harmful effects have been reported. Clarithromycin is an antibiotic that belongs to erythromycin family. In a study of 12 mothers receiving 250 mg twice daily, the C_{max} occurred at 2.2 hours and was reported to be 0.85 mg/L.[3] The estimated average dose of clarithromycin via milk was reported to be 150 µg/kg/day, or 2% of the maternal dose. Clarithromycin is probably compatible with breastfeeding. Observe for diarrhea and thrush in the infant. Lansoprazole is a new proton pump inhibitor. It is very unstable in stomach acid and to a large degree is denatured by acidity of the infant's stomach.[4] A new study shows milk levels of omeprazole are minimal and it is likely milk levels of lansoprazole are small as well. Although there are no studies of lansoprazole in breastfeeding mothers, transfer to milk and its oral absorption (via milk) is likely to be minimal in a breastfed infant. Lansoprazole is secreted in animal milk although no data are available on the amount secreted in human milk. The only likely untoward effects would be reduced stomach acidity.

The drug combination product of amoxicillin + clarithromycin + lansoprazole is probably compatible with breastfeeding.

Pregnancy Risk	C		Lactation Risk	L3	
T ½	= Amoxicillin/clarithromycin/lansoprazole: 1.7 hours/5–7 hours/1.5 hours		M/P	= Amoxicillin/clarithromycin/lansoprazole: 0.014–0.043/>1/	
Vd	= Amoxicillin/clarithromycin/lansoprazole: 0.3/3–4/0.5 l/kg		PB	= Amoxicillin/clarithromycin/lansoprazole: 18%/40–70%/97%	
Tmax	= Amoxicillin/clarithromycin/lansoprazole: 1.5 hours/1.7 hours/1.7 hours		Oral	= Amoxicillin/clarithromycin/lansoprazole: 89%/50%/80%	
MW	= Amoxicillin/clarithromycin/lansoprazole: 365/748/369		pKa	= Amoxicillin/clarithromycin/lansoprazole: 9.48/12.94/8.85	

Adult Concerns: Hypersensitivity reactions, diarrhea, headache, alteration of taste, abdominal pain, dark stools, vaginitis, oral candidiasis.

Pediatric Concerns:

Drug Interactions: Do not administer the combined drug product with the following drugs: cisapride, pimozide, astemizole, terfenadine, ergotamine or dihydroergotamine. Amoxicillin interactions: Efficacy of oral contraceptives may be reduced. Disulfiram and probenecid may increase plasma levels of amoxicillin. Allopurinol may increase the risk of amoxicillin skin rash. Clarithromycin interactions: Clarithromycin increases serum theophylline by as much as 20%. Increases plasma levels of carbamazepine, cyclosporin, digoxin, ergot alkaloids, tacrolimus, triazolam, zidovudine, terfenadine, astemizole, cisapride (serious arrhythmias). Fluconazole increases clarithromycin serum levels by 25%. Numerous other drug-drug interactions are unreported, but probably occur. Lansoprazole interactions: Decreased absorption of ketoconazole, itraconazole, and other drugs dependent on acid for absorption. Theophylline clearance is increased slightly. Reduced lansoprazole absorption when used with sucralfate(30%).

Relative Infant Dose:

Adult Dose: Amoxicillin/clarithromycin/lansoprazole: 1 gm/500 mg/30 mg once daily for 10–14 days.

Alternatives:

References:
1. Pharmaceutical manufacturer prescribing information, 2010.
2. Kafetzis DA, Siafas CA, Georgakopoulos PA, Papadatos CJ. Passage of cephalosporins and amoxicillin into the breast milk. Acta Paediatr Scand 1981; 70(3): 285–288.
3. Sedlmayr T, Peters F, Raasch W, Kees F. Clarithromycin, a new macrolide antibiotic. Effectiveness in puerperal infections and pharmacokinetics in breast milk. Geburtshilfe Frauenheilkd 1993 July; 53(7): 488–91.
4. Pharmaceutical manufacturer prescribing information, 2010.

AMOXICILLIN + CLAVULANATE   L1

Trade: Augmentin, Augmentin ES-600, Augmentin XR, Amoclan
Other Trades: Clavulin, Alti-Amoxi Clav, Apo-Amoxi Clav
Category: Antibiotic

Amoxicillin and Clavulanate potassium is a combination drug product. Its indications include acute otitis media, sinusitis, community acquired pneumonia, urinary tract infections and infections of the skin and subcutaneous tissues. The addition of clavulanate extends the spectrum of amoxicillin by inhibiting beta lactamase enzymes.

Small amounts of amoxicillin (0.9 mg/L milk) are secreted in breastmilk. No harmful effects were reported in one report.[1] In another study of 67 breastfeeding mothers, 27 mothers were treated with amoxicillin + clavulanic acid and 40 mothers were treated with only amoxicillin. In the amoxicillin + clavulanic acid group, 22.3% of the infants had mild adverse effects. Only 7.5% of the control group (amoxicillin-only) infants had adverse effects. However, the authors suggest that this difference in untoward effects is not clinically significant.[2] The reported side effects included constipation (1), rash (4), diarrhea (4), and irritability (6). This amounts to less than 0.5% of a typical infant dose of amoxicillin.

Therefore, it may be stated that amoxicillin + clavulanate combination is compatible with breastfeeding.

Pregnancy Risk	B		Lactation Risk	L1
T ½	= Amoxicillin/clavulanate: 1.7 hours/1 hour		M/P	= Amoxicillin/clavulanate: 0.014–0.043
Vd	= Amoxicillin/clavulanate: 0.3/ l/kg		PB	= Amoxicillin/clavulanate: 18%/22–30%
Tmax	= Amoxicillin/clavulanate: 1.5 hours/1 hour		Oral	= Amoxicillin/clavulanate: 89%/75%
MW	= Amoxicillin/clavulanate: 365/199		pKa	= Amoxicillin/clavulanate: 9.48/15.52

Adult Concerns: Diarrhea, rash, thrush, irritability, or diarrhea.

Pediatric Concerns: None reported but observe for diarrhea, rash.

Drug Interactions: Efficacy of oral contraceptives may be reduced. Disulfiram and probenecid may increase plasma levels of amoxicillin. Allopurinol may increase the risk of amoxicillin skin rash.

Relative Infant Dose: 0.9%

Adult Dose: 875 mg BID

Alternatives:

References:

1. Kafetzis DA, Siafas CA, Georgakopoulos PA, Papadatos CJ. Passage of cephalosporins and amoxicillin into the breast milk. Acta Paediatr Scand 1981; 70(3): 285–288.
2. Benyamini L et al. The Safety of Amoxicillin/Clavulanic Acid and Cefuroxime During Lactation. Ther Drug Monit 2005 Aug; 27(4): 499–502.

AMPHOTERICIN B   L3

Trade: Fungizone, Amphotec

Other Trades: Abelcet, Fungilin, Ambisome, Resteclin, Abelcet, Amphocel

Category: Antifungal

Amphotericin B is an intravenous antifungal effective for the treatment of a range of different organisms, including *Candida albicans*. Amphotericin is significantly toxic when given intravenously, and is reserved for life-threatening infections. No data are available on its transfer to human milk; however, it is virtually unabsorbed orally (<9%), has high protein binding, has a large molecular weight, and is commonly used in pediatrics.[1,2] It is unlikely the amount in milk would be clinically relevant to a breastfeeding infant.

Pregnancy Risk	B	Lactation Risk	L3
T ½	= 15 days	M/P	=
Vd	= 4 l/kg	PB	= >90%
Tmax	= <1 hour	Oral	= <9%
MW	= 924	pKa	= 11.83

Adult Concerns: Adverse effects include anemia, thrombocytopenia, congestive heart failure, thrombophlebitis, paresthesias, hypokalemia, hyperthermia, nephrotoxicity, hepatotoxicity, pulmonary toxicity, erythematous reactions, and anaphylaxis.

Pediatric Concerns: None reported. Unlikely to be absorbed orally.

Drug Interactions: Antagonism with azole antifungals. Enhanced renal toxicity with cyclosporin. Enhanced digitalis toxicity due to hypokalemia.

Relative Infant Dose:

Adult Dose: 0.25 to 1.0 mg/kg daily IV

Alternatives:

References:
1. Pharmaceutical manufacturer prescribing information, 2002.
2. Mactal-Haaf C, Hoffman M, Kuchta A. Use of anti-infective agents during lactation, Part 3: Antivirals, antifungals, and urinary antiseptics. J Hum Lact 2001 May; 17(2): 160–166.

AMPICILLIN   L1

Trade: Polycillin, Omnipen

Other Trades: Ampicyn, Austrapen, Apo-Ampi, Novo-Ampicillin, NuAmpi, Penbriton, Amfipen, Britcin, Vidopen

Category: Penicillin antibiotic

Ampicillin is an antibiotic of the penicillin family. Low milk/plasma ratios of 0.2 have been reported.[1] In a study by Matsuda of 3 breastfeeding patients who received 500 mg of ampicillin orally, levels in milk peaked at 6 hours and averaged only 0.14 mg/L of milk.[2] The milk/plasma ratio was reported to be 0.03 at 2 hours. In a group of 9 breastfeeding women sampled at various times and who received doses of 350 mg TID orally, milk concentrations ranged from 0.06 to 0.17 mg/L with peak milk levels at 3–4 hours after the dose.[3] Milk/plasma ratios varied between 0.01 and 0.58. The highest reported milk level (1.02 mg/L) was in a patient receiving 700 mg TID. Ampicillin was not detected in the plasma of any infant. Ampicillin is one of the most commonly used prophylactic antibiotics in pediatric neonatal nurseries. Neonatal half-life is 2.8 to 4 hours. Possible rash, sensitization, diarrhea, or candidiasis could occur, but unlikely. May alter gastrointestinal flora.

Pregnancy Risk	B	Lactation Risk	L1
T ½	= 1.3 hours	M/P	= 0.58
Vd	= 0.38 l/kg	PB	= 8–20
Tmax	= 1–2 hours	Oral	= 50%
MW	= 349	pKa	= 11.97

Adult Concerns: Diarrhea, rash, fungal overgrowth, agranulocytosis, pseudomembranous colitis, anaphylaxis.

Pediatric Concerns: None reported but observe for diarrhea.

Drug Interactions: Efficacy of oral contraceptives may be reduced. Disulfiram and probenecid may increase plasma levels of ampicillin. Allopurinol may increase the risk of ampicillin skin rash.

Relative Infant Dose: 0.2%–0.5%

Adult Dose: 250–500 mg four times daily

Alternatives: Amoxicillin

References:
1. Kafetzis DA, Siafas CA, Georgakopoulos PA, Papadatos CJ. Passage of cephalosporins and amoxicillin into the breast milk. Acta Paediatr Scand 1981; 70(3): 285–288.
2. Matsuda S. Transfer of antibiotics into maternal milk. Biol Res Pregnancy Perinatol 1984; 5(2): 57–60.
3. Branebjerg PE, Heisterberg L. Blood and milk concentrations of ampicillin in mothers treated with pivampicillin and in their infants. J Perinat Med 1987; 15(6): 555–558.

AMPICILLIN + SULBACTAM   L1

Trade: Unasyn

Other Trades: Dicapen

Category: Antibiotic

Ampicillin sodium and Sulbactam sodium is a drug combination product indicated for use in pelvic inflammatory disease and in infections of the skin and subcutaneous tissues.

Small amounts of ampicillin may transfer (1 mg/L).[1] Possible rash, sensitization, diarrhea, or candidiasis could occur, but unlikely. This drug may alter gastrointestinal flora. Ampicillin is considered compatible with breastfeeding.

The absorption of sulbactam from GI tract is poor.[2] After a dose of 0.5 to 1 gram, sulbactam is secreted into milk at an average concentration of 0.52 µg/mL. This would lead to a maximal dose of 0.7 mg/kg/day in a breastfeeding infant, which equates to less than 1% of the maternal dose. Therefore, untoward effects are unlikely in a breastfeeding infant.[3]

Pregnancy Risk	B	Lactation Risk	L1
T ½	= Ampicillin/sulbactam: 1.3 hours/	M/P	= Ampicillin/sulbactam: 0.58/
Vd	= Ampicillin/sulbactam: 0.38/ l/kg	PB	= Ampicillin/sulbactam: 8–20%/
Tmax	= Ampicillin/sulbactam: 1–2 hours/	Oral	= Ampicillin/sulbactam: 50%/
MW	= Ampicillin/sulbactam: 349/233	pKa	= Ampicillin/sulbactam: 11.97/

Adult Concerns: Diarrhea, rash, fungal overgrowth, agranulocytosis, pseudomembranous colitis, anaphylaxis.

Pediatric Concerns: None reported but observe for diarrhea.

Drug Interactions: Efficacy of oral contraceptives may be reduced. Disulfiram and probenecid may increase plasma levels of amoxicillin. Allopurinol may increase the risk of amoxicillin skin rash.

Relative Infant Dose: 0.5%–1.5%

Adult Dose: 1.5–3 gm four times daily

Alternatives:

References:
1. Kafetzis DA, Siafas CA, Georgakopoulos PA, Papadatos CJ. Passage of cephalosporins and amoxicillin into the breast milk. Acta Paediatr Scand 1981; 70(3): 285–288.
2. Sweetman S (Ed), Martindale: The complete drug reference. London: Pharmaceutical Press. Electronic version. 2010
3. Foulds G, Miller RD, Knirsch AK, Thrupp LD. Sulbactam kinetics and excretion into breast milk in postpartum women. Clin Pharmacol Ther 1985; 38(6): 692–696.

AMPRENAVIR   L3

Trade: Agnerase

Other Trades:

Category: Protease inhibitor, Antiretroviral

Amprenavir is a protease inhibitor most often used in combination with reverse transcriptase inhibitors in the treatment of HIV. It is currently not known whether this drug is excreted into human milk, though it has been shown to be present in the milk of lactating rats.[1] Due to the risk of postnatal transmission of HIV to the infant, it is recommended that mothers infected with the disease abstain from breastfeeding.[2]

Pregnancy Risk	C	Lactation Risk	L3
T ½	= 7–10 hours	M/P	=
Vd	= 430 l/kg	PB	= 90%
Tmax	= 1–2 hours	Oral	= Unknown
MW	= 505.64	pKa	=

Adult Concerns: Hyperglycemia, rash, myocardial infarction, dyslipidemia, paresthesia, headache, nausea, vomiting, diarrhea, depression, seizure

Pediatric Concerns:

Drug Interactions: Amprenavir is a CYP3A4 inhibitor, and as such can decrease the metabolism of drugs that rely on that enzyme.

Relative Infant Dose:

Adult Dose: 1200 mg BID

Alternatives:

References:
1. Product Information: AGENERASE(R) oral solution, amprenavir oral solution. GlaxoSmithKline, Research Triangle Park, NC, 2005b.
2. Panel on Treatment of HIV-Infected Pregnant Women and Prevention of Perinatal Transmission: Recommendations for Use of Antiretroviral Drugs in Pregnant HIV-1–Infected Women for Maternal Health and Interventions to Reduce Perinatal HIV Transmission in the United States. Antiretroviral Pregnancy Registry. Wilmington, NC. 2010. Available from URL: http: //aidsinfo. nih. gov/contentfiles/PerinatalGL. pdf. As accessed 2010–05–24.

ANAGRELIDE   L4

Trade: Agrylin
Other Trades:
Category: Platelet-reducing agent

Anagrelide hydrochloride is used in the treatment of essential thrombocythemia and thrombocythemia associated with chronic myelogenous leukemia, polycythemia vera, and other myeloproliferative disorders. It inhibits the release of arachidonic acid from phospholipase, possibly by inhibiting phospholipase A2.[1] We do not have any data on its use in breastfeeding mothers, but some probably enters milk and would be orally absorbed by the infant. Since this drug is used for prolonged periods, untoward effects such as reduction of blood platelets (thrombocytopenia) and cardiovascular disorders in the infant are a possibility. While the risks of this drug are rather remote, chronic use in breastfeeding mothers should be discouraged or the infant closely monitored.

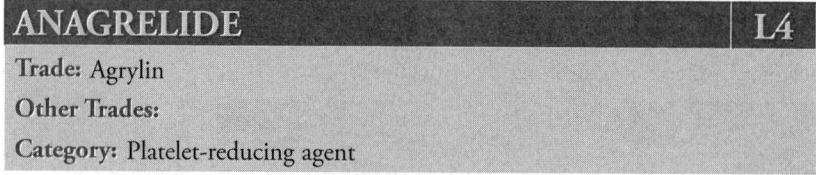

Pregnancy Risk	C	Lactation Risk	L4
T ½	= 1.3 hours	M/P	=
Vd	=	PB	=
Tmax	= 1 hour	Oral	= 70%
MW	= 310	pKa	=

Adult Concerns: Adverse reactions include palpitation, edema, headache, diarrhea, weakness, and dyspnea.

Pediatric Concerns: No data are available, but chronic use is discouraged.

Drug Interactions: May increase adverse effects of drotrecogin alfa, and adverse effects of anagrelide may be increased when taken with NSAIDs, salicylates, or treprostinil.

Relative Infant Dose:

Adult Dose: 0.5 mg 4 times a day or 1 mg twice a day

Alternatives:

References:
1. Pharmaceutical manufacturer prescribing information, 1999.

ANAKINRA   L3

Trade: Kineret
Other Trades: Kineret
Category: Anti-rheumatic

Anakinra is a recombinant form of the human interleukin-1 receptor antagonist (IL-1RA) and is used to reduce the inflammatory stimuli that mediate various inflammatory and immunological responses common in rheumatoid arthritis.[1] It is a large molecular weight protein (17,300 daltons) administered subcutaneously. Due to its size, it is very unlikely to enter milk after the first week postpartum. In addition, it is not likely to be orally bioavailable in an infant. However, we do not have data on its transfer to human milk and if used the infant should be observed for increased risk of gastrointestinal infections.

Pregnancy Risk	B	Lactation Risk	L3
T ½	= 4–6 hours	M/P	=
Vd	=	PB	= Nil
Tmax	= 3–7 hours	Oral	= Nil
MW	= 17,300	pKa	=

Adult Concerns: Adverse events include a high risk of serious infections (2%), URI, headache, nausea, and diarrhea.

Pediatric Concerns: None reported via milk. This agent is too large to enter milk effectively after the first week postpartum.

Drug Interactions: Concurrent use with TNF blocking agents not recommended. A higher rate of adverse reactions observed when used concurrently with etanercept.

Relative Infant Dose:

Adult Dose: 100 mg SC daily.

Alternatives:

References:
1. Pharmaceutical manufacturer prescribing information, 2003.

ANASTROZOLE L5

Trade: Arimidex
Other Trades: Arimidex
Category: Treatment of hormone receptor-positive early breast cancer.

Anastrozole is a potent and selective non-steroidal aromatase inhibitor indicated for the treatment of postmenopausal women with hormone receptor-positive early breast cancer. It significantly lowers serum estradiol concentrations and has no detectable effect on formation of adrenal corticosteroids or aldosterone. Orally administered anastrozole is well absorbed into the systemic circulation with 83 to 85% of the drug recovered in urine and feces. Anastrozole has a mean terminal elimination half-life of approximately 50 hours in postmenopausal women.[1] The major circulating metabolite of anastrozole, triazole, lacks pharmacologic activity. As with other aromatase inhibitors, this product, even in low concentrations in milk, could permanently bind to specific receptors, and potentially suppress estrogen formation completely in a breastfed infant.

Mothers should discontinue breastfeeding for at least 15 days after consuming this medication.

Pregnancy Risk	X	Lactation Risk	L5
T ½	= 50 hours	M/P	=
Vd	=	PB	= 40%
Tmax	= 2 hours	Oral	= Complete
MW	= 293.4	pKa	=

Adult Concerns: Blurred vision, chest pain or discomfort, dizziness, headache, nervousness, pounding in the ears, shortness of breath, slow or fast heartbeat, swelling of the feet or lower legs.

Pediatric Concerns: None yet reported, but this drug should not be used in breastfeeding mothers.

Drug Interactions: Tamoxifen may reduce plasma levels of anastrozole by 27% although they still may be used together.

Relative Infant Dose:

Adult Dose: 1 mg daily

Alternatives:

References:
1. Pharmaceutical manufacturer prescribing information, 2008.

ANIDULAFUNGIN   L3

Trade: Eraxis
Other Trades:
Category: Antifungal

Anidulafungin is an injectable antifungal used in the treatment of Candida infections. It inhibits the formation of 1,3-beta-D-glucan, an essential polysaccharide in the cell wall of *Candida albicans*. This leads to cell lysis.[1] No data are available on levels in human milk, but due to the large molecular weight, its high protein binding, and its large volume of distribution, it is highly unlikely that it will transfer into breastmilk. Lastly, it would not be orally bioavailable in the infant.

Pregnancy Risk	C	Lactation Risk	L3
T ½	= 27 hours	M/P	=
Vd	= 0.43–0.71 l/kg	PB	= >99%
Tmax	=	Oral	= Nil
MW	= 1140.3	pKa	= 11.03

Adult Concerns: Adverse reactions include hypokalemia, diarrhea, and increased transaminase.

Pediatric Concerns: No data are available.

Drug Interactions:

Relative Infant Dose:

Adult Dose: 100 mg IV daily for 14 days

Alternatives: Fluconazole

References:
1. Pharmaceutical manufacturer prescribing information, 2007.

ANTHRALIN   L3

Trade: Anthra-Derm, Drithocreme, Dritho-Scalp, Micanol
Other Trades: Dithranol, Anthraforte, Anthranol, Anthrascalp, Alphodith
Category: Anti-psoriatic

Anthralin is a synthetic tar derivative used topically for suppression of psoriasis. Anthralin, when applied topically, induces burning and inflammation of the skin but is one of the most effective treatments for psoriasis. Purple-brown staining of skin and permanent staining of clothing and porcelain bathroom fixtures is frequent. Anthralin when applied topically is absorbed into the surface layers of the skin and only minimal amounts enter the systemic circulation. That absorbed is rapidly excreted via the kidneys almost instantly; plasma levels are very low to undetectable.[1] No data are available on its transfer into human milk. Most anthralin is eliminated by washing off and desquamation of dead surface cells.[2] For this reason, when placed directly on lesions on the areola or nipple, breastfeeding should be discouraged. Another similar anthraquinone is Senna (laxative), which even in high doses does not enter milk. While undergoing initial intense treatment, it would perhaps be advisable to interrupt breastfeeding temporarily, but this may be overly conservative. Observe the infant for diarrhea. It has been used in children over 2 years of age for psoriasis.

Pregnancy Risk	C	Lactation Risk	L3
T ½	= Brief	M/P	=
Vd	=	PB	=
Tmax	=	Oral	= Complete
MW	= 226	pKa	=

Adult Concerns: Pruritus, skin irritation and inflammation. Purple-brown staining of skin and permanent staining of clothing and porcelain bathroom fixtures is frequent. Anthralin may have carcinogenic properties following high doses in mice. This may have no relevance to humans at all.

Pediatric Concerns: Diarrhea, nausea, vomiting via milk, but no reports have been published.

Drug Interactions:

Relative Infant Dose:

Adult Dose: Apply topical BID

Alternatives:

References:
1. Goodfield MJ, Hull SM, Cunliffe WJ. The systemic effect of dithranol treatment in psoriasis. Acta Derm Venereol 1994; 74(4): 295–297.
2. Shroot B. Mode of action of dithranol, pharmacokinetics/dynamics. Acta Derm Venereol Suppl (Stockh) 1992; 172: 10–12.

ANTHRAX (BACILLUS ANTHRACIS)   L5

Trade: Anthrax Infection, Bacillus Anthracis

Other Trades:

Category: Anthrax infection

Anthrax is an acute infection usually involving skin, lungs, and gastrointestinal tract. Anthrax is caused by the gram-positive, spore-forming bacterium bacillus anthracis. The spore may persist in nature for many years and infect grazing animals such as sheep, goats, and cattle. The most common forms of the disease are inhaled, oral, and cutaneous.

The Centers for Disease Control has recently published guidelines for treating or prophylaxing exposed breastfeeding mothers.[1] Thus far, all of the anthrax strains released by bioterrorists have been sensitive to ciprofloxacin, doxycycline, and the penicillin family. In breastfeeding women, amoxicillin (80 mg/kg/day in 3 divided doses) is an option for antimicrobial prophylaxis when B. anthracis is known to be penicillin- susceptible and no contraindication to maternal amoxicillin use is indicated. The American Academy of Pediatrics also considers ciprofloxacin and tetracyclines (which include doxycycline) to be usually compatible with breastfeeding because the amount of either drug absorbed by infants is small, but little is known about the safety of long-term use. Until culture sensitivity tests have been completed, the breastfeeding mother should be treated with ciprofloxacin (see ofloxacin or levofloxacin as alternates) or doxycycline (< 3 weeks). Once cultures show that the anthrax strain is sensitive to penicillins, then the mother can switch to amoxicillin for long term use up to 60 days or more. Due to possible dental staining following prolonged exposure, this author would not suggest long-term use (60 days) of doxycycline in a breastfeeding mother. The CDC offers several alternative antibiotics such as rifampin, vancomycin, imipenem, clindamycin, and clarithromycin in those patients with allergic conditions.[2] Check the CDC web sites for the most current recommendations.[3] Due to the risks posed by infection with anthrax, mothers who test positive for this infection should probably not breastfeed their infants until after treatment and testing negative for this species.

Pregnancy Risk	Possibly Hazardous	Lactation Risk	L5
T ½	=	M/P	=
Vd	=	PB	=
Tmax	=	Oral	=
MW	=	pKa	=

Adult Concerns: Inhalation anthrax: Flu like symptoms progressing to respiratory distress. Usually fatal. GI anthrax: Fever, nausea, vomiting blood, severe diarrhea. Cases are fatal 25–60% of the time.

Pediatric Concerns:

Drug Interactions:

Relative Infant Dose:

Adult Dose:

Alternatives:

References:

1. http://www.cdc.gov
2. Update: Investigation of bioterrorism-related anthrax and interim guidelines for exposure management and antimicrobial therapy, October 2001 MMWR Morb Mortal Wkly Rep 2001; 50(42): 909–919.
3. Centers for Disease Control Web site: http://www.bt.cdc.gov/. 2004.

ANTHRAX VACCINE   L3

Trade: Anthrax Vaccine, BioThrax

Other Trades:

Category: Vaccination

The anthrax vaccine for humans licensed for use in the United States is a cell-free filtrate vaccine, which means it uses dead bacteria as opposed to live bacteria. The vaccine is reported to be 93% effective in protecting against cutaneous anthrax.[1] The vaccine should only be administered to healthy men and women from 18 to 65 years of age since investigations to date have been conducted exclusively in that population. Because it is not known whether the anthrax vaccine can cause fetal harm, pregnant women should not be vaccinated. There are no data or indications relative to its use in breastfeeding mothers. While it consists primarily of protein fragments of anthrax bacteria, it is very unlikely any would transfer into milk or even be bioavailable in the infant.

The CDC states that, "No data suggest increased risk for side effects or temporally related adverse events associated with receipt of anthrax vaccine by breastfeeding women or breastfed children. Administration of nonliving vaccines (e.g., anthrax vaccine) during breast-feeding is not medically contraindicated. " According to the Advisory Committee on Immunization Practices (ACIP), while vaccination of breastfeeding women with the anthrax vaccine is generally not recommended, it may be administered as post exposure prophylaxis along with antibiotics after an incident of high risk exposure to Bacillus anthracis, or it may also be administered in a setting where the mother faces an occupational risk of exposure to anthrax.[2]

Pregnancy Risk	D	Lactation Risk	L3
T ½	=	M/P	=
Vd	=	PB	=
Tmax	=	Oral	=
MW	=	pKa	=

Adult Concerns: Mild local reactions occur in 30% of recipients and consist of slight tenderness and redness at the injection site. A moderate local reaction can occur if the vaccine is given to anyone with a past history of anthrax infection. Severe local reactions are very infrequent and consist of extensive swelling of the forearm in addition to the local reaction. Systemic reactions occur in fewer than 0.2% of recipients and are characterized by flu-like symptoms.

Pediatric Concerns: None reported via milk.

Drug Interactions:

Relative Infant Dose:

Adult Dose: 0.5 mL injection (IM)

Alternatives:

References:
1. Centers for Disease Control Web site: http: //www. bt. cdc. gov/. 2004.
2. Advisory Committee on Immunization Practices (ACIP): Use of Anthrax Vaccine in the United States. MMWR Recomm Rep 2010; 59(RR-6): 1–30.

ANTIHEMOPHILIC FACTOR-VON WILLEBRAND FACTOR COMPLEX   L3

Trade: Alphanate, Humate-P, Wilate

Other Trades: Humate-P

Category: Antihemophilic agent

This antihemophilic agent is used in hemophilia A and factor VIII deficiency to prevent and treat hemorrhagic episodes. It is also used to treat bleeding and as prophylaxis during procedures in patients with von Willebrand disease.[1] No data are available on the excretion of this antihemophilic agent into breast milk, however, it is highly unlikely due to the large molecular weight. Further, it is minimally bioavailable when ingested orally.

Pregnancy Risk	C	Lactation Risk	L3
T ½	= 10–12 hours	M/P	=
Vd	= 0.36–0.57 l/kg	PB	=
Tmax	=	Oral	= Nil
MW	= 264,726	pKa	=

Adult Concerns: Adverse reactions include epistaxis, body pain, nausea, dyspnea, cardiorespiratory arrest, and chills.

Pediatric Concerns: No data available in infants.

Drug Interactions: None reported.

Relative Infant Dose:

Adult Dose: 15–80 IU/kg (individualize)

Alternatives:

References:
1. Pharmaceutical manufacturer prescribing information, 2006.

ANTIPYRINE   L4

Trade: Antipyrine
Other Trades:
Category: Analgesic, antipyretic

In a group of 7 breastfeeding mothers who were receiving a single oral dose of 18 mg/kg of antipyrine in solution, peak levels in milk ranged from 10–30 mg/L. In five women peak concentrations were attained in milk and saliva by 1 hour and in the other two women by 3 hours.[1] Antipyrine half-life varied from 5.6 to 20.3 hours for saliva and from 5.7 to 21.7 hours for milk. The average amount of antipyrine available to the nursing infant was estimated at 6.4 mg/24 hours (range 3.0–11.1 mg). According to the authors, this is approximately 0.25% to 1.07% of the maternal dose (not weight-adjusted). The authors suggested that lactation may influence antipyrine drug metabolism. This product is no longer used in the USA due to high incidence of fatal bone marrow toxicity.

Pregnancy Risk	C	Lactation Risk	L4
T ½	=	M/P	= 1.0
Vd	= 0.56 l/kg	PB	= <1%
Tmax	= 1–2 hours	Oral	=
MW	= 188	pKa	= 1.4

Adult Concerns: Severe bone marrow toxicity.

Pediatric Concerns: None reported but due to better medications, this product should never be used.

Drug Interactions:

Relative Infant Dose: 8.3%–25%

Adult Dose: 18 mg/kg/day

Alternatives: ibuprofen, acetaminophen

References:
1.   Berlin CM, Jr., Vesell ES. Antipyrine disposition in milk and saliva of lactating women. Clin Pharmacol Ther 1982; 31(1): 38–44.

APREPITANT   L3

Trade: Emend

Other Trades: Ivemend

Category: Antiemetic

Aprepitant is a neurokinin-1 receptor antagonist. It is used as an anti-emetic agent for the prevention of nausea and vomiting following chemotherapy or surgeries.[1] Side effect profiles appear minimal. Levels in milk will likely be minimal due to moderately large molecular weight. Currently there is no data available on the transfer of aprepitant into human milk although it will likely be minimal.

Pregnancy Risk	B	Lactation Risk	L3
T ½	= 9–13 hours	M/P	=
Vd	= 70 L l/kg	PB	= >95%
Tmax	= 3 hours	Oral	= 60–65%
MW	= 534.43	pKa	=

Adult Concerns: Constipation, diarrhea, loss of appetite, headache, hiccoughs and fatigue are the commonly reported side-effects. Tachycardia, Stevens-Johnson Syndrome, neutropenia and hypersensitivity reactions occur rarely. Caution to be exercised in those with compromised liver function.

Pediatric Concerns:

Drug Interactions: Use of aprepitant with the following drugs is contra-indicated: pimozide, terfenadine, astemizole, cisapride. Aprepitant causes toxicity of the following co-administered drugs: etoposide, docetaxel, paclitaxel, ifosfamide, imatinib, vinristine and vinblastine. Aprepitant decreases plasma levels and efficacy of warfarin and tolbutamide. The efficacy of coadministered hormonal contraceptives is decreased during and for up to 28 days following cessation of aprepitant administration. During this time, an alternate form of contraception is advised.

Relative Infant Dose:

Adult Dose: Chemotherapy-induced N/V: 125 mg 1 hour prior, 80 mg on days 2 and 3. Post-operative N/V: 40 mg 3 hours before surgery.

Alternatives:

References:
1. Pharmaceutical manufacturer prescribing information, 2011.

ARFORMOTEROL   L3

Trade: Brovana
Other Trades:
Category: Beta-2 agonist

Arformoterol tartrate is used for long-term treatment of bronchoconstriction in COPD. It is the (R,R)- enantiomer of the racemic formoterol, which relaxes bronchial smooth muscle by selective action on beta 2-receptors without affecting the cardiovascular system.[1] The average steady-state peak plasma concentration is 4.3 pg/mL which means levels in milk would be incredibly low if even present. There have been no studies on the transfer of arformoterol tartrate into human breastmilk. However, due to the extremely low plasma levels, any transfer into milk would be minimal to nil. Just like all the other beta agonists used in asthma, it is unlikely that this product would pose a problem to a breastfeeding infant.

Pregnancy Risk	C	Lactation Risk	L3
T ½	= 26 hours	M/P	=
Vd	=	PB	= 52–65%
Tmax	= 0.5–3 hours	Oral	=
MW	= 494.5	pKa	= 14.21

Adult Concerns: Adverse reactions include chest pain, edema, rash, diarrhea, back pain, sinusitis, and dyspnea.

Pediatric Concerns: No data are available.

Drug Interactions: Alpha-/beta-blockers may decrease the bronchodilatory effect, atomoxetine may enhance the tachycardic effect. Betahistine may diminish the bronchodilator effect of beta agonists. Sympathomimetics may enhance the adverse effects of arformoterol.

Relative Infant Dose:

Adult Dose: 15 µg twice daily.

Alternatives: Formoterol, albuterol

References:
1. Pharmaceutical manufacturer prescribing information, 2006.

ARGATROBAN   L4

Trade: Argatroban
Other Trades:
Category: Synthetic direct thrombin inhibitor: anticoagulant

Argatroban is a synthetic inhibitor of thrombin and is derived from L-arginine.[1] It reversibly binds to the thrombin active site and exerts an anticoagulant effect by inhibiting thrombin-catalyzed reactions. It is primarily indicated as an anticoagulant for treatment of thrombosis in patients with heparin-induced thrombocytopenia. It is primarily in the extracellular fluid as evidenced by its low volume of distribution. No data are available on its transfer to human milk but it is reported to be present in rodent milk. It is not known if this product is orally bioavailable, but probably not. The presence of this product in milk could potentially induce gastrointestinal hemorrhage in weak or susceptible infants including newborns, premature infants, infants with necrotizing enterocolitis, and other infants. Extreme caution is recommended until we know levels present in milk and more about its gastrointestinal stability and absorption.

Pregnancy Risk	B	Lactation Risk	L4
T ½	= 39–51 minutes	M/P	=
Vd	= 0.174 l/kg	PB	= 54%
Tmax	= 1–3 hours	Oral	= Unknown
MW	= 526	pKa	= 10.28

Adult Concerns: Hemorrhage.

Pediatric Concerns: None reported via milk.

Drug Interactions: Prolongation of prothrombin times when co-administered with heparin, warfarin and potentially aspirin. Angelica, Bilberry, Arnica, Astragalus, and Anise may increase the risk of bleeding.

Relative Infant Dose:

Adult Dose: Initial: 25 µg/kg/min. Highly variable.

Alternatives:

References:
1. Pharmaceutical manufacturer Prescribing Information, 2003.

ARGININE   L3

Trade: L-Arginine, Arginine, Juven

Other Trades:

Category: Amino Acid; test for Growth Hormone release

L-Arginine is a naturally occurring basic amino acid. It is classified as a semi essential amino acid and is a potent stimulant of pituitary growth hormone and insulin release.[1] Found in most foods, it can also easily be synthesized by humans. L-Arginine participates in many biochemical reactions, but is most well known for its ability to stimulate endothelium-derived relaxing factor now known as nitric oxide (NO). NO plays critical roles in many diverse physiological processes including neurotransmission, vasorelaxation, and immune responses. Arginine plays an important role in wound healing removing ammonia from the body, immune function, and the release of hormones. There are unconfirmed reports that L-arginine may promote tumor growth in patients with malignancies who receive supplements. Numerous other studies do not show this effect at all. L-Arginine is not overly toxic. Doses as high as 30 gm/day have been generally well tolerated in adults with the most common adverse effects of nausea and diarrhea being reported. Arginine administered to seriously ill patients is known to increase mortality.

We presently have no reports of its transfer into human milk available. Most importantly, we do not know if high doses of oral L-Arginine subsequently increase Arginine levels in milk, although it would seem likely. As this product has limited usefulness in most patients, its use at high doses in breastfeeding mothers should be avoided until milk levels are reported. The wound healing product Juven contains high concentrations of arginine (7 gm), L-glutamine(7 gm), Potassium(270 mg), HMB(1.2 gm), and Calcium(200 mg). Caution is urged with this product in breastfeeding mothers as maternal plasma levels of these amino acids increase 2–3 fold. We do not know what happens in the mothers' breastmilk, or in her infant.

Pregnancy Risk	B	Lactation Risk	L3
T ½	= 0.7–1.3	M/P	=
Vd	= 33 l/kg	PB	=
Tmax	= 1.5 hours	Oral	= 68%
MW	= 174	pKa	= 2.18 and 9.0

Adult Concerns: Allergic reactions have been reported upon the administration of L-Arginine. When infused intravenously, local irritation, nausea and vomiting are reported. Hyperkalemia has occurred. Use cautiously in patients with liver and/or renal disease.

Pediatric Concerns: None reported via milk.

Drug Interactions: Potentially fatal hyperkalemia when used with spironolactone.

Relative Infant Dose:

Adult Dose: 1–2 gm/day but highly variable. Doses as high as 30 gm/d have been used short-term.

Alternatives:

References:
1. Pharmaceutical manufacturer Prescribing Information, 2003.

ARIPIPRAZOLE   L3

Trade: Abilify, Abilitat
Other Trades:
Category: Antipsychotic

Aripiprazole is a second-generation antipsychotic, now a first-line treatment for schizophrenia. In a small study of a single patient receiving 10 mg/day initially and then 15 mg subsequently, levels of aripiprazole in milk were reported to be 13 and 14 µg/L on two consecutive days (15 and 16 after initiation of therapy).[1] Maternal plasma levels at the same time were 71 and 71 µg/L. Levels were drawn in the morning before aripiprazole administration. Thus it appears from this brief report that they were drawn approximately 24 hours post dose. Several reports (personal communication) of somnolence have been reported to this author. The infant should be monitored for somnolence.

Pregnancy Risk	C	Lactation Risk	L3
T ½	= 75 hours	M/P	= 0.2
Vd	= 4.9 l/kg	PB	= 99%
Tmax	= 3–5 hours	Oral	= 87%
MW	= 448	pKa	=

Adult Concerns: Adverse reactions include headache, dizziness, akathisia, sedation, tremor, anxiety, insomnia and restlessness.

Pediatric Concerns: Several cases of somnolence in breastfed infants have been unofficially reported.

Drug Interactions: Carbamazepine may reduce levels of aripiprazole. Fluoxetine, itraconazole, ketoconazole, paroxetine, quinidine, and ranolazine have been reported to increase plasma levels of aripiprazole.

Relative Infant Dose: 1%

Adult Dose: 10–15 mg/day

Alternatives: Risperidone, olanzapine, quetiapine

References:
1. Schlotterbeck P, Leube D, Kircher T, Hiemke C, Grunder G. Aripiprazole in human milk . Int J Neuropsychopharmacol. 2007; 10: 433.

ARMODAFINIL   L4

Trade: Nuvigil
Other Trades:
Category: Wakefulness-Promoting Agent

Armodafinil is a wakefulness-promoting agent used in the treatment of narcolepsy.[1] It is not known whether armodafinil or its metabolites are transferred in human milk. Because many drugs are excreted in human milk, caution should be exercised when armodafinil is prescribed to nursing mothers.

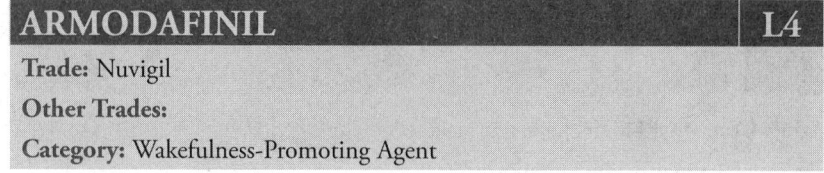

Pregnancy Risk	C	Lactation Risk	L4
T ½	= 15 hours	M/P	=
Vd	= 0.6 l/kg	PB	= 60
Tmax	= 2–4 hours	Oral	=
MW	= 273	pKa	=

Adult Concerns: Rash, Stevens-Johnsons syndrome, angioedema, anaphylaxis, nausea, headache, insomnia, dizziness, anxiety, diarrhea, dry mouth.

Pediatric Concerns:

Drug Interactions: CYP3A4 inducers such as carbamazepine, phenobarbital, rifampin or CYP3A4 inhibitors such as ketoconazole, erythromycin can alter plasma levels.

Relative Infant Dose:

Adult Dose: 150–250 mg daily

Alternatives:

References:
1.   Pharmaceutical manufacturer prescribing information, 2010.

ARTICAINE   L3

Trade:

Other Trades:

Category: Local anesthetic

Articaine is a local anesthetic with an intermediate-duration. It has a structure similar to lidocaine, etidocaine, and prilocaine. It has an ester bond mid-structure that permits it to be rapidly hydrolyzed by blood and tissue esterases.[1] Although its potency is approximately equal to or slightly more than that of lidocaine, it may be less toxic due to its more rapid metabolism. No data are available on its use in breastfeeding mothers. As with lidocaine, however, its transfer into human milk is probably minimal. If ingested, it would be rapidly hydrolyzed by gastric esterases.

Pregnancy Risk	C	Lactation Risk	L3
T ½	= 1.8	M/P	=
Vd	=	PB	= 60–80%
Tmax	=	Oral	=
MW	=	pKa	= 7.8

Adult Concerns: Headache, pain, facial edema, gingivitis.

Pediatric Concerns: None reported.

Drug Interactions:

Relative Infant Dose:

Adult Dose: 20–204 mg (varies)

Alternatives:

References:
1.   Pharmaceutical manufacturer prescribing information, 2006.

ASCORBIC ACID   L1/L5

Trade: Ascorbicap, Cecon, Cevi-Bid, Ce-Vi-Sol, Vitamin C

Other Trades:

Category: Vitamin C

Ascorbic acid is an essential vitamin, commonly referred to as vitamin C. Vitamin C is popularly used for various reasons, the most common being prevention and treatment of infections, fatigue and cancer. Without supplementation, 75 mg/day is excreted in the urine of the average individual due to overabundance. Renal control of vitamin C is significant and maintains plasma levels at 0.4 to 1.5 mg/dL regardless of dose.

Ascorbic acid is secreted into human milk in well-controlled sequence and mature milk. In a large number of studies, ascorbic acid levels in milk ranged from 35 to 200 mg/L depending on the oral intake of the mother.[1] Excessive Vitamin C intake in the mother only modestly changes the controlled secretion into breastmilk. The recommended daily allowance for the mother is 100 mg/day. Maternal supplementation is only required in undernourished mothers.

In a study of 25 lactating women given 90 mg of ascorbic acid for 1 day, followed by 250, 500, or 1000 mg/day for 2 days, the levels of vitamin C in maternal milk were not significantly influenced.[2] Mean vitamin C intakes of infants ranged between 49 ± 9 and 86 ± 11 mg/day and were not statistically different among the five levels of maternal vitamin C intake. This lack of change in vitamin C content in milk suggests a regulatory mechanism for vitamin C levels. In cases where supplementation has reached 1000 to 1500 mg/day, reported milk levels were only slightly increased to 100 and 105 mg/L.[2,3] Whereas the half-life in normal non-supplemented patients is 16 days, high oral doses can induce the metabolism of ascorbic thereby reducing the half-life of ascorbic acid to as little as 3.4 hours. Pregnant women should not use excessive ascorbic acid due to metabolic induction in the maternal or fetal liver, followed by a metabolic rebound scurvy early postpartum in the neonate.

Intravenous vitamin C is used extensively by complementary and alternative medicine (CAM) practitioners. From surveys conducted at annual CAM conferences in 2006 and 2008, it was found that average doses administered were in the order of 28 grams intravenously, but doses ranged from as low as 1 gram to as high as 200 grams.[4] While plasma concentrations following oral administration are strictly controlled by the kidneys between the ranges of 70–85 µmol/L, plasma concentrations are 30–70 times higher with intravenous vitamin C use.[5] Intravenous vitamin C may produce concentrations as high as 15,000 µmol/L. Recent trials in animals and *in vitro* studies have indicated that high plasma concentrations of vitamin C in the order of 1000 µmol/L has anti-cancer properties.[6–10] Although similarly high plasma concentrations were achieved with IV vitamin C use in humans, the anti-tumor role of high vitamin C doses in humans is still in question.[11] Adverse effects with IV vitamin C have been rarely reported and include minor side-effects such as lethargy, fatigue, vein irritation, nausea and vomiting. Three cases of renal failure in those with pre-existing renal disease and two cases of hemolysis in those with G6PD deficiency have been reported.[12–16] Intravenous vitamin C appears to have a moderately safe profile, but avoid use in mothers with pre-existing renal impairment, history of kidney stones, G6PD deficiency or paroxysmal nocturnal hematuria. The use of intravenous vitamin C in breastfeeding women has not been studied. The very high plasma concentrations achieved with IV vitamin C use would probably result in high concentrations in milk as well. This might predispose infants to a higher risk of kidney stones with excessive vitamin C exposure. Mothers of infants with compromised renal function and G6PD deficiency should avoid excessively high doses of vitamin C.

Ascorbic acid should not routinely be administered to breastfed infants unless to treat clinical scurvy. Even following high maternal oral doses, ascorbic acid levels only rise moderately in milk. Recommend normal RDA (100 mg/day) in mothers, and avoid excessively high oral doses. Avoid intravenous vitamin C during breastfeeding, or in those cases where it is used, mothers should avoid breastfeeding, pump and discard milk, for a minimum of 12–24 hours after therapy.

Pregnancy Risk	A/C in third trimester	Lactation Risk	L1 low dose / L5 IV dose
T ½	= 16 days (3.4 h in heavy users)	M/P	=
Vd	=	PB	= 25%
Tmax	= 2–3 hours	Oral	= Complete
MW	= 176	pKa	= 9.07

Adult Concerns: Renal stones with large doses. Faintness, flushing, dizziness, nausea, vomiting, gastritis. Side-effects of IV vitamin C doses: lethargy, fatigue, local vein irritation, nausea, vomiting, hypersensitivity reactions, hypoglycemia, heartburn, dizziness, palpitations, renal stones, renal failure.

Pediatric Concerns: None reported via breastmilk, but excessive use prepartum is strongly discouraged.

Drug Interactions: Ascorbic acid decreases propranolol peak concentrations. Aspirin decreases ascorbate levels and increases aspirin levels. Reduced effect of warfarin when used with ascorbic acid. Urinary acidification results in decreased retention of many basic drugs, including tricyclic antidepressants, amoxapine, amphetamines. Do not use with aluminum antacids. Ascorbic acid reduces renal elimination of aluminum leading to encephalopathy, seizures, coma.

Relative Infant Dose:

Adult Dose: 45–60 mg orally daily.

Alternatives:

References:
1. Picciano MF. Handbook of milk composition. Jensen RG, ed. San Diego: Academic Press; 1995.
2. Byerley LO, Kirksey A. Effects of different levels of vitamin C intake on the vitamin C concentration in human milk and the vitamin C intakes of breast-fed infants. Am J Clin Nutr 1985 Apr; 41(4): 665–71.
3. Kirksey A. and Rahmanifar A. Vitamin and mineral composition of preterm human milk: Implications for the nutritional management of the preterm infant. In "Vitamins and Minerals in Pregnancy and Lactation". H. Berger, ed. Pp 301–329, Raven Press.
4. Padayatty SJ, Sun AY, Chen Q, Espey MG, Drisko J, Levine M. Vitamin C: intravenous use by complementary and alternative medicine practitioners andadverse effects. PLoS One. 2010 Jul 7; 5(7): e11414.
5. Padayatty SJ, Sun H, Wang Y, Riordan HD, Hewitt SM, Katz A, Wesley RA, Levine M. Vitamin C pharmacokinetics: implications for oral and intravenous use. AnnIntern Med. 2004 Apr 6; 140(7): 533–7.
6. Chen Q, Espey MG, Sun AY, Lee JH, Krishna MC, Shacter E, et al. Ascorbate in pharmacologic concentrations selectively generates ascorbate radical and hydrogen peroxide in extracellular fluid in vivo. Proc Natl Acad Sci U S A. 2007; 104: 8749–54.
7. Chen Q, Espey MG, Sun AY, Pooput C, Kirk KL, Krishna MC, et al. Pharmacologic doses of ascorbate act as a prooxidant and decrease growth of aggressive tumor xenografts in mice. Proc Natl Acad Sci U S A. 2008; 105: 11105–9.

8. Verrax J, Calderon PB. Pharmacologic concentrations of ascorbate are achieved by parenteral administration and exhibit antitumoral effects. Free Radic Biol Med. 2009; 47: 27–9.
9. Leung PY, Miyashita K, Young M, Tsao CS. Cytotoxic effect of ascorbate and its derivatives on cultured malignant and nonmalignant cell lines. Anticancer Res. 1993; 13: 475–80.
10. Sakagami H, Satoh K, Hakeda Y, Kumegawa M. Apoptosis-inducing activity of vitamin C and vitamin K. Cell Mol Biol (Noisy-le-grand). 2000; 46: 129–43.
11. Hoffer LJ, Levine M, Assouline S, Melnychuk D, Padayatty SJ, Rosadiuk K,Rousseau C, Robitaille L, Miller WH Jr. Phase I clinical trial of i. v. ascorbicacid in advanced malignancy. Ann Oncol. 2008 Nov; 19(11): 1969–74. Epub 2008 Jun 9. Erratum in: Ann Oncol. 2008 Dec; 19(12): 2095.
12. Lawton JM, Conway LT, Crosson JT, Smith CL, Abraham PA. Acute oxalate nephropathy after massive ascorbic acid administration. Arch Intern Med. 1985; 145: 950–951.
13. Wong K, Thomson C, Bailey RR, McDiarmid S, Gardner J. Acute oxalate nephropathy after a massive intravenous dose of vitamin C. Aust N Z J Med. 1994; 24: 410–411.
14. McAllister CJ, Scowden EB, Dewberry FL, Richman A. Renal failure secondary to massive infusion of vitamin C. JAMA. 1984; 252: 1684.
15. Campbell GD, Jr, Steinberg MH, Bower JD. Ascorbic acid-induced hemolysis in G-6-PD deficiency. Ann Intern Med. 1975; 82: 810.
16. Rees DC, Kelsey H, Richards JD. Acute haemolysis induced by high dose ascorbic acid in glucose-6– phosphate dehydrogenase deficiency. BMJ. 1993; 306: 841–42.

ASENAPINE   L3

Trade: Saphris
Other Trades:
Category: Antispsychotic, atypical

Asenapine is a new atypical antipsychotic used to treat schizophrenia, mania or bipolar disorder. According to the manufacturer[1], asenapine appears in rat milk. There are no data in human subjects but levels when determined will probably be low as with other members of this family. Galactorrhea may occur on asenapine, attributed to hyperprolactinemia from this family of drugs. Elevated prolactin levels may be associated with a decrease in fertility.

Pregnancy Risk	C	Lactation Risk	L3
T ½	= 24 hr	M/P	=
Vd	= 20 to 25 l/kg	PB	= 95%
Tmax	= 0.5–1.5 hr	Oral	= Sublingual–35%
MW	= 285.768	pKa	=

Adult Concerns: Somnolence or insomnia, dyspepsia, elevated prolactin levels, weight gain, tardive dyskinesia.

Pediatric Concerns: None reported but observe for sedation.

Drug Interactions: Increased levels when coadministered with fluvoxamine or imipramine. Decreased plasma levels of asenapine when coadministered with paroxetine or carbamazepine.

Relative Infant Dose:

Adult Dose: 5 mg twice daily

Alternatives: Risperidone, quetiapine, aripiprazole

References:
1. Pharmaceutical manufacturer prescribing information, 2010.

ASPARAGINASE   L3

Trade: Elspar, L-asparaginase, Colaspase, L-ASP, Crasnitin

Other Trades: Kidrolase

Category: Anticancer drug

Asparaginase is used for a number of different cancers. Asparaginase contains the enzyme L-asparagine amidohydrolase derived from E. Coli. Asparaginase removes asparagine from leukemic cells, thus requiring that these cells obtain it from an exogenous source for survival, which cancer cells are unable to do. Fortunately, normal cells are able to synthesize asparagine.[1] It does not have active metabolites and does not pass the blood brain barrier (<1%). No data are available on its transfer to human milk. But due to its long half-life and large volume of distribution, some asparaginase may be present in milk.

Withhold breastfeeding for a minimum of 7 days.

Pregnancy Risk	C	Lactation Risk	L3
T ½	= 8–49 hours	M/P	=
Vd	= 245 l/kg	PB	=
Tmax	= 1 hour	Oral	= Nil
MW	= 31732	pKa	=

Adult Concerns: Joint pain, puffy face, skin rash or itching, severe stomach pain with nausea and vomiting, dyspnea, severe allergic reaction, pancreatitis.

Pediatric Concerns:

Drug Interactions: Asparaginase increases activity of live viruses/vaccines. Increased risk with yellow fever, rotavirus, measles, mumps, influenza and any other live virus vaccine.

Relative Infant Dose:

Adult Dose: 6000 IU/m² IM 3 times/week

Alternatives:

References:
1. Pharmaceutical manufacturer prescribing information, 2005.

ASPARTAME   L1

Trade:

Other Trades:

Category: Artificial sweetener

Aspartame consists of two linked amino acids, aspartic acid and phenylalanine. Once in the GI tract, it is rapidly metabolized to phenylalanine and aspartic acid. Maternal ingestion of 50 mg/kg aspartame will approximately double (2.3 to 4.8

μmol/dL) aspartate milk levels. Phenylalanine milk levels similarly increased from 0.5 to 2.3 μmol/dL. This dose is 3–4 times the normal dose used. These milk levels are too low to produce significant side effects in normal infants.[1,2] Contraindicated in infants with diagnosed phenylketonuria.

Pregnancy Risk	B	Lactation Risk	L1
T ½	= 3–4 days	M/P	=
Vd	=	PB	=
Tmax	=	Oral	= Complete
MW	= 294	pKa	= 12.18

Adult Concerns: Only contraindicated in infants with Phenylketonuria.

Pediatric Concerns: None reported except contraindicated in infants with documented phenylketonuria.

Drug Interactions:

Relative Infant Dose:

Adult Dose:

Alternatives:

References:
1. Levels of free amino acids in lactating women following ingestion of the sweetener aspartame Nutr Rev 1980; 38(5): 183–184.
2. Stegink LD, Filer LJ, Jr., Baker GL. Plasma, erythrocyte and human milk levels of free amino acids in lactating women administered aspartame or lactose. J Nutr 1979; 109(12): 2173–2181.

ASPIRIN   L3

Trade: Ecotrin, Bayer, Ascriptin, Aspergum, Aspirtab, Easprin, Ecpirin, Entercote

Other Trades:

Category: Salicylate analgesic

Aspirin or acetylsalicylic acid is used for its analgesic properties. Extremely small amounts are transferred into breastmilk. Few harmful effects have been reported. In one study, salicylic acid (active metabolite of Aspirin) penetrated poorly into milk (dose=454 mg ASA), with peak levels of only 1.12 to 1.60 μg/mL, whereas maternal peak plasma levels were 33 to 43.4 μg/mL.[1] In another study of a rheumatoid arthritis patient who received 4 gm/day aspirin, none was detectable in her milk (<5mg/100cc).[2] Extremely high doses in the mother could potentially produce slight bleeding in the infant. Because aspirin is implicated in Reye Syndrome, it is a poor choice of analgesic to use in breastfeeding mothers. However, in rheumatic fever patients, it is still one of the anti-inflammatory drugs of choice and a risk-vs-benefit assessment must be done in this case. In a study of a patient consuming aspirin chronically, salicylate concentrations in milk peaked at 3 hours at a concentration of 10 mg/L following a maternal dose of 975 mg.[3] Maternal plasma levels peaked at 2.25 hours at 108 mg/L. The milk/plasma ratio was reported to be 0.08. In a study of 8 women following the use of 1 gram oral doses of aspirin, average milk levels of salicylic acid (active metabolite of aspirin) were 2.4 mg/L at 3 hours.[4] The metabolite salicyluric acid, reached a peak of 10.2 mg/L at 9 hours. Averaging total salicylates and salicyluric acid metabolites, the author suggests the relative infant dose would be 9.4% of the maternal dose.

While the direct use of aspirin in infants and children is definitely implicated in Reye syndrome, the use of the 82 mg/day dose in breastfeeding mothers is unlikely to increase the risk of this syndrome. Unfortunately we do not at present know of any dose-response relationship between aspirin and Reye syndrome other than in older children where even low plasma levels of aspirin were implicated in Reye syndrome during viral syndromes such as flu or chickenpox. Therefore, the use of aspirin in breastfeeding mothers is questionable, but the risk is probably low. Consider ibuprofen or acetaminophen as better choices for pain relief in lactating women. Never use these products if the infant has a viral syndrome.

Pregnancy Risk	C/D in 3rd trimester	Lactation Risk	L3
T½	= 2.5–7 hours	M/P	= 0.03–0.08
Vd	= 0.15 l/kg	PB	= 88–93%
Tmax	= 1–2 hours	Oral	= 80–100%
MW	= 180	pKa	=

Adult Concerns: Gastrointestinal ulceration, distress, esophagitis, nephropathy, hepatotoxicity, tinnitus, platelet dysfunction.

Pediatric Concerns: One 16 day old infant developed metabolic acidosis. Mother was consuming 3.9 grams/day of aspirin. Thrombocytopenia, petechiae and anorexia were reported in an infant of 5 months following exposure to maternal/milk aspirin. Aspirin has definitely been associated with Reye syndrome in infants with viral fevers.

Drug Interactions: May decrease serum levels of other NSAIDs as well as GI distress. Aspirin may antagonize effect of probenecid. Aspirin may increase methotrexate serum levels, and increase free valproic acid plasma levels and valproate toxicity. May increase anticoagulant effect of warfarin.

Relative Infant Dose: 2.5%–10.8%

Adult Dose: 325–900 mg QID

Alternatives: Ibuprofen, Acetaminophen

References:
1. Findlay JW, DeAngelis RL, Kearney MF, Welch RM, Findlay JM. Analgesic drugs in breast milk and plasma. Clin Pharmacol Ther 1981; 29(5): 625–633.
2. Erickson SH, Oppenheim GL. Aspirin in breast milk. J Fam Pract 1979; 8(1): 189–190.
3. Bailey DN, Welbert RT, Naylor A. A study of salicylate and caffeine excretion in the breast milk of two nursing mothers. J Anal Toxicol. 1982; 6: 64–8.
4. Putter J, Satravaha P, Stockhausen H. Quantitative analysis of the main metabolites of acetylsalicylic acid. Comparative analysis in the blood and milk of lactating women. Z Geburtshilfe Perinatol. 1974; 178: 135–8.

ASPIRIN + OXYCODONE   L3

Trade: Percodan, Endodan
Other Trades:
Category: Analgesic for pain.

Aspirin + oxycodone is a combined drug product used for the management of moderate to severe pain.[1]

Extremely small amounts of aspirin are transferred into breastmilk. Few harmful effects have been reported. In one study, salicylic acid (active metabolite of aspirin) penetrated poorly into milk (dose=454 mg ASA), with peak levels of only 1.12 to 1.60 µg/mL, whereas maternal peak plasma levels were 33 to 43.4 µg/mL.[2] In another study of a rheumatoid arthritis patient who received 4 gm/day aspirin, none was detectable in her milk (<5mg/100cc).[3] Extremely high doses in the mother could potentially produce slight bleeding in the infant. Because aspirin is implicated in Reye Syndrome, it is a poor choice of analgesic to use in breastfeeding mothers. However, in rheumatic fever patients, it is still one of the anti-inflammatory drugs of choice and a risk-vs-benefit assessment must be done in this case. In a study of a patient consuming aspirin chronically, salicylate concentrations in milk peaked at 3 hours at a concentration of 10 mg/L following a maternal dose of 975 mg.[4] Maternal plasma levels peaked at 2.25 hours at 108 mg/L. The milk/plasma ratio was reported to be 0.08. In a study of 8 women following the use of 1 gram oral doses of aspirin, average milk levels of salicylic acid (active metabolite of aspirin) were 2.4 mg/L at 3 hours.[5] The metabolite salicyluric acid, reached a peak of 10.2 mg/L at 9 hours. Averaging total salicylates and salicyluric acid metabolites, the author suggests the relative infant dose would be 9.4% of the maternal dose. The direct use of aspirin in infants and children is implicated in Reye syndrome, especially when used in the presence of a viral illness. Therefore the use of aspirin in breastfeeding mothers is questionable, but the risk is probably low. Never use these products if the infant has a viral syndrome.

Small amounts of oxycodone are secreted in breastmilk. Following a dose of 5–10 mg every 4–7 hours, maternal levels peaked at 1–2 hours, and analgesia persisted for up to 4 hours.[6] Reported milk levels ranged from <5 to 226 µg/L. Maternal plasma levels were 14–35 µg/L. The authors suggest a milk/plasma ratio of approximately 3.4. Although active metabolites were not measured, the authors suggest that an exclusively breastfed infant would receive a maximum 8% of the maternal dosage of oxycodone. No reports of untoward effects in infants have been found although sedation is a possibility in some infants.

In another study, 50 post-cesarean women received 30 mg oxycodone rectally, and 10 mg orally up to every 2 hours as needed. Milk/plasma ratios were calculated to be 3.2–3.4. Only one infant had a detectable level of oxycodone in the plasma, with a concentration of 6.6–7.4 ng/mL.[7] These plasma and milk levels suggest that oxycodone concentrates in the milk compartment, however, the authors suggest that at doses less than 90 mg/day for up to 3 days, maternal use of oxycodone poses only a minimal threat to breastfeeding infants. This study did not measure plasma or milk concentrations at steady state or during peak plasma concentrations, therefore, levels may have been higher at times.

In a recent retrospective study, the rate of CNS depression in breastfeeding infants was compared between 3 cohorts of breastfeeding women receiving oxycodone, codeine and acetaminophen, respectively, for alleviation of postpartum pain.[8] The mothers were receiving doses which were within the recommended adult dosages. The rates of infant CNS depression in the three groups was as follows: oxycodone group–20.1%; codeine group–16.7%; acetaminophen group–0.5%. While in the oxycodone group, symptoms appeared in mothers receiving median doses of 0.4 mg/kg/day (28 mg for a 70 kg individual), symptoms in the codeine group appeared at a median dose of 1.4 mg/kg/day (98 mg/day for a 70 kg individual). It was found that higher doses of oxycodone or codeine were more likely to be associated with CNS depression. Further, maternal sedation was more likely with the use of oxycodone than with the use of codeine. Based on these findings, the authors conclude that oxycodone should not be considered a safer alternative to codeine in breastfed infants.

Relative infant dose: aspirin/oxycodone: 2.5–10.8%/1.5–3.5%

Observe for signs of sedation in the breastfed infant while using aspirin + oxycodone. Avoid its use in premature infants and in infants with a viral syndrome. Consider ibuprofen or acetaminophen as better choices for the relief of painful conditions in breastfeeding mothers.

Pregnancy Risk	D	Lactation Risk	L3
T ½	= Aspirin/oxycodone: 2.5–7 hours/3–6 hours	M/P	= Aspirin/oxycodone: 0.03–0.08/3.4
Vd	= Aspirin/oxycodone: 0.15/1.8–3.7 l/kg	PB	= Aspirin/oxycodone: 88–93%/
Tmax	= Aspirin/oxycodone: 1–2 hours/1–2 hours	Oral	= Aspirin/oxycodone: 80–100%/50%
MW	= Aspirin/oxycodone: 180/315	pKa	= Aspirin/oxycodone: /8.5

Adult Concerns: Nausea, vomiting, headache, pruritus, constipation, heartburn, sedation, gastric hemorrhage, respiratory, circulatory and CNS depression with high doses.

Pediatric Concerns:

Drug Interactions: Aspirin interactions: May decrease serum levels of other NSAIDs as well as GI distress. Aspirin may antagonize effect of probenecid. Aspirin may increase methotrexate serum levels, and increase free valproic acid plasma levels and valproate toxicity. May increase anticoagulant effect of warfarin. Oxycodone interactions: Oxycodone may enhance the effect of skeletal muscle relaxants and cause respiratory depression. Use with caution while using with other CNS depressants such as other opioid analgesics, general anesthetics, sedatives, alcohol etc. due to additive effect.

Relative Infant Dose: aspirin/oxycodone: 2.5–10.8%/1.5–3.5%

Adult Dose: Aspirin/oxycodone: 325 mg/4.8 mg every 6 hours or as needed. Do not exceed 12 tablets in a 24 hour period.

Alternatives: Ibuprofen, acetaminophen

References:
1. Pharmaceutical manufacturer prescribing information, 2010.
2. Findlay JW, DeAngelis RL, Kearney MF, Welch RM, Findlay JM. Analgesic drugs in breast milk and plasma. Clin Pharmacol Ther 1981; 29(5): 625–633.
3. Erickson SH, Oppenheim GL. Aspirin in breast milk. J Fam Pract 1979; 8(1): 189–190.
4. Bailey DN, Welbert RT, Naylor A. A study of salicylate and caffeine excretion in the breast milk of two nursing mothers. J Anal Toxicol. 1982; 6: 64–8.
5. Putter J, Satravaha P, Stockhausen H. Quantitative analysis of the main metabolites of acetylsalicylic acid. Comparative analysis in the blood and milk of lactating women. Z Geburtshilfe Perinatol. 1974; 178: 135–8.
6. Marx CM, Pucin F, Carlson JD. et. al. Oxycodone excretion in human milk in the puerperium. Drug Intel Clin 1986; 20: 474.
7. Seaton S, Reeves M, McLean S. Oxycodone as a component of multimodal analgesia for lactating mothers after Caesarean section: Relationships between maternal plasma, breast milk and neonatal plasma levels. Aust NZ J Obstet Gyn 2007; 47: 181–85.
8. Lam J, Kelly L, Ciszkowski C, Landsmeer ML, Nauta M, Carleton BC, Hayden MR, Madadi P, Koren G. Central nervous system depression of neonates breastfed by mothers receiving oxycodone for postpartum analgesia. J Pediatr. 2012Jan; 160(1): 33–37. e2.

ATENOLOL   L3

Trade: Tenoretic, Tenormin

Other Trades: Anselol, Noten, Tenlol, Tensig, Apo-Atenolol, Tenormin, Antipress

Category: Beta adrenergic blocker, antihyertensive

Atenolol is a potent cardio-selective beta-blocker. Data conflict on the secretion of atenolol into breastmilk. One author reports an incident of significant bradycardia, cyanosis, low body temperature, and low blood pressure in breastfeeding infant of mother consuming 100 mg atenolol daily while a number of others have failed to detect plasma levels in the neonate or untoward side effects.[1] Data seem to indicate that atenolol secretion into breastmilk is highly variable but may be as high as 10 times greater than for propranolol. In one study, women taking 50–100 mg/day were found to have milk/plasma ratios of 1.5–6.8. However, even with high M/P ratios, the calculated intake per day (at peak levels) for a breastfeeding infant would only be 0.13 mg.[2] In a study by White et al, breastmilk levels in one patient were 0.7, 1.2 and 1.8 mg/L of milk at doses of 25, 50 and 100 mg daily respectively.[3] In another study, the estimated daily intake for an infant receiving 500 mL milk per day, would be 0.3 mg.[4] In these five patients who received 100 mg daily, the mean milk concentration of atenolol was 630 µg/L. In a study by Kulas et al the amount of atenolol transferred into milk varied from 0.66 mg/L with a maternal dose of 25 mg, 1.2 mg/L with a maternal dose of 50 mg, and 1.7 mg/L with a maternal dose of 100 mg per day.[5] Although atenolol is approved by the AAP, some caution is recommended due to the milk/plasma ratios and the reported problem with one infant.

Pregnancy Risk	D	Lactation Risk	L3
T ½	= 6.1 hours	M/P	= 1.5–6.8
Vd	= 1.3 l/kg	PB	= 5%
Tmax	= 2–4 hours	Oral	= 50–60%
MW	= 266	pKa	= 9.6

Adult Concerns: Persistent bradycardia, hypotension, heart failure, dizziness, fatigue, insomnia, lethargy, confusion, impotence, dyspnea, wheezing in asthmatics.

Pediatric Concerns: One report of bradycardia, cyanosis, low body temperature, and hypotension in a breastfeeding infant of mother consuming 100 mg atenolol daily, but other reports do not suggest clinical effects on breastfed infants.

Drug Interactions: Decreased effect when used with aluminum salts, barbiturates, calcium salts, cholestyramine, NSAIDs, ampicillin, rifampin, and salicylates. Beta blockers may reduce the effect of oral sulfonylureas (hypoglycemic agents). Increased toxicity/effect when used with other antihypertensives, contraceptives, MAO inhibitors, cimetidine, and numerous other products. See drug interaction reference for complete listing.

Relative Infant Dose: 6.6%

Adult Dose: 50–100 mg daily

Alternatives: Propranolol, Metoprolol

References:
1. Schimmel MS, Eidelman AI, Wilschanski MA, Shaw D, Jr., Ogilvie RJ, Koren G, Schmimmel MS, Eidelman AJ. Toxic effects of atenolol consumed during breast feeding. J Pediatr 1989; 114(3): 476–478.
2. Liedholm H, Melander A, Bitzen PO, Helm G, Lonnerholm G, Mattiasson I, Nilsson B, Wahlin-Boll E. Accumulation of atenolol and metoprolol in human breast milk. Eur J Clin Pharmacol 1981; 20(3): 229–231.
3. White WB, Andreoli JW, Wong SH, Cohn RD. Atenolol in human plasma and breast milk. Obstet Gynecol 1984; 63(3 Suppl): 42S-44S.
4. Thorley KJ, McAinsh J. Levels of the beta-blockers atenolol and propranolol in the breast milk of women treated for hypertension in pregnancy. Biopharm Drug Dispos 1983; 4(3): 299–301.
5. Kulas J, Lunell NO, Rosing U, Steen B, Rane A. Atenolol and metoprolol. A comparison of their excretion into human breast milk. Acta Obstet Gynecol Scand Suppl 1984; 118: 65–69.

ATOMOXETINE   L4

Trade: Strattera
Other Trades:
Category: Stimulant for treatment of ADHD

Atomoxetine is a selective norepinephrine reuptake inhibitor that is presently indicated for the treatment of Attention-Deficit/Hyperactivity Disorder (ADHD).[1] Atomoxetine metabolism is highly variable. One group of poor metabolizers (7%) may have extended half-lives (22 h) and higher plasma levels, while another group of normal metabolizers has a half-life of about 5 hours. No data are available on the transfer of Atomoxetine into human milk. Because this is a lipophilic, neuroactive drug, there is some potential risk coincident with its use in a breastfeeding mother, and mothers should probably be cautioned about its use while breastfeeding.

Pregnancy Risk	C	Lactation Risk	L4
T ½	= 5.2 hours	M/P	=
Vd	= 0.85 l/kg	PB	= 98%
Tmax	= 1–2 hours	Oral	= 63–94%
MW	= 291	pKa	=

Adult Concerns: Adverse events include abdominal pain, dyspepsia, vomiting, decreased appetite, dizziness, headache, and cough.

Pediatric Concerns: None reported via milk but no studies are available. If used, reduced weight gain, insomnia, and hyperactivity could occur in the infant.

Drug Interactions: Levels may be increased by inhibitors of CYP2D6 (paroxetine, fluoxetine, quinidine, etc). Albuterol may increase heart rate in patients treated with atomoxetine. Atomoxetine may increase plasma levels of midazolam. Do not use with or within two weeks of the use of a monoamine oxidase inhibitor (MAOI). Do not use in patients with narrow angle glaucoma.

Relative Infant Dose:

Adult Dose: 0.5–1.2 mg/kg/day

Alternatives: Methylphenidate

References:
1. Pharmaceutical manufacturer prescribing information, 2003.

ATORVASTATIN   L3

Trade: Lipitor
Other Trades: Caduet, Lipitor
Category: Cholesterol-lowering agent

Atorvastatin is a typical HMG Co-A reductase inhibitor for lowering plasma cholesterol levels. It is known to transfer into animal milk, but human studies are not available.[1] Due to its poor oral absorption and high protein binding, it is unlikely that clinically relevant amounts would transfer into human milk. Nevertheless, atherosclerosis is a chronic process and discontinuation of lipid-lowering drugs during pregnancy and lactation should have little to no impact on the outcome of long-term therapy of primary hypercholesterolemia. Cholesterol and other products of cholesterol biosynthesis are essential components for fetal and neonatal development and the use of cholesterol-lowering drugs would not be advisable under most circumstances. Cholesterol helps cells adjust to temperature changes and helps insulate nerve cells. Also helps synthesize hormones such as estrogen, testosterone and progesterone. Cholesterol also helps in synthesizing bile which aides in digestion. Cholesterol also helps in making Vitamin D.

Pregnancy Risk	X	Lactation Risk	L3
T ½	= 14 hours	M/P	=
Vd	= 8 l/kg	PB	= 98%
Tmax	= 1–2 hours	Oral	= 12–30%
MW	= 1209	pKa	= 11.82

Adult Concerns: Liver dysfunction, rhabdomyolysis with acute renal failure.

Pediatric Concerns: None reported, but the use of these products in lactating women is not recommended.

Drug Interactions: Increased risk of myopathy when used with cyclosporin, fibric acid derivatives, niacin, erythromycin, and azole antifungals (Diflucan, etc). Decreased plasma levels of atorvastatin when used with antacids, or colestipol.

Relative Infant Dose:

Adult Dose: 10–80 mg daily

Alternatives:

References:
1. Pharmaceutical manufacturer prescribing information, 1999.

ATOVAQUONE   L3

Trade: Mepron

Other Trades: Meprone

Category: Antiprotozoal

Atovaquone is used to treat Pneumocystis pneumonia (PCP; type of pneumonia most likely to affect people with human immunodeficiency virus [HIV]).[1] It is one of the two components (along with proguanil) in the drug Malarone used to treat Malaria. Atovaquone is in a class of medications called antiprotozoal agents. The elimination half-life of atovaquone is much shorter in pediatric patients (1–2 days) than in adult patients (2–3 days). Elimination half-life ranges from 32 to 84 hours for atovaquone.

Pregnancy Risk	C	Lactation Risk	L3
T ½	= 1.5–4 days	M/P	=
Vd	= 0.6 l/kg	PB	= >99%
Tmax	=	Oral	= 36–62%
MW	= 366.84	pKa	=

Adult Concerns: Fever, headache, insomnia, rash, diarrhea, nausea, vomiting, abdominal pain

Pediatric Concerns:

Drug Interactions: Atovaquone increases the concentration of Eptoposide. It may also increase the concentration of hypoglycemic agents. In addition, atovaquone decreases the concentration of Indinavir, Rifamycin derivatives, Ritonavir, Tetracyclines.

Relative Infant Dose:

Adult Dose: 750 mg twice a day

Alternatives:

References:
1.   Pharmaceutical manufacturer prescribing information,2011.

ATOVAQUONE + PROGUANIL   L3

Trade: Malarone

Other Trades: Malarone

Category: Antimalarials

Atovaquone and Proguanil hydrochloride is a drug combination indicated for use in falciparum malaria.[1] Atovaquone + Proguanil drug combination is a fixed combination of atovaquone (250 mg) and proguanil (100 mg) (adult dose). The pediatric chewable tablet contains atovaquone (62.5) and proguanil (25 mg). It is used both to prevent and treat malaria, particularly malaria resistant to certain other drugs. Both adult and pediatric formulations are available for treating pediatric patients down to 11 kg. No data are available on transfer of atovaquone into breastmilk. Only trace quantities of proguanil were found in human milk. Further, while the pharmacokinetics of proguanil is similar in adults and pediatric patients, the elimination half-life of atovaquone is much shorter in pediatric patients (1–2 days) than in adult patients (2–3 days). Elimination half-life ranges from 32 to 84 hours for atovaquone and 12 to 21 hours for proguanil; the half-life of cycloguanil is approximately 14 hours. For current information contact the CDC web site at (www.cdc.gov). According to the CDC, breastfeeding mothers with infants less than 11 kg should use mefloquine instead of atovaquone + proguanil.[2]

	Atovaquone	Proguanil
T½	32-84 hours	12-21 hours
ORAL BIOAVAILABILITY	23%	Complete
PROTEIN BINDING	> 99%	75%

Pregnancy Risk	C		Lactation Risk	L3
T ½	= Atovaquone/proguanil: 1.5–4 days/12–21 hours		M/P	= Atovaquone/proguanil:
Vd	= Atovaquone/proguanil: 0.6/23.1–35.7 l/kg		PB	= Atovaquone/proguanil: >99%/75%
Tmax	= Atovaquone/proguanil: /2–4 hours		Oral	= Atovaquone/proguanil: 36–62%/60%
MW	= Atovaquone/proguanil: 366.84/254		pKa	= Atovaquone/proguanil:

Adult Concerns: Headache, fever, myalgia, abdominal pain, cough, diarrhea, dyspepsia, back pain, gastritis have been reported.

Pediatric Concerns: None reported via milk.

Drug Interactions: Major reductions in plasma levels of atovaquone have been reported following the use of tetracycline (40%), metoclopramide, rifampin (50%), or rifabutin (34%).

Relative Infant Dose:

Adult Dose: Atovaquone (250 mg); Proguanil (100 mg) daily.

Alternatives: Mefloquine

References:
1. Pharmaceutical manufacturer prescribing information, 2011.
2. http://www.cdc.gov/ncidod/dpd/parasites/malaria/default.htm. 2004.

ATROPINE   L3

Trade: Belladonna, Atropine

Other Trades: Atropt, Atropine Minims, Atropisol, Isopto-Atropine, Eyesule

Category: Anticholinergic, drying agent

Atropine is a powerful anticholinergic that is well distributed throughout the body.[1] Only small amounts are believed to be secreted in milk.[2] Effects may be highly variable. Slight absorption together with enhanced neonatal sensitivity creates hazardous potential. Use caution. Avoid if possible but not definitely contraindicated.

Pregnancy Risk	C	Lactation Risk	L3
T ½	= 4.3 hours	M/P	=
Vd	= 2.3–3.6 l/kg	PB	= 14–22%
Tmax	= 1 hour	Oral	= 90%
MW	= 289	pKa	= 9.8

Adult Concerns: Dry, hot skin. Decreased flow of breastmilk. Decreased bowel motility, drying of secretions, dilated pupil, and increased heart rate.

Pediatric Concerns: No reports are available, although caution is urged. Anticholinergics have been found in sheep to reduce prolactin production.

Drug Interactions: Phenothiazines, levodopa, antihistamines, may decrease anticholinergic effects of atropine. Increased toxicity when admixed with amantadine and thiazide diuretics.

Relative Infant Dose:

Adult Dose: 0.6 mg every 6 hours

Alternatives:

References:
1. Drug Facts and Comparisons 1995 ed. ed. St. Louis: 1995.
2. Wilson J. Drugs in Breast Milk. New York: ADIS Press 1981.

ATROPINE + DIPHENOXYLATE | L3

Trade: Lomocot, Lomotil, Lonox, Vi-Atro, Lofene

Other Trades: Lofenoxal

Category: Antidiarrheal

Atropine sulfate and diphenoxylate hydrochloride is a drug combination product used for the treatment of diarrhea. There are no reports on the transfer of this combined drug product in breastmilk.

Atropine is a powerful anticholinergic that is well distributed throughout the body.[1] Only small amounts are believed to be secreted in milk.[2] Effects may be highly variable. Slight absorption together with enhanced neonatal sensitivity creates hazardous potential. Use caution. Avoid if possible but not definitely contraindicated.

Diphenoxylate belongs to the opiate family (meperidine) and acts on the intestinal tract inhibiting gastrointestinal motility and excessive gastrointestinal propulsion.[3] The drug has no analgesic activity. Although no reports on its transfer to human milk are available, it is probably secreted in breastmilk in very small quantities.[4] Some authors consider diphenoxylate to be contraindicated, but this is questionable.

Pregnancy Risk	C	Lactation Risk	L3
T ½	= Atropine/diphenoxylate: 4.3 hours/2.5 hours	M/P	=
Vd	= Atropine/diphenoxylate: 2.3–3.6/3.8 l/kg	PB	= Atropine/diphenoxylate: 14–22%/
Tmax	= Atropine/diphenoxylate: 1 hour/2 hours	Oral	= Atropine/diphenoxylate: 90%/90%
MW	= Atropine/diphenoxylate: 289/453	pKa	= Atropine/diphenoxylate: 9.8/7.1

Adult Concerns: Nausea, vomiting, sedation, dizziness occur more commonly. Some of the serious and rare side-effects are pancreatitis, toxic megacolon and hypersensitivity reactions. Gastrointestinal: Abdominal discomfort, nausea and vomiting. Neurologic: Dizziness, Sedated, Somnolence. Psychiatric: Euphoria. Other: Malaise, Serious. Gastrointestinal: Pancreatitis, toxic megacolon. Immunologic: Anaphylaxis

Pediatric Concerns:

Drug Interactions: Do not co-administer with alcohol, barbiturates, benzodiazepines and monoamine oxidase inhibitors.

Relative Infant Dose:

Adult Dose: Atropine/diphenoxylate: 0.25/2.5 mg, two tablets 4 times daily. Do not exceed 20 mg/day diphenoxylate.

Alternatives:

References:
1. Drug Facts and Comparisons 1995 ed. ed. St. Louis: 1995.
2. Wilson J. Drugs in Breast Milk. New York: ADIS Press 1981.
3. Drug Facts and Comparisons 1994 ed. ed. St. Louis: 1994.
4. Stewart JJ. Gastrointestinal drugs. In Wilson, J. T., ed. Drugs in Breast Milk. Balgowlah, Australia ADIS Press 1981; 71.

AZAPROPAZONE   L2

Trade:

Other Trades: Rheumox

Category: Analgesic

Azapropazone is a partial NSAID and anti-inflammatory. Unlike other NSAIDs its main effect is to stabilize the lysosomal membrane and only to a limited extent does it suppress prostaglandin synthetase. In a study of 4 patients, each received 600 mg IV within 2 hours after giving birth and thereafter, they received 600 mg twice daily.[1] Milk levels of azapropazone were measured on days 4 and 6 postpartum. The amount of azapropazone excreted in the breast milk within 12 h ranged from 0.2 mg to 1.3 mg (mean 0.8 mg in 12 h) or an average milk concentration of 2.43 µg/mL. The volume of milk produced during this 12 hour period averaged 329 mL. The relative infant dose over 24 hours would be 2.1% of the maternal dose. The authors did not report side effects in the infants.

Pregnancy Risk	C/D in 3rd trimester	Lactation Risk	L2
T ½	= 13–14 hours	M/P	=
Vd	= 0.17 l/kg	PB	= 99%
Tmax	= 3–6 hours orally	Oral	= 83%
MW	=	pKa	=

Adult Concerns: Adverse effects include diarrhea, vomiting, nausea, gastrointestinal distress, gastrointestinal bleeding, headache, edema, GI ulceration, and other typical side effects of NSAID drugs.

Pediatric Concerns: None reported via milk in one study.

Drug Interactions: Increased azapropazone levels when mixed with cimetidine. Enhanced anticoagulant effect when mixed with coumarins, and other anticoagulants. Reduced excretion of lithium, and methotrexate when admixed with azapropazone. May block antihypertensive effects of beta-blockers, calcium channel blockers and other antihypertensives.

Relative Infant Dose: 2.1%

Adult Dose: 600 mg twice daily.

Alternatives: Celecoxib

References:
1. Bald R, Bernbeck-Betthauser EM, Spahn H, Mutschler E. Excretion of azapropazone in human breast milk. Eur J Clin Pharmacol 1990; 39(3): 271–273.

AZATHIOPRINE   L3

Trade: Imuran

Other Trades: Thioprine, Imuran

Category: Immunosuppressive agent

Azathioprine is a powerful immunosuppressive agent that is metabolized to 6–Mercaptopurine (6–MP).

In two mothers receiving 75 mg azathioprine, the concentration of 6–MP in milk varied from 3.5–4.5 µg/L in one mother and 18 µg/L in the second mother.[1] Both levels were peak milk concentrations at 2 hours following the dose. The authors conclude that these levels would be too low to produce clinical effects in a breastfed infant. Using this data for 6–MP, an infant would absorb only 0.1% of the weight-adjusted maternal dose, which is probably too low to produce adverse effects in a breastfeeding infant. Plasma levels in treated patients is maintained at 50 ng/mL or higher. One infant continued to breastfeed during therapy and displayed no immunosuppressive effects.

In another study of two infants who were breastfed by mothers receiving 75–100 mg/day azathioprine, milk levels of 6–MP were not measured. But both infants had normal blood counts, no increase in infections, and above-average growth rate.[2] However, caution is recommended. Four mothers who were receiving 1.2–2.1 mg/kg/day of azathioprine throughout pregnancy and continued postpartum were studied while breastfeeding. Using high-performance liquid chromatography, the mothers' blood concentrations of 6–TGN and 6–MMPN (the metabolites of azathioprine) ranged from 234–291 and 284 to 1178 pmol/100 million RBC, respectively. Neither 6–TGN nor 6–MMPN could be detected in the exposed infants. The authors suggest that breastfeeding while taking azathioprine may be safe in mothers with 'normal' TPMT enzyme activity (the enzyme responsible for metabolizing 6–TGN).[3] Four case reports were performed with mothers taking between 50 to 100 mg/day of azathioprine. No adverse events were reported in any of the infants, and milk concentrations in two mothers proved to be undetectable.[4] Ten women at steady state on 75 to 150 mg/day azathioprine provided milk samples on days 3–4, days 7–10 and day 28 after delivery, between 3 and 18 hours after azathioprine administration. 6–MP was detected in only one case, at 1.2 and 7.6 ng/mL at 3 and 6 hours after azathioprine intake on day 28. However, 6–MP and 6–TGN were undetectable in the infants blood. There were no signs of immunosuppression, even in three preterm neonates. The authors suggest that azathioprine therapy should not deter mothers from breastfeeding.[5] Another study of three mothers taking azathioprine while breastfeeding (doses of 100–175 mg) reported normal blood cell counts in all three infants, and only a low amount of 6–TGN in one infant on day 3. At age 3 weeks, this level decreased below the detectable range.[6]

In a group of 8 lactating women who received azathioprine (75–200 mg/day), levels in milk ranged from 2–50 µg/L.[7] After 6 hours an average of 10% of the peak values were measured. The authors estimate the infants dose to be <0.008 mg/kg body weight/24 hours. They suggest that breastfeeding during treatment with azathioprine seems safe and should be recommended. In a 31-year-old mother with Crohn's disease being treated with 100 mg/day azathioprine, peripheral blood levels of 6–MP and 6–TGN in the infant were undetectable at day 8 or after 3 months of therapy.[8] The infant was reported to be normal after 6 months. In a recent study of the long-term follow up (median 3.3 years) of fetal and breastfeeding exposure to azathioprine (n = 11 infants), there were no differences in rates of infectious disease in azathioprine-treated groups compared to non-treated controls. The authors suggest that breastfeeding following exposure to azathioprine does not increase the risk of infections.[9]

In summary, the transport of 6-mercaptopurine into human milk is apparently quite low. However, this is a strong immunosuppressant and some caution is still recommended if it is used in a breastfeeding mother. Monitor the infant closely for signs of immunosuppression, leukopenia, thrombocytopenia, hepatotoxicity, pancreatitis, and other symptoms of 6-mercaptopurine exposure. The risks to the infant are probably low. Recent long-term data suggest that the rate of infections in treated groups is no different from non-treated controls.

Pregnancy Risk	D	Lactation Risk	L3
T ½	= 0.6 hour	M/P	=
Vd	= 0.9 l/kg	PB	= 30%
Tmax	= 1–2 hours	Oral	= 41–44%
MW	= 277	pKa	= 8.2

Adult Concerns: Bone marrow suppression, megaloblastic anemia, infections, skin cancers, lymphoma, nausea, vomiting, hepatoxicity, pulmonary dysfunction and pancreatitis.

Pediatric Concerns: None reported in several case reports, but caution is urged. Recent long-term data suggest that the rate of infections in treated groups is no different from non-treated controls.

Drug Interactions: Increased toxicity when used with allopurinol. Reduce azathioprine dose to ⅓rd to ¼th of normal. Use with ACE inhibitors has produced severe leukopenia. It is best to avoid the following drugs when using mercaptopurine or azathioprine: Neuromuscular blocking agents (such as rocuronium, mivacurium, vercuronium, atracurium, tubocurarine), Warfarin, D-penicillamine, Cotrimoxazole, Captopril, Cimetidine, Indomethacin and live vaccines.

Relative Infant Dose: 0.07%–0.3%

Adult Dose: 1–2.5 mg/kg/day

Alternatives:

References:
1. Coulam CB, Moyer TP, Jiang NS, Zincke H. Breast-feeding after renal transplantation. Transplant Proc 1982; 14(3): 605–609.
2. Grekas DM, Vasiliou SS, Lazarides AN. Immunosuppressive therapy and breast-feeding after renal transplantation. Nephron 1984; 37(1): 68.
3. Gardiner SJ, Gearry RB, Roberts RL, Zhang M, Barclay ML, Begg EJ. Exposure to thiopurine drugs through breast milk is low based on metabolite concentrations in mother-infant pairs. Br J Clin Pharmacol 2006; 62(4): 453–456.

4. Moretti ME, Verjee Z, Ito S, Koren G. Breast-Feeding During Maternal Use of Azathioprine. Ann Pharmacother 2006; 40: 2269–2272.
5. Sau A, Clarke S, Bass J, Kaiser A, Marinaki A, Nelson-Piercy C. Azathioprine and breastfeeding- is it safe? BJOG 2007; 114: 498–501.
6. Bernard N, Garayt C, Chol F, Vial T, Descotes J. Prospective clinical and biological follow-up of three breastfed babies from azathioprine-treated mothers. Fundam clin Pharmacol 2007; 21 (suppl. 1): 62–63. Abstract.
7. Christensen LA, Dahlerup JF, Nielsen MJ, Fallingborg JF, Schmiegelow K. Azathioprine treatment during lactation. Aliment Pharmacol Ther. 2008 Nov 15; 28(10): 1209–13. Epub 2008 Aug 30.
8. Zelinkova Z, De Boer IP, Van Dijke MJ, Kuipers EJ, Van Der Woude CJ. Azathioprine treatment during lactation. Aliment Pharmacol Ther. 2009 Jul; 30(1): 90–1;
9. Angelberger S, Reinisch W, Messerschmidt A, Miehsler W, Novacek G, Vogelsang H, Dejaco C. Long-term follow-up of babies exposed to azathioprine in utero and via breastfeeding. J Crohns Colitis. 2011 Apr; 5(2): 95–100. Epub 2010 Dec 9.

AZELAIC ACID | L3

Trade: Azelex, Finevin, Finacea

Other Trades: Skinoren

Category: Topical treatment of acne

Azelaic acid is a dicarboxylic acid derivative normally found in whole grains and animal products. Azelaic acid, when applied as a cream, produces a significant reduction of Propionibacterium acnes (implicated in the causation of acne) and has an anti-keratinizing effect as well. Small amounts of azelaic acid are normally present in human milk.[1] Azelaic acid is only modestly absorbed via skin (<4%), and it is rapidly metabolized. The amount absorbed does not change the levels normally found in plasma nor milk. Due to its poor penetration into plasma and rapid half-life (45 min), it is not likely to penetrate milk or produce untoward effects in a breastfed infant.

Pregnancy Risk	B	Lactation Risk	L3
T ½	= 45 minutes	M/P	=
Vd	=	PB	=
Tmax	=	Oral	=
MW	= 188	pKa	= 4.98

Adult Concerns: Pruritus, burning, stinging, erythema, dryness, peeling and skin irritation.

Pediatric Concerns: None reported via milk. Normal constituent of milk.

Drug Interactions:

Relative Infant Dose:

Adult Dose: Apply topically twice a day

Alternatives:

References:
1. Pharmaceutical manufacturer prescribing information, 1999.

AZELASTINE   L3

Trade: Astelin, Optivar, Astepro
Other Trades: Azep, Rhinolast, Optilast
Category: Antihistamine

Azelastine (Astelin) is an antihistamine for oral, intranasal and ophthalmic administration.[1] It is effective in treating seasonal and perennial rhinitis and non allergic vasomotor rhinitis. Ophthalmically, it is effective for allergic conjunctivitis (itchy eyes). Oral bioavailability is 80%, and intranasal bioavailability is only 40%. No data are available on the transfer of azelastine into human milk. The doses used intranasally and ophthalmically are so low that it is extremely unlikely to produce clinically relevant levels in human milk. Oral administration could potentially lead to slightly higher levels but azelastine is relatively devoid of serious side effects and it is doubtful that any would occur in a breastfed infant. However, this is an extremely bitter product. It is possible that even miniscule amounts in milk could alter the taste of milk leading to rejection by the infant.

Pregnancy Risk	C	Lactation Risk	L3
T ½	= 22 hours	M/P	=
Vd	= 14.5 l/kg	PB	= 88%
Tmax	= 2–3 hours	Oral	= 80%
MW	= 418	pKa	= 9.5

Adult Concerns: Intranasal: nasal burning and bitter taste, headache, somnolence. Orally: drowsiness and bitter taste. Ophthalmic: transient eye burning/stinging, headache, and bitter taste.

Pediatric Concerns: None reported via milk. Levels in milk are unlikely to pose a problem. May impart bitter taste to milk, infant may reject milk.

Drug Interactions: Avoid use in asthmatics. Cimetidine significantly increases plasma levels of azelastine.

Relative Infant Dose:

Adult Dose: Variable: 1–2 sprays(137 µg/spray) per nostril BID.

Alternatives: Loratadine, cetirizine

References:
1.   Pharmaceutical manufacturer prescribing information, 2003.

AZITHROMYCIN   L2

Trade: Zithromax
Other Trades: Zithromax
Category: Antibiotic, macrolide

Azithromycin belongs to the macrolide family. It has an extremely long half-life, particularly in tissues.[1] Azithromycin is concentrated for long periods in phagocytes, which are known to be present in human milk. In one study of a patient who received 1 gm initially followed by 500 mg doses each at 24 hr intervals, the concentration of azithromycin in breastmilk varied from 0.64 mg/L (initially) to 2.8 mg/L on day 3.[2] The predicted dose of azithromycin received by the infant would be approximately 0.4 mg/kg/day. This would suggest that the level of azithromycin ingested by a breastfeeding infant is not clinically relevant. New pediatric formulations of azithromycin have been recently introduced. Pediatric dosing is 10 mg/kg STAT followed by 5 mg/kg per day for up to 5 days.

Pregnancy Risk	B	Lactation Risk	L2
T ½	= 48–68 hours	M/P	=
Vd	= 23–31 l/kg	PB	= 7–51%
Tmax	= 3–4 hours	Oral	= 37%
MW	= 749	pKa	= 12.90

Adult Concerns: Diarrhea, loose stools, abdominal pain, vomiting, nausea.

Pediatric Concerns: None reported via breastmilk. Pediatric formulations are available.

Drug Interactions: Aluminum and magnesium-containing antacids may slow, but not reduce absorption of azithromycin. Increased effect/toxicity when used with tacrolimus, alfentanil, astemizole, terfenadine, loratadine, carbamazepine, cyclosporine, digoxin, disopyramide, triazolam.

Relative Infant Dose: 5.9%

Adult Dose: 250–500 mg daily.

Alternatives:

References:
1. Pharmaceutical manufacturer prescribing information, 1996.
2. Kelsey JJ, Moser LR, Jennings JC, Munger MA. Presence of azithromycin breast milk concentrations: a case report. Am J Obstet Gynecol 1994; 170(5 Pt 1): 1375–1376.

AZTREONAM   L2

Trade: Azactam
Other Trades: Azactam
Category: Antibiotic

Aztreonam is a monobactam antibiotic whose structure is similar but different from the penicillins and is used for documented gram-negative sepsis. Following a single 1 gm IV dose, breastmilk level was 0.18 mg/L at 2 hours and 0.22 mg/L at 4 hours.[1] An infant would ingest approximately 33 µg/kg/day or <0.03% of the maternal dose per day (not weight adjusted). The manufacturer reports that less than 1% of a maternal dose is transferred into milk.[2] Due to poor oral absorption (<1%), no untoward effects would be expected in nursing infants, aside from changes in gastrointestinal flora. Aztreonam is commonly used in pediatric units. In another study of a patient early postpartum receiving a 1 gm intravenous injection, aztreonam levels in milk at 6 hours were 0.4 µg/mL to 1.0 µg/mL.[3]

Pregnancy Risk	B	Lactation Risk	L2
T ½	= 1.7 hours	M/P	= 0.005
Vd	= 0.26–0.36 l/kg	PB	= 60%
Tmax	= 0.6–1.3 hours	Oral	= <1%
MW	= 435	pKa	= 2.87

Adult Concerns: Changes in gastrointestinal flora, diarrhea, rash, elevations of hepatic function tests.

Pediatric Concerns: None reported via milk in two cases.

Drug Interactions: Check hypersensitivity to penicillins and other beta-lactams. Requires dosage adjustment in renal failure.

Relative Infant Dose: 0.2%–1%

Adult Dose: 1–2 gm BID or QID

Alternatives:

References:
1. Fleiss PM, Richwald GA, Gordon J, Stern M, Frantz M, Devlin RG. Aztreonam in human serum and breast milk. Br J Clin Pharmacol 1985; 19(4): 509–511.
2. Pharmaceutical manufacturer prescribing information, 1996.
3. Ito K, Hirose R, Tamaya T, Yamada Y, Izumi K. Pharmacokinetic and clinical studies on aztreonam in the perinatal period. Jpn J Antibiot. 1990 Apr; 43(4): 719–26.

BACITRACIN   L2

Trade: Baci-Rx BaciiM

Other Trades: Baciject

Category: Antibacterial

Bacitracin is a polypeptide antibiotic with bactericidal activity primarily against gram-positive organisms.[1] There are no adequate and well-controlled studies or case reports in breastfeeding women. It is unknown if bacitracin is distributed in human milk but it is unlikely. The minimal transcutaneous absorption after topical use should limit the amount of medication available for transfer into milk.

Pregnancy Risk	C	Lactation Risk	L2
T ½	= 1.5 hours	M/P	=
Vd	= Nil	PB	= Minimal
Tmax	= 1–2 hours	Oral	= Nil
MW	= 1460	pKa	= 3.95

Adult Concerns: Percutaneous absorption is negligible. Oral absorption is nil, so oral use produces virtually no toxicity. Nephrotoxic but only following parenteral injection.

Pediatric Concerns: Little expected due to poor oral absorption.

Drug Interactions: Numerous drug interaction but only following IM use, which is virtually never done. None reported following topical use.

Relative Infant Dose:

Adult Dose: 25000 units 4 times a day for 7–10 days

Alternatives:

References:
1. Pharmaceutical manufacturer prescribing information, 2010.

BACLOFEN   L2

Trade: Lioresal, Atrofen

Other Trades: Clofen, Lioresal, Novo-Baclofen, Apo-Baclofen

Category: Skeletal muscle relaxant

Baclofen inhibits spinal reflexes and is used to reverse spasticity associated with multiple sclerosis or spinal cord lesions. Animal studies indicate baclofen inhibits prolactin release and may inhibit lactation. Small amounts of baclofen are secreted into milk. In one mother given a 20 mg oral dose, total consumption by infant over a 26 hour period is estimated to be 22 µg, about 0.1% of the maternal dose (authors estimate).[1] Milk levels ranged from 0.6 µmol/L (138 µg/L C_{max}) to 0.052 µmol/L at 26 hours. The maternal plasma and milk half-lives were 3.9 hours and 5.6 hours, respectively. It is quite unlikely that baclofen administered intrathecally would be secreted into milk in clinically relevant quantities. When infant is exposed in utero, a serious discontinuation syndrome in the infant may result.

Pregnancy Risk	C	Lactation Risk	L2
T ½	= 3–4 hours	M/P	=
Vd	= 0.84 l/kg	PB	= 30%
Tmax	= 2–3 hours	Oral	= Complete
MW	= 214	pKa	=

Adult Concerns: Drowsiness, excitement, dry mouth, urinary retention, tremor, rigidity, and wide pupils. Abrupt discontinuation is hazardous and should be avoided. Muscle rigidity, exaggerated spasticity, multiple system organ failure and death have been reported.

Pediatric Concerns: None reported. Exposure in utero may result in hazardous discontinuation syndrome following delivery.

Drug Interactions: Decreased effect when used with lithium. Increased effect of opiate analgesics, CNS depressants, alcohol (sedation), tricyclic antidepressants, clindamycin (neuromuscular blockade), guanabenz, MAO inhibitors.

Relative Infant Dose: 6.9%

Adult Dose: 5–25 mg TID

Alternatives:

References:
1. Eriksson G, Swahn CG. Concentrations of baclofen in serum and breast milk from a lactating woman. Scand J Clin Lab Invest 1981; 41(2): 185–187.

BALSALAZIDE   L3

Trade: Colazal
Other Trades:
Category: Anti-inflammatory drug for ulcerative colitis

Balsalazide disodium is a prodrug that is metabolized to mesalamine (5-aminosalicylic acid).[1] Balsalazide is delivered intact to the colon where it is cleaved by bacterial enzymes to release the active drug mesalamine. The oral absorption of balsalazide is very low. Less than 1% of the parent drug is recovered in the urine. The transfer of the active metabolite mesalamine is documented to be about 7–8%. At least one case of watery diarrhea has been reported with mesalamine. Some caution is recommended, but this agent can probably be used with supervision in breastfeeding mothers.

Pregnancy Risk	B	Lactation Risk	L3
T ½	=	M/P	=
Vd	=	PB	= 99%
Tmax	= 1–2 hours	Oral	= <1%
MW	= 437	pKa	=

Adult Concerns: Headache, abdominal pain, nausea, diarrhea, vomiting, respiratory infection, arthralgia have been reported.

Pediatric Concerns: Watery diarrhea with mesalamine in one breastfeeding infant. Close observation recommended but it can probably be used relatively safely in breastfeeding mothers.

Drug Interactions: May increase risk of myelosuppression when admixed with mercaptopurine, azathioprine. Tamarind may increase absorption of salicylates and cause salicylate toxicity.

Relative Infant Dose:

Adult Dose: 6.75 grams/day

Alternatives: Mesalamine, olsalazine

References:
1. Pharmaceutial manufacturer Prescribing information, 2009.

BARIUM SULFATE   L1

Trade: Barocet, Prepcat, EntroEase, Entrobar, Baricon, Anatrast, Intropaste,
    Tonopaque, Barosperse
Other Trades: Volumen
Category: Radiological Contrast Agent

Barium sulfate is used as a radiocontrast agent for X-ray imaging. Barium sulfate is available in a wide variety of concentrations, from 1.5% to 210%, under many trade names. It is not absorbed orally; therefore, none will enter the maternal milk compartment or cause harm to a breastfeeding infant. No interruption in breastfeeding is necessary.[1]

Pregnancy Risk	Possibly Hazardous	Lactation Risk	L1
T ½	=	M/P	=
Vd	=	PB	=
Tmax	=	Oral	= none
MW	= 233.4	pKa	=

Adult Concerns: Hypersensitivity, constipation, cramping. Serious side effects: Emboli formation (venous intravasation), peritonitis (bowel perforation), pneumonitis (lung aspiration).

Pediatric Concerns: None reported via breast milk.

Drug Interactions:

Relative Infant Dose:

Adult Dose:

Alternatives:

References:
1. Pharmaceutical manufacturer prescribing information, 2008.

BECLOMETHASONE   L2

Trade: Vanceril, Beclovent, Beconase, Becotide, Qvar

Other Trades: Aldecin, Becotide, Propaderm, Vanceril, Beconase, Becloforte, Beclovent

Category: Intranasal, intrapulmonary steroid

Beclomethasone is a potent steroid that is generally used via inhalation in asthma or via intranasal administration for allergic rhinitis. Due to its potency, only very small doses are generally used and, therefore, minimal plasma levels are attained. Intranasal absorption is generally minimal.[1,2] Due to small doses administered, absorption into maternal plasma is extremely small. Therefore, it is unlikely that these doses would produce clinical significance in a breastfeeding infant. See corticosteroids.

Pregnancy Risk	C	Lactation Risk	L2
T ½	= 15 hours	M/P	=
Vd	=	PB	= 87%
Tmax	= 0.5–0.7 hours	Oral	= 90% (oral)
MW	= 409	pKa	= 13.60

Adult Concerns: When administered intranasally or via inhalation, adrenal suppression is very unlikely. Complications include headaches, hoarseness, bronchial irritation, oral candidiasis, cough. When used orally, complications may include adrenal suppression.

Pediatric Concerns: None reported via milk and inhalation or intranasal use. Oral doses could suppress the adrenal cortex, and induce premature closure of the epiphysis, but would require high doses.

Drug Interactions: Corticosteroids have few drug interactions.

Relative Infant Dose:

Adult Dose: 504–840 µg daily.

Alternatives:

References:
1. Pharmaceutical manufacturer prescribing information, 2009.
2. McEvoy GE. AFHS Drug Information. New York, NY: 2008.

BENAZEPRIL   L2

Trade: Lotensin

Other Trades: Lotensin

Category: Antihypertensive, ACE inhibitor

Benazepril hydrochloride belongs to the ACE inhibitor family. Oral absorption is rather poor (37%). The active component (benazeprilat) reaches a peak at approximately 2 hours after ingestion.[1] In a patient receiving 20 mg daily for 3 days, milk levels averaged 0.15 ng/L.[1] Peak benazepril levels (C_{max}) were 0.92 ng/L. Thus, the levels in milk are almost unmeasurable. The manufacturer suggests a newborn infant ingesting only breast milk would receive less than 0.1% of the mg/kg maternal dose of benazepril and benazeprilat. My calculations suggest much less, or a maximum of 0.00005% of the weight-adjusted maternal dose.

Pregnancy Risk	C/D in 2nd and 3rd trimester	Lactation Risk	L2
T ½	= 10–11 hours	M/P	= 0.01
Vd	= . 124 l/kg	PB	= 96.7%
Tmax	= 0.5–1 hr.	Oral	= 37%
MW	= 424	pKa	= 18.01

Adult Concerns: Significant fetal morbidity, hypotension. Contraindicated in 3rd trimester of pregnancy.

Pediatric Concerns: Levels in milk are reportedly exceedingly low. Unlikely to cause problems.

Drug Interactions: Decreased bioavailability with antacids. Reduced hypotensive effect with NSAIDS. Phenothiazines increase hypotensive effect. Allopurinol dramatically increase hypersensitivities (Steven-Johnson Syn.). ACE inhibitors dramatically increase digoxin levels. Lithium levels may be significantly increased with ACE use. Elevated potassium levels with oral potassium supplements.

Relative Infant Dose:

Adult Dose: 20–40 mg daily.

Alternatives: Enalapril, Captopril

References:
1. Pharmaceutical manufacturer prescribing information, 2005.

BENDROFLUMETHIAZIDE | L4

Trade: Naturetin

Other Trades: Aprinox, Naturetin, Aprinox, Berkozide, Centyl, Urizid

Category: Thiazide diuretic

Bendroflumethiazide is a thiazide diuretic sometimes used to suppress lactation. In one study, the clinician found this thiazide to effectively inhibit lactation.[1] Use with caution. Not generally recommended in breastfeeding mothers.

Pregnancy Risk	C	Lactation Risk	L4
$T\frac{1}{2}$	= 3–3.9 hours	M/P	=
Vd	= 1.48 l/kg	PB	= 94%
Tmax	= 2–4 hours	Oral	= Complete
MW	= 421	pKa	= 10.10

Adult Concerns: Diuresis, fluid loss, leukopenia, hypotension, dizziness, headache, vertigo, reduced milk production.

Pediatric Concerns: None reported, but may inhibit lactation.

Drug Interactions: Enhanced hyponatremia and hypotension when used with ACE inhibitors. May elevate lithium levels.

Relative Infant Dose:

Adult Dose: 2.5–10 mg daily.

Alternatives: Hydrochlorothiazide

References:
1. Healy M. Suppressing lactation with oral diuretics. The Lancet 1961; 1353–1354.

BENOXINATE | L3

Trade:

Other Trades:

Category: Local anesthetic

Benoxinate hydrochloride is a derivative of para-aminobenzoic acid and is structurally similar to procaine. The anesthetic activity of benoxinate is ten times that of cocaine and twice that of tetracaine (amethocaine).[1] Its transfer into milk is probably minimal. Further, the ophthalmic dose would be minuscule and unlikely to produce significant plasma levels.

Pregnancy Risk	C	Lactation Risk	L3
T ½	=	M/P	=
Vd	=	PB	=
Tmax	= 1–15 minutes	Oral	=
MW	= 344	pKa	=

Adult Concerns: Conjunctivitis, keratitis, corneal damage due to prolonged, chronic use of benoxinate. Hypersensitivity reactions.

Pediatric Concerns:

Drug Interactions:

Relative Infant Dose:

Adult Dose:

Alternatives:

References:
1. Pharmaceutical manufacturer prescribing information, 2010.

BENOXINATE + FLUORESCEIN   L3

Trade: Fluress, Flurox, Flurate, Altafluor

Other Trades:

Category: Local anesthetic, disclosing agent

Benoxinate hydrochloride and Fluorescein sodium is a drug combination product of a local anesthetic (benoxinate) with a disclosing agent (fluorescein). It is indicated for use in short ophthalmic procedures. This ophthalmic preparation is mainly used in detecting corneal epithelial defects.[1]

Benoxinate is a derivative of para-aminobenzoic acid and is structurally similar to procaine. The anesthetic activity of benoxinate is ten times that of cocaine and twice that of tetracaine (amethocaine).[2] Its transfer into milk is probably minimal. Further, the ophthalmic dose would be minuscule and unlikely to produce significant plasma levels.

Fluorescein is a yellow, water-soluble dye. A 2% fluorescein ophthalmic solution or an impregnated fluorescein strip is used topically to detect corneal abrasions, for fitting of hard contact lenses, and intravenously for fluorescein angiography. In a study of one patient who received an intravenous dose of fluorescein (5 mL of 10% fluorescein= 500 mg), breastmilk levels were monitored for over 76 hours.[3] Concentrations of 372 µg/L at 6 hours and 170 µg/L at 76 hours after the dose were reported. In this patient, the half-life of fluorescein in breastmilk appeared quite long, approximating 62 hours. While the authors conclude that this is a high dose via milk, in another patient who received slightly more (910 mg IV), the patient's plasma levels of fluorescein monoglucuronide were 37,000 µg/L.[4] Using this data, it would appear that an approximation of the milk/plasma ratio would be about 0.018, which suggests that very little of the absolute maternal dose enters milk. Nevertheless, fluorescein-induced phototoxicity remains a possibility in an infant fed breastmilk containing fluorescein. One case of severe fluorescein phototoxicity has been reported in an infant receiving fluorescein intravenously.[5] If the infant is not undergoing phototherapy, it would appear that there is little risk to a breastfeeding infant. However, in the ophthalmic product, the systemic dose would be minuscule and is unlikely to produce clinically relevant levels in milk.

There is virtually no risk to a breastfeeding infant following the maternal use of this combination anesthetic/diagnostic product ophthalmically. The systemic dose would simply be too low.

Pregnancy Risk	C	Lactation Risk	L3
T ½	= Benoxinate/fluorescein: /4.4 hours	M/P	= Benoxinate/fluorescein:
Vd	= Benoxinate/fluorescein: /0.5 l/kg	PB	= Benoxinate/fluorescein: /70–85%
Tmax	= Benoxinate/fluorescein: 1–15 min/1 hour	Oral	= Benoxinate/fluorescein: /50%
MW	= Benoxinate/fluorescein: 344/376	pKa	= Benoxinate/fluorescein: /9.32

Adult Concerns: Hypersensitivity, prolonged ophthalmic use may cause corneal opacification and visual loss, use with caution in hyperthyroidism.

Pediatric Concerns:

Drug Interactions:

Relative Infant Dose:

Adult Dose: 1–2 drops into each eye before operation

Alternatives:

References:
1. Pharmaceutical manufacturer prescribing information, 2011.
2. Pharmaceutical manufacturer prescribing information, 2010. (Prod Info Novesine(R) Wander 1%, 1998a); (Fachinfo Benoxinat SE Thilo(R) Augentropfen, 1998).
3. Maquire AM, Bennett J. Fluorescein elimination in human breast milk. Arch Ophthalmol 1988; 106(6): 718–719.
4. Kearns GL, Williams BJ, Timmons OD. Fluorescein phototoxicity in a premature infant. J Pediatr 1985; 107(5): 796–798.
5. Kearns GL, Williams BJ, Timmons OD. Fluorescein phototoxicity in a premature infant. J Pediatr 1985; 107(5): 796–798.

BENZOCAINE   L2

Trade: Orajel, Americaine, Anacaine, Anasol, Benzodent, Ciggerex, Dent's

Other Trades:

Category: Local Anesthetic

Benzocaine is a local anaesthetic.[1] It temporarily relieves pain associated with minor cuts, minor burns, scrapes itching. There are no adequate and well-controlled studies or case reports in breast feeding women. Due to its poor bioavailability after topical application, concentrations achieved in maternal plasma are probably too low to produce any significant clinical effects in the breastfed infant. Dental procedure benzocaine usage is minimal and should pose no harm to the breastfed infant. Maternal plasma and milk levels do not seem to approach high concentrations and the oral bioavailability in the infant would be quite low (<35%). Probably safe during breastfeeding when used topically or orally.

Pregnancy Risk	C	Lactation Risk	L2
T ½	=	M/P	=
Vd	=	PB	=
Tmax	=	Oral	= Poor
MW	=	pKa	= 2.51

Adult Concerns: Burning, contact dermatitis, edema, erythema, pruritus, rash, stinging, tenderness, urticaria

Pediatric Concerns:

Drug Interactions: Co-administration with hyaluronidase may increase risk of toxic systemic reactions. Do not use concomitantly with St. John's wort due to increased risk for severe fall in blood pressure. Avoid concomitant use with sulfonamides (sulfisoxazole, sulfasalazine, sulfapyridine, sulfamethoxazole, sulfadoxine) since this may inhibit action and decrease their efficacy.

Relative Infant Dose:

Adult Dose: Apply topical 3–4 times a day.

Alternatives:

References:
1.   Pharmaceutical manufacturer prescribing information,2010.

BENZONATATE   L3

Trade: Tessalon Perles

Other Trades:

Category: Antitussive

Benzonatate is a non-narcotic cough suppressant similar to the local anesthetic tetracaine. It anesthetizes stretch receptors in respiratory passages, dampening their activity and reducing the cough reflex.[1] There are little pharmacokinetic data on this product and no data on transfer into human milk. Because low-dose codeine is almost equally effective as an antitussive, and because we know that codeine only marginally transfers into human milk, it is probably a preferred antitussive in breastfeeding mothers. While new data suggests that hypermetabolizers may increase the risks of using codeine in a breastfeeding mother,[2] used in small doses as an antitussive, codeine would still be preferred over benzonatate in breastfeeding women. In addition, benzonatate in overdose (as little as 2 capsules in a child), is a very dangerous product, leading to seizures with cardiac arrest and death, particularly in children.

Pregnancy Risk	C		Lactation Risk	L3
T ½	= <8 hours		M/P	=
Vd	=		PB	=
Tmax	= 20 minutes		Oral	= Good
MW	= 603		pKa	=

Adult Concerns: Sedation, headache, dizziness, constipation, nausea, pruritus have been reported. Para-aminobenzoic acid (PABA) is a metabolite of benzonatate. Severe allergic reactions have been reported in patients who are allergic to PABA. Severe sensitivity reactions to benzonatate have resulted in respiratory side effects such as bronchospasm, laryngospasm and cardiac arrest. Excessive absorption following chewing of capsules may result in the rapid numbness of mouth and throat and in extreme cases pulmonary aspiration may occur. Do not overdose and do not chew capsules.

Pediatric Concerns: None reported via milk. Dangerous in overdose. Use with great caution.

Drug Interactions:

Relative Infant Dose:

Adult Dose: 100 mg TID

Alternatives: Codeine

References:
1. Pharmaceutical manufacturer prescribing information, 2005.
2. Koren G, Cairns J, Chitayat D, Gaedigk A, Leeder SJ. Pharmacogenetics of morphine poisoning in a breastfed neonate of a codeine-prescribed mother. Lancet 2006 Aug 19; 368(9536): 704.

BENZOYL PEROXIDE   L2

Trade: Acne, Acne 10 Gel, Benzac, Banzagel, Benziq

Other Trades:

Category: OTC Acne

Benzoyl peroxide is an organic peroxide commonly used in many products for the treatment of acne, for bleaching hair and teeth, and many other uses. Thus far, there are no data on its transfer into human milk. Benzoyl peroxide if ingested would be largely destroyed, almost instantly by tissue and stomach esterases. None would likely ever be absorbed systemically. Because only about 5% of topically applied benzoyl peroxide is absorbed (but rapidly destroyed in tissues), it is thought to be of low risk to a nursing infant.[1]

Pregnancy Risk	C		Lactation Risk	L2
T ½	=		M/P	=
Vd	=		PB	=
Tmax	=		Oral	= Nil
MW	= 242.23		pKa	=

Adult Concerns: Erythema, irritation, allergy contact sensitization.

Pediatric Concerns:

Drug Interactions:

Relative Infant Dose:

Adult Dose: Apply topically sparingly once a day; can increase to 2–3 times a day if needed

Alternatives:

References:
1. Leachman SA, Reed BR. The use of dermatologic drugs in pregnancy and lactation. Dermatol Clin. 2006; 24(2): 167–97.

BENZOYL PEROXIDE + CLINDAMYCIN | L2

Trade: Duac, Acanya, Duac CS, Benzaclin

Other Trades:

Category: Antiacne

Benzoyl peroxide and Clindamycin phosphate is a drug combination product used for treatment of acne vulgaris. It is meant for topical application.

Benzoyl peroxide is an organic peroxide commonly used in many products for the treatment of acne, for bleaching hair and teeth, and many other uses. Thus far, there are no data on its transfer into human milk. Benzoyl peroxide if ingested would be largely destroyed, almost instantly by tissue and stomach esterases. None would likely ever be absorbed systemically. Because only about 5% of topically applied benzoyl peroxide is absorbed (but rapidly destroyed in tissues), it is thought to be of low risk to a nursing infant.[1]

Lotions or ointments of clindamycin meant for topical application contain clindamycin phosphate equivalent to 10 mg/mL. Transcutaneous absorption is minimal (<1–4%) and reported plasma levels are low to nil. Some does appear in urine of treated patients. Due to low maternal plasma levels, virtually none should be expected in breast milk. With the rise of resistant Staphlococcal infections, clindamycin use in infants has risen enormously. The amount in milk is unlikely to harm a breastfeeding infant.

Benzoyl peroxide + clindamycin phosphate drug combination for topical use is considered compatible with breastfeeding.

Pregnancy Risk	C		Lactation Risk	L2
T½	= Benzoyl peroxide/ clindamycin: /2.4 hours		M/P	= Benzoyl peroxide/ clindamycin: /0.47
Vd	= Benzoyl peroxide/ clindamycin: /2 l/kg		PB	= Benzoyl peroxide/ clindamycin: /94%
Tmax	= Benzoyl peroxide/ clindamycin:		Oral	= Benzoyl peroxide/ clindamycin: nil/90%
MW	= Benzoyl peroxide/ clindamycin: 242.23/425		pKa	= Benzoyl peroxide/ clindamycin: /7.45

Adult Concerns: Dry skin is the most common side-effect reported. Colitis and diarrhea rarely occur.

Pediatric Concerns: Topical application should be of minimal risk to a breastfeeding infant.

Drug Interactions: Concurrent use with erythromycin may decrease each others' effects.

Relative Infant Dose:

Adult Dose: Apply topically to affected areas twice daily.

Alternatives: Clindamycin topical ointment, clindamycin + tretinoin

References:
1. Leachman SA, Reed BR. The use of dermatologic drugs in pregnancy and lactation. Dermatol Clin. 2006; 24(2): 167–97.

BENZTROPINE   L3

Trade: Cogentin

Other Trades:

Category: Anticholinergic for relief of antipsychotic agent-induced extrapyramidal reactions

Benztropine mesylate is commonly used for the relief of parkinsonian signs (extrapyramidal reactions) commonly seen following the use of antipsychotic agents.[1] Benztropine has about one-half the anticholinergic effects of atropine, and has antihistamine effects. Its transfer into human milk has not been studied. Some caution is recommended if this product is used in breastfeeding mothers as some animal studies suggest anticholinergics reduce prolactin levels. The infant should be observed for drying symptoms, including dry mouth, reduced tearing, urinary retention, elevated body temperature, reduced sweating, tachycardia, and constipation.

Pregnancy Risk	C		Lactation Risk	L3
T ½	= Long		M/P	=
Vd	=		PB	= 95%
Tmax	= 1–2 hours		Oral	= 29%
MW	= 307		pKa	= 10.0

Adult Concerns: Side effects are typically those of anticholinergics and include confusion, drug-induced psychosis, hyperpyrexia, paralytic ileus, exaggeration of glaucoma and intraocular pressure, reduced sweating and hyperpyrexia.

Pediatric Concerns: None reported but observe for anticholinergic symptoms including drying, constipation, reduced urine output.

Drug Interactions: Concomitant use with other products with anticholinergic symptoms may be hazardous.

Relative Infant Dose:

Adult Dose: 1–2 mg daily.

Alternatives:

References:
1. Pharmaceutical manufacturer prescribing information, 2009.

BEPRIDIL   L4

Trade: Vascor, Bepadin
Other Trades:
Category: Antihypertensive, calcium channel blocker

Bepridil hydrochloride is a calcium channel blocker that is known to have anti-anginal properties, but poorly characterized type 1 antiarrhythmic and anti-hypertensive properties. It is not related chemically to other calcium channel blockers such as diltiazem hydrochloride, nifedipine and verapamil hydrochloride.

Following therapy with bepridil, milk levels were reported to approach ⅓rd of serum levels.[1,2] As with some calcium channel blockers, this family has been found to produce embryotoxic effects and should be used cautiously in pregnant women. Long half-life, enhanced oral absorption, and potency of this compound would increase the danger in nursing infant. Caution is recommended if used in nursing mothers. There are numerous other preferred calcium channel blockers.

Pregnancy Risk	C		Lactation Risk	L4
T ½	= 42 hours		M/P	= 0.33
Vd	= 8 l/kg		PB	= >99%
Tmax	= 2–3 hours		Oral	= 60%
MW	= 367		pKa	= 6.3

Adult Concerns: Bepridil is contraindicated in patients with history of serious ventricular arrhythmias, patients with sick sinus syndrome or patients with second- or third-degree AV block, patients with low blood pressure (less than 90 mm Hg systolic), patients with uncompensated cardiac insufficiency, patients with congenital QT interval prolongation and patients taking other drugs that prolong QT interval.

Pediatric Concerns: None reported, but other calcium channel blockers may be preferred. See nifedipine.

Drug Interactions: H_2 blockers may enhance oral absorption of bepridil. Beta blockers may enhance hypotensive effect. Bepridil may increase plasma levels of carbamazepine, cyclosporin, digitalis, quinidine, theophylline when used concomitantly with these products.

Relative Infant Dose:

Adult Dose: 300 mg daily.

Alternatives: Nifedipine, Nimodipine, Verapamil

References:
1. Pharmaceutical manufacturer prescribing information, 2010.
2. Drug Facts and Comparisons St. Louis: 2010.

BESIFLOXACIN   L3

Trade: Besivance

Other Trades:

Category: Ophthalmic quinolone antibiotic

Besifloxacin hydrochloride ophthalmic suspension, is a quinolone antimicrobial indicated for the treatment of bacterial conjunctivitis. No data are available on the transfer of this fluoroquinolone antibiotic into human milk, but levels are likely quite low. Plasma concentrations of besifloxacin following ophthalmic use indicated the maximum plasma besifloxacin concentration in each patient was less than 1.3 ng/mL.[1] The mean besifloxacin C_{max} was 0.37 ng/mL on day 1 and 0.43 ng/mL on day 6. The average elimination half-life of besifloxacin in plasma following multiple dosing was estimated to be 7 hours. While there are not studies available, plasma levels are so low that the amount likely present in milk is probably miniscule.

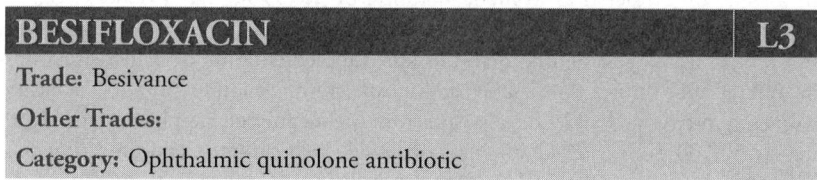

Pregnancy Risk	C		Lactation Risk	L3
T ½	= 7 hours		M/P	=
Vd	=		PB	=
Tmax	=		Oral	=
MW	=		pKa	=

Adult Concerns: Most common side effects: conjunctival redness. Rare side effects: blurred vision, eye pain, eye irritation, eye pruritus and headache.

Pediatric Concerns:

Drug Interactions:

Relative Infant Dose:

Adult Dose: Instill one drop TID for 7 days

Alternatives:

References:
1. Pharmaceutical manufacturer prescribing information, 2009

BETA-CAROTENE   L3

Trade: B-Caro-T, A-Caro-25, Lumitene
Other Trades:
Category: Vitamin A

Beta-carotene is a provitamin A which requires conversion to the active form of vitamin A (retinol) in the liver and intestinal mucosa.[1] Beta-carotene conversion in the liver is regulated by the concentration of retinol in the body. Recommended daily vitamin A intake is equivalent to 8000 IU or 4.8 mg of beta-carotene. Large doses of beta-carotene are used in the treatment of vitamin A deficiency (up to 162,000 IU) and cutaneous lesions of porphyria (up to 540,000 IU).[2]

In a study of 21 lactating women, ingestion of 31–35 mg/day (51,667–58,333 IU) of beta-carotene did not significantly increase beta-carotene concentrations in breast milk, suggesting that beta-carotene supplementation does increase levels in milk at least during the first 27 days postpartum.[3] Another study of lactating women approximately 279 days postpartum, beta-carotene supplementation (30 mg or 50,000 IU for 28 days) increased milk beta-carotene concentration 6.4 times (max around 190 µg/L); however, milk retinoid concentration did not increase significantly.[4]

There are no reports of adverse effects in breastfed infant from maternal beta-carotene supplementation.

Pregnancy Risk	C	Lactation Risk	L3
T ½	=	M/P	=
Vd	=	PB	=
Tmax	=	Oral	= 30%
MW	= 537	pKa	=

Adult Concerns: Carotenodermia, diarrhea, bruising, dizziness.

Pediatric Concerns:

Drug Interactions:

Relative Infant Dose:

Adult Dose: 30–300 mg/day

Alternatives:

References:
1. Polifka JE, Dolan CR, Donlan MA, Friedman JM. Clinical teratology counseling and consultation report: high dose beta-carotene use during early pregnancy. Teratology. 1996 Aug; 54(2): 103–7.
2. Lewis J. M., 0. Bodansky, M. C. C. Lillienfeld, and H. Schneider(1947) Supplements of vitamin A and of carotene during pregnancy. Their effect on the levels of vitamin A and carotene in the blood of mother and of newborn infant. Am. J. Dis. Child. 73-143–15.

3. Gossage CP, Deyhim M, Yamini S, Douglass LW, Moser-Veillon PB. Carotenoid composition of human milk during the first month postpartum and the response to beta-carotene supplementation. Am J Clin Nutr. 2002 Jul; 76(1): 193–7.
4. Canfield LM, Giuliano AR, Neilson EM, Blashil BM, Graver EJ, Yap HH. Kinetics of the response of milk and serum beta-carotene to daily beta-carotene supplementation in healthy, lactating women. Am J Clin Nutr. 1998 Feb; 67(2): 276–83. Erratum in: Am J Clin Nutr 1998 Jun; 67(6): 1286.

BETAHISTINE   L4

Trade: Serc, Hiserc, Betaserc

Other Trades:

Category: Antivertigo

Betahistine hydrochloride is an anti-vertigo drug used for the treatment of Meniere's disease. It is a histamine analogue and has agonistic action on the histamine-1 receptors. It also causes the release of histamine from nerve terminals. Therefore, its pharmacological effects are similar to that of histamine. Some of its side-effects in adults are skin rash, pruritus, dizziness, hypotension, exacerbation of peptic ulcers and precipitation of asthma. Betahistine is completely absorbed after oral absorption and it has very low protein binding. No studies are available of its transfer into human milk, but it is very likely. Due to the possibility of major side effects in the breastfed infant, it is advisable to avoid the use of this drug in lactating women. Consider alternatives such as dimenhydrinate, diphenhydramine or meclizine.

Pregnancy Risk	Hazardous	Lactation Risk	L4
T ½	= 3–4 hours	M/P	=
Vd	=	PB	= Very low
Tmax	= 1 hour	Oral	= Complete
MW	= 136.19	pKa	=

Adult Concerns: Nausea, vomiting, diarrhea, skin rash, pruritus, flushing, headache, dizziness, hypotension. Exacerbation of asthma and peptic ulcers.

Pediatric Concerns:

Drug Interactions:

Relative Infant Dose:

Adult Dose:

Alternatives: Dimenhydrinate, diphenhydramine, meclizine

References:

BETAMETHASONE   L3

Trade: Betameth, Celestone

Other Trades: Betnovate, Beben, Betadermetnesol, Celestone, Diprolene, Dipr, Betnelan, Diprosone

Category: Synthetic corticosteroid

Betamethasone is a potent long-acting steroid and is about 25 times as potent as hydrocortisone. It generally produces less sodium and fluid retention than other steroids.[1] In small doses, most steroids are certainly not contraindicated in nursing mothers. Whenever possible use low-dose alternatives such as aerosols or inhalers. Following administration, wait at least 4 hours if possible prior to feeding infant to reduce exposure. With high doses (>40 mg/day), particularly for long periods, steroids could potentially produce problems in infant growth and development, although we have absolutely no data in this area, or which doses would pose problems. Brief applications of high dose steroids are probably not contraindicated as the overall exposure is low. With prolonged high dose therapy, the infant should be closely monitored for growth and development.

Pregnancy Risk	D/C in 2nd and 3rd trimester	Lactation Risk	L3
T ½	= 5.6 hours	M/P	=
Vd	=	PB	= 64%
Tmax	= 10–36 minutes	Oral	= Complete
MW	= 392	pKa	= 13.48

Adult Concerns: Gastric distress, gastric ulceration, glaucoma, thinning of skin.

Pediatric Concerns: None reported, used in pediatric patients.

Drug Interactions: Numerous, see drug reference. Decreased effect when used with barbiturates, phenytoin, rifampin. Macrolide antibiotics have been reported to cause a significant decrease in corticosteroid clearance. May produce hyperglycemia.

Relative Infant Dose:

Adult Dose: 2.4–4.8 mg BID or TID

Alternatives:

References:
1. Pharmaceutical manufacturer prescribing information, 2010.

BETAXOLOL   L3

Trade: Kerlone, Betoptic

Other Trades: Betoptic

Category: Beta blocker antihypertensive

Betaxolol is a long-acting, cardioselective beta blocker primarily used for glaucoma but can be used orally for hypertension. One report by the manufacturer reports side effects which occurred in one nursing infant.[1] Many in this family of drugs readily transfer into human milk (see atenolol, acebutolol), others do so poorly (propranolol, metoprolol).[2] Betaxolol when used ophthalmically, is apparently poorly absorbed systemically as no evidence of beta blockade can be found in patients following its use ophthalmically. Since maternal plasma levels with ophthalmic are low, levels in mature milk should be low as well, although there are currently no studies to confirm this. In a study of 28 women consuming 10 mg betaxolol during the perinatal period, the milk/plasma ratio in 3 patients was 3.0.[3] Note this was done early postnatally in colostrum and may not at all reflect postnatal levels in mature milk. In one case where the drug was administered 3 hours prior to delivery, colostrum levels were 48 µg/L at 24 hours postpartum and 3 µg/L at 72 hours postpartum. Nothing in this study should reflect levels in mature milk.

Pregnancy Risk	C	Lactation Risk	L3
T ½	= 14–22 hours	M/P	= 2.5–3.0
Vd	= 4.9 l/kg	PB	= 50%
Tmax	= 3 hours	Oral	= 89%
MW	= 307	pKa	= 9.4

Adult Concerns: Hypotension, bradycardia, fatigue.

Pediatric Concerns: No data are available on its transfer to milk. However, when used ophthalmically, no systemic beta blockade was noted, suggesting plasma levels are low to nil. Milk levels are likely low as well.

Drug Interactions: Decreased effect when used with aluminum salts, barbiturates, calcium salts, cholestyramine, NSAIDs, ampicillin, rifampin, and salicylates. Beta blockers may reduce the effect of oral sulfonylureas (hypoglycemic agents). Increased toxicity/effect when used with other antihypertensives, contraceptives, MAO inhibitors, cimetidine, and numerous other products. See drug interaction reference for complete listing.

Relative Infant Dose:

Adult Dose: 10 mg daily.

Alternatives: Propranolol, Metoprolol

References:
1. Pharmaceutical manufacturer prescribing information, 1995.
2. Beresford R and Heel RC: Betaxolol: a review of its pharmacodynamic and pharmacokinetic properties, and therapeutic efficacy in hypertension. Drugs 1986; 31: 6–28.
3. Morselli PL, Boutroy MJ, and Thenot JP: Pharmacokinetics of antihypertensive drugs in the neonatal period. Dev Pharmacol Ther 1989; 13: 190–198.

BETHANECHOL   L4

Trade: Urabeth, Urecholine

Other Trades: Urocarb, Duvoid, Urecholine, Myotonine

Category: Cholinergic stimulant-agonist for urinary retention

Bethanechol chloride is a cholinergic stimulant useful for urinary retention.

Although poorly absorbed from gastrointestinal tract, no reports on entry into breastmilk are available. However, it could conceivably cause abdominal cramps, colicky pain, nausea, salivation, bronchial constriction, or diarrhea in infants. There are several reports of discomfort in nursing infants.[1] Use with great caution.

Pregnancy Risk	C	Lactation Risk	L4
T ½	= 1–2 hours	M/P	=
Vd	=	PB	=
Tmax	= 60–90 minutes (oral)	Oral	= Poor
MW	= 197	pKa	=

Adult Concerns: Gastric distress such as colicky pain, cramping, nausea, salivation, breathing difficulties, diarrhea, hypotension, heart block, headache, urinary urgency. Contraindicated in patients with asthma, bradycardia, hypotension, epilepsy, etc.

Pediatric Concerns: Gastrointestinal distress, discomfort, diarrhea.

Drug Interactions: Bethanechol when used with ganglionic blockers may lead to significant hypotension. Bethanechol effects may be antagonized by procainamide and quinidine.

Relative Infant Dose:

Adult Dose: 10–50 mg BID-QID

Alternatives:

References:
1. Shore MF. Drugs can be dangerous during pregnancy and lactation. Can Pharmaceut J 1970; 103: 358.

BEVACIZUMAB   L3

Trade: Avastin

Other Trades:

Category: Immune modulator, VEGF inhibitor

Bevacizumab is a monoclonal IgG antibody that binds to vascular endothelial growth factor, preventing it from binding to endothelial receptors, thus blocking angiogenesis. This slows the growth of all tissues, including metastatic tissues. It is used in colorectal, lung, breast, prostate, and ovarian cancers, as well as for age-related macular degeneration.[1] There have been no studies reporting the concentration of bevacizumab in human milk; however, due to the large molecular weight, it is very unlikely that it would pass into the milk compartment. Nonetheless, caution should be used in a rapidly growing breastfeeding infant. This product should be avoided in breastfeeding mothers, if possible. Even if small amounts were to penetrate milk, the gastric complications of this product in the infant could be significant. Mothers should be advised to discontinue breastfeeding following the use of this product. Recently, a number of reports have described the off-label use of intravitreous injected bevacizumab for the treatment of macular degeneration. It has an approximate molecular weight of 149 kilodaltons. While we have no reports on its use in breastfeeding mothers, size alone would largely exclude it from the milk compartment. When used intravitreous, the dose (1.25 mg) is much lower than via systemic administration (5–10 mg/kg), and it is largely sequestered in the eye[2], thus plasma levels (and milk) would be exceedingly low. The intravitreous use of this drug is probably compatible with breastfeeding. The systemic use of this drug would not be compatible with breastfeeding.

As of December 2010, the FDA removed the indication for bevacizumab (Avastin) in metastatic breast cancer. We do not know if this will result in withdrawal. The FDA concluded that following 3 clinical trials, that patients treated with bevacizumab did not live any longer and were at greater risk for life-threatening adverse effects.

Pregnancy Risk	C	Lactation Risk	L3
T ½	= 20 days	M/P	=
Vd	= 0.046 l/kg	PB	=
Tmax	=	Oral	= Nil
MW	= 149,000	pKa	=

Adult Concerns: Adverse reactions include: gastrointestinal perforations, surgery and wound healing complications, hemorrhage, venous thromboembolic events, neutropenia and infection, slight proteinuria, congestive heart failure, hypertension, diarrhea, leukopenia.

Pediatric Concerns: None reported via milk. Reduced growth in epiphyseal growth plates in monkey studies.

Drug Interactions: None yet reported.

Relative Infant Dose:

Adult Dose: 5–15 mg/kg every 2–3 weeks

Alternatives:

References:
1. Pharmaceutical manufacturer prescribing information, 2009.
2. Julien S, Heiduschka P, Hofmeister S, Schraermeyer U. Immunohistochemical localisation of intravitreally injected bevacizumab at the posterior pole of the primate eye: implication for the treatment of retinal vein occlusion. Br J Ophthalmol. Oct 2008; 92(10): 1424–1428.

BIMATOPROST   L3

Trade: Lumigan, Latisse
Other Trades: Lumigan
Category: Antiglaucoma agent

Bimatoprost is used in open-angle glaucoma or ocular hypertension to reduce intraocular pressure. It is a synthetic structural analog of prostaglandin, and it mimics the effects of naturally occurring prostamides. Bimatoprost increases the outflow of aqueous humor through the trabecular meshwork and uveoscleral routes.[1] No breastfeeding data are available. However, after intraocular administration, plasma levels peak at 10 minutes, then fall rapidly to undetectable levels within 1.5

hours. Combined with low plasma levels and high protein binding, it is unlikely this product would produce measurable levels in human milk.

Pregnancy Risk	C	Lactation Risk	L3
T ½	= 45 minutes	M/P	=
Vd	= 0.67 l/kg	PB	= 88%
Tmax	= 10 minutes	Oral	=
MW	= 415	pKa	= 14.85

Adult Concerns: Adverse effects include conjunctival hyperemia, growth of eyelashes, and ocular pruritus.

Pediatric Concerns: No data are available.

Drug Interactions: Increased intraocular pressure is seen when used with latanoprost.

Relative Infant Dose:

Adult Dose: 1 drop every evening

Alternatives:

References:
1. Pharmaceutical manufacturer prescribing information, 2004

BIOTIN   L1

Trade:

Other Trades:

Category: Vitamin B$_7$

Biotin, also known as vitamin H or B$_7$, is a coenzyme that assists in many metabolic chemical conversions, and assists in the metabolism of fatty acids, leucine and in gluconeogenesis. It is also required for normal neuronal and hematopoietic function. Symptoms of biotin deficiency include thinning of hair, skin rash, and depression. The recommended daily dose of biotin for a pregnant female is 30 µg/day, while that of a lactating female is 35 µg/day. An infant less than 6 months old needs 0.9 µg/kg/day, while an infant over 6 months should get 6 µg/day.[1] Levels of biotin in human milk range from 5 to 9 µg/L, indicating that there is active transport of biotin into milk.[2] No adverse effects have been found, nor has a toxic upper intake been established.

Pregnancy Risk	Probably Safe	Lactation Risk	L1
T ½	=	M/P	=
Vd	=	PB	=
Tmax	=	Oral	= Complete
MW	= 244	pKa	= 13.55

Adult Concerns: None.

Pediatric Concerns: None. Recommended dietary factor.

Drug Interactions:

Relative Infant Dose:

Adult Dose: 35 micrograms per day

Alternatives:

References:
1. Dietary Reference Intakes for Thiamin, Riboflavin, Niacin, Vitamin B_6, Folate, Vitamin B_{12}, Pantothenic Acid, Biotin, and Choline. Food and Nutrition Board. Institute of Medicine. Washington DC: National Academy Press; 1998.
2. Picciano MF. Handbook of milk composition. Jensen RG, ed. San Diego: Academic Press; 1995.

BISACODYL   L2

Trade:

Other Trades:

Category: Laxative

Bisacodyl is a stimulant laxative that selectively stimulates colon contractions and defecation. It has only limited secretion into breastmilk due to poor gastric absorption and subsequently minimal systemic levels.[1] Little or no known harmful effects on infants.

Pregnancy Risk	C	Lactation Risk	L2
T ½	= 16 hours	M/P	=
Vd	=	PB	=
Tmax	=	Oral	= <5%
MW	= 361	pKa	=

Adult Concerns: Diarrhea, gastrointestinal cramping, rectal irritation.

Pediatric Concerns: None reported via milk.

Drug Interactions: By speeding the emptying of gastrointestinal tract it may reduce efficacy of warfarin, and other products by reducing absorption. Decreased effect of bisacodyl when coadministered with cimetidine, famotidine, ranitidine, or nizatidine. Numerous drug interactions, check other references.

Relative Infant Dose:
Adult Dose: 10–15 mg daily.

Alternatives:

References:
1. Vorherr H. Drug excretion in breast milk. Postgrad Med 1974; 56(4): 97–104.

BISMUTH SUBGALLATE | L3

Trade:

Other Trades:

Category: Deodorizer

Bismuth subgallate is used as an internal deodorant commonly used by people who have fecal incontinence and those who have had an ileostomy, colostomy and bariatric surgery (duodenal switch, gastric bypass, biliopancreatic diversion). It is used to deodorize embarrassing flatulence odor. Bismuth subgallate has poor oral bioavailability of less than 1%.[1] Since it is poorly absorbed, bismuth subgallate is unlikely to be present in breastmilk.

Pregnancy Risk	Probably Safe	Lactation Risk	L3
T ½	=	M/P	=
Vd	=	PB	=
Tmax	=	Oral	= <1%
MW	= 394	pKa	=

Adult Concerns: Common adverse effects: Reversible darkening of stool and tongue, constipation.

Pediatric Concerns:

Drug Interactions:

Relative Infant Dose:

Adult Dose: 200–400 mg four times daily. Not to exceed 8 capsules per day.

Alternatives:

References:
1. Dresow B, Fischer R, Gabbe EE, Wendel J, Heinrich HC. Bismuth absorption from 205Bi-labelled pharmaceutical bismuth compounds used in the treatment of peptic ulcer disease. Scand J Gastroenterol. 1992 Apr; 27(4): 333–6. Abstract.

BISMUTH SUBSALICYLATE | L3

Trade:

Other Trades:

Category: Antisecretory, antimicrobial salt

Bismuth subsalicylate is present in many diarrhea mixtures. Although bismuth salts are poorly absorbed from the maternal GI tract, significant levels of salicylate could be absorbed from these products.[1] While to date, bismuth subsalicylate and other non-acetylated salicylates have not been associated with Reye's syndrome, this drug should not be routinely used in breastfeeding women. Some forms (Parepectolin, Infantol Pink) may contain a tincture of opium (morphine).

Pregnancy Risk	C/D in 2nd and 3rd trimester	Lactation Risk	L3
T ½	= Highly variable	M/P	=
Vd	=	PB	=
Tmax	=	Oral	= Poor
MW	= 362	pKa	=

Adult Concerns: Constipation, salicylate poisoning (tinnitus). May enhance risk of Reye 's syndrome in children.

Pediatric Concerns: Risk of Reye syndrome in neonates, but has not been reported with this product in a breastfed infant.

Drug Interactions: May reduce effects of tetracyclines, and uricosurics. May increase toxicity of aspirin, warfarin, hypoglycemics.

Relative Infant Dose:

Adult Dose: 524 every 30 minutes to one hour as needed up to 8 doses per 24 hour

Alternatives:

References:
1. Findlay JW, DeAngelis RL, Kearney MF, Welch RM, Findlay JM. Analgesic drugs in breast milk and plasma. Clin Pharmacol Ther 1981; 29(5): 625–633.

BISOPROLOL   L3

Trade: Zebeta

Other Trades: Emcor, Monocor

Category: Beta-adrenergic antihypertensive

Bisoprolol fumarate is a typical beta-blocker used to treat hypertension. The manufacturer states that small amounts (<2%) are secreted into milk of animals.[1] Others in this family of drugs are known to produce problems in breastfeeding infants (see atenolol, acebutolol). Propranolol and metoprolol are ideal alternatives.

Pregnancy Risk	C	Lactation Risk	L3
T ½	= 9–12 hours	M/P	=
Vd	=	PB	= 30%
Tmax	= 2–3 hours	Oral	= 80%
MW	= 325	pKa	= 9.5

Adult Concerns: Bradycardia, hypotension, fatigue, excessive fluid loss.

Pediatric Concerns: None reported with this product, but other beta blockers have produced hypotension, hypoglycemia. See metoprolol as an alternative.

Drug Interactions: Decreased effect when used with aluminum salts, barbiturates, calcium salts, cholestyramine, NSAIDs, ampicillin, rifampin, and salicylates. Beta blockers may reduce the effect of oral sulfonylureas (hypoglycemic agents).

Increased toxicity/effect when used with other antihypertensives, contraceptives, MAO inhibitors, cimetidine, and numerous other products. See drug interaction reference for complete listing.

Relative Infant Dose:

Adult Dose: 5–10 mg daily.

Alternatives: Propranolol, Metoprolol

References:
1.   Pharmaceutical manufacturer prescribing information, 1995.

BISOPROLOL + HYDROCHLOROTHIAZIDE   L3

Trade: Ziac

Other Trades:

Category: Cardioselective beta-blocker + thiazide

Bisoprolol fumarate and Hydrochlorothiazide is a drug combination of an adrenergic beta-blocker (bisoprolol) with a thiazide diuretic (hydrochlorothiazide). It is indicated for treatment of hypertension.[1] No reports of the transfer of this drug combination into human milk are currently available.

Bisoprolol is a typical beta-blocker used to treat hypertension. The manufacturer states that small amounts (<2%) are secreted into milk of animals. Others in this family of drugs are known to produce problems in breastfeeding infants (see atenolol, acebutolol). Propranolol and metoprolol are ideal alternatives.

Hydrochlorothiazide (HCTZ) is a typical thiazide diuretic. In one study of a mother receiving a 50 mg dose each morning, milk levels were almost 25% of maternal plasma levels.[2] The dose ingested (assuming milk intake of 600 mL) would be approximately 50 μg/day, a clinically insignificant amount. The concentration of HCTZ in the infant's serum was undetectable (<20 ng/mL). Some authors suggest that HCTZ can produce thrombocytopenia in nursing infant, although this is remote and unsubstantiated. Thiazide diuretics could potentially reduce milk production by depleting maternal blood volume although it is seldom observed. Most thiazide diuretics are considered compatible with breastfeeding if doses are kept low.

Pregnancy Risk	C	Lactation Risk	L3
T ½	= Bisoprolol/HCTZ: 9–12 hours/5.6–14.8 hours	M/P	= Bisoprolol/HCTZ: /0.25
Vd	= Bisoprolol/HCTZ: /3 l/kg	PB	= Bisoprolol/HCTZ: 30%/58%
Tmax	= Bisoprolol/HCTZ: 2–3 hours/2 hours	Oral	= Bisoprolol/HCTZ: 80%/72%
MW	= Bisoprolol/HCTZ: 325/297	pKa	= Bisoprolol/HCTZ: 9.5/7.9,9.2

Adult Concerns: Diarrhea, dizziness, fatigue, headache, heart failure, glaucoma, bronchospasm

Pediatric Concerns:

Drug Interactions: Decreases efficacy of rifampin when used concomitantly, hypersensitivity reactions, decreases clearance of lithium causing lithium toxicity, may decrease serum levels of protein-bound iodine.

Relative Infant Dose:

Adult Dose: Bisoprolol/HCTZ: 2.5–40 mg/12.5–50 mg once daily

Alternatives: Propranolol, Metoprolol

References:
1. Pharmaceutical manufacturer prescribing information, 2011.
2. Miller ME, Cohn RD, Burghart PH. Hydrochlorothiazide disposition in a mother and her breast-fed infant. J Pediatr 1982; 101(5): 789–791.

BLACK COHOSH   L4

Trade:

Other Trades:

Category: Herbal estrogenic compound

The roots and rhizomes of this herb are used medicinally. Traditional uses include the treatment of dysmenorrhea, dyspepsia, rheumatism, and as an antitussive. It has also been used as an insect repellent. The standardized extract, called Remifemin, has been used in Germany for menopausal management.[1]

Black cohosh contains a number of alkaloids including N-methylcytosine, other tannins, and terpenoids. It is believed that the isoflavones or formononetin components may bind to estrogenic receptors.[2] Intraperitoneal injection of the extract selectively inhibits release of luteinizing hormone with no effect on the follicle-stimulating hormone (FSH), or prolactin.[3] The data seems to suggest that this product interacts strongly at certain specific estrogen receptors and might be useful as estrogen replacement therapy in postmenopausal women although this has not been well studied. More studies are needed to address its usefulness in postmenopausal women and osteoporotic states.[1]

Other effects of black cohosh include: hypotension, hypocholesterolemic activity, and peripheral vasodilation in vasospastic conditions (due to acetin content). Overdose may cause nausea, vomiting, dizziness, visual disturbances, bradycardia, and perspiration. Large doses may induce miscarriage. This product should not be used in pregnant women.[4] No data are available on the transfer of Black Cohosh into human milk, but due to its estrogenic activity, it could lower milk production although this is not known at this time. Caution is recommended in breastfeeding mothers. Use for more than 6 months is not recommended.[5]

Pregnancy Risk	X		Lactation Risk	L4
T ½	=		M/P	=
Vd	=		PB	=
Tmax	=		Oral	=
MW	=		pKa	=

Adult Concerns: Large doses may induce miscarriage. . . this product should not be used in pregnant women. Other effects of black cohosh include: hypotension, hypocholesterolemic activity, and peripheral vasodilation in vasospastic conditions. Overdose may cause nausea, vomiting, dizziness, visual disturbances, bradycardia, and perspiration.

Pediatric Concerns: None reported via milk.

Drug Interactions:

Relative Infant Dose:

Adult Dose: 20–40 mg twice daily

Alternatives:

References:
1. Murray M. Am. J. Nat. Med. 4[3], 3–5.1997.
2. Jarry H. et al Planta Medica 1885; 4: 316–319.
3. Jarry H. et al Planta Medica 1885; 1: 46–49.
4. Newall C. Black Cohosh Herbal Medicines. Pharmaceutical Press 1996; 80: 81.
5. The Complete German Commission E Monographs. Ed. M. Blumenthal Amer Botanical Council 1998.

BLEOMYCIN   L4

Trade: Blenoxane, Bleocin, Bleo-cell, Bleo-S

Other Trades:

Category: anticancer drug

Bleomycin sulfate is used for a number of different cancers including: testicular, head and neck cancer, Hodgkin's and non-Hodgkin's lymphomas, and cervical cancer. Seventy percent of the dose is recovered in urine 24 hours after dosing.[1] The elimination of bleomycin is described by two bioexponential curves with a terminal T(beta) of 134–238 minutes. In patients with severely reduced kidney function, the T(beta) increases to 13.5 hours. No data are available on its transfer to milk, but its transfer to milk in clinically relevant levels is remote as its molecular weight is 1415 daltons. Secondly, its oral bioavailability is probably low to nil.

Withhold breastfeeding for at least 24 hours. Extend this recommendation in mothers with poor renal function.

Pregnancy Risk	D	Lactation Risk	L4
T ½	= T(beta) 134–238 minutes	M/P	=
Vd	= 0.35–0.45 l/kg	PB	= 1%
Tmax	= Within 30 minutes	Oral	=
MW	= 1415.56	pKa	= 11.98

Adult Concerns: Nausea, vomiting, weight loss, stomatitis, dermatitis, mucositis, alopecia, fever

Pediatric Concerns:

Drug Interactions:

Relative Infant Dose:

Adult Dose: Varies depending on indication

Alternatives:

References:
1. Grochow LB, Ames MM. A clinician's guide to chemotherapy pharmacokinetics and pharmacodynamics. 1st ed. Baltimore, MD: Williams and Wilkins; 1998.

BLESSED THISTLE | L3

Trade: Blessed Thistle

Other Trades:

Category: Anorexic, antidiarrheal, febrifuge

Blessed thistle contains an enormous array of chemicals, polyenes, steroids, terpenoids, and volatile oils. It is believed useful for diarrhea, hemorrhage, fevers, as an expectorant, as a bacteriostatic, for loss of appetite, indigestion, for promoting lactation, and other antiseptic properties. Traditionally it has been used for loss of appetite, flatulence, cough and congestion, gangrenous ulcers, and dyspepsia. It has been documented to be antibacterial against: B. subtilis, Brucella abortus, B. bronchiseptica, E. coli, Proteus species, P. aeruginosa, Staph. aureus, and Strep. faecalis.

The antibacterial and anti-inflammatory properties are due to its cnicin component.[1] While it is commonly use as a galactagogue, no data could be found supporting its use in this application in the German E commission, nor a number of other herbal references. It is virtually nontoxic (GRAS status), and there are only occasional suggestions that high doses may induce gastrointestinal symptoms.[2] Some sources mention that it is an abortifacient, do not use in pregnant patients.

Pregnancy Risk	Possibly Hazardous	Lactation Risk	L3
T ½	=	M/P	=
Vd	=	PB	=
Tmax	=	Oral	=
MW	=	pKa	=

Adult Concerns: Virtually nontoxic, but may be an abortifacient. In doses > 5 grams per cup, it has been associated with stomach irritation, nausea and vomiting. It also may induce allergies in individuals sensitive to ragweed, daisies, marigolds, and chrysanthemums.

Pediatric Concerns: None reported via milk but it lacks justification as a galactagogue.

Drug Interactions:

Relative Infant Dose:

Adult Dose: 1.5–3 grams as a tea up to three times daily

Alternatives:

References:
1. Vanhaelen-Fastre R. Cnicus benedictus: Seperation of antimicrobial constituents. Plant Med Phytother 1968; 2: 294–299.
2. Newall C. Black Cohosh Herbal Medicines. Pharmaceutical Press 1996; 80: 81.

BLUE COHOSH   L5

Trade: Blue ginseng, Squaw root, Papoose root, Yellow ginseng

Other Trades:

Category: Uterine stimulant

Blue Cohosh is also known as blue ginseng, squaw root, papoose root, or yellow ginseng. It is primarily used as a uterotonic drug to stimulate uterine contractions. In one recent paper, an infant born of a mother who ingested Blue Cohosh root for 3 weeks prior to delivery, suffered from severe cardiogenic shock and congestive heart failure.[1] Subsequent studies have found it cardiotoxic in animals. Blue Cohosh root contains a number of chemicals, including the alkaloid methylcytosine and the glycosides caulosaponin and caulophyllosaponin. Methylcytosine is pharmacologically similar to nicotine and may result in elevated blood pressure, gastric stimulation, and hyperglycemia. Caulosaponin and caulophyllosaponin are uterine stimulants. They also, apparently, produce severe ischemia of the myocardium due to intense coronary vasoconstriction. This product should not be used in pregnant women. No data are available concerning its transfer into human milk. Do not use in pregnant or breastfeeding mothers at any time.

Pregnancy Risk	X		Lactation Risk	L5
T ½	=		M/P	=
Vd	=		PB	=
Tmax	=		Oral	=
MW	=		pKa	=

Adult Concerns: The leaves and seeds contain alkaloids and glycosides that can cause severe stomach pain when ingested. Poisoning have been reported. Symptoms include irritation of mucous membranes, diarrhea, cramping, chest pain, and hyperglycemia. Due to these life-threatening side effects pregnant women should be advised not to ingest any blue cohosh product during pregnancy.

Pediatric Concerns: One case of severe neonatal acute myocardial infarction, congestive heart failure, and shock in a newborn one month prior to delivery. Do not use in breastfeeding mothers. In another case, seizures, renal failure and respiratory distress were reported in an infant whose mother took black and blue cohosh at 42 weeks gestation.

Drug Interactions:

Relative Infant Dose:

Adult Dose:

Alternatives:

References:

1. Jones TK, Lawson BM. Profound neonatal congestive heart failure caused by maternal consumption of blue cohosh herbal medication. J Pediatr 1998; 132(3 Pt 1): 550–552.

BOCEPREVIR | L4

Trade: Victrelis

Other Trades:

Category: Antiviral Hepatitis C

Boceprevir is an antiviral drug for treatment of chronic hepatitis C virus (HCV). It functions by inhibiting hepatitis C virus replication in infected cells. It is usually used in combination with ribavirin and interferon alfa.

There are no studies of its use in breastfeeding women. In one animal study peak serum concentration of boceprevir and metabolite in nursing pups is about 1% of maternal serum concentration.[1]

However, its current use in breastfeeding patients for treatment of Hepatitis C infections when combined with ribavirin for periods up to one year may be more problematic as high concentrations of ribavirin could accumulate in the breastfed infant. (see ribavirin)

Pregnancy Risk	B/X (with ribavirin)	Lactation Risk	L4
T ½	= 3.4 hours	M/P	=
Vd	= 11 l/kg	PB	= 75%
Tmax	= 2 hours	Oral	= 65%
MW	= 520	pKa	=

Adult Concerns: Fatigue, insomnia, chills, anemia, neutropenia, thrombocytopenia, nausea, vomiting, headache, abnormal taste, xerostomia, arthralgia, thromboembolic events.

Pediatric Concerns:

Drug Interactions: Boceprevir is contraindicated in combination with high affinity CYP3A4/5 substrates and CYP3A4/5 inducers.

Relative Infant Dose:

Adult Dose: 800 mg TID

Alternatives:

References:
1. Pharmaceutical manufacturer prescribing information, 2011.

BORAGE   L5

Trade: Borage, Borage oil, Beebread, Bee plant, Burrage, Starflower, Ox

Other Trades:

Category: Herbal expectorant, tonic, galactogogue

Borage is also called Beebread, Bee Plant, Burrage, Starflower. Borage oil or other products may contain the powerful and dangerous pyrrolizidine-type alkaloids. Native Borage oil contains, amabiline, which is hepatotoxic pyrrolizidine alkaloid. The use of this product in pregnant or breastfeeding women is contraindicated unless it is certified to be free of amabiline. Ingestion of 1–2 grams of borage oil per day could provide doses of unsaturated pyrrolizidine alkaloids equal to10 µg, which is in excess of the 1 µg/day limit recommended by the German Federal Health Agency.

Pregnancy Risk	X		Lactation Risk	L5
T ½	=		M/P	=
Vd	=		PB	=
Tmax	=		Oral	=
MW	=		pKa	=

Adult Concerns: May contain amabiline, which is hepatotoxic pyrrolizidine alkaloid.

Pediatric Concerns: Caution, do not use in pregnant or breastfeeding women unless the oil is certified to be amabiline-free.

Drug Interactions:

Relative Infant Dose:

Adult Dose: 1–4 grams

Alternatives:

References:
1. Newall C, Anderson LA, Phillipson JD. Borage. In. Herbal Medicine. A guide for the healthcare professionals. The Pharmaceutical Press, London; 1996.

BOSENTAN   L4

Trade: Tracleer

Other Trades: Tracleer

Category: Endothelin antagonist

Bosentan is used in the treatment of pulmonary artery hypertension. It blocks endothelin receptors on vascular endothelium and smooth muscle, thus blocking vasoconstriction.[1] No data are available on the transfer into human milk, but bosentan is highly protein bound (98%), large molecular weight product, and therefore only small amounts are likely to be found unbound in the plasma. As a result, the amount in the milk compartment would probably be very low. However, this product is highly teratogenic, is 50% bioavailable orally, and has a high incidence of liver toxicity in patients. Great caution is recommended with this product in breastfeeding mothers until we have published milk levels.

Pregnancy Risk	X	Lactation Risk	L4
T ½	= 5 hours	M/P	=
Vd	= 0.26 l/kg	PB	= 98%
Tmax	= 3–5 hours	Oral	= 50%
MW	= 569	pKa	= 15.10

Adult Concerns: Headache, hypotension, palpitations, flushing, anemia, lower extremity edema, elevated liver enzymes (upto 11%), cirrhosis of liver, liver failure (in upto 11% of those on bosentan).

Pediatric Concerns: No data are available. May be dosed down to children weighing at least 10 kg.

Drug Interactions: Bosentan induces CYP2C9 and CYP3A4. Administration of inhibitors of these enzymes, such as amiodarone, fluconazole, itraconazole, or tetoconazole, may produce significant elevations in bosentan plasma concentrations and increase the risk of toxicity. It also may decrease levels of hormonal contraceptives, and increase metabolism of oral anticoagulants and sildenafil. Rifampin may decrease levels of bosentan.

Relative Infant Dose:

Adult Dose: 125 mg BID

Alternatives:

References:
1. Pharmaceutical manufacturer prescribing information, 2009.

BOTULINUM TOXIN | L3

Trade: Botox, Onabotulinumtoxin A, Botulism, *Clostridium botulinum*
Other Trades:
Category: Botulism poisoning and cosmetic procedures

Botulism is a syndrome produced by the deadly toxin secreted by the bacteria *Clostridium botulinum*. Botulinum toxins are neuromuscular blocking agents that produce muscular paralysis. Although the bacteria is wide spread, its colonization in food or the intestine of infants produces a deadly toxin. The syndrome is characterized by GI distress, weakness, malaise, light-headedness, sore throat, and nausea. Dry mouth is almost universal. In most adult poisoning, the bacteria is absent; only the toxin is present. In most pediatric poisoning, the stomach is colonized by the bacterium, often from contaminated honey.

In one published report, a breastfeeding woman severely poisoned by botulism toxin continued to breastfeed her infant throughout the illness.[1] Four hours after admission, her milk was tested and was free of botulinum toxin or C. botulinum bacteria, although she was still severely ill. The infant showed no symptoms of poisoning. It is apparent from this case that neither botulinum bacteria, nor the toxin is secreted in breastmilk.

Onabotulinumtoxin A (Botox): The pharmaceutical product Botox contains a purified Botulinum A toxin.[2] It is commonly used for numerous cosmetic as well as other procedures such as for treatment of rectal tears, spasticity, cerebral palsy, strabismus, etc. When injected into the muscle, it produces a partial chemical denervation resulting in paralysis of the muscle. When injected properly, and directly into the muscle, the toxin does not enter the systemic circulation. Thus levels in maternal plasma, and milk are very unlikely. Waiting a few hours for dissipation of any toxin would all but eliminate any risk to the infant. Also, avoid use of generic or unknown sources of botulinum toxin, as some are known to produce significant plasma levels in humans.

Pregnancy Risk	C		Lactation Risk	L3
T ½	=		M/P	=
Vd	=		PB	=
Tmax	=		Oral	=
MW	=		pKa	=

Adult Concerns: Gastrointestinal distress, weakness, malaise, dizziness, sore throat, nausea, dry mouth, hypersensitivity reactions. The effects of botulinum toxin may sometimes spread from the site of injection and involve other organs of the body, sometimes to cause life-threatening respiratory difficulties. These side–effects may occur hours to weeks after the injection. More pronounced in children, rather than adults.

Pediatric Concerns: None reported in one case of poisoning. No data on its use in breastfeeding mothers.

Drug Interactions: Do not use concomitantly with aminoglycosides or other muscle-relaxants due to possibility of enhanced muscle relaxing action.

Relative Infant Dose:

Adult Dose: 1.25–5 units IM injection. Do not exceed 360 units in a 3 month period.

Alternatives:

References:
1. Middaugh J. Botulism and breast milk. N Engl J Med 1978; 298(6): 343.
2. Pharmaceutical manufactures prescribing information, 2005.

BRIMONIDINE   L3

Trade: Alphagan

Other Trades: Enidin, Combigan, Dom-Brimonidine

Category: Use to treat ocular hypertension

Brimonidine is an alpha adrenergic receptor antagonist used to reduce intraocular pressure in open-angle glaucoma by reducing aqueous humor production and increasing uveoscleral outflow.[1] No data are available on its transfer into human milk. If used in breastfeeding mothers, observe the infant closely for alpha adrenergic blockage although this is unlikely. See side effects.

Pregnancy Risk	B	Lactation Risk	L3
T ½	= 2 hours	M/P	=
Vd	=	PB	=
Tmax	= 0.5–2.5 hours	Oral	=
MW	= 442	pKa	= 7.4

Adult Concerns: Oral dryness, ocular hyperemia, burning and stinging, headache, blurring, fatigue/drowsiness, ocular allergies and pruritus. Brimonidine may produce mild hypotension, palpitations, and syncope.

Pediatric Concerns: No studies available. Use with caution.

Drug Interactions: Use cautiously with CNS depressants, tricyclic antidepressants, beta-blockers, antihypertensives, and/or digitalis. Do not use with MAO inhibitors.

Relative Infant Dose:

Adult Dose: One drop in eye three times daily.

Alternatives:

References:
1. Pharmaceutical manufacturer prescribing information, 2011.

BROMOCRIPTINE   L5

Trade: Parlodel

Other Trades: Kripton, Bromolactin, Apo-Bromocriptine

Category: Inhibits prolactin secretion

Bromocriptine mesylate is an anti-parkinsonian, synthetic ergot alkaloid which inhibits prolactin secretion and hence physiologic lactation. Most of the dose of bromocriptine is absorbed by first-pass by the liver, leaving less than 6% to remain in the plasma. Maternal serum prolactin levels remain suppressed for up to 14 hours after a single dose. The FDA approved indication for lactation suppression has been withdrawn, and it is no longer approved for this purpose due to numerous maternal deaths, seizures, and strokes. Observe for transient hypotension or vomiting. It is sometimes used in hyperprolactinemic patients who have continued to breastfeed although the incidence of maternal side-effects is significant and newer products are preferred.[1,2] Several studies have shown the possibility of breastfeeding during bromocriptine therapy for pituitary tumors with no untoward effects in infants.[3,4] Caution is recommended as profound maternal postpartum hypotension has been reported. While bromocriptine is no longer recommended for suppression of lactation, a newer product cabergoline (Dostinex), is considered much safer for suppression of prolactin production.

Pregnancy Risk	B		Lactation Risk	L5
T ½	= 50 hours		M/P	=
Vd	= 3.4 l/kg		PB	= 90–96%
Tmax	= 1–3 hours		Oral	= <28%
MW	= 654		pKa	= 11.13

Adult Concerns: Most frequent side effects include nausea (49%), headache (19%), and dizziness (17%), peripheral vasoconstriction. Rarely, significant hypotension, shock, myocardial infarction. Transient hypotension and hair loss. A number of deaths have been associated with this product and it is no longer cleared for postpartum use to inhibit lactation.

Pediatric Concerns: No reports of direct toxicity to infant via milk but use with caution. Inhibits lactation. May be useful in patients with hyperprolactinemia who wish to continue breastfeeding, although cabergoline is probably preferred.

Drug Interactions: Amitriptyline, butyrophenones, imipramine, methyldopa, phenothiazines, reserpine, may decrease efficacy of bromocriptine at reducing serum prolactin. May increase toxicity of other ergot alkaloids.

Relative Infant Dose:

Adult Dose: 1.25–2.5 mg BID-TID

Alternatives: Cabergoline

References:
1. Meese MG. Reassessment of bromocriptine use for lactation suppression. P and T 1992; 17: 1003–1004.
2. Spalding G. Bromocriptine (Parlodel) for suppression of lactation. Aust N Z J Obstet Gynaecol 1991; 31(4): 344–345.
3. Canales ES, Garcia IC, Ruiz JE, Zarate A. Bromocriptine as prophylactic therapy in prolactinoma during pregnancy. Fertil Steril 1981; 36(4): 524–526.
4. Verma S, Shah D, Faridi MMA. Breastfeeding a Baby with Mother on Bromocriptine. Indian J Pediatr 2006; 73(5): 435–436.

BROMPHENIRAMINE   L3

Trade: Lodrane, Bidhist, Colhist, Dimetane Extentabs, Dimetapp, LoHist-12, ND-Stat, VaZol

Other Trades:

Category: Antihistamine

Brompheniramine is a popular antihistamine sold as Dimetane or numerous other products, some that include pseudoephedrine. Although untoward effects appear limited, some reported side effects from Dimetapp preparations are known.

Although only insignificant amounts of brompheniramine appear to be secreted into breastmilk, there are a number of reported cases of irritability, excessive crying, and sleep disturbances that have been reported in breastfeeding infants.[1] Note, many sinus products may contain pseudoephedrine, and should be avoided in breastfeeding mothers if possible.

Pregnancy Risk	C	Lactation Risk	L3
T ½	= 24.9 hours	M/P	=
Vd	= 11.7 l/kg	PB	=
Tmax	= 3.1 hours	Oral	= Complete
MW	= 319	pKa	= 3.9

Adult Concerns: Drowsiness, dry mucosa, excessive crying, irritability, sleep disturbances.

Pediatric Concerns: Irritability, excessive crying, and sleep disturbances have been reported.

Drug Interactions: May enhance toxicity of other CNS depressants, MAO inhibitors, alcohol and tricyclic depressants.

Relative Infant Dose:

Adult Dose: 4 mg every 4–6 hours

Alternatives: Loratadine, Cetirizine

References:
1. Paton DM, Webster DR. Clinical pharmacokinetics of H_1-receptor antagonists (the antihistamines). Clin Pharmacokinet 1985; 10(6): 477–497.

BUDESONIDE + FORMOTEROL   L3

Trade: Symbicort

Other Trades:

Category: Antiasthma, Anti-Inflammatory/Bronchodilator Combination

Budesonide and Formoterol fumarate is a drug combination product of an anti-inflammatory (budesonide) agent along with a bronchodilator (formoterol). It is FDA approved for treatment of asthma and chronic obstructive pulmonary disease (COPD).[1] The transfer of this combination product into breastmilk has not been studied.

Budesonide is a potent corticosteroid used intranasally for allergic rhinitis, inhaled for asthma, and orally for Crohn's disease.[2] As such, the lung bioavailability is estimated to be 34% of the inhaled dose.[3] Once absorbed systemically, budesonide is a weak systemic steroid and should not be used to replace other steroids. In one 5 year study of children aged 2–7 years, no changes in linear growth, weight, and bone age were noted following inhalation.[4] Adrenal suppression at these doses is extremely remote. Using normal doses, it is unlikely that clinically relevant concentrations of inhaled budesonide would ever reach the milk nor be systemically bioavailable to a breastfed infant. One study tested breastmilk samples from 8 women before and after their first morning dose of 200 or 400 μg inhaled budesonide (Pulmicort Turbuhaler). Average milk level of budesonide (Cav) was 0.105–0.219 nmol/L with doses of 200 and 400 µg twice daily, respectively. Maternal plasma levels of budesonide reported (Cav) were 0.246–0.437 nmol/L at the doses above. Milk/plasma ratios were 0.428 and 0.502 at the doses above. Plasma samples from infants 1–1.5 hours after feeding showed levels below the limit of quantification. Therefore, the estimated daily infant dose is 0.3% of the mother's daily dose or approximately 0.0068–0.0142 µg/kg/day.[3] Relative Infant Dose for budesonide is 0.29%.

Formoterol is a long-acting selective beta-2 adrenoceptor agonist used for asthma and COPD. Following inhalation of a 120 µg dose, the maximum plasma concentration of 92 pg/mL occurred within 5 minutes.[5] No data are available on its transfer into human milk, but the extremely low plasma levels would suggest that milk levels would be incredibly low, if even measurable. Studies of oral absorption in adults suggests that while absorption is good, plasma levels are still below detectable levels and may require large oral doses prior to attaining measurable plasma levels.[6,7] It is not likely the amount present in human milk would be clinically relevant to a breastfed infant.

Pregnancy Risk	C	Lactation Risk	L3
T ½	= Budesonide/formoterol: 2.8 hours/10 hours	M/P	= Budesonide/formoterol: 0.5/
Vd	= Budesonide/formoterol: 4.3/ l/kg	PB	= Budesonide/formoterol: 85–90%(oral)/64%
Tmax	= Budesonide/formoterol: 32–43 min/5 min	Oral	= Budesonide/formoterol: 10.7%/good
MW	= Budesonide/formoterol: 430/840	pKa	= Budesonide/formoterol: 14.9/

Adult Concerns: Oral candidiasis, vomiting, headache, nasal congestion, nasopharyngitis, sinusitis are the commonly reported side-effects. Less common are hypokalemia, cataract, glaucoma. The use of long-acting beta-adrenergic bronchodilators such as formoterol has been associated with an increased risk of asthma-related hospitalization and asthma-related deaths.

Pediatric Concerns:

Drug Interactions: Concomitant administration with CYP3A4 inhibitors such as ketoconazole, ritonavir, atazanavir, clarithromycin, indinavir, itraconazole, nefazodone, nelfinavir, saquinavir, telithromycin, may increase plasma levels and subsequent systemic exposure to budesonide. Monoamine oxidase inhibitors and tricyclic anti-depressants may enhance the action of formoterol. Caution while using concurrently with beta-blockers to avoid precipitation of brochospasm. Use with diuretics may cause hypokalemia.

Relative Infant Dose:

Adult Dose: Budesonide/formoterol: 80–160 µg/4.5 µg twice daily.

Alternatives:

References:

1. Pharmaceutical manufacturer prescribing information, 2010.

2. Pharmaceutical manufacturer prescribing information, 2007.
3. Falt A, Bengtsson T, Gyllenberg A, Lindberg B, Strandgarden K. Negligible Exposure of Infants to Budesonide Via Breast Milk. J Allergy Clin Immunol 2007; 120(4): 798–802.
4. Volovitz B, Amir J, Malik H, Kauschansky A, Varsano I. Growth and pituitary-adrenal function in children with severe asthma treated with inhaled budesonide. N Engl J Med 1993; 329(23): 1703–1708.
5. Pharmaceutical manufacturer prescribing information, 2001.
6. Tattersfield AE. Long-acting beta 2-agonists. Clin Exp Allergy 1992; 22(6): 600–605.
7. Maesen FP, Smeets JJ, Gubbelmans HL, Zweers PG. Bronchodilator effect of inhaled formoterol vs salbutamol over 12 hours. Chest 1990; 97(3): 590–594.

BUDESONIDE INHALED | L1

Trade: Rhinocort, Pulmicort, Pulmicort Respules, Pulmicort Flexhaler, Pulmicort Turbuhaler, Entocort EC

Other Trades: Pulmicort Nebbuamp, Rhinocort Turbuhaler

Category: Corticosteroid

Budesonide is a potent corticosteroid used intranasally for allergic rhinitis, inhaled for asthma, and in capsule form for Crohn's disease.[1] As such, the lung bioavailability is estimated to be 34% of the inhaled dose.[3] Once absorbed systemically, budesonide is a weak systemic steroid and should not be used to replace other steroids. In one 5 year study of children aged 2–7 years, no changes in linear growth, weight, and bone age were noted following inhalation.[2] Adrenal suppression at these doses is extremely remote. Using normal doses, it is unlikely that clinically relevant concentrations of budesonide would ever reach the milk nor be systemically bioavailable to a breastfed infant. One study tested breastmilk samples from 8 women before and after their first morning dose of 200 or 400 µg inhaled budesonide (Pulmicort Turbuhaler). Average milk level of budesonide (Cav) was 0.105–0.219 nmol/L with doses of 200 and 400 µg twice daily, respectively. Maternal plasma levels of budesonide reported (Cav) were 0.246–0.437 nmol/L at the doses above. Milk/plasma ratios were 0.428 and 0.502 at the doses above. Plasma samples from infants 1–1.5 hours after feeding showed levels below the limit of quantification. Therefore, the estimated daily infant dose is 0.3% of the mother's daily dose or approximately 0.0068–0.0142 µg/kg/day.[3]

Pregnancy Risk	B	Lactation Risk	L1
T ½	= 2.8 hours	M/P	= 0.50
Vd	= 4.3 l/kg	PB	= 85–90% (oral)
Tmax	= 32–43 min (Inh)	Oral	= 10.7% (oral)
MW	= 430	pKa	= 14.91

Adult Concerns: Adverse effects following intranasal use include irritation, pharyngitis, cough, bleeding, candidiasis, dry mouth. No adrenal suppression has been reported. Side effects following oral use include: headache, acne, bruising, and nausea.

Pediatric Concerns: None reported via milk. Pediatric use down to age 6 is permitted, but it is used in infants routinely.

Drug Interactions: Ketoconazole (inhibitor of CYP3A4) causes an 8 fold increase of the systemic exposure to budesonide. Avoid using with ketoconazole, itraconazole, ritonavir, indinavir, erythromycin, and others that may inhibit this drug-metabolizing system.

Relative Infant Dose: 0.3%

Adult Dose: Intranasal: 200–400 µg BID; Oral: 9 mg daily.

Alternatives:

References:
1. Pharmaceutical manufacturer prescribing information, 2007.
2. Falt A, Bengtsson T, Gyllenberg A, Lindberg B, Strandgarden K. Negligible Exposure of Infants to Budesonide Via Breast Milk. J Allergy Clin Immunol 2007; 120(4): 798–802.
3. Volovitz B, Amir J, Malik H, Kauschansky A, Varsano I. Growth and pituitary-adrenal function in children with severe asthma treated with inhaled budesonide. N Engl J Med 1993; 329(23): 1703–1708.

BUDESONIDE ORAL   L3

Trade: Entocort EC

Other Trades: Pulmicort, Pulmicort Spacer

Category: Corticosteroid

Budesonide has a high topical corticosteroid activity and a substantial first pass elimination. Thus plasma levels are generally quite low.

The new oral formulation of budesonide (Entocort EC) is used for Crohn's disease and is placed in special granules that pass the stomach before releasing the drug in controlled-release manner in the duodenum. Plasma budesonide has a high clearance rate due to high uptake by the liver. Plasma levels are low and brief, and its ability to suppress normal cortisol levels is about half that of prednisone. Because of its high first-pass clearance, it is rather unlikely to produce high or even significant levels in milk, nor be orally bioavailable to a significant degree in breastfeeding infants.

Pregnancy Risk	C	Lactation Risk	L3
T ½	= 2–3.6 hours	M/P	=
Vd	= 3.9 l/kg	PB	= 85–90%
Tmax	= 30–600 minutes	Oral	= 9–21%
MW	= 430	pKa	= 14.91

Adult Concerns: Use with caution in patients with tuberculosis, hypertension, diabetes mellitus, osteoporosis, peptic ulcer, glaucoma or cataracts, or with a family history of diabetes or glaucoma, or with any other condition where glucocorticosteroids may have unwanted effects. If use chronically, systemic glucocorticosteroid effects such as hypercorticism and adrenal suppression may occur.

Pediatric Concerns: None yet reported in breastfed infants. Unlikely.

Drug Interactions: Budesonide is metabolized via CYP3A4. Co-administration of ketoconazole results in an eight-fold increase in AUC of budesonide. Grapefruit juice, an inhibitor of gut mucosal CYP3A, approximately doubles the systemic exposure of oral budesonide. Conversely, induction of CYP3A4 can result in the lowering of budesonide plasma levels. Oral contraceptives containing ethinyl estradiol, which are also metabolized by CYP3A4, do not affect the pharmacokinetics of budesonide. Budesonide does not affect the plasma levels of oral contraceptives (ie, ethinyl estradiol).

Relative Infant Dose:

Adult Dose: 9 mg daily

Alternatives: Azathioprine, prednisone, methylprednisolone

References:
1. Pharmaceutical manufacturer prescribing information, 2010.

BUMETANIDE   L3

Trade: Bumex

Other Trades: Burinex

Category: Loop diuretic

Bumetanide is a potent loop diuretic similar to furosemide.[1] As with all diuretics, some reduction in breastmilk production may result but it is rare. It is not known if bumetanide transfers into human milk. If needed furosemide may be a better choice, as the oral bioavailability of furosemide in neonates is minimal.

Pregnancy Risk	C	Lactation Risk	L3
T ½	= 1–1.5	M/P	=
Vd	= . 129–. 357 l/kg	PB	= 97%
Tmax	= 1 hour (oral)	Oral	= 59–89%
MW	= 364	pKa	= 9.62

Adult Concerns: Dehydration, hepatic cirrhosis, ototoxicity, potassium loss. See furosemide.

Pediatric Concerns: None reported via milk.

Drug Interactions: Numerous interactions exist, this is a partial list of the most important. NSAIDS may block diuretic effect. Lithium excretion may be reduced. Increased effect with other antihypertensives. May induce hypoglycemia when added to sulfonylurea users. Clofibrate may induce an exaggerated diuresis. Increased ototoxicity with aminoglycoside antibiotics. Increased anticoagulation with anticoagulants.

Relative Infant Dose:

Adult Dose: 0.5–2 mg one to two times a day

Alternatives: Furosemide

References:
1. Pharmaceutical manufacturer prescribing information, 1999.

BUPIVACAINE   L2

Trade: Marcaine, Sensorcaine
Other Trades: Marcain, Marcaine, Sensorcaine
Category: Epidural, local anesthetic

Bupivacaine is the most commonly employed regional anesthetic used in delivery because its concentrations in the fetus are the least of the local anesthetics. In one study of five patients, levels of bupivacaine in breastmilk were below the limits of detection (<0.02 mg/L) at 2 to 48 hours postpartum.[1] These authors concluded that bupivacaine is a safe drug for perinatal use in mothers who plan to breastfeed. In a study of 27 patients who received an average of 183.3 mg lidocaine and 82.1 mg bupivacaine via an epidural catheter, lidocaine plasma levels at 2, 6, and 12 hours post administration were 0.86, 0.46, and 0.22 mg/L respectively.[2] Levels of bupivacaine in milk at 2, 6, and 12 hours were 0.09, 0.06, 0.04 mg/L respectively. The milk/serum ratio based upon area under the curve values (AUC) were 1.07 and 0.34 for lidocaine and bupivacaine respectively. Based on AUC data of lidocaine and bupivacaine milk levels, the average milk concentration of these agents over 12 hours was 0.5 and 0.07 mg/L. Most of the infants had a maximal APGAR score.

Pregnancy Risk	C	Lactation Risk	L2
T ½	= 2.7 hours	M/P	=
Vd	= 0.4–1.0 l/kg	PB	= 95%
Tmax	= 30–45 minutes	Oral	=
MW	= 288	pKa	= 8.1

Adult Concerns: Sedation, bradycardia, respiratory depression.

Pediatric Concerns: None reported via milk.

Drug Interactions: Increases effect of hyaluronidase, beta blockers, MAO inhibitors, tricyclic antidepressants, phenothiazines, and vasopressors.

Relative Infant Dose: 0.9%

Adult Dose: 25–100 mg once

Alternatives:

References:
1. Naulty JS. Bupivacaine in breast milk following epidural anesthesia for vaginal delivery. Regional Anesthesia 1983; 8(1): 44–45.
2. Ortega D, Viviand X, Lorec AM, Gamerre M, Martin C, Bruguerolle B. Excretion of lidocaine and bupivacaine in breast milk following epidural anesthesia for cesarean delivery. Acta Anaesthesiol Scand 1999; 43(4): 394–397.

BUPRENORPHINE   L2

Trade: Buprenex, Subutex
Other Trades: Temgesic, Subutex
Category: Narcotic analgesic

Buprenorphine is a potent, long-acting narcotic agonist and antagonist and may be useful as a replacement for methadone treatment in addicts. It is also recently approved for the treatment of opiate dependence. Its elimination half-life varies from paper to paper, but new recent sublingual studies suggests it ranges from 23–30 hours.[1]

In one patient who received 4 mg/day to facilitate withdrawal from other opiates, the amount of buprenorphine transferred via milk was only 3.28 µg/day, an amount that was clinically insignificant.[2] No symptoms were noted in this breastfed infant. In another study of continuous epidural bupivacaine and buprenorphine in post cesarean women for 3 days[3], it was suggested that buprenorphine may suppress the production of milk (and infant weight gain) although this was not absolutely clear. In another study of one patient on buprenorphine maintenance for 7 months, and who received 8 mg daily sublingually over 4 days, milk levels of buprenorphine and norbuprenorphine ranged from 1.0 to 14.7 ng/mL and 0.6 to 6.3 ng/mL, respectively.[4] Plasma concentrations of both analytes ranged from 0.2 to 20.1 ng/mL (buprenorphine) and 1.2 to 4.4 ng/mL (norbuprenorphine) over 4 days of study. Using peak levels only, the concentration of buprenorphine and norbuprenorphine were 1.47 and 0.63 µg/100 mL of breast milk, respectively. Assuming an intake of 150 mL/kg/day, the authors estimated the daily dose would be less than 10 µg for a 4 kg infant, a dose that is probably far subclinical. In a recent study[5] of 7 women who were taking a median of 0.32 mg/kg/day buprenorphine, the median area under the curve estimates of milk levels were 0.12 mg.h/L for buprenorphine and 0.10 mg.h/L for norbuprenorphine. Levels of buprenorphine and norbuprenorphine in the infant plasma were approximately 4.5% and 11.7% of maternal levels. In another study of 7 women who received a mean buprenorphine dose of 7 mg/day (2.4–24 mg), the mean milk concentrations of buprenorphine and norbuprenorphine were 3.65 µg/L and 1.94 µg/L respectively.[6] The authors calculated the relative infant dose to be 0.38% for buprenorphine, and 0.18% for norbuprenorphine. The authors concluded that the doses of buprenorphine and norbuprenorphine received by the infant though lactational exposure are clinically insignificant.

Based on these studies it may be concluded that although experience with the use of buprenorphine in breastfeeding women is limited, there is no evidence that the use of this drug will have an adverse effect in the breastfed infant. The relative infant dose of buprenorphine is 0.09–1.9%.

Pregnancy Risk	C	Lactation Risk	L2
T ½	= 23–30 hours sublingual	M/P	= 1.7
Vd	= 97 l/kg	PB	= 96%
Tmax	= 15–30 minutes	Oral	= 31%
MW	= 504	pKa	= 8.24, 9.92

Adult Concerns: Typical opiate side effects include pruritus, sedation, analgesia, hallucinations, euphoria, dizziness, respiratory depression.

Pediatric Concerns: Low weight gain and reduced breast milk levels in one study, and no effects in two other studies.

Drug Interactions: May enhance effects of other opiates, benzodiazepines, and barbiturates.

Relative Infant Dose: 0.09%–1.9%

Adult Dose: 0.3 mg (IV) every 6 hours PRN; 2–8 mg PO

Alternatives: Methadone

References:
1. McAleer SD, Mills RJ, Polack T et al. Pharmacokinetics of high-dose buprenorphine following single administration of sublingual tablet formulations in opioid naive healthy male volunteers under a naltrexone block. Drug Alcohol Depend. 2003; 72: 75–83.
2. Marquet P, Chevrel J, Lavignasse P, Merle L, Lachatre G. Buprenorphine withdrawal syndrome in a newborn. Clin Pharmacol Ther 1997; 62(5): 569–571.
3. Hirose M, Hosokawa T, Tanaka Y. Extradural buprenorphine suppresses breast feeding after caesarean section. Br J Anaesth 1997; 79(1): 120–121.
4. Grimm D, Pauly E, Poschl J et al. Buprenorphine and Norbuprenorphine Concentrations in Human Breast Milk Samples Determined by Liquid Chromatography-Tandem Mass Spectrometry. Ther Drug Monit. 2005; 27: 526–530.
5. Lindemalm S, Nydert P, Svensson JO, Stahle L, Sarman I. Transfer of buprenorphine into breast milk and calculation of infant drug dose. J Hum Lact. May 2009; 25(2): 199–205.
6. Ilett K, Hackett LP, Gower S, Doherty D, Hamilton D, and Bartu AE. Estimated Dose Exposure of the Neonate to Buprenorphine and Its Metabolite Norbuprenorphine via Breastmilk During Maternal Buprenorphine Substitution Treatment. Breastfeeding Medicine. -Not available-, ahead of print. doi: 10.1089/bfm. 2011.0096.

BUPRENORPHINE + NALOXONE | L3

Trade: Suboxone

Other Trades:

Category: Suppression of opiate withdrawal in drug addiction programs.

Buprenorphine hydrochloride and Naloxone hydrochloride is a combination drug product indicated for use in opioid dependence.[1] Buprenorphine and naloxone are combined in a sublingual tablet that contains a partial opioid agonist (buprenorphine) and an opioid antagonist (naloxone) in a 4:1 (buprenorphine: naloxone) ratio. Buprenorphine reduces the patients' craving for opioids, and naloxone discourages the use of other opioids by blocking the opiate receptor. Naloxone is poorly absorbed orally and buprenorphine is only 31% absorbed. It is unlikely breast milk levels will be significant.[2]

In one patient who received 4 mg/day buprenorphine to facilitate withdrawal from other opiates, the amount of buprenorphine transferred via milk was only 3.28 µg/day, an amount that was clinically insignificant.[3] No symptoms were noted in this breastfed infant. In another study of continuous epidural bupivacaine and buprenorphine in post cesarean women for 3 days[4], it was suggested that buprenorphine may suppress the production of milk (and infant weight gain) although this was not absolutely clear.

In another study of one patient on buprenorphine maintenance for 7 months, and who received 8 mg daily sublingually over 4 days, milk levels of buprenorphine and norbuprenorphine ranged from 1.0 to 14.7 ng/mL and 0.6 to 6.3 ng/mL, respectively.[5] Plasma concentrations of both analytes ranged from 0.2 to 20.1 ng/mL (buprenorphine) and 1.2 to 4.4 ng/mL (norbuprenorphine) over 4 days of study. Using peak levels only, the concentration of buprenorphine and norbuprenorphine were 1.47 and 0.63 µg/100 mL of breast milk, respectively. Assuming an intake of 150 mL/kg/day, the authors estimated the daily dose would be less than 10 µg for a 4 kg infant, a dose that is probably far subclinical.

In a recent study of 7 women[6] who were taking a median of 0.32 mg/kg/day buprenorphine, the median area under the curve estimates of milk levels were 0.12 mg. h/L for buprenorphine and 0.10 mg. h/L for norbuprenorphine. Levels of buprenorphine and norbuprenorphine in the infant plasma were approximately 4.5% and 11.7% of maternal levels.

In another study of 7 women[6] who received a mean buprenorphine dose of 7 mg/day (2.4–24 mg), the mean milk concentrations of buprenorphine and norbuprenorphine were 3.65 µg/L and 1.94 µg/L respectively. The authors calculated the relative infant dose to be 0.38% for buprenorphine, and 0.18% for norbuprenorphine. The authors concluded that the doses of buprenorphine and norbuprenorphine received by the infant though lactational exposure are clinically insignificant. Based on these studies it can be concluded that although experience with the use of buprenorphine in breastfeeding women is limited, there is no evidence that the use of this drug will have an adverse effect in the breastfed infant. The relative infant dose of buprenorphine is 0.09–1.9%.

Naloxone is commonly used for the treatment of opiate overdose, and now to prevent opiate abuse in patients undergoing withdrawal treatment. Naloxone is poorly absorbed orally and plasma levels in adults are undetectable (<0.05 ng/mL) two hours after oral doses. Following intravenous use (0.4 mg), plasma naloxone levels averaged <0.084 µg/mL. Side effects are minimal except in narcotic-addicted patients. The AAP has advised that naloxone should not be administered (directly) to infants of narcotic-dependent mothers. Its use in breastfeeding mothers would be unlikely to cause problems as its milk levels would likely be low and its oral absorption is minimal to nil.

In summary, it is unlikely that the breastmilk levels of buprenorphine and naloxone will be significant. Therefore the use of buprenorphine + naloxone combination is probably safe during breastfeeding.

Pregnancy Risk	C		Lactation Risk	L3	
T ½	= Buprenorphine/naloxone: 26 hours/64 min		M/P	= Buprenorphine/naloxone:	
Vd	= Buprenorphine/naloxone: 97–187/2.6–2.8 l/kg		PB	= Buprenorphine/naloxone: 96%/45%	
Tmax	= Buprenorphine/naloxone: day 3/		Oral	= Buprenorphine/naloxone: 15%/nil	
MW	= Buprenorphine/naloxone: 504/399		pKa	= Buprenorphine/naloxone: 8.24,9.92/7.9	

Adult Concerns: Palpitations, peripheral edema, sweating, abdominal pain, constipation, nausea, vomiting, hypersensitivity reactions. Hepatitis especially in those with pre-existing liver disease. Respiratory depression especially when used concomitantly with other CNS depressants. Abuse potential and withdrawal symptoms on discontinuation of drug.

Pediatric Concerns: None reported but data is limited at these doses.

Drug Interactions: Precipitation of withdrawal symptoms when used with other opioids such as hydrocodone, oxycodone, methadone, codeine. Altered efficacy when used with anti-HIV medications such as ritonavir, indinavir; when used with antibiotics such as ketoconazole and rifampin; and when used with anti-convulsants such as phenytoin and carbamazepine.

Relative Infant Dose:

Adult Dose: 16 mg buprenorphine/4 mg naloxone daily for maintenance therapy.

Alternatives:

References:
1. Pharmaceutical manufacturer prescribing information, 2006.
2. McAleer SD, Mills RJ, Polack T et al. Pharmacokinetics of high-dose buprenorphine following single administration of sublingual tablet formulations in opioid naive healthy male volunteers under a naltrexone block. Drug Alcohol Depend. 2003; 72: 75–83.
3. Marquet P, Chevrel J, Lavignasse P, Merle L, Lachatre G. Buprenorphine withdrawal syndrome in a newborn. Clin Pharmacol Ther 1997; 62(5): 569–571.
4. Hirose M, Hosokawa T, Tanaka Y. Extradural buprenorphine suppresses breast feeding after caesarean section. Br J Anaesth 1997; 79(1): 120–121.
5. Grimm D, Pauly E, Poschl J et al. Buprenorphine and Norbuprenorphine Concentrations in Human Breast Milk Samples Determined by Liquid Chromatography-Tandem Mass Spectrometry. Ther Drug Monit. 2005; 27: 526–530.
6. Lindemalm S, Nydert P, Svensson JO, Stahle L, Sarman I. Transfer of buprenorphine into breast milk and calculation of infant drug dose. J Hum Lact. May 2009; 25(2): 199–205.

BUPRENORPHINE TRANSDERMAL   L2

Trade: Butrans

Other Trades:

Category: Narcotic analgesic

Buprenorphine is a potent, long-acting narcotic agonist and antagonist and may be useful as a replacement for methadone treatment in addicts. It is also recently approved for the treatment of opiate dependence.[1] In one patient who received 4 mg/day to facilitate withdrawal from other opiates, the amount of buprenorphine transferred via milk was only 3.28 µg/day, an amount that was clinically insignificant.[2] No symptoms were noted in this breastfed infant. In another study of continuous epidural bupivacaine and buprenorphine in post cesarean women for 3 days[3], it was suggested that buprenorphine may suppress the production of milk (and infant weight gain) although this was not absolutely clear. In another study of one patient on buprenorphine maintenance for 7 months, and who received 8 mg daily sublingually over 4 days, milk levels of buprenorphine and norbuprenorphine ranged from 1.0 to 14.7 ng/mL and 0.6 to 6.3 ng/mL, respectively.[4] Plasma concentrations of both analytes ranged from 0.2 to 20.1 ng/mL (buprenorphine) and 1.2 to 4.4 ng/mL (norbuprenorphine) over 4 days of study. Using peak levels only, the concentration of buprenorphine and norbuprenorphine were 1.47 and 0.63 µg/100 mL of breast milk, respectively. Assuming an intake of 150 mL/kg/day, the authors estimated the daily dose would be less than 10 µg for a 4 kg infant, a dose that is probably far subclinical. In a recent study [5] of 7 women who were taking a median of 0.32 mg/kg/day buprenorphine, the median area under the curve estimates of milk levels were 0.12 mg.h/L for buprenorphine and 0.10 mg. h/L for norbuprenorphine. Levels of buprenorphine and norbuprenorphine in the infant plasma were approximately 4.5% and 11.7% of maternal levels.

Based on these studies it can be concluded that although experience with the use of buprenorphine in breastfeeding women is limited, there is no evidence that the use of this drug will have an adverse effect in the breastfed infant.

Pregnancy Risk	C	Lactation Risk	L2
T ½	= 26 hours	M/P	=
Vd	= 97–187 l/kg	PB	= 96%
Tmax	= Day 3	Oral	= 15%
MW	= 504	pKa	= 8.24, 9.92

Adult Concerns: Headache, dizziness, somnolence, nausea, constipation, vomiting, pruritus at the site of application.

Pediatric Concerns: Low weight gain and reduced breast milk levels in one study, and no effects in two other studies.

Drug Interactions: Atazanavir may increase the concentration of buprenorphine. Buprenorphine may enhance the effects of selective serotonin reuptake inhibitors. They may also enhance the effects of thiazide diuretics. The combination of benzodiazepines and buprenorphine alters the usual ceiling effect on buprenorphine-induced respiratory depression, making the respiratory effects of buprenorphine appear similar to those of full opioid agonists. Use with caution in patients taking benzodiazepines or other drugs that act on the central nervous system. Buprenorphine transdermal, like other opioids, may interact with skeletal muscle relaxants to enhance neuromuscular blocking action and increase respiratory depression.

Relative Infant Dose: 0.09%–1.9%

Adult Dose: 5 μg/hour applied once every 7 days

Alternatives:

References:
1. McAleer SD, Mills RJ, Polack T et al. Pharmacokinetics of high-dose buprenorphine following single administration of sublingual tablet formulations in opioid naive healthy male volunteers under a naltrexone block. Drug Alcohol Depend. 2003; 72: 75–83.
2. Marquet P, Chevrel J, Lavignasse P, Merle L, Lachatre G. Buprenorphine withdrawal syndrome in a newborn. Clin Pharmacol Ther 1997; 62(5): 569–571.
3. Hirose M, Hosokawa T, Tanaka Y. Extradural buprenorphine suppresses breast feeding after caesarean section. Br J Anaesth 1997; 79(1): 120–121.
4. Grimm D, Pauly E, Poschl J et al. Buprenorphine and Norbuprenorphine Concentrations in Human Breast Milk Samples Determined by Liquid Chromatography-Tandem Mass Spectrometry. Ther Drug Monit. 2005; 27: 526–530.
5. Lindemalm S, Nydert P, Svensson JO, Stahle L, Sarman I. Transfer of buprenorphine into breast milk and calculation of infant drug dose. J Hum Lact. May 2009; 25(2): 199–205.

BUPROPION   L3

Trade: Wellbutrin, Zyban, Aplenzin
Other Trades: Wellbutrin, Zyban
Category: Antidepressant, smoking deterrent

Bupropion is an older antidepressant with a structure unrelated to tricyclics. One report in the literature indicates that bupropion probably accumulates in human milk although the absolute dose transferred appears minimal as in three infants studied, no bupropion was detected in the plasma compartment. Following one 100 mg dose in a mother, the milk/plasma ratio ranged from 2.51 to 8.58, clearly suggesting a concentrating mechanism for this drug in human milk.[1] However, plasma levels of bupropion (or its metabolites) in the infant were undetectable, indicating that the dose transferred to the infant was low, and accumulation in infant plasma apparently did not occur under these conditions (infant was fed 7.5 to 9.5 hours after dosing). The peak milk bupropion level (0.189 mg/L) occurred two hours after a 100 mg dose. This milk level would provide 0.66% of the maternal dose, a dose that is likely to be clinically insignificant to a breastfed infant.

In a recent study of two breastfeeding patients consuming 75 mg twice daily and 150 mg (sustained release) daily respectively, no bupropion or metabolite were detected in either breastfed infant.[2] In the first patient at 17 weeks postpartum, plasma levels were drawn at 2 hours post-dose and bupropion or hydroxybupropion levels were undetectable. In the second patient at 29 weeks postpartum, bupropion and hydroxybupropion were undetectable as well. The limit of detection for bupropion was 5–10 ng/mL and for hydroxybupropion was 100–200 ng/mL. Seizures in a 6-month-old breastfed infant were reported four days following administration of 150 mg/day bupropion in the mother.[3] The mother discontinued bupropion and continued breastfeeding. No further seizures were reported. Due to persistent case reports to the author, bupropion may, in some women, suppress milk production. Some caution is recommended concerning changes to milk supply. In a study of 10 breastfeeding patients who received 150 mg bupropion SR daily for 2 days and then 300 mg bupropion SR daily thereafter for 5 more days, milk concentrations of bupropion averaged 45 µg/L.[4] The average infant dose via milk was 6.75 µg/kg/day. The reported relative infant dose was 0.14% of the weight-normalized maternal dose. When the active metabolites present in milk were added, the Relative Infant Dose would be 2% of the maternal dose. No side effects were noted in any of the infants. In a study of 4 mothers consuming 150 to 300 mg/day of bupropion SR, peak and trough blood levels were highly variable, but averaged 64 ng/mL at peak and 9.2 ng/mL at trough.[5] Bupropion was detected in urine in only 1 of 4 infants (infant was 6 week premature). The average milk/serum ratio was 1.3.

Pregnancy Risk	C	Lactation Risk	L3
T½	= 8–24 hours	M/P	= 2.51–8.58
Vd	= 40 l/kg	PB	= 75–88%
Tmax	= 2 hours	Oral	= 85%
MW	= 240	pKa	= 8.0

Adult Concerns: Seizures, restlessness, agitation, sleep disturbances. Probably contraindicated in patients with seizure disorders.

Pediatric Concerns: Thus far plasma levels in breastfed infants are undetectable. One case of seizure in a 6 month-old infant.

Drug Interactions: May increase clearance of diazepam, carbamazepine, phenytoin. May increase effects of MAO inhibitors.

Relative Infant Dose: 0.2%–2%

Adult Dose: 100 mg TID

Alternatives: Sertraline, Paroxetine

References:
1. Briggs GG, Samson JH, Ambrose PJ, Schroeder DH. Excretion of bupropion in breast milk. Ann Pharmacother 1993; 27(4): 431–433.
2. Baab SW, Peindl KS, Piontek CM, Wisner KL. Serum bupropion levels in 2 breastfeeding mother-infant pairs. J Clin Psychiatry. 2002; 63: 910–911.
3. Chaudron LH and Schoenecker CJ. Bupropion and breastfeeding: a case of possible infant seizure. (Letter) J. Clin. Psychiatry 2004: 64(6): 881–882
4. Haas JS, Kaplan CP, Barenboim D, Jacob P, III, Benowitz NL. Bupropion in breast milk: an exposure assessment for potential treatment to prevent postpartum tobacco use. Tob Control 2004 Mar; 13(1): 52–6.
5. Davis MF, Miller HS, Nolan PE, Jr. Bupropion levels in breast milk for 4 mother-infant pairs: more answers to lingering questions. J Clin Psychiatry. Feb 2009; 70(2): 297–298.

BUSPIRONE   L3

Trade: BuSpar

Other Trades: BuSpar, Apo-Buspirone, Novo-Buspirone

Category: Antianxiety medication

Buspirone is an antianxiety agent used in the treatment of generalized anxiety disorder. No data exists on excretion into human milk. It is secreted into animal milk, so the same would be expected in human milk.[1] Buspirone is mg for mg equivalent to diazepam in its anxiolytic properties but does not produce significant sedation or addiction as the benzodiazepine family. Its metabolite is partially active but has a brief half-life (4.8 hours) as well. Compared to the benzodiazepine family, this product would be a better choice for treatment of anxiety in breastfeeding women. Without accurate breastmilk levels, it is not known if the product is safe for breastfeeding women or the levels the infant would ingest daily. The rather brief half-life of this product and its metabolite would not likely lead to buildup in the infants plasma.

Pregnancy Risk	B	Lactation Risk	L3
T ½	= 2–3 hours	M/P	=
Vd	= 5.3 l/kg	PB	= 95%
Tmax	= 60–90 minutes	Oral	= 90%
MW	= 386	pKa	= 1.22, 7.32

Adult Concerns: Dizziness, nausea, drowsiness, fatigue, excitement, euphoria.

Pediatric Concerns: None reported.

Drug Interactions: Cimetidine may increase the effect of buspirone. Increased toxicity may occur when used with MAO inhibitors, phenothiazines, CNS depressants, digoxin and haloperidol.

Relative Infant Dose:

Adult Dose: 5 mg TID

Alternatives:

References:
1. Pharmaceutical manufacturer prescribing information, 1996.

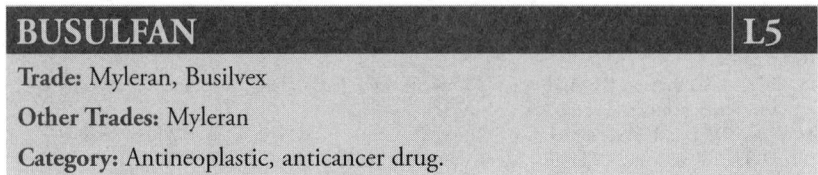

BUSULFAN   L5

Trade: Myleran, Busilvex

Other Trades: Myleran

Category: Antineoplastic, anticancer drug.

Busulfan is an alkylating agent used in chronic myeloid leukemia and bone marrow transplant. Oral absorption varies enormously but is probably 100%. Its elimination is described by a monoexponential curve with a plasma elimination half-life of approximately 2.6 hours. Volume of distribution varies but is reported to be two to three fold higher in young children.[1] No data are available on the transfer of busulfan into human milk. However, approximately 20% enters the CNS, which suggests similar amounts could enter the milk compartment. Busulfan is a potent antineoplastic agent that can produce severe bone marrow suppression, anemia, loss of blood cells, and elevated risk of infection.[1] It is not known if busulfan is distributed to human milk. No data are available concerning breastmilk concentrations, but this agent would be extremely toxic to growing infants and continued breastfeeding would not be justified. Use of this drug during breastfeeding is definitely not recommended.

Breastfeeding should be interrupted for a minimum of 24 hours following exposure to this agent.

Pregnancy Risk	D	Lactation Risk	L5
T ½	= 2.6 hours	M/P	=
Vd	= 0.94 l/kg	PB	= 14%
Tmax	= 0.5–2 hours	Oral	= Complete
MW	= 246	pKa	=

Adult Concerns: Severe bone marrow suppression, anemia, leukopenia, pulmonary fibrosis, cholestatic jaundice.

Pediatric Concerns: Extremely cytotoxic, use is not recommended in nursing women. Withhold breastfeeding for at least 24 hours following its use.

Drug Interactions: Antifungals may decrease the concentration of busulfan. Echinacea may decrease the effects of busulfan.

Relative Infant Dose:

Adult Dose: 1 mg/kg/dose every 6 hours (16 doses total)

Alternatives:

References:
1. Pharmaceutical manufacturer prescribing information, 2005.

BUTALBITAL COMPOUND   L3

Trade: Fioricet, Fiorinal, Bancap, Two-Dyne
Other Trades: Tecnal, Fiorinal
Category: Mild analgesic, sedative

Mild analgesic with acetaminophen (325mg) or aspirin, caffeine (40 mg), and butalbital (50 mg). Butalbital is a mild, short-acting barbiturate that probably transfers into breastmilk to a limited degree although it is unreported.[1] No data are available on the transfer of butalbital to breastmilk, but it is likely minimal.

Pregnancy Risk	C	Lactation Risk	L3
T ½	= 40–140 hours	M/P	=
Vd	= 0.8 l/kg	PB	= 26%
Tmax	= 40–60 minutes	Oral	= Complete
MW	= 224	pKa	= 12.15

Adult Concerns: Sedation.

Pediatric Concerns: Sedation.

Drug Interactions: Decreased effect when used with phenothiazines, haloperidol, cyclosporin, tricyclic antidepressants, and oral contraceptives. Increased effect when used with alcohol, benzodiazepines, CNS depressants, valproic acid, methylphenidate.

Relative Infant Dose:

Adult Dose: 50–100 mg every 4 hours

Alternatives:

References:
1. McEvoy GE. (ed): AFHS Drug Information. New York, NY: 2003.

BUTENAFINE   L3

Trade: Mentax, Lotrimin Ultra
Other Trades:
Category: Antifungal

Butenafine is a topical antifungal available in OTC medications.[1] It absorbs well into the skin, but does not appear to absorb greatly into the systemic circulation. It is unlikely that it would enter the milk compartment when applied through the topical route. There are currently no adequate and well-controlled studies or case reports in breastfeeding women.

Pregnancy Risk	C	Lactation Risk	L3
T ½	= 35 hours and >150 (biphasic)	M/P	=
Vd	=	PB	=
Tmax	= 6–15 hours	Oral	=
MW	= 353.93	pKa	=

Adult Concerns: Contact dermatitis, burning sensation, erythema, pruritus, local irritation.

Pediatric Concerns:

Drug Interactions:

Relative Infant Dose:

Adult Dose: Apply topically once daily for 2 weeks

Alternatives:

References:
1. Pharmaceutical manufacturer prescribing information, 2009.

BUTOCONAZOLE   L3

Trade: Gynazole-1, Mycelex-3
Other Trades: Femstat One
Category: Anti-fungal

Butoconazole nitrate is an imidazole derivative that has fungicidal activity *in vitro* against Candida species and has been demonstrated to be clinically effective against vaginal infections due to *Candida albicans*.[1] It is not known whether this drug is excreted in human milk. Absorption of the drug vaginally is 1.7%. Peak plasma levels 13.6–18.6 ng/mL. While it is not known whether this drug is excreted in human milk, vaginal absorption is low and plasma levels even lower. It is not likely this would produce untoward effects in a breastfed infant.

Pregnancy Risk	C	Lactation Risk	L3
T ½	= 12–24 hours	M/P	=
Vd	=	PB	=
Tmax	= 12–24 hours	Oral	= 5.5% (vaginal)
MW	= 474.8	pKa	=

Adult Concerns: Local irritation, burning, cramping, abdominal pain.

Pediatric Concerns:

Drug Interactions:

Relative Infant Dose:

Adult Dose: Insert one applicator as a single dose

Alternatives: Ketoconazole, clotrimazole, miconazole

References:
1.   Pharmaceutical manufacturer prescribing information, 2009.

BUTORPHANOL   L2

Trade: Stadol
Other Trades: Stadol
Category: Potent narcotic analgesic

Butorphanol is a potent narcotic analgesic. It is available as IV, IM, and a nasal spray. In one study of twelve breastfeeding women, six of whom received a single 2 mg IM dose, and 6 received a single 8 mg oral dose, the milk/serum ratio was constant over time and was 0.7 (intramuscular) and 1.9 (oral).[1] The average milk concentrations following a 2 mg IM dose, were 1.5, 0.7, and 0.3 µg/L at 2, 4 and 8 hours respectively. Following an oral dose of 8 mg, milk levels were 3.6, 1.8, and 1.1 µg/L at 3, 5, and 8 hours respectively. The elimination half-life in milk was approximately 2 hours. The estimated dose via milk is 0.1 µg/kg following an 8 mg oral dose, or 0.04 µg/kg following a 2 mg IM dose. The authors estimate that the infant would receive a maximum of only 4 micrograms butorphanol per day.

Levels received by infants are considered very low to insignificant. Butorphanol undergoes first-pass extraction by the liver, thus only 17% of the oral dose reaches the plasma. Butorphanol has been frequently used in labor and delivery in women who subsequently nursed their infants, although, it has been noted to produce a sinusoidal fetal heart rate pattern and dysphoric or psychotomimetic responses in infants. Butorphanol use in breastfeeding mothers is however, of minimum risk to the normal term infant.

Pregnancy Risk	C	Lactation Risk	L2
T ½	= 4.56 hours	M/P	= 0.7(IM)–1.9 (oral)
Vd	= 6.9 l/kg	PB	= 80%
Tmax	= 1 hour	Oral	= 17%
MW	= 327	pKa	= 8.6

Adult Concerns: Sedation, respiratory depression. There have been rare reports of infant respiratory distress/apnea following the administration of butorphanol injection during labor. The reports of respiratory distress/apnea have been associated with administration of a dose within 2 hours of delivery, use of multiple doses, use with additional analgesic or sedative drugs, or use in preterm pregnancies. In a study of 119 patients, the administration of 1 mg of IV butorphanol injection during labor was associated with transient sinusoidal fetal heart rate patterns, but was not associated with adverse neonatal outcomes.

Pediatric Concerns: None reported via milk but sedation is possible in newborns.

Drug Interactions: May produce increased toxicity when used with CNS depressants, other opiates, phenothiazines, barbiturates, benzodiazepines, MAO inhibitors.

Relative Infant Dose: 0.5%

Adult Dose: 1–4 mg IM every 3–4 hours

Alternatives: Ibuprofen, acetaminophen, hydrocodone

References:
1. Pittman KA, Smyth RD, Losada M, Zighelboim I, Maduska AL, Sunshine A. Human perinatal distribution of butorphanol. Am J Obstet Gynecol 1980; 138(7 Pt 1): 797–800.

C-1 ESTERASE INHIBITOR   L3

Trade: Cinryze, Berinert

Other Trades:

Category: Serine Proteinase Inhibitor

C-1 esterase inhibitor is one of the serine proteinase inhibitors normally found in human blood. This endogenous C-1 inhibitor regulates the fibrinolytic system and also regulates the activation of the complement and intrinsic coagulation pathways. C-1 esterase inhibitor is used prophylactically in adolescents and adults with Hereditary Angioedema (HAE) to prevent recurrent episodes of angioedema.[1] In a study by Martinez-Saguer et al, no adverse effects were noted in 35 infants whose mothers were treated during pregnancy and lactation.[2] Due to the large molecular weight (105,000 kd) of C-1 esterase inhibitor, it is not expected to be found in large amounts in breastmilk. This constituent of plasma would also be unstable in the gastrointestinal tract of the infant.

Pregnancy Risk	C	Lactation Risk	L3
T ½	= single dose 56.36 hours; double dose 62 ± 38 hours	M/P	=
Vd	=	PB	=
Tmax	= single dose 3.9 ± 7.3; double dose 2.7 ± 1.9	Oral	= nil
MW	= 104,000 to 105,00	pKa	=

Adult Concerns: Most common side effects are upper respiratory infections, sinusitis, rash and headache; less common side effects are bronchitis, limb injury, back pain, pain in extremity and pruritus.

Pediatric Concerns:

Drug Interactions:

Relative Infant Dose:

Adult Dose: 1000 units every 3 to 4 days IV for prophylaxis; administered 1 ml per minute

Alternatives:

References:
1. Pharmaceutical manufacturer prescribing information
2. Martinez-Saguer I, Rusicke E, Aygoren-Pursun E, Heller C, Klingebiel T, and Kreuz W. Characterization of acute hereditary angioedema attacks during pregnancy and breast-feeding and their treatment with C1 inhibitor concentrate. Am J Obstet Gynecol 2010; 203: 131. e1–7.

CABERGOLINE   L4

Trade: Dostinex
Other Trades: Dostinex
Category: Inhibits prolactin secretion

Cabergoline is a long-acting synthetic ergot alkaloid derivative which produces a dopamine agonist effect similar to but much safer than bromocriptine. Cabergoline directly inhibits prolactin secretion by the pituitary.[1] It is primarily indicated for pathological hyperprolactinemia, but in several European studies, it has been used for inhibition of postpartum lactation.[2]

The dose regimen used for the inhibition of physiologic lactation is cabergoline 1 mg administered as a single dose on the first day postpartum. For the suppression of established lactation, cabergoline 0.25 mg is taken every 12 hours for 2 days for a total of 1 mg. Single doses of 1 mg have been found to completely inhibit postpartum lactation.[3] Transfer into human milk is not reported. In patients with hyperprolactinemia, it is possible to carefully administer doses to lower the prolactin to safe ranges, but high enough to retain lactation. In such cases, the infant should be observed for potential ergot side effects, if any. In addition, mothers treated with cabergoline early postpartum, may in some cases recover their milk supply following pumping and extensive breastfeeding.

Pregnancy Risk	B	Lactation Risk	L4
T ½	= 63–69 hours	M/P	=
Vd	=	PB	= 40–42%
Tmax	= 2–3 hours	Oral	= Complete
MW	= 451	pKa	= 17.07

Adult Concerns: Headache, dizziness, fatigue, orthostatic hypotension, nose bleed, inhibition of lactation.

Pediatric Concerns: Transfer via milk is unknown. Completely suppresses lactation and should not be used in mothers who are breastfeeding.

Drug Interactions: Do not use with other dopamine antagonists such as the phenothiazines (Thorazine,etc), butyrophenones (Haldol), thioxanthines, and metoclopramide (Reglan).

Relative Infant Dose:

Adult Dose: 0.25–1 mg twice a week

Alternatives:

References:
1. Caballero-Gordo A, Lopez-Nazareno N, Calderay M, Caballero JL, Mancheno E, Sghedoni D. Oral cabergoline. Single-dose inhibition of puerperal lactation. J Reprod Med 1991; 36(10): 717–721.
2. Single dose cabergoline versus bromocriptine in inhibition of puerperal lactation: randomised, double blind, multicentre study. European Multicentre Study Group for Cabergoline in Lactation Inhibition BMJ 1991; 302(6789): 1367–1371.
3. Bravo-Topete EG, Mendoza-Hernandez F, Cejudo-Alvarez J, Briones-Garduno C. Cabergoline for inhibition of lactation. Cir Cir 2004; 72(1): 5–9.

CAFFEINE   L2

Trade:

Other Trades:

Category: CNS stimulant

Caffeine is a naturally occurring CNS stimulant present in many foods and drinks. While the half-life in adults is 4.9 hours, the half-life in neonates is as high as 97.5 hours. The half-life decreases with age to 14 hours at 3–5 months and 2.6 hours at 6 months and older. The average cup of coffee contains 100–150 mg of caffeine depending on preparation and country of origin.

Peak levels of caffeine are found in breast milk 60–120 minutes after ingestion. In a study of 5 patients following an ingestion of 150 mg caffeine, peak concentrations of caffeine in serum ranged from 2.39 to 4.05 µg/mL and peak concentrations in milk ranged from 1.4 to 2.41 mg/L with a milk/serum ratio of 0.52.[1] The average milk concentration at 30, 60, and 120 minutes post dose was 1.58, 1.49, and 0.926 mg/L respectively. In another study of 7 breastfeeding mothers who consumed 750 mg caffeine/day for 5 days, and were 11– 22 days postpartum, the average milk concentration was 4.3 mg/L.[2] Values ranged significantly from non detectable to 15.7 mg/L. The mean concentration of caffeine in sera of the infants on day 5 was 1.4 µg/mL (range non detectable to 2.8 µg/mL). In two patients whose milk levels were 13.4 and 28 mg/L, the respective infant serum levels were 0.25 and 3.2 µg/mL. In a study of 6 breastfeeding mothers who received one dose of 100 mg PO, peak levels (C_{max}) in maternal serum ranged from 0.5 to 1 hour and 0.75 to 2 hours in milk.[3] The maternal plasma C_{max} ranged from 3.6 to 6.15 µg/mL, while the C_{max} for their milk ranged from 1.98 to 4.3 mg/L. The average concentration of caffeine in milk was 2.45 mg/L at 1 hour. The average milk/plasma ratio (AUC) was 0.812 for both breasts. This elegant study shows that caffeine rapidly enters milk and that the decay of caffeine in milk is similar to that of plasma. In infants from 4 to 7 kg body weight, the estimated dose to the infant would be 1.77 to 3.10 mg/d following a 100 mg maternal dose. In a group of mothers who ingested from 35 to 336 mg of caffeine daily, the level of caffeine in milk ranged from 2.09 to 7.17 mg/L.[4] The author estimates the dose to infant is at 0.01 to 1.64 mg/d or 0.06% to 1.5% of the maternal dose. An interesting review of the nutritional effects of caffeine ingestion on infants is provided by Nehlig.[5] There is some evidence that chronic coffee drinking may reduce the iron content of milk. Irritability and insomnia may occur and have been reported.[6] Occasional use of caffeine is not contraindicated, but persistent, chronic use may lead to high plasma levels in the infant particularly during the neonatal period.

Pregnancy Risk	C	Lactation Risk	L2
T ½	= 4.9 hours	M/P	= 0.52–0.76
Vd	= 0.4–0.6 l/kg	PB	= 36%
Tmax	= 60 minutes	Oral	= 100%
MW	= 194	pKa	= 0.8

Adult Concerns: Agitation, irritability, poor sleeping patterns.

Pediatric Concerns: Rarely, irritability and insomnia.

Drug Interactions: Reduces vasodilation of adenosine. Reduces bioavailability of alendronate by 60%. Cimetidine reduces caffeine clearance by 50%. Fluoroquinolone antibiotics increases half-life of caffeine by 5 to 8 hours.

Relative Infant Dose: 6%–25.9%

Adult Dose:

Alternatives:

References:
1. Tyrala EE, Dodson WE. Caffeine secretion into breast milk. Arch Dis Child 1979; 54(10): 787–800.
2. Ryu JE. Caffeine in human milk and in serum of breast-fed infants. Dev Pharmacol Ther 1985; 8(6): 329–337.
3. Stavchansky S, Combs A, Sagraves R, Delgado M, Joshi A. Pharmacokinetics of caffeine in breast milk and plasma after single oral administration of caffeine to lactating mothers. Biopharm Drug Dispos 1988; 9(3): 285–299.
4. Berlin CM, Jr., Denson HM, Daniel CH, Ward RM. Disposition of dietary caffeine in milk, saliva, and plasma of lactating women. Pediatrics 1984; 73(1): 59–63.
5. Nehlig A, Debry G. Consequences on the newborn of chronic maternal consumption of coffee during gestation and lactation: a review. J Am Coll Nutr 1994; 13(1): 6–21.
6. Munoz LM, Lonnerdal B, Keen CL, Dewey KG. Coffee consumption as a factor in iron deficiency anemia among pregnant women and their infants in Costa Rica. Am J Clin Nutr. 1988; 48: 645–51. PMID: 3414579

CALCIPOTRIENE   L3

Trade: Dovonex, Taclonex Scalp, Sorilux Foam

Other Trades: Dovonex

Category: Synthetic Vitamin D_3 used for treatment of psoriasis

Calcipotriene is a synthetic vitamin D_3 derivative used topically for the treatment of plaque psoriasis.[1] Only 5–6% is transcutaneously absorbed into the systemic circulation (via ointment). It is rapidly bound to plasma proteins, and excreted by the liver via bile. Less than 1% is absorbed from the scalp when the solution is used. It is unlikely plasma levels of calcipotriene would be elevated at all, and milk levels would be virtually nil because vitamin D transport to milk is normally quite low. Calcipotriene is active however, and if used over wide areas of the body could (but unlikely) lead to some absorption. However, hypercalcemia in treated patients has been reported only rarely.

Taclonex Scalp Topical Suspension contains 52.18 µg of calcipotriene hydrate and 0.643 mg of betamethasone dipropionate.

Sorilux Foam is a vitamin D analog indicated for the topical treatment of plaque psoriasis in patients aged 18 years and older.

Pregnancy Risk	C		Lactation Risk	L3
T ½	=		M/P	=
Vd	=		PB	=
Tmax	=		Oral	= Variable
MW	= 430		pKa	= 15.29

Adult Concerns: Adverse events include skin irritation, rare but reversible hypercalcemia, rash, pruritus, and worsening of psoriasis. .

Pediatric Concerns: None reported via milk but no studies are available. Adverse effects in a breastfed infant are unlikely if the surface area treated is moderate to low.

Drug Interactions: Vitamin D Analogs may increase the concentration of Aluminum Hydroxide. It may also increase the effect of cardiac glycosides. It may increase the concentration of Sucralfate. Thiazide diuretics may increase the hypercalcemic effects of Vitamin D Analogs.

Relative Infant Dose:

Adult Dose: Apply to skin lesions twice daily.

Alternatives:

References:
1. Pharmaceutical manufacturer Package Insert, 2009.

CALCITONIN   L3

Trade: Calcimar, Salmonine, Osteocalcin, Miacalcin
Other Trades: Calcitare, Calsynar, Miacalcic, Caltine, Calcimar
Category: Calcium metabolism

Calcitonin is a large polypeptide hormone (32 amino acids) secreted by the parafollicular cells of the thyroid that inhibits osteoclastic bone resorption, thus, maintaining calcium homeostasis in mammals.[1] It is used for control of postmenopausal osteoporosis and other calcium metabolic diseases. Calcitonins are destroyed by gastric acids, requiring parenteral (SC, IM) or intranasal dosing. Calcitonin is unlikely to penetrate human milk due to its large molecular weight. Further, its oral bioavailability is nil due to destruction in the gastrointestinal tract. It has been reported to inhibit lactation in animals although this has not been reported in humans.[2]

Pregnancy Risk	C		Lactation Risk	L3
T ½	= 43 minutes		M/P	=
Vd	= 0.15–0.3 l/kg		PB	= 30–40%
Tmax	= 23 minutes		Oral	= None
MW	= 3454.93		pKa	=

Adult Concerns: Nausea, facial flushing, back pain, headache, arthralgia, shivering, edema, metallic taste, and increased urinary frequency.

Pediatric Concerns: None reported via milk. Unlikely to enter milk. Calcitonins have been reported to inhibit lactation in animals.

Drug Interactions: It is reported that ketoprofen inhibits the calciuric and uricosuric effect of porcine calcitonin. May have additive effect with plicamycin.

Relative Infant Dose:

Adult Dose: 50–100 units (salmon) three times weekly

Alternatives:

References:

1. Pharmaceutical manufacturer prescribing information, 1997.
2. Fiore CE, Petralito A, Mazzarino MC, Liuzzo A, Malaponte G, Mangiafico RA, Gibiino S. Effects of ketoprofen on the calciuric and uricosuric activities of calcitonin in man. J Endocrinol Invest 1981; 4(1): 81–84.

CALCITRIOL   L3

Trade: Rocaltrol

Other Trades: Rocaltrol

Category: Vitamin D analog

Vitamin D typically undergoes a series of metabolic steps to become active. Calcitriol (1,25 dihydro cholecalciferol) is believed to be the active metabolite of vitamin D metabolism. Calcitriol is the most potent of the synthetic vitamin D analogs. It is indicated for treatment of hypocalcemia in patients undergoing chronic renal dialysis, and renal osteodystrophy. Calcitriol is also indicated in patients with severe liver dysfunction and who are unable to hydroxylate dihydrotachysterol to its active form. Because calcitriol works more quickly, it is useful in the treatment of patients with severe hypocalcemia. Calcitriol is well absorbed from the GI tract with a peak at 3–6 hours.[1] It is 99.9% protein bound to a specific alpha-globulin vitamin D binding protein. The elimination half-life is about 5–8 hours in adults and 27 hours in pediatric age patients. However, plasma levels are quite low, averaging approximately 40 pg/mL. Transfer of calcitriol into human milk is reported to be 2.2 pg/mL.[2] It is not likely that normal doses of this vitamin D analog would lead to clinically relevant levels in human milk, particularly since vitamin D transfers only minimally into human milk anyway. While plasma levels of vitamin D are normally quite low in human milk (<20 IU/L), at least one study now suggests that supplementing a mother with extraordinarily high levels of vitamin D_2 can elevate milk levels, and subsequently lead to hypercalcemia in a breastfed infant.[3] See Vitamin D for new data.

Pregnancy Risk	C		Lactation Risk	L3
T ½	= 5–8 hours		M/P	=
Vd	=		PB	= 99.9%
Tmax	= 3–6 hours		Oral	= Complete
MW	= 416		pKa	= 15.29

Adult Concerns: Overdosage of any form of vitamin D is dangerous and could lead to severe hypercalcemia, hypercalciuria, and hyperphosphatemia. Hypercalcemia may subsequently lead to vascular calcification, nephrocalcinosis, and other soft-tissue calcification. Early symptoms include weakness, headache, somnolence, nausea, vomiting, dry mouth, constipation, muscle pain, bone pain and metallic taste. Late symptoms include polyuria, polydipsia, anorexia, weight loss, nocturia, conjunctivitis (calcific), pancreatitis, photophobia, rhinorrhea, pruritus, hyperthermia, decreased libido, elevated BUN, albuminuria, hypercholesterolemia, elevated liver aminotransferases, ectopic calcification, hypertension, cardiac arrhythmias and, rarely, overt psychosis.

Pediatric Concerns: None reported via milk, but caution recommended at higher doses.

Drug Interactions: Cholestyramine, colestipol may reduce the oral absorption of calcitriol. Hypercalcemia may result from adding thiazide diuretics in patients receiving calcitriol. Ketoconazole, may reduce calcitriol concentrations in plasma. A functional antagonism can occur by adding corticosteroids to calcitriol. Avoid high-dose calcium supplements. Magnesium-containing antacid and calcitriol injection should not be used concomitantly, because such use may lead to the development of hypermagnesemia.

Relative Infant Dose:

Adult Dose: Variable, but 0.25–0.5 µg/day initially.

Alternatives: Vitamin D

References:
1. Pharmaceutical manufacturer prescribing information, 2003.
2. Teva Pharmaceuticals USA manufacturer prescribing information, 2008.
3. Greer FR, Hollis BW, Napoli JL. High concentrations of vitamin D_2 in human milk associated with pharmacologic doses of vitamin D_2. J Pediatr 1984; 105(1): 61–64.

CALCIUM SALT   L3

Trade:

Other Trades:

Category: Calcium supplement

Calcium salts comes in different forms such as calcium carbonate, calcium lactate, calcium gluconate, calcium citrate and etc. Calcium salt is used as an antacid and for treatment and prevention of calcium deficiency or hyperphosphatemia (such as osteoporosis or mild to moderate renal insufficiency). Recommended dietary allowance for calcium in breastfeeding women is 1000 mg/day. Milk-alkali syndrome during pregnancy has been associated with excessive intake of calcium carbonate antacids.[1] Calcium supplementation does not provide lactation benefits during late pregnancy or lactation.[2,3] Symptoms of milk-alkali syndrome (hypercalcemia) are nausea, vomiting, weight loss, thirst, muscle weakness and confusion.

Pregnancy Risk	Probably Safe	Lactation Risk	L3
T ½	=	M/P	=
Vd	=	PB	=
Tmax	=	Oral	=
MW	=	pKa	=

Adult Concerns: Constipation, headache, nausea, vomiting, dry mouth, flatulence, hypercalcemia, hypophosphatemia, milk-alkali syndrome.

Pediatric Concerns:

Drug Interactions: Antacids may decrease the concentration of ACE Inhibitors.

It may decrease the concentration of HMG-CoA Reductase Inhibitors. It may also decrease the absorption of Allopurinol. It may decrease the effect of Calcium Channel Blockers. It may decrease the bioavailability of Corticosteroids.

Relative Infant Dose:

Adult Dose: 1000 mg daily

Alternatives:

References:
1. Ulliam ME, Linas SL: Themilk-alkali syndrome in pregnancy. Casereport. Miner Electrolyte Metab14: 208–10, 1988.
2. Karandish M, Djazayery A, MahmoodiM, Behrooz A, Moremazi F: The Effect OfCalcium Supplementation During PregnancyOn Breast Milk Calcium Concentration: ADouble Blind Placebo Controlled ClinicalTrial. J Pediatr Gastroenterol Nutr2004; 39(Suppl 1): S472.
3. Prentice A, Jarjou LM, Cole TJ, etal: Calcium requirements of lactatingGambian mothers: effects of a calciumsupplement on breast-milk calciumconcentration, maternal bone mineralcontent, and urinary calcium excretion. Am J Clin Nutr 1995; 62: 58–67.

CALENDULA | L3

Trade:

Other Trades:

Category: Herbal wound healing

Calendula, grown worldwide, has been used topically to promote wound healing and to alleviate conjunctivitis and other ocular inflammations. It consists of a number of flavonol glycosides and saponins, but the active ingredients are unknown.[1] Despite these claims, there are almost no studies regarding its efficacy in any of these disorders. Further, there are no suggestions of overt toxicity, with exception of allergies. It should not be used in pregnant patients.[2] Although it may have some uses externally, its internal use as an antiphlogistic and spasmolytic is largely obsolete.

No data are available on its transfer into human milk.

Pregnancy Risk	X	Lactation Risk	L3
T ½	=	M/P	=
Vd	=	PB	=
Tmax	=	Oral	= Good
MW	=	pKa	=

Adult Concerns: Allergies, anaphylactoid shock.

Pediatric Concerns: None reported via milk.

Drug Interactions: Caution when using calendula with sedative drugs. Calendula has been reported to increase hexobarbital sleep time in animal modes.

Relative Infant Dose:

Adult Dose: One cup of the tea (1–2 grams of the dried flowers) three times daily.

Alternatives:

References:

1. Bissett NG. In: Herbal Drugs and Phytopharmaceuticals. Medpharm Scientific Publishers, CRC Press, Boca Raton, 1994.
2. Natural Medicines Comprehensive Database, 2010.

CAMPHOR   L3

Trade:

Other Trades:

Category: Antipruritic, cooling agent

Camphor is transparent waxy product with a strong odor and is derived from the wood of Cinnamomum camphora. Used in medicine for centuries, it can be absorbed transcutaneously producing a cooling sensation. It is commonly added to topical products to produce antipruritic and cooling effects.[1] It is available in balm, cream, gel, liquid and ointment forms. When ingested in large amounts, it may be toxic producing CNS stimulation, nausea, vomiting, and hepatotoxicity.

There are no adequate and well-controlled studies in breastfeeding women. Used topically, on small areas of the body, it is probably relatively safe to use in breastfeeding mothers.

Pregnancy Risk	C	Lactation Risk	L3
T ½	=	M/P	=
Vd	= 2–4 l/kg	PB	=
Tmax	=	Oral	= Complete
MW	= 152	pKa	=

Adult Concerns: Confusion, contact eczema, hallucinations, nausea and vomiting, seizures, tremors, vertigo, warmth, and headache.

Pediatric Concerns: Neonatal respiratory failure and death have been reported from oral ingestion, not from breastfeeding.

Drug Interactions:

Relative Infant Dose:

Adult Dose:

Alternatives:

References:
1. Pharmaceutical manufacturer prescribing information,2011.

CANDESARTAN   L3

Trade: Atacand, Amias

Other Trades:

Category: Antihypertensive agent

Candesartan is a specific blocker of the receptor site (AT1) for angiotensin II. It is typically used as an antihypertensive similar to the ACE inhibitor family.[1] Both the ACE inhibitor family and the specific AT1 receptor blockers such as candesartan are contraindicated in the 2nd and 3rd trimesters of pregnancy due to severe hypotension, neonatal skull hypoplasia, irreversible renal failure, and death in the newborn infant. Never use in pregnant women past the first trimester.

Some of the ACE inhibitors can be used in breastfeeding mothers postpartum without major risk, in some cases with due caution. However, no data are available on candesartan in human milk although the manufacturer states that it is present in rodent milk. Some caution is recommended in the neonatal period and particularly when used in mothers with premature infants.

Pregnancy Risk	C/D in 2nd and 3rd trimester	Lactation Risk	L3
T ½	= 9 hours	M/P	=
Vd	= 0.13 l/kg	PB	= >99%
Tmax	= 3–4 hours	Oral	= 15%
MW	= 611	pKa	= 8.15

Adult Concerns: Headache, back pain, pharyngitis, and dizziness have been reported. The use of ACE inhibitors and angiotensin receptor blockers during pregnancy or the neonatal period is extremely dangerous and has resulted in hypotension, neonatal skull hypoplasia, anuria, renal failure and death. Other side effects include asthenia, fever, paresthesia, vertigo, dyspepsia, gastroenteritis, tachycardia, palpitations, hyperglycemia, hypertriglyceridemia, hyperuricemia, myalgia, platelet/bleeding and clotting disorders, anxiety, depression, somnolence, dyspnea, rash, increased sweating and hematuria.

Pediatric Concerns: None reported via milk. Caution is recommended in the early postpartum period. Do not expose infants and children < 1 year of age to candesartan. The consequences of administering drugs that act directly on the renin-angiotensin system (RAS) can have effects on the development of immature kidneys.

Drug Interactions: Caution when used concomitantly with NSAIDs, especially in hose with compromised renal function. Concomitant use with lithium may result in increased plasma lithium levels and subsequent lithium toxicity.

Relative Infant Dose:

Adult Dose: 4–32 mg daily

Alternatives: Captopril, Enalapril

References:
1. Pharmaceutical manufacturer prescribing information, 2010.

CANDIN   L3

Trade:

Other Trades:

Category: Skin test antigen

Candin is a *Candida albicans* skin test antigen used to evaluate for cellular immune response in those suspected to have reduced cellular immunity.[1] This product is prepared from the culture filtrate and strains of C. albicans. When administered intradermally in immunocompetent individuals, a delayed type hypersensitivity response is elicited within 48 hours. An induration of >=5 mm at the site of injection represents adequate cellular immunity. There are currently no studies done on its use in breastfeeding women. However, since only very little amounts of the antigen is used for this test (0.1 mL), plasma concentrations attained after its injection are probably too low to cause significant transfer into breastmilk.

Pregnancy Risk	C		Lactation Risk	L3
T ½	=		M/P	=
Vd	=		PB	=
Tmax	=		Oral	=
MW	=		pKa	=

Adult Concerns: Redness, swelling, itching, excoriation at the site of injection. Severe hypersensitivity reactions may occur. Use caution while administering in those with bleeding disorders.

Pediatric Concerns:

Drug Interactions: Corticosteroid therapy may alter the test results.

Relative Infant Dose:

Adult Dose: 0.1 mL intradermal.

Alternatives:

References:
1. Pharmaceutical manufacturer prescribing information, 2000.

CANNABIS   L5

Trade: Marijuana, Tetrahydrocannabinol
Other Trades:
Category: Sedative, hallucinogen

Studies concerning the use of Cannabis in pregnant women appear to be inconsistent in their results. Cannabis should not be used during pregnancy or breastfeeding, despite possible application for stimulating hunger in "failure-to-thrive" infants.

Commonly called marijuana, the active component delta-9–THC (Tetrahydrocannabinol) is rapidly distributed to the brain and adipose tissue. It is stored in fat tissues for long periods (weeks to months). Small to moderate secretion into breastmilk has been documented.[1] In one mother who consumed marijuana once daily, milk levels were reportedly 105 µg/L. In another mother who consumed marijuana 7–8 time daily, milk levels of THC were 340 µg/L.[1] Analysis of breastmilk in a chronic heavy user revealed an eight fold accumulation in breastmilk compared to plasma although the dose received is apparently insufficient to produce significant side effects in the infant. Studies have shown significant absorption and metabolism in infants although long term sequela are conflicting. In one study of 27 women who smoked marijuana routinely during breastfeeding, no differences were noted in outcomes on growth, mental, and motor development.[2]

In another study, marijuana in breastmilk was shown to be associated with a slight decrease in infant motor development at one year of age, especially when used during the first month of lactation.[3] This study's data was conflicted however, by the use of marijuana during the first trimester of pregnancy. Interestingly, in this study, maternal use of marijuana during pregnancy and lactation had no detectable effect on infant mental development at one year of age.[3]

Another study of low-risk, predominantly middle-class infants found that the use of marijuana during lactation produced no effect.[4] Prenatal exposure to marijuana was not significantly related to any growth measures at birth, although a smaller head circumference observed at all ages reached statistical significance among the early adolescents (9–12 years of age) born to the heavy marijuana users. Studies in animals suggests that marijuana inhibits prolactin production and could inhibit lactation. One study with 16 women found that plasma prolactin levels were significantly lowered with marijuana smoking during the luteal phase of the menstrual cycle.[5] This drug should not be used by nursing mothers. Infants exposed to marijuana via breastmilk will test positive in urine screens for long periods of time (2–3 weeks).

One article reports that binding of THC to cannabinoid receptors may regulate a variety of hormone secretions from the anterior pituitary and have profound effects on the Hypothalmic-Pituitary-Gonadal (HPG) axis. The main effect is inhibiting the release of gonadotropin, prolactin, growth hormone, and thyroid-stimulating hormone and stimulating the release of corticotropin. Thus, major changes in the reproductive system, lactation, metabolism, and stress systems are possible.[6]

Pregnancy Risk	C	Lactation Risk	L5
T ½	= 25–57 hours	M/P	= 8
Vd	= 4–19 l/kg	PB	= 99.9%
Tmax	=	Oral	= 6–20%
MW	= 314	pKa	=

Adult Concerns: Sedation, weakness, poor feeding patterns. Possible decreased milk production.

Pediatric Concerns: Sedation. Urine will be drug screen positive for weeks.

Drug Interactions:

Relative Infant Dose:

Adult Dose:

Alternatives:

References:
1. Perez-Reyes M, Wall ME. Presence of delta9-tetrahydrocannabinol in human milk. N Engl J Med 1982; 307(13): 819–820.
2. Tennes K, Avitable N, Blackard C, Boyles C, Hassoun B, Holmes L, Kreye M. Marijuana: prenatal and postnatal exposure in the human. NIDA Res Monogr 1985; 59: 48–60.
3. Astley SJ, Little RE. Maternal Marijuana Use During Lactation and Infant Development at One Year. Neurotoxicol Teratol 1990; 12: 161–168.

4. Fried PA, Watkinson B, Gray R. Growth from birth to early adolescence in offspring prenatally exposed to cigarettes and marijuana. Neurotoxicol Teratol. 1999 ; 21: 513–25.
5. Mendelson, J. H., N. K. Mello, et al. (1985). "Acute effects of marihuana smoking on prolactin levels in human females. " J Pharmacol Exp Ther 232(1): 220–222.
6. Murphy, L. L., R. M. Munoz, et al. (1998). "Function of cannabinoid receptors in the neuroendocrine regulation of hormone secretion. " Neurobiol Dis 5(6 Pt B): 432–446.

CAPECITABINE   L5

Trade: Xeloda

Other Trades:

Category: Anticancer drug

Capecitabine is an antineoplastic agent commonly used in the treatment of colon cancer. It is converted enzymatically to the active drug 5–Fluorouracil.[1] Capecitabine is readily absorbed orally and rapidly metabolized in most tissues to 5–FU in about two hours following administration.

5–Fluorouracil is well absorbed orally, but poorly absorbed transcutaneously. Milk levels have not yet been published. Breastfeeding is probably fine if exposure is due to topical application over small to moderate areas (not large areas). If used orally, or intravenously in significant doses, a suitable waiting period should be used to avoid exposure of the infant. Because it has only a 12 minute half-life, a few hours, or better, 24 hours would probably reduce any risk from this agent. The injection into the intraocular space would prolong the release of 5FU into the plasma. But the dose is so low, it is unlikely to cause significant exposure to a breastfeeding infant via breastmilk.

Pregnancy Risk	D	Lactation Risk	L5
T ½	= 38–45 minutes	M/P	=
Vd	=	PB	= <60%
Tmax	= 1.5 hours	Oral	=
MW	= 359.4	pKa	= 12.59

Adult Concerns: Diarrhea, pain, blistering, peeling, redness, or swelling of palms of hands and/or bottoms of feet; sores, or ulcers in mouth or on lips.

Pediatric Concerns:

Drug Interactions: Echinacea may decrease the effects of immunosuppressants. It may increase the concentration of phenytoin. It may increase the concentration of Vitamin K Antagonists, such as Warfarin. Tacrolimus may enhance the adverse effects of immunosuppressants.

Relative Infant Dose:

Adult Dose: 1000 mg/m² twice daily for two weeks every 21 days

Alternatives:

References:
1. Pharmaceutical manufacturer prescribing information, 2005.

CAPSAICIN   L3

Trade: Pepper Spray
Other Trades:
Category: Analgesic, topical

Capsaicin is an alkaloid derived from peppers from the Solanaceae family. It is commonly found in Pepper Spray devices. Used topically, it increases, depletes, and then suppresses substance P release from sensory neurons, thus preventing pain sensation. Substance P is the principal chemomediator of pain from the periphery to the CNS.[1,2] After repeated application (days to weeks), it depletes substance P and prevents reaccumulation in the neuron. Very little or nothing is known about the kinetics of this product. It is approved for use in children >2 years of age. No data are available on transfer into human milk. However, topical application to the nipple or areola should be avoided unless it is thoroughly removed prior to breastfeeding.

Pregnancy Risk	C	Lactation Risk	L3
T ½	= 1.64 hours	M/P	=
Vd	=	PB	=
Tmax	=	Oral	= None
MW	= 305	pKa	= 9.5

Adult Concerns: Local irritation, burning, stinging, erythema. Cough and infrequently neurotoxicity. Avoid use near eyes, or on the nipple.

Pediatric Concerns: None reported. Avoid transfer to eye and other sensitive surfaces via hand contact.

Drug Interactions: May increase risk of cough with ACE inhibitors.

Relative Infant Dose:

Adult Dose: Apply to affected area 3–4 times a day

Alternatives:

References:
1. Bernstein JE. Capsaicin in dermatologic disease. Semin Dermatol 1988; 7(4): 304–309.
2. Watson CP, Evans RJ, Watt VR. The post-mastectomy pain syndrome and the effect of topical capsaicin. Pain 1989; 38(2): 177–186.

CAPTOPRIL   L2

Trade: Capoten
Other Trades: Acenorm, Enzace, Capoten, Apo-Capto, Novo-Captopril, Acepril
Category: Antihypertensive drug (ACE inhibitor)

Captopril is a typical angiotensin converting enzyme inhibitor (ACE) used to reduce hypertension. In one report of 12 women treated with 100 mg three times daily, maternal serum levels averaged 713 μg/L while breast milk levels averaged

4.7 µg/L at 3.8 hours after administration.[1] Data from this study suggest that an infant would ingest approximately 0.002% of the free captopril consumed by its mother (300 mg) on a daily basis. No adverse effects have been reported in this study. Use with care in mothers with premature infants.

Pregnancy Risk	C/D in 2nd and 3rd trimester	Lactation Risk	L2
T ½	= 2.2 hours	M/P	= 0.012
Vd	= 0.7 l/kg	PB	= 30%
Tmax	= 1 hour	Oral	= 60–75%
MW	= 217	pKa	= 3.7, 9.8

Adult Concerns: Hypotension, bradycardia, decreased urine output and possible seizures. A decrease in taste acuity or metallic taste.

Pediatric Concerns: None reported but observe for hypotension.

Drug Interactions: Probenecid increases plasma levels of captopril. Captopril and diuretics have additive hypotensive effects. Antacids reduce bioavailability of ACE inhibitors. NSAIDS reduce hypotension of ACE inhibitors. Phenothiazines increase effects of ACE inhibitors. Allopurinol may increase risk of Steven-Johnson's syndrome when admixed with captopril. ACEIs increase digoxin and lithium plasma levels. May elevate potassium levels when potassium supplementation is added.

Relative Infant Dose:

Adult Dose: 50 mg TID

Alternatives: Enalapril, benazepril

References:
1. Devlin R. Selective resistance to the passage of captopril into human milk. Clin Pharmacol Ther 27: 250, 1980.

CARBAMAZEPINE   L2

Trade: Tegretol, Epitol, Carbatrol
Other Trades: Teril, Apo-Carbamazepine, Mazepine, Tegretol
Category: Anticonvulsant

Carbamazepine (CBZ) is a unique anticonvulsant commonly used for grand mal, clonic-tonic, simple and complex seizures. It is also used in manic depression and a number of other neurologic syndromes. It is one of the most commonly used anticonvulsants in pediatric patients.

In a brief study by Kaneko, with maternal plasma levels averaging 4.3 µg/mL, milk levels were 1.9 mg/L.[1] In a study of 3 patients who received from 5.8 to 7.3 mg/kg/day carbamazepine, milk levels were reported to vary from 1.3 to 1.8 mg/L while the epoxide metabolite varied from 0.5 to 1.1 mg/L.[2] No adverse effects were noted in any of the infants.

In another study by Niebyl, breast milk levels were 1.4 mg/L in the lipid fraction and 2.3 mg/L in the skim fraction in a mother receiving 1000 mg daily of carbamazepine.[3] This author estimated a daily intake of 2 mg carbamazepine daily (0.5 mg/kg) in an infant ingesting 1 liter of milk per day. In a study of CBZ and its epoxide metabolite (ECBZ) in milk, 16 patients received an average dose of 13.8 mg/kg/day.[4] The average maternal serum levels of CBZ and ECBZ were 7.1 and 2.6 μg/mL respectively. The average milk levels of CBZ and ECBZ were 2.5 and 1.5 mg/L respectively. The relative percent of CBZ and ECBZ in milk were 36.4% and 53% of the maternal serum levels. A total of 50 milk samples in 19 patients were analyzed. Of these, the lowest CBZ concentration in milk was 1.0 mg/L; the highest was 4.8 mg/L. The CBZ level was determined in 7 infants 4–7 days postpartum. All infants have CBZ levels below 1.5 μg/mL.

In a study of 7 women receiving 250–800 mg/d carbamazepine, the CBZ level ranged from 2.8–4.5 mg/L in milk to 3.2–15.0 mg/L in plasma.[5] The levels of ECBZ ranged from 0.5–1.7 mg/L in milk to 0.8–4.8 mg/L in plasma. The amount of CBZ transferred to the infant is apparently quite low. Although the half-life of CBZ in infants appears shorter than in adults, infants should still be monitored for sedative effects.

We have one report of a mother consuming 400 mg daily of carbamazepine, in which the infant at 9 days, had elevated liver function tests (GGT).[6] Serum carbamazepine levels in the infant at 2 days and 63 days of life, were 1.8 and 1.1 mg/L respectively. CBZ-induced hepatic dysfunction in neonates may be associated with exposure to CBZ via breast milk.

Infants of epileptic mothers treated with CBZ throughout pregnancy and breastfeeding should be carefully monitored for possible adverse effects.

Pregnancy Risk	D	Lactation Risk	L2
T ½	= 18–54 hours	M/P	= 0.69
Vd	= 0.8–1.8 l/kg	PB	= 74%
Tmax	= 4–5 hours	Oral	= 100%
MW	= 236	pKa	= 7.0

Adult Concerns: Sedation, nausea, respiratory depression, tachycardia, vomiting, diarrhea, blood dyscrasias. The US FDA warns that patients of Asian ancestry should be screened for the human leukocyte antigen (HLA) allele HLA-B*1502 before receiving carbamazepine therapy. The risk for Stevens Johnson syndrome (SJS) and toxic epidermal necrolysis (TEN) is higher among these patients.

Pediatric Concerns: None reported via milk.

Drug Interactions: Carbamazepine may induce the metabolism of warfarin, cyclosporin, doxycycline, oral contraceptives, phenytoin, theophylline, benzodiazepines, ethosuximide, valproic acid, corticosteroids, and thyroid hormones. Macrolide antibiotics, isoniazid, verapamil, danazol, diltiazem may inhibit metabolism of carbamazepine and increase plasma levels.

Relative Infant Dose: 3.8%–5.9%

Adult Dose: 800–1200 mg daily divided TID or QID

Alternatives:

References:
1. Kaneko S, Sato T, Suzuki K. The levels of anticonvulsants in breast milk. Br J Clin Pharmacol 1979; 7(6): 624–627.
2. Pynnonen S, Kanto J, Sillanpaa M, Erkkola R. Carbamazepine: placental transport, tissue concentrations in foetus and newborn, and level in milk. Acta Pharmacol Toxicol (Copenh) 1977; 41(3): 244–253.
3. Niebyl JR, Blake DA, Freeman JM, Luff RD. Carbamazepine levels in pregnancy and lactation. Obstet Gynecol 1979; 53(1): 139–140.
4. Froescher W, Eichelbaum M, Niesen M, Dietrich K, Rausch P. Carbamazepine levels in breast milk. Ther Drug Monit 1984; 6(3): 266–271.
5. Shimoyama R, Ohkubo T, Sugawara K. Monitoring of carbamazepine and carbamazepine 10,11-epoxide in breast milk and plasma by high-performance liquid chromatography. Ann Clin Biochem 2000; 37 (Pt 2): 210–215.
6. Merlob P, Mor N, Litwin A. Transient hepatic dysfunction in an infant of an epileptic mother treated with carbamazepine during pregnancy and breastfeeding. Ann Pharmacother. 1992 Dec; 26(12): 1563–5.

CARBAMIDE PEROXIDE　　　　　　　　　　　　L1

Trade: Debrox, Auro ear drops, Audiologist's choice, Auraphene-B, Cankaid, Dent's ear wax drops, Dewax, E-R-O

Other Trades:

Category: Antibacterial, whitening agent

Carbamide peroxide, also called urea peroxide, is stable while immersed in glycerin, but upon contact with moisture, releases hydrogen peroxide and nascent oxygen, both strong oxidizing agents.[1] It is used to disinfect infected lesions, for the removal of earwax, and for whitening of teeth and dental appliances. Hydrogen peroxide is rapidly metabolized by hydroperoxidases, peroxidases, and catalase present in all tissues, plasma, and saliva. Its transfer to the plasma is minimal if at all. It would be all but impossible for any to reach breastmilk unless under extreme overdose.

Pregnancy Risk	C	Lactation Risk	L1
T½	=	M/P	=
Vd	=	PB	=
Tmax	=	Oral	=
MW	= 94	pKa	=

Adult Concerns: Dermal irritation, mucous membrane irritation, inflammation. Overgrowth of Candida and other opportunistic infections.

Pediatric Concerns: Possibly toxic in major oral overdose. Exposure to small amounts may lead to inflamed membranes.

Drug Interactions: There are no known significant interactions.

Relative Infant Dose:

Adult Dose: Apply several drops on affected area for 4 times a day after meals and at bedtime.

Alternatives:

References:
1. Pharmaceutical manufacturer prescribing information, 2011.

CARBENICILLIN   L1

Trade: Geopen, Geocillin, Carindacillin
Other Trades: Carbapen, Geopen
Category: Extended spectrum penicillin antibiotic

Carbenicillin is an extended spectrum penicillin antibiotic. Only limited levels are secreted into breastmilk (0.26 mg/L or about 0.001% of adult dose).[1] In a study of 2–3 women who received 1000 mg IM, the maximum milk level occurred at 4 hours and averaged 0.24 mg/L.[2] The average milk/plasma ratio reported was 0.045 at 4 hours. Due to its poor oral absorption (<10%) the amount absorbed by a nursing infant would be minimal.

Pregnancy Risk	B	Lactation Risk	L1
T½	= 1 hour	M/P	= 0.02
Vd	= 0.206 l/kg	PB	= 30–60%
Tmax	= 1–3 hours	Oral	= <10–30%
MW	= 378	pKa	= 3.86

Adult Concerns: Rash, thrush, diarrhea, headache, hyperthermia.

Pediatric Concerns: None reported via milk.

Drug Interactions: Co-administration of aminoglycosides (within 1 hour) may inactivate both drugs. Increased half-life with probenecid.

Relative Infant Dose: 0.3%

Adult Dose: 382–764 mg every 6 hours

Alternatives:

References:
1. Pharmaceutical manufacturer prescribing information, 1996.
2. Matsuda S. Transfer of antibiotics into maternal milk. Biol Res Pregnancy Perinatol 1984; 5(2): 57–60.

CARBETAPENTANE   L5

Trade: Exhall, Expectuss
Other Trades:
Category: Antitussive

One report indicated that carbetapentane may be excreted in human milk in quantities large enough to cause respiratory problems in the infant[1]. Carbetapentane found in maternal serum, milk, and in the child's serum and urine.[1] The 4 week-old infant that was exclusively breastfed by his mother developed acute respiratory failure. Symptoms ended once carbetapentane was identified and breastfeeding was discontinued.[1]

Pregnancy Risk	C		Lactation Risk	L5
T ½	=		M/P	=
Vd	=		PB	=
Tmax	=		Oral	=
MW	= 333		pKa	=

Adult Concerns: Drowsiness, nausea, vomiting, anaphylaxis, leukopenia, allergic reaction.

Pediatric Concerns:

Drug Interactions: There are no known interactions.

Relative Infant Dose:

Adult Dose: 1–2 tablets every 12 hours

Alternatives:

References:
1. Stier BJ, Sieverding L, Moeller H: Pentoxyverine poisoning via maternal milk in a fully breast-fed newborn infant. Dtsch Med Wochenschr 113: 898–900, 198

CARBIDOPA   L3

Trade: Lodosyn

Other Trades: Kinson, Sinacarb, Sinemet

Category: Inhibits levodopa metabolism

Carbidopa inhibits the metabolism of levodopa in parkinsonian patients therefore extending the half-life of levodopa. Its effect on lactation is largely unknown, but skeletal malformations have occurred in pregnant rabbits.[1,2] Use discretion in administering to pregnant or lactating women. Warning: Carbidopa and levodopa are known to suppress prolactin production in normal, and breastfeeding mothers.[3,4,5,6,7]

Pregnancy Risk	C		Lactation Risk	L3
T ½	= 1–2 hours		M/P	=
Vd	=		PB	= 36%
Tmax	=		Oral	= 40–70%
MW	= 226.23		pKa	= 9.29

Adult Concerns: Gastrointestinal distress, nausea, vomiting, diarrhea.

Pediatric Concerns:

Drug Interactions: May interact with tricyclic antidepressants leading to hypertensive reactions.

Relative Infant Dose:

Adult Dose: 70–100 mg daily; maximum daily dose 200 mg

Alternatives:

References:

1. Pharmaceutical manufacturer prescribing information, 1996.
2. McEvoy GE. (ed): AFHS Drug Information. New York, NY: 2003.
3. Thulin PC, Woodward WR, Carter JH, Nutt JG. Levodopa in human breast milk: clinical implications. Neurology. 1998 Jun; 50(6): 1920–1.
4. Ayalon D, Peyser MR et al. Effect of L-dopa on galactopoiesis and gonadotropin levels in the inappropriate lactation syndrome. Obstet Gynecol. 1974; 44: 159–70.
5. Leblanc H, Yen SS. The effect of L-dopa and chlorpromazine on prolactin and growth hormone secretion in normal women. Am J Obstet Gynecol. 1976; 126: 162–4.
6. Board JA, Fierro RJ et al. Effects of alpha- and beta-adrenergic blocking agents on serum prolactin levels in women with hyperprolactinemia and galactorrhea. Am J Obstet Gynecol. 1977; 127: 285–7.
7. Rao R, Scommegna A, Frohman LA. Integrity of central dopaminergic system in women with postpartum hyperprolactinemia. Am J Obstet Gynecol. 1982; 143: 883–7.

CARBIMAZOLE   L3

Trade: NeoMercazole

Other Trades: Neo-Mercazole

Category: Thyroid inhibitor

Carbimazole, a prodrug of methimazole, is rapidly and completely converted to the active metabolite methimazole in the plasma. Only methimazole is detected in plasma, urine and thyroid tissue. See breastfeeding specifics for methimazole.

In a study, Rylance et al suggests that subclinical levels of methimazole enter milk subsequent to a maternal dose of 30 mg/day carbimazole.[1] Free methimazole measured in milk on 10 occasions averaged 43 µg/L. Plasma methimazole in twins was 45 to 52 ng/mL. Thyroid suppression is believed to occur only when plasma levels exceed 50–100 ng/mL. No thyroid suppression was noted in these two twins. Peak transfer into milk occurred at 2–4 hours, and the lowest at 6 hours after the dose. The authors suggest that breastfeeding is permissible if the maternal dose is less than 30 mg/day. In another study of 5 five lactating women receiving 40 mg/d, the mean concentration of methimazole in milk was 182 µg/L, with a mean milk/serum ratio of 0.98.[2] The mean total amount of methimazole excreted in milk over 8 h was 34 µg. The limited data above suggests that the transfer of carbimazole is too low to affect thyroid function in breastfeeding infants. However, close monitoring of infant thyroid function is probably advisable. See propylthiouracil as alternative. However, close monitoring of infant thyroid function is probably advisable.

Pregnancy Risk	D	Lactation Risk	L3
T ½	= 6–13 hours	M/P	= 0.3–0.7
Vd	=	PB	=
Tmax	= 4 hours	Oral	= Complete
MW	= 186	pKa	=

Adult Concerns: Hypothyroidism, hepatic dysfunction, bleeding, drowsiness, skin rash, nausea, vomiting, fever.

Pediatric Concerns: None reported via milk, but propylthiouracil is generally preferred in breastfeeding women.

Drug Interactions: Use with iodinated glycerol, lithium, and potassium iodide may increase toxicity.

Relative Infant Dose: 2.3%–5.3%

Adult Dose: 15–60 mg daily taken in 2–3 divided doses

Alternatives: Propylthiouracil

References:
1. Rylance GW, Woods CG, Donnelly MC, Oliver JS, Alexander WD. Carbimazole and breastfeeding. Lancet 1987; 1(8538): 928.
2. Johansen K, Andersen AN, Kampmann JP, Molholm Hansen JM, Mortensen HB. Excretion of methimazole in human milk. Eur J Clin Pharmacol 1982; 23(4): 339–341.

CARBINOXAMINE   L2

Trade: Palgic, Arbinoxa

Other Trades:

Category: Antihistamine

Carbinoxamine is an antihistamine used over-the-counter.[1] Usage during breastfeeding is probably safe. The main adverse effect is sedation. The use of this sedating antihistamine in breastfeeding mothers is not ideal. Non-sedating antihistamines are generally preferred.

Because of the higher risk of antihistamines for infants generally and for newborns and premature infants in particular, use of carbinoxamine maleate is contraindicated in nursing mothers

Pregnancy Risk	C	Lactation Risk	L2
T ½	= 10–20 hours	M/P	=
Vd	=	PB	=
Tmax	=	Oral	=
MW	= 407	pKa	= 8.1

Adult Concerns: Sedation, urticaria, hypotension, epigastric distress, thickening of bronchial secretions, dizziness, disturbed coordination.

Pediatric Concerns:

Drug Interactions: MAO inhibitors and alcohol

Relative Infant Dose:

Adult Dose: 4–8 mg 3–4 times a day

Alternatives:

References:
1. Pharmaceutical manufacturer prescribing information, 2011.

CARBON MONOXIDE   L3

Trade:

Other Trades:

Category: Poisonous gas; air pollutant

Carbon monoxide (CO) is an odorless, colorless gas. It is a gaseous component of the atmospheric air. In fact, it is the most abundant air pollutant in the lower atmosphere, produced from the incomplete combustion of carbonaceous fuels such as gasoline, natural gas, oil, coal, and wood, and other materials such as tobacco.

Acute CO poisoning due to environmental exposure in mother or baby should be considered an emergency and treated immediately. It should be noted the effects of CO toxicity in an infant are more than those in an adult. An infant or child experiences an earlier onset of hypoxia as compared to an adult. Further, an infant up to the age of 6 months has fetal hemoglobin. Fetal hemoglobin has a 2.5–3 times higher affinity for carbon monoxide as compared to adult hemoglobin, causing the infant carboxyhemoglobin levels to be 10–15% higher than maternal levels.[1,2,3] Therefore, the hypoxia that occurs in an infant is more severe than that which occurs in an adult for the same amount of exposure. Chronic CO poisoning generally occurs when incomplete combustion of fuels occurs in poorly ventilated, closed spaces. Some of the most common sources of exposure in infants is when heavy smoking occurs in poorly ventilated areas, or when gas ranges or vehicles are turned on in unventilated garages. Some of the other common sources of chronic CO exposure are gas furnaces, water and space heaters, wood and coal stoves or fireplaces, regularly used in poorly ventilated spaces. Chronic CO exposure over prolonged periods has been known to cause neurological, neurodevelopmental and cognitive effects. Symptoms may include personality changes, mental confusion, and movement disorders.

There are no studies of transfer of CO in human milk following maternal exposure. Following CO exposure, almost all of it is absorbed into the bloodstream via lungs, where it forms carboxyhemoglobin (COHb). The remaining 1% is oxidized by metabolic processes to produce carbon dioxide. The half-life of COHb is 4–5 hours, which is significantly decreased following exposure to oxygen. It is not known if COHb enters human milk, but it is highly unlikely that COHb would be capable of entry into human milk as there is no binding protein. Therefore, it would be almost impossible for a breastfed infant to be exposed to CO strictly through breastmilk. Further, even if it is assumed that some does enter breastmilk, the absorption of CO following oral absorption would probably be negligible to nil. Although, there are no data on the oral absorption of CO in humans, a study conducted in monkeys where the oral and nasal cavities were exposed to large amounts of smoke containing CO, the amount of CO absorbed through the nasal and oral mucosa was found to be nil.[4]

Therefore, a mother exposed to high levels of CO may safely continue to breastfeed once she is treated with oxygen or released from care. Although, the exposed mother may suffer some long-term effects of acute CO poisoning for up to 1–3 months, such clinical effects are not expected in the breastfed infant.

Pregnancy Risk	Hazardous	Lactation Risk	L3
T ½	= 4–5 hours	M/P	=
Vd	=	PB	=
Tmax	=	Oral	=
MW	= 28.01	pKa	=

Adult Concerns: Acute CO poisoning: Headache, nausea, malaise, and fatigue. Increasing exposures causes increase in heart rate, hypotension and cardiac arrhythmias. Central nervous system involvement is manifested with delirium, hallucinations, dizziness, ataxia, confusion and seizures. Delayed neurological manifestation up to 1–3 months following CO exposure have been reported. Some of these manifestations include mood disturbances, amnesia, dementia, memory loss, ataxia, speech disturbances and personality disorders. Chronic CO poisoning: Persistent headaches, light-headedness, depression, confusion, memory loss, nausea and vomiting. Chronic exposure to carbon monoxide causes accelerated development of atherosclerosis and increases the risk for heart disease and myocardial infarction.

Pediatric Concerns: Manifestations of CO exposures in children and infants are more subtle and difficult to recognize. Excessive sleepiness or somnolence, change in mental status or mental confusion should arouse suspicion of CO poisoning.

Drug Interactions:

Relative Infant Dose:

Adult Dose:

Alternatives:

References:
1. Hill EP, Hill JR, Power GG et al (1977) Carbon monoxide ex-changes between the human fetus and mother: a mathematical model. Am J Physiol 232: H311–H323
2. Londo LD, Hill EP (1977) Carbon monoxide uptake and elimina-tion in fetal and maternal sheep. Am J Physiol 232: H324–H330
3. Yildiz H, Aldemir E, Altuncu E, Celik M, Kavuncuoglu S. A rare cause of perinatal asphyxia: maternal carbon monoxide poisoning. Arch Gynecol Obstet. 2010 Feb; 281(2): 251–4. Epub 2009 Jun 6.
4. Schoenfisch WH, Hoop KA, Struelens BS. Carbon monoxide absorption through the oral and nasal mucosae of cynomolgus monkeys. Arch Environ Health. 1980 may-Jun; 35(3): 152–4.

CARBOPLATIN   L5

Trade: Carboplat, Carbosin, Emorzim, Novoplat, Paraplatin

Other Trades: Paraplatin-AQ

Category: Anticancer drug

Carboplatin is a platinum derivative anticancer agent similar to cisplatin. Platinum agents have high affinity for plasma proteins.[1] Approximately 90% of carboplatin is covalently bound to plasma proteins after 24 hours. Estimates of plasma half-life are as high as 49 hours. Once bound and distributed, it has a large volume of distribution of 20–30 liters. However, carboplatin is apparently more rapidly cleared when compared to cisplatin. After 24 hours, only 23–35% of the platinum is still present, which is much less than with cisplatin. However, the T(beta) is still long, about five days.[2] About 65% is eliminated renally in the first 24 hours, and the remaining 35% is retained for long periods in other tissues. See cisplatin for levels present in human milk. In a study of one mother undergoing carboplatin chemotherapy (233 mg/week) for papillary thyroid cancer, milk levels were determined at 4, 28, 172, and 316 hours following infusion. The AUC0–316h was 127.92 mg. h/L.[3] The the Cave was 0.404 mg/L with an RID of 1.82%. Levels were demonstrable in milk even 300 hours after final infusion.

Two options are suggested. One, the breastmilk should be tested for platinum levels and not used as long as they are measurable. Or two, without measuring platinum levels, breastfeeding should be interrupted for at least 20 days for low doses as above, or much longer(permanently) for higher doses.

Pregnancy Risk	D	Lactation Risk	L5
T ½	= 2.6–5.9 hours (carboplatin) >=5 days (platinum from carboplatin)	M/P	=
Vd	= 0.229 l/kg	PB	= 0% (carboplatin)
Tmax	=	Oral	= None
MW	= 371.3	pKa	=

Adult Concerns: Nausea and vomiting; unusual tiredness or weakness, pain at the site of injection

Pediatric Concerns:

Drug Interactions: Aminoglycosides enhance the ototoxic effect of carboplatin. Echinacea decreases the effect of immunosuppressants. Tacrolimus may enhance the toxic effect of carboplatin.

Relative Infant Dose: 1.8%

Adult Dose: Varies depending on indication

Alternatives:

References:
1. Pharmaceutical manufacturer prescribing information, 2005.
2. Grochow LB, Ames MM. A clinician's guide to chemotherapy pharmacokinetics and pharmacodynamics. 1st ed. Baltimore, MD: Williams and Wilkins; 1998.
3. Griffin SJ, Milla M, Baker TE, Hale TW. Transfer of carboplatin and paclitaxel into human breastmilk. Submitted, 2012.

CARBOPROST   L3

Trade: Hemabate

Other Trades: Hemabate

Category: Oxytocic prostaglandin for postpartum hemorrhage

Carboprost tromethamine is a prostaglandin analogue (15-methyl prostaglandin F2-alpha) which stimulates the myometrial contractions in a gravid uterus simulating labor.[1] It is a commonly used oxytocic agent used to prevent postpartum hemorrhage. No data are available on its transfer to human milk. Prostaglandins have brief half-lives and little distribution out of the plasma compartment. Even then, rather large intramuscular doses only produce picogram concentrations in the plasma of recipients. It is not likely it will penetrate milk in clinically relevant amounts.

Pregnancy Risk	C	Lactation Risk	L3
T ½	= <1 hour	M/P	=
Vd	=	PB	=
Tmax	= 15–30 minutes	Oral	= None
MW	= 489	pKa	= 14.51

Adult Concerns: Adverse events include vomiting, diarrhea, leukocytosis, hypertension, headache, dystonic reactions, fever, uterine rupture, bronchoconstriction, and flushing of the skin.

Pediatric Concerns: None reported via milk. Commonly used in obstetrics without complications in breastfeeding mothers.

Drug Interactions: May augment other oxytocics.

Relative Infant Dose:

Adult Dose: 100–250 mg initially.

Alternatives:

References:
1. Pharmaceutical manufacturer prescribing information, 2003.

CARBOXYMETHYL CELLULOSE   L2

Trade:

Other Trades:

Category: Ocular lubricant / Laxative

Carboxymethyl cellulose is a polysaccharide polymer most often used as an ophthalmic lubricant and orally as a laxative. There are no controlled studies in breastfeeding women. Carboxymethyl cellulose has been used in the standardized feeding regimens as a laxative for premature neonates.[1] Though it lacks data regarding it safety in lactation, due to its inert nature and low oral bioavailability, carboxymethyl cellulose is probably compatible with breastfeeding.

Pregnancy Risk	Probably safe	Lactation Risk	L2
T ½	=	M/P	=
Vd	=	PB	=
Tmax	=	Oral	= Poor
MW	=	pKa	=

Adult Concerns: None reported.

Pediatric Concerns:

Drug Interactions:

Relative Infant Dose:

Adult Dose: Instill 1–2 drops in eye(s)

Alternatives:

References:
1. Patole S, McGlone L, Muller R. Virtual elimination of necrotising enterocolitis for 5 years–reasons? Med Hypotheses. 2003 Nov-Dec; 61(5–6): 617–22.

CARISOPRODOL   L3

Trade: Soma Compound, Solol, Vanadom

Other Trades: Soma, Carisoma

Category: Muscle relaxant, CNS depressant

Carisoprodol is a commonly used skeletal muscle relaxant that is a CNS depressant. It is metabolized to an active metabolite called meprobamate. As Soma Compound it also contains 325 mg of aspirin. In a study of one breastfeeding mother receiving 2100 mg/day, the average milk concentration of carisoprodol and meprobamate was 0.9 mg/L and 11.6 mg/L respectively.[1] No adverse effects on the infant were noted.

Pregnancy Risk	C	Lactation Risk	L3
T ½	= 8 hours	M/P	= 2–4
Vd	=	PB	= 60%
Tmax	=	Oral	= Complete
MW	= 260	pKa	= 15.56

Adult Concerns: Nausea, vomiting, hiccups, sedation, weakness, mild withdrawal symptoms after chronic use.

Pediatric Concerns: None reported, but observe for sedation.

Drug Interactions: Increased toxicity when added to alcohol, CNS depressants, MAO inhibitors.

Relative Infant Dose: 0.5%–6.3%

Adult Dose: 350 mg TID-QID

Alternatives:

References:
1. Nordeng H, Zahlsen K, Spigset O. Transfer of carisoprodol to breast milk. Ther Drug Monit 2001; 23(3): 298–300.

CARMUSTINE   L5

Trade: BCNU, Bicnu, Carmubris, Nitrumon, Gliadel

Other Trades: Gliadel

Category: Anticancer drug

Carmustine is an alkylating agent of the nitrosourea type. Among its indications are brain tumors, gastric carcinoma, Hodgkin's lymphomas, and other syndromes.

With a rather low molecular weight (214), it is best known for its ability to enter the CNS by crossing the blood-brain barrier.[1] This would suggest its ability to enter the milk compartment is significant. No data are available on its transfer to milk, however, initial transfer may be significant. The metabolism of this product is somewhat obscure, and may account to some degree for its lasting side effects. Further, the half-life is highly varied among patients (15–20 fold). Because of the prolonged and delayed side effect profiles (pulmonary injury) associated with this drug, mothers should delay breastfeeding for a minimum of 24–48 hours.

Withhold breastfeeding for a minimum of 24–48 hours.

Pregnancy Risk	D	Lactation Risk	L5
T ½	= (beta) 12–45 minutes	M/P	=
Vd	= 3.3 l/kg	PB	= 80%
Tmax	=	Oral	= 5–28%
MW	= 214.05	pKa	=

Adult Concerns: Cough, pain or redness at the injection site, shortness of breath, diarrhea, discoloration of the skin along the injection site

Pediatric Concerns:

Drug Interactions: Decreased effect with use of cardiac glycosides or echinacea. The metabolism of Carmustine may be decreased with the use of Cimetidine. Adverse effects are increased with the use of Tacrolimus.

Relative Infant Dose:

Adult Dose: IV: 150–200 mg/m² every 6 weeks or 75–100 mg/m² for two days every 6 weeks

Alternatives:

References:
1. Pharmaceutical manufacturer prescribing information, 2005.

CARNITINE   L2

Trade: Carnitor, L-Carnitine
Other Trades:
Category: Dietary supplement

Carnitine is biosynthesized from lysine and methionine and its main function is to facilitate fatty acid metabolism. Carnitine supplementation comes in the form of L-carnitine, acetyl l-carnitine, and propionyl l-carnitine. Carnitine supplementation is used for primary carnitine deficiency in hemodialysis patients.[1] L-carnitine is present in some formulas and many foods. Carnitine is present in breastmilk with a concentration of 45 µmol/L.[2] Carnitine levels in breastmilk are not dependent on dietary carnitine supplementation, but rather is transported into milk by the mother.[2] Another study suggests that the levels of carnitine in breastmilk are constant around 56–69.8 µmol/L for the first 21 days and reduces to 35.2 µmol/L around 40–50 days postpartum.[3] Because carnitine is naturally present in breastmilk and its concentration is not affected by supplementation, the risk to the infant is probably remote from exogenous sources.

Pregnancy Risk	B		Lactation Risk	L2
T ½	= 17.4 hours		M/P	=
Vd	=		PB	=
Tmax	=		Oral	= 15%
MW	= 161		pKa	=

Adult Concerns: Diarrhea, abdominal pain, hypertension, headache, hypercalcemia, weakness, cough, infection, rash.

Pediatric Concerns: None reported. Natural component of breastmilk.

Drug Interactions:

Relative Infant Dose:

Adult Dose: 990 mg 2–3 times/day (oral)

Alternatives:

References:
1. An Evidence-based Systematic Review of L-Carnitine by the Natural Standard Research Collaboration. www. naturalstandard. com. Last accessed July 13, 2011.
2. Mitchell ME, Snyder EA. Dietary carnitine effects on carnitine concentrations in urine and milk in lactating women. Am J Clin Nutr. 1991 Nov; 54(5): 814–20.
3. Sandor A, Pecsuvac K, Kerner J, Alkonyi I. On carnitine content of the human breast milk. Pediatr Res. 1982 Feb; 16(2): 89–91. Abstract.

CARTEOLOL   L3

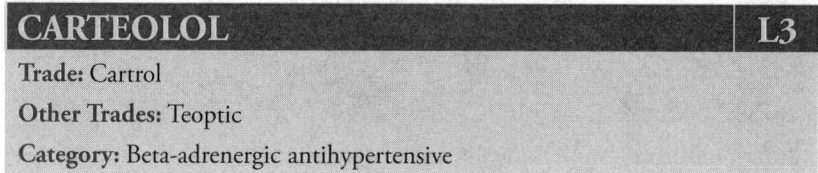

Trade: Cartrol

Other Trades: Teoptic

Category: Beta-adrenergic antihypertensive

Carteolol is a typical beta-blocker used for hypertension. Carteolol is reported to be excreted in breastmilk of lactating animals.[1] No data are available on levels in human milk.

Pregnancy Risk	C		Lactation Risk	L3
T ½	= 6 hours		M/P	=
Vd	= 4.05 l/kg		PB	= 23–30%
Tmax	=		Oral	= 80%
MW	= 292		pKa	= 14.19

Adult Concerns: Hypotension, bradycardia, lethargy, and sedation.

Pediatric Concerns: None reported but observe for hypoglycemia, hypotension, bradycardia, lethargy.

Drug Interactions: Decreased effect when used with aluminum salts, barbiturates, calcium salts, cholestyramine, NSAIDs, ampicillin, rifampin, and salicylates. Beta blockers may reduce the effect of oral sulfonylureas (hypoglycemic agents).

Increased toxicity/effect when used with other antihypertensives, contraceptives, MAO inhibitors, cimetidine, and numerous other products. See drug interaction reference for complete listing.

Relative Infant Dose:

Adult Dose: 2.5–5 mg daily.

Alternatives: Propranolol, Metoprolol

References:
1. Pharmaceutical manufacturer prescribing information, 2010.

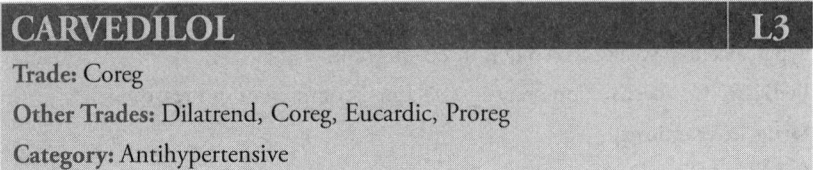

CARVEDILOL   L3

Trade: Coreg

Other Trades: Dilatrend, Coreg, Eucardic, Proreg

Category: Antihypertensive

Carvedilol is a nonselective beta-adrenergic blocking agent (with partial alpha-1 blocking activity) with high lipid solubility and no intrinsic sympathomimetic activity.[1] There are no data available on the transfer of this drug into human milk. However, due to its high lipid solubility, some may transfer. As with any beta-blocker, some caution is recommended until milk levels are reported.

Pregnancy Risk	C	Lactation Risk	L3
T ½	= 7–10 hours	M/P	=
Vd	= 1.64 l/kg	PB	= >98%
Tmax	= 1–1.5 hours; Extended release-5 hours	Oral	= 25–35%
MW	= 406.47	pKa	= 15.00

Adult Concerns: Postural hypotension, fatigue, dizziness, lightheadedness, bradycardia, bronchospasm. Use with caution in asthmatics.

Pediatric Concerns: None reported via milk. Observe for hypotension, bradycardia, hypoglycemia.

Drug Interactions: Severe bradycardia may result when used with amiodarone. Digoxin may prolong AV conduction time. Severe hypotension when added with calcium channel blockers. Severe hypertension, bradycardia when used with epinephrine.

Relative Infant Dose:

Adult Dose: 6.25–12.5 mg BID

Alternatives: Propranolol, metoprolol.

References:
1. Pharmaceutical manufacturer prescribing information, 2010.

CASCARA SAGRADA | L3

Trade:

Other Trades:

Category: Laxative

Cascara sagrada is a strong laxative. Trace amounts appear to be secreted into breastmilk.[1,2] No exact estimates have been published. May cause loose stools and diarrhea in neonates.

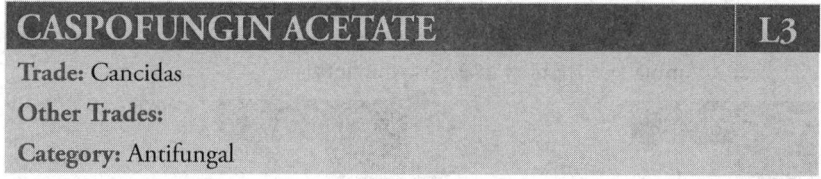

Pregnancy Risk	C	Lactation Risk	L3
T ½	=	M/P	=
Vd	=	PB	=
Tmax	=	Oral	=
MW	=	pKa	=

Adult Concerns: Diarrhea, gastrointestinal cramping.

Pediatric Concerns: May loosen stools in infants.

Drug Interactions: Decreased effect of oral anticoagulants.

Relative Infant Dose:

Adult Dose: 5 mL daily.

Alternatives:

References:
1. O'Brien TE. Excretion of drugs in human milk. Am J Hosp Pharm 1974; 31(9): 844–854.
2. Vorherr H. Drug excretion in breast milk. Postgrad Med 1974; 56(4): 97–104.

CASPOFUNGIN ACETATE | L3

Trade: Cancidas

Other Trades:

Category: Antifungal

Caspofungin is a unique semisynthetic lipopeptide that is active against Aspergillus fumigatus. It has a large polycyclic structure with a molecular weight of 1213 daltons. The half-life of this product is unique with a polyphasic elimination curve with 3 distinct phases. The half-life varies from 11 hours in one phase to 40–50 hours in the last phase.[1] This is a new product and limited data are available on its use, particularly in pediatrics. The pharmaceutical manufacturer states that it was found in rodent milk; no data are available for human milk. Nevertheless, the oral bioavailability is reported as poor and it is unlikely an infant would absorb enough to be clinically relevant, but this is only speculative.

Pregnancy Risk	C	Lactation Risk	L3
T ½	= >11 hours	M/P	=
Vd	= 0.138 l/kg	PB	= 97% to albumin
Tmax	=	Oral	= Poor
MW	= 1213	pKa	= 5.1, 10.7

Adult Concerns: Fever, nausea, vomiting, flushing, phlebitis, anemia, headache, etc.

Pediatric Concerns: None reported via milk. Not cleared for pediatric patients.

Drug Interactions: Cyclosporin increases AUC of caspofungin. Do not use with cyclosporin unless potential benefits outweigh risk. Caspofungin reduces plasma levels of tacrolimus.

Relative Infant Dose:

Adult Dose: 70 mg STAT, 50 mg/d

Alternatives:

References:
1. Pharmaceutical manufacturer prescribing information, 2001.

CASTOR OIL   L3

Trade: Purge

Other Trades:

Category: Laxative

Castor oil is converted to ricinoleic acid in the gut.[1] It is indicated for use in constipation and for pre-operative bowel preparation. Its transfer into milk is unknown. Caution should be used. Usage in excess amounts could produce diarrhea, insomnia and tremors in exposed infants.

Pregnancy Risk	X	Lactation Risk	L3
T ½	=	M/P	=
Vd	=	PB	=
Tmax	= 2–3 hours	Oral	= Unknown
MW	= 932	pKa	=

Adult Concerns: Insomnia, tremors, diarrhea.

Pediatric Concerns: Observe for diarrhea, insomnia, tremors in infants.

Drug Interactions: There are no known significant interactions.

Relative Infant Dose:

Adult Dose: N/A

Alternatives:

References:
1. Pharmaceutical manufacturer prescribing information, 2009.

CEFACLOR   L1

Trade: Ceclor

Other Trades: Keflor, Ceclor, Apo-Cefaclor, Distaclor

Category: Cephalosporin antibiotic

Cefaclor is a commonly used pediatric cephalosporin antibiotic. Small amounts are known to be secreted into human milk. Following a single dose of 250 mg orally in two mothers, the levels in milk were undetectable in one, and ranged from 0.15 to 0.19 mg/L from 2 to 4 hours postdose. Following a 500 mg oral dose in 5 mothers, milk levels averaged 0.16 to 0.21 mg/L. Average levels were 0.18, 0.20, 0.21, and 0.16 µg/mL at 2, 3, 4, and 5 hours respectively.[1] Trace amounts were detected at 1 hour. Observe for changes in gut flora or diarrhea.

Pregnancy Risk	B		Lactation Risk	L1
T ½	= 0.5–1 hr.		M/P	=
Vd	= 0.35 l/kg		PB	= 23.5%
Tmax	= 0.5–1 hr.		Oral	= 100%
MW	= 386		pKa	= 11.26

Adult Concerns: Diarrhea, gastrointestinal irritation, rash, penicillin allergy, delayed serum sickness at 14 days.

Pediatric Concerns: None reported via milk. Observe for changes in gut flora and diarrhea.

Drug Interactions: Probenecid may increase levels of cephalosporins by reducing renal clearance.

Relative Infant Dose: 0.4%–0.8%

Adult Dose: 250–500 mg every 8 hours

Alternatives:

References:
1. Takase Z. Clinical and laboratory studies of cefaclor in the field of obstetrics and gynecology. Chemotherapy 1979; 27: (Suppl)668.

CEFADROXIL   L1

Trade: Ultracef, Duricef

Other Trades: Duricef, Baxan

Category: Cephalosporin antibiotic

Cefadroxil is a typical first-generation, cephalosporin antibiotic. Small amounts are known to be secreted into milk. Milk concentrations following a 1000 mg oral dose were 0.10 mg/L at 1 hour and 1.24 mg/L at 5 hours.[1] Milk/serum ratios were 0.009 at 1 hour and 0.019 at 3 hours.

In a study of 2–3 patients who received an oral dose of 500 mg cefadroxil, milk levels peaked at 4 hours at an average of 0.4 mg/L which is only about 1.3% of the maternal dose.[2] The milk/plasma ratio was 0.085.

Pregnancy Risk	B	Lactation Risk	L1
T ½	= 1.5 hours	M/P	= 0.009–0.019
Vd	= 0.2 l/kg	PB	= 20%
Tmax	= 1–2 hours	Oral	= 100%
MW	= 381	pKa	= 9.48

Adult Concerns: Diarrhea, allergic rash.

Pediatric Concerns: None reported via milk. Observe for gastrointestinal symptoms such as diarrhea.

Drug Interactions: Probenecid may decrease clearance. Furosemide, aminoglycosides may enhance renal toxicity.

Relative Infant Dose: 0.8%–1.3%

Adult Dose: 0.5–1 gm BID

Alternatives:

References:
1. Kafetzis DA, Siafas CA, Georgakopoulos PA, Papadatos CJ. Passage of cephalosporins and amoxicillin into the breast milk. Acta Paediatr Scand 1981; 70(3): 285–288.
2. Matsuda S. Transfer of antibiotics into maternal milk. Biol Res Pregnancy Perinatol 1984; 5(2): 57–60.

CEFAZOLIN   L1

Trade: Ancef, Kefzol

Other Trades: Cefamezin, Ancef, Kefzol

Category: Cephalosporin antibiotic

Cefazolin is a typical first-generation, cephalosporin antibiotic that has adult and pediatric indications. It is only used IM or IV, never orally. In 20 patients who received a 2 gm STAT dose over 10 minutes, the average concentration of cefazolin in milk 2, 3, and 4 hours after the dose was 1.25, 1.51, and 1.16 mg/L respectively.[1] A very small milk/plasma ratio (0.023) indicates insignificant transfer into milk. Cefazolin is poorly absorbed orally; therefore, the infant would absorb a minimal amount. Plasma levels in infants are reported to be too small to be detected.

Pregnancy Risk	B	Lactation Risk	L1
T ½	= 1.2–2.2 hours	M/P	= 0.023
Vd	= 0.143 l/kg	PB	= 89%
Tmax	= 1–2 hours	Oral	= Poor
MW	= 455	pKa	= 10.87

Adult Concerns: Allergic rash, thrush, diarrhea.

Pediatric Concerns: None reported via milk. Observe for gastrointestinal symptoms such as diarrhea.

Drug Interactions: Probenecid may decrease clearance. Furosemide, aminoglycosides may enhance renal toxicity.

Relative Infant Dose: 0.8%

Adult Dose: 250–2000 mg TID

Alternatives:

References:
1. Yoshioka H, Cho K, Takimoto M, Maruyama S, Shimizu T. Transfer of cefazolin into human milk. J Pediatr 1979; 94(1): 151–152.

CEFDINIR   L1

Trade: Omnicef

Other Trades:

Category: Antibiotic

Cefdinir is a broad-spectrum cephalosporin antibiotic. The manufacturer reports that following administration of a 600 mg oral doses, no cefdinir was detected in human milk.[1]

Pregnancy Risk	B		Lactation Risk	L1
T ½	= 1.7 hours		M/P	=
Vd	= 0.35 l/kg		PB	= 70%
Tmax	= 3 hours		Oral	= 21%
MW	= 395		pKa	= 3.27

Adult Concerns: Similar to other cephalosporins, and include diarrhea, vaginal moniliasis, nausea, and rash. Allergic reactions are possible.

Pediatric Concerns: None reported via milk. Milk levels virtually undetectable. Observe for diarrhea.

Drug Interactions: Reduced oral absorption following use of antacids. Probenecid will decrease renal excretion and a 54% increase in peak levels, and a 50% prolongation of clearance.

Relative Infant Dose:

Adult Dose: 14 mg/kg/day

Alternatives:

References:
1. Pharmaceutical manufacturer prescribing information, 2010.

CEFDITOREN   L2

Trade: Spectracef

Other Trades:

Category: Cephalosporin antibiotic

Cefditoren is a new third generation cephalosporin antibiotic that is indicated in the treatment of acute bacterial exacerbations of chronic bronchitis, pharyngitis, tonsillitis, and uncomplicated skin infections.[1] It is moderately active against penicillin-resistant pneumococcus. It is cleared for use in children <12 years of age. No data are available on breastmilk levels.

Pregnancy Risk	B	Lactation Risk	L2
T ½	= 1.3–2 hours	M/P	=
Vd	= 9.3 l/kg	PB	= 88%
Tmax	= 1–3 hours	Oral	= 14%
MW	= 620	pKa	= 11.38

Adult Concerns: Diarrhea, nausea, headache, vaginal moniliasis.

Pediatric Concerns: No data reported in breastfed infants.

Drug Interactions: Concentrations of Cefditoren may be decreased with use of antacids, H₂–Antagonists, and Proton Pump Inhibitors. Probenecid may increase the concentrations of Cefditoren.

Relative Infant Dose:

Adult Dose: 200–400 mg BID for 10–14 days depending on indication

Alternatives: Cephalexin

References:
1. Pharmaceutical manufacturer prescribing information, 2010.

CEFEPIME   L2

Trade: Maxipime

Other Trades: Maxipime

Category: Cephalosporin antibiotic

Cefepime is a new 'fourth-generation' parenteral cephalosporin. Cefepime is secreted in human milk in small amounts averaging 0.5 mg/L.[1,2] In a mother consuming 2 gm/day, an infant would ingest approximately 75 µg/kg/day or only approximately 0.3% of the maternal dose. This amount is too small to produce any clinical symptoms other than possible changes in gut flora.

Pregnancy Risk	B	Lactation Risk	L2
T ½	= 2 hours	M/P	= 0.8
Vd	= 0.3 l/kg	PB	= 16–19%
Tmax	= 0.5–1.5 hours	Oral	= Poor
MW	= 571	pKa	= 11.15

Adult Concerns: Headache, blurred vision, dyspepsia, diarrhea, transient elevation of liver enzymes.

Pediatric Concerns: None reported via milk.

Drug Interactions: May produce additive nephrotoxic effects when used with aminoglycosides.

Relative Infant Dose: 0.3%

Adult Dose: 1–2 gm BID

Alternatives:

References:
1. Pharmaceutical manufacturer prescribing information, 1997.
2. Sanders CC. Cefepime: the next generation? Clin Infect Dis 1993; 17(3): 369–379.

CEFIXIME | L2

Trade: Suprax

Other Trades: Suprax

Category: Cephalosporin antibiotic

Cefixime is an oral, third-generation cephalosporin used in treating infections. It is poorly absorbed (30–50%) by the oral route. It is secreted to a limited degree in the milk although in one study of a mother receiving 100 mg, it was undetected in the milk from 1–6 hours after the dose.[1]

Pregnancy Risk	B	Lactation Risk	L2
T ½	= 7 hours	M/P	=
Vd	= 0.1 l/kg	PB	= 70%
Tmax	= 2–6 hours	Oral	= 30–50%
MW	= 453	pKa	= 3.26

Adult Concerns: Allergic rash, diarrhea, thrush.

Pediatric Concerns: None reported. Observe for gastrointestinal symptoms such as diarrhea.

Drug Interactions: Probenecid may decrease clearance. Furosemide, aminoglycosides may enhance renal toxicity.

Relative Infant Dose:

Adult Dose: 200 mg BID

Alternatives:

References:
1. Pharmaceutical manufacturer prescribing information, 2010.

CEFOPERAZONE | L2

Trade: Cefobid

Other Trades: Cefobid

Category: Cephalosporin antibiotic

Cefoperazone sodium is a broad-spectrum, third-generation cephalosporin antibiotic. It is poorly absorbed from the gastrointestinal tract and is only available in IV and IM injectable forms. Cefoperazone is extremely labile in acid environments, which would account both for its destruction and its lack of absorption via the gastrointestinal tract. Following an IV dose of 1000 mg, milk levels ranged from 0.4 to 0.9 mg/L.[1] In a study of 2–3 women who received 1000 mg IV, the maximum milk concentration was 0.4 mg/L at 6 hours.[2] The average milk/plasma ratio was 0.12 at 4 hours. Cefoperazone is extremely acid labile and would be destroyed in the gastrointestinal tract of an infant. It is unlikely that significant absorption would occur.

Pregnancy Risk	B	Lactation Risk	L2
T ½	= 2 hours	M/P	= 0.12
Vd	= 0.143–0.186 l/kg	PB	= 82–93%
Tmax	= 73–153 minutes (IV)	Oral	= Poor
MW	= 645	pKa	= 9.47

Adult Concerns: Diarrhea, allergic rash, thrush.

Pediatric Concerns: None reported. Observe for gastrointestinal symptoms such as diarrhea.

Drug Interactions: Probenecid may decrease clearance. Furosemide, aminoglycosides may enhance renal toxicity.

Relative Infant Dose: 0.4%–1%

Adult Dose: 1–2 gm BID

Alternatives:

References:
1. Pfizer/Roerig Laboratories. Personal Communication. 1996.
2. Matsuda S. Transfer of antibiotics into maternal milk. Biol Res Pregnancy Perinatol 1984; 5(2): 57–60.

CEFOTAXIME   L2

Trade: Claforan

Other Trades: Claforan

Category: Cephalosporin antibiotic

Cefotaxime is poorly absorbed orally and is only available in IV or IM injectable forms. Milk levels following a 1000 mg IV maternal dose were 0.26 mg/L at 1 hour, 0.32 mg/L at 2 hours, and 0.30 mg/L at 3 hours.[1] No effect on infant or lactation were noted. Milk/serum ratio at 3 hours was 0.160. In a group of 2–3 patients receiving 1000 mg IV, none to trace amounts were found in milk after 6 hours.[2]

Pregnancy Risk	B	Lactation Risk	L2
T ½	= 1 hour	M/P	= 0.027–0.16
Vd	= 0.22–0.29 l/kg	PB	= 40%
Tmax	= 30 minutes	Oral	= Poor
MW	= 455	pKa	= 11.04

Adult Concerns: Diarrhea, allergic rash, thrush.

Pediatric Concerns: None reported. Observe for GI symptoms such as diarrhea.

Drug Interactions: Probenecid may decrease clearance. Furosemide, aminoglycosides may enhance renal toxicity.

Relative Infant Dose: 0.3%

Adult Dose: 1–2 gm every BID

Alternatives:

References:
1. Kafetzis DA, Lazarides CV, Siafas CA, Georgakopoulos PA, Papadatos CJ. Transfer of cefotaxime in human milk and from mother to foetus. J Antimicrob Chemother 1980; 6 Suppl A: 135–141.
2. Matsuda S. Transfer of antibiotics into maternal milk. Biol Res Pregnancy Perinatol 1984; 5(2): 57–60.

CEFOTETAN　　　　　　　　　　　　　　　　　L2

Trade: Cefotan

Other Trades: Apatef, Cefotan

Category: Cephalosporin antibiotic

Cefotetan is a third generation cephalosporin that is poorly absorbed orally and is only available in IM and IV injectable forms. The drug is distributed into human milk in low concentrations. Following a maternal dose of 1000 mg IM every 12 hours in 5 patients, breastmilk concentrations ranged from 0.29 to 0.59 mg/L.[1] Plasma concentrations were almost 100 times higher. In a group of 2–3 women who received 1000 mg IV, the maximum average milk level reported was 0.2 mg/L at 4 hours with a milk/plasma ratio of 0.02.[2] In a study of 7 women who received a 1 gram dose IV, levels were undetectable in 2. In the remaining 5, milk levels ranged from 0.22–0.34 mg/L. The mean peak level was 0.34 mg/L at 4 hours.[3]

Pregnancy Risk	B	Lactation Risk	L2
T ½	= 3–4.6 hours	M/P	=
Vd	= 0.147 l/kg	PB	= 76–91%
Tmax	= 1.5–3 hours	Oral	= Poor
MW	= 576	pKa	= 4.06

Adult Concerns: Diarrhea, allergic rash, thrush.

Pediatric Concerns: None reported. Observe for gastrointestinal symptoms such as diarrhea.

Drug Interactions: Probenecid may decrease clearance. Furosemide, aminoglycosides may enhance renal toxicity.

Relative Infant Dose: 0.2%–0.3%

Adult Dose: 1–2 gm BID

Alternatives:

References:
1. Novelli A. The penetration of intramuscular cefotetan disodium into human extra-vascular fluid and maternal milk secretion. Chemotherapia 1983; 11(5): 337–342.
2. Matsuda S. Transfer of antibiotics into maternal milk. Biol Res Pregnancy Perinatol 1984; 5(2): 57–60.
3. Cho N, Fukunaga K, Kuni K. Fundamental and clinical studies on cefotetan (YM09330) in the field of obstetrics and gynecology. Chemotherapy. 1982; 30 (suppl 1): 832–42.

CEFOXITIN   L1

Trade: Mefoxin

Other Trades: Mefoxin

Category: Cephalosporin antibiotic

Cefoxitin is a cephalosporin antibiotic with a spectrum similar to the second generation family. It is transferred into human milk in very low levels. In a study of 18 women receiving 2000–4000 mg doses, only one breast milk sample contained cefoxitin (0.9 mg/L), all the rest were too low to be detected.[1]

In another study of 2–3 women who received 1000 mg IV, only trace amounts were reported in milk over 6 hours.[2] In a group of 5 women who received an IM injection of 2000 mg, the highest milk levels were reported at 4 hours after dose.[3] The maternal plasma levels varied from 22.5 at 2 hours to 77.6 µg/mL at 4 hours. Maternal milk levels ranged from <0.25 to 0.65 mg/L. Observe for changes in gut flora.

In a group of 18 women, 25 milk samples were obtained following doses of 2–4 grams IV.[4] In only one case was cefoxitin found in milk (0.9 mg/L). In another group of 15 women receiving 1 gram IV one month postpartum, milk levels at 2 hours averaged 0.05 mg/L.[5]

Pregnancy Risk	B	Lactation Risk	L1
T ½	= 0.7–1.1 hour	M/P	=
Vd	= 0.11–0.17 l/kg	PB	= 85–99%
Tmax	= 20–30 minutes (IM)	Oral	= Poor
MW	= 427	pKa	= 10.97

Adult Concerns: Diarrhea, allergic rash, thrush.

Pediatric Concerns: None reported. Observe for gastrointestinal symptoms such as diarrhea.

Drug Interactions: Probenecid may decrease clearance. Furosemide, aminoglycosides may enhance renal toxicity.

Relative Infant Dose: 0.1%–0.3%

Adult Dose: 1–2 gm TID

Alternatives:

References:

1. Roex AJ, van Loenen AC, Puyenbroek JI, Arts NF. Secretion of cefoxitin in breast milk following short-term prophylactic administration in caesarean section. Eur J Obstet Gynecol Reprod Biol 1987; 25(4): 299–302.
2. Matsuda S. Transfer of antibiotics into maternal milk. Biol Res Pregnancy Perinatol 1984; 5(2): 57–60.
3. Dresse A, Lambotte R, Dubois M, Delapierre D, Kramp R. Transmammary passage of cefoxitin: additional results. J Clin Pharmacol 1983; 23(10): 438–440.

4. Roex AJ, van Loenen AC, Puyenbroek JI, Arts NF. Secretion of cefoxitin in breast milk following short-term prophylactic administration in caesarean section. Eur J Obstet Gynecol Reprod Biol. 1987 Aug; 25(4): 299–302.
5. Zhang Y, Zhang Q, Xu Z.ʳTissue and body fluid distribution of antibacterial agents in pregnant and lactating women]. Zhonghua Fu Chan Ke Za Zhi. 1997 May; 32(5): 288–92. Chinese.

CEFPODOXIME PROXETIL   L2

Trade: Vantin

Other Trades: Orelox

Category: Cephalosporin antibiotic

Cefpodoxime is a cephalosporin antibiotic that is subsequently metabolized to an active metabolite. Only 50% is orally absorbed. In a study of 3 lactating women, levels of cefpodoxime in human milk were 0%, 2%, and 6% of maternal serum levels at 4 hours following a 200 mg oral dose.[1] At 6 hours post-dosing, levels were 0%, 9%, and 16% of concomitant maternal serum levels. Pediatric indications down to 6 months of age are available.

Pregnancy Risk	B	Lactation Risk	L2
T ½	= 2.09–2.84 hours	M/P	= 0–0.16
Vd	= 0.151 l/kg	PB	= 22–33%
Tmax	= 2–3 hours	Oral	= 50%
MW	= 558	pKa	= 11.09

Adult Concerns: Diarrhea, allergic rash, thrush.

Pediatric Concerns: None reported. Observe for gastrointestinal symptoms such as diarrhea.

Drug Interactions: Probenecid may decrease clearance. Furosemide, aminoglycosides may enhance renal toxicity. Antacids and H_2 blockers reduce gastrointestinal absorption of cefpodoxime.

Relative Infant Dose:

Adult Dose: 100–400 mg BID

Alternatives:

References:
1. Pharmaceutical manufacturer prescribing information, 1996.

CEFPROZIL   L1

Trade: Cefzil

Other Trades:

Category: Oral cephalosporin antibiotic

Cefprozil is a typical second-generation, cephalosporin antibiotic. Following an oral dose of 1000 mg, the breastmilk concentrations were 0.7, 2.5, and 3.5 mg/L at 2, 4, and 6 hours post-dose respectively. The peak milk concentration occurred at 6 hours and was lower thereafter.[1] Milk/plasma ratios varied from 0.05 at 2 hours to 5.67 at 12 hours. However, the milk concentration at 12 hours was small (1.3 µg/mL). Using the highest concentration found in breastmilk (3.5 mg/L), an infant consuming 800 mL of milk daily would ingest about 2.8 mg of cefprozil daily. Because the dose used in this study is approximately twice that normally used, it is reasonable to assume that an infant would ingest less than 1.7 mg per day, an amount clinically insignificant. Pediatric indications for infants 6 months and older are available.

Pregnancy Risk	B		Lactation Risk	L1
T ½	= 78 minutes		M/P	= 0.05–5.67
Vd	= 0.23 l/kg		PB	= 36%
Tmax	= 1.5 hours		Oral	= Complete
MW	=		pKa	= 9.48

Adult Concerns: Diarrhea, allergic rash, and thrush.

Pediatric Concerns: None reported. Observe for gastrointestinal symptoms such as diarrhea.

Drug Interactions: Probenecid may decrease clearance. Furosemide, aminoglycosides may enhance renal toxicity.

Relative Infant Dose: 3.7%

Adult Dose: 250 mg BID

Alternatives:

References:
1. Shyu WC, Shah VR, Campbell DA, Venitz J, Jaganathan V, Pittman KA, Wilber RB, Barbhaiya RH. Excretion of cefprozil into human breast milk. Antimicrob Agents Chemother 1992; 36(5): 938–941.

CEFTAROLINE   L3

Trade: Teflara
Other Trades:
Category: Antibacterial

Ceftaroline is a fifth generation cephalosporin used in the treatment of community-acquired pneumonia and acute skin and skin structure infections, such as Methicillin-resistant *Staphylococcus aureus* (MRSA).[1]

While there are no data on the transfer of this drug into human milk, cephalosporins rarely cause adverse effects in breastfed infants. Occasionally disruption of the infant's gastrointestinal flora, resulting in diarrhea or thrush have been reported with cephalosporins.

Pregnancy Risk	B	Lactation Risk	L3
T ½	= 2.66 hours	M/P	=
Vd	= 0.29 l/kg	PB	= 20%
Tmax	= 0.92 hour	Oral	=
MW	= 762.8	pKa	=

Adult Concerns: Most common adverse effects are diarrhea, nausea, and rash.

Pediatric Concerns: Possibly diarrhea, thrush

Drug Interactions: No clinical drug-drug interactions have been conducted with ceftaroline. There is minimal potential for drug-drug interactions between ceftaroline and CYP450 substrates, inhibitors, or inducers; drugs known to undergo active renal secretion; and drugs that may alter renal blood flow.

Relative Infant Dose:

Adult Dose: 600 mg IV every 12 hours

Alternatives:

References:
1.　Pharmaceutical manufacturer prescribing information, 2010.

CEFTAZIDIME　　L1

Trade: Ceftazidime, Fortaz, Tazidime, Ceptaz
Other Trades: Fortum, Fortaz, Ceptaz
Category: Cephalosporin antibiotic

Ceftazidime is a broad-spectrum, third-generation, cephalosporin antibiotic. It has poor oral absorption (<10%). In a group of 11 lactating women who received 2000 mg (IV) every 8 hours for 5 days, concentrations of ceftazidime in milk averaged 3.8 mg/L before the dose and 5.2 mg/L at 1 hour after the dose and 4.5 mg/L 3 hours after the dose.[1] There is, however, no progressive accumulation of ceftazidime in breastmilk, as evidenced by the similar levels prior to and after seven doses. The therapeutic dose for neonates is 30–50 mg/kg every 12 hours.

Pregnancy Risk	B	Lactation Risk	L1
T ½	= 1.4–2 hours	M/P	=
Vd	= 0.230 l/kg	PB	= 5–24%
Tmax	= 69–90 minutes	Oral	= <10%
MW	= 547	pKa	= 3.16

Adult Concerns: Diarrhea, allergic rash, thrush.

Pediatric Concerns: None reported. Observe for gastrointestinal symptoms such as diarrhea.

Drug Interactions: Probenecid may decrease clearance. Furosemide, aminoglycosides may enhance renal toxicity.

Relative Infant Dose: 0.9%

Adult Dose: 500–2000 mg BID

Alternatives:

References:
1.   Blanco JD, Jorgensen JH, Castaneda YS, Crawford SA. Ceftazidime levels in human breast milk. Antimicrob Agents Chemother 1983; 23(3): 479–480.

CEFTIBUTEN   L2

Trade: Cedax

Other Trades: Cedax

Category: Cephalosporin antibiotic

Ceftibuten is a broad-spectrum, third generation oral cephalosporin antibiotic. No data yet available on penetration into human breastmilk.[1] Small to moderate amounts may penetrate into milk, but ceftibuten is cleared for pediatric use.[2] Its strength is in its activity against gram negative species. Its weakness is in staphylococci and strep. pneumonia coverage (which causes many inner ear infections).

Pregnancy Risk	B	Lactation Risk	L2
T ½	= 2.4 hours	M/P	=
Vd	= 0.21 l/kg	PB	= 65%
Tmax	= 2.6 hours	Oral	= High
MW	= 410	pKa	= 3.68

Adult Concerns: Diarrhea, vomiting, loose stools, abdominal pain.

Pediatric Concerns: None reported. Observe for gastrointestinal symptoms such as diarrhea.

Drug Interactions: Probenecid may decrease clearance. Furosemide, aminoglycosides may enhance renal toxicity.

Relative Infant Dose:

Adult Dose: 400 mg daily.

Alternatives:

References:
1.   Pharmaceutical manufacturer prescribing information, 1996.
2.   Barr WH, Affrime M, Lin CC, Batra V. Pharmacokinetics of ceftibuten in children. Pediatr Infect Dis J 1995; 14(7 Suppl): S93–101.

CEFTIZOXIME   L1

Trade: Cefizox, Baxam

Other Trades: Cefizox

Category: Cephalosporin antibiotic

Ceftizoxime is a third generation cephalosporin used for many infections, similar to ceftriaxone and others. In a study of 18 patients who received 1 gm IV daily, milk levels of ceftizoxime averaged 0.52 mg/L. The maximum reported concentration was 2.38 mg/L.[1] In studies of 5 and 7 women (1 gm IV), milk levels averaged 0.43 and 0.54 mg/L.[2,3] In a study of 6 women who received 1 gm IV, milk levels of 0.25 mg/L were reported at 1 hour post dose.[4] In four good studies, ceftizoxime produced only negligible levels in milk. Observe for changes in gut flora and diarrhea.

Pregnancy Risk	B	Lactation Risk	L1
T ½	= 2.3 hours	M/P	=
Vd	= 0.5 l/kg	PB	= 28–50%
Tmax	= <1 hour	Oral	= Minimal
MW	= 383	pKa	= 11.00

Adult Concerns: Skin rash in allergic patients, nausea, vomiting, diarrhea.

Pediatric Concerns: None in three studies as milk levels are low. Some changes in gut flora could occur as with any antibiotic.

Drug Interactions: A decreased response to typhoid vaccine. H_2 antagonists (ranitidine, famotidine, etc) may reduce oral bioavailability of ceftizoxime.

Relative Infant Dose: 0.3%–0.6%

Adult Dose: 1 gm IV daily

Alternatives: Ceftriaxone

References:
1. Matsuda S, Shimizu T, Ichinoe K, Cho N, Noda K, Ninomiya K, et al.[Pharmacokinetic and clinical studies of ceftizoxime in the perinatal period. The Chemotherapy Research Group for Mothers and Children]. Jpn J Antibiot 1988 Aug; 41(8): 1129–41.
2. Cho N, Fukunaga K, Kunii K, Tezuka K, Kobayashi I.[Studies of ceftizoxime in perinatal period]. Jpn J Antibiot 1988 Aug; 41(8): 1142–54.
3. Ito K, Izumi K, Takagi H, Yokoyama Y, Tamaya T, Baba Y, et al.[Pharmacokinetic and clinical studies of ceftizoxime in obstetrical and gynecological field (2)]. Jpn J Antibiot 1988 Aug; 41(8): 1155–63.
4. Gerding DN, Peterson LR. Comparative tissue and extravascular fluid concentrations of ceftizoxime. J Antimicrob Chemother 1982 Nov; 10 Suppl C: 105–16.: 105–16.

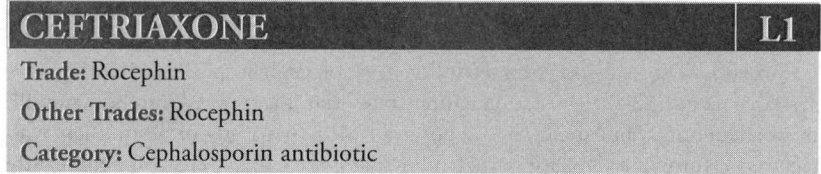

CEFTRIAXONE   L1

Trade: Rocephin

Other Trades: Rocephin

Category: Cephalosporin antibiotic

Ceftriaxone is a very popular third-generation broad-spectrum cephalosporin antibiotic. Small amounts are transferred into milk (3–4% of maternal serum level). Following a 1 gm IM dose, breastmilk levels were approximately 0.5–0.7 mg/L between 4–8 hours.[1,2] The estimated mean milk levels at steady state were 3–4 mg/L. Another source indicates that following a 2 gm/day dose and at steady state, approximately 4.4% of dose penetrates into milk.[3] In this study, the maximum breast milk concentration was 7.89 mg/L after prolonged therapy (7 days). Poor oral absorption of ceftriaxone would further limit systemic absorption by the infant. The half-life of ceftriaxone in human milk varies from 12.8 to 17.3

hours (longer than maternal serum). Even at this high dose, no adverse effects were noted in the infant. Ceftriaxone levels in breastmilk are probably too low to be clinically relevant, except for changes in gastrointestinal flora. Ceftriaxone is not commonly used in neonates.

Pregnancy Risk	B	Lactation Risk	L1
T ½	= 7.3 hours	M/P	= 0.03
Vd	= 0.192 l/kg	PB	= 95%
Tmax	= 1 hour	Oral	= Poor
MW	= 555	pKa	= 3.96

Adult Concerns: Diarrhea, allergic rash, pseudomembranous colitis, thrush.

Pediatric Concerns: None reported. Observe for gastrointestinal symptoms such as diarrhea.

Drug Interactions: Probenecid may decrease clearance. Furosemide, aminoglycosides may enhance renal toxicity.

Relative Infant Dose: 4.1%–4.2%

Adult Dose: 1–2 gm every 12–24 hours depending on indication

Alternatives:

References:
1. Kafetzis DA, Siafas CA, Georgakopoulos PA, Papadatos CJ. Passage of cephalosporins and amoxicillin into the breast milk. Acta Paediatr Scand 1981; 70(3): 285–288.
2. Kafetzis DA, Brater DC, Fanourgakis JE, Voyatzis J, Georgakopoulos P. Ceftriaxone distribution between maternal blood and fetal blood and tissues at parturition and between blood and milk postpartum. Antimicrob Agents Chemother 1983; 23(6): 870–873.
3. Bourget P, Quinquis-Desmaris V, Fernandez H. Ceftriaxone distribution and protein binding between maternal blood and milk postpartum. Ann Pharmacother 1993; 27(3): 294–297.

CEFUROXIME   L2

Trade: Ceftin, Zinacef, Kefurox

Other Trades: Zinnat, Zinacef

Category: Cephalosporin antibiotic

Cefuroxime is a broad-spectrum second-generation cephalosporin antibiotic that is available orally and IV. The manufacturer states that it is secreted into human milk in small amounts, but the levels are not available.[1] In a study of 38 mothers who received cefuroxime, 2.6% reported mild side effects that were not significantly different from controls (9%).[2] Following a single dose of 750 mg in 5 women, the mean peak level reported in milk was 370 µg/L.[3] In another group of 8 women who received a single dose of 750 mg, milk levels at peak (8 hours) were 1.45 mg/L.[4] Cefuroxime has a very bitter taste. The IV salt form, cefuroxime sodium, is very poorly absorbed orally. Only the axetil salt form is orally bioavailable.

Pregnancy Risk	B	Lactation Risk	L2
T ½	= 1.4 hours	M/P	=
Vd	= 0.326 l/kg	PB	= 33–50%
Tmax	= 2–3 hours	Oral	= 30–50%
MW	= 424	pKa	= 10.98

Adult Concerns: Nausea, vomiting, diarrhea, gastrointestinal distress, skin rash, allergies.

Pediatric Concerns: None reported. Observe for GI symptoms such as diarrhea, rash.

Drug Interactions: Probenecid may decrease clearance. Furosemide, aminoglycosides may enhance renal toxicity.

Relative Infant Dose: 0.6%–2%

Adult Dose: 250–500 mg BID

Alternatives:

References:
1. Pharmaceutical manufacturer prescribing information, 1995.
2. Benyamini L et al. The Safety of Amoxicillin/Clavulanic Acid and Cefuroxime During Lactation. Ther Drug Monit 2005 Aug; 27(4): 499–502.
3. Takase Z, Shirofuji H, Uchida M. Fundamental and clinical studies of cefuroxime in the field of obstetrics and gynecology. Chemotherapy (Tokyo). 1979; 27 (Suppl 6): 600–2.
4. Voropaeva SD, Emelyanova AI, Ankirskaya AS et al. Cefuroxime efficacy in obstetrics and gynecology. Antibiotiki. 1981; 27: 697–701.

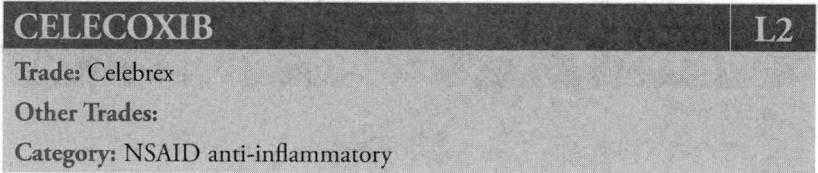

CELECOXIB   L2

Trade: Celebrex

Other Trades:

Category: NSAID anti-inflammatory

Celecoxib is an NSAID that specifically blocks the cyclooxygenase (COX-2) enzyme. It is primarily used for arthritic or inflammatory pain. In a case report of a patient receiving 100 mg twice daily, the authors report a milk level of 133 and 101 ng/mL in left and right breasts 4.75 hours after the dose.[1] They estimated (using the C_{max} levels) the M/P ratio to be 0.27 to 0.59 and that the infant's exposure would be approximately 20 µg/kg/day. In data from our laboratories in 5 women receiving 200 mg once daily, the mean milk/plasma AUC ratio was 0.23.[2] The average concentration of celecoxib (AUC) in milk was 66 µg/L. The absolute infant dose averaged 9.8 µg/kg/day. Using this data, the relative infant dose was 0.30% of the maternal dose. Plasma levels of celecoxib in two infants studied were undetectable. In another study, blood and milk were sampled for 48 hours after celecoxib 200 mg orally in six lactating volunteers. The median infant dose was 0.23% of the maternal dose after adjusting for weight. Therefore, the authors suggest that the relative dose that infants are exposed to via milk is very low and breastfeeding would probably not be a threat to the infant.[3]

Pregnancy Risk	C	Lactation Risk	L2
T ½	= 11.2 hours	M/P	= 0.23
Vd	= 5.71 l/kg	PB	= 97%
Tmax	= 2.8 hours	Oral	= 99%
MW	= 381	pKa	= 11.1

Adult Concerns: Gastrointestinal distress, diarrhea, dyspepsia, headache, aggravated hypertension and asthma.

Pediatric Concerns: None reported via milk. Plasma levels in 2 infants were undetectable. Milk levels are very low.

Drug Interactions: Celecoxib may significantly diminish antihypertensive effects of ACE inhibitors, and the natriuretic effect of furosemide. Fluconazole may increase plasma levels of celecoxib two-fold. Celecoxib may increase lithium levels by 17%.

Relative Infant Dose: 0.3%–0.7%

Adult Dose: 100–400 mg daily

Alternatives: Ibuprofen

References:
1. Knoppert DC, Stempak D, Baruchel S, Koren G. Celecoxib in human milk: a case report. Pharmacotherapy 2003; 23(1): 97–100.
2. Hale TW, McDonald R, Boger J. Transfer of celecoxib into human milk. J Hum Lact 2004 Nov; 20(4): 397–403.
3. Gardiner SJ, Doogue MP, Zhang M, Begg EJ. Quantification of infant exposure to celecoxib through breast milk. Br J Clin Pharmacol 2006; 61(1): 101–104.

CEPHALEXIN   L1

Trade: Keflex

Other Trades: Ibilex, Apo-Cephalex, Ceporex, Novo-Lexin

Category: Cephalosporin antibiotic

Cephalexin is a typical first-generation, cephalosporin antibiotic. Only minimal concentrations are secreted into human milk. Following a 1000 mg maternal oral dose, milk levels at 1, 2, 3, 4, and 5 hours ranged from 0.20, 0.28, 0.39, 0.50, and 0.47 mg/L respectively.[1] Milk/serum ratios varied from 0.008 at 1 hour to 0.140 at 3 hours. These levels are probably too low to be clinically relevant. In a group of 2–3 patients who received 500 mg orally, milk levels averaged 0.7 mg/L at 4 hours although the average milk level was 0.36 mg/L over 6 hours.[2] The milk/plasma ratio was 0.25. In another case report of a mother taking probenecid along with cephalexin to prolong the half-life of cephalexin, the baby developed severe diarrhea. The average milk concentration of probenecid and cephalexin was 964 µg/L and 0.745 µg/L, respectively. This corresponds to a relative infant dose of 0.7% for probenecid and 0.5% for cephalexin. The authors concluded that when using this combination of drugs in breast feeding women, clinicians should expect the possibility of adverse gastrointestinal effects in the infant.[3] Safe in breastfeeding. Watch infant for diarrhea.

Pregnancy Risk	B		Lactation Risk	L1
T ½	= 50–80 minutes		M/P	= 0.008–0.14
Vd	= 0.25 l/kg		PB	= 10%
Tmax	= 1 hour		Oral	= Complete
MW	= 347		pKa	= 11.91

Adult Concerns: Diarrhea, allergic rash, thrush.

Pediatric Concerns: Diarrhea in the groups exposed to probenecid plus cephalexin.

Drug Interactions: Probenecid may decrease clearance. Furosemide, aminoglycosides may enhance renal toxicity.

Relative Infant Dose: 0.5%–1.5%

Adult Dose: 250–1000 mg every 6 hours

Alternatives:

References:
1. Kafetzis DA, Siafas CA, Georgakopoulos PA, Papadatos CJ. Passage of cephalosporins and amoxicillin into the breast milk. Acta Paediatr Scand 1981; 70(3): 285–288.
2. Matsuda S. Transfer of antibiotics into maternal milk. Biol Res Pregnancy Perinatol 1984; 5(2): 57–60.
3. Ilett K, Hackett P, Ingle B, Bretz PJ. Transfer of Probenecid and Cephalexin into Breast Milk. Ann Pharmacother 2006; 40: 986–988.

CEPHALOTHIN   L1

Trade: Keflin

Other Trades: Ceporacin, Keflin

Category: Cephalosporin antibiotic

Cephalothin is a first-generation, cephalosporin antibiotic for use by IM or IV administration. Following a 1000 mg IV maternal dose, milk levels varied from 0.27, 0.41, 0.47, 0.36, and 0.28 mg/L at 0.5, 1, 2, 3, and 4 hours respectively.[1] Milk/serum ratios varied from 0.06 at 1 hour to 0.51 at 3 hours.

Pregnancy Risk	B		Lactation Risk	L1
T ½	= 30–50 minutes		M/P	= 0.06–0.5
Vd	=		PB	= 70%
Tmax	= 1–2 hours		Oral	= Poor
MW	= 396		pKa	= 11.75

Adult Concerns: Diarrhea, allergic rash, thrush.

Pediatric Concerns: None reported. Observe for diarrhea.

Drug Interactions: Probenecid may decrease clearance. Furosemide, aminoglycosides may enhance renal toxicity.

Relative Infant Dose: 0.3%–0.5%

Adult Dose: 500–2000 mg every 4–6 hours

Alternatives: Cephalexin, amoxicillin, dicloxacillin

References:
1. Kafetzis DA, Siafas CA, Georgakopoulos PA, Papadatos CJ. Passage of cephalosporins and amoxicillin into the breast milk. Acta Paediatr Scand 1981; 70(3): 285–288.

CEPHAPIRIN   L1

Trade: Cefadyl

Other Trades: Cefadyl

Category: Cephalosporin antibiotic

Cephapirin is a typical first-generation, cephalosporin antibiotic for IM or IV administration. Following a 1000 mg IV maternal dose, milk levels varied from 0.26, 0.41, 0.43, 0.33, and 0.27 mg/L at 0.5, 1, 2, 3, and 4 hours respectively.[1] These are too low to be clinically relevant. Milk/serum ratios varied from 0.068 at 1 hour to 0.48 at 3 hours.

Pregnancy Risk	B	Lactation Risk	L1
T½	= 24–36 minutes	M/P	= 0.068–0.48
Vd	= 0.23 l/kg	PB	= 54%
Tmax	= 1–2 hours	Oral	= Poor
MW	= 445	pKa	= 11.54

Adult Concerns: Diarrhea, allergic rash, thrush.

Pediatric Concerns: None reported. Observe for GI symptoms such as diarrhea.

Drug Interactions: Probenecid may decrease clearance. Furosemide, aminoglycosides may enhance renal toxicity.

Relative Infant Dose: 0.3%–0.4%

Adult Dose: 500–1000 mg every 6 hours

Alternatives:

References:
1. Kafetzis DA, Siafas CA, Georgakopoulos PA, Papadatos CJ. Passage of cephalosporins and amoxicillin into the breast milk. Acta Paediatr Scand 1981; 70(3): 285–288.

CEPHRADINE   L1

Trade: Velosef, Anspor

Other Trades: Velosef, Nicef

Category: Cephalosporin antibiotic

Cephradine is typical first-generation cephalosporin antibiotic. In a group of 6 lactating women receiving 500 mg orally every 6 hours for 2 days, milk levels averaged about 0.6 mg/L.[1] In another study group by this same author, the average milk level was 1.0 mg/L.[2] These levels are too low to be clinically relevant.

Pregnancy Risk	B	Lactation Risk	L1
T ½	= 0.7–2 hours	M/P	= 0.2
Vd	= 0.29 l/kg	PB	= 8–17%
Tmax	= 1 hour	Oral	= Complete
MW	= 349	pKa	= 11.99

Adult Concerns: Diarrhea, allergic rash, thrush, liver dysfunction.

Pediatric Concerns: None reported. Observe for gastrointestinal symptoms such as diarrhea.

Drug Interactions: Probenecid may decrease clearance. Furosemide, aminoglycosides may enhance renal toxicity.

Relative Infant Dose: 0.3%–0.5%

Adult Dose: 250–500 mg every 6–12 hours

Alternatives:

References:
1. Mischler TW, Corson SL, Larranaga A, Bolognese RJ, Neiss ES, Vukovich RA. Cephradine and epicillin in body fluids of lactating and pregnant women. J Reprod Med 1978; 21(3): 130–136.
2. Mischler TW. et. al. Presence of cephradine in body fluids of lactating and pregnant women. Clin Pharmacol Ther 1974; 15: 214.

CERTOLIZUMAB PEGOL   L3

Trade: Cimzia

Other Trades:

Category: Monoclonal Antibody

Certolizumab Pegol is a pegylated, humanized monoclonal anti-TNF antigen binding fragment that blocks tumor necrosis factor-alpha (TNF-alpha).[1] Certolizumab is used for the treatment of rheumatoid arthritis and Crohn's disease. No human studies have been done but animal studies have shown minimal transfer of Certolizumab into milk and no antibodies were detected in the nursing pups. The molecular weight, 91 kilodaltons, is a large molecule and not likely to transfer into milk.

Pregnancy Risk	B	Lactation Risk	L3
T ½	= 14 days	M/P	=
Vd	= 0.086–0.114 l/kg	PB	=
Tmax	= 54–171 hours	Oral	= 80%
MW	= 91 kiloDaltons	pKa	=

Adult Concerns: Infections, nausea, vomiting, headache, dizziness, hypertension, fever, arthralgia, fatigue, injection site reactions, renal failure, seizure, peripheral neuropathy, myocardial infarction, malignancy.

Pediatric Concerns:

Drug Interactions: Certolizumab may increase the adverse effects of Abacept and Anakinra. Rituximab may increase the immunosuppressant effects of Certolizumab Pegol.

Relative Infant Dose:

Adult Dose: 400 mg SQ every 2 weeks until response, then every 4 weeks

Alternatives:

References:
1. Pharmaceutical manufacturer prescribing information, 2011.

CETIRIZINE	L2

Trade:

Other Trades:

Category: Antihistamine

Cetirizine is a popular new antihistamine useful for seasonal allergic rhinitis. It is a metabolite of hydroxyzine and is one of the most potent of the antihistamines. It is rapidly and extensively absorbed orally and due to a rather long half-life is used only once daily. It penetrates the CNS poorly and therefore produces minimal sedation. Compared to other new antihistamines, cetirizine is not very toxic in overdose and produces few cardiovascular changes at higher doses.[1] Further, as with many other antihistamines, cetirizine has very few drug interactions, alcohol being the main one. Studies in dogs suggests that only 3% of the dose is transferred into milk.

Pregnancy Risk	B		Lactation Risk	L2
T ½	= 8.3 hours		M/P	=
Vd	= 0.429–0.571 l/kg		PB	= 93%
Tmax	= 1.7 hour		Oral	= 70%
MW	= 389		pKa	= 1.6, 2.9, 8.3

Adult Concerns: Sedation, fatigue, dry mouth.

Pediatric Concerns: None reported but observe for sedation.

Drug Interactions: Increased sedation with other CNS sedatives, alcohol.

Relative Infant Dose:

Adult Dose: 5–10 mg daily.

Alternatives:

References:
1. Pharmaceutical manufacturer prescribing information, 1996.
2. Pharmaceutical Manufacturer. Personal Communication. 1996.

CETUXIMAB   L4

Trade: Erbitux
Other Trades:
Category: anticancer drug

Cetuximab is a recombinant, human/mouse chimeric monoclonal antibody (152 kDa) that binds specifically to the human epidermal growth factor receptor, resulting in inhibition of cell growth, induction of apoptosis, and decreased matrix metalloproteinase and vascular endothelial growth factor production. Following a two-hour infusion of 400 mg/m², the mean elimination half-life was 97 hours (range 41–213 hours).[1] The volume of the distribution (Vd) for cetuximab appeared to be independent of dose and approximated the vascular space of 2–3 L/m². The manufacturer recommends mothers discontinue breastfeeding for 60 days, which would correspond with the longer half-life of this product.

Although no data are available on its transfer into human milk, some transfer into colostrum should be expected. The amount in mature milk would likely be exceedingly low as IgG levels in mature milk are low anyway (4 mg/dL). When admixed and diluted with the plasma compartment IgG, few if any, molecules of cetuximab would enter mature milk. Withhold breastfeeding for approximately 60 days.

Pregnancy Risk	C	Lactation Risk	L4
T ½	= 114 hours	M/P	=
Vd	= 2–3 L/m²	PB	=
Tmax	=	Oral	=
MW	= 145781.6	pKa	=

Adult Concerns: Pimples or skin rash, bloating or swelling of the face, arms, hands, lower legs, or feet, body aches or pain, chills, congestion, cough or hoarseness, deep cracks, grooves, or lines in the skin, difficult or labored breathing, dizziness, fever, headache, lower back or side pain, nausea, vomiting; painful or difficult urination, pale skin, rapid weight gain, runny nose, tender, swollen glands in the neck, tightness in the chest, tingling of the hands or feet, difficulty in swallowing, bleeding or bruising, tiredness or weakness, weight gain or loss, weakness, wheezing.

Pediatric Concerns:

Drug Interactions: There are no known significant interactions.

Relative Infant Dose:

Adult Dose: 250 mg/m² infused over 60 minutes weekly

Alternatives:

References:
1. Pharmaceutical manufacturer prescribing information, 2005.

CEVIMELINE   L3

Trade: Evoxac
Other Trades:
Category: Treatment of dry mouth; Alzheimer's disease

Cevimeline is a cholinergic agonist agent, which binds to muscarinic receptors and can increase secretion of exocrine glands such as salivary and sweat glands, and increase tone in the gastrointestinal and urinary tracts. It is indicated for the treatment of patients with Sjogren's Syndrome.[1] This drug has a large volume of distribution which suggests that most of the compound is stored in peripheral tissues, not the plasma compartment. Many such drugs produce lower milk levels. No data are available on its transfer into human milk. Due to its strong cholinergic effects, some caution is recommended in breastfeeding mothers. Observe closely for excess salivation, diarrhea, excess sweating, nausea, and urinary frequency and infection.

Pregnancy Risk	C	Lactation Risk	L3
T ½	= 3–5 hours	M/P	=
Vd	= 6 l/kg	PB	= <20%
Tmax	= 1–2 hours	Oral	= Complete
MW	= 244	pKa	=

Adult Concerns: Diaphoresis (excessive perspiration), nausea, rhinitis, urinary frequency, headache, diarrhea, and gastric cramping are reported.

Pediatric Concerns: No reports in breastfeeding mothers available.

Drug Interactions: None reported.

Relative Infant Dose:

Adult Dose: 30 mg TID

Alternatives: Oral pilocarpine

References:
1. Pharmaceutical manufacturer prescribing information, 2010.

CHAMOMILE, GERMAN   L3

Trade:
Other Trades:
Category: Anti-inflammatory, carminative

Chamomile has been used since Roman times and is primarily used for its anti-inflammatory, carminative, antispasmodic, mild sedative, and antiseptic properties. It has been used for flatulent dyspepsia, travel sickness, diarrhea, gastrointestinal irritation.[1] It has been used topically for hemorrhoids and mastitis. Chamomile contains coumarins, flavonoids such as quercetin, rutin, and others. Anti-allergic and anti-inflammatory effects have been well documented and are due to the azulene components of the volatile oil which inhibit histamine release.[2] Matricin is reported to be a significant anti-inflammatory agent. In humans, German chamomile has been reported to exhibit anti-inflammatory, anti-peptic, and anti-spasmodic effects on the stomach.[2] Reports of allergic reactions to chamomile include two cases of anaphylaxis, although this is probably rare.[3,4,5] Asthmatics should probably avoid this product. German chamomile is reported to be uterotonic and teratogenic in rats, rabbits, and dogs although the dose of alpha-bisabolol used in these studies was excessively high.[6] Some authors suggest this product should be avoided in pregnant and breastfeeding mothers[7], but the German Commission E considers it safe.[8]

Pregnancy Risk	Possibly Hazardous	Lactation Risk	L3
T ½	=	M/P	=
Vd	=	PB	=
Tmax	=	Oral	=
MW	=	pKa	=

Adult Concerns: Reports of allergic reactions to chamomile are common, including two cases of anaphylaxis. Asthmatics should avoid this product. German chamomile is reported to be uterotonic and teratogenic in rats, rabbits, and dogs. This product should be avoided in pregnant and lactating patients.

Pediatric Concerns: None reported via milk, but hypersensitization is possible.

Drug Interactions: Do not use with benzodiazepines, CNS depressants, oral contraceptives, tamoxifen and warfarin.

Relative Infant Dose:

Adult Dose: 400–1600 mg daily in divided doses

Alternatives:

References:
1. Berry M. The chamomiles. Pharm J 1995; 254: 191–193.
2. Mann C, Staba EJ. The chemistry, pharmacology, and commercial formulations of chamomile. In: Herbs, spices, and medicinal plants: Recent advances in botany, horticulture, and pharmacology. Vol. 1. Arizona: Oryx Press, 1986.
3. Hausen BM. The sensitizing capacity of Compositae plants. Planta Med 1984; 50: 229–234.
4. Casterline CL. Allergy to chamomile tea. JAMA 1980; 244(4): 330–331.
5. Benner MH, Lee HJ. Anaphylactic reaction to chamomile tea. J Allergy Clin Immunol 1973; 52(5): 307–308.
6. Habersang S, Leuschner F, Isaac O, Thiemer K. Pharmacological studies with compounds of chamomile. IV. Studies on toxicity of (-)-alpha-bisabolol (author's transl)]. Planta Med 1979; 37(2): 115–123.
7. Newall C, Anderson LA, Phillipson JD. Chamomile, German. In. Herbal Medicine. A guide for the healthcare professionals. The Pharmaceutical Press, London, 1996.
8. The Complete German Commission E Monographs. Ed. M. Blumenthal Amer Botanical Council 1998.

CHLORAL HYDRATE   L3

Trade: Aquachloral, Noctec

Other Trades: Dormel, Elix-Noctec, Nortec, Novo-Chlorhydrate

Category: Sedative, hypnotic

Chloral hydrate is a sedative hypnotic. Small to moderate amounts are known to be secreted into milk. Mild drowsiness was reported in one infant following administration of dichloralphenazone (1300 mg/d), which is metabolized to the same active metabolite as chloral hydrate. Infant growth and development were reported to be normal. In a study of 50 postpartum women using a 1.3 gm rectal suppository, the average milk concentration of chloral hydrate at 1 hour was 3.2 mg/L.[1] The maximum milk level found in this study was 15 mg/L in one patient. The oral pediatric sedative dose of chloral hydrate is generally 5–15 mg/kg/dose every 8 hours.[2]

Pregnancy Risk	C	Lactation Risk	L3
T ½	= 7–10 hours	M/P	=
Vd	= 0.6 l/kg	PB	= 35–41%
Tmax	= 30–60 minutes	Oral	= Complete
MW	= 165	pKa	= 10.0

Adult Concerns: Irritating to mucous membrane, laryngospasm, gastrointestinal irritation, paradoxical excitement, delirium, hypotension, respiratory depression and sedation.

Pediatric Concerns: None reported via milk, but observe for sedation.

Drug Interactions: May potentiate effects of warfarin, CNS depressants such as alcohol, etc. Use with furosemide (IV) may induce flushing, hypotension.

Relative Infant Dose: 2.6%

Adult Dose: 250 mg TID

Alternatives: Alprazolam, Midazolam

References:
1. Bernstine JB, Meyer AE, Bernstine RL. Maternal blood and breast milk estimation following the administration of chloral hydrate during the puerperium. J Obstet Gynaecol Br Emp 1956; 63(2): 228–231.
2. Johnson KB. ed. The Harriet Lane Handbook, Thirteenth Edition. Mosey, 1993.

CHLORAMBUCIL   L5

Trade: Leukeran, Linfolysin, Alti-Chlorambucil

Other Trades:

Category: anticancer drug

Chlorambucil is a derivative of nitrogen mustard with molecular weight of 304.[1] Administered orally, it is well absorbed (Oral= > 56%). It is eliminated rapidly with a half-life of 1–2 hours. Only trace levels are found in CNS. Milk levels are unpublished, but probably low due to high protein binding, and amine structure. Withhold breastfeeding for at least 24 hours.

Pregnancy Risk	D	Lactation Risk	L5
T ½	= 1–1.9 hours	M/P	=
Vd	= 0.14–0.24 l/kg	PB	= 99%
Tmax	= 1 hour	Oral	= Rapid and complete; reduced 10%-20% with food
MW	= 304.2	pKa	= 5.8

Adult Concerns: Black, tarry stools, blood in urine, cough or hoarseness, fever or chills, lower back or side pain, painful or difficult urination, pinpoint red spots on skin, unusual bleeding or bruising

Pediatric Concerns:

Drug Interactions: Adverse effects may be increased by Denosumab and Pimecrolimus. Chlorambucil may enhance adverse effects of Leflunomide and Natalizumab. Roflumilast may increase the immunosuppressant effects of Chlorambucil.

Relative Infant Dose:

Adult Dose: 0.1 mg/kg/day for 3–6 weeks or 0.4 mg/kg biweekly

Alternatives:

References:
1. Grochow LB, Ames MM. A clinician's guide to chemotherapy pharmacokinetics and pharmacodynamics. 1st ed. Baltimore, MD: Williams and Wilkins; 1998.

CHLORAMPHENICOL   L4

Trade: Chloromycetin

Other Trades: Chlorsig, Ak-Chlor, Chloromycetin, Chloroptic, Sopamycetin, Biocetin

Category: Antibiotic

Chloramphenicol is a broad-spectrum antibiotic. In one study of 5 women receiving 250 mg chloramphenicol orally four times daily, the concentration of chloramphenicol in milk ranged from 0.54 to 2.84 mg/L.[1] In the same study but in another group receiving 500 mg orally four times daily, the concentration of chloramphenicol in milk ranged from 1.75 to 6.10 mg/L. In a group of patients being treated for typhus, milk levels were lower than maternal plasma levels.[2] With maternal plasma levels of 49 and 26 mg/L in two patients, the milk levels were 26 and 16 mg/L respectively. In a study of 2–3 patients who received a single 500 mg oral dose, the average milk concentration at 4 hours was 4.1 mg/L.[3] The milk/plasma ratio at 4 hours was 0.84. Safety in infants is highly controversial. Milk levels are too low to produce overt toxicity in infants but could produce allergic sensitization to subsequent exposures. Generally, chloramphenicol is considered contraindicated in nursing mothers although it is occasionally used in infants.

This antibiotic can be extremely toxic, particularly in newborns, and should not be used for trivial infections. Blood levels should be constantly monitored and kept below 20 µg/mL.

Pregnancy Risk	C	Lactation Risk	L4
T ½	= 4 hours	M/P	= 0.5–0.6
Vd	= 0.57 l/kg	PB	= 53%
Tmax	= 1 hour	Oral	= Complete
MW	= 323	pKa	= 5.5

Adult Concerns: Numerous blood dyscrasias, aplastic anemia, fever, skin rashes.

Pediatric Concerns: None reported via milk.

Drug Interactions: Phenobarbital and rifampin may reduce plasma levels of chloramphenicol. Chloramphenicol inhibits metabolism of chlorpropamide, phenytoin, and oral anticoagulants.

Relative Infant Dose: 3.2%–8.5%

Adult Dose: 50–100 mg/kg daily divided every 6 hours

Alternatives:

References:
1. Havelka J, Hejzlar M, Popov V, Viktorinova D, Prochazka J. Excretion of chloramphenicol in human milk. Chemotherapy 1968; 13(4): 204–211.
2. Smadel JE. et. al. Chloramphenicol in the treatment of tsutsugamushi disease. J Clin Invest 1949; 28: 1196–1215.
3. Matsuda S. Transfer of antibiotics into maternal milk. Biol Res Pregnancy Perinatol 1984; 5(2): 57–60.

CHLORDIAZEPOXIDE   L3

Trade: Apo-Chlordiazepoxide, Librium, Libritabs, Solium

Other Trades: Limbitrol, Apo-Chlordiazepoxide, Librium, Medilium, Librium

Category: Antianxiety, benzodiazepine sedative

Chlordiazepoxide is an older benzodiazepine that belongs to Valium family. It is secreted in breastmilk in moderate but unreported levels.[1] See Diazepam.

Pregnancy Risk	D	Lactation Risk	L3
T ½	= 6.6–25 hours	M/P	=
Vd	= 3.3 l/kg	PB	= 90–98%
Tmax	= 1–4 hours	Oral	= Complete
MW	= 300	pKa	= 4.8

Adult Concerns: Sedation.

Pediatric Concerns: Observe for sedation.

Drug Interactions: Increased CNS sedation when used with other sedative-hypnotics. May increase risk when used with anticoagulants, alcohol, tricyclic antidepressants, MAO inhibitors.

Relative Infant Dose:

Adult Dose: 15–100 mg every 6–8 hours

Alternatives: Alprazolam

References:
1. Pharmaceutical manufacturer prescribing information, 2010.

CHLORDIAZEPOXIDE + CLIDINIUM — L3

Trade: Librax, Clinoxide

Other Trades: Apo-chlorax, Pro-Chlorax, Corium

Category: Anticholinergic/spasmolytic

Chlordiazepoxide hydrochloride and Clidinium bromide is a drug combination product. Its indications include its use as an adjunct in acute enterocolitis, irritable bowel syndrome and peptic ulcer disease.

Chlordiazepoxide has antianxiety effects while clidinium bromide has anticholinergic properties giving pronounced antispasmodic and antisecretory effects on the gastrointestinal tract. This combination should not be used in patients with glaucoma or benign bladder neck obstruction. Chlordiazepoxide is secreted in breastmilk in moderate but unreported levels.[1] However, its transfer into breastmilk should be similar to that of diazepam.

Clidinium is incompletely absorbed from the small intestine and is rapidly hydrolyzed in the liver to form its quaternary amino-alcohol. As a quaternary ammonium compound it is fully ionized, and as such has very limited lipid solubility, thus limiting its volume of distribution. It is currently unknown if clidinium is excreted into breast milk. Other antimuscarinic drugs have shown some data regarding transfer into milk, but so far no substantial evidence has been found to support that claim.[2]

Pregnancy Risk	D	Lactation Risk	L3
T ½	= Chlordiazepoxide/clidinium: 6.6–25 hours/1.2–20 hours	M/P	= Chlordiazepoxide/clidinium:
Vd	= Chlordiazepoxide/clidinium: 3.3/ l/kg	PB	= Chlordiazepoxide/clidinium: 90–98%
Tmax	= Chlordiazepoxide/clidinium: 1–4 hours/	Oral	= Chlordiazepoxide/clidinium: completely/incompletely absorbed
MW	= Chlordiazepoxide/clidinium: 300/432.4	pKa	= Chlordiazepoxide/clidinium: 4.8/

Adult Concerns: Sedation, constipation, dry mouth, headache, drowsiness, nervousness, mental confusion, weakness, insomnia, dizziness, and blurred vision.

Pediatric Concerns:

Drug Interactions: May increase sedation when used with other benzodiazepines and sedatives.

Relative Infant Dose:

Adult Dose: 1–2 capsules 3–4 times daily, before meals and at bedtime

Alternatives: Lorazepam

References:
1. Pharmaceutical manufacturer prescribing information, 2010.
2. AHFS Drug Information. © Copyright, 1959–2011, Selected Revisions May 2008. American Society of Health-System Pharmacists, Inc. Bethesda, Maryland.

CHLORHEXIDINE   L4

Trade: Hibiclens, Peridex, Periogard

Other Trades:

Category: Lozenge antimicrobial

Chlorhexidine in various forms is a topical antimicrobial used in topical detergents, oral lozenges and mouthwashes.[1] Pharmacokinetic studies with a 0.12% chlorhexidine gluconate oral rinse indicate approximately 30% of the active ingredient is retained in the oral cavity following rinsing. The drug retained in the oral cavity is slowly released into the oral fluids and swallowed. Studies conducted on human subjects and animals demonstrate chlorhexidine gluconate is poorly absorbed from the gastrointestinal tract. In a study of 200 mothers in which 100 each received breast sprays containing water or 0.2% chlorhexidine in alcohol, the chlorhexidine/alcohol spray group showed greater compliance to breastfeeding and lower incidence of trauma and discomfort. No adverse effects occurred that could be attributed to the medications.[2] In another case report, a mother used chlorhexidine spray (430 µg/spray) on her breasts to prevent mastitis starting with the third feed when the baby was 12 hours old. After 48 hours, the baby developed bradycardia. Some episodes over the next 2 days required atropine therapy, which subsequently increased the heart rate. An electrocardiogram confirmed sinus bradycardia. The chlorhexidine spray was discontinued and the bradycardia became less severe and less frequent. By day 6, bradycardia was no longer present. Each spray of chlorhexidine contains 430 µg and over 24 hours the baby could have ingested 2.5 mg.[3]

The differences between the two studies could be attributed to the difference in the amount of chlorhexidine available to the infants. Regardless, chlorhexidine should not be used on a breastfeeding mother's nipples.

Pregnancy Risk	B	Lactation Risk	L4
T ½	= <4 hours	M/P	=
Vd	= Poor l/kg	PB	= 87%
Tmax	= <12 hours	Oral	= Poor
MW	= 505	pKa	= 10.8

Adult Concerns: Staining of teeth and dentures. Keep out of eyes. Changes in taste, increased plaque, staining of tongue.

Pediatric Concerns: Bradycardia in one infant exposed to chlorhexidine on the nipple.

Drug Interactions: There are no known significant interactions.

Relative Infant Dose:

Adult Dose: Swish 15 ml in mouth for 30 seconds and then spit. Do not swallow.

Alternatives:

References:

1. Lacy C. Drug information handbook. Lexi-Comp Inc. Cleveland, OH, 1996.
2. Herd B, Feeney JG. Two aerosol sprays in nipple trauma. Practicioner 1986; 230: 31–38.
3. Quinn MW, Bini RM. Bradycardia associated with chlorhexidine spray. Arch Dis Child 1989; 64(6): 892–3.

CHLOROQUINE   L2

Trade: Aralen, Novo-Chloroquine

Other Trades: Chlorquin, AralenAvloclor

Category: Antimalarial

Chloroquine is an antimalarial drug. In a group of 6 women who received 5 mg/kg IM during delivery, and then again at 17 days postpartum, milk levels averaged 0.227 mg/L and ranged from 0.192 to 0.319 mg/L.[1] The milk/blood ratio ranged from 0.268 to 0.462. Based on these levels, the infant would consume approximately 34 µg/kg/day, an amount considered safe. If an infant consumed 500 mL/day of milk, it would receive an average of 113.5 µg of chloroquine per day. Other studies have shown absorption to vary from 2.2 to 4.2% of maternal dose.[2] The breastmilk concentration of chloroquine in this study averaged 0.58 mg/L following a single dose of 600 mg. In a recent study, the milk samples of 16 postpartum women were collected from day 3 to day 17–21 following delivery and examined for the concentrations of chloroquine and its metabolite, desethylchloroquine. The average concentration in milk (AUC) during the sampling period was 167 µg/L for chloroquine and 54 µg/L for desethylchloroquine.[3] The absolute and relative infant doses were 34 µg/kg/day and 15 µg/kg/day, and 2.3% and 1.0% for chloroquine and desethylchloroquine respectively. The authors suggested that chloroquine was compatible with breastfeeding. The current recommended pediatric dose for patients exposed to malaria is 8.3 mg/kg per week which greatly exceeds that present in breastmilk. In a recent study, chloroquine was reported to reduce HIV transmission into human milk.[4] It was found that chloroquine may reduce levels of HIV RNA in breastmilk.[5]

Data suggests that the transfer into milk is probably too low to affect an infant and that the relative infant dose of chloroqine and desethylchloroquin is about 2.3% and 1% respectively. Therefore, this drug is probably safe to use during breastfeeding.

Pregnancy Risk	C	Lactation Risk	L2
T ½	= 72–120 hours	M/P	= 0.358
Vd	= 116–285 l/kg	PB	= 61%
Tmax	= 1–2 hours	Oral	= Complete
MW	= 320	pKa	= 8.4, 10.8

Adult Concerns: Ocular disturbances including blindness, skin lesions, headache, fatigue, nervousness, hypotension, neutropenia, aplastic anemia.

Pediatric Concerns: None reported but close observation is required. Observe for diarrhea, gastrointestinal distress, hypotension.

Drug Interactions: Decreased oral absorption if used with kaolin and magnesium trisilicate. Increased toxicity if used with cimetidine.

Relative Infant Dose: 0.6%–1.1%

Adult Dose: 300–600 mg every day

Alternatives:

References:
1. Akintonwa A, Gbajumo SA, Mabadeje AF. Placental and milk transfer of chloroquine in humans. Ther Drug Monit 1988; 10(2): 147–149.
2. Edstein MD, Veenendaal JR, Newman K, Hyslop R. Excretion of chloroquine, dapsone and pyrimethamine in human milk. Br J Clin Pharmacol 1986; 22(6): 733–735.
3. Law I, Ilett KF, Hackett LP, et. al. Transfer of chloroquine and desethylchloroquine across the placenta and into milk in Melanesian mothers. Br J Clin Pharmacol 2008, 65(5): 674–679.
4. Semrau K, Kuhn L, Kasonde P, et al. Impact of chloroquine on viral load in breast milk. Trop Med Int Health. Jun 2006; 11(6): 800–803.
5. Semrau K, Kuhn L, Kasonde P, Sinkala M, Kankasa C, Shutes E, Vwalika C, Ghosh M, Aldrovandi G, Thea DM. Impact of chloroquine on viral load in breast milk. Trop Med Int Health. 2006 Jun; 11(6): 800–3.

CHLOROTHIAZIDE   L3

Trade: Diuril

Other Trades: Chlotride, Saluric

Category: Diuretic

Chlorothiazide is a typical thiazide diuretic. In one study of 11 lactating women, each receiving 500 mg of chlorothiazide, the concentrations in milk samples taken one, two, and three hours after the dose were all less than 1 mg/L with a milk/plasma ratio of 0.05.[1] Although thiazide diuretics are reported to produce thrombocytopenia in nursing infants, it is remote and unsubstantiated. Most thiazide diuretics are considered compatible with breastfeeding if doses are kept low and milk production is unaffected.

Pregnancy Risk	C		Lactation Risk	L3
T ½	= 1.5 hours		M/P	= 0.05
Vd	= 0.3 l/kg		PB	= 95%
Tmax	= 1 hour		Oral	= 20%
MW	= 296		pKa	= 6.7, 9.5

Adult Concerns: Fluid loss, dehydration, lethargy.

Pediatric Concerns: None reported but observe for reduced milk production.

Drug Interactions: NSAIDs may reduce hypotensive effect of chlorothiazide. Cholestyramine resins may reduce absorption of chlorothiazide. Diuretics reduce efficacy of oral hypoglycemics. May reduce lithium clearance leading to high levels. May elevate digoxin levels.

Relative Infant Dose: 2.1%

Adult Dose: 500–2000 mg every 12–24 hours

Alternatives:

References:
1. Werthmann MW, Jr., Krees SV. Excretion of chlorothiazide in human breast milk. J Pediatr 1972; 81(4): 781–783.

CHLORPHENIRAMINE   L3

Trade: Aller-Chlor, C. P. M., Chlor-Phen, Chlor-Trimeton Allergy, Teldrin HBP

Other Trades:

Category: Antihistamine

Chlorpheniramine is a commonly used antihistamine. Although no data are available on secretion into breastmilk, it has not been reported to produce side effects. Sedation is the only likely side effect.[1]

Pregnancy Risk	B		Lactation Risk	L3
T ½	= 12–43 hours		M/P	=
Vd	= 5.9 l/kg		PB	= 70%
Tmax	= 2–6 hours		Oral	= 25–45%
MW	= 275		pKa	= 9.2

Adult Concerns: Sedation, dry mouth.

Pediatric Concerns: None reported but observe for sedation.

Drug Interactions: May increase sedation when used with other CNS depressants such as opiates, tricyclic antidepressants, MAO inhibitors.

Relative Infant Dose:

Adult Dose: 4 mg every 4–6 hours

Alternatives: Cetirizine, Loratadine

References:
1. Paton DM, Webster DR. Clinical pharmacokinetics of H_1-receptor antagonists (the antihistamines). Clin Pharmacokinet 1985; 10(6): 477–497.

CHLORPROMAZINE   L3

Trade: Thorazine, Ormazine

Other Trades: Chlorpromanyl, Largactil, Novo-Chlorpromazine, Chloractil

Category: Tranquilizer

Chlorpromazine is a powerful CNS tranquilizer. Small amounts are known to be secreted into milk. Following a 1200 mg oral dose, samples were taken at 60, 120, and 180 minutes.[1] Breastmilk concentrations were highest at 120 minutes and were 0.29 mg/L at that time. The milk/plasma ratio was less than 0.5. Ayd[2] suggests that in one group of 16 women who took chlorpromazine during and after pregnancy, and while breastfeeding, the side effects were minimal and infant development was normal. In a group of 4 breastfeeding mothers receiving unspecified amounts of chlorpromazine, milk levels varied from 7 to 98 μg/L.[3] Maternal serum levels ranged from 16 to 52 μg/L. Only the infant who ingested milk with a chlorpromazine level of 92 μg/L showed drowsiness and lethargy.

Chlorpromazine has a long half-life and is particularly sedating. Long-term use of this product in a lactating mother may be risky to the breastfed infant. There are consistent reports of phenothiazine products increasing the risk of apnea and SIDS. Observe for sedation and lethargy and avoid if possible.

Pregnancy Risk	C	Lactation Risk	L3
T ½	= 30 hours	M/P	= <0.5
Vd	= 10–35 l/kg	PB	= 95%
Tmax	= 1–2 hours	Oral	= Complete
MW	= 319	pKa	= 9.3

Adult Concerns: Sedation, lethargy, extrapyramidal jerking motion, apnea, SIDS.

Pediatric Concerns: One report of lethargy and sedation. Observe for apnea.

Drug Interactions: Additive effects when used with other CNS depressants. May increase valproic acid plasma levels.

Relative Infant Dose: 0.3%

Adult Dose: 200 mg daily.

Alternatives:

References:
1. Blacker KH, Weinstein BJ. et. al. Mothers milk and chlorpromazine. Am J Psychol 1962; 114: 178–179.
2. Ayd FJ. Excretion of psychotropic drugs in breast milk. In: International Drug Therapy Newsletter. Ayd Medical Communications 8[November-December]. 1973.
3. Wiles DH, Orr MW, Kolakowska T. Chlorpromazine levels in plasma and milk of nursing mothers. Br J Clin Pharmacol 1978; 5(3): 272–273.

CHLORPROPAMIDE   L3

Trade: Diabinese
Other Trades: Apo-Chlorpropamide, Diabinese, Novopropamide, Melitase
Category: Oral hypoglycemic

Chlorpropamide stimulates the secretion of insulin in some patients. Following one 500 mg dose, the concentration of chlorpropamide in milk after 5 hours was approximately 5 mg/L of milk.[1] This study lacked details and may not be accurate. May cause hypoglycemia in infants although effects are largely unknown and unreported.

Pregnancy Risk	C	Lactation Risk	L3
T ½	= 33 hours	M/P	=
Vd	= 0.1–0.3 l/kg	PB	= 96%
Tmax	= 3–6 hours	Oral	= Complete
MW	= 277	pKa	= 4.8

Adult Concerns: Hypoglycemia, diarrhea, edema.

Pediatric Concerns: None actually reported, but observe for hypoglycemia although unlikely.

Drug Interactions: Thiazides and hydantoins reduce hypoglycemic effect of chlorpropamide. Chlorpropamide may increase disulfiram effects when used with alcohol. Increases anticoagulant effect when used with warfarin. Sulfonamides may decrease chlorpropamide clearance.

Relative Infant Dose: 10.5%

Adult Dose: 250–500 mg daily.

Alternatives: Metformin

References:
1. Pharmaceutical manufacturer prescribing information, 2010.

CHLORPROTHIXENE   L3

Trade: Taractan
Other Trades: Tarasan
Category: Sedative, tranquilizer.

Sedative commonly used in psychotic or disturbed patients. Chlorprothixene is poorly absorbed orally (<40%) and has been found to increase serum prolactin levels in mothers. Although the milk/plasma ratios are relatively high, only modest levels of chlorprothixene are actually secreted into human milk. In one patient taking 200 mg/day, maximum milk concentrations of the parent and metabolite were 19 µg/L and 28.5 µg/L respectively.[1]

Pregnancy Risk	C	Lactation Risk	L3
T ½	= 8–12 hours	M/P	= 1.2–2.6
Vd	= 11–23 l/kg	PB	= >99%
Tmax	= 4.25 hours	Oral	= <40%
MW	= 316	pKa	= 8.8

Adult Concerns: Sedation, hypotension, pseudoparkinsonian jerking, constipation.

Pediatric Concerns: None reported, but observe for sedation.

Drug Interactions: May reduce effect of guanethidine. May increase effects of alcohol and other CNS sedatives.

Relative Infant Dose: 0.3%

Adult Dose: 25–50 mg three times daily

Alternatives:

References:
1. Matheson I, Evang A, Overo KF, Syversen G. Presence of chlorprothixene and its metabolites in breast milk. Eur J Clin Pharmacol 1984; 27(5): 611–613.

CHLORTHALIDONE   L4

Trade: Thalitone, Hydone, Hygroton
Other Trades:
Category: Diuretic

Chlorthalidone is a typical thiazide diuretic commonly used as a antihypertensive. In a group of 7 women receiving 50 mg orally daily, milk levels 3 days postpartum ranged from 90 to 860 µg/liter. The infant was estimated to have received approximately 180 µg per day.[1] The relative infant dose (RID) would range from 1.9%–18%, but the authors estimate the RID at 6%. Chlorthalidone has a long half-life, and clearance from the infant may be slow possibly leading to accumulation. Hydrochlorothiazide may be more appropriate in breastfeeding women. When a child is exposed to chlorthalidone in pregnancy as well as through the mother's milk, the possibility for accumulation increases. The above study has estimated that a 3.5 kg infant would be born with about 250 µg of chlorthalidone in its blood if the mother was exposed to the drug throughout pregnancy. In the event that the child is also breastfed while the drug is present in the mother, an additional 180 µg per day may be administered. Due to the rapid accumulation that could occur in this situation, it may be appropriate to discontinue breastfeeding for a few days postpartum.[1]

Pregnancy Risk	B	Lactation Risk	L4
T ½	= 40–60 hours	M/P	=
Vd	= 3.9 l/kg	PB	= 75%
Tmax	= 2–6 hours	Oral	= 75%
MW	= 338	pKa	= 9.22

Adult Concerns: Anorexia, photosensitivity, hypokalemia, epigastric pain, hypercalcemia, agranulocytosis, gout.

Pediatric Concerns: Potential for long half-life in breastfed infant.

Drug Interactions: Chlorthalidone will increase the hypotensive effects of ACE Inhibitors and other antihypertensive medications. NSAIDs may decrease the effects of chlorthalidone. Phosphodiesterase 5 inhibitors may increase the effects of chlorthalidone.

Relative Infant Dose: 1.9%–18.1%

Adult Dose: 25–100 mg/day

Alternatives: Hydrochlorthiazide, furosemide

References:
1. Mulley BA, Parr GD, Pau WK, Rye RM, Mould JJ, Siddle NC. Placental transfer of chlorthalidone and its elimination in maternal milk. Eur J Clin Pharmacol. 1978 May 17; 13(2): 129–31.

CHLORZOXAZONE | L4

Trade: Paraflex, Parafon Forte DSC, Relaxazone, Remular-S, Lorzone

Other Trades:

Category: centrally acting skeletal muscle relaxant

Chlorzoxazone is a centrally acting skeletal muscle relaxant used for muscle pain/spasms. The parent drug is metabolized into 6-hydroxychlorzoxazone (metabolite). The average peak plasma levels achieved with a 750 mg dose was 36.3 µg/mL. Seventy-four percent of the drug is excreted renally in the first 10 hours of dosing.[1] No studies were located on the transfer of chlorzoxazone into breastmilk. Because of the low molecular weight, and being 100% orally bioavailable, chlorzoxazone is not recommended for breastfeeding mothers. A preferred medication would be Metaxalone.

Pregnancy Risk	C	Lactation Risk	L4
T ½	= 1.1 hours	M/P	=
Vd	= 13.7 l/kg	PB	=
Tmax	= 1 to 2 hours	Oral	= 100%
MW	= 169.57	pKa	=

Adult Concerns: Gastrointestinal hemorrhage, hepatotoxicity, anaphylaxis

Pediatric Concerns:

Drug Interactions: Concurrent use with other CNS depressants such as barbiturates (phenobarbital), benzodiazepines (diazepam, alprazolam) or opioids (hydrocodone, oxycodone) may result in enhanced respiratory depression.

Relative Infant Dose:

Adult Dose: 500–750 mg three to four times daily.

Alternatives: Metaxalone

References:
1. Pharmaceutical manufacturer prescribing information, 2010.

CHOLERA VACCINE   L3

Trade: Cholera Vaccine, Dukoral
Other Trades:
Category: Cholera vaccination.

Cholera vaccine is available in an oral preparation and a sterile injectable solution containing equal parts of phenol inactivated Ogawa and Inaba serotypes of Vibrio cholerae bacteria.

Maternal immunization with cholera vaccine significantly increases levels of anti-cholera antibodies (IgA, IgG) in their milk.[1] It is not contraindicated in nursing mothers. Breastfed infants are generally protected from cholera transmission. Immunization is approved from the age of 6 months and older.

Pregnancy Risk	C	Lactation Risk	L3
T ½	=	M/P	=
Vd	=	PB	=
Tmax	=	Oral	=
MW	=	pKa	=

Adult Concerns: Malaise, fever, headache, pain at injection site.

Pediatric Concerns: None reported.

Drug Interactions: Decreased effect when used with yellow fever vaccine. Wait at least 3 weeks between.

Relative Infant Dose:

Adult Dose: Two doses of 0.5 mL injections (IM or SC) 1 week to 1 month apart

Alternatives:

References:
1. Merson MH, Black RE, Sack DA, Svennerholm AM, Holmgren J. Maternal cholera immunization and secretory IgA in breast milk. Lancet 1980; 1(8174): 931–932.

CHOLESTYRAMINE   L1

Trade: Questran, Cholybar
Other Trades: Questran, Novo-Cholamine
Category: Cholesterol binding resin

Cholestyramine is a bile salt chelating resin. Used orally in adults, it binds bile salts and prevents reabsorption of bile salts in the gut, thus reducing cholesterol plasma levels.[1] This resin is not absorbed from the maternal gastrointestinal tract. Therefore, it is not secreted into breastmilk.

Pregnancy Risk	C	Lactation Risk	L1
T ½	= 6 minutes	M/P	=
Vd	=	PB	=
Tmax	= 21 days	Oral	=
MW	=	pKa	=

Adult Concerns: Constipation, skin rash, nausea, vomiting, malabsorption, intestinal obstruction.

Pediatric Concerns: None reported via milk. Observe mother for vitamin deficiency states.

Drug Interactions: Decreases oral absorption of vitamins, digoxin, warfarin, thyroid hormones, thiazide diuretics, propranolol, phenobarbital, amiodarone, methotrexate, NSAIDs, and many other drugs.

Relative Infant Dose:

Adult Dose: 16–32 grams daily

Alternatives:

References:
1. Pharmaceutical manufacturer prescribing information, 2010.

CHONDROITIN SULFATE   L3

Trade:

Other Trades:

Category: Biologic polymer used for arthritis

Chondroitin sulfate is a biological polymer that acts as a flexible connecting matrix between the protein filaments in cartilage. It is derived largely from natural sources such as shark or bovine cartilage and is chemically composed of a high-viscosity mucopolysaccharide (glycosaminoglycan) polymer found in most mammalian cartilaginous tissues.[1] Thus far, chondroitin has been found to be nontoxic. Its molecular weight averages 50,000 daltons, which is far too large to permit its entry into human milk. Combined with a poor oral bioavailability and large molecular weight, it is unlikely to pose a problem for a breastfed infant.

Pregnancy Risk	C	Lactation Risk	L3
T ½	=	M/P	=
Vd	=	PB	=
Tmax	=	Oral	= 0–13%
MW	= 50,000	pKa	=

Adult Concerns: Virtually nontoxic and poorly absorbed orally.

Pediatric Concerns: None reported via milk.

Drug Interactions: There are no known significant interactions.

Relative Infant Dose:

Adult Dose: 200–400 mg 2–3 times daily

Alternatives:

References:
1. Review of Natural Products Facts and Comparisons, St Louis, MO 1996.

CHORIONIC GONADOTROPIN | L3

Trade: A. P. L., Chorex-5, Profasi, Gonic, Pregnyl, Novarel, Ovidrel

Other Trades: Pregnyl, Profasik, APL, Humegon Pregnyl, Profasi HPProfasi

Category: Placental hormone

Human chorionic gonadotropin (HCG) is a large polypeptide hormone produced by the human placenta with functions similar to luteinizing hormone (LH). Its function is to stimulate the corpus luteum of the ovary to produce progesterone, thus sustaining pregnancy.[1,2] During pregnancy, HCG secreted by the placenta maintains the corpus luteum, supporting estrogen and progesterone secretion and preventing menstruation. It is used for multiple purposes including pediatric cryptorchidism, male hypogonadism, and ovulatory failure. HCG has no known effect on fat mobilization, appetite, sense of hunger, or body fat distribution. HCG has not been found to be effective in treatment of obesity. Due to the large molecular weight of HCG (36,000 to 47,000 Daltons), it would be extremely unlikely to penetrate into human milk. Further, it would not be orally bioavailable due to destruction in the gastrointestinal tract.

Choriogonadotropin alfa (Ovidrel) is a biosynthetic form of the human chorionic gonadotropin, of recombinant origin.

Pregnancy Risk	X	Lactation Risk	L3
T ½	= 5.6 hours	M/P	=
Vd	=	PB	=
Tmax	= 6 hours	Oral	=
MW	= 47,000	pKa	=

Adult Concerns: Headache, irritability, restlessness, depression, fatigue, edema, gynecomastia, pain at injection site.

Pediatric Concerns: None reported via milk. Absorption unlikely due to gastric digestion and poor penetration into milk.

Drug Interactions:

Relative Infant Dose:

Adult Dose: 5000–10000 units X 1

Alternatives:

References:
1. Drug Facts and Comparisons 1996 ed. ed. St. Louis: 1996.
2. Pharmaceutical manufacturer prescribing information, 1997.

CHROMIUM   L3

Trade: Chromium Picrolinate
Other Trades:
Category: Metal supplement

Trace metal, required in glucose metabolism. Less than 1% is absorbed following oral administration. Chromium levels are depleted in multiparous women. Chromium levels in neonates are approximately 2.5 times that of mother due to concentrating mechanism during gestation. Because chromium is difficult to measure, levels reported vary widely.

One article reports that breastmilk levels are less than 2% of the estimated safe and adequate daily intake of 10 μg (which is probably excessive and needs review).[1] Most importantly, breastmilk levels are independent of dietary intake in mother and do not apparently increase with increased maternal intake. Chromium is apparently secreted into breastmilk by a well-controlled pumping mechanism. Hence, breastmilk levels of chromium are independent of maternal plasma levels. Increased maternal plasma levels may not alter milk chromium levels.

Pregnancy Risk	C		Lactation Risk	L3
T ½	=		M/P	=
Vd	=		PB	=
Tmax	=		Oral	= <1%
MW	= 52		pKa	=

Adult Concerns: Chromium poisoning if used in excess.

Pediatric Concerns: None reported.

Drug Interactions:

Relative Infant Dose:

Adult Dose: 200 μg/day

Alternatives:

References:
1. Anderson RA, Bryden NA, Patterson KY, Veillon C, Andon MB, Moser-Veillon PB. Breast milk chromium and its association with chromium intake, chromium excretion, and serum chromium. Am J Clin Nutr 1993; 57(4): 519–523.

CICLESONIDE   L3

Trade: Omnaris
Other Trades:
Category: Corticosteroid

Ciclesonide is a topical corticosteroid used presently for allergic rhinitis. Ciclesonide is a pro-drug that is enzymatically hydrolyzed to a pharmacologically active metabolite, C21-desisobutyryl-ciclesonide (des-ciclesonide or RM1). Ciclesonide and its metabolite, des-ciclesonide, has negligible oral bioavailability (<1%) as it is poorly absorbed, and has a high first-pass absorption by the liver.[1] While we have no data on its use in breastfeeding mothers, as with the other nasal steroids, this product poses little risk.

Pregnancy Risk	C	Lactation Risk	L3
T ½	= 6–7 hours	M/P	=
Vd	= 12.1 l/kg	PB	= 99%
Tmax	= 1.04 hours	Oral	= <1%
MW	= 540	pKa	= 15.56

Adult Concerns: Headache, nose bleed, nasopharyngitis, ear pain.

Pediatric Concerns: None yet reported.

Drug Interactions: Ketoconazole may produce a 3.6-fold increase in desciclesonide AUC at steady state.

Relative Infant Dose:

Adult Dose: 100 µg/day in each nostril

Alternatives: Budesonide, fluticasone, mometasone

References:
1.   Pharmaceutical manufacturer prescribing information, 2010.

CICLOPIROX OLAMINE   L3

Trade: Loprox
Other Trades: Loprox
Category: Antifungal

Ciclopirox is a broad-spectrum antifungal and is active in numerous species including tinea, *Candida albicans*, and *Trichophyton rubrum*. An average of 1.3% ciclopirox is absorbed when applied topically although only 0.01% of the dose is found in the urine.[1] Topical application produces minimal systemic absorption; it is unlikely that topical use would expose the nursing infant to significant risks. The risk to a breastfeeding infant associated with application directly on the nipple is not known and it should not be used on the nipple. Ciclopirox and miconazole are comparable in the treatment of vaginal candidiasis.

Pregnancy Risk	B	Lactation Risk	L3
T ½	= 1.7 hours	M/P	=
Vd	=	PB	= 98%
Tmax	= 6 hours	Oral	=
MW	= 268	pKa	= 7.2

Adult Concerns: Pruritus and burning following topical therapy.

Pediatric Concerns: None via milk.

Drug Interactions: There are no know significant interactions.

Relative Infant Dose:

Adult Dose: Apply topically BID

Alternatives: Fluconazole, Miconazole.

References:
1.   Pharmaceutical manufacturer prescribing information, 2011.

CILASTATIN   L3

Trade:

Other Trades:

Category: Dehydropeptidase inhibitor

Cilastatin is a derivative of heptenoic acid which inhibits renal dehydropeptidase I. It is used in combination with imipenem, to reduce imipenem's degradation by dehydropeptidase at the brush border of proximal renal tubular cells.[1] Cilastatin is not well absorbed from the gastrointestinal tract. It is able to cross the placental barrier and gets distributed in milk. However currently there are no evidence of adverse reactions or teratogenicity in animal studies.

Pregnancy Risk	Probably Safe	Lactation Risk	L3
T ½	=	M/P	=
Vd	=	PB	=
Tmax	=	Oral	=
MW	= 358	pKa	= 4.38

Adult Concerns: Nausea, diarrhea, vomiting, abdominal pain, decreased white blood cells, decreased hemoglobin, seizures.

Pediatric Concerns:

Drug Interactions:

Relative Infant Dose:

Adult Dose:

Alternatives:

References:
1.   McEvoy GE. (ed): AFHS Drug Information. New York, NY: 2003.

CILASTATIN + IMIPENEM   L2

Trade: Primaxin IM, Primaxin IV

Other Trades: Primaxin

Category: Antibiotic

Cilastatin and Imipenem is a combination drug product. Its indications include urinary tract infections, female genital tract infections, infections of the bone or joint, infections of the skin and subcutaneous tissues, lower respiratory tract infections and bacterial systemic infections.

Imipenem is structurally similar to penicillins and acts similarly. Cilastatin is added to extend the half-life of imipenem. Both imipenem and cilastatin are poorly absorbed orally and must be administered IM or IV.[1,2] Imipenem is destroyed by gastric acidity. Transfer into breastmilk is probably minimal but no data are available. Changes in gastrointestinal flora could occur but is probably remote.

Pregnancy Risk	C	Lactation Risk	L2
T ½	= 0.85–1.3 hours	M/P	=
Vd	=	PB	= 20–35%
Tmax	= Immediate (IV)	Oral	= Poor
MW	= 317	pKa	= Imipenem (15), Cilastin (4.38)

Adult Concerns: Nausea, diarrhea, vomiting, abdominal pain, decreased white blood cells, decreased hemoglobin, seizures.

Pediatric Concerns: No studies available. Probably similar to other penicillins.

Drug Interactions: May have increased toxicity when used with other beta lactam antibiotics. Probenecid may increase toxic potential.

Relative Infant Dose:

Adult Dose: 500–750 mg BID

Alternatives:

References:
1. Pharmaceutical manufacturer prescribing information, 1995.
2. McEvoy GE. (ed): AFHS Drug Information. New York, NY: 2003.

CIMETIDINE   L1

Trade: Tagamet, Tagamet HB
Other Trades:
Category: Reduces gastric acid production

Cimetidine is an antisecretory, histamine-2 antagonist that reduces stomach acid secretion. Cimetidine is apparently actively transported into human milk as evidenced by a higher milk/plasma ratio. In a study of 12 women who received single oral doses of 100, 600, and 1200 mg cimetidine, the observed milk/serum ratio was 5.65, 5.84, and 5.83 respectively.[1] The reported maximum concentration in milk were 2.5, 16.2, and 37.2 mg/L respectively. In another study of one patient ingesting 600 mg daily, the reported milk level was 5.6 mg/L.[2] The maximum potential dose from lactation would be approximately 5.58 mg/kg/d, which is still quite small. The pediatric dose administered IV for therapeutic treatment of pediatric gastroesophageal reflux averages 8–20 mg/kg/24 hours. Other choices for breastfeeding mothers should preclude the use of this drug however. See famotidine, nizatidine. Short-term use (days) would not be incompatible with breastfeeding.

Pregnancy Risk	B	Lactation Risk	L1
T ½	= 2 hours	M/P	= 4.6–11.76
Vd	= 1.3 l/kg	PB	= 19%
Tmax	= 0.75–1.5 hours	Oral	= 60–70%
MW	= 252	pKa	= 6.8

Adult Concerns: Headache, dizziness, somnolence.

Pediatric Concerns: None reported via milk. Frequently used in pediatric patients.

Drug Interactions: Cimetidine inhibits the metabolism of many drugs and may potentially increase their plasma levels. Such drugs include lidocaine, theophylline, phenytoin, metronidazole, triamterene, procainamide, quinidine, propranolol, warfarin, tricyclic antidepressants, diazepam, cyclosporin.

Relative Infant Dose: 9.8%–32.6%

Adult Dose: 800 mg every HS

Alternatives: Famotidine, Nizatidine

References:
1. Oo CY, Kuhn RJ, Desai N, McNamara PJ. Active transport of cimetidine into human milk. Clin Pharmacol Ther 1995; 58(5): 548–555.
2. Somogyi A, Gugler R. Cimetidine excretion into breast milk. Br J Clin Pharmacol 1979; 7(6): 627–629.

CINACALCET   L3

Trade: Sensipar

Other Trades:

Category: Calcimimetic

Cinacalcet is a calcium regulator/calcium-sensing receptor agonist used in the management of hypercalcemia when it occurs in the setting of parathyroid carcinoma, primary hyperparathyroidism and secondary hyperparathyroidism in dialysis patients.[1] There are no adequate and well-controlled studies or case reports in breast feeding women. It is relatively large in molecular weight (357) and has poor oral absorption (20%). Levels in milk are probably low.

Pregnancy Risk	C	Lactation Risk	L3
T ½	= 30–40 hours	M/P	=
Vd	= 14.28 l/kg	PB	= 93–97%
Tmax	= 2–6 hours	Oral	= 20–25%
MW	= 357	pKa	= 8.72

Adult Concerns: Hypocalcemia, nausea, vomiting, headache, dizziness, fatigue, dehydration, paraesthesia, anorexia, myalgia, fracture, diarrhea, anemia, upper respiratory infection, hypertension.

Pediatric Concerns:

Drug Interactions: Cinacalcet is metabolized by CYP3A4. Therefore, concurrent use with CYP3A4 inhibitors such as ketoconazole, itraconazole, indinavir, ritonavir may increase cinacalcet plasma levels. Cinacalcet is a strong inhibitor of CYP2D6, therefore caution while using concomitantly with agents such as carvedilol, metoprolol, amitriptyline, desipramine, doxepin, clarithromycin, clomipramine. Caution while using concomitantly with clozapine, prolonged QT may occur. For a complete list, see drug interactions reference.

Relative Infant Dose:

Adult Dose: 30 mg once daily

Alternatives:

References:
1. Pharmaceutical manufacturer prescribing information, 2011.

CINNARIZINE   L3

Trade:
Other Trades: Arlevert, Stugeron
Category: Antiemetic

Cinnarizine is an antiemetic used for motion sickness, and is not available in the USA. It is an H_1 histamine antagonist, and reduces the vascular response to epinephrine, norepinephrine, serotonin, angiotensin, dopamine, and other vasoactive hormones. It is primarily used for vestibular disorders of the inner ear and the vomiting center of the hypothalamus. No data are available on its use in breastfeeding mothers.

Pregnancy Risk	C	Lactation Risk	L3
T ½	= 3–6 hours	M/P	=
Vd	=	PB	= 91%
Tmax	= 1–3 hours	Oral	=
MW	= 368	pKa	= 1.95, 7.5

Adult Concerns: Adverse effects include drowsiness, headache, sweating, and weight gain.

Pediatric Concerns: Fatigue and slight hair loss have been reported from direct use of cinnarizine in children. No reports of complications via breastmilk.

Drug Interactions: Concurrent use with procarbazine or other CNS depressants such as barbiturates, benzodiazepines, sedatives may cause enhanced CNS depression.

Relative Infant Dose:

Adult Dose: 30 mg

Alternatives:

References:

CIPROFLOXACIN   L3

Trade: Cipro, Ciloxan

Other Trades: Ciproxin, Cipro

Category: Fluoroquinolone antibiotic

Ciprofloxacin is a fluoroquinolone antibiotic primarily used for gram negative coverage and is presently the drug of choice for anthrax treatment and prophylaxis. Because it has been implicated in arthropathy in newborn animals, it is not normally used in pediatric patients. Levels secreted into breastmilk (2.26 to 3.79 mg/L) are somewhat conflicting. They vary from the low to moderate range to levels that are higher than maternal serum up to 12 hours after a dose. In one study of 10 women who received 750 mg every 12 hours, milk levels of ciprofloxacin ranged from 3.79 mg/L at 2 hours post-dose to 0.02 mg/L at 24 hours.[1] In another study of a single patient receiving one 500 mg tablet daily at bedtime, the concentrations in maternal serum and breast milk were 0.21 μg/mL and 0.98 μg/mL respectively.[2] Plasma levels were undetectable (<0.03 μg/mL) in the infant. The dose to the 4-month-old infant was estimated to be 0.92 mg/day or 0.15 mg/kg/day. No adverse effects were noted in this infant.

There has been one reported case of severe pseudomembranous colitis in an infant of a mother who self-medicated with ciprofloxacin for 6 days.[3] In a patient 17 days postpartum, who received 500 mg orally, ciprofloxacin levels in milk were 3.02, 3.02, 3.02 and 1.98 mg/L at 4, 8, 12, and 16 hours post dose respectively.[4] In another study of the direct application of ciprofloxacin to infants, 10 infants aged 4 days to 1-month-old were given ciprofloxacin 10 to 40 mg/kg/day in 2 divided doses by slow IV infusion over 30 minutes for 10 to 20 days. Eight infants survived and 2 had greenish discoloration of the teeth at age 12–23 months. The discoloration requires further evaluation to determine the association with ciprofloxacin therapy.[5]

If used in lactating mothers, observe the infant closely for gastrointestinal symptoms such as diarrhea. Current studies seem to suggest that the amount of ciprofloxacin present in milk is quite low. Ciprofloxacin is becoming increasingly popular for use in pediatric patients.[6] Ciprofloxacin is available in several ophthalmic preparations (Ciloxan), where the absorption and clinical dose is minimal. As the absolute dose presented to the nursing mother is minimal, ophthalmic formulations would not be contraindicated in breastfeeding mothers.

Pregnancy Risk	C	Lactation Risk	L3
T ½	= 4.1 hours	M/P	= >1
Vd	= 1.4 l/kg	PB	= 40%
Tmax	= 0.5–2.3 hours	Oral	= 50–85%
MW	= 331	pKa	= 7.1

Adult Concerns: Nausea, vomiting, diarrhea, abdominal cramps, gastrointestinal bleeding. Several cases of tendon rupture have been noted.

Pediatric Concerns: Pseudomembranous colitis in one infant. Observe for diarrhea. Tooth discoloration in several infants reported.

Drug Interactions: Decreased absorption with antacids. Quinolones cause increased levels of caffeine, warfarin, cyclosporine, theophylline. Cimetidine, probenecid, azlocillin increase ciprofloxacin levels. Increased risk of seizures when used with foscarnet.

Relative Infant Dose: 2.1%–6.3%

Adult Dose: 500 mg BID

Alternatives: Norfloxacin, Ofloxacin

References:

1. Giamarellou H, Kolokythas E, Petrikkos G, Gazis J, Aravantinos D, Sfikakis P. Pharmacokinetics of three newer quinolones in pregnant and lactating women. Am J Med 1989; 87(5A): 49S-51S.
2. Gardner DK, Gabbe SG, Harter C. Simultaneous concentrations of ciprofloxacin in breast milk and in serum in mother and breast-fed infant. Clin Pharm 1992; 11(4): 352–354.
3. Harmon T, Burkhart G, Applebaum H. Perforated pseudomembranous colitis in the breast-fed infant. J Pediatr Surg 1992; 27(6): 744–746.
4. Cover DL, Mueller BA. Ciprofloxacin penetration into human breast milk: a case report. DICP 1990; 24(7–8): 703–704.
5. Lumbiganon P, Pengsaa K, Sookpranee T. Ciprofloxacin in Neonates and its Possible Adverse Effect on the Teeth. Pediatr Infect Dis J 1991; 10(8): 619–620.
6. Ghaffar F, McCracken GH. Quinolones in Pediatrics. In: Hooper DC, Rubinstein E, editors. Quinolone Antimicrobial Agents. Washington, D. C.: ASM Press, 2003: 343–354.

CISPLATIN   L5

Trade: Cisplatin, Abiplatin, Bioplatino, Cis-Gry, C-Platin, Placis

Other Trades:

Category: Anticancer drug

Cisplatin is a platinum-containing anticancer agent. Platinum agents have high affinity for plasma proteins. Approximately 90% of cisplatin is covalently bound to plasma proteins within four hours. Following administration of radioactive cisplatin, cisplatin levels were eliminated in a biphasic manner.[1] T(alpha) was 25 to 49 minutes. T(beta) was 58 to 73 hours. Other estimates of the terminal elimination half-life of total plasma cisplatin range between five to ten days. The volume of distribution is high, about 0.5 L/kg.[2] Platinum penetrates into tissues and is irreversibly bound to tissue proteins. Platinum can be found in these tissues for years afterward.

Plasma and breastmilk samples were collected from a 24 year-old woman treated for three prior days with cisplatin (30 mg/meter).[3] On the third day, 30 minutes prior to chemotherapy, platinum levels in milk were 0.9 mg/L and plasma levels were 0.8 mg/L, giving a milk: plasma ratio of 1:1. In another study, no cisplatin was found in breastmilk, following a dose of 100 mg/m².[4] Other studies suggest that milk levels are ten-fold lower than serum levels in an older lactating woman (milk: plasma ratio= -0.1).[5] These studies generally support the recommendation that mothers should not breastfeed while undergoing cisplatin therapy or withhold breastfeeding for many days (>20–30 days).

Two options are suggested. One, the breastmilk should be tested for platinum levels and not used as long as they are measurable. Two, without measuring platinum levels, breastfeeding should be permanently interrupted for this infant.

Pregnancy Risk	D	Lactation Risk	L5
T ½	= (beta) < 130 hours	M/P	=
Vd	= 0.5 l/kg	PB	= >90%
Tmax	=	Oral	= poor
MW	= 300.051	pKa	= 6.56

Adult Concerns: Joint pain, loss of balance, ringing in ears, swelling of feet or lower legs, trouble in hearing, unusual tiredness or weakness

Pediatric Concerns: Hazardous. Do not use.

Drug Interactions: Cisplatin may reduce plasma levels of various anticonvulsants.

Relative Infant Dose:

Adult Dose: Highly variable.

Alternatives:

References:
1. DeConti RC, Toftness BR, Lange RC, et al: Clinical and pharmacological studies with cis-diamminedichloroplatinum (II). Cancer Res 1973; 33: 1310–1315.
2. Grochow LB, Ames MM. A clinician's guide to chemotherapy pharmacokinetics and pharmacodynamics. 1st ed. Baltimore, MD: Williams and Wilkins; 1998.
3. Ben-Baruch G, Menczer J, Goshen R, et al: Cisplatin excretion in human milk. J Natl Cancer Inst 1992; 84: 451–452.
4. de Vries EGE, van der Zee AGJ, Uges DRA, et al: Excretion of cisplatin into breast milk. Lancet 1989; 1: 497.
5. Egan PC, Costanza ME, Dodion P, et al: Doxorubicin and cisplatin excretion into human milk. Cancer Treat Rep 1985; 69: 1387–1389.

CITALOPRAM   L2

Trade: Celexa

Other Trades: Celexa, Cipramil, Talam, Talohexal,

Category: Antidepressant, SSRI

Citalopram is an SSRI antidepressant. These medications are the drugs of choice for use in depressive and anxiety disorders during pregnancy and lactation. In general, these medications are more compatible with breastfeeding than tricyclic antidepressants.[1] In one study of a 21-year-old patient receiving 20 mg citalopram per day, citalopram levels in milk peaked at 3–9 hours following administration.[2] Peak milk levels varied during the day, but the mean daily concentration was 298 nM (range 270–311 nM). The milk/serum ratio was approximately 3. The metabolite, desmethylcitalopram, was present in milk in low levels (23–28 nM). The concentration of metabolite in milk varied little during the day. Assuming a milk intake of 150 mL/kg/day baby, approximately 272 nM (88 µg or 16 ng/kg) of citalopram was passed to the baby each day. This amounts to only 0.4% of the dose administered to the mother. At three weeks, maternal serum levels of citalopram were 185 nM, compared to the infants plasma level of just 7 nM. No untoward effects were noted in this breastfed infant. In another study[3], a milk/serum ratio of 1.16 to 1.88 was reported. This study suggests the infant would ingest 4.3 μg/kg/day and a relative dose of 0.7 to 5.9% of the weight-adjusted maternal dose.

In another study of 7 women receiving an average of 0.41 mg/kg/day citalopram, the average peak level (C_{max}) of citalopram was 154 μg/L and 50 μg/L for desmethylcitalopram (metabolite is 8 times less potent than citalopram).[4] However, average milk concentrations (AUC) were lower and averaged 97 μg/L for citalopram and 36 μg/L for desmethylcitalopram during the dosing interval. The mean peak milk/plasma AUC ratio was 1.8 for citalopram. Low concentrations of citalopram (around 2–2.3 μg/L) were detected in only three of the seven infant plasmas. No adverse effects were found in any of the infants. The authors estimate the daily intake to be approximately 3.7% of the maternal dose.

In a study of a single patient receiving 40 mg/day of citalopram, the concentration in milk and serum were 205 μg/L and 98.9 ng/mL respectively.[5] Infant serum levels were 12.7 ng/mL. This infant was noted to have 'uneasy' sleep patterns, which were reduced upon lowering the maternal dose.

In a recent study of women (n=31) who were consuming citalopram while breastfeeding, no significant difference was noted in infant side effect profiles as compared to depressed and non-depressed control patients who were not consuming citalopram.[6] In one infant, colic, decreased feeding and irritability/restlessness was reported. In another infant, irritability and restlessness was reported. The authors recommend continued breastfeeding while consuming citalopram. Another case occurred during which the infant exhibited irregular breathing, apnea, sleep disorders, and hypotonia. These adverse effects have been associated with SSRI use, and infants may need to be monitored if such effects persist. In this case, symptoms resolved spontaneously after 3 weeks.[7] Eleven mothers taking citalopram and their babies were monitored during pregnancy and lactation. Plasma and milk samples were taken that suggested citalopram and its metabolite concentrations in milk were 2–3 times higher than in maternal plasma, but infant plasma levels were very low or undetectable.[8]

One case reported an infant experiencing neonatal withdrawal syndrome after in utero exposure. The mother was taking 20–30 mg/day. The symptoms started upon delivery, and the child was discharged at day 7 with no medical treatment needed.[9] Measurements were taken in a breastfed infant at periodic intervals up to 53 days after delivery. Serum concentrations of citalopram were taken from both the infant and the mother and the ratios were compared. The infant's serum showed 1.4–1.8% of the mother's citalopram concentrations, with absolute ranges of 3.7–7.1 nM.[7] This analysis further showed that the concentrations of citalopram in breastmilk were roughly twice that found in the mother's serum.

While the original anecdotal data suggested that symptoms such as somnolence, colic, restlessness may occur in breastfed infants exposed to citalopram, the majority of new data suggests these symptoms are minimal and may not be associated with therapy. All this newer data suggests that the risks of this product are probably quite low. However, recent data on escitalopram suggests it is a better alternative.

Pregnancy Risk	C	Lactation Risk	L2
T ½	= 36 hours	M/P	= 1.16–3
Vd	= 12 l/kg	PB	= 80%
Tmax	= 2–4 hours	Oral	= 80%
MW	= 405	pKa	= 9.59

Adult Concerns: Diarrhea, headache, anxiety, dizziness, insomnia, constipation, nausea, vomiting, and tremor. Tachycardia, hypotension have been reported. Increased salivation and flatulence. Amenorrhea, cough, rash, pruritus, polyuria have been reported. Doses higher than 40 mg have been reported to induce prolonged QT syndrome and a higher risk of developing Torsade de Pointes.

Pediatric Concerns: There have been two cases of excessive somnolence, decreased feeding, and weight loss in breastfed infants. However, the majority of studies show no or limited side effects in breastfed infants.

Drug Interactions: Increased citalopram levels when used with macrolide antibiotics (erythromycin), and azole antifungals such as fluconazole, itraconazole, ketoconazole, etc. Carbamazepine may reduce plasma levels of citalopram. Serious reactions may occur if citalopram is administered too soon after monoamine oxidase inhibitor use. Beta blocker (metoprolol) levels may increase by two-fold when admixed with citalopram.

Relative Infant Dose: 3.6%

Adult Dose: 20–40 mg daily

Alternatives: Sertraline, escitalopram

References:
1. Briggs G, Freeman RK, Yaffe SJ. Drugs in Pregnancy and Lactation: A Reference Guide to fetal and Neonatal Risk. 6th ed. Philadelphia: Lippincott Williams and Wilkins; 2002.
2. Jensen PN, Olesen OV, Bertelsen A, Linnet K. Citalopram and desmethylcitalopram concentrations in breast milk and in serum of mother and infant. Ther Drug Monit 1997; 19(2): 236–239.
3. Spigset O, Carieborg L, Ohman R, Norstrom A. Excretion of citalopram in breast milk. Br J Clin Pharmacol 1997; 44(3): 295–298.
4. Rampono J, Kristensen JH, Hackett LP, Paech M, Kohan R, Ilett KF. Citalopram and demethylcitalopram in human milk; distribution, excretion and effects in breast fed infants. Br J Clin Pharmacol 2000; 50(3): 263–268.
5. Schmidt K, Olesen OV, Jensen PN. Citalopram and breast-feeding: serum concentration and side effects in the infant. Biol Psychiatry 2000; 47(2): 164–165.
6. Lee A, Woo J, Ito S. Frequency of infant adverse events that are associated with citalopram use during breast-feeding. Am J Obstet Gynecol 2004 Jan; 190(1): 218–21.
7. Frannsen EJF, et al. Citalopram Serum and Milk Levels in Mother and Infant During Lactation. Ther Drug Monit. Vol. 28(1). February 2006.2–4.
8. Heikkinen T, Ekblad U, Kero P, Ekblad S, Laine K. Citalopram in pregnancy and lactation. Clin Pharmacol Ther 2002; 72(2): 184–191.
9. Nordeng H, Lindemann R, Perminov KV, Reikvam A. Neonatal withdrawl syndrome after in utero exposure to selective serotonin reuptake inhibitors. Acta Paediatr 2001; 90: 288–91.

CLADRIBINE   L5

Trade: Leustatin, Leustat, Litak
Other Trades:
Category: anticancer drug

Cladribine is an antimetabolite, antineoplastic, purine nucleoside analog used for various forms of leukemia, multiple sclerosis, etc. Oral absorption ranges from 37–55%. The manufacturer reports a biphasic or triphasic elimination for this drug. For patients with normal renal function, the manufacturer reports the mean terminal half-life was 5.4 hours. Others report cladribine plasma concentrations after intravenous administration declines multi-exponentially, with an average half-life of 6.7±2.5 hours.[1] In general, the apparent volume of distribution of cladribine is approximately <9L/kg, indicating extensive sequestration in body tissues. Cladribine penetrates into cerebrospinal fluid which suggests it might enter milk as well. One report indicates that concentrations are approximately 25% of those in plasma. Other reports suggest that the terminal half-life is much longer, as high as 19 hours. Following a two-hour infusion in 12 adult patients receiving cladribine 0.14 mg/kg/day, cladribine has an alpha half-life of 35 ± 12 minutes and a beta half-life of 6.7 ± 2.5 hours. No data are available on its transfer into human milk, but the mother should pump and discard her milk for at least 48 hours.

Withhold breastfeeding for a minimum period of 48 hours. Adjust longer for patients with poor renal clearance.

Pregnancy Risk	D	Lactation Risk	L5
T ½	= (beta) 5.4–6.7 hours	M/P	=
Vd	= 0.7–9 l/kg	PB	= 20%
Tmax	=	Oral	= 55%
MW	= 285.7	pKa	= 14.78

Adult Concerns: Black, tarry stools, blood in urine, cough or hoarseness, fever or chills, lower back or side pain, painful or difficult urination, pinpoint red spots on skin, unusual bleeding or bruising

Pediatric Concerns:

Drug Interactions: Denosumab may increase the effects of cladribine. Echinacea may decrease the effects of cladribine. Cladribine may increase the effects of leflunomide, natalizumab, pimecrolimus, roflumilast, and tacrolimus. Live vaccines such as MMR, varicella, influenza, typhoid, rotavirus vaccines should not be administered while a patient is on cladribine therapy.

Relative Infant Dose:

Adult Dose: 0.09 mg/kg/day days 1–7; may be repeated every 28–35 days

Alternatives:

References:
1. Pharmaceutical manufacturer prescribing information, 2005.

CLARITHROMYCIN   L1

Trade: Biaxin
Other Trades: Klacid, Biaxin, Klaricid
Category: Antibiotic

Antibiotic that belongs to erythromycin family. In a study of 12 mothers receiving 250 mg twice daily, the C_{max} occurred at 2.2 hours and was reported to be 0.85 mg/L.[1] The estimated average dose of clarithromycin via milk was reported to be 150 µg/kg/day, or 2% of the maternal dose. Clarithromycin is probably compatible with breastfeeding. Observe for diarrhea and thrush in the infant.

Pregnancy Risk	C	Lactation Risk	L1
T ½	= 5–7 hours	M/P	= >1
Vd	= 3–4 l/kg	PB	= 40–70%
Tmax	= 1.7 hours	Oral	= 50%
MW	= 748	pKa	= 12.94

Adult Concerns: Diarrhea, nausea, dyspepsia, abdominal pain, metallic taste.

Pediatric Concerns: None reported via milk. Pediatric indications are available.

Drug Interactions: Clarithromycin increases serum theophylline by as much as 20%. Increases plasma levels of carbamazepine, cyclosporin, digoxin, ergot alkaloids, tacrolimus, triazolam, zidovudine, terfenadine, astemizole, cisapride (serious arrhythmias). Fluconazole increases clarithromycin serum levels by 25%. Numerous other drug-drug interactions are unreported, but probably occur.

Relative Infant Dose: 2.1%

Adult Dose: 250–500 mg BID

Alternatives:

References:
1. Sedlmayr T, Peters F, Raasch W, Kees F.[Clarithromycin, a new macrolide antibiotic. Effectiveness in puerperal infections and pharmacokinetics in breast milk]. Geburtshilfe Frauenheilkd 1993 July; 53(7): 488–91.

CLAVULANATE   L3

Trade:
Other Trades:
Category: Antibiotic penicillin

Clavulanate is a beta-lactamase inhibitor used in combination with amoxicillin or ticarcillin.[1] Its chemical structure is similar to beta lactam antibiotic such as penicillin. In a study of 67 breastfeeding mothers, 27 mothers were treated with amoxicillin/clavulanic acid and 40 mothers were treated with only amoxicillin.[2] In the amoxicillin/ clavulanic acid group, 22.3% of the infants had mild adverse effects. Only 7.5% of the control group (amoxicillin-only) infants had adverse effects. However, the authors suggest that this difference in untoward effects is not clinically significant.

Pregnancy Risk	C	Lactation Risk	L3
T ½	= 1 hour	M/P	=
Vd	=	PB	= 22–30%
Tmax	= 1 hour	Oral	= 75%
MW	= 199.1608	pKa	= 15.52

Adult Concerns: Rash, Nausea, Diarrhea, Urticaria, and Vomiting. Rarely hepatotoxicity may occur.

Pediatric Concerns: Urticaria in breastfed infant was reported when mother was using amoxicillin/clavulanate.

Drug Interactions:

Relative Infant Dose:

Adult Dose:

Alternatives:

References:
1. Saudagar PS, Survase SA, Singhal RS. Clavulanic acid: a review. Biotechnol Adv. 2008 Jul-Aug; 26(4): 335–51. Epub 2008 Mar 26. Review.
2. Benyamini L et al. The Safety of Amoxicillin/Clavulanic Acid and Cefuroxime During Lactation. Ther Drug Monit 2005 Aug; 27(4): 499–502.

CLEMASTINE   L4

Trade: Tavist, Dayhist Allergy

Other Trades:

Category: Antihistamine

Clemastine is a long-acting antihistamine. Following a maternal dose of 1 mg twice daily a 10-week-old breastfeeding infant developed drowsiness, irritability, refusal to feed, and neck stiffness.[1] Levels in milk and plasma (20 hours post dose) were 5–10 µg/L (milk) and 20 µg/L (plasma) respectively.

Pregnancy Risk	B	Lactation Risk	L4
T ½	= 10–12 hours	M/P	= 0.25–0.5
Vd	= 11.4 l/kg	PB	= 95%
Tmax	= 2–5 hours	Oral	= 100%
MW	= 344	pKa	=

Adult Concerns: Drowsiness, headache, fatigue, nervousness, appetite increase, depression.

Pediatric Concerns: Drowsiness, irritability, refusal to feed, and neck stiffness in one infant. Increased risk of seizures.

Drug Interactions: Increased toxicity when mixed with CNS depressants, anticholinergics, monoamine oxidase inhibitors, tricyclic antidepressants, phenothiazines.

Relative Infant Dose: 5.2%

Adult Dose: 1.34 to 2.68 mg BID or TID

Alternatives: Cetirizine, Loratadine

References:
1. Kok TH, Taitz LS, Bennett MJ, Holt DW. Drowsiness due to clemastine transmitted in breast milk. Lancet 1982; 1(8277): 914–915.

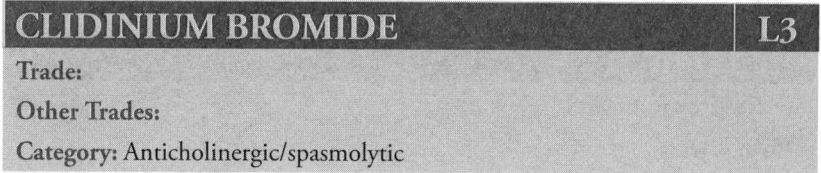

CLIDINIUM BROMIDE   L3

Trade:

Other Trades:

Category: Anticholinergic/spasmolytic

Clidinium bromide has anticholinergic properties giving pronounced antispasmodic and antisecretory effects on the gastrointestinal tract. In the United States, it is only available as an oral formulation in combination with chlordiazepoxide.

Clidinium is incompletely absorbed from the small intestine and is rapidly hydrolyzed in the liver to form its quaternary amino-alcohol.[1] As a quaternary ammonium compound it is fully ionized, and as such has very limited lipid solubility. This in turn does not allow clidinium to cross the blood-brain barrier. High ionization does however, cause it to exert a high nicotinic effect when compared to some other antimuscarinic agents. Due to potential risks associated with this drug and the lack of data concerning its use, it is only advisable to use during pregnancy when there is a clear indication that the benefit to the mother outweighs the risk to the infant.

It is currently unknown if clidinium is excreted into breast milk. Other antimuscarinic drugs have shown some data regarding transfer into milk, but so far no substantial evidence has been found to support that claim.

Pregnancy Risk	C	Lactation Risk	L3
T ½	= 1.2/20 hr, biphasic	M/P	=
Vd	=	PB	=
Tmax	=	Oral	= Incompletely absorbed
MW	= 432.4	pKa	=

Adult Concerns: Constipation, dry mouth, headache, drowsiness, nervousness, mental confusion, weakness, insomnia, dizziness, blurred vision, palpitations, allergic urticaria, decreased sweating, lactation suppression, urinary hesitancy, increased intraocular tension, cycloplegia, mydriasis, and impotence.

Pediatric Concerns:

Drug Interactions: Amantadine, antiarrhythmics, antihistamines, tricyclic antidepressants, antiparkinsonian agents, and meperidine may increase the adverse effects of clidinium. Clidinium may also increase gastrointestinal transit time, leading to possible toxicity of potassium chloride and slower absorption of acetaminophen. Ketoconazole absorption may be reduced when used in combination with clidinium. Intraocular pressure may increase when administering clidinium with corticosteroids. Clidinium may increase digoxin concentrations.

Relative Infant Dose:

Adult Dose: 2.5–5 mg 3–4 times daily

Alternatives:

References:
1. AHFS Drug Information. © Copyright, 1959–2011, Selected Revisions May 2008. American Society of Health-System Pharmacists, Inc. Bethesda, Maryland.

CLINDAMYCIN   L2

Trade: Cleocin Pediatric, Cleocin HCL

Other Trades:

Category: Antibiotic

Clindamycin hydrochloride is a broad-spectrum antibiotic frequently used for anaerobic infections. In one study of two nursing mothers and following doses of 600 mg IV every 6 hours, the concentration of clindamycin in breastmilk was 3.1 to 3.8 mg/L at 0.2 to 0.5 hours after dosing.[1]

Following oral doses of 300 mg every 6 hours, the breastmilk levels averaged 1.0 to 1.7 mg/L at 1.5 to 7 hours after dosing. In another study of 2–3 women who received a single oral dose of 150 mg, milk levels averaged 0.9 mg/L at 4 hours with a milk/plasma ratio of 0.47.[2] An alteration of gastrointestinal flora is possible even though the dose is low.

One case of bloody stools (pseudomembranous colitis) has been associated with clindamycin and gentamicin therapy on day 5 postpartum, but this is considered rare.[3] In this case, the mother of a newborn infant was given 600 mg IV every 6 hours. In rare cases, pseudomembranous colitis can appear several weeks later. In a study by Steen, in 5 breastfeeding patients who received 150 mg three times daily for 7 days, milk concentrations ranged from <0.5 to 3.1 mg/L with the majority of levels being <0.5 mg/L.[4] There are a number of pediatric clinical uses of clindamycin (anaerobic infections, bacterial endocarditis, pelvic inflammatory disease, and bacterial vaginosis). The current pediatric dosage recommendation is 10–40 mg/kg/day divided every 6–8 hours.[5] In a study of 15 women who received 600 mg clindamycin intravenously, levels of clindamycin in milk averaged 1.03 mg/L at two hours following the dose.[6]

Lotions or ointments of clindamycin meant for topical application contain clindamycin phosphate equivalent to 10 mg/mL. Transcutaneous absorption is minimal (<1–4%) and reported plasma levels are low to nil. Some does appear in urine of treated patients. Due to low maternal plasma levels, virtually none should be expected in breast milk. With the rise of resistant *Staphylococcal* infections, clindamycin use in infants has risen enormously. The amount in milk is unlikely to harm a breastfeeding infant.

Pregnancy Risk	B	Lactation Risk	L2
T ½	= 2.4 hours	M/P	= 0.47
Vd	= 2 l/kg	PB	= 94%
Tmax	= 45–60 minutes	Oral	= 90%
MW	= 425	pKa	= 7.45

Adult Concerns: Diarrhea, rash, pseudomembranous colitis, nausea, vomiting, gastrointestinal cramps.

Pediatric Concerns: One case of pseudomembranous colitis has been reported. But this is rare in infants. It is unlikely the levels in breastmilk would be clinically relevant. Commonly used in pediatric infections. Observe for diarrhea.

Drug Interactions: Increased duration of muscle blockade when administered with neuromuscular blockers such as tubocurarine and pancuronium. Antagonism has been demonstrated between clindamycin and erythromycin *in vitro*. Because of possible clinical significance, these two drugs should not be administered concurrently.

Relative Infant Dose: 0.9%–1.8%

Adult Dose: 150–450 mg every 6 hours

Alternatives:

References:
1. Smith JA. et. al. Clindamycin in human breast milk. Can Med Assn J 1975; 112: 806.
2. Matsuda S. Transfer of antibiotics into maternal milk. Biol Res Pregnancy Perinatol 1984; 5(2): 57–60.
3. Mann CF. Clindamycin and breast-feeding. Pediatrics 1980; 66(6): 1030–1031.
4. Steen B, Rane A. Clindamycin passage into human milk. Br J Clin Pharmacol 1982; 13(5): 661–664.
5. Johnson KB. ed. The Harriet Lane Handbook. Thirteenth ed. Mosby Publishing, 1993.
6. Zhang Y, Zhang Q, Xu Z. Tissue and body fluid distribution of antibacterial agents in pregnant and lactating women. Zhonghua Fu Chan Ke Za Zhi. 1997; 32: 288–92.

CLINDAMYCIN + TRETINOIN   L2

Trade: Veltin, Ziana

Other Trades:

Category: Antibiotic, Antiacne

Clindamycin phosphate and Tretinoin is a combination drug product indicated for acne vulgaris.

Lotions or ointments of clindamycin meant for topical application contain clindamycin phosphate equivalent to 10 mg/mL. Transcutaneous absorption is minimal (<1–4%) and reported plasma levels are low to nil. Some does appear in urine of treated patients. Due to low maternal plasma levels, virtually none should be expected in breast milk. With the rise of resistant *Staphylococcal* infections, clindamycin use in infants has risen enormously. The amount in milk is unlikely to harm a breastfeeding infant.[1-6]

The blood concentrations of tretinoin measured 2–48 hours following application are essentially zero. Absorption of Retin-A via topical sources is reported to be minimal, and breastmilk would likely be minimal to none.[7] However, if it is used orally, transfer into milk is likely and should be used with great caution in a breastfeeding mother.

The topical application of clindamycin/tretinoin drug combination appears to be of minimal risk in breastfeeding.

Pregnancy Risk	B		Lactation Risk	L2
T ½	= Clindamycin/tretinoin: 2.4 hours/ 2 hours	M/P	= Clindamycin/tretinoin: 0.47/
Vd	= Clindamycin/tretinoin: 2/0.44 l/kg	PB	= Clindamycin/tretinoin: 94%/
Tmax	= Clindamycin/tretinoin: 45–60 min/	Oral	= Clindamycin/tretinoin: 90%/70%
MW	= Clindamycin/tretinoin: 425/300	pKa	= Clindamycin/tretinoin: 7.45/4.79

Adult Concerns: Diarrhea, rash, pseudomembranous colitis, nausea, vomiting, gastrointestinal cramps.

Pediatric Concerns: One case of pseudomembranous colitis has been reported. But this is rare in infants. It is unlikely the levels in breastmilk would be clinically relevant. Commonly used in pediatric infections. Observe for diarrhea.

Drug Interactions: Increased duration of muscle blockade when administered with neuromuscular blockers such as tubocurarine and pancuronium. Antagonism has been demonstrated between clindamycin and erythromycin *in vitro*. Because of possible clinical significance, these two drugs should not be administered concurrently.

Relative Infant Dose: 1%–7.3%

Adult Dose: 150–450 mg every 6 hours

Alternatives:

References:
1. Smith JA. et. al. Clindamycin in human breast milk. Can Med Assn J 1975; 112: 806.
2. Matsuda S. Transfer of antibiotics into maternal milk. Biol Res Pregnancy Perinatol 1984; 5(2): 57–60.
3. Mann CF. Clindamycin and breast-feeding. Pediatrics 1980; 66(6): 1030–1031.
4. Steen B, Rane A. Clindamycin passage into human milk. Br J Clin Pharmacol 1982; 13(5): 661–664.
5. Johnson KB. ed. The Harriet Lane Handbook. Thirteenth ed. Mosby Publishing, 1993.
6. Zhang Y, Zhang Q, Xu Z. Tissue and body fluid distribution of antibacterial agents in pregnant and lactating women. Zhonghua Fu Chan Ke Za Zhi. 1997; 32: 288–92.
7. Lucek RW, Colburn WA. Clinical pharmacokinetics of the retinoids. Clin Pharmacokinet 1985; 10(1): 38–62.

CLINDAMYCIN TOPICAL   L2

Trade: Cleocin T, ClindaDerm, ClindaMax, Clindagel
Other Trades: Clindatech, Dalacin T
Category: Antibiotic

Clindamycin is a broad-spectrum antibiotic frequently used for anaerobic infections.[1]

Lotions or ointments of clindamycin meant for topical application contain clindamycin phosphate equivalent to 10 mg/mL. Transcutaneous absorption is minimal (<1–4%) and reported plasma levels are low to nil. Some does appear in urine of treated patients. Due to low maternal plasma levels, virtually none should be expected in breast milk. With the rise of resistant *Staphylococcal* infections, clindamycin use in infants has risen enormously. The amount in milk is unlikely to harm a breastfeeding infant.

Pregnancy Risk	B	Lactation Risk	L2
T ½	= 1.5–2.6 hours	M/P	=
Vd	=	PB	=
Tmax	= 10–14 hours	Oral	= None
MW	=	pKa	=

Adult Concerns: Headache, nausea, diarrhea, vomiting, abdominal pain, erythema, burning, itching, dryness, hypersensitivity.

Pediatric Concerns: One case of pseudomembranous colitis has been reported from oral clindamycin. But this is rare in infants. It is unlikely the levels in breastmilk would be clinically relevant. Commonly used in pediatric infections. Observe for diarrhea.

Drug Interactions:

Relative Infant Dose:

Adult Dose: Apply topical twice daily

Alternatives:

References:

1. Pharmaceutical manufacturer prescribing information, 2010.

CLINDAMYCIN VAGINAL   L2

Trade: Cleocin Vaginal, Cleocin Phosphate IV
Other Trades: Dalacin Vaginal Cream
Category: Antibiotic

Clindamycin is a broad-spectrum antibiotic frequently used for anaerobic infections. Clindamycin when administered by intravenously has been found in breastmilk. One case of bloody stools (pseudomembranous colitis) has been associated with oral clindamycin. However, only about 5% of clindamycin is absorbed into the maternal circulation, when applied vaginally (100 mg/dose), which would amount to approximately 5 mg clindamycin/day.[1] It is unlikely that clindamycin when administered via a vaginal gel would produce any significant danger to a breastfeeding infant.

Pregnancy Risk	B	Lactation Risk	L2
T ½	= 2.9 hours	M/P	=
Vd	=	PB	= 94%
Tmax	= 10–14 hours	Oral	= 90%
MW	= 425	pKa	=

Adult Concerns: Diarrhea, rash, gastrointestinal cramps, colitis, rarely bloody diarrhea. Transient neutropenia (leukopenia), eosinophilia, agranulocytosis, and thrombocytopenia have been reported. No direct etiologic relationship to concurrent clindamycin therapy could be made in any of these reports.

Pediatric Concerns: Unlikely to harm a breastfeeding infant.

Drug Interactions: Clindamycin has been shown to have neuromuscular blocking properties that may enhance the action of other neuromuscular blocking agents.

Relative Infant Dose: 0%

Adult Dose: 100 mg intravaginally every HS for 3 days

Alternatives:

References:
1.   Pharmaceutical manufacturer prescribing information, 2010.

CLOBAZAM   L3

Trade: Frisium
Other Trades: Frisium
Category: Benzodiazepine anxiolytic

Clobazam is a typical benzodiazepine very similar to diazepam.[1] It is primarily an anxiolytic, but it is sometimes used to treat refractory seizures.

Clobazam is known to be excreted into breastmilk in minimal quantities. The milk: plasma ratio of clobazam is 0.13–0.36.[2] Based on this, short-term use of clobazam is probably compatible with breastfeeding, and will not cause untoward effects in the infant.[3] However, the median half-life for tolerance is only 3.5 months, so it would not be suitable for long-term therapy of seizures. It has a rather long half-life averaging 17–31 hours for the parent drug in young adults and 11–77 hours for the active metabolite desmethylclobazam. As with diazepam, it could possibly reach elevated levels in a breastfeeding infant over time.

Therefore, it may be concluded that short-term use of clobazam is probably compatible with breastfeeding, but long-term use is best avoided.

Pregnancy Risk	C	Lactation Risk	L3
T ½	= 17–31 hours	M/P	= 0.13–0.36
Vd	= 0.87–1.8 l/kg	PB	= 90%
Tmax	= 1–2 hours	Oral	= 87%
MW	= 301	pKa	= 9

Adult Concerns: Sedation, drowsiness, hangover, weakness, insomnia.

Pediatric Concerns: Typical benzodiazepine, use caution. See Diazepam.

Drug Interactions: May increase effects of opiates, CNS depressants. Macrolide (erythromycin) antibiotics may increase levels of clobazam. Clobazam may increase levels of carbamazepine.

Relative Infant Dose:

Adult Dose: 20–30 mg/day

Alternatives: Alprazolam

References:
1. Pharmaceutical manufacturer prescribing information, 2010.
2. Hajdu P and Wernicke OA: Untersuchung zur Uberprufung des Ubertritts von Frisium in die Muttermilch (Internal Report). Hoechst, 1978, 1978.
3. Anon: Breastfeeding and Maternal Medication. World Health Organization, Geneva, Switzerland, 1995.

CLOBETASOL   L5

Trade: Clobevate, Clobex, Cormax, Olux-E, Olux, Temovate E, Temovate

Other Trades: Taro-Clobetasol, Dermovate, Gen-Clobetasol, Novo-Clobetasol

Category: Topical Corticosteroid

Clobetasol propionate is a very high potency topical corticosteroid used for the short-term relief of inflammation of moderate to severe corticosteroid responsive dermatoses including psoriasis.[1] Because this is such a high potency steroid, oral absorption by an infant could be hazardous. Do not use this on the nipple or areola of a breastfeeding mother. There are reports of excretion of corticosteroids into the breastmilk when they are administered systemically. When infants are exposed to corticosteroids through the milk there is a risk of growth suppression, though the risk for such an effect is most common with prolonged use of high dose corticosteroids.[2]

Pregnancy Risk	C	Lactation Risk	L5
T ½	=	M/P	=
Vd	=	PB	=
Tmax	= 2 months	Oral	=
MW	= 467	pKa	= 15.14

Adult Concerns: Adverse reactions include adrenal suppression, application site burning, cracking, dryness, irritation, and glucosuria.

Pediatric Concerns: Use is not recommended in children under 12 years of age. Do not use on the nipple or areola of the breast of a breastfeeding mother.

Drug Interactions: Clobetasol propionate may decrease the effects of aldesleukin and corticorelin. Clobetasol may increase the toxic effects of deferasirox.

Relative Infant Dose:

Adult Dose: Apply twice daily

Alternatives: Hydrocortisone, mometasone ointments or creams

References:
1. Pharmaceutical manufacturer prescribing information, 2002.
2. Product Information: Temovate(R), clobetasol. Glaxo Dermatology Products, Research Triangle Park, NC, 1998a.

CLOFAZIMINE   L3

Trade: Lamprene

Other Trades: Lamprene

Category: Antimicrobial for leprosy

Clofazimine exerts a slow bactericidal effect on Mycobacterium leprae. In a study of 8 female leprosy patients on clofazimine (50 mg/day or 100 mg on alternate days) for 1–18 months, blood samples were taken at 4–6 hours after the dose.[1] Average plasma and milk levels were 0.9 mg/L and 1.33 mg/L (range= 0.8 to 1.7 mg/L), respectively. The milk/plasma ratio varied from 1.0 to 1.7 with a mean of 1.48. A red tint and pigmentation has been reported in breastfed infants.[2,3]

Pregnancy Risk	C	Lactation Risk	L3
T ½	= 70 days	M/P	= 1.0–1.7
Vd	= 21 l/kg	PB	=
Tmax	= 4–12 hours	Oral	= 45–70%
MW	= 473	pKa	= 8.37

Adult Concerns: Reversible red-brown discoloration of skin and eyes. Gastrointestinal effects include nausea, abdominal cramps and pain, nausea and vomiting. Splenic infarction, crystalline deposits of clofazimine in multiple organs and tissues.

Pediatric Concerns: Levels in milk are moderate to high. Reddish discoloration of milk and infant may occur. No toxicity in infants has been reported however.

Drug Interactions: Dapsone may decrease the effects of clofazimine. Isoniazid may increase the plasma and urine concentrations of clofazimine.

Relative Infant Dose: 14%–28.2%

Adult Dose: 100–200 mg daily.

Alternatives:

References:

1. Venkatesan K, Mathur A, Girdhar A, Girdhar BK. Excretion of clofazimine in human milk in leprosy patients. Lepr Rev 1997; 68(3): 242–246.
2. Farb H, West DP, Pedvis-Leftick A. Clofazimine in pregnancy complicated by leprosy. Obstet Gynecol 1982; 59(1): 122–123.
3. Freerksen E, Seydel JK. Critical comments on the treatment of leprosy and other mycobacterial infections with clofazimine. Arzneimittelforschung 1992; 42(10): 1243–1245.

CLOFEDANOL / CHLOPHEDIANOL   L3

Trade:

Other Trades: Ulone

Category: Antitussive

Clofedanol or chlophedianol is an antitussive agent indicated for treatment of dry cough.[1] Structurally it is similar to diphenhydramine, hence some anticholinergic and antihistamine actions should be expected. There are no controlled studies in breastfeeding women and very little kinetic data are available. This drug should probably be avoided until we know more about its clinical effects.

Pregnancy Risk	Probably Safe	Lactation Risk	L3
T ½	=	M/P	=
Vd	=	PB	=
Tmax	=	Oral	=
MW	= 290	pKa	=

Adult Concerns: Drying and sedation.

Pediatric Concerns:

Drug Interactions:

Relative Infant Dose:

Adult Dose: 12.5 mg dose

Alternatives:

References:
1. Pharmaceutical manufacturer prescribing information, 2010.

CLOMIPHENE   L4

Trade: Clomid, Serophene, Milophene

Other Trades: Clomid, Serophene

Category: Ovulation stimulator for ovulatory failure

Clomiphene appears to stimulate the release of the pituitary gonadotropins, follicle-stimulating hormone (FSH), and luteinizing hormone (LH), which result in development and maturation of the ovarian follicle, ovulation, and subsequent development and function of the corpus luteum. It has both estrogenic and anti-estrogenic effects. LH and FSH peak at 5–9 days after completing clomiphene therapy.

In a study of 60 postpartum women (1–4 days postpartum), clomiphene was effective in totally inhibiting lactation early postnatally and in suppressing established lactation (day 4).[1] Only 7 of 40 women receiving clomiphene to inhibit lactation had signs of congestion or discomfort. In the 20 women who received clomiphene to suppress established lactation (on day 4), a rapid amelioration of breast engorgement and discomfort was produced. After 5 days of treatment, no signs of lactation were present. In another study of 177 postpartum women, clomiphene was very effective at inhibiting lactation.[2]

Bromocriptine, stilboestrol, clomiphene, testosterone and a placebo were given to 75 postpartum women for the suppression of puerperal lactation. An additional 15 women who breastfed their babies served as a control group.[3] Blood samples were taken for the determination of serum prolactin levels by a specific homologous double antibody radioimmunoassay. Concurrently, the clinical effectiveness of the various treatments was assessed. High levels of prolactin were found at the time of delivery. Bromocriptine effectively reduced serum prolactin and prevented lactation; stilboestrol increased serum prolactin and partially suppressed lactation; clomiphene citrate and testosterone propionate both lowered serum prolactin levels and partially suppressed lactation. The placebo showed almost no effect on serum prolactin.

Clomiphene appears in one study to be very effective in suppressing lactation when used up to 4 days postpartum. However, in another study of 10 puerperal women who received 100 mg of clomiphene orally for 7 days, beginning on day one postpartum, no change in maternal plasma prolactin or in milk production occurred in this group over the seven days of the study.[4]

Its efficacy in reducing milk production in women, months after lactation is established, is unknown but believed to be minimal.

Pregnancy Risk	X	Lactation Risk	L4
T ½	= 5–7 days	M/P	=
Vd	= >57 l/kg	PB	=
Tmax	= 6 hours	Oral	= Complete
MW	= 406	pKa	= 12.4

Adult Concerns: Dizziness, insomnia, light-headedness, hot flashes, ovarian enlargement, depression, headache, alopecia. May inhibit lactation early postpartum.

Pediatric Concerns: Transfer and effect on infant is unreported, but may suppress early lactation.

Drug Interactions:

Relative Infant Dose:

Adult Dose: 50 mg daily.

Alternatives:

References:
1. Masala A, Delitala G, Alagna S, Devilla L, Stoppelli I, Lo DG. Clomiphene and puerperal lactation. Panminerva Med 1978; 20(3): 161–163.

2. Zuckerman H, Carmel S. The inhibition of lactation by clomiphene. J Obstet Gynaecol Br Commonw 1973; 80(9): 822–823.
3. Weinstein D, Ben-David M, Polishuk WZ. Serum prolactin and the suppression of lactation. Br J Obstet Gynaecol. 1976 Sep; 83(9): 679–82.
4. Canales ES, Lasso P, Soria J, Z√°rate A. Effect of clomiphene on prolactin secretion and lactation in puerperal women. Br J Obstet Gynaecol. 1977 Oct; 84(10): 758–9.

CLOMIPRAMINE   L2

Trade: Anafranil

Other Trades: Placil, Anafranil, Apo-Clomipramine

Category: Anti-obsessional, antidepressant drug

Clomipramine is a tricyclic antidepressant frequently used for obsessive-compulsive disorder.[1] In one patient taking 125 mg/day, on the 4th and 6th day postpartum, milk levels were 342.7 and 215.8 µg/L respectively.[2] Maternal plasma levels were 211 and 208.4 µg/L at day 4 and 6 respectively. Milk/plasma ratio varies from 1.62 to 1.04 on day 4 to 6 respectively. Neonatal plasma levels continued to drop from a high of 266.6 ng/mL at birth to 127.6 ng/mL at day 4, to 94.8 ng/mL at day 6, to 9.8 ng/mL at 35 days. In a study of four breastfeeding women who received doses of 75 to 125 mg/day, plasma levels of clomipramine in the breastfed infants were below the limit of detection, suggesting minimal transfer to the infant via milk.[3] No untoward effects were noted in any of the infants.

Pregnancy Risk	C	Lactation Risk	L2
T ½	= 19–37 hours	M/P	= 0.84–1.62
Vd	= 17 l/kg	PB	= 96%
Tmax	=	Oral	= Complete
MW	= 315	pKa	= 9.5

Adult Concerns: Drowsiness, fatigue, dry mouth, seizures, constipation, sweating, reduced appetite.

Pediatric Concerns: None reported in several studies.

Drug Interactions: Decreased effect when used with barbiturates, carbamazepine and phenytoin. Increased sedation when used with alcohol, CNS depressants (hypnotics). Increased dangers when used with monoamine oxidase inhibitors. Additive anticholinergic effects when used with other anticholinergics.

Relative Infant Dose: 2.8%

Adult Dose: 50 mg BID

Alternatives: Sertraline, Paroxetine, Fluoxetine

References:
1. Pharmaceutical manufacturer prescribing information, 2010.
2. Schimmell MS, Katz EZ, Shaag Y, Pastuszak A, Koren G. Toxic neonatal effects following maternal clomipramine therapy. J Toxicol Clin Toxicol 1991; 29(4): 479–484.
3. Wisner KL, Perel JM, Foglia JP. Serum clomipramine and metabolite levels in four nursing mother-infant pairs. J Clin Psychiatry 1995; 56(1): 17–20.

CLONAZEPAM   L3

Trade: Klonopin
Other Trades: Paxam, Rivotril, Apo-Clonazepam, PMS-Clonazepam
Category: Anticonvulsant, sedative

Clonazepam is a typical benzodiazepine sedative, anticonvulsant. In one case report, milk levels varied between 11 and 13 µg/L (the maternal dose was omitted).[1] Milk/maternal serum ratio was approximately 0.33. In this report, the infant's serum level of clonazepam dropped from 4.4 µg/L at birth to 1.0 µg/L at 14 days while continuing to breastfeed, suggesting increasing clearance with time. In this case, excessive periodic breathing and apnea and cyanosis occurred in this infant (36 weeks gestation) at 6 hours until 10 days postpartum. The infant was exposed in utero as well as postpartum via breastmilk. In another study of a mother treated with 2 mg clonazepam twice daily recorded peak milk concentrations of 10.7 µg/L at 4 hours post dose, and a maximum infant dose of 2.5% of the weight-adjusted maternal dose. The infant's serum level of clonazepam at days 2–4 was 4.7 µg/L.[2] In a group of 11 mothers receiving 0.25 to 2 mg clonazepam daily, 10 of 11 breastfed infants had no detectable (limit of detection: 5–14 µg/L) clonazepam or metabolites in their serum.[3] One infant (1.9 weeks old) had a serum concentration of 22 µg/L. Maternal dose was 0.5 mg daily.

These data suggest the low incidence of toxicity with this medication in breastfeeding infants.

Pregnancy Risk	D	Lactation Risk	L3
T ½	= 18–50 hours	M/P	= 0.33
Vd	= 1.5–4.4 l/kg	PB	= 50–86%
Tmax	= 1–4 hours	Oral	= Complete
MW	= 316	pKa	= 1.5, 10.5

Adult Concerns: Apnea, sedation, ataxia, hypotonia. Behavioral disturbances (in children) include aggressiveness, irritability, agitation.

Pediatric Concerns: Apnea, cyanosis and hypotonia was reported in one infant at 6 hours postnatally to a woman consuming clonazepam throughout pregnancy. Maternal and cord serum levels of clonazepam were 32 ng/mL and 19 ng/mL respectively. The infant had prolonged apnea and hypotonia. The infant had repeated periodic breathing episodes up to 10 weeks of age.[1] In another group of 11 mothers consuming clonazepam, none of the infants had any reported side effects.[3]

Drug Interactions: Phenytoin and barbiturates may increase clearance of clonazepam. CNS depressants may increase sedation.

Relative Infant Dose: 2.8%

Adult Dose: 0.5–1 mg TID

Alternatives: Lorazepam

References:

1. Fisher JB, Edgren BE, Mammel MC, Coleman JM. Neonatal apnea associated with maternal clonazepam therapy: a case report. Obstet Gynecol 1985; 66(3 Suppl): 34S-35S.
2. Soderman P, Matheson I. Clonazepam in breast milk. Eur J Pediatr 1988; 147(2): 212–213.
3. Birnbaum CS, Cohen LS, Bailey JW et al. Serum concentrations of antidepressants and benzodiazepines in nursing infants: a case series. Pediatrics. 1999; 104: e11.

CLONIDINE   L3

Trade: Catapres

Other Trades: Catapres, Dixarit, Apo-Clonidine, Novo-Clonidine

Category: Antihypertensive

Clonidine is an antihypertensive that reduces sympathetic nerve activity from the brain. Clonidine is excreted in human milk minimally. In a study of 9 nursing women receiving between 241.7 and 391.7 µg/day of clonidine, milk levels varied from approximately 1.8 µg/L to as high as 2.8 µg/L on postpartum day 10–14.[1] In another report following a maternal dose of 37.5 µg twice daily, maternal plasma was determined to be 0.33 ng/mL and milk level was 0.60 µg/L.[2] Clinical symptoms of neonatal toxicity are unreported and are unlikely in normal full term infants.

Clonidine may reduce prolactin secretion and could conceivably reduce milk production early postpartum. Transdermal patches produce maternal plasma levels of 0.39, 0.84, and 1.12 ng/mL using the 3.5, 7, and 10.5 cm^2 patches respectively. The 3.7 cm^2 patch would produce maternal plasma levels equivalent to the 37.5 µg oral dose and would likely produce milk levels equivalent to the above study.

Pregnancy Risk	C		Lactation Risk	L3
T ½	= 20–24 hours		M/P	= 2
Vd	= 3.2–5.6 l/kg		PB	= 20–40%
Tmax	= 3–5 hours		Oral	= 75–100%
MW	= 230		pKa	= 8.3

Adult Concerns: Drowsiness, dry mouth, hypotension, constipation, dizziness.

Pediatric Concerns: None reported, but may induce hypotension in infant. May reduce milk production by reducing prolactin secretion.

Drug Interactions: Tricyclic antidepressants inhibit hypotensive effect of clonidine. Beta blockers may potentiate slow heart rate when administered with clonidine. Discontinue beta blockers several days to week prior to using clonidine.

Relative Infant Dose: 0.9%–7.1%

Adult Dose: 0.1–0.3 mg BID

Alternatives:

References:
1. Hartikainen-Sorri AL, Heikkinen JE, Koivisto M. Pharmacokinetics of clonidine during pregnancy and nursing. Obstet Gynecol 1987; 69(4): 598–600.
2. Bunjes R, Schaefer C, Holzinger D. Clonidine and breast-feeding. Clin Pharm 1993; 12(3): 178–179.

CLOPIDOGREL   L3

Trade: Plavix
Other Trades: Plavix
Category: Platelet aggregation inhibitor

Clopidogrel selectively inhibits platelet adenosine diphosphate-induced platelet aggregation. It is used to prevent ischemic events in patients at risk (e. g. cardiovascular disease, strokes, myocardial infarction). Aspirin is generally preferred as it is less expensive, quite tolerable, and very effective.

Clopidogrel is only used in those patients who are aspirin-intolerant. It is not known if it transfers into human milk, but it does enter rodent milk.[1] Although the plasma half-life is rather brief (6–8 hours), it's metabolite (thiol derivative) covalently bonds to platelet receptors with a half-life of 11 days. Because it produces an irreversible inhibition of platelet aggregation, any present in milk could inhibit an infant's platelet function for a prolonged period. However, thiol derivative of clopidogrel has but a 0.5–0.7 hour half-life. Thus patients could return to breastfeeding within 24 hours after stopping the use of clopidogrel.

Because aspirin affects platelet aggregation similarly, and its milk levels are quite low, it would appear to be an ideal alternative to clopidogrel. However, aspirin also inhibits platelet aggregation for long periods as well and may increase the risk of Reye' s syndrome in infants. The choice between using clopidogrel and aspirin must be made on clinical grounds and following a risk vs. benefit assessment until we know more about the levels secreted into human milk.

Pregnancy Risk	B	Lactation Risk	L3
T ½	= 8 hours	M/P	=
Vd	=	PB	= 9%
Tmax	= 1 hour	Oral	= 50%
MW	= 420	pKa	= 5.3

Adult Concerns: Contraindicated in individuals with bleeding phenomenon.

Pediatric Concerns: None reported via milk. The transfer of clinically relevant amounts to the infant is remote, but we do not have any data thus far suggesting milk levels and clinical dose transferred to the infant.

Drug Interactions: At high concentrations, clopidogrel inhibits Cytochrome P450 2C9, and may inhibit metabolism of phenytoin, tamoxifen, tolbutamide, warfarin, torsemide, fluvastatin, and many NSAIDs.

Relative Infant Dose:

Adult Dose: 75 mg daily

Alternatives:

References:
1. Pharmaceutical manufacturer prescribing information, 2010.

CLORAZEPATE   L3

Trade: Tranxene, Tranxene-SD

Other Trades: Apo-Clorazepate, Novo-Clopate

Category: Benzodiazepine sedative

Clorazepate is a typical benzodiazepine. The primary metabolite, nordiazepam, is the same as from diazepam. Clorazepate has a brief half-life of less than 2 hours, and is rapidly converted to the active drug, nordiazepam, and oxazepam. The active metabolite has a prolonged half-life of 40–50 hours.[1] In 7 mothers who were breastfeeding early postnatally, and who received 20 mg IM clorazepate, levels of nordiazepam ranged from 7.5–15.5 µg/L 48 hours after the dose and 6–12 µg/L 4 days following the dose.[2]

Pregnancy Risk	D	Lactation Risk	L3
T ½	= 40–50 hours (metab)	M/P	=
Vd	= 1.7 l/kg	PB	= 98%
Tmax	= 1 hour	Oral	= 97%
MW	= 408	pKa	= 3.5; 12.5

Adult Concerns: Adverse reactions include drowsiness, dizziness, blurred vision, dry mouth, headache, fatigue, ataxia, slurred speech, and mental confusion.

Pediatric Concerns: Poor suckling, sedation, lethargy, constipation have been reported for diazepam.

Drug Interactions: This drug is additive for almost all CNS sedatives. They may prolong the sleeping time after hexobarbital, ethyl alcohol, and other hypnotic sedatives including barbiturates, narcotics, phenothiazines, monoamine oxidase inhibitors, etc. Cimetidine may increase plasma levels of clorazepate.

Relative Infant Dose:

Adult Dose: 15–60 mg/day.

Alternatives: Lorazepam, midazolam

References:
1. Pharmaceutical manufacturer prescribing information, 2010.
2. Rey E, Giraux P, d'Athis P, Turquais JM, Chavinie J, Olive G. Pharmacokinetics of the placental transfer and distribution of clorazepate and its metabolite nordiazepam in the feto-placental unit and in the neonate. Eur J Clin Pharmacol. 1979 Apr 17; 15(3): 181–5.

CLOTRIMAZOLE   L1

Trade: Gyne-Lotrimin, Mycelex, Lotrimin, FemCare, Trivagizole

Other Trades: Hiderm, Clonea, Canesten, Clotrimaderm, Myclo

Category: Antifungal

Clotrimazole is a broad-spectrum antifungal agent. It is generally used for candidiasis and various tinea species (athletes foot, ring worm). Clotrimazole is available in oral lozenges, topical creams, intravaginal tablets and creams. No data are available on penetration into breastmilk. However, after intravaginal administration, only 3–10% of the drug is absorbed (peak serum level= 0.01 to 0.03 µg/mL) and even less by oral lozenge.[1] Hence, following vaginal administration it seems unlikely that levels absorbed by a breastfeeding infant would be high enough to produce untoward effects. Safety of clotrimazole lozenges in children younger than 3 years of age has not been established. The risk of contact dermatitis with this agent may be higher.[2]

Pregnancy Risk	B (for topical/vaginal)/C oral	Lactation Risk	L1
T ½	= 3.5–5 hours	M/P	=
Vd	=	PB	=
Tmax	= 3 hours (oral)	Oral	= Poor
MW	= 345	pKa	= 4.7

Adult Concerns: Nausea and vomiting from oral administration. Itching, burning, and stinging following topical application. The following have been reported: erythema, stinging, blistering, peeling, edema, pruritus, urticaria, burning, and general irritation of the skin. Elevated liver enzymes in >10% of those treated. Contact dermatitis has been reported in breastfeeding women.

Pediatric Concerns: None reported via milk. Limited oral absorption probably limits clinical relevance in breastfed infants.

Drug Interactions: May inhibit amphotericin activity. Clotrimazole is reported to increase cyclosporin plasma levels. May enhance hypoglycemic effect of oral hypoglycemic agents. Clotrimazole inhibits cytochrome P450 and may inhibit metabolism of any number of other medications.

Relative Infant Dose:

Adult Dose: 500 mg intravaginally every HS

Alternatives: Fluconazole, Miconazole

References:
1. McEvoy GE. (ed): AFHS Drug Information. New York, NY: 2003.
2. Newman J. Personal communication. 1999.

CLOXACILLIN   L2

Trade: Tegopen, Cloxapen

Other Trades: Alclox, Apo-Cloxi, Novo-Cloxin, Orbenin, Kloxerate-DC

Category: Penicillin antibiotic

Cloxacillin is an oral penicillinase-resistant penicillin frequently used for peripheral (non-CNS) *Staphylococcus aureus* and *Staphylococcus epidermidis* infections, particularly mastitis. Following a single 500 mg oral dose of cloxacillin in lactating women, milk concentrations of the drug were zero to 0.2 mg/L one and two hours after the dose respectively and 0.2 to 0.4 mg/L after 6 hours.[1] Usual dose for adults is 250–500 mg four times daily for at least 10–14 days.[2] As with most penicillins, it is unlikely these levels would be clinically relevant.

Pregnancy Risk	B	Lactation Risk	L2
T ½	= 0.7–3 hours	M/P	=
Vd	= 6.6–10.8 l/kg	PB	= 90–96%
Tmax	= 0.5–2 hours	Oral	= 37–60%
MW	= 436	pKa	= 13.65

Adult Concerns: Rash, diarrhea, nephrotoxicity, fever, shaking, chills.

Pediatric Concerns: None reported but observe for gastrointestinal symptoms such as diarrhea.

Drug Interactions: Efficacy of oral contraceptives may be reduced. Disulfiram, probenecid may increase cloxacillin levels. Increased effect of oral anticoagulants.

Relative Infant Dose: 0.4%–0.8%

Adult Dose: 250–500 mg every 6 hours

Alternatives:

References:
1. Matsuda S. Transfer of antibiotics into maternal milk. Biol Res Pregnancy Perinatol 1984; 5(2): 57–60.
2. McEvoy GE. (ed): AFHS Drug Information. New York, NY: 2003.

CLOZAPINE   L3

Trade: Clozaril

Other Trades: Clozaril

Category: Antipsychotic, sedative

Clozapine is an atypical antipsychotic, sedative drug somewhat similar to the phenothiazine family. In a study of one patient receiving 50 mg/day clozapine at delivery, the maternal and fetal plasma were reported to be 14.1 ng/mL and 27 ng/mL respectively.[1] After 24 hours postpartum, the maternal plasma level was 14.7 ng/mL and maternal milk levels were 63.5 ng/mL. On day 7 postpartum and receiving a dose of 100 mg/day clozapine, the maternal plasma and milk levels were 41.1 ng/mL and 115.6 µg/L respectively. From this data it is apparent that clozapine concentrates in milk with a milk/plasma ratio of 4.3 at a dose of 50 mg/day and 2.8 at a dose of 100 mg/day. The change from day 1 to day 7 suggests that clozapine entry into mature milk is less.

Pregnancy Risk	B	Lactation Risk	L3
T ½	= 8–12 hours	M/P	= 2.8–4.3
Vd	= 5 l/kg	PB	= 95%
Tmax	= 2.5 hours	Oral	= 90%
MW	= 327	pKa	= 3.7, 7.6

Adult Concerns: Drowsiness, dizziness/vertigo, salivation, constipation, tachycardia, nausea, gastrointestinal distress, extrapyramidal symptoms, tardive dyskinesia, agranulocytosis.

Pediatric Concerns: None reported but use with great caution.

Drug Interactions: Decreased effect of epinephrine, phenytoin. Increased sedation with CNS depressants. Increased effect with guanabenz, anticholinergics. Increased toxicity with cimetidine, monoamine oxidase inhibitors, tricyclic antidepressants.

Relative Infant Dose: 1.4%

Adult Dose: 300–600 mg daily.

Alternatives:

References:
1. Barnas C, Bergant A, Hummer M, Saria A, Fleischhacker WW. Clozapine concentrations in maternal and fetal plasma, amniotic fluid, and breast milk. Am J Psychiatry 1994; 151(6): 945.

COAGULATION FACTOR VIIa | L2

Trade: NovoSeven, Septrin

Other Trades: NovoSeven

Category: Promotes coagulation in hemophilia

Recombinant human coagulation factor VIIa (rFVIIa) is intended to promote coagulation by activating the extrinsic pathway of the coagulation cascade.[1] It is a vitamin K-dependent glycoprotein consisting of 406 amino acids and a molecular weight of 50,000 daltons. The recombinant human coagulation factor VIIa is structurally similar to human plasma-derived Factor VIIa normally found in human plasma.

This is a large molecular weight protein that is very unlikely to enter milk. It is structurally similar to human plasma derived factor VIIa normally found in humans anyway.

Pregnancy Risk	C	Lactation Risk	L2
T ½	= 1.7–2.7 hours	M/P	=
Vd	= 0.103 l/kg	PB	=
Tmax	=	Oral	= Nil
MW	= 50,000	pKa	=

Adult Concerns: Adverse reactions include fever, allergic reaction, purpura, rash, hemorrhage, hemarthrosis and hypertension.

Pediatric Concerns: None reported via milk. It is unlikely to enter milk.

Drug Interactions: Do not use simultaneously with activated prothrombin complex.

Relative Infant Dose:

Adult Dose: 90 µg/kg/2 hours until hemostasis is achieved.

Alternatives:

References:
1. Pharmaceutical manufacturer prescribing information, 2010.

COAL TAR — L2

Trade: Neutrogena T/Gel, Neutrogena T/Derm, Betatar Gel, Cutar Emulsion, DHS Tar, Denorex, Doak Tar, Duplex T

Other Trades:

Category: Anti-psoriatic, anti-seborrheic, keratolytic

Coal tar is an anti-psoriatic, anti-seborrheic and keratolytic agent, FDA approved for treatment of dandruff, psoriasis and seborrheic dermatitis.

One case report describes a woman who used coal tar to treat atopic dermatitis for 50 days while breast feeding her 3-month-old baby. The patient used 2 different coal tar ointments with a maximum estimated dose of 993 mg of pyrene and 464 mg of benzapyrene topically. The patient applied coal tar daily to all areas of the body excluding the face and breasts. Levels of coat tar constitutents in breast milk were undetectable (0.0035 and 0.54 respectively). Interestingly, urine samples of the breastfed child contained elevated levels of coal tar metabolite, 1-hydroxypyrene. The authors suggest that the infant obtained the pyrene via skin-to-skin or skin-to-mouth contact with the mother because the mother's breastmilk contained no detectable pyrene or benzo[a]pyrene, and only low levels of 1-hydroxypyrene.[1] In summary, patients should be advised that coal tar is not likely transferred through breast milk but may be transferred to the baby by skin-to-skin absorption or skin-to-mouth contact.

Pregnancy Risk	C	Lactation Risk	L2
T ½	=	M/P	=
Vd	=	PB	=
Tmax	=	Oral	=
MW	= 110	pKa	= 10

Adult Concerns: Contact dermatitis, smelly, irritating, may irritate herpes lesions, folliculitis.

Pediatric Concerns: None reported, but avoid skin to skin contact with the infant as some absorption in the infant has been reported (via skin to skin).

Drug Interactions:

Relative Infant Dose:

Adult Dose:

Alternatives:

References:

1. Scheepers PT, van Houtum JL, Anzion RB et al. Uptake of pyrene in a breast-fed child of a mother treated with coal tar. Pediatr Dermatol. 2009; 26: 184–7.

COBALT-57 + VITAMIN B$_{12}$ L4

Trade: Vitamin B$_{12}$-radiolabelled, Cyanocobalamin-radiolabelled, Schilling test, Vitamin B$_{12}$ absorption test

Other Trades:

Category: Radiopharmaceutical agent

Cobalt-57 (Co-57) is a radioactive isotope of cobalt that emits radiation in the form of beta and gamma rays. When tagged with vitamin B$_{12}$, radiolabeled vitamin B$_{12}$ is obtained which is used in the Schilling test. The Schilling test is used to diagnose pernicious anemia, caused due to the inability to absorb vitamin B$_{12}$. In this test, the patient is administered oral capsules of radiolabeled vitamin B$_{12}$ (Co-57 vitamin B$_{12}$), and the amount of radioactivity excreted in the urine over 24 hours is measured. A decreased excretion of Co-57 vitamin B$_{12}$ (<14%) suggests the possibility of pernicious anemia.

When radiopharmaceutical agents such as the one under discussion are administered to a lactating mother, the agent may get excreted in breastmilk, thereby potentially exposing the breastfed infant to radiation.

Pomeroy, Sawyer and Evans studied the amount of radioactivity excreted in milk following the use of Co-57 vitamin B$_{12}$ in a 20 year-old lactating mother who was 3 weeks postpartum.[1] The maternal dose administered was 18.6 kBq. Breastmilk samples were collected every time the baby was breastfed in the first 24 hours, one sample was collected at 48 hours and one at 72 hours. It was found that there was an initial delay of a few hours in the first appearance of radioactivity in breastmilk, following this radioactivity in breastmilk peaked at 24 hours, and eventually decreased to initial levels by the end of 72 hours. Assuming that the infant consumed 0.85 L of breastmilk per day, the total amount of radioactivity ingested by the infant was found to be 360 Bq. The authors estimated that in a 4 kg baby, this would amount to an effective radioactive exposure to the infant of 0.025 mSv. This is less than 1 mSv, which is the minimal amount of radiation exposure to an infant deemed safe and acceptable by many authorities. The authors of this study conclude that preferably the Schilling test should be avoided in a lactating mother. But if an occasion arises where such a test is found to be necessary, then the mother should feed the baby just prior to administration of oral Co-57 vitamin B$_{12}$. Due to the initial delay of a few hours in the first appearance of radioactivity in breastmilk, the authors suggest that the baby may receive the first feed immediately following the test, but should avoid breastfeeding at the 24 hour peak. The authors further inform that in this published case, the mother was diagnosed to have vitamin B$_{12}$ malabsorption; however, in a mother with normal vitamin B$_{12}$ absorption, more amount of radioactivity is expected to enter the milk.

Based on this study, it is best to avoid the Schilling test in a breastfeeding mother. but if an occasion arises where it is deemed necessary in a lactating mother, it would be advisable to interrupt breastfeeding for a period of 72 hours following a Schilling test.

Pregnancy Risk	Hazardous	Lactation Risk	L4
T ½	= 271.79 days (Co-57); 6 days (vitamin B$_{12}$)	M/P	=
Vd	=	PB	=
Tmax	=	Oral	=
MW	= 59	pKa	=

Adult Concerns:

Pediatric Concerns:

Drug Interactions:

Relative Infant Dose: 0.02%

Adult Dose: 1 µCi (37 kBq)

Alternatives:

References:
1. Pomeroy KM, Sawyer LJ, Evans MJ. Estimated radiation dose to breast feeding infant following maternal administration of ^{57}Co labelled to vitamin B$_{12}$. NuclMed Commun. 2005 Sep; 26(9): 839–41.

COCAINE   L5

Trade: Crack

Other Trades:

Category: Powerful CNS stimulant, local anesthetic

Cocaine is a local anesthetic and a powerful central nervous system stimulant. It is well absorbed from all locations including the stomach, nasal passages, intrapulmonary tissues via inhalation, and even via ophthalmic instillation. Adverse effects include agitation, nervousness, restlessness, euphoria, hallucinations, tremors, tonic-clonic seizures, and myocardial arrhythmias.

Although the pharmacologic effects of cocaine are relatively brief (20–30 min.) due to redistribution out of the brain, cocaine is slowly metabolized and excreted over a prolonged period. Urine samples can be positive for cocaine metabolites for up to 7 days or longer in adults. Breastfeeding infants will likewise become urine positive for cocaine for even longer periods. Even after the clinical effects of cocaine have subsided, the breastmilk will still probably contain significant quantities of benzoylecgonine, the inactive metabolite of cocaine. The infant could still test positive for urine cocaine metabolites for long periods (days). The ingestion of small amounts of cocaine by infants via inhalation of smoke (environmental) is likely.

Studies of exact estimates of cocaine transmission to breastmilk have not been reported. Significant secretion into breastmilk is suspected with a probable high milk/plasma ratio. A mother of an 11 day-old infant applied cocaine powder to her nipples as an analgesic. Three hours following breastfeeding, she discovered the infant choking, blue and gasping for air. Upon arrival at the emergency room, the infant was hypertensive, tachycardic, ashen and cyanotic. The infant subsequently seized repeatedly.[1]

Another case report of a mother who used cocaine 3 days before delivery, reported a milk level 6 days later of 8 ng/mL. The authors propose that if this mother consumed 0.5 gm of cocaine, then the infant would have likely received 0.48 mg of cocaine, or 1.62% of the maternal dose per kilogram.[2]

In a study of 11 mothers who admitted prior use during pregnancy, cocaine was detected in six milk samples.[3] The highest cocaine concentration found was over 12 µg/mL. Topical application to nipples is EXTREMELY dangerous and is definitely contraindicated. Oral, intranasal, and smoking of crack cocaine is dangerous and definitely contraindicated.

Breastfeeding mothers should avoid cocaine absolutely. In those individuals who have ingested cocaine, a minimum pump and discard period of 24 hours is recommended for clearance. In addition, mothers who consume cocaine will continue to transfer the inactive metabolite of cocaine into their breast milk for many days, and the infant will become drug-screen-positive, even if not exposed to the parent, cocaine.

Pregnancy Risk	C/X in third trimester	Lactation Risk	L5
T ½	= 0.8 hour	M/P	=
Vd	= 1.6–2.7 l/kg	PB	= 91%
Tmax	= 15 minutes	Oral	= Complete
MW	= 303	pKa	= 8.6

Adult Concerns: Nausea, vomiting, CNS excitement, hypertension, tachycardia, arrhythmias, seizures.

Pediatric Concerns: Choking, vomiting, diarrhea, tremulousness, hyperactive startle reflex, gasping, agitation, irritability, hypertension, tachycardia. Extreme danger.

Drug Interactions: Increased toxicity when used with monoamine oxidase inhibitors.

Relative Infant Dose:

Adult Dose: N/A

Alternatives:

References:
1. Chaney NE, Franke J, Wadlington WB. Cocaine convulsions in a breast-feeding baby. J Pediatr 1988; 112(1): 134–135.
2. Sarkar M, Djulus J, Koren G. When a Cocaine-Using Mother Wishes to Breastfeed. Ther Drug Monit 2005; 27(1): 1–2.
3. Winecker RE, Goldberger BA, Tebbett IRet al. Detection of cocaine and its metabolites in breast milk. J Forensic Sci. 2001; 46: 12221–3.

CODEINE   L3

Trade: Empirin #3 #4, Tylenol #3 #4

Other Trades: Actacode, Codalgin, Codral, Panadeine, Veganin, Paveral, Penntuss, Kaodene, Teropin

Category: Analgesic

Codeine is considered a mild opiate analgesic whose action is probably due to its metabolism to small amounts (about 7%) of morphine. The amount of codeine secreted into milk is low and dose dependent. Infant response is higher during neonatal period (first or second week).

Four cases of neonatal apnea have been reported following administration of 60 mg codeine every 4–6 hours to breastfeeding mothers although codeine was not detected in serum of the infants tested.[1] Apnea resolved after discontinuation of maternal codeine. Tylenol # 3 tablets contain 30 mg and Tylenol #4 tablets contain 60 mg of codeine in the USA.

In another study, following a dose of 60 mg, milk concentrations averaged 140 µg/L of milk with a peak of 455 µg/L at 1 hour.[2] Following 12 doses in 48 hours, the authors estimate the dose of codeine in milk (2000 mL milk) was 0.7 mg. There are few reported side effects following codeine doses of 30 mg, and it is believed to produce only minimal side effects in newborns.

In a study of 7 mothers consuming 60 mg codeine, codeine and morphine levels were studied in breastmilk of 17 samples, and neonatal plasma of 24 samples from 11 healthy, term neonates. Milk codeine levels ranged from 33.8 to 314 µg/L 20 to 240 minutes after codeine; morphine levels ranged from 1.9 to 20.5 µg/L. Infant plasma samples one to four hours after feeding had codeine levels ranging from <0.8 to 4.5 µg/L; morphine ranged from <0.5 to 2.2 µg/L. The authors suggest that moderate codeine use during breastfeeding (< or = four 60 mg doses) is probably safe.[3]

In a recent report, an infant death was reported following the use of codeine (initially two tablets every 12 h, reduced to half that dose from day 2 to 2 weeks because of maternal somnolence and constipation) in a mother.[4] Morphine levels in milk were reported to be 87 µg/L while the average reported milk levels in most mothers range from 1.9 to 20.5 µg/L at doses of 60 mg every 6 hours. Genotype analysis of this specific mother indicated that she was an ultra-rapid metabolizer of codeine. This genotype (which is very rare) leads to increased formation of morphine from codeine.

Ultimately, each infant's response to exposure to codeine should be independently determined. In the vast majority of mothers, codeine taken in moderation should be safe for their breastfed infant. However, any report of overt somnolence, apnea, poor feeding, grey skin, should be reported to the physician and could be associated with exposure to codeine.

A similar drug called dihydrocodeine has the following kinetics: Peak concentration: 1.2 to 1.8 hours, half-life: 3.5 to 5 hours and oral bioavailability: 20%. Observe baby for sedation and constipation.

Pregnancy Risk	C	Lactation Risk	L3
T ½	= 2.9 hours	M/P	= 1.3–2.5
Vd	= 3.5 l/kg	PB	= 7%
Tmax	= 0.5–1 hour	Oral	= Complete
MW	= 299	pKa	= 8.2

Adult Concerns: Sedation, respiratory depression, constipation.

Pediatric Concerns: Several rare cases of neonatal apnea have been reported, but at higher doses. Codeine analgesics are so commonly used postpartum, that side effects are extremely rare and seldom reported. Observe for sedation, apnea in premature or weakened infants.

Drug Interactions: Cigarette smoking increases effect of codeine. Increased toxicity/sedation when used with CNS depressants, phenothiazines, tricyclic antidepressants, other opiates, guanabenz, monoamine oxidase inhibitors, neuromuscular blockers.

Relative Infant Dose: 8.1%

Adult Dose: 15–60 mg every 4–6 hours

Alternatives: Hydrocodone, oxycodone

References:
1. Davis JM, Bhutari VK. Neonatal apnea and maternal codeine use. Ped Res 1985; 19(4): 170A abstract.
2. Findlay JW, DeAngelis RL, Kearney MF, Welch RM, Findlay JM. Analgesic drugs in breast milk and plasma. Clin Pharmacol Ther 1981; 29(5): 625–633.
3. Meny RG, Naumburg EG, Alger LS, Brill-Miller JL, Brown S. Codeine and the breastfed neonate. J Hum Lact 1993 Dec; 9(4): 237–40.
4. Koren G, Cairns J, Chitayat D, Gaedigk A, Leeder SJ. Pharmacogenetics of morphine poisoning in a breastfed neonate of a codeine-prescribed mother. Lancet 2006 Aug 19; 368(9536): 704.

COENZYME Q10   L3

Trade: Ubiquinone, CoQ10, Ubidecarenone

Other Trades:

Category: Cofactor in electron transport chain

Coenzyme Q10, also known as ubiquinone and ubidecarenone, is a cofactor in the mitochondrial electron-transport chain in the synthesis of ATP within the cell. It may also possess antioxidant and membrane-stabilizing properties. Although it is a naturally occurring cofactor, it is generally synthesized within the cell. Those cells that have the highest metabolic activity such as the heart and the liver have the highest CoQ10 concentrations.

The clinical uses of ubiquinone are quite interesting and include congestive heart disease, hypertension, periodontal disease, obesity, immune deficiencies, and angina.[1] Ubiquinone is slowly absorbed requiring 5–10 hours to reach a peak. Following oral doses of 100 mg, peak blood levels of 1 µg/mL have been reported.[2] With doses of 300 mg/day, mean plasma levels were 5.4 µg/mL after 4 days. No data are available on ubiquinone levels in milk. However, ubiquinone is very lipid soluble and has a long plasma half-life; transfer to milk is likely. If one were to assume a milk/plasma ratio of 1.0 and a significant maternal dose of 300 mg/d, then the average daily intake via milk in an infant would be approximately 16% of the weight-adjusted maternal dose. Were these numbers correct, it is not likely that this dose would be overtly toxic to an infant. Although ubiquinone is relatively non-toxic in adults, there are no data on the relative toxicity of this substance in infants. Most references suggest that pregnant and lactating women should avoid supplementation with this cofactor.

Pregnancy Risk	Probably Safe	Lactation Risk	L3
T ½	= 34 hours	M/P	=
Vd	=	PB	=
Tmax	= 5–10 hours	Oral	= Complete
MW	= 863	pKa	=

Adult Concerns: Caution when using in patients with biliary obstruction. Caution when using with hypolipidemic agents, oral hypoglycemic agents, insulin, in patients with hepatic and renal insufficiency. Most common adverse effects include nausea, epigastric pain, diarrhea, heartburn, appetite suppression.

Pediatric Concerns: None reported but high dose supplementation should be avoided.

Drug Interactions: Do not use with oral hypoglycemics, hypolipidemic agents. May decrease INR in patients taking warfarin.

Relative Infant Dose:

Adult Dose:

Alternatives:

References:
1. Gaby AR. Coenzyme Q10, in Pizzorno JE. Churchill Livingstone(eds): Textbook of Natural Medicine. 1999.
2. Greenberg S, Frishman WH. Co-enzyme Q10: a new drug for cardiovascular disease. J Clin Pharmacol 1990; 30(7): 596–608.

COLCHICINE   L4

Trade: Colchicine, Colcrys

Other Trades: Colgout, Colchicine

Category: Analgesic in gouty arthritis

Colchicine is an old product primarily used to reduce pain associated with inflammatory gout. Although it reduces the pain, it is not a true analgesic but simply reduces the inflammation associated with uric acid crystals by inhibiting leukocyte and other cellular migration into the region. However, it is quite toxic, and routine blood counts should be done while under treatment. Blood dyscrasias, hepatomegaly, and bone marrow depression are all possible, particularly in infants. Although the plasma half-life is only 20 minutes, it deposits in blood leukocytes and many other tissues thereby extending the elimination half-life to over 60 hours.

Little or no consistent data on breastmilk levels are available. In one study published, even the authors questioned the percent recovery in the breastmilk, so the data must be considered questionable. Nevertheless, the milk concentration varied from 1.2 to 2.5 µg/L (16–19 days postpartum) in one patient receiving 0.6 mg of colchicine twice daily.[1]

In an older study of a mother taking 1 mg once daily, average milk concentrations were 30 µg/L in the 8 hours following maternal drug ingestion, leading to a maximum of 10% of the weight-adjusted maternal dose in the infant. The authors suggest that if a mother chooses to breastfeed, she should wait 8 hours post dose before feeding, or pumping.[2] The use of colchicine in breastfeeding mothers is probably not advisable, as we have many other analgesics and anti-inflammatories that are superior for the treatment of gouty symptoms.

Pregnancy Risk	C	Lactation Risk	L4
T ½	= 12–30 minutes	M/P	=
Vd	= 10–12 l/kg	PB	= 10–31%
Tmax	= 1–2 hours	Oral	= Complete
MW	= 399	pKa	= 1.7, 12.4

Adult Concerns: Nausea, vomiting, diarrhea, myopathy, leukopenia, bone marrow suppression.

Pediatric Concerns: None reported in one case reviewed. Caution recommended and other alternative analgesics.

Drug Interactions: Colchicine is a P-gp and CYP3A4 substrate. Life-threatening and fatal drug interactions have been reported in patients who were administered colchicine concurrently with P-gp and strong CYP3A4 inhibitors. Cyclosporine, amprenavir, aprepitant, diltiazem, erythromycin, fluconazole, fosamprenavir, grapefruit juice, verapamil, atazanavir, clarithromycin, indinavir, itraconazole, ketoconazole, nefazodone, nelfinavir, ritonavir, saquinavir, telithromycin may significantly increase levels of colchicine. Colchichine reduces vitamin B-12 absorption. Avoid alcohol.

Relative Infant Dose: 4.7%–31.5%

Adult Dose: 0.5–0.6 mg 1–4 times a week

Alternatives: Indomethacin

References:
1. Milunsky JM. Breast-feeding during colchicine therapy for familial Mediterranean fever. J Pediatr 1991; 119(1 (Pt 1)): 164.
2. Guillonneau M, Aigrain EJ, Galliot M, Binet M, Darbois Y. Colchicine is excreted at high concentrations in human breast milk. Eur J Obstet Gynaecol Reprod Biol 1995; 61: 177–178.

COLESEVELAM   L1

Trade: WelChol
Other Trades:
Category: Cholesterol lower agent

Colesevelam hydrochloride is a non-absorbed, polymeric, lipid-lowering agent that prevents the absorption of bile acids from the intestines.[1] As bile acids are the precursors for cholesterol production, hepatic cholesterol production is lowered. Colesevelam is almost totally unabsorbed from the gastrointestinal tract (only 0.05%) and is unlikely to enter milk at all (see cholestyramine). The only potential problem of using this product in breastfeeding mothers is the lowering of maternal plasma cholesterol levels, and the possible lowering of milk cholesterol levels. Milk cholesterol is particularly important in infant neurodevelopment.

Pregnancy Risk	B		Lactation Risk	L1
T ½	=		M/P	=
Vd	=		PB	=
Tmax	=		Oral	= None
MW	=		pKa	=

Adult Concerns: Constipation, dyspepsia and myalgia are the most commonly reported.

Pediatric Concerns: None reported via milk. It is totally unabsorbed so none would penetrate milk.

Drug Interactions: Apparently does not inhibit absorption of many drugs tested (as is seen with cholestyramine). May decrease absorption of verapamil.

Relative Infant Dose:

Adult Dose: 625 mg 3–6 times daily.

Alternatives: Cholestyramine

References:
1.   Pharmaceutical manufacturer prescribing information, 2010.

COLESTIPOL   L3

Trade: Colestid
Other Trades:
Category: Bile Acid Sequestrant

Colestipol is a bile acid sequestrant that is used to inhibit absorption of cholesterol by binding to bile acid complexes and promoting excretion.[1] As bile acids are the precursors for cholesterol production, hepatic cholesterol production is lowered. Colestipol is almost totally unabsorbed from the gastrointestinal tract and is unlikely to enter milk at all. Only problem is that it may lower milk cholesterol levels, which is important for the growth and neurodevelopment of the infant. Caution should be exercised when micronized colestipol hydrochloride tablets are administered to a nursing mother. Colestipol is known to interfere with the absorption of fat-soluble vitamins A, D, E and K. This may have an effect on nursing infants.

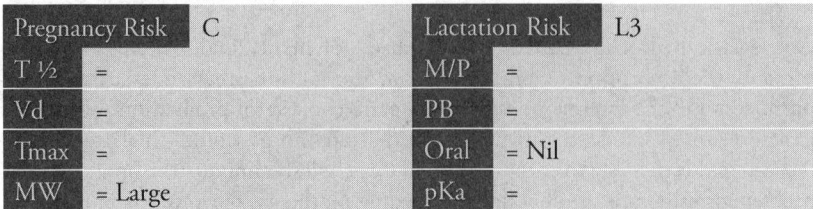

Pregnancy Risk	C	Lactation Risk	L3
T ½	=	M/P	=
Vd	=	PB	=
Tmax	=	Oral	= Nil
MW	= Large	pKa	=

Adult Concerns: Constipation, abdominal discomfort, intestinal gas, indigestion, diarrhea, bloating

Pediatric Concerns:

Drug Interactions: The absorption of tetracycline, furosemide, penicillin G, hydrochlorothiazide, and gemfibrozil was significantly decreased when given simultaneously with colestipol hydrochloride

Relative Infant Dose:

Adult Dose:

Alternatives:

References:
1. Pharmaceutical manufacturer prescribing information, 2009.

COMFREY   L5

Trade: Russian comfrey, Knitbone, Bruisewort, Blackwort, Slippery root
Other Trades:
Category: Herbal poultice

Comfrey has been claimed to heal gastric ulcers, hemorrhoids, and suppress bronchial congestion and inflammation.[1] The product contains allantoin, tannin, and a group of dangerous pyrrolizidine alkaloids. Ointments containing Comfrey have been found to be anti-inflammatory, probably due to the allantoin content. Some of the topically applied pyrrolizidine alkaloids are absorbed transcutaneously.

However, when administered orally to animals, most members of this family (Boraginaceae) have been noted to induce severe liver toxicity including elevated liver enzymes and liver tumors (hepatocellular adenomas).[2,3] Bladder tumors were noted at low concentrations. Russian Comfrey has been found to induce liver damage and pancreatic islet cell tumors.[4] A number of significant human toxicities have been reported including several deaths, all associated with the ingestion of Comfrey teas or yerba mate tea.[5] Even when applied to the skin, pyrrolizidine alkaloids were noted in the urine of rodents. Lactating rats excreted pyrrolizidine alkaloids into breastmilk.

Comfrey and members of this family are exceedingly dangerous and should not be used topically, ingested orally, or used in any form in breastfeeding or pregnant mothers.

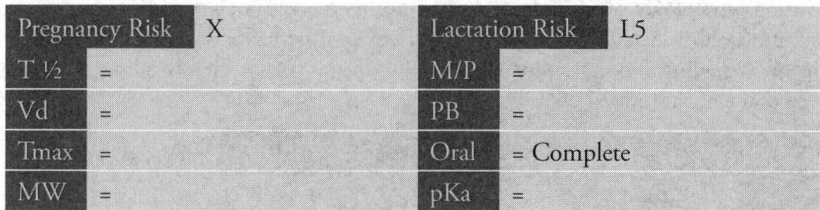

Pregnancy Risk	X		Lactation Risk	L5
T ½	=		M/P	=
Vd	=		PB	=
Tmax	=		Oral	= Complete
MW	=		pKa	=

Adult Concerns: Liver toxicity, hepatic carcinoma, hepatocellular adenomas, hepatonecrosis.

Pediatric Concerns: Passes into animal milk. Absorbed topically. Too dangerous for breastfeeding mothers and infants in any form.

Drug Interactions:

Relative Infant Dose:

Adult Dose:

Alternatives:

References:
1. Review of Natural Products Facts and Comparisons, St Louis, MO 1996.
2. Hirono I, Mori H, Haga M. Carcinogenic activity of Symphytum officinale. J Natl Cancer Inst 1978; 61(3): 865–869.
3. Yeong ML, Wakefield SJ, Ford HC. Hepatocyte membrane injury and bleb formation following low dose comfrey toxicity in rats. Int J Exp Pathol 1993; 74(2): 211–217.
4. Yeong ML, Clark SP, Waring JM, Wilson RD, Wakefield SJ. The effects of comfrey derived pyrrolizidine alkaloids on rat liver. Pathology 1991; 23(1): 35–38.
5. McGee J, Patrick RS, Wood CB, Blumgart LH. A case of veno-occlusive disease of the liver in Britain associated with herbal tea consumption. J Clin Pathol 1976; 29(9): 788–794.

CONJUGATED ESTROGENS   L3

Trade: Estratab, Premarin, Menext, Elestrin

Other Trades: Estrace, Estraderm, Delestrogen, Estinyl, Estring, Evorel

Category: Estrogen hormone

Conjugated estrogens consist primarily of estrone (>50%), equilin (15–25%) and equilenin. In this form the estrogen molecules are conjugated or attached to hydrophilic side groups such as sulfates. These are commonly found in the product, Premarin. Although small amounts may pass into breastmilk, the effects of estrogens on the infant appear minimal. Early postpartum use of estrogens may reduce volume of milk produced and the protein content, but it is variable and depends on dose and the individual.[1,2,3,4] Breastfeeding mothers should attempt to wait until lactation is firmly established (6–8 weeks) prior to use of estrogen-containing oral contraceptives. In one study of six lactating women who received 50 or 100 mg vaginal suppositories of estradiol, the plasma levels peaked at 3 hours.[5] These doses are extremely large and are not used clinically. In another study of 11 women, the mean concentration of estradiol in breastmilk was found to be 113 picograms/mL.[6] This is very close to that seen when the woman begins ovulating during lactation. If oral contraceptives are used during lactation, the transfer of estradiol to human milk will be low and will not exceed the transfer during physiologic conditions when the mother has resumed ovulation. However, suppression of lactation is still the major concern with the use of these products in breastfeeding mothers. If at all possible, do not use in breastfeeding mothers. See oral contraceptives.

Pregnancy Risk	X	Lactation Risk	L3
T ½	= 60 minutes	M/P	= 0.08
Vd	=	PB	= 98%
Tmax	= Rapid	Oral	= Complete, vaginal 77%
MW	= 272	pKa	= 19.38

Adult Concerns: Estrogen use has been associated with breast tenderness, increased risk of thromboembolic disorders, headache, nausea, vomiting, etc.

Pediatric Concerns: None reported. Infantile feminization is unlikely at normal dosages.

Drug Interactions: Rifampin reduces the serum levels of estrogen. Exogenous estrogens increase toxicity of hydrocortisone, and thromboembolic events with anticoagulants such as warfarin.

Relative Infant Dose:

Adult Dose: 10 mg TID

Alternatives: Norethindrone

References:
1. Booker DE, Pahl IR. Control of postpartum breast engorgement with oral contraceptives. Am J Obstet Gynecol 1967; 98(8): 1099–1101.
2. Kamal I, Hefnawi F, Ghoneim M, Abdallah M, Abdel RS. Clinical, biochemical, and experimental studies on lactation. V. Clinical effects of steroids on the initiation of lactation. Am J Obstet Gynecol 1970; 108(4): 655–658.
3. Kora SJ. Effect of oral contraceptives on lactation. Fertil Steril 1969; 20(3): 419–423.
4. Koetsawang S, Bhiraleus P, Chiemprajert T. Effects of oral contraceptives on lactation. Fertil Steril 1972; 23(1): 24–28.
5. Laukaran VH. The effects of contraceptive use on the initiation and duration of lactation. Int J Gynaecol Obstet 1987; 25 Suppl: 129–142.
6. Nilsson S, Nygren KG, Johansson ED. Transfer of estradiol to human milk. Am J Obstet Gynecol 1978; 132(6): 653–657.

CORTICOTROPIN   L3

Trade: ACT, Acthar, ACTH

Other Trades: Acthar

Category: Stimulates cortisol release

ACTH or adrenocorticotropic hormone is secreted by the anterior pituitary gland in the brain and stimulates the adrenal cortex to produce and secrete adrenocortical hormones (cortisol, hydrocortisone). Corticotropin is a sterile preparation of ACTH with pharmacological actions similar to that of endogenous ACTH.[1]

As a peptide product, ACTH is easily destroyed in the infants' gastrointestinal tract. None would be absorbed by the infant. ACTH stimulates the endogenous production of cortisol, which theoretically can transfer to the breastfed infant. However, the use of ACTH in breastfeeding mothers largely depends on the dose and duration of exposure and the risks to the infant. Brief exposures are probably not contraindicated.

Pregnancy Risk	C	Lactation Risk	L3
T ½	= 15 minutes	M/P	=
Vd	=	PB	=
Tmax	=	Oral	= Nil
MW	=	pKa	=

Adult Concerns: Hypersensitivity reactions, increased risk of infection, embryocidal effects, other symptoms of hypercorticalism.

Pediatric Concerns: None reported via milk.

Drug Interactions:

Relative Infant Dose:

Adult Dose: 80 U injection (IM or SC)

Alternatives:

References:
1. Pharmaceutical manufacturer prescribing information,2011.

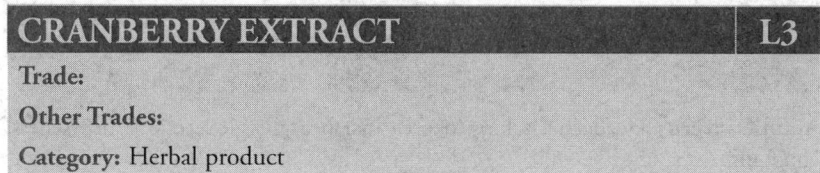

CRANBERRY EXTRACT   L3

Trade:
Other Trades:
Category: Herbal product

Purported use of cranberry extract are for urine deodorizer (urinary incontinent), prevention of urinary tract infections, and etc.[1] There are no adequate and well-controlled studies or case reports in breastfeeding women. See Phenazopyridine.

Pregnancy Risk	Probably Safe	Lactation Risk	L3
T ½	=	M/P	=
Vd	=	PB	=
Tmax	=	Oral	=
MW	=	pKa	=

Adult Concerns: Kidney stones.

Pediatric Concerns:

Drug Interactions:

Relative Infant Dose:

Adult Dose: 500 mL/day

Alternatives:

References:
1. Cranberry. In: Natural Medicines Comprehensive Database[Internet Database]. Stockton, CA: Therapeutic Research Faculty. Date last updated (2011, July 5).

CROMOLYN SODIUM   L1

Trade: Nasalcrom, Gastrocrom, Intal

Other Trades: Cromese, Opticrom, Rynacrom, Nalcrom, Rhynacrom, Vistacrom, Intal

Category: Antiasthmatic, antiallergic

Cromolyn sodium is an extremely safe drug that is used clinically as an antiasthmatic, antiallergic, and to suppress mast cell degranulation and allergic symptoms. No data on penetration into human breastmilk are available, but it has an extremely low pKa, and minimal levels would be expected.[1] Less than 0.001% of a dose is distributed into milk of the monkey. No harmful effects have been reported on breastfeeding infants. Less than 1% of this drug is absorbed from the maternal (and probably the infant's) gastrointestinal tract, so it is unlikely to produce untoward effects in nursing infants. This product is frequently used in pediatric patients and poses no risk for an infant when used in a breastfeeding mother.

Pregnancy Risk	B	Lactation Risk	L1
T ½	= 80–90 minutes	M/P	=
Vd	=	PB	=
Tmax	= <15 minutes	Oral	= <1%
MW	= 512	pKa	= Low

Adult Concerns: Headache, itching, nausea, diarrhea, allergic reactions, hoarseness, coughing.

Pediatric Concerns: None reported via milk. Probably quite safe.

Drug Interactions:

Relative Infant Dose:

Adult Dose: 20 mg QID via inhalation

Alternatives:

References:
1. Pharmaceutical manufacturer prescribing information, 2010.

CYCLIZINE   L3

Trade: Cyclivert

Other Trades:

Category: Antinausea

Cyclizine is an antihistamine commonly used to treat nausea and vomiting due to motion sickness.[1] There are no controlled studies in breastfeeding women, however, other studies of antihistamine medications suggest only low amounts were found in breastmilk (see diphenhydramine). This product has been used extensively in the treatment of nausea and vomiting of pregnancy without fetal complications.

Pregnancy Risk	B	Lactation Risk	L3
T ½	= 20 hours	M/P	=
Vd	=	PB	=
Tmax	=	Oral	=
MW	= 266	pKa	= 7.7

Adult Concerns: Dry mouth, drowsiness, headache, urinary retention, nausea.

Pediatric Concerns:

Drug Interactions:

Relative Infant Dose:

Adult Dose: 50 mg

Alternatives:

References:
1. Pharmaceutical manufacturer prescribing information, 2011.

CYCLOBENZAPRINE   L3

Trade: Flexeril, Cycoflex, Fexmid

Other Trades: Flexeril, Novo-Cycloprine

Category: Muscle relaxant, CNS depressant

Cyclobenzaprine is a centrally acting skeletal muscle relaxant that is structurally and pharmacologically similar to the tricyclic antidepressants. Cyclobenzaprine is used as an adjunct to rest and physical therapy for the relief of acute, painful musculoskeletal conditions.[1] Studies have not conclusively shown whether the skeletal muscle relaxation properties are due to the sedation or placebo effects. At least one study has found it no more effective than placebo. It is not known if cyclobenzaprine is secreted in milk, but one must assume that its secretion would be similar to the tricyclics (see amitriptyline, desipramine). There are no pediatric indications for this product.

Pregnancy Risk	B	Lactation Risk	L3
T ½	= 24–72 hours	M/P	=
Vd	= High l/kg	PB	= 93%
Tmax	= 3–8 hours	Oral	= Complete
MW	= 275	pKa	= 8.47

Adult Concerns: Drowsiness, dry mouth, dizziness, nausea, vomiting, unpleasant taste sensation. Tachycardia, hypotension, arrhythmias.

Pediatric Concerns: None reported, but caution is urged.

Drug Interactions: Do not use concurrently or within 14 days of cessation of monoamine oxidase inhibitors. Additive effect with tricyclic antidepressants. Enhances effect of alcohol, barbiturates, and other CNS depressants.

Relative Infant Dose:

Adult Dose: 20–60 mg daily.

Alternatives: Metaxalone

References:
1. Pharmaceutical manufacturer prescribing information, 2010.

CYCLOPENTOLATE   L3

Trade: AK-Pentolate, Cyclogyl, Cylate, Ocu-Pentolate, Pentolair
Other Trades: Ak-Pentolate, Diopentolate, Cyclogyl, Minims Cyclopentolate
Category: Anticholinergic for the induction of mydriasis

Cyclopentolate is used to dilate the pupils to facilitate refraction, eye examinations and other diagnostic purposes in the eye.[1] Cyclopentolate is commonly used by ophthalmologists and optometrists because it works rapidly, and briefer than atropine. It is a potent anticholinergic and some is absorbed systemically. Children and particularly infants would be extremely susceptible to this agent. Several cases of pediatric seizures[2] and one case of necrotizing enterocolitis[3], has been reported following the ophthalmic use of this agent in children and an infant respectively. While no data are available on the transfer of this agent into human milk, it is rather unlikely that significant quantities would enter as maternal plasma levels are so low, and milk levels would be even lower.

Plasma levels are approximately 3000 times lower than ophthalmic levels. Only 3–18% of muscarinic receptors were occupied after 55–124 minutes following administration. In healthy volunteers peak plasma concentration of cyclopentolate, 2.06 nM, occurred at 53 minute, maximum receptor occupancy being 5.9%.[4] After topical application plasma receptor occupancy was not high enough to cause any significant changes in heart rate and in P-Q interval time. None of the subjects experienced subjectively or objectively adverse effects to be attributed to cyclopentolate. In another study, peak plasma drug concentrations of about 3 ng/mL occurred within 30 min after all formulations.[5] The mean elimination half-life of cyclopentolate was 111 min when all subjects and formulations were considered together.

Some caution is recommended with this product. A waiting period of perhaps 6 hours following its use would be sufficient to reduce risks.

Pregnancy Risk	C	Lactation Risk	L3
T ½	= 111 minutes	M/P	=
Vd	=	PB	=
Tmax	= 25–75 minutes	Oral	=
MW	=	pKa	= 8.4

Adult Concerns: While systemic side effects are rare, children, especially infants, are more susceptible than adults. Systemic effects are consistent with other anticholinergics and include blurred vision, dry mouth, dry eye, urinary retention, seizures in infants and children, sedation, drowsiness, hyperpyrexia have all been reported.

Pediatric Concerns: None via milk, but caution is recommended. A brief interruption of breastfeeding is advised to reduce risk.

Drug Interactions: Additive with belladonna alkaloids and procainamide. May negate effects of cisapride on peristaltic contractions.

Relative Infant Dose:

Adult Dose: 1–2 drops in each eye.

Alternatives: Atropine

References:
1. Pharmaceutical manufacturer prescribing information, 2010.
2. Fitzgerald DA, Hanson RM, West C, Martin F, Brown J, Kilham HA. Seizuresassociated with 1% cyclopentolate eyedrops. J Paediatr Child Health. 1990Apr; 26(2): 106–7.
3. Bauer CR, Trottier MC, Stern L. Systemic cyclopentolate (Cyclogyl) toxicity inthe newborn infant. J Pediatr. 1973 Mar; 82(3): 501–5.
4. Haaga M, Kaila T, Salminen L, Ylitalo P. Systemic and ocular absorption andantagonist activity of topically applied cyclopentolate in man. PharmacolToxicol. 1998 Jan; 82(1): 19–22.
5. Lahdes K, Huupponen R, Kaila T, Monti D, Saettone MF, Salminen L. Plasmaconcentrations and ocular effects of cyclopentolate after ocular application ofthree formulations. Br J Clin Pharmacol. 1993 May; 35(5): 479–83.

CYCLOPHOSPHAMIDE   L5

Trade: Neosar, Cytoxan, Carloxan

Other Trades: Cycloblastin, Endoxan, Procytox, Endoxana

Category: anticancer drug

Cyclophosphamide is a powerful and toxic antineoplastic drug, used in many treatments, including breast cancer. The oral bioavailability of CP is 75% and reaches a peak at one to two hours. The elimination half-life (T½ beta) is 7.5 hours.[1] The active metabolites stay in the plasma compartment with brief half-lives of four hours or less. Transport of CP and its metabolites into the CNS is exceedingly low. This would suggest milk levels will be low as well when they are ultimately determined. The kinetics of this agent are highly variable depending on renal function, creatinine clearance, liver function, etc.

A number of reports in the literature indicate that cyclophosphamide can transfer into human milk as evidenced by the production of leukopenia and bone marrow suppression in at least 2 breastfed infants. In one case of a mother who received 800 mg/week of cyclophosphamide, the infant was significantly neutropenic following 6 weeks of exposure via breastmilk.[2] In another mother who was receiving 10 mg/kg intravenously daily for seven days for a total of 3.5 gm, major leukopenia was also reported in her breastfed infant.[3] Thus far, no reports have provided quantitative estimates of cyclophosphamide in milk. Withhold breastfeeding for a period of at least 72 hours.

Pregnancy Risk	D	Lactation Risk	L5
T ½	= 7.5 hours	M/P	=
Vd	= 0.7 l/kg	PB	= 13%
Tmax	= 2–3 hours	Oral	= 75%
MW	= 261	pKa	=

Adult Concerns: Leukopenia, infections, anemia, gastrointestinal distress, nausea, vomiting, diarrhea, hemorrhagic colitis.

Pediatric Concerns: Leukopenia and bone marrow suppression in at least 3 breastfed infants.

Drug Interactions: Cyclophosphamide may reduce digoxin serum levels. Increased bone marrow suppression when used with allopurinol, and cardiotoxicity when used with doxorubicin. May prolong effect of neuromuscular blocking agents. Chloramphenicol increases half-life of cyclophosphamide. Numerous others, see complete review.

Relative Infant Dose:

Adult Dose: 1–5 mg/kg daily.

Alternatives:

References:
1. Pharmaceutical manufacturer prescribing information, 2005.
2. Amato D, Niblett JS. Neutropenia from cyclophosphamide in breast milk. Med J Aust 1977; 1(11): 383–384.
3. Durodola JI. Administration of cyclophosphamide during late pregnancy and early lactation: a case report. J Natl Med Assoc 1979; 71(2): 165–166.

CYCLOSERINE   L3

Trade: Seromycin
Other Trades: Closina, Cycloserine
Category: Anti-tuberculosis drug

Cycloserine is an antibiotic primarily used for treating tuberculosis. It is also an effective against various *staphylococcal* infections. It is a small molecule with a structure similar to the amino acid, D-alanine and interferes with the bacterial cell wall synthesis. Following 250 mg oral dose given four times daily to mothers, milk levels ranged from 6 to 19 mg/L, an average of 13.4 mg/L.[1] This is approximately 2 mg/kg/day. The normal antitubercular dose in infants is 10–20 mg/kg/day. Levels of cycloserine in human milk are significant. Mothers should probably withhold breastfeeding for 24 hours.

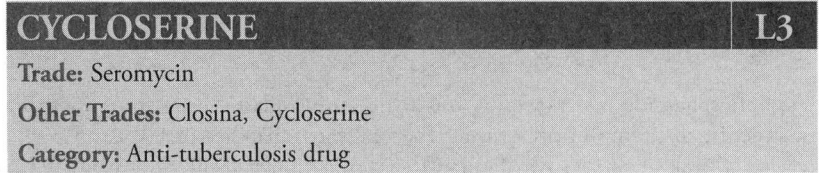

Pregnancy Risk	C	Lactation Risk	L3
T ½	= 12+ hours	M/P	= 0.72
Vd	=	PB	=
Tmax	= 3–4 hours	Oral	= 70–90%
MW	= 102	pKa	= 20

Adult Concerns: Drowsiness, CNS confusion, dizziness, headache, lethargy, depression, seizures. Precautions urged in epilepsy, depression, severe anxiety.

Pediatric Concerns: None reported.

Drug Interactions: Increased toxicity with alcohol, isoniazid. Phenytoin levels may be elevated due to inhibition of metabolism.

Relative Infant Dose: 14.1%

Adult Dose: 250 mg BID

Alternatives:

References:
1. Charles E, McKenna MH, Morton RF. Studies on the absorption, diffusion, and excretion of cycloserine. Antibiot Annu 1955; 3: 169–172.

CYCLOSPORINE   L3

Trade: Sandimmune, Neoral, Restasis
Other Trades: Neoral, Sandimmune
Category: Immunosuppressant

Cyclosporine is an immunosuppressant used to reduce organ rejection following transplant and in autoimmune syndromes such as arthritis, etc. In a recent report of 7 breastfeeding mothers treated with cyclosporine, the levels of cyclosporine in breastmilk ranged from 50 to 227 µg/L. Corresponding plasma levels in the breastfed infants were undetectable (<30 ng/mL) in all infants. In this study, the infants received less than 300 µg per day via breastmilk.[1] In another, following a dose of 320 mg/day, the milk level at 22 hours post dose was 16 µg/L and the milk/plasma ratio was 0.28.[2] In another report of a mother receiving 250 mg twice daily, the maternal plasma level of cyclosporine was measured at 187 µg/L, and the breastmilk level was 167 µg/L.[3] None was detected in the plasma of the infant. In a study of a breastfeeding transplant patient who received 300 mg twice daily, maternal serum levels were 193, 273, and 123 ng/mL at 23 days, 6.5 and 9.7 weeks postpartum.[4] Corresponding milk cyclosporine levels were 160, 286, and 79 µg/L respectively. Using the higher milk level, an infant would receive less than 0.4% of the weight-adjusted maternal dose. In another mother receiving cyclosporine (3 mg/kg/day), the concentration of cyclosporine in milk averaged 596 µg/L, or a dose of about <0.1 mg/kg to the infant.[5] The infant's trough blood level was always <3 µg/L while the mother's was 260 µg/L. No untoward effects were noted in the infant. In a more recent study of 5 patients receiving 5.3, 4.0, 5, 4.11, and 5 mg/kg/day cyclosporine respectively, the average concentration of cyclosporine in the mothers was 403 µg/L, 465 µg/L, 97.6 µg/L, 117.7 µg/L, and 84–144 µg/L (range) respectively.[6] Hind milk levels were much higher in one case, probably due to the high lipid content. In mother one, the cyclosporine blood levels in the infant were 131 µg/L and 117 µg/L on two occasions which were near a therapeutic trough. In none of the other infants, were blood levels of cyclosporine determinable (<25 µg/L). This study clearly suggests that some infants could potentially attain near-therapeutic levels from ingesting breastmilk. From this data the relative infant dose would be approximately 0.78% of the weight-normalized maternal dose.

These studies together suggest cyclosporine transfer to milk is generally low, but the latter study suggests that some infants may receive more than has been expected from the prior studies. Therefore cyclosporine use in breastfeeding mothers should be followed by close observation of the infant to probably include monitoring of the infants plasma levels.[7]

Pregnancy Risk	C	Lactation Risk	L3
T ½	= 6–27 hours	M/P	= 0.28–0.4
Vd	= 3.1–4.3 l/kg	PB	= 93%
Tmax	= 3.5 hours	Oral	= 28% pediatric
MW	=	pKa	= 9.3

Adult Concerns: Kidney toxicity, edema, tremor, seizures, elevated liver enzymes, hypertension, hirsutism. Use during pregnancy does not pose a major risk. Infections and possible lymphomas may result.

Pediatric Concerns: In 14 reported cases, milk levels were low and infant plasma levels low to undetectable. However one case of near-clinical levels in an infant have been reported.

Drug Interactions: Rifampin, phenytoin, phenobarbital decrease plasma concentrations of cyclosporine. Ketoconazole, fluconazole, and itraconazole increase plasma concentrations of cyclosporine. Do not use with St. John's wort or statin drugs.

Relative Infant Dose: 0.4%–3%

Adult Dose: 5–15 mg/kg daily, but highly variable

Alternatives:

References:
1. Nyberg G, Haljamae U, Frisenette-Fich C, Wennergren M, Kjellmer I. Breast-feeding during treatment with cyclosporine. Transplantation 1998; 65(2): 253–255.
2. Flechner SM, Katz AR, Rogers AJ, Van Buren C, Kahan BD. The presence of cyclosporine in body tissues and fluids during pregnancy. Am J Kidney Dis 1985; 5(1): 60–63.
3. K. D. T. Personal communication. 1997.
4. Munoz-Flores-Thiagarajan KD, Easterling T, Davis C, Bond EF. Breast-feeding by a cyclosporine-treated mother. Obstet Gynecol 2001; 97(5 Pt 2): 816–818.
5. Thiru Y, Bateman DN, Coulthard MG. Successful breast feeding while mother was taking cyclosporin. BMJ 1997; 315(7106): 463.
6. Moretti ME, Sgro M, Johnson DW, Sauve RS, Woolgar MJ, Taddio A, Verjee Z, Giesbrecht E, Koren G, Ito S. Cyclosporine excretion into breast milk. Transplantation 2003; 75(12): 2144–2146.
7. American Academy of Pediatrics, Committee on Drugs. Transfer of drugs and other chemicals into human milk. Pediatrics 2001; 108(3): 776–89.

CYPROHEPTADINE   L3

Trade: Periactin

Other Trades: Periactin, PMS-Cyproheptadine

Category: Antihistamine

Cyproheptadine is a serotonin and histamine antagonist with anticholinergic and sedative effects. It has been used as an appetite stimulant in children and for rashes and pruritus (itching).[1] No data are available on its transfer to human milk. The adverse effect to watch out for is sedation. Switching to a non-sedating antihistamine (loratadine, cetirizine) may be a suitable alternative.

Pregnancy Risk	B	Lactation Risk	L3
T ½	= 16 hours	M/P	=
Vd	=	PB	= 99%
Tmax	=	Oral	=
MW	= 287	pKa	= 9.3

Adult Concerns: Sedation, nausea, vomiting, diarrhea, dizziness, blurred vision, constipation, dry mouth, throat, or nose, restlessness.

Pediatric Concerns: None reported. Observe for sedation.

Drug Interactions: Additive sedation when used with other antihistamines and CNS depressants. Increased toxicity (hallucinations) when used with monoamine oxidase inhibitors.

Relative Infant Dose:

Adult Dose: 4 mg TID-QID

Alternatives: Hydroxyzine, cetirizine, loratadine

References:
1. Pharmaceutical manufacturer prescribing information, 2003.

CYTARABINE   L5

Trade: Cytarabine, Alexan, Arabine, Cytosar-U, Tarabine PFS
Other Trades: Cytosar
Category: Anticancer drug

Cytosine arabinoside or Cytarabine is an antimetabolite and antineoplastic agent commonly used in the treatment of acute lymphoid leukemia in adults and children.[1] Cytarabine is rapidly metabolized by the liver and gastrointestinal mucosa, and it is not effective orally, less than 20% of the orally administered dose is absorbed from the gastrointestinal tract.

Following rapid intravenous injection of cytarabine, the disappearance from plasma is biphasic. There is an initial distributive phase with a half-life of about ten minutes, followed by a second elimination phase with a half-life of about one to three hours.[1] After the distributive phase, more than 80% of the drug can be accounted for by the inactive metabolite 1–β-D-arabinofuranosyluracil (ara-U). Cytarabine is essentially cleared from the body by conversion to ara-U. Within 24 hours about 80 percent of the administered drug is recovered in the urine, approximately 90 percent of which is excreted as ara-U. No data are available on its transfer to milk but levels would probably be quite low.

Withhold breastfeeding for at least 24–48 hours.

Pregnancy Risk	D		Lactation Risk	L5
T ½	= (beta) 1-3 hours		M/P	=
Vd	= 0.6 l/kg		PB	=
Tmax	=		Oral	= <20%
MW	= 243.2		pKa	=

Adult Concerns: Sores in mouth and on lips, joint pain, numbness or tingling in fingers, toes, or face, swelling of feet or lower legs, tiredness, anemia, bone marrow suppression, nausea, vomiting, diarrhea, gastrointestinal hemorrhage, elevated liver enzymes.

Pediatric Concerns:

Drug Interactions: Decreases effect of gentamicin, flucytosine, digoxin. Increases toxicity of alkylating agents, radiation, purine analogs, methotrexate.

Relative Infant Dose:

Adult Dose: 100 mg/m^2 IV daily.

Alternatives:

References:
1. Pharmaceutical manufacturer prescribing information, 2005.

CYTOMEGALOVIRUS INFECTIONS | L3

Trade: Human Cytomegalovirus, CMV

Other Trades:

Category: Viral infection

Cytomegalovirus (CMV) belongs to the family of herpes viruses and is a rather ubiquitous virus. Many infants have been exposed in utero and later in day care centers.[1] Maternal cervical infection is also very common. CMV is found in the breastmilk of virtually all CMV positive women using the newer PCR techniques.[2] The timing of maternal infection is important. If the mother seroconverts early in gestation, the infant is likely to be exposed in utero and develop antibodies to the virus. Symptoms include small for gestational age, jaundice, microcephaly, petechiae, hepatosplenomegaly, and hearing loss. If the mother seroconverts late in gestation, the infant is less likely to be severely affected. In seropositive mothers, the CMV found in breastmilk is not overtly dangerous, and these mothers can breastfeed successfully.[3]

However, if the mother seroconverts postpartum, there is a greater possibility (ranging from 5.7 to 69%) that the infant will be exposed and infected, however none of these infants demonstrated chronic long-term sequelae.[1,4] Most had only minor symptoms.

A recent review of the risks of CMV acquisition in premature infants suggests a new look at this problem.[5] Depending on the population, approximately 74% of mothers delivering premature infants are already CMV-seropositive. Of these infants, none had CMV isolated from their urine. From other studies, the relative risk of contracting CMV is about the same in infants fed milk from seropositive mothers (5.7%)[6] and those fed milk from seronegative mothers or formula ((0–11%).[7] This new data suggests that the relative risk of using milk from seropositive mothers, whether frozen or fresh, is low.

Pregnancy Risk	Possibly Hazardous	Lactation Risk	L3
T ½	=	M/P	=
Vd	=	PB	=
Tmax	=	Oral	=
MW	=	pKa	=

Adult Concerns: Asymptomatic to hepatosplenomegaly. Fever, mild hepatitis.

Pediatric Concerns: CMV transfer into breastmilk is known but apparently of low risk to infants born of CMV positive mothers. Despite high CMV seropositivity rate in mothers of premature infants, the incidence of postnatal transmission of CMV is apparently low.

Drug Interactions:

Relative Infant Dose: 0%

Adult Dose:

Alternatives:

References:
1. Dworsky M, Yow M, Stagno S, Pass RF, Alford C. Cytomegalovirus infection of breast milk and transmission in infancy. Pediatrics 1983; 72(3): 295–299.
2. Hotsubo T, Nagata N, Shimada M, Yoshida K, Fujinaga K, Chiba S. Detection of human cytomegalovirus DNA in breast milk by means of polymerase chain reaction. Microbiol Immunol 1994; 38(10): 809–811.
3. Lawrence RA. Breastfeeding: A guide for the medical profession. St. Louis: Mosby Publishers, 1994.
4. Miron D, Brosilow S, Felszer K, et al. Incidence and clinical manifestations of breast milk acquired Cytomegalovirus infection in low birth weight infants. J Perinatol 2005; 25: 299–303.
5. Schanler RJ. CMV acquisition in premature infants fed human milk: reason to worry? J Perinatol 2005 May; 25(5): 297–8.
6. Miron D, Brosilow S, Felszer K, Reich D, Halle D, Wachtel D, et al. Incidence and clinical manifestations of breast milk-acquired Cytomegalovirus infection in low birth weight infants. J Perinatol 2005 May; 25(5): 299–303.
7. Doctor S, Friedman S, Dunn MS, Asztalos EV, Wylie L, Mazzulli T, et al. Cytomegalovirus transmission to extremely low-birthweight infants through breast milk. Acta Paediatr 2005 Jan; 94(1): 53–8.

DABIGATRAN ETEXILATE   L3

Trade: Pradaxa
Other Trades:
Category: Direct Thrombin Inhibitor

Dabigatran is an inhibitor of platelet function and is used in the treatment of thromboembolic disorders. The drug is not metabolized by the cytochrome P450 system and has a low risk of bleeding. Food delays time to peak. Eighty-five percent of dabigatran is excreted in urine unchanged.[1] There were no studies on the transfer of dabigatran into breast milk found. The oral bioavailability is low at 6.5%;

therefore, minimal transfer into breast milk is expected. Observe for bleeding and bruising in the breastfed infant.[1]

Pregnancy Risk	C	Lactation Risk	L3
T ½	= 12–17 hours	M/P	=
Vd	= 50 to 70 L l/kg	PB	= Low
Tmax	= 0.5–2 hours	Oral	= 6.5%
MW	= 627.7	pKa	=

Adult Concerns: Bleeding, dyspepsia, gastrointestinal bleeding, anemia, elevated liver enzymes, wound secretion, gastroesophageal reflux.

Pediatric Concerns:

Drug Interactions: Avoid concomitant use with P-gp inducers such as rifampin which decreases plasma levels and efficacy of dabigatran. Do not use concomitantly with P-gp inhibitors such as verapamil, amiodarone, quinidine, and clarithromycin, which could cause increased plasma levels and dabigatran toxicity, leading to risk of major bleeding episodes. Exercise caution especially in those with compromised renal function and adjust dose accordingly.

Relative Infant Dose:

Adult Dose: 75 mg bid

Alternatives:

References:
1. Stangier J. Clinical pharmacokinetics and pharmacodynamics of the oral direct thrombin inhibitor dabigatran etexilate. Clin Pharmacokinet. 2008; 47(5): 285–95.

DACTINOMYCIN   L5

Trade: Cosmegen, Actinomycin D
Other Trades:
Category: Anticancer drug

Dactinomycin is one of the actinomycins, a group of antibiotics produced by various species of Streptomyces, and it is used to treat Wilm's tumor, Ewing's sarcoma, and many other malignancies. After single or multiple IV doses, dactinomycin is rapidly distributed into and extensively bound to body tissues. Results of a study with radioactive actinomycin D in patients with malignant melanoma indicate that dactinomycin is minimally metabolized, is concentrated in nucleated cells, and does not appreciably penetrate the blood brain barrier (<10%). Approximately 30% of the dose is recovered in urine and feces in one week.[1] The terminal plasma half-life for radioactivity was approximately 36 hours. Dactinomycin is concentrated in nucleated cells. Concentrations are highest in bone marrow and tumor cells relative to plasma. It has a molecular weight of 1255, which would probably reduce its entry into the milk compartment. No data are available on its transfer to human milk, but it is probably quite low. That withstanding, it is extremely cytotoxic. Mothers should abstain from breastfeeding for at least 10 days.

Pregnancy Risk	D	Lactation Risk	L5
T ½	= 36 hours	M/P	=
Vd	=	PB	=
Tmax	=	Oral	=
MW	= 1255.4	pKa	= 11.10

Adult Concerns: Black, tarry stools, blood in urine, cough or hoarseness, fever or chills, lower back or side pain, painful or difficult urination, pinpoint red spots on skin, unusual bleeding or bruising, diarrhea, difficulty in swallowing, heartburn, sores in mouth and on lips, stomach pain, unusual tiredness or weakness

Pediatric Concerns:

Drug Interactions: Do not administer live vaccines such as MMR vaccine, varicella vaccine, influenza live vaccine or rotavirus vaccine while patient is on concurrent dactinomycin therapy. Dactinomycin should not be administered concomitantly with radiation therapy or with regional perfusion therapy.

Relative Infant Dose:

Adult Dose: Do not exceed 15 µg/kg/day IV for five days per 2-week cycle.

Alternatives:

References:
1. Pharmaceutical manufacturer prescribing information, 2005.

DALFOPRISTIN + QUINUPRISTIN | L3

Trade: Synercid
Other Trades:
Category: Antimicrobial

Dalfopristin and Quinupristin is a drug combination indicated for complicated infections of the skin and subcutaneous tissues. It is a streptogramin antibacterial agent for intravenous use only. Mainly indicated for the treatment of vancomycin-resistant *enterococcus faecium* as well as for treatment of susceptible *Staphylococcus aureus*. It has some use against methicillin-resistant organisms. No data are available on its transfer to human milk. However, due to its acidity and large molecular weight, milk levels will probably be low.

Pregnancy Risk	B	Lactation Risk	L3
T ½	= Dalfopristin/quinupristin: 0.7 hours/0.85 hours (1.3–1.5 hours for the combination)	M/P	=
Vd	= Dalfopristin/quinupristin: 0.24/0.45 l/kg	PB	= Dalfopristin/quinupristin: 50–56%/23–32%
Tmax	=	Oral	= Dalfopristin/quinupristin: nil
MW	= Dalfopristin/quinupristin: 690.85/1022	pKa	=

Adult Concerns: This product is well-tolerated. Infusion site problems such as pain and erythema have been reported. Headache, gastrointestinal disturbances, and elevated liver enzymes reported. Arthralgia, myalgia have been reported.

Pediatric Concerns: None reported via milk.

Drug Interactions: Dalfopristin + qunupristin drug combination inhibits cytochrome P450 3A4. Thus numerous interactions with other drugs metabolized by this enzyme. A partial list includes: cyclosporin, midazolam, nifedipine, and terfenadine. Check numerous other drug interactions with alternate drug source.

Relative Infant Dose:

Adult Dose: 7.5 mg/kg every 8–12 hours

Alternatives:

References:
1. Pharmaceutical manufacturer prescribing information, 2002.

DALTEPARIN SODIUM   L2

Trade: Fragmin, Low Molecular Weight Heparin
Other Trades: Fragmin
Category: Anticoagulant

Dalteparin is a low molecular weight polysaccharide fragment of heparin (LMWH) used clinically as an anticoagulant. In a study of two patients who received 5000–10,000 IU of dalteparin, none was found in human milk.[1] In another study of 15 post-caesarian patients early postpartum (mean=5.7 days), blood and milk levels of dalteparin were determined 3–4 hours post-treatment.[2] Following subcutaneous doses of 2500 IU, maternal plasma levels averaged 0.074 to 0.308 IU/mL. Breastmilk levels of dalteparin ranged from <0.005 to 0.037 IU/mL of milk. The milk/plasma ratio ranged from 0.025 to 0.224. Using this data, an infant ingesting 150 mL/kg/day of milk, would ingest approximately 5.5 IU/kg/day. Due to the polysaccharide nature of this production, oral absorption is unlikely. Further, because this study was done early postpartum, it is possible that the levels in 'mature' milk would be lower. The authors suggest that "it appears highly unlikely that puerperal thromboprophylaxis with LMWH has any clinically relevant effect on the nursing infant".

Pregnancy Risk	B	Lactation Risk	L2
T ½	= 2.3 hours	M/P	= 0.025–0.224
Vd	= 0.06 l/kg	PB	=
Tmax	= 2–4 hours (SC)	Oral	= None
MW	= 4000	pKa	=

Adult Concerns: Anticoagulant effects in adults when administered subcutaneously.

Pediatric Concerns: Transfer to milk is low. Oral bioavailability is minimal. Side effects remote. No adverse effects were reported.

Drug Interactions: Increased risk of major bleeding episodes when used concurrently with oral anticoagulants, platelet inhibitors or thrombolytic agents.

Relative Infant Dose:

Adult Dose: 2500 units daily

Alternatives: Enoxaparin.

References:
1. Harenberg J, Leber G, Zimmermann R, Schmidt W.[Prevention of thromboembolism with low-molecular weight heparin in pregnancy]. Geburtshilfe Frauenheilkd 1987; 47(1): 15–18.
2. Richter C, Sitzmann J, Lang P, Weitzel H, Huch A, Huch R. Excretion of low molecular weight heparin in human milk. Br J Clin Pharmacol 2001; 52(6): 708–710.

DANAZOL   L5

Trade: Danocrine

Other Trades: Azol, Danocrine, Cyclomen, Danol

Category: Synthetic androgen, antigonadotropic agent

Danazol suppresses the pituitary-ovarian axis by inhibiting ovarian steroidogenesis resulting in decreased secretion of estradiol and may increase androgens.[1] Danazol is believed to reduce plasma prolactin levels in individuals. The mechanisms through which Danazol treatment affects prolactin release has not been fully delineated, but it is probably due to the hypo-estrogenic status resulting from the medication. Danazol is primarily used for treating endometriosis. Due to its effect on pituitary hormones and its androgenic effects, it may reduce the rate of breastmilk production although this has not been documented. No data on its transfer to human milk are available, however its use should be avoided in breastfeeding mothers.

Pregnancy Risk	X	Lactation Risk	L5
T ½	= 4.5 hours	M/P	=
Vd	=	PB	=
Tmax	= 2 hours	Oral	= Complete
MW	= 337	pKa	= 13.10

Adult Concerns: Breast size reduction, androgenic effects, hirsutism, acne, weight gain, edema, testicular atrophy, thrombocytopenia, thrombocytosis, hot flashes, breakthrough menstrual bleeding.

Pediatric Concerns: None reported, but caution is urged. May suppress prolactin production.

Drug Interactions: Decreased insulin requirements. May increase anticoagulation with warfarin therapy.

Relative Infant Dose:

Adult Dose: 50–200 mg BID

Alternatives:

References:
1. Pharmaceutical manufacturer prescribing information, 2010.

DANTROLENE   L4

Trade: Dantrium
Other Trades: Dantrium
Category: Skeletal muscle relaxant

Dantrolene produces a direct skeletal muscle relaxation and is indicated for spasticity resulting from upper motor neuron disorders such as multiple sclerosis, cerebral palsy, etc.[1] It is not indicated for rheumatic disorders or musculoskeletal trauma.

In one study, a mother received IV dantrolene (160 mg) for symptoms of malignant hyperthermia, after the umbilical cord was clamped just after the delivery of her baby.[2] Concentrations of dantrolene in breastmilk ranged from 1.2 mg/L on day 2 to 0.05 mg/L on day 4. The relative infant dose is calculated at 7.9% of the maternal dose. The highest concentration in breast milk was detected 36 hours after the first IV bolus of dantrolene. Based on the elimination half-life determined in this study (9.02 hours), the authors suggest that breastfeeding is safe 2 days after discontinuation of IV dantrolene administration in the mother. The infant should be monitored for nausea, vomiting, fatigue, and muscle weakness, which are all known side effects of therapeutic doses in adults.[2]

Pregnancy Risk	C		Lactation Risk	L4
T ½	= 8.7 hours		M/P	=
Vd	=		PB	=
Tmax	= 5 hours		Oral	= 35%
MW	= 314		pKa	= 14.89

Adult Concerns: Adverse effects are quite common and include weakness, dizziness, diarrhea, slurred speech, drooling, and nausea. Significant risk for hepatotoxicity. Visual and auditory hallucinations. Dantrolene should be used with caution in patients with impaired pulmonary function, particularly those with obstructive pulmonary disease, and in patients with severely impaired cardiac function due to myocardial disease. It should be used with caution in patients with a history of previous liver disease or dysfunction.

Pediatric Concerns: None reported, but caution is urged. A suitable waiting period for breastfeeding is recommended.

Drug Interactions: Increased toxicity with estrogens, CNS sedatives, MAO inhibitors, phenothiazines, calcium channel blockers, warfarin, and tolbutamide.

Relative Infant Dose: 7.9%

Adult Dose: 1–2 mg/kg TID-QID

Alternatives:

References:
1. Pharmaceutical manufacturer prescribing information, 2010.
2. Fricker RM, Hoerauf KH, Drewe J, Kress HG. Secretion of Dantrolene into Breast Milk after Acute Therapy of a Suspected Malignant Hyperthermia Crisis during Cesarean Section. Anesthesiology 1998; 89(4): 1023–1025.

DAPSONE   L4

Trade: Dapsone, Aczone
Other Trades: Maloprim, Avlosulfon
Category: Sulfone antibiotic

Dapsone is a sulfone antibiotic useful for treating leprosy, tuberculoid leprosy, dermatitis herpetiformis, and *Pneumocystis carinii* pneumonia. In one case report of a mother consuming 50 mg daily while breastfeeding, both the mother and infant had symptoms of hemolytic anemia.[1] Plasma levels of dapsone in mother and infant were 1622 ng/mL and 439 ng/mL respectively. Breastmilk levels were reported to be 1092 µg/L. In another study of 3 patients receiving 100 mg/day, milk levels averaged 580 µg/L, but these were not steady state levels.[2] The authors estimated the dose via milk was 4.6 to 14.3% of the maternal dose.

Dapsone gel 5% has just been released for the treatment of acne. After application twice daily for 14 days, the dapsone AUC 0–24 hours was 415 ng-h/mL for dapsone gel, 5%, whereas following a single 100 mg dose of oral dapsone the AUC was 52,641 ng-h/mL. Apparently the transcutaneous absorption of dapsone is minimal.

Dapsone is one of those drugs which apparently has all the proper kinetic parameters to enter milk, high lipophilicity, low molecular weight, high volume of distribution, high pKa, etc. While it is approved by the AAP, this is one exception that should be used very cautiously, if at all. Its topical use is probably of minimal risk to the infant.

Pregnancy Risk	C	Lactation Risk	L4
T ½	= 28 hours	M/P	=
Vd	= 1–2 l/kg	PB	= 70–90%
Tmax	= 4–8 hours	Oral	= 86–100%
MW	= 248	pKa	= 1.3

Adult Concerns: Adverse effects reported include hemolytic anemia (particularly in G6PD deficient persons), methemoglobinemia, aplastic anemia, psychotic episodes, peripheral neuropathy, acute renal failure, nephrotic syndrome, hepatotoxicity, exfoliative dermatitis, erythema multiforme, toxic epidermal necrolysis, and hypersensitivity reactions

Pediatric Concerns: Hemolytic anemia in one breastfeeding patient. Caution is recommended.

Drug Interactions: Increased dapsone levels when taken with amprenavir, trimethoprim, delavirdine, and probenecid. Dapsone may increase chloramphenicol plasma levels. Rifampin may decrease plasma levels of dapsone. Concomitant administration of zidovudine with drugs like dapsone which are cytotoxic or suppress bone marrow function may increase the risk of hematologic toxicity

Relative Infant Dose: 6.3%–22.5%

Adult Dose: 100 mg daily

Alternatives:

References:
1. Sanders SW, Zone JJ, Foltz RL, Tolman KG, Rollins DE. Hemolytic anemia induced by dapsone transmitted through breast milk. Ann Intern Med 1982; 96(4): 465–466.
2. Edstein MD, Veenendaal JR, Newman K, Hyslop R. Excretion of chloroquine, dapsone and pyrimethamine in human milk. Br J Clin Pharmacol 1986; 22(6): 733–735.

DAPTOMYCIN   L1

Trade: Cubicin

Other Trades:

Category: Antibiotic for resistant *Staphylococcus* infections.

Daptomycin is used intravenously for the treatment of complicated skin infections caused by susceptible strains of *Staphylococcus aureus* (including methicillin-resistant or MRSA strains), *Streptococcus pyogenes*, *Streptococcus agalactiae*, *Streptococcus dysgalactiae*, *Equisimilis*, and *Enterococcus faecalis*.[1]

In a mother 5 months postpartum who received 500 mg IV daily (6.7 mg/kg/day), the highest concentration measured in milk was 44.7 ng/mL at 8 hours following administration.[2] Reported levels in milk were 33.5, 44.7, 40.8, 39.3, and 29.2 ng/mL at 4, 8, 12, 16, and 20 hours respectively. The mother and infant received therapy for 4 weeks, and no adverse events were noted in the mother or infant. In addition, the daptomycin present in milk is poorly absorbed orally.

Pregnancy Risk	B	Lactation Risk	L1
T ½	= 9 hours	M/P	= 0.0012
Vd	= 0.9 l/kg	PB	= 92%
Tmax	= 0.5 hours	Oral	= Unlikely
MW	= 1620	pKa	= 5.3

Adult Concerns: Elevations of creatinine kinase have been reported suggesting skeletal muscle toxicity and blood tests are required weekly during treatment. Gastrointestinal disorders, injection site reactions, fever, headache, insomnia, dizziness, and rash have been infrequently reported.

Pediatric Concerns: None reported via milk in one case exposed for 4 weeks.

Drug Interactions: When used with tobramycin, a small increase (12.7%) in plasma concentration of daptomycin was produced.

Relative Infant Dose: 0.1%

Adult Dose: 4 mg/kg infusions once every 24 hours for 7–14 days.

Alternatives: Nafcillin

References:
1. Pharmaceutical manufacturer prescribing information, 2003.
2. Buitrago MI, Crompton JA, Bertolami S, North DS, Nathan RA. Extremely low excretion of daptomycin into breast milk of a nursing mother with methicillin-resistant *Staphylococcus aureus* pelvic inflammatory disease. Pharmacotherapy. 2009 Mar; 29(3): 347–51.

DARBEPOETIN ALFA   L3

Trade: Aranesp
Other Trades: Aranesp
Category: Colony stimulating factor

Darbepoetin alfa is used to treat anemia in patients with chronic renal failure, and patients receiving chemotherapy. It stimulates erythropoiesis much the same way as endogenous erythropoietin. Administration can be either IV or subcutaneous, with peak serum levels following subcutaneous dosing occurring after 34 hours.[1] No data are available concerning levels in breast milk. However, this is a large molecular weight protein that is unlikely to enter the milk compartment, or be orally bioavailable to an infant.

Pregnancy Risk	C	Lactation Risk	L3
T ½	= 21 hours	M/P	=
Vd	= 0.06 l/kg	PB	=
Tmax	=	Oral	= Nil
MW	= 37,000	pKa	=

Adult Concerns: Adverse effects include hypertension, hypotension, edema, fatigue, diarrhea, and infection.

Pediatric Concerns: No data are available. Because of its large molecular weight, it is unlikely that this protein will enter breast milk.

Drug Interactions: No data are available.

Relative Infant Dose:

Adult Dose: IV: 0.45 µg/kg once weekly; SQ: 2.25 µg/kg once weekly

Alternatives:

References:
1. Pharmaceutical manufacturer prescribing information, 2010.

DARIFENACIN   L3

Trade: Enablex
Other Trades:
Category: Anticholinergic agent used for overactive bladder

Darifenacin is an anticholinergic agent used for the treatment of overactive bladder with symptoms of urgent urinary incontinence, urgency, and frequency.[1] It is not known if darifenacin is transferred into human milk, although its chemistry would probably limit its transfer into milk. However, some caution is recommended as this is a strong anticholinergic muscarinic agent and could cause urinary retention, dry mouth, mydriasis, constipation, and other gastrointestinal symptoms in a breastfed infant.

Pregnancy Risk	C	Lactation Risk	L3
T ½	= 12.3 hours	M/P	=
Vd	= 2.3 l/kg	PB	= 98%
Tmax	= 6.5 hours	Oral	= 15–19%
MW	= 507	pKa	= 9.20

Adult Concerns: Observe for typical anticholinergic symptoms which include dry mouth, blurred vision, dry eyes, dyspepsia, abdominal pain, urinary tract infection, constipation, urinary retention, and heat prostration due to decreased sweating. Do not use in patients with narrow angle glaucoma.

Pediatric Concerns: None reported in infants. No data available. Use with some caution and observe for anticholinergic symptoms.

Drug Interactions: Darifenacin is primarily metabolized by CYP2D6 and CYP3A4. Use with great caution with drugs that affect these enzyme systems such as ketoconazole, itraconazole, fluconazole, ritonavir, nelfinavir, clarithromycin, nefazodone and many others. Check drug-drug interaction reference.

Relative Infant Dose:

Adult Dose: 7.5 mg daily

Alternatives:

References:
1. Pharmaceutical manufacturer prescribing information, 2010.

DAUNORUBICIN   L5

Trade: Cerubidin, Daunoblastina, Daunoblastin, DaunoXome, Cerubidine
Other Trades:
Category: Anticancer drug

This is a typical anthracycline agent used in many forms of cancer, including acute myelogenous, and lymphocytic leukemias, and others. As with doxorubicin, it is widely distributed to many body tissues. It is eliminated from the plasma compartment with a triphasic elimination curve. Its last elimination T½ (gamma) ranges from 11.2 to 47.4 hours, depending on the dose. It is rapidly metabolized to daunorubicinol which achieves a C_{max} at 24 hours.[1] Daunorubicinol has a half-life of approximately 20–37 hours. No data are available on the transfer of this anthracycline into human milk. However, a close congener, doxorubicin, has been measured in milk, and the levels are low, but prolonged. Withhold breastfeeding for a minimum of seven to ten days.

Pregnancy Risk	D	Lactation Risk	L5
T ½	= 18.5 hours, (daunorubicinol) 20–40 hours	M/P	=
Vd	= 1725 L/m^2	PB	= 97%
Tmax	=	Oral	=
MW	= 527	pKa	= 11.02

Adult Concerns: Cough or hoarseness, fever or chills, irregular heartbeat, lower back or side pain, pain at injection site, painful or difficult urination, shortness of breath, swelling of feet and lower legs.

Pediatric Concerns: None reported, but this agent is extremely toxic and breastfeeding should be withheld for a minimum of 7–10 days.

Drug Interactions: Do not use daunorubicin in patients who have previously received it due to increased risk of cardiotoxicity. Use of daunorubicin concurrently with cyclophosphamide also increases risk of cardiotoxicity. Caution while using concurrently with myelosuppression agents. Use with hepatotoxic agents like methotrexate increases risk of liver toxicity.

Relative Infant Dose:

Adult Dose: 45–100 mg/m^2/day IV

Alternatives:

References:
1. Pharmaceutical manufacturer prescribing information, 2008.

DEET | L3

Trade: DEET, 6–12 Plus, Off!, Deep Woods Off!, Cutter Insect Repellent, Muskol, Diethyl-m-Toluamide, Diethyltoluamide

Other Trades:

Category: Insect repellant

N,N-Diethyl-meta-toluamide (DEET) is used worldwide as an insect repellent. The U. S. EPA estimates that 30% of the U. S. population applies DEET every year. In use for more than 45 years, the reports of adverse effects in humans have been relatively rare, even though it has been used in billions of applications. Case reports of toxicity are invariably moderate to low, but some cases of death have been reported.

Skin absorption is significant and generally occurs within 2 hours of application. DEET is very lipophilic and has a large volume of distribution (2.7–6.21) and remains in the skin and adipose tissue for long periods, slowly leaking into the plasma compartment and being eliminated. Between 5 and 17% of an applied dose is absorbed in 6 hours, and most is eliminated from the plasma compartment within 4 hours via hepatic metabolism and excretion in urine.[1] Animal data suggests highest concentrations in the lacrimal gland, liver, kidney, and nasal mucosa

No data are available on the transfer of DEET into human milk, but due to its lipophilicity, some probably enters the milk compartment. Avoid the use of concentrated solutions (>25%) over large surface areas of the body if you are breastfeeding or pregnant. A brief waiting period of 4 hours or more may be useful in avoiding transfer of high levels into milk, but this is probably unnecessary under conditions of normal use. While there are numerous reports of DEET toxicity, most involve the use of concentrated solutions over large body areas, and repeated applications over many days.

The American Academy of Pediatrics recommends DEET concentrations of 10% or less for children and infants. Infants less than 2 months of age should not be exposed to this agent. Most commercial preparations for infants and children contain 5–7% DEET. DEET should be applied only to exposed skin. Avoid use on children's hands, so that the child does not ingest DEET directly. Mothers should avoid chronic use over large body areas, and should use lower concentrations.

Pregnancy Risk	Probably Safe	Lactation Risk	L3
T ½	= 2.5 hours	M/P	=
Vd	=	PB	=
Tmax	= 1–2 hours	Oral	= Complete; 9–56% cutaneous
MW	= 191	pKa	=

Adult Concerns: Dyspnea, disorientation, seizures, tremors, ataxia and incoordination, depression, hypersalivation, have been reported. DEET has not been found to be a human teratogen, or induce malignancies.

Pediatric Concerns: Avoid use of solutions containing more than 10% DEET in children and avoid application over large surface areas.

Drug Interactions: Avoid use with other emollients, skin lotions, or alcohol which could increase the transcutaneous absorption of DEET.

Relative Infant Dose:

Adult Dose:

Alternatives:

References:
1. Robbins PJ, Cherniack MB. 1986. Review of the biodistribution and toxicity of the insect repellent N,N-diethyl-m-toluamide (DEET). J Toxicol Environ Health 18: 502–525.
2. Selim S, Hartnagel R EJR, Osimitz TG, Gabriel KL, Schoenig GP. 1995. Absorption, metabolism, and excretion of N,N-diethyl-m-toluamide: Following dermal application to human volunteers. Fundam Appl Toxicol 25 (1): 95–100.

DEFERASIROX   L3

Trade: Exjade
Other Trades:
Category: Iron chelating agent

Deferasirox is an orally bioavailable chelating agent that is selective for iron. It forms a complex with the iron that is unabsorbed and subsequently excreted in the feces. While deferasirox has a very low affinity for other metals such as zinc and copper, it still decreases serum concentrations of these metals. It is used in chronic iron overload due to blood transfusions.[1] No data are available on the concentrations in the breast milk compartment, however it is unlikely that high concentrations would be in breast milk due to high protein binding. Should the mother breastfeed, the infant's ferritin and iron levels should be monitored. Modest oral iron supplementation in the infant would block absorption of any deferasirox.

Pregnancy Risk	B	Lactation Risk	L3
T ½	= 8–16 hours	M/P	=
Vd	= 14.4 l/kg	PB	= 99%
Tmax	= 2–4 hours	Oral	= 70%
MW	= 373	pKa	= 8.41

Adult Concerns: Adverse reactions include diarrhea, vomiting, nausea, headache, abdominal pain, pyrexia, and cough.

Pediatric Concerns: No data available in infants. May test infant ferritin and iron levels and supplement with iron drops if necessary.

Drug Interactions: Deferasirox should not be taken with aluminum-containing antacids or with other iron chelator therapies.

Relative Infant Dose:

Adult Dose: 20 mg/kg daily

Alternatives: Deferoxamine

References:
1. Pharmaceutical manufacturer prescribing information, 2010.

DEFEROXAMINE   L3

Trade: Desferal, Desferrioxamine
Other Trades: Desferal
Category: Iron chelator

Deferoxamine is an iron-chelating agent, commonly used to facilitate the increased clearance of iron from the plasma compartment. It is indicated for the treatment of acute iron intoxication and of chronic iron overload due to transfusion-dependent anemias.[1] No data are available on its transfer into human milk, but levels in milk are likely low. Further, oral bioavailability of this product is virtually nil and it is not likely to harm a breastfeeding infant.

Pregnancy Risk	C	Lactation Risk	L3
T ½	= 3–6 hours	M/P	=
Vd	= 1.33 l/kg	PB	=
Tmax	=	Oral	= Nil
MW	= 656	pKa	= 8.39

Adult Concerns: Adverse events include flushing, pain at injection site, erythema, urticaria, hypotension and shock. Other side effects which occur with chronic administration include allergy-type reactions, pruritus, rash, anaphylactoid reactions, ocular and otic effects, abdominal discomfort, leg cramps, etc. Ocular disturbances include blurring of vision, cataracts after prolonged administration in chronic iron overload, decreased visual acuity including visual loss, visual defects, scotoma, impaired peripheral, color, and night vision, optic neuritis, cataracts, corneal opacities, and retinal pigmentary abnormalities. The auditory abnormalities reported have been tinnitus and hearing loss including high frequency sensorineural hearing loss. In most cases, both ocular and auditory disturbances were reversible upon immediate cessation of treatment

Pediatric Concerns: None reported via milk but no studies are available. Oral bioavailability is low to nil so it is not likely to be hazardous. However, observe for iron deficiency anemia.

Drug Interactions: Temporary loss of consciousness has been reported when used with prochlorperazine. Vitamin C is commonly added to deferoxamine therapy to enhance availability of iron for absorption.

Relative Infant Dose:

Adult Dose: 1 gm followed by 500 mg every 4 hours times two. Highly variable.

Alternatives:

References:
1. Pharmaceutical manufacturer prescribing information, 2010.

DEHYDROEPIANDROSTERONE (DHEA)   L5

Trade: DHEA

Other Trades:

Category: Dietary supplement

Dehydroepiandrosterone (DHEA) is a metabolic precursor to testosterone and estrogen. The use of DHEA-S for labor induction has been associated with a decrease in milk production postpartum with no changes in prolactin levels [1]. This may be due to the biotransformation of DHEA-S to estrogens. The use of DHEA during lactation is not recommended due to possible androgen effects.

Pregnancy Risk	Possibly Hazardous	Lactation Risk	L5
T½	=	M/P	=
Vd	=	PB	=
Tmax	=	Oral	=
MW	= 288.4	pKa	= 19.96

Adult Concerns: Acne, hirsutism, decreased HDL, insomnia, headache, irregular menses.

Pediatric Concerns:

Drug Interactions:

Relative Infant Dose:

Adult Dose:

Alternatives:

References:
1. Aisaka K, Ando S, Kokubo K, Sasaki S, Yoshida K. Comprehensive approach to the clinical study of the administration of dehydroepiandrosterone-sulfate (DHA-S) during the induction of labor]. Nippon Sanka Fujinka Gakkai Zasshi 1986; 38: 1605–12. English abstract.

DELAVIRDINE   L5

Trade: Rescriptor

Other Trades:

Category: Antiretroviral agent used in HIV infections. Antiretroviral drug

Delavirdine is an antiretroviral agent that is commonly used in the treatment of human immunodeficiency virus (HIV). There are no adequate and well-controlled studies or case reports in breastfeeding women. Breastfeeding is not recommended in mothers who have HIV.[1,2]

Pregnancy Risk	C	Lactation Risk	L5
T ½	= 2–11 hours	M/P	=
Vd	=	PB	= 98–99%
Tmax	= 1 hour	Oral	= 60–100%
MW	=	pKa	= 12.41

Adult Concerns: Fever, headache, nausea, vomiting, diarrhea, rash, symptoms of depression, elevated liver enzymes, anxiety, bronchitis, abdominal pain, increased prothrombin time, Steven-Johnson syndrome, acute renal failure.

Pediatric Concerns:

Drug Interactions: Concomitant use of the following drugs is contra-indicated: Astemizole, terfenadine, ergot derivatives, cisapride, pimozide, alprazolam, midazolam, triazolam. Concomitant use with the following drugs decreases plasma levels and efficacy of delavirdine: Phenytoin, phenobarbital, carbamazepine, rifabutin, rifampin, St. John's wort, nelfinavir, antacids, corticosteroids. Delavirdine causes toxicity of the following co-administered drugs: Statins, amprenavir, indinavir, ritonavir, lopinavir, saquinavir, amphetamines, trazodone, antiarrhythmics, warfarin, clarithromycin, calcium channel blockers, sildenafil, immunosuppressants, fluticasone, methadone, ethinyl estradiol.

Relative Infant Dose:

Adult Dose: 400 mg three times daily.

Alternatives:

References:
1. World Health Organization: Global Programme on AIDS. Consensus statement from the WHO/UNICEF consultation on HIV transmission and breast-feeding. Geneva: WHO, 1992.
2. Latham MC, Greiner T: Breastfeeding versus formula feeding in HIV infection. Lancet 352: 737, 1998

DENOSUMAB   L4

Trade: Prolia, Xgeva
Other Trades:
Category: Monoclonal antibody.

Denosumab is a monoclonal antibody used in the treatment of postmenopausal osteoporosis and to prevent osteopenia in those on breast cancer and prostate cancer therapy. Also used to prevent bone metastasis. Denosumab is an IgG2 monoclonal antibody which inhibits the human RANKL (receptor activator of nuclear factor kappa-B ligand), thereby interfering with the action of the bone-resorbing osteoclasts.[1]

Pregnancy studies done in mice have shown that the removal of the gene for RANKL, and subsequent absence of RANKL in pregnant mice resulted in impaired mammary gland development and absence of postpartum milk production. There are currently no studies available on the transfer of denosumab into human breastmilk. The manufacturer advises against its use in nursing mothers. Due to its high molecular weight, transfer is unlikely, or if any transfer does occur, oral absorption in the infant's gut is not probable. However, this assumption is only theoretical, and currently there are no established data to confirm this. Until, more is known about this drug and its transfer into human milk, the use of this drug in lactating women is justified only if the potential benefits to the mother outweigh the potential risks to the infant.

Pregnancy Risk	C	Lactation Risk	L4
T ½	= 25.4–28 days	M/P	=
Vd	=	PB	=
Tmax	= 10 days	Oral	= 62% (subcutaneous)
MW	= 147,000	pKa	=

Adult Concerns: Hypercholesterolemia, nausea, vomiting, arthralgia, cystitis, upper respiratory tract infections. Serious but rare side effects include rash, pancreatitis, hypocalcemia, hypophosphatemia, dyspnea, aseptic necrosis of jaw bone. Contra-indicated in hypocalcemia.

Pediatric Concerns:

Drug Interactions:

Relative Infant Dose:

Adult Dose: 60 mg every 6 months, subcutaneous.

Alternatives:

References:
1. Pharmaceutical manufacturer prescribing information, 2011.

DESIPRAMINE   L2

Trade: Pertofrane, Norpramin
Other Trades: Pertofran, Norpramin, Pertofrane, Novo-Desipramine
Category: Tricyclic antidepressant

Desipramine is a prototypal tricyclic antidepressant. In one case report, a mother taking 200 mg of desipramine at bedtime had milk/plasma ratios of 0.4 to 0.9 with milk levels ranging between 17–35 µg/L.[1] Desipramine was not found in the infant's blood although these levels are probably too low to measure.

In another study of a mother consuming 300 mg of desipramine daily, the milk levels were 30% higher than the maternal serum.[2] The milk concentrations of desipramine were reported to be 316 to 328 µg/L with peak concentrations occurring at 4 hours post-dose. Assuming an average milk concentration of 280 µg/L an infant would receive approximately 42 µg/kg/day. No untoward effects have been reported.

Pregnancy Risk	C	Lactation Risk	L2
T ½	= 7–60 hours	M/P	= 0.4–0.9
Vd	= 22–59 l/kg	PB	= 82%
Tmax	= 4–6 hours	Oral	= 90%
MW	= 266	pKa	= 9.5

Adult Concerns: Anticholinergic side effects, such as drying of secretions, dilated pupils, sedation, constipation, fatigue, peculiar taste.

Pediatric Concerns: None reported in several studies.

Drug Interactions: Do not use with monoamine oxidase inhibitors or within two weeks of therapy. Increased effects occur following use with stimulants, and benzodiazepines. Decreased effects occur with barbiturates, carbamazepine, and phenytoin use.

Relative Infant Dose: 0.3%–0.9%

Adult Dose: 100–200 mg daily.

Alternatives: Amoxapine, Imipramine, Sertraline

References:
1. Sovner R, Orsulak PJ. Excretion of imipramine and desipramine in human breast milk. Am J Psychiatry 1979; 136(4A): 451–452.
2. Stancer HC, Reed KL. Desipramine and 2-hydroxydesipramine in human breast milk and the nursing infant's serum. Am J Psychiatry 1986; 143(12): 1597–1600.

DESLORATADINE   L2

Trade: Clarinex
Other Trades: Clarinex
Category: Antihistamine

Desloratadine is the active metabolite of loratadine and its half-life is longer than the parent compound. While we do not have specific data on desloratadine, we do have a good report on the prodrug loratadine.

During 48 hours following administration of 'loratadine', the amount of loratadine transferred via milk was 4.2 µg, which was 0.01% of the administered dose.[1] Through 48 hours, only 6.0 µg of desloratadine (active metabolite)(7.5 µg loratadine equivalents) were excreted into breast milk, or 0.029% of the administered dose of loratadine or its active metabolite were transferred via milk to the infant. A 4 kg infant would receive only 0.46% of the loratadine dose received by the mother on a mg/kg basis (2.9 µg/kg/day). It is very unlikely this dose would present a hazard to infants. Desloratadine does not transfer into the CNS of adults, so it is unlikely to induce sedation even in infants. The half-life in neonates is not known although it is likely quite long. Pediatric formulations are available.

Pregnancy Risk	C	Lactation Risk	L2
T ½	= 27 hours	M/P	=
Vd	=	PB	= 87%
Tmax	= 3 hours	Oral	= Good
MW	= 310	pKa	= 4.2, 9.7

Adult Concerns: Sedation, dry mouth, fatigue, nausea, tachycardia, palpitations.

Pediatric Concerns: None reported via milk. Levels of loratadine have been reported and are low. No adverse effects have been reported in breastfeeding infants with loratadine or desloratadine.

Drug Interactions: Clarithromycin, erythromycin, and ketoconazole may increase plasma levels of desloratadine but they do not appear to be hazardous.

Relative Infant Dose: 0.03%

Adult Dose: 5 mg daily

Alternatives: Loratadine, cetirizine

References:
1. Pharmaceutical manufacturer prescribing information, 2010.

DESMOPRESSIN ACETATE   L2

Trade: DDAVP, Stimate
Other Trades: Minirin, DDAVP, Rhinyle, Desmospray
Category: Synthetic antidiuretic hormone.

Desmopressin acetate (DDAVP) is a small synthetic octapeptide antidiuretic hormone.[1] Desmopressin increases reabsorption of water by the collecting ducts in the kidneys resulting in decreased urinary flow (ADH effect). Generally used in patients who lack pituitary vasopressin, it is primarily used intranasally or intravenously. Unlike natural vasopressin, desmopressin has no effect on growth hormone, prolactin, or luteinizing hormone. Following intranasal administration, less than 10–20% is absorbed through the nasal mucosa. This peptide has been used in lactating women without effect on nursing infants.[2,3]

In a study of one breastfeeding mother receiving 10 µg twice daily of DDAVP (desmopressin), maternal plasma levels peaked at 40 minutes after the dose at approximately 7 ng/L, while milk levels were virtually unchanged at 1–1.5 ng/L.[4] Because DDAVP is easily destroyed in the gastrointestinal tract by trypsin, the oral absorption of these levels in milk would be nil.

Pregnancy Risk	B	Lactation Risk	L2
T ½	= 75.5 minutes	M/P	= 0.2
Vd	=	PB	=
Tmax	= 40 minutes	Oral	= 0.16%
MW	= 1069	pKa	= 4.8

Adult Concerns: Reduced urine production, edema, fluid retention.

Pediatric Concerns: None reported. It is probably not absorbed orally.

Drug Interactions: Lithium, demeclocycline may decrease ADH effect. Chlorpropamide, fludrocortisone may increase ADH effect.

Relative Infant Dose: 0.08%

Adult Dose: 10–40 µg intranasally daily.

Alternatives:

References:
1. Pharmaceutical manufacturer prescribing information, 2010.
2. Hime MC, Richardson JA. Diabetes insipidus and pregnancy. Case report, incidence and review of literature. Obstet Gynecol Surv 1978; 33(6): 375–379.
3. Hadi HA, Mashini IS, Devoe LD. Diabetes insipidus during pregnancy complicated by preeclampsia. A case report. J Reprod Med 1985; 30(3): 206–208.
4. Burrow GN, Wassenaar W, Robertson GL, Sehl H. DDAVP treatment of diabetes insipidus during pregnancy and the postpartum period. Acta Endocrinol (Copenh) 1981; 97(1): 23–25.

DESOGESTREL   L3

Trade:

Other Trades:

Category: Potent Progestin

Desogestrel is a potent progestin used in hormonal contraceptives. Progesterone is a naturally occurring steroid (progestin) that is secreted by the ovary, placenta, and adrenal gland. Oral administration is hampered by rapid and extensive intestinal and liver metabolism leading to poorly sustained serum concentrations and poor bioavailability.[1] As progesterone is virtually unabsorbed orally, the vaginal route has become the most established way to deliver natural progesterone because it is easily administered, avoids liver first-pass metabolism, and has no systemic side-effects. Absorption through the vagina produces higher uterine levels and is called the 'uterine first-pass effect'. A study by Levine[2] suggests the area under the curve is about 38 times less with oral administration as with progesterone vaginal gel. Thus fewer systemic effects are noted.

With the use of progesterone in breastfeeding mothers, two principles are of paramount interest. What effect does it have on milk production and the components of milk? Does it transfer into milk in high enough levels to affect the infant directly? In general, there is significant confusion in the literature as to the effect of progestins on milk composition, but the compositional changes do not appear major, volume is normal or higher, and some authors report minor changes in lipid and protein content.[3-5] However, the majority of the studies are with other progestins (e. g. medroxyprogesterone). Shaaban studied the effect of an intravaginal progesterone ring (10 mg/d) in 120 women and found no changes in growth and development of the infant or breastfeeding performance of the study participants.[6] The author suggests the ring adds a measure of safety because the amount of steroid present in milk would be effectively absorbed from the infant's gut. Another new study also suggests no impact on breastfeeding from the intravaginal progesterone ring.[7]

The effect of progestins on milk production is poorly studied. Early postpartum, while progestin receptors are still present in the breast, administering progestins may actually suppress milk production just as it does in the pregnant women. This has been seen occasionally in patients early postpartum. Several days to a week later, most progestin receptors disappear from the lactocyte and breast tissues become relatively immune to the effects of progestins. Thus it is advisable to wait as long as possible postpartum prior to instituting therapy with progesterone to avoid reducing the milk supply.

The direct effect of progesterone therapy on the nursing infant is generally unknown, but it is believed minimal to none as natural progesterone is poorly bioavailable to the infant via milk. Several cases of gynecomastia in infants have been reported but are extremely rare.

Pregnancy Risk	X	Lactation Risk	L3
T ½	= 13–18	M/P	=
Vd	=	PB	= 99%
Tmax	= 6 hours	Oral	= Low
MW	= 314	pKa	= 13.04

Adult Concerns: Bloating, cramps, pain, dizziness, headache, nausea, breast pain, constipation, diarrhea, nausea, somnolence, breast enlargement.

Pediatric Concerns: None reported, not bioavailable.

Drug Interactions:

Relative Infant Dose:

Adult Dose:

Alternatives:

References:

1. Levy T, Gurevitch S, Bar-Hava I, Ashkenazi J, Magazanik A, Homburg R, Orvieto R, Ben Rafael Z. Pharmacokinetics of natural progesterone administered in the form of a vaginal tablet. Hum Reprod 1999; 14(3): 606–610.
2. Naqvi HM, Baseer A. Milk composition changes--a simple and non-invasive method of detecting ovulation in lactating women. J Pak Med Assoc 2001; 51(3): 112–115.
3. Rodriguez-Palmero M, Koletzko B, Kunz C, Jensen R. Nutritional and biochemical properties of human milk: II. Lipids, micronutrients, and bioactive factors. Clin Perinatol 1999; 26(2): 335–359.
4. Costa TH, Dorea JG. Concentration of fat, protein, lactose and energy in milk of mothers using hormonal contraceptives. Ann Trop Paediatr 1992; 12(2): 203–209.
5. Sas M, Gellen JJ, Dusitsin N, Tunkeyoon M, Chalapati S, Crawford MA, Drury PJ, Lenihan T, Ayeni O, Pinol A. An investigation on the influence of steroidal contraceptives on milk lipid and fatty acids in Hungary and Thailand. WHO Special Programme of Research, Development and Research Training in Human Reproduction. Task Force on oral contraceptives. Contracep 1986; 33(2): 159–178.
6. Shaaban MM. Contraception with progestogens and progesterone during lactation. J Steroid Biochem Mol Biol 1991; 40(4–6): 705–710.
7. Massai R, Quinteros E, Reyes MV, Caviedes R, Zepeda A, Montero JC, et al. Extended use of a progesterone-releasing vaginal ring in nursing women: a phase II clinical trial. Contracep 2005 Nov; 72(5): 352–7.

DESOGESTREL + ETHINYL ESTRADIOL   L3

Trade: Mircette, Cyclessa, Ortho-Cept, Apri, Kariva, Desogen, Reclipsen, Velivet

Other Trades: Marvelon

Category: Low dose oral contraceptive

Desogestrel and Ethinyl Estradiol is a combination drug product indicated for use as a oral contraceptive. This is a combination of a lower-dose estrogen with a progestin. It contains a potent progestin desogestrel in combination with 10 or 20 micrograms/day of ethinyl estradiol (EE).[1] While most oral contraceptives contain 40 micrograms of EE or more, the reduced level estrogen in this product may be less inhibitory of milk production as is occasionally seen with the higher dose products. Small amounts of estrogens and progestins are known to pass into milk, but long-term follow-up of children whose mothers used combination hormonal contraceptives while breastfeeding has shown no deleterious effects on infants. Estrogen-containing contraceptives may interfere with milk production by decreasing the quantity and quality of milk production.

The effect of progestins on milk production is poorly studied. Early postpartum, while progestin receptors are still present in the breast, administering progestins may actually suppress milk production. This has been seen occasionally in patients early postpartum. Several days to a week later, most progestin receptors disappear from the lactocyte and breast tissues become relatively immune to the effects of progestins. Thus it is advisable to wait as long as possible postpartum prior to instituting therapy with progesterone to avoid reducing the milk supply. The direct effect of progesterone therapy on the nursing infant is generally unknown, but it is believed minimal to none as natural progesterone is poorly bioavailable to the infant via milk. Several cases of gynecomastia in infants have been reported but are extremely rare.[2-6]

Although small amounts may pass into breastmilk, the effects of estrogens on the infant appear minimal. In one study, ethinyl estradiol was not detected in breastmilk after administration of 50 µg/day.[6] After administration of 500 µg/day, amount in milk were measured around 300 pg/mL.[6] Early postpartum use of estrogens may reduce volume of milk produced and the protein content, but it is variable and depends on dose and the individual.[7-11] Breastfeeding mothers should attempt to wait until lactation is firmly established (6–8 weeks) prior to use of estrogen-containing oral contraceptives.

Oral contraceptives, particularly those containing estrogens, tend to decrease the volume of milk produced.[12] The earlier oral contraceptives are started, the greater the negative effect on lactation.[13,14] It is recommended that women wait at least 6–8 weeks postpartum to establish good milk flow, prior to beginning oral contraceptives.

Pregnancy Risk	X	Lactation Risk	L3
T ½	= Desogestrel/ethinyl estradiol: 22.3–51.9 hours/17.7–38.7 hours	M/P	=
Vd	=	PB	= Desogestrel/ethinyl estradiol: 99%/98.3%
Tmax	= Desogestrel/ethinyl estradiol: 1.1–1.6 hours/1.2–1.5 hours	Oral	= Desogestrel/ethinyl estradiol: 100%/92–98%
MW	=	pKa	=

Adult Concerns: Observe for reduced milk production. Breakthrough bleeding is more common with this product. Fluid retention has been reported. Other side-effects include chloasma, weight change, bloating, nausea, vomiting, migraine, depression, breast tenderness. Serious and rare side-effects include deep venous thrombosis, hypertension, liver disease, gall bladder disease.

Pediatric Concerns: Reduced milk supply is possible. Do not use early postpartum.

Drug Interactions: Reduced efficacy when used with rifampin, barbiturates, phenytoin, carbamazepine, griseofulvin, ampicillin, and tetracyclines.

Relative Infant Dose:

Adult Dose: One daily.

Alternatives: Norethindrone

References:
1. Pharmaceutical Manufacturer package insert, 2010.
2. Rodriguez-Palmero M, Koletzko B, Kunz C, Jensen R. Nutritional and biochemical properties of human milk: II. Lipids, micronutrients, and bioactive factors. Clin Perinatol 1999; 26(2): 335-359.

3. Costa TH, Dorea JG. Concentration of fat, protein, lactose and energy in milk of mothers using hormonal contraceptives. Ann Trop Paediatr 1992; 12(2): 203–209.
4. Sas M, Gellen JJ, Dusitsin N, Tunkeyoon M, Chalapati S, Crawford MA, Drury PJ, Lenihan T, Ayeni O, Pinol A. An investigation on the influence of steroidal contraceptives on milk lipid and fatty acids in Hungary and Thailand. WHO Special Programme of Research, Development and Research Training in Human Reproduction. Task Force on oral contraceptives. Contracep 1986; 33(2): 159–178.
5. Shaaban MM. Contraception with progestogens and progesterone during lactation. J Steroid Biochem Mol Biol 1991; 40(4–6): 705–710.
6. Massai R, Quinteros E, Reyes MV, Caviedes R, Zepeda A, Montero JC, et al. Extended use of a progesterone-releasing vaginal ring in nursing women: a phase II clinical trial. Contracep 2005 Nov; 72(5): 352–7.
7. Nilsson S, Nygren KG, Johansson ED. Ethinyl estradiol in human milk and plasma after oral administration. Contraception. 1978 Feb; 17(2): 131–9.
8. Booker DE, Pahl IR. Control of postpartum breast engorgement with oral contraceptives. Am J Obstet Gynecol 1967; 98(8): 1099–1101.
9. Kamal I, Hefnawi F, Ghoneim M, Abdallah M, Abdel RS. Clinical, biochemical, and experimental studies on lactation. V. Clinical effects of steroids on the initiation of lactation. Am J Obstet Gynecol 1970; 108(4): 655–658.
10. Kora SJ. Effect of oral contraceptives on lactation. Fertil Steril 1969; 20(3): 419–423.
11. Koetsawang S, Bhiraleus P, Chiemprajert T. Effects of oral contraceptives on lactation. Fertil Steril 1972; 23(1): 24–28.
12. Booker DE, Pahl IR. Control of postpartum breast engorgement with oral contraceptives. Am J Obstet Gynecol 1967; 98(8): 1099–1101.
13. Laukaran VH. The effects of contraceptive use on the initiation and duration of lactation. Int J Gynaecol Obstet 1987; 25 Suppl: 129–142.
14. Kora SJ. Effect of oral contraceptives on lactation. Fertil Steril 1969; 20(3): 419–423.

DESONIDE | L3

Trade: Desonate, DesOwen, LoKara, Verdeso

Other Trades: Desocort, PMS-Desonide

Category: Topical Corticosteroid

Corticosteroids when systemically absorbed is excreted in the breast milk. Absorption varies when applied topically depending on potency.[1] Low potency agents are generally preferred for infants due to high body surface area to weight ratio. No studies are available to show whether topical corticosteroids are distributed in detectable quantities in human milk. Systemic adverse effects may occur when applied on large areas of the body, used for prolonged periods of time, and used with occlusive dressings. Apply sparingly and caution should be used when breast feeding.[2,3]

In one case report, daily topical administration of a corticosteroid with a high mineralocorticoid activity to the mother's nipples since birth resulted in a prolonged QT interval, hypokalemia, hypertension, and decreased growth in the 2-month-old infant. Infant's blood pressure remained high for 6 months, but normalized after a year.[4]

Pregnancy Risk	C	Lactation Risk	L3
T ½	= Unknown	M/P	=
Vd	=	PB	=
Tmax	=	Oral	=
MW	= 416.5	pKa	= 14.91

Adult Concerns: Serious systemic reactions–Adreno-cortical suppression, cushing syndrome, hyperglycemia. Common side effects are allergic contact dermatitis, dry skin, pruritus, stinging of skin, and burning sensation

Pediatric Concerns: Adreno-cortical suppression, cushing's syndrome, and intracranial hypertension

Drug Interactions: May diminish effects of aldesleukin, corticorelin, and enhance toxic effects of deferasirox

Relative Infant Dose:

Adult Dose: 0.05%

Alternatives:

References:
1. Lexi-Comp OnlineTM Lexi-Drugs OnlineTM Hudson, Ohio: Lexi-Comp, Inc. ; 2007; May 26, 2011.
2. AHFS drug information 2007. McEvoy GK, ed. Desonide. Bethesda, MD: American Society of Health-Systems Pharmacists; 2007: 3529–30.
3. AHFS drug information 2007 McEvoy GK, ed. Topical corticosteroids general statement. Bethesda, MD: American Society of Health-System Pharmacists; 2005: 3423–5.
4. De Stefano B, Bongo IG, Borgna-Pignatti C et al. Factitious hypertension with mineralocorticoid excess in an infant. Helv Paediatr Acta. 1983; 38: 185–9

DESVENLAFAXINE   L3

Trade: Pristiq
Other Trades:
Category: Antidepressant, SSRI, SSNRI

Desvenlafaxine (O-desmethylvenlafaxine) is an active metabolite of venlafaxine with similar antidepressant activity. There is some data on the transmission of desvenlafaxine into human milk following the use of its precursor, venlafaxine.[1,2] In a study of 6 women receiving an average of 244 mg/day venlafaxine, the mean maximum concentration of desvenlafaxine in milk was 796 ng/mL. Desvenlafaxine was detected in the plasma of 4 of the infants ranging from 3 to 38 ng/mL.[1] All the infants were healthy and unaffected. The milk/plasma ratio for venlafaxine and desvenlafaxine were 2.5 and 2.7 respectively. In a group of 13 women who consumed from 37.5 to 300 mg/day (mean=194.3 mg/day) of venlafaxine, levels of desvenlafaxine in milk ranged from 318 to 1912.7 ng/mL with a mean of 919 ng/mL.[2] The relative infant dose for desvenlafaxine using the highest levels reported (C_{max}) ranged from 6.8% to 9.3%. A recent literature review revealed a few reports of milk levels following desvenlafaxine therapy; these are briefed below. The milk levels of desvanlafaxine were measured in a 35-year-old breastfeeding mother who had been on 250 mg desvenlafaxine daily for 2 months prior to the initiation of this study.[3] Assuming a milk ingestion of 0.15 /day, the absolute infant dose was found to be 294 µg/kg/day and the relative infant dose was calculated to be 7.8%. No untoward effects were noted or reported in the breastfed infant.

Yet another study by Ilett and Hackett, of the transfer of desvenlafaxine into human milk was done in 10 women who were being treated with 50–150 mg daily dose of desvenlafaxine for postpartum depression.[4] The mean relative infant dose in this study was calculated to be 6.8% (5.5–8.1%), with a mean milk/plasma ratio of

2.24. Interestingly, in this study, it was found that the peak concentrations (C_{max}) in milk occurred at 3.28 hours, which did not parallel with the C_{max} in maternal plasma which is 7.5 hours. This suggests that milk concentration kinetics do not always correlate with plasma concentration kinetics. The authors of this study suggest that the relative infant dose of desvenlafaxine remains almost the same, whether received from direct desvenlafaxine therapy or as an active metabolite of venlafaxine therapy; but desvenlafaxine therapy may be preferable since the absolute infant dose of total antidepressant activity following desvenlafaxine therapy only is 41–45% of that following venlafaxine therapy.

Therefore, desvenlafaxine does enter the milk in moderate amounts, however no side-effects have been reported following its lactational exposure. The total anti-depressant dose to the infant following desvenlafaxine therapy is only 41–45% of that following venlafaxine therapy, and may therefore be preferred over venlafaxine for the treatment of postpartum depression.

Pregnancy Risk	C	Lactation Risk	L3
T ½	= 11 hours	M/P	= 2.7
Vd	= 3.4 l/kg	PB	= 30%
Tmax	= 7.5 hours	Oral	= 80%
MW	= 263	pKa	= 14.46

Adult Concerns: While these are a function of dose, the following are common side effects of desvenlafaxine: nausea, suicidal ideation, palpitations, dry mouth, diarrhea, constipation, fatigue, anorexia, dizziness, somnolence, headache, anorgasmia, erectile dysfunction, and ejaculation disorder.

Pediatric Concerns: None reported.

Drug Interactions: Do not use with monoamine oxidase inhibitors.

Relative Infant Dose: 5.9%–9.3%

Adult Dose: 50–400 mg/day

Alternatives: Sertraline, paroxetine, venlafaxine, fluoxetine

References:
1. Ilett KF, Hackett LP, Dusci LJ, et al. Distribution and excretion of venlafaxine and O-desmethylvenlafaxine in human milk. British Journal of Clinical Pharmacology. 1998; 45(5): 459–462.
2. Newport DJ, Ritchie JC, Knight BT, Glover BA, Zach EB, Stowe ZN. Venlafaxine in human breast milk and nursing infant plasma: determination of exposure. J Clin Psychiatry. Sep 2009; 70(9): 1304–1310.
3. Ilett KF, Watt F, Hackett LP, Kohan R, Teoh S. Assessment of infant dose through milk in a lactating woman taking amisulpride and desvenlafaxine for treatment-resistant depression. Ther Drug Monit. 2010 Dec; 32(6): 704–7.
4. Rampono J, Teoh S, Hackett LP, Kohan R, Ilett KF. Estimation of desvenlafaxine transfer into milk and infant exposure during its use in lactating women with postnatal depression. Arch Womens Ment Health. 2011 Feb; 14(1): 49–53.

DEXAMETHASONE   L3

Trade: Decadron, AK-Dex, Maxidex

Other Trades: AK-Dex

Category: Corticosteroid anti-inflammatory

Dexamethasone is a long-acting corticosteroid, similar in effect to prednisone, although more potent. Dexamethasone 0.75 mg is equivalent to a 5 mg dose of prednisone.[1] While the elimination half-life is brief, only 3–6 hours in adults, its metabolic effects last for up to 72 hours. No data are available on the transfer of dexamethasone into human milk. It is likely similar to that of prednisone which is extremely low. Doses of prednisone as high as 120 mg fail to produce clinically relevant milk levels. This product is commonly used in pediatrics for treating immune syndromes such as arthritis and, particularly, acute onset asthma or other bronchoconstrictive diseases. It is not likely that the amount in milk would produce clinical effects unless used in high doses over prolonged periods.

Pregnancy Risk	C	Lactation Risk	L3
T ½	= 3.3 hours	M/P	=
Vd	= 2 l/kg	PB	=
Tmax	= 1–2 hours	Oral	= 78%
MW	= 392	pKa	= 13.48

Adult Concerns: In pediatrics: shortened stature, gastrointestinal bleeding, gastrointestinal ulceration, edema, osteoporosis, glaucoma, and other symptoms of hyperadrenalism.

Pediatric Concerns: None reported via milk. Avoid high doses over prolonged periods of time.

Drug Interactions: Barbiturates, phenytoin, rifampin may reduce the corticosteroid effect of dexamethasone. Dexamethasone may decrease effects of vaccines, salicylates, and toxoids.

Relative Infant Dose:

Adult Dose: 0.5–9 mg daily

Alternatives: Prednisone

References:
1. Pharmaceutical manufacturer prescribing information, 1999.

DEXBROMPHENIRAMINE   L3

Trade:

Other Trades:

Category: Antihistamine

Dexbrompheniramine is a first-generation antihistamine with anticholinergic properties. Due to the fact that dexbrompheniramine is well-absorbed and has a long half-life, it is likely secreted into human milk. One case report of a 3-month-old nursing infant suggests that it causes irritability, excessive crying, and difficulty sleeping; symptoms resolved after discontinuation of dexbrompheniramine 6 mg.[1] Since there are also anticholinergic effects, milk production may be impacted adversely. However, there have been no reports of decreased milk production in the literature.

Pregnancy Risk	B	Lactation Risk	L3
T ½	= 25 hours	M/P	=
Vd	=	PB	=
Tmax	= 5 hours	Oral	= Well absorbed
MW	=	pKa	= 3.59, 9.12

Adult Concerns: Maculopapular rash, dry mouth, drowsiness, dizziness, nervousness, insomnia

Pediatric Concerns: Irritability, excessive crying, disrupted sleep patterns

Drug Interactions: Alcohol, amphetamines, anticholinergics, antacids, monoamine oxidase inhibtors

Relative Infant Dose:

Adult Dose:

Alternatives:

References:
1. Mortimer, E. A., Jr. (1977). "Drug toxicity from breast milk?" Pediatrics 60(5): 780–781.

DEXCHLORPHENIRAMINE   L3

Trade: Polaramine
Other Trades:
Category: Antihistamine

Dexchlorpheniramine is structurally similar to chlorpheniramine but is the pharmacologically active dextrorotatory isomer of chlorpheniramine. Chlorpheniramine is a commonly used antihistamine in over-the-counter medications. Although no data are available on its secretion into breastmilk, it has not been reported to produce side effects. Sedation is the only likely side effect.[1] We suggest you use non-sedating antihistamines if at all possible. See alternatives.

Pregnancy Risk	B	Lactation Risk	L3
T ½	= 3–6 hours	M/P	=
Vd	=	PB	= 72%
Tmax	= 1 hour	Oral	= Complete
MW	=	pKa	= 9.2

Adult Concerns: Sedation, dry mouth.

Pediatric Concerns: No reported complications but we suggest you use non-sedating antihistamines if at all possible.

Drug Interactions: Avoid use with alcohol and other sedative products.

Relative Infant Dose:

Adult Dose:

Alternatives: Cetirizine, loratadine

References:
1. Paton DM, Webster DR. Clinical pharmacokinetics of H_1-receptor antagonists (the antihistamines). Clin Pharmacokinet 1985; 10(6): 477–497.

DEXLANSOPRAZOLE   L2

Trade: Kapidex, Dexilant

Other Trades:

Category: Suppresses gastric acid secretion

Dexlansoprazole is a proton pump inhibitor and is the active metabolite of lansoprazole. Due to poor stability at acid pH and short half-life, these products are encased in prolonged release formulations that open in the small intestine over a prolonged period of time. Structurally similar to omeprazole and lansoprazole, it is very unstable in stomach acid and to a large degree would be largely denatured by acidity of the infant's stomach.[1] A new study shows milk levels of omeprazole in milk are minimal (see omeprazole) and it is likely milk levels of dexlansoprazole are small as well. Although there are no studies of dexlansoprazole in breastfeeding mothers, transfer to milk and its oral absorption (via milk) is likely to be minimal in a breastfed infant.

Pregnancy Risk	B	Lactation Risk	L2
T ½	= 1–2 hours	M/P	=
Vd	=	PB	= 98.8%
Tmax	= 1–2 hours	Oral	= Poor
MW	= 369	pKa	= 17.30

Adult Concerns: Reduced stomach acidity, diarrhea, nausea, elevated liver enzymes.

Pediatric Concerns: None reported via milk. It is unlikely to be absorbed while dissolved in milk due to instability in acid.

Drug Interactions: Decreased absorption of ketoconazole, itraconazole, and other drugs dependent on acid for absorption. Theophylline clearance is increased slightly. Reduced lansoprazole absorption when used with sucralfate (30%).

Relative Infant Dose:

Adult Dose: 30–60 mg daily

Alternatives: Omeprazole, lansoprazole, famotidine, ranitidine

References:
1. Pharmaceutical manufacturer prescribing information, 2010.

DEXMETHYLPHENIDATE   L3

Trade: Focalin
Other Trades:
Category: CNS stimulant, treatment of ADHD

Dexmethylphenidate hydrochloride, the more pharmacologically active d-enantiomer of racemic methylphenidate, is a CNS stimulant that is used mainly in the treatment of ADHD. It is available in extended release formulations which would extend its biological half-life.[1] In a study of 3 women receiving an average of 52 (35–80) mg/day of methylphenidate, the average drug in milk was 19 (13–28) µg/L.[2] The milk/plasma ratio averaged 2.8 (2–3.6). The absolute infant dose averaged 2.9 (2–4.25) µg/kg/day. The average relative infant dose was 0.9% (0.7–1.1). In the one infant studied, plasma levels were <1 µg/L. These levels are probably too low to be clinically relevant. Another case reported a mother taking 15 mg/day with breast milk concentrations averaging 2.5 ng/mL. The daily infant dose was estimated at 0.38 µg/kg, which corresponds to 0.16% of the maternal dose.[3] No drug was detected in breast milk 20–21 hours after the maternal dose.

A mother taking 80 mg/day was determined to have a milk-to-plasma ratio of 2.7, giving an absolute infant dose of 2.3 µg/kg/day, or 0.2% of the maternal dose. Methylphenidate was not detected in the infant's plasma.[4] No adverse effects were noted in any of the infants.

While we do not have individual studies with dexmethylphenidate, one should assume they will be similar to the above studies with methylphenidate. These levels are significantly less than for dextroamphetamine. Infants should be observed for agitation, and reduced weight gain although these are quite unlikely at these levels.

Pregnancy Risk	C	Lactation Risk	L3
T ½	= 2–4.5 hours for immediate release	M/P	=
Vd	= 1.54–3.76 l/kg	PB	=
Tmax	= 1–1.5 hours for immediate release. 1.5 hour for first peak, 6.5 hours for second peak, for extended release.	Oral	= 22–25%
MW	= 270	pKa	= 8.9

Adult Concerns: Dizziness, headache, restlessness, anxiety, xerostomia.

Pediatric Concerns: None yet reported via milk, however, observe for excitation, poor feeding and appetite, insomnia.

Drug Interactions: MAO inhibitors, phenytoin, tricyclic antidepressants, anticoagulants. Dexmethylphenidate should not be used concurrently with monoamine oxidase inhibitors. Caution to be exercised when used concurrently with pressor agents and it may decrease efficacy of anti-hypertensives. Co-administration with antacids may alter its release and absorption. Concomitant therapy with dexmethylphenidate may increase plasma levels and cause subsequent toxicity of the following drugs: warfarin and other coumarin derivatives, phenobarbital, phenytoin, primidone, imipramine, clomipramine, desipramine.

Relative Infant Dose:

Adult Dose: 20–40 mg per day

Alternatives: Methylphenidate

References:
1. Pharmaceutical manufacturer prescribing information, 2010.
2. Hackett LP, Ilett KF, Kristensen JH, Kohan R, Hale TW. Infant dose and safety of breastfeeding for dexamphetamine and methylphenidate in mothers with attention deficit hyperactivity disorder. Proceedings of the 9th International Congress of Therapeutic Drug Monitoring and Clinical Toxicology, Louisville, USA, April 23–28, 2005, Therapeutic Drug Monitoring 2005; 27: 220. (Abstract # 40).
3. Spigset O, Brede WR, Zahlsen K. Excretion of methylphenidate in Breast Milk. Am J Psychiatry 2007; 164(2): 348.
4. Hackett LP, Kristensen JH, Hale TW, Paterson R, Ilett, KF. Methylphenidate and Breast-Feeding. Ann Pharmacother 2006; 40(10): 1890–1891.

DEXTROAMPHETAMINE | L3/L5

Trade: Dexedrine, Amphetamine, Oxydess, Adderall, Adderall XR, ProCentra, Dextrostat, Liquadd

Other Trades: Dexamphetamine, Dexten

Category: Powerful CNS stimulant

Dextroamphetamine is a potent and long-acting amphetamine. Following a 20 mg daily dose of racemic amphetamine administered at 10: 00, 12: 00, 14: 00, and 16: 00 hours each day (total= 80 mg/day) to a breastfeeding mother, amphetamine concentrations were determined in milk at 10 days and 42 days postpartum. Samples were taken at 20 min prior to the 10: 00 hour dose and immediately prior to the 14: 00 hour dose. Milk levels were 55 and 118 μg/L respectively.[1] Corresponding maternal plasma levels were 20 and 40 ng/mL at the same times. Milk/plasma ratios at these times were 2.8 and 3.0 respectively. At 42 days, breastmilk levels of amphetamine were 68 and 138 μg/L while maternal plasma levels were 9 and 21 ng/mL respectively. Milk/plasma ratios in the 42-day samples were 7.5 and 6.6 respectively. Although the milk/plasma ratios appear high, using a daily milk intake of 150 mL/kg/day, the relative infant dose would be only 1.8% of the weight-normalized maternal dose, which probably accounts for the fact that the infant in this study was unaffected.

In another study of 4 mothers who received 15–45 mg/day dextroamphetamine, the average absolute infant dose was 21 (11–39) μg/kg/day.[2] The authors suggest the relative infant dose was 5.7% (4–10.6). Plasma levels in the infants ranged from undetectable to 18 μg/L. No untoward effects were noted in any of the 4 infants.

The above data suggest that with normal therapeutic doses, the dose of dextroamphetamine in milk is probably subclinical. However, abuse of this medication is common. Doses are unknown and sometimes extraordinarily high. Thus mothers should be strongly advised to withhold breastfeeding for 24 hours following the non-clinical use of dextroamphetamine.

This drug is also available as continuous release formulations (Adderall XR). With continuous release formulations, plasma levels are virtually identical to the twice daily dosing system. Thus if a patient is using XR 20 mg, plasma levels are identical to the 10 mg twice daily.

Pregnancy Risk	C	Lactation Risk	L3 in clinical doses/L5 if abused
T ½	= 6–8 hours	M/P	= 2–5.2
Vd	= 3.2–5.6 l/kg	PB	= 16–20%
Tmax	= 1–2 hours	Oral	= Complete
MW	= 368	pKa	= 9.9

Adult Concerns: Nervousness, insomnia, anorexia, hyperexcitability.

Pediatric Concerns: Possible insomnia, irritability, anorexia, reduced weight gain, or poor sleeping patterns in infants. However in these studies, none of the infants were affected.

Drug Interactions: May precipitate hypertensive crisis in patients on monoamine oxidase inhibitors and arrhythmias in patients receiving general anesthetics. Increased effect/toxicity with tricyclic antidepressants, phenytoin, phenobarbital, norepinephrine, meperidine.

Relative Infant Dose: 1.8%–6.9%

Adult Dose: 5–60 mg daily

Alternatives: Methylphenidate

References:
1. Steiner E, Villen T, Hallberg M, Rane A. Amphetamine secretion in breast milk. Eur J Clin Pharmacol 1984; 27(1): 123–124.
2. Ilett KF, Hackett LP, Kristensen JH, Kohan R. Transfer of dexamphetamine into breast milk during treatment for attention deficit hyperactivity disorder. Br J Clin Pharmacol 2006; 63(3): 371–375.

DEXTROMETHORPHAN   L1

Trade: Robitussin, Pediacare, Creomulsion, Vicks 44 Cough Relief, Dexalone, Hold DM, Babee Cof Syrup, Benylin Pediatric Formula

Other Trades:

Category: Antitussive, Cough preparation

Dextromethorphan is a weak antitussive commonly used in infants and adults. It is a congener of codeine and appears to elevate the cough threshold in the brain. It does not have addictive, analgesic, or sedative actions, and it does not produce respiratory depression at normal doses.[1] It is the safest of the antitussives and is routinely used in children and infants. No data on its transfer to human milk are available. It is very unlikely that enough would transfer via milk to provide clinically significant levels in a breastfed infant.

Pregnancy Risk	C	Lactation Risk	L1
T ½	= <4 hours	M/P	=
Vd	=	PB	=
Tmax	= 1–2 hours	Oral	= Complete
MW	= 271	pKa	= 8.3

Adult Concerns: Drowsiness, fatigue, dizziness, hyperpyrexia.

Pediatric Concerns: None reported.

Drug Interactions: May interact with monoamine oxidase inhibitors producing hypotension, hyperpyrexia, nausea, coma.

Relative Infant Dose:

Adult Dose: 10–20 mg every 4 hours

Alternatives: Codeine

References:
1. Pender ES, Parks BR. Toxicity with dextromethorphan-containing preparations: a literature review and report of two additional cases. Pediatr Emerg Care 1991; 7(3): 163–165.

DIATRIZOATE   L2

Trade: Angiovist, Cardiografin, Cystografin, Hypaque, Reno-M, Renografin, Urovist, Sinografin, Retrografin

Other Trades: Renografin-30, Renografin-60, Renografin-Dip, Gastrografin

Category: Iodinated Contrast Agent

Diatrizoate is an iodinated radiopaque medium used in a wide variety of X-rays. These radiocontrast agents contain iodine in the range of 8.5 to 59.87% iodine.[1] However, the iodine is covalently bound to the molecule and is poorly released after injection, most being eliminated in the urine rapidly. Reported levels in breastmilk are very low. In a study of a single patient who received 18.5 grams of iodine in the form of sodium and meglumine salts of diatrizoate, diatrizoate levels were undetectable (Level of Detection <2 mg/L).[2] In another woman who received 93 grams of Iodine as diatrizoate, total iodine transferred into breast milk in the first 24 hours was 0.03% or 31 mg.[3] Based on kinetic data, the American College of Radiology suggests that it is safe for mothers to continue breastfeeding after receiving iodinated X-ray contrast media.[4]

Pregnancy Risk	D	Lactation Risk	L2
T ½	= 120 minutes	M/P	=
Vd	=	PB	= 0–10%
Tmax	=	Oral	= 0.04–1.2%
MW	= 614	pKa	= 11.84

Adult Concerns: Pain at injection site, flushing, nephrosis, taste alteration, nausea, vomiting, dizziness, cough, paresthesia, hypersensitivity, edema.

Pediatric Concerns: None reported via breast milk.

Drug Interactions: Concurrent use of diatrizoate with metformin may cause lactic acidosis and renal failure. Concomitant use with propranolol should be avoided due to increased risk of hypersensitivity reaction. Concomitant use with diltiazem may result in hypotension.

Relative Infant Dose:

Adult Dose:

Alternatives:

References:
1. Pharmaceutical manufacturer prescribing information, 2002.
2. Fitz John, T. P., Williams, D. G., Laker, M. F., and Owen, J. P. Intravenous urography during lactation. Br. J Radiol. 55(656): 603–605, 1982.
3. Texier, F., Roque, d. O., and Etling, N. [Stable iodine level in human milk after pulmonary angiography]. Presse Med.%19; 12(12): 769, 1983.
4. ACR Committee on Drugs and Contrast Media. Administration of contrast medium to breastfeeding mothers. 2004; 42–43.

DIAZEPAM   L3

Trade: Valium

Other Trades: Antenex, Ducene, Valium, Apo-Diazepam, Meval, Novo-Dipam, Vivol, Sedapam

Category: Sedative, anxiolytic drug

Diazepam is a powerful CNS depressant and anticonvulsant. Published data on milk and plasma levels are highly variable and many are poor studies. In 3 mothers receiving 10 mg three times daily for up to 6 days, the maternal plasma levels of diazepam averaged 491 ng/mL (day 4) and 601 ng/mL (day 6).[1] Corresponding milk levels were 51 ng/mL (day 4) and 78 ng/mL (day 6). The milk/plasma ratio was approximately 0.1. In a case report of a patient taking 6–10 mg of diazepam daily, her milk levels varied from 7.5 to 87 µg/L.[2] In a study of 9 mothers receiving diazepam postpartum, milk levels of diazepam varied from approximately 0.01 to 0.08 mg/L.[3] Other reports suggest slightly higher values. Taken together, most results suggest that the dose of diazepam and its metabolite, desmethyldiazepam, to a suckling infant will be on average 0.78–9.1% of the weight-adjusted maternal dose of diazepam.[4] The active metabolite, desmethyldiazepam, in general has a much longer half-life in adults and pediatric patients and may tend to accumulate on longer therapy. The excretion of diazepam, N-desmethyldiazepam, temazepam and oxazepam in breast milk was studied during withdrawal of a 22-year-old patient from combined high dose of 80 mg diazepam and 30 mg oxazepam therapy.[5] The mean milk/plasma ratio of diazepam and its metabolite desmthyldiazepam was found to be 0.2 and 0.13 respectively. The milk concentration of diazepam during therapy ranged between 67–307 µg/L and that of desmethyldiazepam was 42–141 µg/L; with the milk concentrations being barely 6 µg/L 8 days following cessation of therapy. No diazepam was detected in infant's plasma and only low levels of desmethyldiazepam were present in infant's plasma. No untoward effects were reported in the breastfed infant. The authors conclude that very low levels of benzodiazepines get transferred into breastmilk and are unlikely to be clinically relevant in the breastfed infant.

Some reports of lethargy, sedation, and poor suckling have been found. The acute use such as in surgical procedures is not likely to lead to significant accumulation. Long-term, sustained therapy may prove troublesome. The benzodiazepine family, as a rule, is not ideal for breastfeeding mothers due to relatively long half-lives and the development of dependence. However, it is apparent that the shorter-acting benzodiazepines (lorazepam, alprazolam) are safest during lactation provided their use is short-term or intermittent, low dose, and after the first week of life.[6]

Pregnancy Risk	D	Lactation Risk	L3
T ½	= 43 hours	M/P	= 0.2–2.7
Vd	= 0.7–2.6 l/kg	PB	= 99%
Tmax	= 1–2 hours	Oral	= Complete
MW	= 285	pKa	= 3.4

Adult Concerns: Adverse reactions include drowsiness, dizziness, blurred vision, dry mouth, headache, fatigue, ataxia, slurred speech, and mental confusion.

Pediatric Concerns: Some reports of lethargy, sedation, poor suckling have been found.

Drug Interactions: May increase sedation when used with CNS depressants such as alcohol, barbiturates, opioids. Cimetidine may decrease metabolism and clearance of diazepam. Cisapride can dramatically increase plasma levels of diazepam. Valproic acid may displace diazepam from binding sites, thus increasing sedative effects. SSRIs (fluoxetine, sertraline, paroxetine) can dramatically increase diazepam levels by altering clearance, thus leading to sedation .

Relative Infant Dose: 7.1%

Adult Dose: 2–10 mg 2–4 times daily.

Alternatives: Lorazepam, midazolam

References:
1. Erkkola R, Kanto J. Diazepam and breast-feeding. Lancet 1972; 1(7762): 1235–1236.
2. Wesson DR, Camber S, Harkey M, Smith DE. Diazepam and desmethyldiazepam in breast milk. J Psychoactive Drugs 1985; 17(1): 55–56.
3. Cole AP, Hailey DM. Diazepam and active metabolite in breast milk and their transfer to the neonate. Arch Dis Child 1975; 50(9): 741–742.
4. Spigset O. Anaesthetic agents and excretion in breast milk. Acta Anaesthesiol Scand 1994; 38(2): 94–103.
5. Dusci LJ, Good SM, Hall RW, Ilett KF. Excretion of diazepam and its metabolites in human milk during withdrawal from combination high dose diazepam and oxazepam. Br J Clin Pharmacol. 1990 Jan; 29(1): 123–6.
6. Maitra R, Menkes DB. Psychotropic drugs and lactation. N Z Med J 1996; 109(1024): 217–218.

DIBUCAINE   L3

Trade: Nupercainal
Other Trades:
Category: Local anesthetic

Dibucaine is a long-acting local anesthetic generally used topically. It is primarily used topically in creams and ointments, and due to toxicity, has been banned in USA for IV or IM injections.[1] No data are available on transfer to breastmilk. Dibucaine is effective for sunburn, topical burns, rash, rectal hemorrhoids, and other skin irritations. Long-term use and use over large areas of the body are discouraged. Although somewhat minimal, some dibucaine can be absorbed from irritated skin. Do not use dibucaine ointment on the nipple. Two toddlers developed seizures following a dose of 15 mg/kg of 1% dibucaine ointment.

Pregnancy Risk	C	Lactation Risk	L3
T ½	=	M/P	=
Vd	=	PB	=
Tmax	=	Oral	=
MW	= 379	pKa	= 8.8

Adult Concerns: Rash or allergic symptoms.

Pediatric Concerns: None reported via milk. Do not use dibucaine ointment on the nipple. Two toddlers developed seizures following a dose of 15 mg/kg of 1% dibucaine ointment.

Drug Interactions: Avoid use with St. John's wort as concurrent use may cause shock.

Relative Infant Dose:

Adult Dose:

Alternatives:

References:
1. Pharmaceutical manufacturer prescribing information, 1995.

DICLOFENAC   L2

Trade: Cataflam, Voltaren, Pennsaid, Zipsor, Flector patch, Cambia
Other Trades: Voltaren, Fenac, Voltaren, Apo-Diclo, Novo-Difenac, Voltarol
Category: NSAID analgesic for arthritis

Diclofenac is a typical nonsteroidal analgesic (NSAID). Diclofenac is available in both sustained release formulations (Voltaren), as well as in immediate release formulations (Cataflam). In one study of six postpartum mothers receiving three 50 mg doses on day 1, followed by two 50 mg doses on day 2, the levels of diclofenac in breastmilk were approximately 5 µg/L of milk, although the limit of detection was reported as <19 ng/mL.[1]

In another patient on long-term treatment with diclofenac, milk levels of 0.1 μg/mL milk were reported which would amount to 0.015 mg/kg/day ingested.[2] These amounts are probably far too low to affect an infant.

Pregnancy Risk	C/D in 3rd trimester	Lactation Risk	L2
T ½	= 1.1 hours	M/P	=
Vd	= 0.55 l/kg	PB	= 99.7%
Tmax	= 1 hour (Cataflam)	Oral	= Complete
MW	= 318	pKa	= 4.0

Adult Concerns: Gastrointestinal distress, diarrhea, nausea, vomiting.

Pediatric Concerns: None reported via milk. Milk levels are extremely low.

Drug Interactions: May prolong prothrombin time when used with warfarin. Antihypertensive effects of ACE inhibitors may be blunted or completely abolished by NSAIDs. Some NSAIDs may block antihypertensive effects of beta blockers, diuretics. Used with cyclosporin, may dramatically increase renal toxicity. May increase digoxin, phenytoin, lithium levels. May increase toxicity of methotrexate. May increase bioavailability of penicillamine. Probenecid may increase NSAID levels.

Relative Infant Dose:

Adult Dose: 75 mg BID

Alternatives: Ibuprofen

References:
1. Sioufi A. et. al. Recent findings concerning clinically relevant pharmacokinetics of diclofenac sodium. In: Kass(ed), Voltaren-new findings. Hans Huber Publishers, Bern, 1982.
2. Pharmaceutical manufacturer prescribing information

DICLOXACILLIN   L1

Trade: Pathocil, Dycill, Dynapen

Other Trades: Diclocil, Dicloxsig, Dynapen

Category: Penicillin antibiotic

Dicloxacillin is an oral penicillinase-resistant penicillin frequently used for peripheral (non CNS) infections caused by *Staphylococcus aureus* and *Staphylococcus epidermidis* infections, particularly mastitis. Following oral administration of a 250 mg dose, milk concentrations of the drug were 0.1, and 0.3 mg/L at 2 and 4 hours after the dose respectively.[1] Levels were undetectable after 1–6 hours. Compatible with breastfeeding. Observe for diarrhea or Candida diaper rash.

Pregnancy Risk	B	Lactation Risk	L1
T ½	= 0.6–0.8 hour	M/P	=
Vd	=	PB	= 96%
Tmax	= 0.5–2 hours	Oral	= 35–76%
MW	= 470	pKa	= 13.64

Adult Concerns: Elimination is delayed in neonates. Rash, diarrhea.

Pediatric Concerns: None reported via milk. Observe for diarrhea and Candida

Drug Interactions: May increase effect of oral anticoagulants. Disulfiram, probenecid may increase levels of penicillin. May reduce efficacy of oral contraceptives.

Relative Infant Dose: 0.6%–1.4%

Adult Dose: 125–250 mg every 6 hours

Alternatives: Amoxicillin + clavulanate

References:
1. Matsuda S. Transfer of antibiotics into maternal milk. Biol Res Pregnancy. 1984; 5: 57–60.

DICYCLOMINE   L4

Trade: Bentyl, Antispas, Spasmoject
Other Trades: Merbentyl, Bentylol, Formulex, Lomine
Category: Anticholinergic, drying agent.

Dicyclomine is a tertiary amine antispasmodic. It belongs to the family of anticholinergics such as atropine and the belladonna alkaloids. It was previously used for infant colic but due to overdoses and reported apnea, it is seldom recommended for this use. Infants are exceedingly sensitive to anticholinergics, particularly in the neonatal period. Following a dose of 20 mg in a lactating woman, a 12 day-old infant reported severe apnea. The manufacturer reports milk levels of 131 µg/L with corresponding maternal serum levels of 59 µg/L.[1] The reported milk/plasma level was 2.22.

Pregnancy Risk	B	Lactation Risk	L4
T ½	= 9–10 hours	M/P	= 2.22
Vd	=	PB	=
Tmax	= 1–1.5 hours	Oral	= 67%
MW	= 345	pKa	= 9.0

Adult Concerns: Apnea, dry secretions, urinary hesitancy, dilated pupils.

Pediatric Concerns: Severe apnea in one 12 day old infant. Observe for anticholinergic symptoms, drying, constipation, rapid heart rate.

Drug Interactions: Decreased effect with antacids, phenothiazines, haloperidol. Increased toxicity when used with other anticholinergics, amantadine, opiates, antiarrhythmics, antihistamines, tricyclic antidepressants.

Relative Infant Dose: 6.9%

Adult Dose: 20–40 mg QID

Alternatives:

References:
1. Pharmaceutical manufacturer prescribing information, 2010.

DIDANOSINE L5

Trade: Videx
Other Trades:
Category: Antiretroviral agent used in HIV infections. Antiretroviral drug

Didanosine is an antiretroviral agent used for the treatment of HIV infection. There are no adequate and well-controlled studies or case reports in breastfeeding women. Breastfeeding is generally not recommended in mothers who have HIV.[1,2]

Pregnancy Risk	B	Lactation Risk	L5
T ½	= 1.3–1.5 hours	M/P	=
Vd	= 0.8–1 l/kg	PB	= <5%
Tmax	= 0.67–2 hours	Oral	= 21–43%
MW	=	pKa	= 9.13

Adult Concerns: Abdominal pain, diarrhea, rash, nausea, vomiting, peripheral neuropathy, headache, elevated liver enzymes, pancreatitis, arrhythmia, increased risk of heart attack, nephrotoxicity, hypersensitivity, hepatitis, leucopenia, anemia, arthralgia, myalgia, hyperuricemia, increased or decreased blood sugar.

Pediatric Concerns:

Drug Interactions: Concurrent use with allopurinol and ribavirin is contraindicated. Concomitant use with ganciclovir and tenofovir may increase plasma levels and risk of toxicity with didanosine. Concurrent use with methodone may decrease plasma levels and efficacy of didanosine. Caution to be exercised while coadministering with the following drugs due to increased risk of pancreatitis and/or neuropathy: hydroxyurea, zalcitabine, valganciclovir.

Relative Infant Dose:

Adult Dose:

Alternatives:

References:
1. World Health Organization: Global Programme on AIDS. Consensus statement from the WHO/UNICEF consultation on HIV transmission and breast-feeding. Geneva: WHO, 1992.
2. Latham MC, Greiner T: Breastfeeding versus formula feeding in HIV infection. Lancet 352: 737, 1998

DIENOGEST L3

Trade:
Other Trades:
Category: Progestin

Dienogest is a synthetic progesterone, generally used in combination with estradiol as oral contraceptive. It is 10 times more potent than levonorgestrel and has minimal androgenic adverse effects. There are no controlled studies in breastfeeding women; however, since it is a type of progesterone, dienogest may have effects similar to that of progesterone. With the use of progesterone in breastfeeding mothers there is significant confusion in the literature as to the effect of progestins on milk composition, but the compositional changes do not appear major, volume is normal or higher, and some authors report minor changes in lipid and protein content.[1-3]

However, the majority of the studies are with other progestins (e. g. medroxyprogesterone). Shaaban studied the effect of an intravaginal progesterone ring (10 mg/day) in 120 women and found no changes in growth and development of the infant or breastfeeding performance of the study participants.[4] The author suggests the ring adds a measure of safety because the amount of steroid present in milk would be effectively absorbed from the infant's gut. Another new study also suggests no impact on breastfeeding from the intravaginal progesterone ring.[5]

The effect of progestins on milk production is poorly studied. Early postpartum, while progestin receptors are still present in the breast, administering progestins may actually suppress milk production just as it does in the pregnant women. This has been seen occasionally in patients early postpartum. Several days to a week later, most progestin receptors disappear from the lactocyte and breast tissues become relatively immune to the effects of progestins. Thus it is advisable to wait as long as possible postpartum prior to instituting therapy with progesterone to avoid reducing the milk supply.

Pregnancy Risk	X	Lactation Risk	L3
T ½	= 9–10 hours	M/P	=
Vd	= 0.571 l/kg	PB	= 90%
Tmax	= 1.5 hours	Oral	= 91%
MW	= 311	pKa	=

Adult Concerns: Headache, acne, breast discomfort, amenorrhea, irregular menstrual bleeding, weight gain.

Pediatric Concerns:

Drug Interactions:

Relative Infant Dose:

Adult Dose: 2–3 mg/day

Alternatives:

References:
1. Rodriguez-Palmero M, Koletzko B, Kunz C, Jensen R. Nutritional and biochemical properties of human milk: II. Lipids, micronutrients, and bioactive factors. Clin Perinatol 1999; 26(2): 335–359.

2. Costa TH, Dorea JG. Concentration of fat, protein, lactose and energy in milk of mothers using hormonal contraceptives. Ann Trop Paediatr 1992; 12(2): 203–209.
3. Sas M, Gellen JJ, Dusitsin N, Tunkeyoon M, Chalapati S, Crawford MA, Drury PJ, Lenihan T, Ayeni O, Pinol A. An investigation on the influence of steroidal contraceptives on milk lipid and fatty acids in Hungary and Thailand. WHO Special Programme of Research, Development and Research Training in Human Reproduction. Task Force on oral contraceptives. Contracep 1986; 33(2): 159–178.
4. Shaaban MM. Contraception with progestogens and progesterone during lactation. J Steroid Biochem Mol Biol 1991; 40(4–6): 705–710.
5. Massai R, Quinteros E, Reyes MV, Caviedes R, Zepeda A, Montero JC, et al. Extended use of a progesterone-releasing vaginal ring in nursing women: a phase II clinical trial. Contracep 2005 Nov; 72(5): 352–7.

DIENOGEST + ESTRADIOL   L3

Trade: Natazia

Other Trades:

Category: Oral contraceptive

Dienogest and Estradiol valerate is a drug combination indicated for its use as an oral contraceptive agent. This combination oral contraceptive contains estradiol valerate as the estrogen component and dienogest as the progestin component in a four-phasic formulation. It is administered as an estrogen step-down and a progestin step-up approach over 26 days of active treatment followed by 2 days of placebo. Combined oral contraceptives lower the risk of becoming pregnant primarily by suppressing ovulation. Other potential mechanisms may include cervical mucus changes that inhibit sperm penetration and endometrial changes that reduce the likelihood of implantation.

When possible, advise the nursing mother to use other forms of contraception until she has weaned her child. Estrogen-containing oral contraceptives may reduce milk production in breastfeeding mothers. This is less likely to occur once breastfeeding is well-established, which usually takes around 6–8 weeks; however, this duration varies in different women, and may be longer in some women. Small amounts of oral contraceptive steroids and/or metabolites are present in breast milk but have not been reported to produce untoward effects in breastfed infants. Avoid if possible in breastfeeding mothers due to reduction of milk supply.

The effect of progestins on milk production is poorly studied. Early postpartum, while progestin receptors are still present in the breast, administering progestins may actually suppress milk production. This has been seen occasionally in patients early postpartum. Several days to a week later, most progestin receptors disappear from the lactocyte and breast tissues become relatively immune to the effects of progestins. Thus it is advisable to wait as long as possible postpartum prior to instituting therapy with progesterone to avoid reducing the milk supply. The direct effect of progesterone therapy on the nursing infant is generally unknown, but it is believed minimal to none as natural progesterone is poorly bioavailable to the infant via milk. Several cases of gynecomastia in infants have been reported but are extremely rare.[1-5]

Breastfeeding women are strongly advised to avoid using combination (containing both estrogen and progesterone) oral contraceptives while breastfeeding because combination oral contraceptives have been shown to interfere with the production of milk and will reduce the duration of breastfeeding.[6-11] It is recommended that women wait at least 6–8 weeks postpartum to establish good milk flow, prior to beginning oral contraceptives.

Pregnancy Risk	X		Lactation Risk	L3
T ½	= dienogest/estradiol: 11 hours/14 hours		M/P	=
Vd	= dienogest/estradiol: 46/1.2 l/kg		PB	= dienogest/estradiol: 90%/60%
Tmax	=		Oral	=
MW	=		pKa	=

Adult Concerns: Irregular uterine bleeding, nausea, breast tenderness, headache have been reported. Do not use oral contraceptives in women who smoke to avoid the risk for cardiovascular events.

Pediatric Concerns: Reduction of milk supply, especially if used early postpartum. Preferably use after 6–8 weeks postpartum, or once lactation is firmly established.

Drug Interactions: Drugs or herbal products that induce certain enzymes, including CYP3A4, may decrease the effectiveness of contraceptives. These include: barbiturates, bosentan, felbamate, griseofulvin, oxcarbazepine, and topiramate. Avoid using carbamazepine, phenytoin, rifampicin, and St. John's wort, rifamicin, ketoconazole, erythromycin. Numerous other contraindications exist, check other resources.

Relative Infant Dose:

Adult Dose: One tablet at the same time everyday.

Alternatives:

References:

1. Rodriguez-Palmero M, Koletzko B, Kunz C, Jensen R. Nutritional and biochemical properties of human milk: II. Lipids, micronutrients, and bioactive factors. Clin Perinatol 1999; 26(2): 335–359.
2. Costa TH, Dorea JG. Concentration of fat, protein, lactose and energy in milk of mothers using hormonal contraceptives. Ann Trop Paediatr 1992; 12(2): 203–209.
3. Sas M, Gellen JJ, Dusitsin N, Tunkeyoon M, Chalapati S, Crawford MA, Drury PJ, Lenihan T, Ayeni O, Pinol A. An investigation on the influence of steroidal contraceptives on milk lipid and fatty acids in Hungary and Thailand. WHO Special Programme of Research, Development and Research Training in Human Reproduction. Task Force on oral contraceptives. Contracep 1986; 33(2): 159–178.
4. Shaaban MM. Contraception with progestogens and progesterone during lactation. J Steroid Biochem Mol Biol 1991; 40(4–6): 705–710.
5. Massai R, Quinteros E, Reyes MV, Caviedes R, Zepeda A, Montero JC, et al. Extended use of a progesterone-releasing vaginal ring in nursing women: a phase II clinical trial. Contracep 2005 Nov; 72(5): 352–7.
6. Costa TH, Dorea JG. Concentration of fat, protein, lactose and energy in milk of mothers using hormonal contraceptives. Ann Trop Paediatr 1992; 12(2): 203–209.
7. McCann MF, Potter LS. Progestin-only oral contraception: a comprehensive review. Contraception. 1994 Dec; 50(6 Suppl 1): S1–195. Review.
8. Peralta O, D?az S, Juez G, Herreros C, Casado ME, Salvatierra AM, Miranda P, Dur?n E, Croxatto HB. Fertility regulation in nursing women: V. Long-term influence of a low-dose combined oral contraceptive initiated at day 90 postpartum upon lactation and infant growth. Contraception. 1983 Jan; 27(1): 27–38.

9. Croxatto HB, D?az S, Peralta O, Juez G, Herreros C, Casado ME, Salvatierra AM, Miranda P, Dur?n E. Fertility regulation in nursing women: IV. Long-term influence of a low-dose combined oral contraceptive initiated at day 30 postpartum upon lactation and infant growth. Contraception. 1983 Jan; 27(1): 13–25.
10. Diaz S, Peralta O, Juez G, Herreros C, Casado ME, Salvatierra AM, Miranda P, Dur?n E, Croxatto HB. Fertility regulation in nursing women: III. Short-term influence of a low-dose combined oral contraceptive upon lactation and infant growth. Contraception. 1983 Jan; 27(1): 1–11.
11. Effects of hormonal contraceptives on breast milk composition and infant growth. World Health Organization (WHO) Task Force on Oral Contraceptives. Stud Fam Plann. 1988 Nov-Dec; 19(6 Pt 1): 361–9.

DIETHYLPROPION   L5

Trade: Tepanil, Tenuate

Other Trades: Tenuate, Dospan

Category: Anorexiant

Diethylpropion belongs to the amphetamine family and is typically used to reduce food intake. No data or literature reports are available of the transfer of this drug into human milk. Manufacturer states that this medication is secreted into breastmilk.[1] Diethylpropion's structure is similar to amphetamines. Upon withdrawal, significant withdrawal symptoms have been reported in adults. Such symptoms could be observed in breastfeeding infants of mothers using this product. The use of this medication during lactation is simply unrealistic and not justified. Weight-loss medications are generally not recommended for breastfeeding women since this may interfere with the nutritive properties of the breastmilk provided to the infant.[2]

Pregnancy Risk	B	Lactation Risk	L5
T ½	= 8 hours	M/P	=
Vd	=	PB	=
Tmax	= 2 hours	Oral	= 70%
MW	= 205	pKa	= 8.2

Adult Concerns: Overstimulation, insomnia, anorexia, jitteriness, rapid heart rate, elevated blood pressure.

Pediatric Concerns: None reported, but observe for anorexia, agitation, insomnia.

Drug Interactions: Increased toxicity with monoamine oxidase inhibitors, CNS depressants, general anesthetics (arrhythmias), other adrenergics.

Relative Infant Dose:

Adult Dose: 25 mg TID

Alternatives:

References:
1. Pharmaceutical manufacturer prescribing information, 2010.
2. Schaefer CSchaefer C: Drugs During Pregnancy and Lactation, Elsevier Science B. V., Amsterdam, The Netherlands, 2001.

DIETHYLSTILBESTROL   L5

Trade: DES

Other Trades: Honvan, Fosfestrol, Honvol, Apstil

Category: Synthetic estrogen

Diethylstilbestrol (DES) is a synthetic estrogen that is seldom used today. It is known to produce a high risk of cervical cancer in female infants exposed during pregnancy.[1,2] It has been shown to cause anatomical abnormalities in males and females, neoplasia, reduced fertility, and immunologic changes. Its effect in the breastfeeding infant is unknown but should be absolutely avoided. DES would probably inhibit milk production. Do not use this estrogen during breastfeeding. Contraindicated.

Pregnancy Risk	X	Lactation Risk	L5
T ½	=	M/P	=
Vd	=	PB	=
Tmax	=	Oral	= Complete
MW	= 268	pKa	= 9.73

Adult Concerns: Decreased breast milk production.

Pediatric Concerns: None reported via milk, but this product is too dangerous for use in breastfeeding mothers.

Drug Interactions:

Relative Infant Dose:

Adult Dose: 15 mg daily.

Alternatives:

References:
1. O'Brien TE. Excretion of drugs in human milk. Am J Hosp Pharm 1974; 31(9): 844–854.
2. Shapiro S, Slone D. The effects of exogenous female hormones on the fetus. Epidemiol Rev 1979; 1: 110–123.

DIFLUNISAL   L3

Trade: Dolobid

Other Trades: Apo-Diflunisal, Dolobid, Novo-Diflunisal

Category: Nonsteroidal anti-inflammatory analgesic

Diflunisal is a derivative of salicylic acid. It is a nonsteroidal anti-inflammatory agent (NSAID). Diflunisal is excreted into human milk in concentrations 2–7% of the maternal plasma levels following 7 days of treatment with 125–250 mg twice daily, although specific milk levels were not reported.[1] Thus levels in the infant would probably be quite low to undetectable. No reports of side-effects have been located.[1] This product is potentially a higher risk NSAID and other less toxic compounds such as ibuprofen should be used.

Pregnancy Risk	C/D in 3rd trimester	Lactation Risk	L3
T ½	= 8–12 hours	M/P	=
Vd	= 0.1–0.2 l/kg	PB	= 99%
Tmax	= 2–3 hours	Oral	= Complete
MW	= 250	pKa	= 12.68

Adult Concerns: Prolonged bleeding time, headache, gastrointestinal distress, diarrhea, gastrointestinal cramping, fluid retention, ulcer complications, worsening hypertension.

Pediatric Concerns: None reported but alternatives are suggested.

Drug Interactions: Antacids reduce effect. Increased toxicity of digoxin, methotrexate, anticoagulants, phenytoin, sulfonylureas, lithium acetaminophen.

Relative Infant Dose: 7.8%–11.5%

Adult Dose: 500 mg BID or TID

Alternatives: Ibuprofen, celecoxib

References:
1. Steelman SL, Breault GO, Tocco D. Pharmacokinetics of MK-647, a novel salicylate. Clin Pharmacol Ther. 1975; 17: 245. Abstract.

DIFLUPREDNATE   L3

Trade: Durezol, Epitopic, Myser

Other Trades:

Category: Adrenal Glucocorticoid

Difluprednate is an adrenal glucocorticoid ophthalmic solution used as an anti-inflammatory agent after ophthalmic surgery. The medication comes in 0.01% and 0.05% strengths. There is limited systemic absorption. One study found no metabolites in the urine of patients using the ophthalmic solution daily for 1 week.[1] Clinical pharmacokinetic studies of difluprednate after repeat ocular instillation of 2 drops of difluprednate (0.01% or 0.05%) QID for 7 days showed that DFB levels in blood were below the quantification limit (50 ng/mL) at all time points for all subjects, indicating the systemic absorption of difluprednate after ocular instillation of Durezol is limited. Due to the limited systemic absorption, levels of difluprednate in milk are probably minimal to nil.

Pregnancy Risk	C	Lactation Risk	L3
T ½	=	M/P	=
Vd	=	PB	=
Tmax	=	Oral	=
MW	= 508.6	pKa	= 14.46

Adult Concerns: Blepharitis, anterior chamber flare, corneal edema, blepharitis, pain, photophobia, conjunctiva edema, posterior capsule opacification, ocular hyperemia, constipation.

Pediatric Concerns:

Drug Interactions:

Relative Infant Dose:

Adult Dose: Instill 1 drop 4 times a day

Alternatives:

References:
1. Difluprednate. In: DRUGDEX Æ System [Internet database]. Greenwood Village, Colo: Thomson Healthcare. Updated periodically. Accessed 06-09-2011.

DIGITOXIN   L3

Trade: Crystodigin

Other Trades: Digitaline

Category: Cardiac stimulant

Digitoxin is a cardiac glycoside and an ionotropic agent (cardiac stimulant). No data available on digitoxin and its transfer to human milk.[1] Digitoxin is occasionally given to infants. High lipid solubility and good oral bioavailability would suggest some transfer into breastmilk. See digoxin.

Pregnancy Risk	C	Lactation Risk	L3
T ½	= 6.7 days	M/P	=
Vd	= 7 (variable) l/kg	PB	= 97%
Tmax	= 4 hours	Oral	= 90–100%
MW	= 765	pKa	= 13.03

Adult Concerns: Nausea, vomiting, anorexia, cardiac arrhythmias.

Pediatric Concerns: None reported thus far.

Drug Interactions: Reduced plasma levels when used with antacids, penicillamine, bran fiber, sucralfate, cholestyramine, rifampin, etc. Increased toxicity when used with diltiazem, ibuprofen, cimetidine, omeprazole, etc.

Relative Infant Dose:

Adult Dose: 0.15 mg daily.

Alternatives:

References:
1. Levy M, Granit L, Laufer N. Excretion of drugs in human milk. N Engl J Med 1977; 297(14): 789.

DIGOXIN   L2

Trade: Lanoxin, Lanoxicaps, Digibind, Digifab

Other Trades: Lanoxin, Novo-Digoxin

Category: Cardiac stimulant

Digoxin is a cardiac stimulant used primarily to strengthen the contractile process. In one mother receiving 0.25 mg digoxin daily, the amount found in breast milk ranged from 0.96 to 0.61 µg/L at 4 and 6 hours post-dose respectively.[1] Mean peak breastmilk levels varied from 0.78 µg/L in one patient to 0.41 µg/L in another. Plasma levels in the infants were undetectable.

In another study of 5 women receiving digoxin therapy, the average breastmilk concentration was 0.64 µg/L.[2] From these studies, it is apparent that a breastfeeding infant would receive less than 1 µg/day of digoxin, too low to be clinically relevant. The small amounts secreted into breastmilk have not produced problems in nursing infants. Poor and erratic gastrointestinal absorption could theoretically reduce absorption in nursing infant.

Digoxin immune fab (ovine), is composed of antigen binding fragments made from antidigoxin antibodies. It is used for life-threatening digoxin toxicity or overdose. The dosage needed can be calculated using the ratio that one vial of Digibind (38 mg) will bind 0.5 mg of digoxin. The molecular weight of these fragments are approximately 46,000 daltons, and thus would not be able to transfer into the milk compartment.[3]

Pregnancy Risk	C	Lactation Risk	L2
T ½	= 39 hours	M/P	= <0.9
Vd	= 5.1–7.4 l/kg	PB	= 25%
Tmax	= 1.5–3 hours	Oral	= 65–85%
MW	= 781	pKa	= 12.98

Adult Concerns: Nausea, vomiting, bradycardia, arrhythmias.

Pediatric Concerns: None reported in several studies.

Drug Interactions: Too numerous to list all. Decreased digoxin effect when used with antacids, bran fiber, sucralfate, sulfasalazine, diuretics, phenytoin, cholestyramine, aminoglutethimide. Increased digoxin effects may result when used with diltiazem, ibuprofen, cimetidine, omeprazole, bepridil, reserpine, amphotericin B, erythromycin, quinine, tetracycline, cyclosporine, etc.

Relative Infant Dose: 2.7%–2.8%

Adult Dose: 0.125–0.5 mg daily.

Alternatives:

References:
1. Loughnan PM. Digoxin excretion in human breast milk. J Pediatr 1978; 92(6): 1019–1020.
2. Levy M, Granit L, Laufer N. Excretion of drugs in human milk. N Engl J Med 1977; 297(14): 789.
3. Pharmaceutical manufacturer prescribing information, 2006.

DILTIAZEM | L3

Trade: Cardizem SR, Dilacor-XR, Cardizem CD, Cartia XT

Other Trades: Cardcal, Coras, Dilzem, Cardizem, Apo-Diltiazem, Apo-Diltiaz, Adizem, Britiazim, Tildiem

Category: Antihypertensive, calcium channel blocker

Diltiazem hydrochloride is an typical calcium channel blocker antihypertensive.[1] In a report of a single patient receiving 240 mg/day on day 14 postpartum, levels in milk were parallel to those of serum (milk/plasma ratio is approximately 1.0).[2] Peak level in milk (and plasma) was slightly higher than 200 µg/L and occurred at 8 hours. While nifedipine is probably a preferred choice calcium channel blocker because of our experience with it, the relative infant dose with this agent is quite small and it is not likely to be problematic.

Pregnancy Risk	C	Lactation Risk	L3
T ½	= 3.5–6 hours	M/P	= 1.0
Vd	= 1.7 l/kg	PB	= 78%
Tmax	= 2–3 hours	Oral	= 40–60%
MW	= 433	pKa	= 7.7

Adult Concerns: Hypotension, bradycardia.

Pediatric Concerns: Hypotension, bradycardia is possible. See nifedipine.

Drug Interactions: H-2 blockers may increase bioavailability of diltiazem. Beta blockers may increase cardio-depressant effect. May increase cyclosporine, and carbamazepine levels. Fentanyl may increase hypotension.

Relative Infant Dose: 0.9%

Adult Dose: 30–90 mg QID

Alternatives: Nifedipine, Nimodipine, Verapamil

References:
1. Pharmaceutical manufacturer prescribing information, 1995.
2. Okada M, Inoue H, Nakamura Y, Kishimoto M, Suzuki T. Excretion of diltiazem in human milk. N Engl J Med 1985; 312(15): 992–993.

DIMENHYDRINATE | L2

Trade: Dramamine, Driminate, Hydrate, Triptone

Other Trades:

Category: Antihistamine for vertigo and motion sickness

Dimenhydrinate is an anti-histamine and an ant-emetic agent used for the treatment and prevention of motion sickness. Consists of 55% diphenhydramine and 45% of 8-chlorotheophylline. Diphenhydramine is considered to be the active ingredient. Small but unreported levels of diphenhydramine are thought to be secreted into breastmilk. In one study following an IM dose of 100 mg, drug levels in milk were undetectable in two individuals, and ranged from 42 to 100 µg/L in two subjects.[1]

While these levels are low, the use of this sedating antihistamine in breastfeeding mothers is not ideal. Non-sedating antihistamines are generally preferred. There are anecdotal reports that diphenhydramine suppresses milk production. There are no data to support this theory.

Pregnancy Risk	B	Lactation Risk	L2
T ½	= 8.5 hours	M/P	=
Vd	=	PB	= 78%
Tmax	= 1–2 hours	Oral	=
MW	= 470	pKa	=

Adult Concerns: Sedation, dry secretions.

Pediatric Concerns: None reported but observe for sedation. See diphenhydramine.

Drug Interactions: May enhance CNS depressants, anticholinergics, tricyclic antidepressants, and monoamine oxidase inhibitors. Increased toxicity of antibiotics, especially aminoglycosides "ototoxicity."

Relative Infant Dose:

Adult Dose: 50–100 mg every 4–6 hours

Alternatives: Cetirizine, loratadine

References:
1. Rindi V. La eliminazione degli antistaminici di sintesi con il latte e l'azione latto-goga de questi. Riv Ital Ginecol. 1951; 34: 147–57.

DIMETHICONE   L3

Trade:

Other Trades:

Category: Silicone

Dimethicone is a silicone compound mainly used in topical creams.[1] There are no adequate and well-controlled studies or case reports in breastfeeding women. Because the drug is not absorbed, the risk to a nursing infant from maternal use of dimethicone is thought to be negligible.

Pregnancy Risk	Probably Safe	Lactation Risk	L3
T ½	=	M/P	=
Vd	=	PB	=
Tmax	=	Oral	=
MW	=	pKa	=

Adult Concerns: Rash due to hypersensitivity reactions to ingredient.

Pediatric Concerns:

Drug Interactions:

Relative Infant Dose:

Adult Dose:

Alternatives:

References:
1. Pharmaceutical manufacturer prescribing information, 2012.

DIMETHYLSULFOXIDE   L3

Trade: DMSO, Rimso-50, DMSO2, MSM
Other Trades:
Category: Solvent used for arthritis, etc.

Dimethylsulfoxide (DMSO) is a solvent that has been found useful for musculoskeletal inflammation and injury, and interstitial cystitis. It has been used topically, orally, and intravenously. DMSO is relatively nontoxic, requiring rather large intravenous doses to induce toxicity (20 gm). Following dermal application of 1 gm/kg (640 mL/70 kg), reported serum concentrations were 560 mg/L within 4–8 hours. By 48 hours only traces were detectable.[1] Daily oral doses of 32 mL/70 kg for 14 days produced peak serum levels of 1850 mg/L. DMSO penetrates to many compartments and it would probably penetrate into milk in significant quantities. Due to the high plasma levels above, it is probable that milk levels would be quite high as well. Although the overall toxicity of this compound is quite minimal, exposing an infant to this agent, which is minimally efficacious, is probably not justified. DMSO is capable of transporting most substances across the skin. When contaminated with other solvents it can become quite dangerous. Only highly purified products should be used.

Methylsulfonylmethane (DMSO$_2$, MSM, "Crystalline DMSO") is the normal oxidation product of DMSO. No data are available on this product, but it is probably distributed and eliminated the same as DMSO above.

Pregnancy Risk	C	Lactation Risk	L3
T ½	= 11–14 hours (dermal)	M/P	=
Vd	= 0.53 l/kg	PB	=
Tmax	= 4–8 hours (topically)	Oral	= Complete
MW	=	pKa	=

Adult Concerns: DMSO imparts a garlic-like breath, taste and body odor to all users. Gastrointestinal disturbances including vomiting and nausea, drowsiness, sedation, neuropathy, dizziness, headache and dermatologic rash have been reported. Hepatotoxicity, milk jaundice and hepatic precoma was reported in two elderly patients receiving IV infusions of 100 gm of 20% DMSO.

Pediatric Concerns: None reported. This agent is not particularly effective, therefore the risks do not justify its use in breastfeeding mothers.

Drug Interactions:

Relative Infant Dose:

Adult Dose: Variable.

Alternatives:

References:

1. Baselt RC. Disposition of toxic drugs and chemicals in man. Foster City, CA: Chemical Toxicology Institute, 2000: 282–283.

DINOPROSTONE   L3

Trade: Prostin E_2, Prepidil, Cervidil
Other Trades: Cervidil, Propress
Category: Prostaglandin E_2

Dinoprostone is a naturally occurring prostaglandin E_2 that is primarily used for induction of labor, for cervical ripening, as an abortifacient, for postpartum bleeding, and for uterine atony.[1] Available as a vaginal gel or insert, it is slowly absorbed into the plasma where it is rapidly cleared and metabolized by most tissues and the lung. Its half-life is brief 2.5 to 5 minutes although absorption from the vaginal mucosa is slow. Neonatal effects from maternal dinoprostone include fetal heart rate abnormalities, and neonatal jaundice. The amount of dinoprostone entering milk is not known, but a brief wash out period would preclude any possible side effects.

However, dinoprostone has been used to suppress lactation. When used orally (2 mg orally/day on day 3 and 4; then 6 mg/day thereafter) it has been found to significantly suppress milk production.[2,3] However, the use of prostaglandin E_2 products for cervical ripening (during delivery) is generally brief and probably does not clinically impact the production of breastmilk many hours or days later.

Pregnancy Risk	X/C during delivery	Lactation Risk	L3
T ½	= 2.5–5 minutes	M/P	=
Vd	=	PB	= High
Tmax	= 0.5–1 hour	Oral	=
MW	= 352.5	pKa	= 14.68

Adult Concerns: Side effects of vaginal dinoprostone are numerous and include abortion, labor induction, blood loss, hypotension, syncope, tachycardia, dizziness, hyperthermia, nausea, vomiting, diarrhea, and taste disorders.

Pediatric Concerns: None reported via milk, but a washout period is suggested.

Drug Interactions: Concurrent use of dinoprostone with oxytocin, methylergonovine and ergonovine is contraindicated.

Relative Infant Dose:

Adult Dose: 10–20 mg X 1–2

Alternatives:

References:

1. Pharmaceutical manufacturer prescribing information, 2010.

2. Caminiti F, De Murtas M, Parodo G, Lecca U, Nasi A. Decrease in human plasma prolactin levels by oral prostaglandin E_2 in early puerperium. J Endocrinol 1980; 87(3): 333–337.
3. Nasi A, De Murtas M, Parodo G, Caminiti F. Inhibition of lactation by prostaglandin E_2. Obstet Gynecol Surv 1980; 35(10): 619–620.

DIPHENHYDRAMINE   L2

Trade:

Other Trades:

Category: Antihistamine, antitussive

Diphenhydramine is an anti-histamine used for allergic conditions. It is also used as a sleep aid and as an anti-emetic agent for the prevention of motion sickness. Small but unreported levels are thought to be secreted into breastmilk. In one study following an IM dose of 100 mg, drug levels in milk were undetectable in two individuals, and ranged from 42 to 100 µg/L in two subjects.[1] While these levels are low, the use of this sedating antihistamine in breastfeeding mothers is not ideal. Non-sedating antihistamines are generally preferred. There are anecdotal reports that diphenhydramine suppresses milk production. There are no data to support this theory.

Pregnancy Risk	B	Lactation Risk	L2
T ½	= 4.3 hours	M/P	=
Vd	= 3–4 l/kg	PB	= 78%
Tmax	= 2–3 hours	Oral	= 43–61%
MW	= 255	pKa	= 8.3

Adult Concerns: Sedation, drowsiness.

Pediatric Concerns: None reported, but observe for sedation. Some suggestions of reduced milk supply but these are unsubstantiated.

Drug Interactions: Increased sedation when used with other CNS depressants. Monoamine oxidase inhibitors may increase anticholinergic side effects.

Relative Infant Dose: 0.7%–1.4%

Adult Dose: 25–50 mg TID or QID

Alternatives: Cetirizine, Loratadine

References:
1. Rindi V. La eliminazione degli antistaminici di sintesi con il latte e l'azione latto-goga de questi. Riv Ital Ginecol. 1951; 34: 147–57.

DIPHENOXYLATE + ATROPINE   L3

Trade: Lomotil, Di-Atro Dimotal, Lomocot, Lonox, Vi-Atro

Other Trades: Tropergen

Category: Antidiarrheal

Diphenoxylate belongs to the opiate family (meperidine) and acts on the intestinal tract inhibiting gastrointestinal motility and excessive gastrointestinal propulsion.

The drug has no analgesic activity. Although no reports on its transfer to human milk are available, it is probably secreted in breastmilk in very small quantities.[1] Some authors consider diphenoxylate to be contraindicated, but this is questionable. Diphenoxylate is never used by itself, but is always used with atropine to prevent abuse.

Pregnancy Risk	C	Lactation Risk	L3
T ½	= 2.5 hours	M/P	=
Vd	= 3.8 l/kg	PB	=
Tmax	= 2 hours	Oral	= 90%
MW	= 453	pKa	= 7.1

Adult Concerns: Anticholinergic effects, such as drying, constipation, and sedation.

Pediatric Concerns: None reported, but observe for dryness, constipation, sedation.

Drug Interactions: Increased toxicity when used with monoamine oxidase inhibitors, CNS depressants, anticholinergics.

Relative Infant Dose:

Adult Dose: 5 mg QID

Alternatives:

References:
1. Stewart JJ. Gastrointestinal drugs. In Wilson, J. T., ed. Drugs in Breast Milk. Balgowlah, Australia ADIS Press 1981; 71.

DIPHTHERIA + TETANUS + PERTUSSIS VACCINE (DTaP/Tdap/DTP)   L2

Trade: DTaP, Acel-Imune(DTaP), Tripedia (DTaP), Daptacel (DTaP), Tdap, Infanrix (DTaP), Boostrix (Tdap), Adacel (Tdap)

Other Trades: Triple Antigen (DTP)

Category: Vaccine

This is a combination vaccine containing the diphtheria and tetanus toxoids, along with acellular pertussis adsorbed vaccine.[1] Those currently licensed for use in the United States by the FDA are DTaP and Tdap. The primary difference between these is that Tdap contains reduced diphtheria toxoid making it suitable for use in adults and those more than 10 years of age. DTaP is used only in those between 6 weeks to 6 years of age. DTP vaccines which contain diphtheria and tetanus toxoids, along with whole-cell pertussis vaccines are used in some countries, but is not licensed for use in the United States due to higher risk of severe adverse reactions, such as seizures, attributed to the whole-cell pertussis content of this vaccine. DTaP is generally recommended at 2,4 and 6 months of age with boosters at 15–20 months and at 4–6 years of age. Tdap is given as a single booster dose after the age of 10 years and is recommended for all adults who are, or anticipate being in close contact with an infant of less than 12 months of age, if not previously immunized with Tdap.[2]

Diphtheria vaccine contains diphtheria toxoid, which is a formalin-inactivated form of diphtheria toxin. Currently, no data are available on the transfer of diphtheria toxoid into human milk. However, diphtheria toxoid is considered compatible with breastfeeding.[3,4] The diphtheria toxoid is a large molecular weight protein toxoid. It is extremely unlikely that proteins of this size would transfer into breastmilk.

There are two types of pertussis vaccines, whole cell and acellular. Whole cell pertussis vaccine is made form inactivated B. pertussis cells. Acellular pertussis vaccines are made from inactivated components of B. pertussis cells. Because pertussis vaccine is an inactivated bacterial product, there is no specific contraindication in breastfeeding following injection with these vaccine. It is extremely unlikely proteins of this size would be secreted in breastmilk.

Tetanus vaccine is made from inactivated tetanus toxoid by formaldehyde.[5] Because tetanus vaccine is an inactivated bacterial product, there is no specific contraindication in breastfeeding following injection with these vaccine. It is extremely unlikely proteins of this size would be secreted in breastmilk.

Because this is an inactivated bacterial product, there is no specific contraindication in breastfeeding following injection with these vaccines.

Pregnancy Risk	B		Lactation Risk	L2
T ½	=		M/P	=
Vd	=		PB	=
Tmax	=		Oral	=
MW	=		pKa	=

Adult Concerns: Swelling, redness, tenderness at the site of injection, fretfulness, drowsiness, anorexia, vomiting, headache. Hypersensitivity reactions to any of the components of the vaccine. Avoid during on-going acute illness. Guillan-Barre syndrome may occur within 6 weeks of receipt of a tetanus-toxoid containing vaccine.

Pediatric Concerns: None reported via breastmilk exposure. Redness, induration and tenderness at site of injection. Inconsolable crying for up to 3 days following vaccination. Fever. Seizures. Lethargy. Shock-like state or hypotonic-hyporesponsive episodes have occurred within 48 hours of receiving pertussis containing vaccines. Hypersensitivity reactions to any of the components of the vaccine. Not recommended in those less than 6 weeks of age and in those more than 7 years of age. Avoid during on-going acute illnesses.

Drug Interactions: Immunological response and efficacy of vaccine is reduced when co-administered with corticosteroids, immunosuppressive agents, anti-cancer agents. Efficacy of vaccine also decreases when administered in immune-deficient states. As with all intramuscular injections, caution to be exercised while administering in an individual on anti-coagulant therapy.

Relative Infant Dose:

Adult Dose: 0.5 mL injection (IM)

Alternatives:

References:
1. Pharmaceutical manufacturer prescribing information, 2010.
2. Centers for Disease Control and Prevention (CDC). Updated recommendations for use of tetanus toxoid, reduced diphtheria toxoid and acellular pertussis vaccine (Tdap) in pregnant women and persons who have or anticipate having close contact with an infant aged <12 months --- Advisory Committee on Immunization Practices
3. Anon: Resource materials: general recommendations on immunization. Am J Prev Med 1994; 10(suppl): 60–82.
4. Schaefer CSchaefer C: Drugs During Pregnancy and Lactation, Elsevier Science B. V., Amsterdam, The Netherlands, 2001.
5. Atkinson W, Wolfe S, Hamborsky J, eds. 2011. Tetanus. "Centers for Disease Control and Prevention. Epidemiology and Prevention of Vaccine-Preventable Diseases". 12th ed. Washington DC: Public Health Foundation.

DIPHTHERIA + TETANUS VACCINE (DT/Td)   L3

Trade: DT, Td, Decavac (Td)

Other Trades: ADT (Td), CDT TM (DT), ADT TM (DT), Diftavax (Td)

Category: Vaccine

This is a combination vaccine containing both the diphtheria and tetanus toxoids. It is indicated for prevention of diphtheria and tetanus. Those currently licensed for use in the United States are DT and Td. The primary difference between these is that Td contains reduced diphtheria toxoid, making it suitable for use in adults and those more than 7 years of age. DT is recommended for those up to 7 years of age.

Diphtheria vaccine contains diphtheria toxoid, which is a formalin-inactivated form of diphtheria toxin. Diphtheria toxoid is almost always administered along with other vaccines such as tetanus toxoid vaccine and pertussis vaccine. Currently, no data are available on the transfer of diphtheria toxoid into human milk. However, diphtheria toxoid is considered compatible with breastfeeding.[1,2,3] The diphtheria toxoid is a large molecular weight protein toxoid. It is extremely unlikely that proteins of this size would transfer into breastmilk.

Tetanus toxoid vaccine contains a large molecular weight protein. It is always given in combination with diphtheria toxoid. Tetanus vaccine is made from inactivated tetanus toxoid by formaldehyde.[4] Tetanus vaccine is part of Tdap, DT, Td, DTaP, Pediarix, Pentacel and DTP vaccines. Because tetanus vaccine is an inactivated bacterial product, there is no specific contraindication in breastfeeding following injection with these vaccine. It is extremely unlikely proteins of this size would be secreted in breastmilk.

The diphtheria toxoid + tetanus toxoid vaccine combination (Td) is considered compatible with breastfeeding.

Pregnancy Risk	C		Lactation Risk	L3
T ½	=		M/P	=
Vd	=		PB	=
Tmax	=		Oral	=
MW	=		pKa	=

Adult Concerns: Swelling, redness, tenderness at the site of injection, fretfulness, drowsiness, anorexia, vomiting, headache. Hypersensitivity reactions to any of the components of the vaccine. Avoid during on-going acute illness. Guillan-Barre syndrome may occur within 6 weeks of receipt of a tetanus-toxoid containing vaccine.

Pediatric Concerns: None reported via breastmilk exposure. Redness, induration and tenderness at site of injection. Inconsolable crying for up to 3 days following vaccination. Fever, seizures, lethargy and a shock-like state or hypotonic-hyporesponsive episodes have occurred within 48 hours of receiving pertussis containing vaccines. Hypersensitivity reactions to any of the components of the vaccine. Not recommended in those less than 6 weeks of age and in those more than 7 years of age. Avoid during on-going acute illnesses.

Drug Interactions: Immunological response and efficacy of vaccine is reduced when coadministered with corticosteroids, immunosuppressive agents, anti-cancer agents. Efficacy of vaccine also decreases when administered in immune-deficient states. As with all intramuscular injections, caution to be exercised while administering in an individual on anti-coagulant therapy.

Relative Infant Dose:

Adult Dose: 0.5 ml injection intramuscular

Alternatives:

References:
1. Anon: Resource materials: general recommendations on immunization. Am J Prev Med 1994; 10(suppl): 60–82.
2. Schaefer CSchaefer C: Drugs During Pregnancy and Lactation, Elsevier Science B. V., Amsterdam, The Netherlands, 2001.
3. Product Information: Infanrix(R), diphtheria and tetanus toxoids and acellular pertussis vaccine adsorbed. GlaxoSmithKline Biologicals, Research Triangle Park, NC, 2003.
4. Atkinson W, Wolfe S, Hamborsky J, eds. 2011. Tetanus. "Centers for Disease Control and Prevention. Epidemiology and Prevention of Vaccine-Preventable Diseases". 12th ed. Washington DC: Public Health Foundation.

DIPHTHERIA VACCINE   L3

Trade: Diphtheria vaccine
Other Trades:
Category: Vaccine

Diphtheria vaccine contains diphtheria toxoid, which is a formalin-inactivated form of diphtheria toxin. Diphtheria toxoid, when injected, induces an immunological response against diphtheria toxin by producing anti-diphtheria antibodies. Adequate titres of anti-diphtheria antibodies in the serum protects the individual from subsequent diphtheria infection. Diphtheria toxoid is almost always administered along with other vaccines such as tetanus toxoid vaccine and pertussis vaccine. The use of diphtheria toxoid, alone is not recommended, especially in those 7 years of age and older, due to the risk of adverse reactions. Diphtheria toxoid alone however, is reserved for use in those pediatric patients in whom the use of tetanus toxoid and/or pertussis vaccine is contraindicated.

Currently, no data are available on the transfer of diphtheria toxoid into human milk. However, diphtheria toxoid is considered compatible with breastfeeding.[1,2] The diphtheria toxoid is a large molecular weight protein toxoid. It is extremely unlikely that proteins of this size would transfer into breastmilk. Remember, the use of combination vaccines of diphtheria, tetanus toxoid, and pertussis (adsorbed DTP/DTaP), is contraindicated in adults and those older than 7 years of age due to increased risk of adverse reactions.[3] But the combination of diphtheria and tetanus toxoid (Td) may be safely used in all adults, including breastfeeding women.

Pregnancy Risk	C	Lactation Risk	L3
T ½	=	M/P	=
Vd	=	PB	=
Tmax	=	Oral	=
MW	=	pKa	=

Adult Concerns: Redness, tenderness and induration at the site of injection.

Pediatric Concerns:

Drug Interactions: Should not be administered while individual is on immunosuppressive agents or on corticosteroids. Avoid administration at the time of ongoing acute infections.

Relative Infant Dose:

Adult Dose:

Alternatives:

References:
1. Anon: Resource materials: general recommendations on immunization. Am J Prev Med 1994; 10(suppl): 60–82.
2. Schaefer C: Drugs During Pregnancy and Lactation, Elsevier Science B. V., Amsterdam, The Netherlands, 2001.
3. Product Information: Infanrix(R), diphtheria and tetanus toxoids and acellular pertussis vaccine adsorbed. Glaxo Smith Kline Biologicals, Research Triangle Park, NC, 2003.

DIPIVEFRIN   L2

Trade: AK-Pro, Propine

Other Trades: Propine, PSM-Dipivefrin

Category: Adrenergic for glaucoma

Dipivefrin is a synthetic prodrug that is metabolized to epinephrine although it is only used topically in the eye. Because of its structure, it is more lipophilic and better absorbed into the eye; hence, it is more potent.[1] Following absorption into the eye, dipivefrin reduces intraocular pressure. It is not known if dipivefrin enters milk, but small amounts may be present. It is unlikely that any dipivefrin or epinephrine present in milk would be orally bioavailable to the infant.

Pregnancy Risk	B	Lactation Risk	L2
T ½	=	M/P	=
Vd	=	PB	=
Tmax	= 1 hour	Oral	= Minimal
MW	=	pKa	=

Adult Concerns: Infrequently, tachycardia, arrhythmias, hypertension have occurred with intraocular epinephrine. Burning, itching, tearing, hyperemia of eyes, redness of the eyes, burning and stinging have been reported.

Pediatric Concerns: None via milk.

Drug Interactions: When admixed with a pilocarpine Ocusert system, a transient increase in myopia was reported.

Relative Infant Dose:

Adult Dose: 1 drop in affected eye every 12 hours.

Alternatives:

References:
1. Pharmaceutical manufacturer prescribing information, 2010.

DIPYRIDAMOLE   L3

Trade: Persantine
Other Trades: Persantin, Apo-Dipyridamole, Novo-Dipiradol
Category: Vasodilator, antiplatelet agent

Dipyridamole is most commonly used in addition to coumarin anticoagulants to prevent thromboembolic complications of cardiac valve replacement. According to the manufacturer, only small amounts are believed to be secreted in human milk.[1] No reported untoward effects have been reported.

Pregnancy Risk	B	Lactation Risk	L3
T ½	= 10–12 hours	M/P	=
Vd	= 2–3 l/kg	PB	= 91–99%
Tmax	= 45–150 minutes	Oral	= Poor
MW	= 505	pKa	= 15.40

Adult Concerns: Headache, dizziness, gastrointestinal distress, nausea, vomiting, diarrhea, flushing.

Pediatric Concerns: No untoward effects have been reported.

Drug Interactions: When used with Heparin, may increase anticoagulation. Theophylline may reduce the hypotensive effect of dipyridamole.

Relative Infant Dose:

Adult Dose: 75–100 mg QID

Alternatives:

References:
1. Pharmaceutical manufacturer prescribing information, 1995.

DIRITHROMYCIN   L3

Trade: Dynabac

Other Trades:

Category: Macrolide antibiotic

Dirithromycin is a macrolide antibiotic similar to erythromycin but is characterized by low serum levels and high tissue levels.[1] Dirithromycin is metabolized to erythromycyclamine which is the active component. No data on the transfer of erythromycyclamine into human milk are available. Due to the kinetics of dirithromycin and its distribution largely to tissues, it is unlikely that major levels in milk will result. Suitable alternatives include azithromycin and clarithromycin.

Pregnancy Risk	C	Lactation Risk	L3
T ½	= 20–50 hours	M/P	=
Vd	= 11 l/kg	PB	= 15–30%
Tmax	= 3.9 hours	Oral	= 6–14%
MW	=	pKa	= 12.97

Adult Concerns: Gastrointestinal distress, abdominal pain, diarrhea, nausea, vomiting, skin rash, headache and dizziness. Changes in liver function have been reported.

Pediatric Concerns: None reported via milk. Suitable alternatives are erythromycin and azithromycin.

Drug Interactions: Increased anticoagulant effect when used with warfarin, dicoumarol, phenindione, and anisindione. Dirithromycin may increase the level of astemizole significantly. May increase digoxin levels. Acute and dangerous toxicity have resulted following use of dirithromycin with ergot alkaloids. Increased serum levels of pimozide and triazolam may result.

Relative Infant Dose:

Adult Dose: 500 mg daily.

Alternatives: Azithromycin, clarithromycin

References:
1. Pharmaceutical manufacturer prescribing information, 2011.

DISOPYRAMIDE   L2

Trade: Norpace, Napamide

Other Trades: Norpace, Rythmodan, Isomide

Category: Antiarrhythmic

Disopyramide is used for treating cardiac arrhythmias similar to quinidine and procainamide. Small levels are secreted into milk. Following a maternal dose of 450 mg every 8 hours for two weeks, the milk/plasma ratio was approximately 1.06 for disopyramide and 6.24 for its active metabolite.[1] Although no disopyramide was measurable in the infant's plasma, the milk levels were 2.6–4.4 mg/L (disopyramide), and 9.6–12.3 mg/L (metabolite). Infant urine collected over an 8-hour period contained 3.3 mg/L of disopyramide. Such levels are probably too small to affect an infant. No side effects were reported.

In another study, in a woman receiving 100 mg five times daily, the maternal serum level was 10.3 µmol/L and the breast milk level was 4.0 µmol/L, giving a milk/serum ratio of 0.4.[2] From these levels, an infant ingesting 1 liter of milk would receive only 1.5 mg per day. Lowest milk levels are at 6–8 hours post-dose.

Pregnancy Risk	C	Lactation Risk	L2
T ½	= 8.3–11.65 hours	M/P	= 0.4–1.06
Vd	= 0.6–1.3 l/kg	PB	= 50%
Tmax	= 2.3 hours	Oral	= 60–83%
MW	= 339	pKa	= 8.4

Adult Concerns: Dry mouth, constipation, edema, hypotension, nausea, vomiting, diarrhea.

Pediatric Concerns: None reported.

Drug Interactions: Increased side effects with drugs such as phenytoin, phenobarbital, rifampin. Increased effects/toxicity with rifamycin. Increased plasma levels of digoxin.

Relative Infant Dose: 3.4%

Adult Dose: 150 mg every 6 hours

Alternatives:

References:
1. MacKintosh D, Buchanan N. Excretion of disopyramide in human breast milk. Br J Clin Pharmacol 1985; 19(6): 856–857.
2. Ellsworth AJ, Horn JR, Raisys VA, Miyagawa LA, Bell JL. Disopyramide and N-monodesalkyl disopyramide in serum and breast milk. DICP 1989; 23(1): 56–57.

DISULFIRAM   L5

Trade: Antabuse

Other Trades: Antabuse

Category: Inhibitor of alcohol metabolism

Disulfiram is an old product that is occasionally used to prevent alcohol consumption in chronic alcoholics.[1,2] Disulfiram inhibits the enzyme, aldehyde dehydrogenase (ADH), which is one of the two enzymes responsible for the metabolism of alcohol. Patients receiving disulfiram, and who ingest alcohol, become extremely nauseated due to elevated plasma levels of acetaldehyde. This also results in flushing, thirst, palpitations, chest pain, vertigo, and hypotension. All sources of alcohol should be avoided including mouthwash, cough syrups, and after-shave.

There are no data on the transfer of disulfiram into human milk, but due to its small molecular weight, it likely penetrates milk to some degree. Because it produces an irreversible inhibition of aldehyde dehydrogenase, any absorbed via milk could potentially produce long-lasting inhibition of the infants' ADH. With the ingestion of any alcohol containing product, the infant could become seriously ill. Further, because the enzyme is permanently inhibited, the individual will be susceptible to alcohol toxicity for up to 2 weeks following discontinuing of the medication. Because so many products contain small amounts of alcohol (cough syrups, etc.), the use of this product in breastfeeding mothers is extremely risky and probably does not justify continued breastfeeding unless the mother is warned and compliant.

Pregnancy Risk	C	Lactation Risk	L5
T ½	=	M/P	=
Vd	=	PB	= 96%
Tmax	= 1–2 hours	Oral	= 80–90%
MW	= 296	pKa	= 13.14

Adult Concerns: Symptoms primarily occur following ingestion of alcohol, and include ectopic heartbeats, tachycardia, chest pain, angina, palpitations, hypertension, headache, severe nausea and vomiting, leg and muscle cramps, dyspnea and shortness of breath.

Pediatric Concerns: None reported via milk, but with ingestion of alcohol could produce profound symptoms in infant.

Drug Interactions: Severe reactions may occur with any product containing alcohol. Concomitant therapy with amitriptyline or metronidazole has resulted in a confusional and psychotic mental state. When used with anisindione or dicumarol, an increased hypoprothrombinemic effect has been documented. Use with bacampicillin has resulted in a disulfiram-type reaction. Significantly increased plasma levels of chlordiazepoxide and diazepam, phenytoin and fosphenytoin when coadministered with disulfiram. An increased half-life and plasma level of desipramine.

Relative Infant Dose:

Adult Dose: 250 mg daily

Alternatives:

References:
1. Pharmaceutical manufacturer prescribing information, 2010.
2. McEvoy GE. (ed): AFHS Drug Information. New York, NY: 2003.

DOBUTAMINE   L2

Trade: Dobutrex

Other Trades: Dobutrex

Category: Adrenergic stimulant

Dobutamine is an isoproterenol derivative that stimulates beta-1 receptors with less effects on beta-2 and alpha receptors in the heart.[1] Dobutamine is a catecholamine pressor agent used in shock and severe hypotension.[2] It is rapidly destroyed in the gastrointestinal tract and are only used IV. It is not known if dobutamine transfers into human milk, but the half-life is so short they would not last long.

Pregnancy Risk	B	Lactation Risk	L2
T ½	= 2 minutes	M/P	=
Vd	= 0.2 l/kg	PB	=
Tmax	=	Oral	=
MW	= 301	pKa	= 10.79

Adult Concerns: Fever, nausea, headache, tachycardia, arrhythmia, palpitation, chest pain, dyspnea.

Pediatric Concerns:

Drug Interactions:

Relative Infant Dose:

Adult Dose: 2.5–20 µg/kg/min IV

Alternatives:

References:
1. Tuttle RR, Mills J. Dobutamine: development of a new catecholamine to selectively increase cardiac contractility. Circ Res. 1975 Jan; 36(1): 185–96.
2. McEvoy GE. (ed): AFHS Drug Information. New York, NY: 2003.

DOCETAXEL   L5

Trade: Taxotere

Other Trades:

Category: Anticancer drug

Docetaxel is an antineoplastic agent derived from the yew plant. It has a large molecular weight of 861 daltons and acts by disrupting the mitotic and interphase cellular functions. Docetaxel's pharmacokinetic profile is consistent with a three-compartment kinetic model, with half-lives for the alpha, beta and gamma of 4 min, 36 min, and 11.1 hours, respectively. Oral bioavailability is just 8%. The initial rapid decline represents distribution to the peripheral compartments, and the late (terminal) phase is due, in part, to a relatively slow efflux of docetaxel from the peripheral compartment. Mean value for steady state volume of distribution is 113 L.[1] Within seven days, urinary and fecal excretion accounted for approximately 6% and 75% of the administered radioactivity, respectively. About 80% of the radioactivity recovered in feces is excreted during the first 48 hours, as metabolites with very small amounts (less than 8%) of unchanged drug. No data are available on its transfer into human milk. Due to its large molecular weight and high protein binding, milk levels are probably quite low. Withhold breastfeeding for a minimum of four to five days.

Pregnancy Risk	D	Lactation Risk	L5
T ½	= 11.1 hours (gamma)	M/P	=
Vd	= 1.6 l/kg	PB	= 95%
Tmax	=	Oral	=
MW	= 807.9	pKa	= 12.02

Adult Concerns: Swelling of abdomen, face, fingers, hands, feet, or lower legs, tiredness or weakness, weight gain.

Pediatric Concerns:

Drug Interactions:

Relative Infant Dose:

Adult Dose:

Alternatives:

References:
1. Pharmaceutical manufacturer prescribing information, 2005.

DOCOSAHEXAENOIC ACID (DHA)　　　L3

Trade:
Other Trades:
Category: N-3 Fatty Acid

Docosahexaenoic Acid (DHA)(C22–6) is a N-3 fatty acid that is a precursor of alpha linolenic acid. Fish that live in cold water are high in DHA content. The central nervous system and retina contain high amounts of DHA. The DHA accumulation in the brain is most rapid during the last trimester of pregnancy and the first year of life. The first year of life is thought to have critical windows when DHA is most important to infant development. Animal studies with nonhuman primates suggest that DHA enhances the development of the brain's neurotransmitter systems such as the dopaminergic and serotoninergic systems. Amounts of DHA vary between cultures with those who have a high intake of oceanic fish having the highest DHA levels. Breast milk contains DHA in varying levels depending on mother's diet. Most infant formulas now contain added DHA.

Large maternal doses should be used with great caution in breastfeeding mothers, diabetics, and patients with bleeding disorders. Because this lipid is selectively transferred into human milk, milk levels could be high and potentially hazardous to an infant. Daily doses in breastfeeding mothers should probably not exceed 300 mg/day (International Society for the Study of Fatty Acids and Lipids).

Pregnancy Risk	Probably Safe	Lactation Risk	L3
T ½	= 20 hours	M/P	=
Vd	=	PB	=
Tmax	=	Oral	= Complete
MW	= 328	pKa	=

Adult Concerns: Nausea, flatulence, bruising, and prolonged bleeding, fishy taste, decreased glucose tolerance, increased blood glucose, reduced plasma insulin in type II diabetics, belching, nosebleeds, nausea, and loose stools.

Pediatric Concerns:

Drug Interactions:

Relative Infant Dose:

Adult Dose: 300 mg/day

Alternatives:

References:
1. Carlson SE. Docosahexaenoic acid supplementation in pregnancy and lactation. Am J Clin Nutr. 2009 Feb; 89(2): 678S-84S. Epub 2008 Dec 30.

DOCOSANOL   L3

Trade:

Other Trades:

Category: Antiviral

Docosanol, also called behenyl alcohol, is a fatty alcohol use in cosmetics as a thickener, emulsifier, and an emollient. It is also approved as an antiviral agent to treatment of oral-facial herpes simplex only. It should not be used in the eyes or on the genitalia. It inhibits lipid-enveloped viruses from entering the cell by fusion between the plasma membrane and the viral envelope.[1] There have been no studies on docosanol in breastmilk, however it is not orally absorbed and therefore probably poses little threat to a nursing infant.

Pregnancy Risk	Probably Safe	Lactation Risk	L3
T ½	=	M/P	=
Vd	=	PB	=
Tmax	=	Oral	= Nil
MW	= 327	pKa	=

Adult Concerns: Adverse effects include headache, rash, and increased redness.

Pediatric Concerns: No data are available but it would be orally unabsorbed in an infant.

Drug Interactions:

Relative Infant Dose:

Adult Dose: Apply topically 5 times daily to lesions until healed.

Alternatives:

References:
1. Pharmaceutical manufacturer prescribing information, 2008.

DOCUSATE   L2

Trade:

Other Trades:

Category: Laxative, stool softener

Docusate is a detergent commonly used as a stool softener. The degree of oral absorption is poor, but some is known to be absorbed and re-secreted in the bile. Although some drug is absorbed by mother via her gastrointestinal tract, transfer into breastmilk is unknown but probably minimal. Watch for loose stools in infant. It is not likely this would be overly detrimental to a breastfed infant.

Pregnancy Risk	C	Lactation Risk	L2
T ½	=	M/P	=
Vd	=	PB	=
Tmax	=	Oral	= Poor
MW	= 444	pKa	=

Adult Concerns: Nausea, diarrhea.

Pediatric Concerns: None reported. Observe for loose stools.

Drug Interactions: Decreased effect of coumadin with high doses of docusate. Increased toxicity with mineral oil, phenolphthalein.

Relative Infant Dose:

Adult Dose: 50–200 mg daily.

Alternatives:

References:
1. Pharmaceutical manufacturer prescribing information, 2003.

DOLASETRON   L3

Trade: Anzemet

Other Trades:

Category: Antinauseant and antiemetic

Dolasetron mesylate and its active metabolite, hydrodolasetron, are selective serotonin 5–HT3 receptor antagonists, primarily in the chemoreceptor trigger zone responsible for control of nausea and vomiting. It is believed that chemotherapeutic agents release serotonin in the gastrointestinal tract that then activates the 5–HT3 receptors on the vagus nerve that initiates the vomiting reflex. This product is used prior to treatment with cancer chemotherapeutic agents, or prior to surgery and general anesthesia.[1]

No data are available on its transfer into milk. The maximum concentration in maternal plasma would be 556 ng/mL, which is quite low. At this plasma level and assuming a 1: 1 milk/plasma ratio, an infant would likely receive far less than a milligram daily. It has been safely used in children 2 years of age at doses of 1.2 mg/kg.

Pregnancy Risk	B	Lactation Risk	L3
T ½	= 8.1 hours	M/P	=
Vd	= 5.8 l/kg	PB	= 77%
Tmax	= 1 hour	Oral	= 75%
MW	= 438	pKa	= 18.25

Adult Concerns: Changes in ECG intervals (PR, QT prolongation, and QRS widening) have been reported but are dose related. Use cautiously in patients with hypokalemia or hypomagnesemia, patients on diuretics, or patients on other antiarrhythmics. Side effects include headache, fatigue, diarrhea, bradycardia.

Pediatric Concerns: None reported via milk.

Drug Interactions: Drug-drug interactions are few, but include rifampin, and cimetidine.

Relative Infant Dose:

Adult Dose: 100 mg orally.

Alternatives:

References:
1. Pharmaceutical manufacturer prescribing information, 2011.

DOMPERIDONE   L1

Trade:

Other Trades: Motilium, Motilidone

Category: Gastrokinetic agent, galactagogue

Domperidone is a peripheral dopamine antagonist (similar to Reglan) generally used for controlling nausea and vomiting, dyspepsia, and gastric reflux. It blocks peripheral dopamine receptors in the gastrointestinal wall and in the CRTZ (nausea center) in the brain stem and is currently used in Canada as an antiemetic.[1] Unlike metoclopramide (Reglan), it does not enter the brain compartment and it has few CNS effects such as depression.

It is also known to produce significant increases in prolactin levels and has proven useful as a galactagogue. Serum prolactin levels have been found to increase from 8.1 ng/mL to 124.1 ng/mL in non-lactating women after one 20 mg dose.[2] Concentrations of domperidone reported in milk vary according to dose. But following a dose of 10 mg three times daily, the average concentration in milk was only 2.6 µg/L.[3]

In a study by da Silva, 16 mothers with premature infants and low milk production (mean= 112.8 mL/day in domperidone group; 48.2 mL/day in placebo group) were randomly chosen to receive placebo (n= 9) or domperidone (10 mg TID) (n= 7) for 7 days.[4] Milk volume increased from 112.8 to 162.2 mL/day in the domperidone group and 48.2 to 56.1 mL/day in the placebo group. Prolactin levels increased from 12.9 to 119.3 µg/L in the domperidone group and 15.6 to 18.1 µg/L in the placebo group. On day 5, the mean domperidone concentration was 6.6 ng/mL in plasma and 1.2 µg/L in breastmilk of the treated group (n= 6). No adverse effects were reported in infants or mothers.

In a new study just released, a group of 6 breastfeeding women were placed in a double blind randomized crossover trial to compare doses of domperidone.[5] In this trial, mothers were studied in a run-in phase (no drug treatment), 30 mg, or 60 mg domperidone daily doses (10 or 20 mg every 8 hours). Milk volume created per hour, and plasma prolactin levels were monitored. With milk production, two mothers did not respond to domperidone treatment. Four other mothers showed a significant increase from 8.7 gm/hour in the run-in phase to 23.6 gm/hour for the 30 mg/day dose, to 29.4 gm/hour for the 60 mg dose. While plasma prolactin levels were increased by domperidone treatment, there was only a slight increase in milk production at the 60 mg dose. Median domperidone concentrations in milk were 0.28 µg/L and 0.49 µg/L for the 30 mg and 60 mg doses respectively. The mean Relative Infant Dose was 0.012% at 30 mg daily and 0.009% at the 60 mg/day dose. The authors suggest that milk production increased at both doses and there was a small trend for a dose-response.

Forty-six mothers who had delivered infants at <31 weeks' gestation, and who experienced lactation failure, were randomly assigned to receive domperidone or placebo for 14 days.[6] Protein, energy, fat, carbohydrate, sodium, calcium, and phosphate levels in breast milk were measured on days 0, 4, 7, and 14, serum prolactin levels were measured on days 0, 4, and 14, and total milk production was recorded daily. By day 14, breast milk volumes has increased by 267% in the domperidone-treated group and by 18.5% in the placebo group. Serum prolactin increased by 97% in the domperidone group and by 17% in the placebo group. Mean breast milk protein declined by 9.6% in the domperidone group and increased by 3.6% in the placebo group. There were no changes in caloric content, fat, carbohydrate, sodium, or phosphate content. Significant increases in milk carbohydrate (2.7% vs -2.7%) and calcium (61.8% vs -4.4%) were noted in the domperidone-treated group. No adverse effects were observed in infants or mothers. The authors concluded that domperidone increases the volume of breast milk of preterm mothers experiencing lactation failure, without substantially altering the nutrient composition.

In a recent study to determine the effect of withdrawal on subsequent milk production, 25 women who initially received domperidone (20 mg 4 times daily) were gently withdrawn stepwise over a period of 2–4 weeks, from 20 mg QID to 10 mg QID to nil.[8] Formula use was reported during this duration. Twenty three of twenty five cases (93%) reported no significant increase in formula use after stopping domperidone. Normal infant growth was reported in all cases. The authors concluded that following a slow withdrawal from domperidone, there is no significant increase in formula supplementation. This clearly suggests that once sufficient milk production is reestablished, it is maintained even without the use of domperidone.

The usual oral dose for controlling gastrointestinal distress is 10–20 mg three to four times daily although for nausea and vomiting the dose can be higher (up to 40 mg). The galactagogue dose is suggested to be 10–20 mg orally 3–4 times daily. The prior studies clearly suggest that doses of 10–20 mg three to four times daily elevate prolactin levels to levels more than adequate to produce milk. Doses higher than this should be avoided in breastfeeding mothers.

The US FDA has issued a warning on this product stating that it could induce arrhythmias in patients. These claims were derived from data many years old where domperidone was used intravenously as an antiemetic during cancer chemotherapy (20 mg stat followed by 10 mg/kg/24 hours).[7] Many of these patients were undergoing extensive chemotherapy, were extremely ill, and hypokalemic to begin with. In addition, intravenous domperidone produces plasma levels many times higher than oral use.

Nevertheless, domperidone is known to prolong the QT interval of the heart in some patients which is highly dose-related. Doses should be kept to less than 10–20 mg three to four times daily. There is no evidence that doses higher than this increase prolactin levels above these lower doses, but they may dramatically increase the risk of prolonged QT interval in patients. In addition, a slow withdrawal is strongly recommended to prevent loss of milk production, and a potential dysphoric withdrawal. Do not use in patients with a preexisting prolonged QT interval.

Pregnancy Risk	C	Lactation Risk	L1
T ½	= 7–14 hours	M/P	= 0.25
Vd	=	PB	= 93%
Tmax	= 30 minutes	Oral	= 13–17%
MW	= 426	pKa	= 13.14

Adult Concerns: Dry mouth, skin rash, itching, headache, thirst, abdominal cramps, diarrhea, drowsiness. Seizures have occurred rarely. Could induce arrhythmias in hypokalemic patients, or patients subject to arrhythmias (prolonged QT interval).

Pediatric Concerns: None reported in breastfed infants. Considered the ideal galactagogue.

Drug Interactions: Cimetidine, famotidine, nizatidine, ranitidine (H-2 blocker) plasma levels may be reduced by domperidone. Prior use of bicarbonate reduces absorption of domperidone. Alfuzosin, artemether, chloroquine, ciprofloxacin, ketoconazole, itraconazole, diltiazem, verapamil, grapefruit juice, erythromycin, clarithromycin, dronedarone, gadobutrol, lumefantrine, nilotinib, pimozide, quinine, tetrabenazine, thioridazine, ziprasidone, amiodarone, arsenic trioxide, astemizole, bepridil, chloroquine, chlorpromazine, cisapride, disopyramide, dofetilide, droperidol, halofantrine, aloperidol, ibutilide, evomethadyl, mesoridazine, methadone, pentamidine, pimozide, probucol, procainamide, sotalol, sparfloxacin, terfenadine enhance QT prolonging effect of domperidone

Relative Infant Dose: 0.01%–0.04%

Adult Dose: 10–20 mg 3–4 times daily

Alternatives: Metoclopramide

References:
1. Hofmeyr GJ, van Iddekinge B. Domperidone and lactation. Lancet 1983; 1(8325): 647.
2. Brouwers JR, Assies J, Wiersinga WM, Huizing G, Tytgat GN. Plasma prolactin levels after acute and subchronic oral administration of domperidone and of metoclopramide: a cross-over study in healthy volunteers. Clin Endocrinol (Oxf) 1980; 12(5): 435–440.
3. Hofmeyr GJ, van Iddekinge B, Blott JA. Domperidone: secretion in breast milk and effect on puerperal prolactin levels. Br J Obstet Gynaecol 1985; 92(2): 141–144.
4. da Silva OP, Knoppert DC, Angelini MM, Forret PA. Effect of domperidone on milk production in mothers of premature newborns: a randomized, double-blind, placebo-controlled trial. CMAJ 2001; 164(1): 17–21.
5. Wan E W-X, Davey K, Page-Sharp M, Hartmann PE, Simmer K, Ilett KF. Dose-effect study of domperidone as a galactagogue in preterm mothers with insufficient milk supply, and its transfer into milk. British Journal of Clinical Pharmacology 2008; 66(2): 283–289.
6. Campbell-Yeo ML, Allen AC, Joseph KS, Ledwidge JM, Caddell K, Allen VM, Dooley KC. Effect of domperidone on the composition of preterm human breast milk. Pediatrics. 2010 Jan; 125(1): e107–14. Epub 2009 Dec 14.
7. Osborne RJ, Slevin ML, Hunter RW, Hamer J. Cardiac arrhythmias during cytotoxic chemotherapy: role of domperidone. Hum Toxicol 1985 Nov; 4(6): 617–26.
8. Livingston V, Blaga Stancheva L, Stringer J. The effect of withdrawing domperidone on formula supplementation. Breastfeeding Med. 2007; 2: 278, Abstract 3.

DONEPEZIL   L3

Trade: Aricept

Other Trades: Aricept

Category: Cholinesterase inhibitor in Alzheimer's disease

Donepezil is a reversible inhibitor of acetylcholinesterase which ultimately increases synaptic levels of acetylcholine by inhibition of its breakdown. It is believed to improve mild to moderate dementia and cognitive function in patients with Alzheimer's disease. While this agent is only 'cleared' for treatment of patients with Alzheimer's disease, numerous other applications probably exist. No data are available on its transfer to human milk. Due to its long half-life, and its ability to affect cholinergic function in all mammals, some caution is recommended in breastfeeding women until data are available.

Pregnancy Risk	C	Lactation Risk	L3
T½	= 70 hours	M/P	=
Vd	= 12 l/kg	PB	= 96%
Tmax	= 3–4 hours	Oral	= 100%
MW	= 415	pKa	= 9.1

Adult Concerns: May impede bladder emptying. Seizures, and convulsions have been reported. Increase gastric acid secretion. Patients at risk would be those subject to ulcers, using concurrent NSAIDs. Diarrhea, nausea, vomiting, muscle cramps, fatigue and loss of appetite have been reported. Should be used cautiously in patients with pulmonary diseases such as asthma.

Pediatric Concerns: None reported via milk.

Drug Interactions: Use cautiously with NSAIDs. Interfere with activity of anticholinergics such as atropine.

Relative Infant Dose:

Adult Dose: 5–10 mg daily.

Alternatives:

References:
1.   Pharmaceutical manufacturer prescribing information, 2003.

DOPAMINE   L2

Trade: Intropin, Revimine

Other Trades:

Category: Adrenergic stimulants

Dopamine is a catecholamine pressor agent used in shock and severe hypotension.[1] It is rapidly destroyed in the gastrointestinal tract and is only used IV. It is not known if it transfers into human milk, but the half-life is so short they would not last long. Dopamine, while in the plasma, significantly (>60%) inhibits prolactin secretion and would likely inhibit lactation while being used.

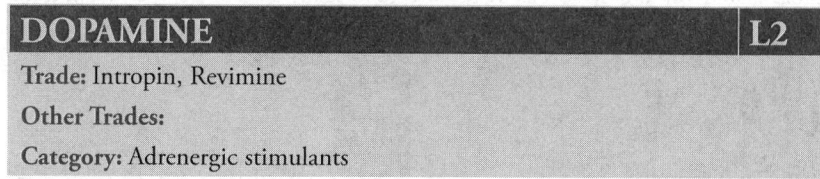

Pregnancy Risk	C		Lactation Risk	L2
T ½	= 2 minutes		M/P	=
Vd	=		PB	=
Tmax	= 5 minutes		Oral	=
MW	= 153		pKa	= 12.93

Adult Concerns: Stimulation, agitation, tachycardia.

Pediatric Concerns: None reported. No gastrointestinal absorption.

Drug Interactions: Caution to be exercised while coadministered dopamine with halogenated anesthetics due to increased cardiovascular risk. Do not administer with phenytoin due to increased risk of hypotension and bradycardia. Concomitant use with other vasopressors and oxytocin may cause hypertension. Effects of dopamine potentiated when coadministered with monoamine oxidase inhibitors and tricyclic antidepressants. Effects of dopamine antagonized when used with beta-blockers like metoprolol.

Relative Infant Dose:

Adult Dose: 1–50 µg/kg/min IV

Alternatives:

References:
1.   McEvoy GE. (ed): AFHS Drug Information. New York, NY: 2003.

DORIPENEM   L3

Trade: Doribax
Other Trades:
Category: Antibiotic

Doripenem is a new carbapenem antibiotic similar in structure to the penicillins.[1] Doripenem is resistant to most beta-lactamases including penicillinases and cephalosporinases produced by gram-positive and gram-negative bacteria. It is cleared for treatment of various resistant bacteria. No data are available on its use in breastfeeding mothers, but levels in milk will likely be low, and the oral bioavailability in infants low as well. Observe for diarrhea and changes in gut flora.

Pregnancy Risk	B	Lactation Risk	L3
T ½	= 1 hour	M/P	=
Vd	= 0.24 l/kg	PB	= 8.1%
Tmax	= 1 hour	Oral	= Poor
MW	= 438	pKa	= 2.8, 7.9

Adult Concerns: Diarrhea, headache.

Pediatric Concerns: None reported but observe for changes in gut flora, diarrhea.

Drug Interactions: Doripenem reduces the plasma levels of valproic acid. Probenecid reduces clearance of doripenem.

Relative Infant Dose:

Adult Dose: 500 mg every 8 hours IV

Alternatives: Piperacillin/tazobactam and imipenem, levofloxacin

References:
1. Pharmaceutical manufacturer prescribing information, 2010.

DORNASE   L3

Trade: Pulmozyme
Other Trades: Pulmozyme
Category: Mucolytic enzyme

Dornase is a mucolytic enzyme used in the treatment of cystic fibrosis. It is a large molecular weight peptide (260 amino acids, 37,000 daltons) that selectively digests DNA.[1] It is poorly absorbed by the pulmonary tissues. Serum levels are undetectable. Even if it were to reach the milk, it would not be orally bioavailable in the infant.

Pregnancy Risk	B	Lactation Risk	L3
T ½	=	M/P	=
Vd	=	PB	=
Tmax	=	Oral	= None
MW	= 37,000	pKa	=

Adult Concerns: Hoarseness, sore throat, facial edema.

Pediatric Concerns: None reported.

Drug Interactions: Co-administration with probenecid increases plasma levels of dornase.

Relative Infant Dose:

Adult Dose: 2.5 mg via inhalation

Alternatives:

References:
1. Pharmaceutical manufacturer prescribing information, 1995.

DORZOLAMIDE   L3

Trade: Trusopt

Other Trades:

Category: Carbonic anhydrase inhibitor for open-angle glaucoma

Dorzolamide is a carbonic anhydrase inhibitor used to treat intraocular hypertension, open-angle glaucoma, etc. It is a unique formulation that exerts its effects directly in the eye. No data are available on its transfer into human milk. However, this product is only slightly absorbed by the mother. This agent is stored for long periods in the red blood cell, although plasma levels are exceedingly low.[1] Milk levels will probably be low to undetectable.

Pregnancy Risk	C	Lactation Risk	L3
T ½	=	M/P	=
Vd	=	PB	= 33%
Tmax	= 2 hours	Oral	=
MW	= 361	pKa	= 19.43

Adult Concerns: Bitter or unusual taste, allergic reactions, contact dermatitis in the throat, vertigo, dizziness, This is a sulfonamide, so do not use in sulfa-allergic patients.

Pediatric Concerns: No breastfeeding studies thus far. Risks are probably minimal.

Drug Interactions: Do not use with topiramate.

Relative Infant Dose:

Adult Dose: One drop in eye three times daily.

Alternatives:

References:
1. Pharmaceutical manufacturer prescribing information, 2005.

DOTHIEPIN   L2

Trade: Prothiaden
Other Trades: Dothep, Prothiaden
Category: Tricyclic antidepressant

This is a new analog of the older tricyclic antidepressant amitriptyline. Dothiepin appears in breastmilk in a concentration of 11 µg/L following a dose of 75 mg/day while the maternal plasma level was 33 µg/L.[1] If the infant ingests 150 mL/kg/day of milk, the total daily dose of dothiepin ingested by the infant in this case would be approximately 1.7 µg/kg/day, approximately 1/650th of the adult dose. In an outcome study of 15 mother/infant pairs 3–5 years postpartum, no overall cognitive differences were noted in dothiepin treated mothers/infants, suggesting that this medication did not alter cognitive abilities in breastfed infants.[2]

In a study by Ilett[3], dothiepin concentrations in the milk of 8 mothers was determined (dose ranged from 25–225 mg/day). The mean post-feeding milk/plasma ratio was 1.59 and the mean post-feeding dothiepin concentration in milk ranged from 20–475 µg/L (median=52 µg/L). Mean daily infant doses on a weight basis (in dothiepin equivalents) was 4.4% for dothiepin and its metabolites. Blood levels in all 5 infants were low (>10 µg/L). No untoward effects were noted in any of the 8 infants following chronic maternal use.

Pregnancy Risk	D	Lactation Risk	L2
T ½	= 14.4–23.9 hours	M/P	= 0.3
Vd	= 20–92 l/kg	PB	=
Tmax	= 3 hours	Oral	= 30%
MW	= 295	pKa	= 8.5

Adult Concerns: Anticholinergic side effects, such as drying of secretions, dilated pupil, sedation, dizziness, drowsiness, urinary retention.

Pediatric Concerns: None reported in numerous studies.

Drug Interactions: Phenobarbital may reduce effect of dothiepin. Dothiepin blocks the hypotensive effect of guanethidine. May increase toxicity of dothiepin when used with clonidine. Dangerous when used with monoamine oxidase inhibitors, other CNS depressants. May increase anticoagulant effect of Coumadin, warfarin. SSRIs (Fluoxetine, sertraline etc) should not be used with or soon after dothiepin or other tricyclic antidepressants due to serotonergic crisis.

Relative Infant Dose: 0.8%–2.2%

Adult Dose: 75–300 mg/day

Alternatives:

References:
1.   Rees JA. Serum and breast milk concentrations of dotheipin. Practitioner 1976; 217: 686.

2. Buist A, Janson H. Effect of exposure to dothiepin and northiaden in breast milk on child development. Br J Psychiatry 1995; 167(3): 370–373.
3. Ilett KF, Lebedevs TH, Wojnar-Horton RE, Yapp P, Roberts MJ, Dusci LJ, Hackett LP. The excretion of dothiepin and its primary metabolites in breast milk. Br J Clin Pharmacol 1992; 33(6): 635–639.

DOXAZOSIN   L4

Trade: Cardura

Other Trades: Carduran, Cardura

Category: Antiadrenergic antihypertensive

Doxazosin mesylate is an alpha-1 adrenergic receptor blocker indicated for use in hypertension and benign prostatic hyperplasia. Studies in lactating animals indicate milk levels that are 20 times that of maternal plasma levels, suggesting a concentrating mechanism in breastmilk.[1] It is not known if this occurs in human milk. Extreme caution recommended.

Pregnancy Risk	C	Lactation Risk	L4
T ½	= 9–22 hours	M/P	= 20
Vd	=	PB	= 98%
Tmax	= 2 hours	Oral	= 62–69%
MW	= 451	pKa	= 6.93

Adult Concerns: Low blood pressure, malaise, and edema.

Pediatric Concerns: None reported, but extreme caution is recommended.

Drug Interactions: Decreased antihypertensive effect with NSAIDs. Increased effect with other diuretics, antihypertensive medications particularly beta blockers.

Relative Infant Dose:

Adult Dose: 2–4 mg daily.

Alternatives: Propranolol, metoprolol

References:
1. Pharmaceutical manufacturer prescribing information, 2010.

DOXEPIN   L5

Trade: Adapin, Sinequan, Silenor

Other Trades: Deptran, Sinequan, Triadapin, Novo-Doxepin

Category: Antidepressant

Doxepin is a tricyclic antidepressant used in the treatment of depression, anxiety, and psychotic depressive disorders. It is also used in the treatment of insomnia and moderate pruritus of atopic dermatitis. Small but significant amounts are secreted in milk. Two published reports indicate absorption by infant varying from significant to modest. One report of dangerous sedation and respiratory arrest in one infant.[1] Doxepin has an active metabolite with long half-life (37 hours). In one study, peak milk doxepin levels were 27 and 29 µg/L 4–5 hours after a dose of

25 mg, and the level of metabolite was 9 μg/L.[2] In this infant, the metabolite was believed responsible for the severe depression. Although the milk concentrations were low, the infant's plasma level of metabolite was similar to the maternal plasma level. It is apparent that the active metabolite of doxepin can concentrate in nursing infants and may be hazardous.

In another case report of a mother ingesting 35 mg/day, the infant was readmitted to the neonatal intensive care unit at day 9 postpartum because of poor sucking and swallowing, muscle hypotonia, vomiting, drowsiness, and jaundice.[3] Doxepin levels in the infant were found in small amounts. Breastmilk levels were reported at 60–100 μg/L with a milk/plasma ratio of 1.0–1.7. Upon withdrawal of breastfeeding the infant rapidly became lively and active. We have numerous other antidepressants that are much safer and are preferred in breastfeeding mothers.

Pregnancy Risk	C	Lactation Risk	L5
T ½	= 8–24 hours	M/P	= 1.08–1.66
Vd	= 9–33 l/kg	PB	= 80–85%
Tmax	= 2 hours	Oral	= Complete
MW	= 279	pKa	= 8.0

Adult Concerns: Respiratory arrest, sedation, dry mouth.

Pediatric Concerns: One report of dangerous sedation and respiratory arrest in an infant. Poor sucking and swallowing, muscle hypotonia, vomiting, drowsiness and jaundice reported in a second infant.

Drug Interactions: Decreased effect of doxepin when used with bretylium, guanethidine, clonidine, levodopa, ascorbic acid and cholestyramine. Increased toxicity when used with carbamazepine, amphetamines, thyroid preparations. Increased toxicity with fluoxetine, thyroid preparations, monoamineoxidase inhibitors, albuterol, CNS depressants such as benzodiazepines and opiate analgesics, anticholinergics, cimetidine.

Relative Infant Dose: 1.2%–3%

Adult Dose: 75–300 mg daily.

Alternatives: Sertraline, paroxetine

References:
1. Matheson I, Pande H, Alertsen AR. Respiratory depression caused by N-desmethyldoxepin in breast milk. Lancet 1985; 2(8464): 1124.
2. Kemp J, Ilett KF, Booth J, Hackett LP. Excretion of doxepin and N-desmethyldoxepin in human milk. Br J Clin Pharmacol 1985; 20(5): 497–499.
3. Frey OR, Scheidt P, von Brenndorff AI. Adverse effects in a newborn infant breast-fed by a mother treated with doxepin. Ann Pharmacother 1999; 33(6): 690–693.

DOXEPIN CREAM   L4

Trade: Zonalon cream, Prudoxin cream

Other Trades: Zonalon

Category: Antipruritic cream

Doxepin cream is an antihistamine-like cream used to treat severe itching. In one study of 19 women, plasma levels ranged from zero to 47 µg/L following transcutaneous absorption.[1] Target therapeutic ranges in doxepin antidepressant therapy is 30–150 ng/mL. Small but significant amounts are secreted in milk. Two published reports indicate absorption by infant varying from significant to modest but only in mothers consuming oral doses.[2,3] This product is probably too hazardous to use in breastfeeding mothers.

Pregnancy Risk	B	Lactation Risk	L4
T ½	= 28–52 hours	M/P	= 1.08, 1.66
Vd	=	PB	= 80–85%
Tmax	= 2 hours	Oral	= Complete
MW	= 279	pKa	=

Adult Concerns: Respiratory arrest, sedation, dry mouth.

Pediatric Concerns: Sedation, respiratory arrest have been reported following oral administration.

Drug Interactions: Decreased effect of doxepin when used with bretylium, guanethidine, clonidine, levodopa, ascorbic acid and cholestyramine. Increased toxicity when used with carbamazepine, amphetamines, thyroid preparations. Increased toxicity with fluoxetine, thyroid preparations, monoamine oxidase inhibitors, albuterol, CNS depressants such as benzodiazepines and opiate analgesics, anticholinergics, cimetidine.

Relative Infant Dose:

Adult Dose: 150–300 mg daily.

Alternatives:

References:
1. Facts and Comparisons. St. Louis: 2010..
2. Kemp J, Ilett KF, Booth J, Hackett LP. Excretion of doxepin and N-desmethyldoxepin in human milk. Br J Clin Pharmacol 1985; 20(5): 497–499.
3. Matheson I, Pande H, Alertsen AR. Respiratory depression caused by N-desmethyldoxepin in breast milk. Lancet 1985; 2(8464): 1124.

DOXERCALCIFEROL   L3

Trade: Hectorol

Other Trades: Hectoral

Category: Vitamin D analog

Doxercalciferol is a vitamin D analog that following metabolic activation becomes 1,25-dihydroxyvitamin D_2. Doxercalciferol is indicated for the treatment of hyperparathyroidism associated with chronic renal failure in patients undergoing hemodialysis. Excessive doses may lead to dangerously elevated plasma calcium levels. No data are available on its transfer into human milk. It is not likely that normal doses would lead to clinically relevant levels in human milk, particularly since vitamin D transfers only minimally into human milk. While plasma levels of vitamin D are normally quite low in human milk (<20 IU/L), at least one study now suggests that supplementing a mother with extremely high levels of vitamin D_2 can significantly elevate milk levels, and subsequently lead to hypercalcemia in a breastfed infant.[1] Some caution with these highly active forms of vitamin D is recommended.

Pregnancy Risk	B	Lactation Risk	L3
T ½	= 32–37 hours	M/P	=
Vd	=	PB	= 99%
Tmax	= 8 hours	Oral	= Complete
MW	=	pKa	=

Adult Concerns: Adverse events include hypercalcemia, hyperphosphatemia, and over suppression of parathyroid hormone. Additional side effects include edema, headache, malaise, dizziness, pruritus, and constipation.

Pediatric Concerns: None reported via milk, but caution is recommended in breastfeeding mothers.

Drug Interactions: Do not use with magnesium antacids, as hypermagnesemia has been reported.

Relative Infant Dose:

Adult Dose: 4 µg three times weekly.

Alternatives: Vitamin D

References:
1. Greer FR, Hollis BW, Napoli JL. High concentrations of vitamin D_2 in human milk associated with pharmacologic doses of vitamin D_2. J Pediatr 1984; 105(1): 61–64.

DOXORUBICIN   L5

Trade: Adriamycin, Adriblastina, Caelyx

Other Trades:

Category: Anticancer drug

Doxorubicin is an anti-cancer agent. Doxorubicin and its metabolite are secreted in significant amounts in breastmilk. Following a dose of 70 mg/m^2, peak milk levels of doxorubicin and metabolite occurred at 24 hours and were 128 and 111 µg/L respectively.[1] The highest milk/plasma ratio was 4.43 at 24 hours.

A classic anthracycline, doxorubicin is one of a number of anthracyclines in this family. Doxorubicin when administered reaches a rapid C_{max} and disappears from the plasma compartment with a 3-exponential decay characterized by 3 differing half-lives, 3–5 minutes, 1–2 hours, and 24–36 hours.[2] A fourth curve has been identified with a half-life of 110 hours which accounts for approximately 30% of the total AUC. The last two elimination curves are probably due to this product's high volume of distribution. In essence, it is distributed and stored in sites remote from the plasma compartment and leaks into the plasma over many days thereafter. However, the peak in milk occurred at 24 hours. Because this product is detectable in plasma (and milk) for long periods, a waiting period of approximately 7–10 days is recommended. The kinetics of this agent are highly variable, depending on renal function, creatinine clearance, liver function, etc. Waiting periods before returning to breastfeeding should be adjusted for this factor. Withhold breastfeeding for at least seven to ten days.

Pregnancy Risk	D	Lactation Risk	L5
T ½	= 24–36 hours	M/P	= 4.43
Vd	= 25 l/kg	PB	= 85%
Tmax	= 24 hours	Oral	= Poor
MW	= 544	pKa	= 11.02

Adult Concerns: Bone marrow suppression, cardiac toxicity, arrhythmias, nausea, vomiting, stomatitis, liver toxicity.

Pediatric Concerns: This product could be extremely toxic to a breastfeeding infant and is not recommended.

Drug Interactions: Doxorubicin may decrease digoxin plasma levels and renal excretion. Allopurinol and verapamil may increase cytotoxicity of doxorubicin.

Relative Infant Dose:

Adult Dose: 20–75 mg/m² IV

Alternatives:

References:
1. Egan PC, Costanza ME, Dodion P, Egorin MJ, Bachur NR. Doxorubicin and cisplatin excretion into human milk. Cancer Treat Rep 1985; 69(12): 1387–1389.
2. Grochow LB, Ames MM. A clinician's guide to chemotherapy pharmacokinetics and pharamcodynamics. 1st ed. Baltimore, MD: Williams and Wilkins; 1998.
3. American Academy of Pediatrics, Committee on Drugs. Transfer of drugs and other chemicals into human milk. Pediatrics 2001; 108(3): 776–89.

DOXYCYCLINE   L3

Trade: Doxychel, Vibramycin, Periostat

Other Trades: Doxylin, Vibra-Tabs, Apo-Doxy, Doxycin, Vibramycin, Vibra-Tabs, Doryx, Doxylar

Category: Tetracycline antibiotic

Doxycycline is a long half-life tetracycline antibiotic. In a study of 15 subjects, the average doxycycline level in milk was 0.77 mg/L following a 200 mg oral dose.[1] One oral dose of 100 mg was administered 24 hours later, and the breastmilk levels were 0.38 mg/L. Following a dose of 100 mg daily in 10 mothers, doxycycline levels in milk on day 2 averaged 0.82 mg/L (range 0.37–1.24 mg/L) at 3 hours after the dose, and 0.46 mg/L (range 0.3–0.91 mg/L) 24 hours after the dose.[2] The relative infant dose in an infant would be < 6% of the maternal weight-adjusted dosage.

Following a single dose of 100 mg in 3 women or 200 mg in 3 women, peak milk levels occurred between 2 and 4 hours following the dose. The average peak milk levels were 0.96 mg/L (100 mg dose) or 1.8 mg/L (200 mg dose). After repeated dosing for 5 days, milk levels averaged 3.6 mg/L at doses of 100 mg twice daily.[3] In another study of 13 women receiving 100–200 mg doses of doxycycline, peak levels in milk were 0.6 mg/L (n=3 @100 mg dose) and 1.1 mg/L (n=11 @ 200 mg dose).[4]

Tetracyclines administered orally to infants are known to bind in teeth, producing discoloration and inhibit bone growth, although doxycycline and oxytetracycline stain teeth the least severe. Although most tetracyclines secreted into milk are generally bound to calcium, thus inhibiting their absorption, doxycycline is the least bound (20%), and may be better absorbed in a breastfeeding infant than the older tetracyclines. While the absolute absorption of older tetracyclines may be dramatically reduced by calcium salts, the newer doxycycline and minocycline analogs bind less and their overall absorption while slowed, may be significantly higher than earlier versions. Prolonged use (months) could potentially alter gastrointestinal flora, and induce dental staining although doxycycline produces the least dental staining. Short term use (three-four weeks) is not contraindicated. No harmful effects have yet been reported in breastfeeding infants but prolonged use is not advised. For prolonged administration such as for exposure to anthrax, check the CDC web site as they have published specific dosing guidelines.

Pregnancy Risk	D	Lactation Risk	L3
T ½	= 15–25 hours	M/P	= 0.3–0.4
Vd	=	PB	= 90%
Tmax	= 1.5–4 hours	Oral	= 90–100%
MW	= 462	pKa	= 4.79

Adult Concerns: Nausea, vomiting, diarrhea, photosensitivity. Doxycycline decreased prothrombin activity.

Pediatric Concerns: None reported, but prolonged exposure may lead to dental staining, and decreased bone growth.

Drug Interactions: Reduced absorption with aluminum, calcium, or magnesium salts, iron or bismuth subsalicylate. Reduced doxycycline half-life when used with barbiturates, phenytoin, and carbamazepine. Concurrent use with methoxyflurane has resulted in fatal renal toxicity. May render oral contraceptives less effective.

Relative Infant Dose: 4.2%–13.3%

Adult Dose: 100 mg daily

Alternatives:

References:
1. Morganti G, Ceccarelli G, Ciaffi G. [Comparative concentrations of a tetracycline antibiotic in serum and maternal milk]. Antibiotica 1968; 6(3): 216–223.
2. Lutziger H. Konzentrationsbestimmungen und klinisch wirksamkeit von doxycyclin (Vibramycin) in uterus, adnexen und muttermilch. Ther Umsch. 1969; 26: 476–80.

3. Tokuda G, Yuasa M, Mihara S et al. Clinical study of doxycycline in obstetrical and gynecological fields. Chemotherapy (Tokyo). 1969; 17: 339–44.
4. Borderon E, Soutoul JH et al. Excretion of antibiotics in human milk. Med Mal Infect. 1975; 5: 373–6.

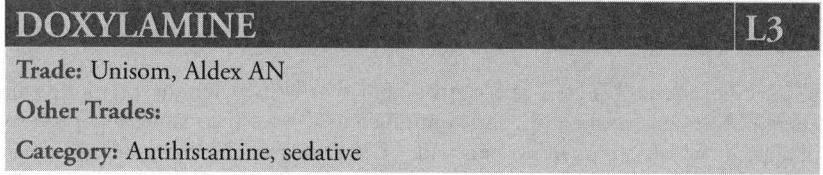

DOXYLAMINE L3

Trade: Unisom, Aldex AN

Other Trades:

Category: Antihistamine, sedative

Doxylamine is an antihistamine similar in structure to diphenhydramine (Benadryl). Because it has strong sedative properties, it is primarily used in over-the-counter sleep aids. Like other such antihistamines, it should be used only cautiously in infants and particularly in premature or term neonates due to paradoxical effects such as CNS stimulation or even sedation.[1,2] Levels in breastmilk are not known but caution is recommended particularly in infants with apnea or other respiratory syndromes.

Pregnancy Risk	A	Lactation Risk	L3
T ½	= 10.1 hours	M/P	=
Vd	= 2.7 l/kg	PB	=
Tmax	= 2.4 hours	Oral	= Complete
MW	= 270	pKa	= 9.2

Adult Concerns: Sedation, paradoxical CNS stimulation, agitation.

Pediatric Concerns: None reported via milk, but observe for sedation and paradoxical CNS stimulation. Do not use in infants with apnea.

Drug Interactions: Increased CNS sedation when added to other antihistamines and CNS sedative-hypnotics.

Relative Infant Dose:

Adult Dose: 25–50 mg orally for insomnia

Alternatives: Diphenhydramine

References:

1. Friedman H, Greenblatt DJ, Scavone JM, Burstein ES, Ochs HR, Harmatz JS, Shader RI. Clearance of the antihistamine doxylamine. Reduced in elderly men but not in elderly women. Clin Pharmacokinet 1989; 16(5): 312–316.
2. Friedman H, Greenblatt DJ. The pharmacokinetics of doxylamine: use of automated gas chromatography with nitrogen-phosphorus detection. J Clin Pharmacol 1985; 25(6): 448–451.

DRONABINOL   L3

Trade: Marinol
Other Trades:
Category: Cannabinoid

Dronabinol (delta-9–THC) is a cannabinoid that is used for the prevention of chemotherapy-induced nausea and vomiting and also for the management of loss of appetite which occurs in patients with HIV. Dronabinol, structurally is similar to a naturally occurring active component of the plant Cannabis sativa (marijuana).

Its oral bioavailability is 10–20% with a high protein binding of 90–99%. It has high lipid solubility and a high volume of distribution with a prolonged half-life. Due to its high lipid solubility and high volume of distribution, it is widely distributed in the body and tends to accumulate in the brain from where it is released slowly. In chronic marijuana users, delta-9–THC has been detected in the plasma up to 1 month after the last use.[1]

Adequate data on the transfer of dronabinol in human milk are not currently available. There are however data on the transfer of delta-9–THC into breastmilk after marijuana use. Bennett reports that the relative infant dose of delta-9–THC available to the infant via breastmilk after smoking of one marijuana joint is 0.8%.[1,2] Peres-Reyes who compared the transfer of THC into breastmilk after maternal marijuana use of one pipe per day versus 7 pipes per day reported that in the mother using high doses of marijuana for prolonged periods during lactation, delta-9–THC is secreted and is concentrated in human milk. It is also at least partially orally bioavailable in the breastfed infant.[3] Another study of 68 breastfed infants revealed that marijuana exposure during the first month postpartum was associated adverse motor development at one year of age.[4]

Peak plasma concentration of THC after a single smoked marijuana cigarette is 100–200 ng/mL which declines to less than 5 ng/mL in 3 hours. The peak plasma concentrations of THC following use of dronabinol in clinical doses ranges from 1.32 to 7.88 ng/mL. This indicates that, although marijuana and dronabinol are structurally similar, the amount of exposure to THC that occurs following clinical doses of dronabinol is minimal compared to the exposure that occurs following the use of a single marijuana cigarette.

Therefore, due to the low oral bioavailability, high protein binding and low peak plasma concentrations of delta-9–THC following usage of clinical doses of dronabinol, if used in clinical doses and short-term, it is probably compatible with breastfeeding. However, until more data are available of chronic, long-term effects of delta-9–THC exposure in breastfed infants, it is best advised that long-term use of dronabinol in breastfeeding mothers should be avoided. Further, caution is recommended as dronabinol has abuse potential, which is enhanced in mothers with a history of abuse of other substances such as alcohol. Long-term use of this product is not recommended in breastfeeding mothers.

Pregnancy Risk	C	Lactation Risk	L3
T ½	= 19–36 hours.	M/P	= 8
Vd	= 10 l/kg	PB	= 90–99%
Tmax	= 2–4 hours	Oral	= 10–20%
MW	= 314.47	pKa	= 10.6

Adult Concerns: Contraindicated in those with allergies to cannabinoid or sesame seed oil. Seizures, sedation, euphoria, mood disturbances, changes in blood pressure, palpitations, syncope, tachycardia, abuse potential are some of the reported side-effects.

Pediatric Concerns:

Drug Interactions: Concomitant administration with the following drugs could cause additive sympathomimetic effects such as hypertension, tachycardia, palpitations, tachyarrhythmias: Amphetamine, cocaine, atropine, scopolamine, amitriptyline, amoxapine, desipramine, other antihistamines, anticholinergics, tricyclic antidepressants. Concomitant use with the following drugs could cause additive CNS depressant effects: phenobarbital and other barbiturates, phenytoin, carbamazepine, diazepam and other benzodiazepines, alcohol, lithium, morphine, oxycodone and other opiates. Co-administration with the following drugs could cause dronabinol toxicity (sedation, headache, diarrhea, constipation): ritonavir. Caution urged while using concurrently with the following: disulfiram, fluoxetine, theophylline.

Relative Infant Dose:

Adult Dose: 2.5–20 mg per day.

Alternatives:

References:
1. Djulus J, Moretti M, Koren G. Marijuana use and breastfeeding. Can Fam Physician. 2005 Mar; 51: 349–50.
2. Bennett PN. Cannabis. Drugs and human lactation. In: Bennett PN and the WHO Working Group, editors. 2nd ed. Amsterdam, Holl: Elsevier; 1997.
3. Perez-Reyes M, Wall ME. Presence of delta9-tetrahydrocannabinol in human milk. N Engl J Med. 1982 Sep 23; 307(13): 819–20.
4. Astley SJ, Little RE. Maternal marijuana use during lactation and infant development at one year. Neurotoxicol Teratol. 1990 Mar-Apr; 12(2): 161–8.

DRONEDARONE   L3

Trade: Multaq

Other Trades: Dronedarone Winthrop, Dronedarone Sanofi

Category: Antiarrhythmic agent

Dronedarone was developed as an antiarrhythmic agent for the first line treatment of atrial fibrillation and atrial flutter. It is structurally related to amiodarone but lacks the iodine component.[1] It is not known whether dronedarone is excreted in human breast milk. Animal studies have shown excretion of dronedarone and its metabolites in breast milk. A study of rats suggests maternal dronedarone administration was associated with minor reduced body-weight gain in the offspring.[1] It is poorly absorbed orally, so the oral absorption by levels in milk are probably subclinical.

Pregnancy Risk	X	Lactation Risk	L3
T ½	= 13–19 hours	M/P	=
Vd	= 20 (based on a 70 kg patient) l/kg	PB	= >98%
Tmax	= 3–6 hours	Oral	= 4% (without food); 15% (with high fat meal)
MW	= 566.8	pKa	= 9.40 (basic function); 9.46 (acidic function)

Adult Concerns: Common side effects are diarrhea, nausea, or weakness. More serious side effects are weight gain, swelling of the arms and/or legs, and shortness of breath.

Pediatric Concerns:

Drug Interactions: CYP3A4 inhibitors (ketoconazole, verapamil, diltiazem, statins, tacrolimus) may increase dronedarone concentration. Concomitant use with digoxin increases therapeutic levels of digoxin in the plasma. Co-administration with warfarin or dabigatran may increase bleeding tendencies. Do not take dronedarone with grapefruit or grapefruit juice. Grapefruit juice increases the bioavailability of dronedarone threefold and can therefore alter the effects of the medication. St. John's wort may decrease dronedarone levels.

Relative Infant Dose:

Adult Dose: 400 mg twice daily with morning and evening meals

Alternatives:

References:
1. Pharmaceutical manufacturer prescribing information, 2010.

DROPERIDOL   L3

Trade: Inapsine
Other Trades: Inapsine, Droleptan
Category: Tranquilizer, antiemetic

Droperidol is a powerful tranquilizer. It is sometimes used as a preanesthetic medication in labor and delivery because of fewer respiratory effects in neonates. In pediatric patients 2–12 years of age, it is sometimes used as an antiemetic (20–75 micrograms/kg IM, IV).[1,2] It apparently crosses the placenta only very slowly. There are no data available on secretion into breastmilk. Due to the potent sedative properties of this medication, caution is urged.

Pregnancy Risk	C	Lactation Risk	L3
T ½	= 2.2 hours	M/P	=
Vd	= 2.0 l/kg	PB	= High
Tmax	= 10–30 minutes (IM)	Oral	=
MW	= 379	pKa	= 7.46

Adult Concerns: Sedation, hypotension, dizziness, chills, shivering, unusual ocular movements.

Pediatric Concerns: None reported via milk, but observe for sedation, hypotension.

Drug Interactions: Can cause peripheral vasodilation and hypotension when used with certain anesthesia medications. Can potentiate effects of other CNS depressants and antidepressants such as barbiturates.

Relative Infant Dose:

Adult Dose: 2.5–10 mg injection (IM)

Alternatives: Haloperidol

References:
1. McEvoy GE. (ed): AFHS Drug Information. 1992.
2. Pharmaceutical manufacturer prescribing information, 1995.

DROSPIRENONE + ETHINYL ESTRADIOL   L3

Trade: Gianvi, Ocella, Yaz, Yasmin, Loryna, Zarah, Vestura

Other Trades: Yaz, Yasmin

Category: Contraceptive

Drospirenone and Ethinyl estradiol is a combination drug product indicated for use in acne vulgaris, premenstrual dysphoric disorder and as an oral contraceptive agent.

Drospirenone (DRSP) in combination with ethinyl estradiol (EE) is used as an oral contraceptive agent. After oral administration of 3 mg DRSP/0.03 mg EE tablets about 0.02% of the drospirenone dose was excreted into the breast milk of postpartum women within 24 hours. This results in a maximal daily dose of about 3 μg drospirenone in an infant. In a study of 6 women who received 3 mg drospirenone with ethinyl estradiol (Yasmin), the time to peak in plasma and milk was 2.5 and 2.8 hour respectively.[1] Average concentrations at C_{max} were 30.8 and 13.5 ng/mL of serum or milk respectively. The mean milk/serum ratios increased from 0.16 to 0.57 at 2 hours following dosing and decreased to 0.16 at 24 hours although the AUC (0–48 h) ratio was only 0.23. The mean drospirenone concentration in breast milk over the 24 hour period was 3.7 ng/mL. Using this average, the relative infant dose would be approximately 1.2% of the maternal dose. The authors estimate in this group of 6 women, the average transfer of drospirenone was 635 ng/day. Although not clear in this study, the lower estimates could be due to lower milk production in this study. Progesterone (in this case, drospirenone) has limited or no ill-effects on infants. May decrease the volume of breastmilk to some degree in some mothers if therapy is initiated too soon after birth and if dose is too high. It is advisable to wait as long as possible postpartum prior to instituting therapy with progesterone to avoid reducing the milk supply.

This combination oral contraceptive also contains ethinyl estradiol which is an estrogenic agent. Estrogens are believed though not proven to strongly inhibit milk production in some women. Some caution is recommended. Although small amounts may pass into breastmilk, the effects of estrogens on the infant appear minimal. Early postpartum use of estrogens may reduce the volume of milk produced and the protein content, but it is variable and depends on dose and the individual.[2,3,4,5] Breastfeeding mothers should attempt to wait until lactation is firmly established (6–8 weeks) prior to use of estrogen-containing oral contraceptives.

Breastfeeding women should be advised to avoid using combination (estrogen-containing) oral contraceptives while breastfeeding because combination oral contraceptives have been found to interfere with the production of milk and will reduce the duration of breastfeeding.[6–10] It is recommended that women wait at least 6–8 weeks postpartum to establish good milk flow, prior to beginning oral contraceptives.

There is present concern about the potential increased risk of blood clots with the use of drospirenone-containing birth control pills. Preliminary results of an FDA-funded study suggest an approximately 1.5-fold increase in the risk of blood clots for women who use drospirenone-containing birth control pills compared to users of other hormonal contraceptives.

Pregnancy Risk	X		Lactation Risk	L3	
T ½	= Drospirenone/ethinyl estradiol: 31 hours/24 hours		M/P	= Drospirenone/ethinyl estradiol: 0.23/0.25	
Vd	= Drospirenone/ethinyl estradiol: 4/4–5 l/kg		PB	= Drospirenone/ethinyl estradiol: 97%/97%	
Tmax	= Drospirenone/ethinyl estradiol: 1.7 hours/1.5 hours		Oral	= Drospirenone/ethinyl estradiol: 76%/40%	
MW	= Drospirenone/ethinyl estradiol: 366.5/296.4		pKa	= Drospirenone/ethinyl estradiol: /17.6	

Adult Concerns: Thromboembolism, thrombophlebitis, edema, migraine, depression, amenorrhea, breast tenderness, decreased lactation.

Pediatric Concerns: In the one study, transfer of drospirenone to milk was low. No untoward effects were noted in the infants.

Drug Interactions: Decreased efficacy noted when used concomitantly with rifampin, phenobarbital, phenytoin carbamazepine, ampicillin, tetracyclines and griseofulvin. Also, use with herbal agents such as St. John's Wort may also decrease its efficacy.

Relative Infant Dose:

Adult Dose: Drospirenone/ethinyl estradiol: 3 mg/0.03 mg, taken as directed.

Alternatives:

References:

1. Blode H, Foidart JM, Heithecker R. Transfer of drospirenone to breast milk after a single oral administration of 3 mg drospirenone + 30 μg ethinylestradiol to healthy lactating women. Eur J Contracept Reprod Health Care 2001; 6(3): 167–171. Estrogens and progestins should not beused during pregnancy.
2. Booker DE, Pahl IR. Control of postpartum breast engorgement with oral contraceptives. Am J Obstet Gynecol 1967; 98(8): 1099–1101.
3. Kamal I, Hefnawi F, Ghoneim M, Abdallah M, Abdel RS. Clinical, biochemical, and experimental studies on lactation. V. Clinical effects of steroids on the initiation of lactation. Am J Obstet Gynecol 1970; 108(4): 655–658.
4. Kora SJ. Effect of oral contraceptives on lactation. Fertil Steril 1969; 20(3): 419–423.
5. Koetsawang S, Bhiraleus P, Chiemprajert T. Effects of oral contraceptives on lactation. Fertil Steril 1972; 23(1): 24–28.
5. Costa TH, Dorea JG. Concentration of fat, protein, lactose and energy in milk of mothers using hormonal contraceptives. Ann Trop Paediatr 1992; 12(2): 203–209.
6. McCann MF, Potter LS. Progestin-only oral contraception: a comprehensive review. Contraception. 1994 Dec; 50(6 Suppl 1): S1–195. Review.
7. Peralta O, D?az S, Juez G, Herreros C, Casado ME, Salvatierra AM, Miranda P, Dur?n E, Croxatto HB. Fertility regulation in nursing women: V. Long-term influence of a low-dose combined oral contraceptive initiated at day 90 postpartum upon lactation and infant growth. Contraception. 1983 Jan; 27(1): 27–38.
8. Croxatto HB, D?az S, Peralta O, Juez G, Herreros C, Casado ME, Salvatierra AM, Miranda P, Dur?n E. Fertility regulation in nursing women: IV. Long-term influence of a low-dose combined oral contraceptive initiated at day 30 postpartum upon lactation and infant growth. Contraception. 1983 Jan; 27(1): 13–25.
9. D?az S, Peralta O, Juez G, Herreros C, Casado ME, Salvatierra AM, Miranda P, Dur?n E, Croxatto HB. Fertility regulation in nursing women: III. Short-term influence of a low-dose combined oral contraceptive upon lactation and infant growth. Contraception. 1983 Jan; 27(1): 1–11.
10. Effects of hormonal contraceptives on breast milk composition and infant growth. World Health Organization (WHO) Task Force on Oral Contraceptives. Stud Fam Plann. 1988 Nov-Dec; 19(6 Pt 1): 361–9.

DULOXETINE   L3

Trade: Cymbalta, Ariclaim, Duceten, Xeristar, Yentreve
Other Trades: Cymbalta
Category: Antidepressant

Duloxetine is a selective serotonin and norepinephrine reuptake inhibitor (SNRI) that is indicated for depression and for patient with neuropathic pain.[1] The primary role of SNRIs is as an alternative in patients with major depressive disorder who have responded poorly to other agents (e. g., tricyclics or SSRIs).

The transfer of duloxetine into breastmilk was studied in 6 women who were at least 12 weeks postpartum and taking 40 mg twice daily for 3.5 days.[2] Paired blood and breastmilk samples were taken at 0, 1, 2, 3, 6, 9, and 12 hours post dose. The milk/plasma ratio was reported to be about 0.267. The daily dose of duloxetine was estimated to be 7 μg/day (range=4–15 μg/day). According to the manufacturer, the weight-adjusted infant dose would be approximately 0.141% of the maternal dose. Further, even this is unlikely absorbed, as duloxetine is unstable under acid conditions of the infants stomach. In a more recent study in a mother consuming duloxetine (60 mg daily), levels in milk were 31 μg/L and 64 μg/L at trough and peak respectively.[3] The milk/plasma ratios were 1.29 (trough) and 1.21 (peak). These authors suggest a relative infant dose of 0.14%.

An investigation was undertaken to study the transfer of duloxetine across placenta as well as breastmilk in a 31-year-old mother who received 60 mg duloxetine daily throughout her pregnancy and continued it during lactation.[4] An assessment of maternal and cord blood concentrations immediately at birth revealed that the placental transfer for duloxetine is low. No withdrawal symptoms or malformations occurred in the infant. Breastmilk samples were obtained at 18 days post-delivery. The first milk sample was obtained just prior to the morning dose, and subsequently 8 more milk samples were obtained over a period of 22.5 hours following the morning dose. A mean milk concentration of 51 µg/L rendered a mean relative infant dose (RID) of 0.81%. This RID for duloxetine is low as compared to some of other commonly used SSRIs/SNRIs such as venlafaxine, desvenlafaxine, citalopram, mirtazepine, fluoxetine. Further, it was found that the concentration of duloxetine in hindmilk was 1.5–2 times that in foremilk, suggesting a lipid co-transport for duloxetine. The authors of this study concluded that the placental and milk transfer of duloxetine is low as compared to a few other SSRIs/SNRIs commonly used. No untoward effects were reported in the infant.

Pregnancy Risk	C	Lactation Risk	L3
T½	= 12 hours	M/P	= 0.267–1.29
Vd	= 23.4 l/kg	PB	= >90%
Tmax	= 6 hours	Oral	= >70%
MW	= 333	pKa	= 9.5

Adult Concerns: Common side effects include nausea, dry mouth, constipation, diarrhea, vomiting, decreased appetite, fatigue, dizziness, somnolence, tremor, sweating, blurred vision, insomnia, erectile dysfunction, and others. Warnings of hepatic injury have been posted by the FDA and include abdominal pain, hepatomegaly, elevation of transaminase levels with or without jaundice.

Pediatric Concerns: Milk levels in one study (6 mothers) are low and the relative infant dose is low. Subsequent study suggests Relative Infant Dose = 0.14%.

Drug Interactions: Numerous drug-drug interactions have been reported. Duloxetine is metabolized by CYP1A2 and CYP2D6. Drugs which inhibit duloxetine metabolism and may increase plasma levels in patients include cimetidine, ciprofloxacin, enoxacin, and other fluoroquinolones, fluvoxamine. Consult a good drug reference for other interactions.

Relative Infant Dose: 0.1%–1.1%

Adult Dose: 40–60 mg/day

Alternatives: Venlafaxine, sertraline, paroxetine

References:
1. Pharmaceutical manufacturer prescribing information,2005.
2. Lobo ED, Loghin C, Knadler MP et al. Pharmacokinetics of duloxetine in breast milk and plasma of healthy postpartum women. Clin Pharmacokinet. 2008; 47: 103–109.

3. Briggs GG, Ambrose PJ, Ilett KF, Hackett LP, Nageotte MP, Padilla G. Use of duloxetine in pregnancy and lactation. Ann Pharmacother. Nov 2009; 43(11): 1898–1902.
4. Boyce PM, Hackett LP, Ilett KF. Duloxetine transfer across the placenta duringpregnancy and into milk during lactation. Arch Womens Ment Health. 2011Apr; 14(2): 169–72.

DYCLONINE HYDROCHLORIDE   L3

Trade: Cepacol Maximum Strength, Sucrets Children's Formula, Sucrets Maximum Strength, Sucrets Regular Strength
Other Trades:
Category: Local anesthetic oral

Dyclonine hydrochloride is a local anesthetic that is used to relieve pain in the oral mucosa. Available evidence is inconclusive for determining the risk associated with breastfeeding and the levels in milk are unknown.[1,2] In general, topical anesthetics are present in the milk, but not at concentrations that would cause a pharmacologic effect in the infant.[3]

Pregnancy Risk	C	Lactation Risk	L3
T ½	= 30–60 minutes	M/P	=
Vd	=	PB	=
Tmax	=	Oral	=
MW	= 289.4	pKa	= 8.2

Adult Concerns: Irritation, numbness, pain, stinging at site of application.
Pediatric Concerns:
Drug Interactions: There are no known significant drug-drug interactions with dyclonine.
Relative Infant Dose:
Adult Dose: One lozenge every 2 hours as needed (max: 10 lozenges/day)
Alternatives:
References:
1. Giuliani M, Grossi GB, Pileri M, et al: Could local anesthesia while breast-feeding be harmful to infants?. J Ped Gastroenterol Nutr 2001; 32: 142–144.
2. Zeisler JA, Gaarder TD, and De Mesquita SA: Lidocaine excretion in breast milk. Drug Intell Clin Pharm 1986; 20: 691–693.
3. Taketomo CK, Hodding JH and Kraus DM: Pediatric Dosage Handbook, 4th ed. Lexi-Comp Inc, Hudson, OH-1998, 1997.

DYPHYLLINE   L3

Trade: Dilor, Lufyllin, Dyphylline
Other Trades: Broncho-Grippol, Silbephylline, Noradran
Category: Anti-asthmatic drug

Dyphylline is a methylxanthine, bronchodilator similar to theophylline. It is apparently secreted into milk in small quantities. Following a 5 mg/kg dose IM, the milk/plasma ratio was 2.08. Using the kinetics provided, the average milk level at 2 hours would have been approximately 14.1 mg/L.[1] No reported untoward effects. Observe infant for irritability, insomnia, and elevated heart rate.

Pregnancy Risk	C	Lactation Risk	L3
T ½	= 3–12.8 hours	M/P	= 2.08
Vd	= 0.6–1.1 l/kg	PB	= 56%
Tmax	= 1–2 hours (oral)	Oral	= Complete
MW	= 254	pKa	= 15.63

Adult Concerns: Irritability, insomnia, tachycardia, arrhythmias, gastrointestinal distress, headache, seizures, hyperglycemia.

Pediatric Concerns: None reported via milk, but observe for irritability, insomnia, tachycardia.

Drug Interactions: Probenecid significantly increases half-life of dyphylline and increases plasma levels.

Relative Infant Dose: 42.3%

Adult Dose: 15 mg/kg QID

Alternatives: Theophylline

References:
1. Jarboe CH, Cook LN, Malesic I, Fleischaker J. Dyphylline elimination kinetics in lactating women: blood to milk transfer. J Clin Pharmacol 1981; 21(10): 405–410.

ECHINACEA   L3

Trade:
Other Trades:
Category: Herbal immunostimulant

Echinacea is a popular herbal remedy in the central US and has been traditionally used topically to stimulate wound healing and internally to stimulate the immune system. The plant contains a complex mixture of compounds and, thus far, no single component appears responsible for its immunostimulant properties. A number of *in vitro* and animal studies have documented the activation of immunologic properties although most of these are via intraperitoneal injections, not orally. Three recent studies have reported echinacea may not be a active against the common cold.[1,2,3] but more studies are presently underway. Thus far, little is known about the toxicity of this plant although its use has been widespread for many years. Apparently, purified Echinacea extract is relatively non-toxic even at high doses.[3,4] No data are available on its transfer into human milk or its effect on lactation. It should not be used for more than 8 weeks.[4]

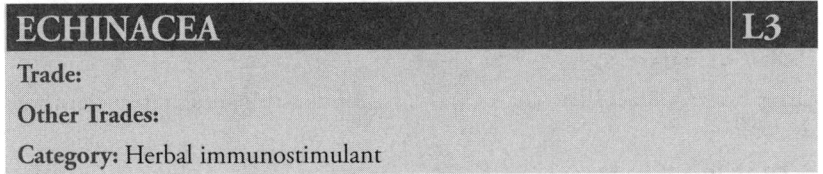

Pregnancy Risk	C	Lactation Risk	L3
T ½	=	M/P	=
Vd	=	PB	=
Tmax	=	Oral	=
MW	=	pKa	=

Adult Concerns: None reported.

Pediatric Concerns: None reported via milk.

Drug Interactions:

Relative Infant Dose:

Adult Dose:

Alternatives:

References:
1. Turner, R. B., Bauer, R., Woelkart, K., Hulsey, T. C., and Gangemi, J. D. An evaluation of Echinacea angustifolia in experimental rhinovirus infections. N. Engl. J Med 7–28–2005; 353(4): 341–348.
2. Taylor, J. A., Weber, W., Standish, L., Quinn, H., Goesling, J., McGann, M., and Calabrese, C. Efficacy and safety of echinacea in treating upper respiratory tract infections in children: a randomized controlled trial. JAMA 12–3–2003; 290(21): 2824–2830.
3. Barrett, B. P., Brown, R. L., Locken, K., Maberry, R., Bobula, J. A., and D'Alessio, D. Treatment of the common cold with unrefined echinacea. A randomized, double-blind, placebo-controlled trial. Ann Intern Med 12–17–2002; 137(12): 939–946.
4. The Complete German Commission E Monographs. Ed. M. Blumenthal Amer Botanical Council 1998.

ECONAZOLE   L3

Trade: Spectazole

Other Trades:

Category: Antifungal, particularly candida infections

Econazole nitrate is a typical azozle antifungal and is indicated for topical application in the treatment of tinea pedis, tinea cruris, and tinea corporis.[1] It is not known whether econazole nitrate is excreted in human milk. Following oral administration of econazole nitrate to lactating rats, econazole and/or metabolites were excreted in milk and were found in nursing pups. Also, in lactating rats receiving large oral doses (40 or 80 times the human dermal dose), there was a reduction in postpartum viability of pups and survival to weaning, however, at these high doses, maternal toxicity was present and may have been a contributing factor. Caution should be exercised when econazole nitrate is administered to a nursing woman.

Pregnancy Risk	C	Lactation Risk	L3
T ½	=	M/P	=
Vd	=	PB	=
Tmax	=	Oral	=
MW	= 381.7	pKa	= 6.0

Adult Concerns: Erythema, burning sensation, stinging, pruritus.

Pediatric Concerns:

Drug Interactions:

Relative Infant Dose:

Adult Dose: Apply topically 1–2 times daily.

Alternatives:

References:
1. Pharmaceutical manufacturer prescribing information, 2009.

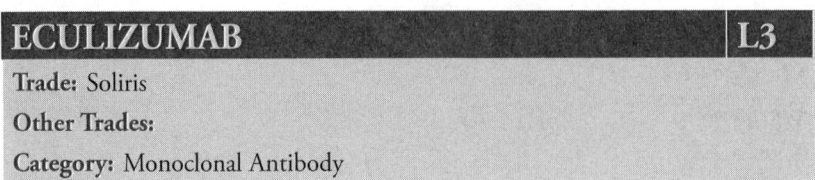

ECULIZUMAB   L3

Trade: Soliris
Other Trades:
Category: Monoclonal Antibody

Eculizumab is a large monoclonal antibody used in the treatment of paroxysmal nocturnal hemoglobinuria to reduce hemolysis, and reducing the need for RBC transfusions.[1] It is a monoclonal antibody with high affinity to complement protein C5. It is extremely unlikely that this antibody would be transported into human milk after the colostral period, and due to its size, it would be largely unable to penetrate the milk compartment after the first week postpartum. Oral bioavailability would be nil.

Pregnancy Risk	C	Lactation Risk	L3
T ½	= 272 hours	M/P	=
Vd	= 7.7 l/kg	PB	=
Tmax	=	Oral	= Nil
MW	= 148,000	pKa	=

Adult Concerns: Headache, nasopharyngitis, back pain, nausea and fatigue.

Pediatric Concerns: None reported via milk.

Drug Interactions:

Relative Infant Dose:

Adult Dose: Variable

Alternatives:

References:
1. Pharmaceutical manufacturer prescribing information, 2008.

EDROPHONIUM   L3

Trade: Enlon, Reversol
Other Trades: Enlon, Tensilon
Category: Cholinergic Agonist

Edrophonium is used to diagnose myasthenia gravis, to differentiate cholinergic crises from myasthenia crises, and to reverse neuromuscular blockers.[1] It inhibits acetylcholinesterase and thus prevents the metabolism of acetylcholine. This product is only used for acute episodes or for diagnosis, as its effects last only briefly (10 minutes) before it is rapidly redistributed to peripheral tissues. It also has a unique structure that would largely preclude its entry into human milk. A brief waiting period of a few hours would reduce any possible risk from this medication in breastfed infants.

Pregnancy Risk	C	Lactation Risk	L3
T ½	= 1.2–2.4 hours	M/P	=
Vd	= 1.1 l/kg	PB	=
Tmax	=	Oral	= Nil
MW	= 166	pKa	=

Adult Concerns: Adverse effects include arrhythmias, dizziness, headache, nausea, weakness, and bronchospasm.

Pediatric Concerns: Can be used in infants at a dose of 0.5 to 1 mg intramuscularly, and in children at a dose of 1 mg if under 34 kg, or 5 mg if over 34 kg. Unlikely to enter milk, or be orally absorbed.

Drug Interactions:

Relative Infant Dose:

Adult Dose: 10 mg IM, or 2 mg IV

Alternatives:

References:
1. Pharmaceutical manufacturer prescribing information, 2009.

EFALIZUMAB   L3

Trade: Raptiva
Other Trades:
Category: Monoclonal antibody

Efalizumab is an immunosuppressant used to treat moderate to severe plaque psoriasis. It binds to CD11a on the surface of leukocytes, thus blocking multiple T cell mediated responses involved in the pathogenesis of psoriasis plaques.[1] No data are available on the transfer of efalizumab into human milk. Because this antibody is quite large (150 kilodaltons), its size alone would prohibit its transfer into human milk in clinically relevant amounts.

Pregnancy Risk	C	Lactation Risk	L3
T ½	= 6.2 days(subcut); 3 days (IV)	M/P	=
Vd	=	PB	=
Tmax	= 1–5 days (subcut)	Oral	= Nil
MW	= 150,000	pKa	=

Adult Concerns: Adverse effects include headache, chills, nausea, lymphocytosis, and leukocytosis.

Pediatric Concerns: No data available.

Drug Interactions: Other immunosuppressants may increase risk of infection.

Relative Infant Dose:

Adult Dose: 1 mg/kg SQ weekly

Alternatives:

References:
1. Pharmaceutical manufacturer prescribing information, 1997

EFAVIRENZ   L4

Trade: Sustiva, Atripla
Other Trades:
Category: Antiretroviral agent used in HIV infections.

Efavirenz is an antiretroviral agent used in the treatment of HIV infection. There are no adequate or well-controlled studies in breastfeeding women. Schneider found that infant plasma concentrations were 13% of the maternal plasma concentration in those who are breastfeeding.[1] Maternal plasma concentrations 6.55 mg/L, 3.51 mg/L skim breast milk, and 0.85 mg/L in infant plasma. Breastfeeding in developed countries is generally not recommended in mothers who have HIV.[2,3]

Pregnancy Risk	D	Lactation Risk	L4
T ½	= 40–55 hours (multiple dose)	M/P	=
Vd	=	PB	= 99.5%
Tmax	= 3–5 hours	Oral	=
MW	= 315.68	pKa	= 10.2

Adult Concerns: Rash, fever, dizziness, nausea, vomiting, diarrhea, cough, fatigue, somnolence, itching, elevated liver enzymes, neutropenia, elevated cholesterol and triglycerides.

Pediatric Concerns: No adverse effects via breast milk reported in one study.

Drug Interactions: Drugs contra-indicated with efavirenz are the following: ergot derivatives, bepridil, midazolam, triazolam, cisapride, pimozide and St. john's wort. Concomitant use reduces efficacy and plasma levels of the following coadministered drugs: amprenavir, ritonavir, lopinavir, saquinavir, indinavir, carbamazepine, bupropion, sertraline, voriconazole, itraconazole, ketoconazole, clarithromycin, rifabutin, diltiazem, atorvastatin, pravastatin, simvastatin.

Relative Infant Dose:

Adult Dose: 600 mg once daily.

Alternatives:

References:
1. Schneider S, Peltier A, Gras A, et al. Efavirenz in human breast milk, mothers', and newborns' plasma. J Acquir Immune Defic Syndr. Aug 1 2008; 48(4): 450–454.
1. World Health Organization: Global Programme on AIDS. Consensus statement from the WHO/UNICEF consultation on HIV transmission and breast-feeding. Geneva: WHO, 1992.
2. Latham MC, Greiner T: Breastfeeding versus formula feeding in HIV infection. Lancet 352: 737, 19981.

EFLORNITHINE HYDROCHLORIDE | L3

Trade: Vaniqa
Other Trades: Vaniqa
Category: Hair growth retardant

Eflornithine hydrochloride is used topically to remove unwanted facial hair in women. It is also available intravenously as an antiprotozoal agent for the treatment of sleeping sickness, although it is not FDA approved for this use. Eflornithine hydrochloride is a suicide inhibitor of ornithine decarboxylase, the rate limiting enzyme in the biosynthesis of major polyamines in nucleated cells. The inhibition of this enzyme leads to a decreased rate of hair growth.[1] No data are available on the transfer of eflornithine into human milk, however, when used topically, this medication is less than 1% absorbed and produces steady state plasma levels of only 5–10 ng/mL, far too low to produce clinically relevant milk levels in milk or an infant. A risk-benefit assessment of this product does not necessarily suggest the benefits are worth the risk for a breastfed infant, even if the risks are quite low.

Pregnancy Risk	C	Lactation Risk	L3
T ½	= 3–3.5 hours	M/P	=
Vd	= 0.3–0.35 l/kg	PB	= None
Tmax	= 4–6 hours	Oral	= 54–58%
MW	= 218	pKa	=

Adult Concerns: Adverse effects include acne, pseudofolliculitis barbae, stinging skin, headache, itching, and tingling skin.

Pediatric Concerns: No data are available.

Drug Interactions: No data available.

Relative Infant Dose:

Adult Dose:

Alternatives:

References:
1. Pharmaceutical manufacturer prescribing information, 2004.

EICOSAPENTAENOIC ACID (EPA) | L3

Trade: EPA
Other Trades:
Category: Omega-3 fatty acid

Eicosapentaenoic acid (EPA) is an omega-3 fatty acid which is usually found in fish or fish oil and usually used in combination with docosahexaenoic acid (DHA). Eicosapentaenoic acid is a polyunsaturated lipid commonly found in human milk. In one study, cod liver oil supplementation increases breastmilk composition of EPA by 0.15% (wt%) and DHA by 0.36% (wt%).[1] Another study suggested that infant serum EPA increased from 0.11% to 0.7% after breastfeeding women were given fish oil supplementations consisting of 3,092 mg/day of total omega-3 fatty acid which contain 2,006 mg of very long-chain omega-3 fatty acid (>C18).[2]

Use caution in patients who have a known hypersensitivity to fish and/or shellfish. EPA may prolong bleeding time. Coagulation studies should be done on patients who concurrently take anticoagulants such as warfarin or coumadin. Also, monitor bleeding time if patients are on aspirin or NSAIDS routinely.

Pregnancy Risk	Probably Safe	Lactation Risk	L3
T ½	=	M/P	=
Vd	=	PB	=
Tmax	=	Oral	=
MW	= 302	pKa	=

Adult Concerns: Nausea, flatulence, skin rash, diarrhea, belching, fishy taste, nose bleed.

Pediatric Concerns:

Drug Interactions:

Relative Infant Dose:

Adult Dose: 159–563 mg per day

Alternatives:

References:
1. Helland IB, Saarem K, Saugstad OD, Drevon CA. Fatty acid composition in maternal milk and plasma during supplementation with cod liver oil. Eur J Clin Nutr. 1998 Nov; 52(11): 839–45.
2. Henderson RA, Jensen RG, Lammi-Keefe CJ, Ferris AM, Dardick KR. Effect of fish oil on the fatty acid composition of human milk and maternal and infant erythrocytes. Lipids. 1992 Nov; 27(11): 863–9.

ELETRIPTAN   L3

Trade: Relpax
Other Trades: Relpax
Category: Anti-migraine

Eletriptan is a selective 5-hyroxytryptamine (5–HT) receptor agonist specifically used to treat migraine attacks. The oral bioavailability of eletriptan is greater than sumatriptan and it is presumably faster acting.

The manufacturer reports that in one study of 8 women given a single dose of 80 mg eletriptan, the mean total amount of eletriptan in breast milk over 24 hours in this group was approximately 0.02% of the administered dose.[1] The milk/plasma ratio was 0.25 but there was great variability. The resulting eletriptan concentration-time profile in milk was similar to that seen in the plasma over 24 hours, with very low concentrations of drug (mean 1.7 ng/mL) still present in the milk 18–24 hours post dose. It is not likely the clinical dose delivered above would harm a breastfed infant.

Pregnancy Risk	C	Lactation Risk	L3
T ½	= 4 hours	M/P	= 0.25
Vd	= 1.97 l/kg	PB	= 85%
Tmax	= 1.5 hours	Oral	= 50%
MW	= 463	pKa	=

Adult Concerns: Nausea, asthenia, somnolence, dizziness, dry mouth, paresthesias, headache and abdominal cramps have been reported.

Pediatric Concerns: None reported via milk in one study.

Drug Interactions: Increased plasma levels of eletriptan could occur if given concomitantly with cyclosporine, ketoconazole, erythromycin, amiodarone, amprenavir, aprepitant, clarithromycin, delavirdine, diltiazem, etc. Enhanced vasospastic reactions when given with ergot alkaloids such as dihydroergotamine, ergotamine, or methysergide.

Relative Infant Dose: 0.02%

Adult Dose: 20–40 mg initially for headache. One repeat dose after 2 hours if needed.

Alternatives: Sumatriptan

References:
1. Pharmaceutical manufacturer prescribing information, 2003.

EMTRICITABINE   L4

Trade: Emtriva

Other Trades: Emtriva

Category: Antiretroviral agent, reverse transcriptase inhibitor

Emtricitabine is a cytosine analogue that acts as a reverse transcriptase inhibitor, which is used in the treatment of HIV infection with at least two other antiretroviral agents.[1] The Centers for Disease Control and Prevention recommend that HIV-1 infected mothers not breastfeed their infants to avoid risking postnatal transmission of HIV-1.

From a study conducted to investigate the concentrations of emtricitabine and tenofovir in the breastmilk samples of 5 HIV-infected women, it was found that breastmilk concentrations of emtricitabine and tenofovir were 2% and 0.03% respectively, of the normal oral dose administered to an infant.[2] These women were treated with emtricitabine 400 mg/tenofovir 600 mg, at the time of delivery, followed by emtricitabine 200 mg/tenofovir 300 mg daily for 7 days postpartum. The breast milk concentrations for emtricitabine were 177–679 ng/mL, while those for tenofovir were 6.8–14.1 ng/mL. Considering this, the relative infant dose for emtricitabine ranges from 0.9–3.6% while those for tenofovir ranges from 0.02–0.5%.

Pregnancy Risk	B	Lactation Risk	L4
T ½	= 10 hours	M/P	=
Vd	=	PB	= <4%
Tmax	= 1–2 hours	Oral	= 93%
MW	= 247	pKa	= 2.65

Adult Concerns: Dizziness, insomnia, abnormal dreams, rash, nausea, vomiting, diarrhea, abdominal pain, weakness, headache, depression, dyspepsia. Emtricitabine is known to cause lactic acidosis and severe hepatomegaly with steatosis.

Pediatric Concerns: Fever, hyperpigmentation of palms and/or soles, nausea, vomiting, diarrhea, gastroenteritis, otitis media, cough, rhinitis, pneumonia, infection.

Drug Interactions: Ganciclovir-Valganciclovir may enhance hematologic toxicity of nucleoside reverse transcriptase inhibitors. Avoid use with lamivudine. Ribavirin enhances hepatotoxic effect of emtricitabine.

Relative Infant Dose:

Adult Dose: 200 mg daily

Alternatives:

References:
1. Pharmaceutical manufacturer prescribing information, 2011.
2. Benaboud S, Pruvost A, Coffie PA, et al: Concentrations of tenofovir and emtricitabine in breast milk of HIV-1-infected women in Abidjan, Cote d'Ivoire, in the ANRS 12109 TEmAA Study, Step 2. Antimicrob Agents Chemother 2011; 55(3): 1315–1317.

EMTRICITABINE + TENOFOVIR   L4

Trade: Truvada, Atripla

Other Trades:

Category: Antiretroviral agent

Emtricitabine and Tenofovir disoproxil fumarate is a combination drug product indicated for use in HIV infections. From a study conducted to investigate the concentrations of emtricitabine and tenofovir in the breastmilk samples of 5 HIV-infected women, it was found that breastmilk concentrations of emtricitabine and tenofovir were 2% and 0.03% respectively, of the normal oral dose administered to an infant.[1] These women were treated with emtricitabine 400 mg/tenofovir 600 mg, at the time of delivery, followed by emtricitabine 200 mg/tenofovir 300 mg daily for 7 days postpartum. The breast milk concentrations for emtricitabine were 177–679 ng/mL, while those for tenofovir were 6.8–14.1 ng/mL. Considering this, the relative infant dose for emtricitabine ranges from 0.9–3.6% while those for tenofovir ranges from 0.02–0.5%.

Emtricitabine is a cytosine analogue that acts as a reverse transcriptase inhibitor. The Centers for Disease Control and Prevention recommend that HIV-1-infected mothers not breast-feed their infants to avoid risking postnatal transmission of

HIV-1. Because of both the potential for HIV-1 transmission and the potential for serious adverse reactions in nursing infants, mothers should be instructed not to breast-feed if they are receiving this medication.

Tenofovir is used in the management of HIV and hepatitis B infections. It interferes with the viral RNA dependent DNA polymerase, inhibiting viral replication.[2] In a recent study in two Rhesus macaques monkeys, and following a subcutaneous dose of 30 mg/kg tenofovir, peak plasma levels were reported to be 18.3 and 30.3 μg/mL.[3] Peak levels in milk were reported to be 0.808 and 0.610 μg/mL. The AUC levels were 68.9 and 12.8 μg. h/mL for plasma and milk in one animal and 56.2 and 12.1 μg. h/mL for plasma and milk in the second animal. Using this peak data, the relative infant dose would only be 0.4% of the maternal dose. In addition, the oral bioavailability of tenofovir (non salt form) is negligible (5%). Thus the overall risk to a breastfeeding infant would probably be low from tenofovir.

In summary, because of both the potential for HIV-1 transmission and the potential for infection of the nursing infant, mothers should be instructed not to breastfeed if they are receiving this medication.

Pregnancy Risk	B	Lactation Risk	L4
T ½	= Emtricitabine/tenofovir: 10 hours/17 hours	M/P	=
Vd	= Emtricitabine/tenofovir: /1.2–1.3 l/kg	PB	= Emtricitabine/tenofovir: <4%/7%
Tmax	= Emtricitabine/tenofovir: 1–2 hours/36–144 min	Oral	= Emtricitabine/tenofovir: 93%/25–40%
MW	= Emtricitabine/tenofovir: 247/636	pKa	= Emtricitabine/tenofovir: 2.65/3.75

Adult Concerns: Lactic acidosis, pancreatitis, peripheral neuropathy, renal effects, weight gain, alteration of blood glucose levels, rash, nausea, vomiting, myalgia.

Pediatric Concerns:

Drug Interactions: Do not use concomitantly with renally eliminated drugs such as acyclovir, ganciclovir, valacyclovir, adefovir etc. Do not use with didanosine to avoid didanosine toxicity.

Relative Infant Dose: 0.9%–3.6%

Adult Dose: Emtricitabine 200 mg/tenofovir 300 mg once daily

Alternatives:

References:
1. Benaboud S, Pruvost A, Coffie PA, et al: Concentrations of tenofovir and emtricitabine in breast milk of HIV-1-infected women in Abidjan, Cote d'Ivoire, in the ANRS 12109 TEmAA Study, Step 2. Antimicrob Agents Chemother 2011; 55(3): 1315–1317.

2. Pharmaceutical manufacturer prescribing information, 2005.
3. K. Van Rompay, M. Hamilton, B. Kearney and N. Bischofberger, Pharmacokinetics of tenofovir in breast milk of lactating rhesus macaques. Antimicrob Agents Chemother 49, 2093–2094 (2005).

ENALAPRIL   L2

Trade: Vasotec

Other Trades: Amprace, Renitec, Vasotec, Innovace

Category: Antihypertensive, ACE inhibitor

Enalapril maleate is an ACE inhibitor used as an antihypertensive. Upon absorption, it is rapidly metabolized by the adult liver to enalaprilat, the biologically active metabolite. In one study of 5 lactating mothers who received a single 20 mg dose, the mean maximum milk concentration of enalapril and enalaprilat was only 1.74 µg/L and 1.72 µg/L respectively.[1] The author suggests that an infant consuming 850 mL of milk daily would ingest less than 2 µg of enalapril daily. The milk/plasma ratios for enalapril and enalaprilat averaged 0.013 and 0.025 respectively. However, this was only a single dose study, and the levels transferred into milk at steady state may be slightly higher.

In a study by Rush of a patient receiving 10 mg/day, the total amount of enalapril and enalaprilat measured in milk during the 24 hour period was 81.9 ng and 36.1 ng respectively or 1.44 µg/L and 0.63 µg/L of milk respectively.[2] Some caution is recommended in using ACE inhibitors in mothers with premature infants due to possible renal toxicity.

Pregnancy Risk	C/D in 2nd and 3rd trimester	Lactation Risk	L2
T ½	= 35 hours (metabolite)	M/P	=
Vd	=	PB	= 60%
Tmax	= 0.5–1.5 hours	Oral	= 60%
MW	= 492	pKa	= 3.0, 5.5

Adult Concerns: Hypotension, bradycardia, headache, fatigue, diarrhea, rash, cough.

Pediatric Concerns: None reported via milk, but observe for hypotension.

Drug Interactions: Bioavailability of ACE inhibitors may be decreased when used with antacids. Capsaicin may exacerbate coughing associated with ACE inhibitor treatment. Pharmacologic effects of ACE inhibitors may be increased. Increased plasma levels of digoxin may result. Increased serum lithium levels may result when used with ACE inhibitors.

Relative Infant Dose: 0.07%–0.2%

Adult Dose: 10–40 mg daily.

Alternatives: Captopril, benazepril

References:

1. Redman CW, Kelly JG, Cooper WD. The excretion of enalapril and enalaprilat in human breast milk. Eur J Clin Pharmacol 1990; 38(1): 99.
2. Rush JE, Snyder BA, Barrish A. et. al. Comment. Clin Nephrol 1991; 35: 234.

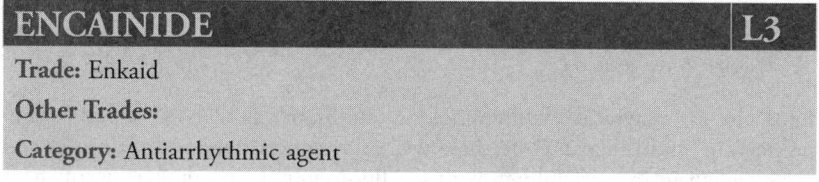

ENCAINIDE — L3

Trade: Enkaid

Other Trades:

Category: Antiarrhythmic agent

Encainide is a local anesthetic-type antiarrhythmic agent. It was voluntarily removed from the market in 1999 but is available on a limited basis for certain patients with life-threatening arrhythmias. The plasma kinetics are highly variable depending on the metabolic capabilities of the maternal liver. The oral bioavailability is extremely variable and varies from 25–65% in extensive metabolizers to 80–90% in poor metabolizers. Half-lives are variable as well according to the metabolic capacity of the individual's liver.[1]

However, encainide and its 3 active metabolites are excreted into human milk. In one patient receiving 50 mg four times daily, milk concentrations of encainide and o-desmethyl encainide were 200–400 µg/L and 100–200 µg/L respectively.[2] The relative infant dose of encainide and active metabolites ranges from 1.5%–3.2%. These milk concentrations are similar to the maternal serum levels.

Pregnancy Risk	B	Lactation Risk	L3
T ½	= 2–36 hours	M/P	= 1
Vd	= 2.7–4.3 l/kg	PB	= 70.5–78%
Tmax	= 1.7 hours	Oral	= Variable
MW	= 352	pKa	=

Adult Concerns: Arrhythmias, chest pain, congestive heart failure, abdominal pain.

Pediatric Concerns: None reported, but extreme caution is recommended.

Drug Interactions: Use with caution when encainide is used with any other drug that affects cardiac conduction. Cimetidine increases plasma concentrations of encainide.

Relative Infant Dose: 1.5%–3.2%

Adult Dose: 50–200 mg daily in 3–4 divided doses.

Alternatives:

References:
1. Pharmaceutical manufacturer prescribing information, 1992.
2. Briggs GG, Freeman RK, Yaffee SJ. Drugs in Pregnancy and Lactation. Philadelphia: Lippincott Williams and Wilkins, 1998.

ENOXACIN   L3

Trade: Penetrex

Other Trades: Enoxin, Comprecin

Category: Antibiotic

Enoxacin is a typical fluoroquinolone antibiotic similar to ciprofloxacin, norfloxacin, and others. While there was prior concern about arthropathy and bone growth in infants/children with the fluoroquinolones, these concerns have been discredited.[1] However, no data are available on the transfer of enoxacin into human milk. It is unlikely that levels in milk will be extensive, however changes in gut flora may occur. Other alternatives include ofloxacin and norfloxacin for which we have breastfeeding information.

Pregnancy Risk	C	Lactation Risk	L3
T ½	= 3–6 hours	M/P	=
Vd	= 2.5 l/kg	PB	= 40%
Tmax	=	Oral	= 90%
MW	= 320.32	pKa	= 6.04

Adult Concerns: Nausea, vomiting, diarrhea, abdominal cramps, gastrointestinal bleeding, increased intracranial pressure, tremor, restlessness, other CNS reactions. Photosensitivity.

Pediatric Concerns: None reported via milk, but caution urged. Changes in gut flora.

Drug Interactions: Decreased absorption with antacids. Quinolones cause increased levels of caffeine, warfarin, cyclosporine, theophylline. Cimetidine, probenecid, azlocillin increase ciprofloxacin levels. Increased risk of seizures when used with foscarnet.

Relative Infant Dose:

Adult Dose: 200–400 mg BID

Alternatives: Ofloxacin, norfloxacin, ciprofloxacin

References:
1. Gurpinar AN, Balkan E, Kilic N, Kiristioglu I, Dogruyol H. The effects of a fluoroquinolone on the growth and development of infants. J Int Med Res. 1997 Sep-Oct; 25(5): 302–6.

ENOXAPARIN   L3

Trade: Lovenox, Low Molecular Weight Heparin

Other Trades: Lovenox, Clexane

Category: Anticoagulant

Enoxaparin is a low molecular weight fraction of heparin used clinically as an anticoagulant. In a study of 12 women receiving 20–40 mg of enoxaparin daily for up to 5 days postpartum for venous pathology (n= 4) or cesarean section (n= 8), no change in anti-Xa activity was noted in the in the 12 breastfed infants.[1]

Because it is a peptide fragment of heparin, its molecular weight is large (2000–8000 daltons). The size alone would largely preclude its entry into human milk at levels clinically relevant. Due to minimal oral bioavailability, any present in milk would not be orally absorbed by the infant. A similar compound, dalteparin, has been studied and milk levels are extremely low as well. See dalteparin.

Pregnancy Risk	B	Lactation Risk	L3
T ½	= 4.5 hours	M/P	=
Vd	= 0.1 l/kg	PB	=
Tmax	= 3–5 hours	Oral	= None
MW	= 8000	pKa	= -2.37

Adult Concerns: Anticoagulant effects in adults when administered subcutaneously.

Pediatric Concerns: No change in clotting factors of 12 infants. Molecular weight is too large to produce clinically relevant milk levels.

Drug Interactions: Anticoagulants and platelet inhibitors. NSAIDS may increase risk of bleeding.

Relative Infant Dose:

Adult Dose: 30 mg BID

Alternatives: Dalteparin

References:
1. Guillonneau M, de Crepy A, Aufrant C, Hurtaud-Roux MF, Jacqz-Aigrain E. L'allaitement est possible en cas de traitement maternel par l'enoxaparien. Arch Pediatr 1996; 3(5): 513–514.

EPHEDRINE   L4

Trade: Vatronol Nose Drops

Other Trades: Adalixin, Bethal, Amsec, Anestan, Anodesyn, Cam

Category: Adrenergic stimulant, anti-asthmatic.

Ephedrine is a mild stimulant that belongs to the adrenergic family and functions similar to the amphetamines. Small amounts of d-isoephedrine, a close congener of ephedrine, is believed to be secreted into milk although no data are available on ephedrine itself.[1] This product is commonly used to support blood pressure of parturients during delivery. On an acute basis, it is not likely to harm a breastfeeding infant. However, it should not be used regularly by breastfeeding mothers.

Pregnancy Risk	C	Lactation Risk	L4
T ½	= 3–5 hours	M/P	=
Vd	=	PB	=
Tmax	= 15–60 minutes	Oral	= 85%
MW	= 165	pKa	= 9.6

Adult Concerns: Anorexia, tachycardia, arrhythmias, agitation, insomnia, hyperstimulation.

Pediatric Concerns: None reported, but observe for anorexia, irritability, crying, disturbed sleeping patterns, excitement.

Drug Interactions: May increase toxicity and cardiac stimulation when used with theophylline. Monoamine oxisade inhibitors or atropine may increase blood pressure.

Relative Infant Dose:

Adult Dose: 25–50 mg injection

Alternatives:

References:
1.　Mortimer EA, Jr. Drug toxicity from breast milk? Pediatrics 1977; 60(5): 780–781.

EPINEPHRINE   L1

Trade: Adrenalin, Sus-Phren, Medihaler, Primatene

Other Trades: Adrenalin, Bronkaid, Epi-pen, Adrenutol, Eppy, Simplene

Category: Stimulant

Epinephrine is a powerful adrenergic stimulant. Although likely to be secreted in milk, it is almost instantly destroyed in the gastrointestinal tract.[1] It is unlikely that any would be absorbed by the infant unless in the early neonatal period.

Pregnancy Risk	C	Lactation Risk	L1
T ½	= 1 hour (inhalation)	M/P	=
Vd	=	PB	=
Tmax	= <1–10 minutes	Oral	= Poor
MW	= 183	pKa	= 12.65

Adult Concerns: Nervousness, tremors, agitation, tachycardia.

Pediatric Concerns: None reported, but observe for brief stimulation.

Drug Interactions: Increase cardiac irritability when used with halogenated inhaled anesthetics, alpha blocking agents. Do not use with monoamine oxidase inhibitors.

Relative Infant Dose:

Adult Dose: 0.1–0.25 mg injection (IV)

Alternatives:

References:
1.　Wilson J. Drugs in Breast Milk. New York: ADIS Press 1981.

EPIRUBICIN   L5

Trade: Ellence, Epi-Cell, Farmorubicina, Pharmarubicin, Rubina

Other Trades:

Category: Anticancer drug

Epirubicin is an anthracycline similar to but less cardiotoxic than doxorubicin. It is used for the treatment of breast, lung, and bladder cancer. The terminal

T½ (gamma) is 31.2 hours, even though the plasma levels are much lower than doxorubicin.[1,2] The volume of distribution is variable among studies, but is similar if not higher than doxorubicin. No data are available on its transfer to milk, but it is probably as low if not lower than doxorubicin. Mothers should be advised to discontinue breastfeeding for at least seven to ten days following the use of this product. Withhold breastfeeding for at least seven to ten days.

Pregnancy Risk	D	Lactation Risk	L5
T ½	= (gamma) 35 hours	M/P	=
Vd	= 33 l/kg	PB	=
Tmax	=	Oral	=
MW	= 543.52	pKa	= 11.02

Adult Concerns: Bleeding, redness, or ulcers in mouth or throat, cough or hoarseness, fever or chills, lower back or side pain, painful or difficult urination, pain or burning in mouth or throat, sores in mouth or on lips.

Pediatric Concerns: Potentially hazardous chemotherapeutic agent. Withhold breastfeeding for 7–10 days.

Drug Interactions: Do not coadminister live vaccines such as rotavirus, influenza, MMR. Use with caution while co-administering with trastuzumab, cimetidine, paclitaxel, calcium channel blockers.

Relative Infant Dose:

Adult Dose:

Alternatives:

References:
1. Grochow LB, Ames MM. A clinician's guide to chemotherapy pharmacokinetics and pharmacodynamics. 1st ed. Baltimore, MD: Williams and Wilkins; 1998.
2. Pharmaceutical manufacturer prescribing information, 2005.

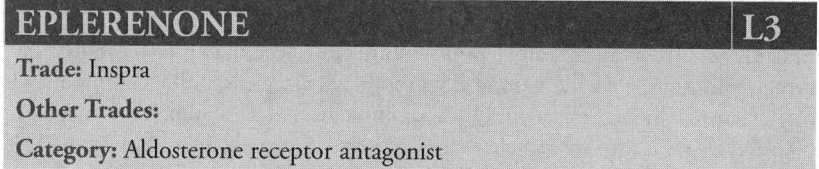

EPLERENONE   L3

Trade: Inspra

Other Trades:

Category: Aldosterone receptor antagonist

Eplerenone blocks the binding of aldosterone by competitively inhibiting the aldosterone receptor and regulating blood pressure as a result. It is similar in structure to spironolactone, but has a lower affinity to steroid receptors, and thus has fewer adverse reactions.[1] It is used to improve survival of stable patients with left ventricular systolic dysfunction (ejection fraction ≤40%) and clinical evidence of congestive heart failure after an acute myocardial infarction. No data are currently available on the transfer on eplerenone into human milk. Until more is known about this drug, caution is urged while administering in breastfeeding women.

Pregnancy Risk	B		Lactation Risk	L3
T ½	= 4–6 hours		M/P	=
Vd	= 1.28 l/kg		PB	= 50%
Tmax	= 1.5 hours		Oral	= 69%
MW	= 414		pKa	=

Adult Concerns: Adverse reactions include angina, heart attack, diarrhea, hyperkalemia, headache, and coughing. Observe for hyperkalemia.

Pediatric Concerns: No data are available.

Drug Interactions: Eplerenone is metabolized via the CYP3A4 pathway, and thus inhibitors of CYP3A4 will increase plasma levels (ketoconazole, saquinavir). Concurrent use of potassium sparing diuretics or ACE inhibitors increase the chance of hyperkalemia when taken with eplerenone. No clinically significant drug-drug pharmacokinetic interactions were observed when eplerenone was administered with cisapride, cyclosporine, digoxin, glyburide, midazolam, oral contraceptives (norethindrone/ethinyl estradiol), simvastatin, or warfarin. St. John's Wort (a CYP3A4 inducer) caused a small (about 30%) decrease in eplerenone AUC.

Relative Infant Dose:

Adult Dose: 25–100 mg QD

Alternatives: Spironolactone

References:
1. Pharmaceutical manufacturer prescribing information, 2005.

EPOETIN ALFA   L3

Trade: Epogen
Other Trades:
Category: Stimulates red blood cell production

Epoetin alfa is a glycoprotein which stimulates red blood cell production.[1] Structurally similar to the natural erythropoietin, it consists of 165 amino acids manufactured by recombinant DNA technology. It has a molecular weight of 30,400 daltons. Large molecular weight proteins in general are poorly transferred into human milk after the first week postpartum. Due to its protein nature, it would not likely be absorbed orally to any degree by the infant.

Pregnancy Risk	C		Lactation Risk	L3
T ½	= 4–13 hours		M/P	=
Vd	=		PB	=
Tmax	= 5–24 hours		Oral	= Nil
MW	= 30,400		pKa	= 4.5–5.5

Adult Concerns: Headache, hypertension, arthralgias, nausea, edema, vomiting and chest pain have been reported in adults.

Pediatric Concerns: None reported via milk.

Drug Interactions: None.

Relative Infant Dose:

Adult Dose: 50–100 Units three times weekly

Alternatives:

References:
1. PM2001. Pharmaceutical manufacturer prescribing information, 2003.

EPOPROSTENOL   L3

Trade: Flolan

Other Trades:

Category: Vasodilator, platelet function inhibitor

Epoprostenol (Prostacyclin; PGX; PGI-2) is a naturally occurring prostaglandin that is a potent inhibitor of platelet aggregation and a vasodilator. It is commonly used to treat primary pulmonary hypertension. It is rapidly metabolized in plasma to a metabolite, which is biologically inactive, and has a half-life of only 3–5 minutes.[1] Prostaglandins are known to be transferred into human milk, but they are believed to be derived from mammary tissue and synthesized with cellular components of breastmilk.[2] With the extraordinarily short half-life of this product, it is unlikely any would penetrate into milk, be retained for very long, or be stable in the infant's gut. Oral absorption by the infant is unlikely.[1–2]

Pregnancy Risk	B	Lactation Risk	L3
T ½	= 6 minutes	M/P	=
Vd	= 357 mL l/kg	PB	=
Tmax	=	Oral	= Nil
MW	= 374	pKa	= 14.80

Adult Concerns: Flushing, headache, nausea, vomiting, hypotension, anxiety, chest pain, dizziness, bradycardia, abdominal pain.

Pediatric Concerns: None reported, unlikely to be absorbed.

Drug Interactions: May decrease clearance of digoxin. Decreased oral clearance of furosemide.

Relative Infant Dose:

Adult Dose: 2 ng/kg per minute

Alternatives:

References:
1. Pharmaceutical manufacturer prescribing information, 2010.
2. Friedman Z. Prostaglandins in breast milk. Endocrinol Exp 1986; 20(2–3): 285–291.

EPROSARTAN   L3/L4

Trade: Teveten
Other Trades:
Category: Antihypertensive, angiotensin receptor blocker

Eprosartan is an angiotensin receptor blocker (ARB) used in the treatment of hypertension.[1] No data are available on its use in breastfeeding mothers. Its use in mothers breastfeeding premature infants or even infants less than 4 months should be avoided due to possible renal toxicity.

Pregnancy Risk	C/X in 2nd and 3rd trimester	Lactation Risk	L3/L4 first 4 months
T ½	= 20 hours	M/P	=
Vd	= 4.4 l/kg	PB	= 98%
Tmax	= 1–2 hours	Oral	= 13%
MW	= 520	pKa	= 4.38

Adult Concerns: Headache, dizziness, fatigue, facial edema, cough have been reported.

Pediatric Concerns: None yet via milk, however do not use in breastfeeding mothers with newborn or premature infants.

Drug Interactions: None yet reported.

Relative Infant Dose:

Adult Dose:

Alternatives: Captopril, enalapril, benazepril

References:
1. Pharmaceutical manufacturer prescribing information, 2010.

EPSTEIN-BARR VIRUS   L3

Trade: Mononucleosis, EBV
Other Trades:
Category: Herpesvirus infection (EBV)

The Epstein-Barr virus (EBV) is one of the causes of infectious mononucleosis. EBV belongs to the herpesvirus family. Symptoms include fever, exudative pharyngitis, lymphadenopathy, hepatosplenomegaly, and atypical lymphocytosis. Close personal contact is generally required for transmission and it is not known if EBV is secreted into human milk, although it is likely. Studies by Kusuhara[1] indicate that the seroprevalence of EBV at 12–23 months was the same in bottle-fed and in breastfed infants. This data suggests that breastmilk is not a significant source of early EBV infections.

Pregnancy Risk	Probably Safe	Lactation Risk	L3
T ½	=	M/P	=
Vd	=	PB	=
Tmax	=	Oral	=
MW	=	pKa	=

Adult Concerns: Symptoms include fever, exudative pharyngitis, lymphadenopathy, hepatosplenomegaly, and atypical lymphocytosis.

Pediatric Concerns:

Drug Interactions:

Relative Infant Dose:

Adult Dose:

Alternatives:

References:
1. Kusuhara K, Takabayashi A, Ueda K, Hidaka Y, Minamishima I, Take H, Fujioka K, Imai S, Osato T. Breast milk is not a significant source for early Epstein-Barr virus or human herpesvirus 6 infection in infants: a seroepidemiologic study in 2 endemic areas of human T-cell lymphotropic virus type I in Japan. Microbiol Immunol 1997; 41(4): 309–312.

EPTIFIBATIDE   L3

Trade: Integrilin
Other Trades: Integrilin
Category: Antiplatelet agent

Eptifibatide is used in the treatment of acute coronary syndrome. It works by blocking the platelet glycoprotein IIb/IIIa receptor, and thus inhibits platelet aggregation.[1] It is a small peptide of approximately 831 daltons and is probably poorly absorbed orally if at all. No data are available on the transfer into human milk, however, due to the large molecular weight of eptifibatide and its poor bioavailability as a peptide, it is unlikely that it would pass into the milk compartment or be absorbed orally by the infant.

Pregnancy Risk	B	Lactation Risk	L3
T ½	= 2.5 hours	M/P	=
Vd	= 0.18 l/kg	PB	= 25%
Tmax	= 5 minutes	Oral	= Nil
MW	= 831	pKa	=

Adult Concerns: Adverse reactions include bleeding, hypotension, and thrombocytopenia.

Pediatric Concerns: No data are available. Unlikely to enter milk.

Drug Interactions: Cephalosporins, antiplatelet agents, heparin, aspirin, and warfarin can all increase the risk of bleeding.

Relative Infant Dose:

Adult Dose: 2 µg/kg/minute

Alternatives:

References:

1. Pharmaceutical manufacturer prescribing information, 1998.

ERGONOVINE   L3

Trade: Ergotrate

Other Trades: Syntometrine, Ergotrate

Category: Postpartum uterine bleeding

Ergonovine maleate and its close congener, methylergonovine maleate, directly stimulate uterine and vascular smooth muscle contractions. They are primarily used to prevent/treat postpartum hemorrhage. Although pharmacologically similar, many clinicians prefer methylergonovine because it produces less hypertension than ergonovine. In a study of 8 postpartum women receiving 0.125 mg three times daily until day 5 when a 0.25 mg tablet was introduced, measurable ergonovine was only found in 4 of 8 patients and averaged 0.8 µg/L.[1] These authors suggested that use of the drug during breastfeeding would not affect the infant.

In addition, the effect of ergonovine on prolactin levels is controversial. In one study methylergonovine did not alter postpartum maternal prolactin levels[2], while in another study[3] a significant reduction in prolactin production was produced by ergonovine. Ergonovine use in lactating women would presumably suppress lactation, whereas methylergonovine may not.

When used at doses of 0.2 mg up to 3–4 times daily, only small quantities of ergonovine are found in milk. Short-term (1 week) low-dose regimens of these agents do not apparently pose problems in nursing mothers or their infants. Methylergonovine is preferred because it does not inhibit lactation and levels in milk are minimal. The prolonged use of ergot alkaloids should be avoided and can lead to severe gangrenous manifestations.

Pregnancy Risk	X	Lactation Risk	L3
T ½	= 0.5–2 hours	M/P	=
Vd	=	PB	=
Tmax	= 30–180 minutes	Oral	= >60%
MW	= 441	pKa	= 15.94

Adult Concerns: Hypertension, seizures, vomiting, diarrhea, cold extremities.

Pediatric Concerns: None reported, but long term exposure is not recommended. Methylergonovine is commonly recommended early postpartum for breastfeeding mothers to reduce uterine bleeding.

Drug Interactions:

Relative Infant Dose: 1.9%

Adult Dose: 0.2 mg injection (IM) every 2–4 hours

Alternatives: Methylergonovine

References:

1. Erkkola R, Kanto J, Allonen H, Kleimola T, Mantyla R. Excretion of methylergometrine (methylergonovine) into the human breast milk. Int J Clin Pharmacol Biopharm 1978; 16(12): 579–580.
2. Del Pozo E, Brun DR, Hinselmann M. Lack of effect of methyl-ergonovine on postpartum lactation. Am J Obstet Gynecol 1975; 123(8): 845–846.
3. Canales ES, Garrido JT, Zarate A, Mason M, Soria J. Effect of ergonovine on prolactin secretion and milk let-down. Obstet Gynecol 1976; 48(2): 228–229.

ERGOTAMINE   L4

Trade: Wigraine, Cafergot, Ergostat, Ergomar, DHE-45

Other Trades: Cafergot, Ergodryl, Migral, Ergomar, Gynergen, Lingraine

Category: Anti-migraine, inhibits prolactin

Ergotamine tartrate is a potent vasoconstrictor generally used in acute phases of migraine headache. It is never used chronically for prophylaxis of migraine. Although early reports suggest ergotamine compounds are secreted in breastmilk[1] and cause symptoms of ergotism (vomiting, and diarrhea) in infants, other authors[2] suggest that the short term use of ergotamine (0.2 mg postpartum) generally presents no problem to a nursing infant. This is likely, due to the fact that less than 5% of ergotamine is orally absorbed in adults. However, excessive dosing and prolonged administration may inhibit prolactin secretion and hence lactation. Although the initial plasma half-life is only 2 hours, ergotamine is stored for long periods in various tissues producing long-lasting effects (terminal half-life= 21 hours). Use during lactation should be strongly discouraged.

Pregnancy Risk	X	Lactation Risk	L4
T ½	= 21 hours	M/P	=
Vd	=	PB	=
Tmax	= 0.5–3 hours	Oral	= <5%
MW	= 581	pKa	= 11.64

Adult Concerns: Ergotism, peripheral artery insufficiency, nausea, vomiting, paresthesia, cold skin temperatures, headache.

Pediatric Concerns: One case of ergotism reported and included symptoms such as vomiting and diarrhea. Long term exposure is contraindicated.

Drug Interactions: Rifamycin and other macrolide antibiotics may enhance ergot toxicity.

Relative Infant Dose:

Adult Dose: 2 mg every 30 minutes

Alternatives: Propranolol, Sumatriptan

References:
1. Fomina PL. Untersuchungen uber den ubergang des aktiven agens des Muttrkorns in die milch stillender Mutter. Arch Gynecol 1934; 157: 275.
2. White G, White M. Breastfeeding and drugs in human milk. Vet and Human Tox 1984; 26: supplement 1.

ERLOTINIB　　　　　　　　　　　　　　　　　　L4

Trade: Tarceva

Other Trades:

Category: Anticancer drug

Erlotinib is a human epidermal growth factor receptor inhibitor. It is an antineoplastic used for the treatment and maintenance therapy of advanced non-small cell lung cancer after the failure of other chemotherapy treatment. It is also used in conjunction with gemcitabine to treat cancer of the pancreas.

Erlotinib is about 60% absorbed after oral administration, and its bioavailability is substantially increased by food to almost 100%.[1] Its half-life is about 36 hours. Bioavailability of erlotinib following a 150 mg oral dose is about 60%, and peak plasma levels occur four hours after dosing. Following absorption, erlotinib is approximately 93% protein bound to albumin and alpha-1 acid glycoprotein (AAG). Erlotinib has an apparent volume of distribution of 232 liters.

No data are available on its transfer to human milk. While administering in breastfeeding women, weigh the potential benefits against the potential risks. Because this drug is a inhibitor of epidermal growth factor, it could have profound effects on a rapidly growing infant. Its entry into milk is likely minimal due to its size and pKa, but because of its enormous volume of distribution, mothers should withhold breastfeeding for a minimum of 10–15 days. Withhold breastfeeding for a minimum of 10–15 days.

Pregnancy Risk	D	Lactation Risk	L4
T ½	= 36 hours	M/P	=
Vd	= 3.3 l/kg	PB	= 93%
Tmax	= 4 hours	Oral	=
MW	= 429.9	pKa	= 5.42

Adult Concerns: Burning, tingling, numbness or pain in the hands, arms, feet, or legs, cough or hoarseness, diarrhea, difficult or labored breathing, fever or chills, lower back or side pain, painful or difficult urination, rash, sensation of pins and needles, shortness of breath, stabbing chest pain, chest tightness, wheezing.

Pediatric Concerns:

Drug Interactions: Concomitant use with the following drugs increases plasma levels and potential toxicity of erlotinib: ketoconazole, atazanavir, clarithromycin, indinavir, itraconazole, nefazodone, nelfinavir, ritonavir, saquinavir, telithromycin, troleandomycin, voriconazole and grapefruit or grapefruit juice. Co-administration with the following drugs decreases plasma levels and efficacy of erlotinib: rifampin, rifabutin, rifapentine, phenytoin, carbamazepine, phenobarbital and St. John's

Wort. Coadministration with proton-pump inhibitors such as omeprazole, rabeprazole, pantoprazole also decreases efficacy of erlotinib by decreasing its oral bioavailability. Cigarette smoking has been found to decrease its efficacy and therapeutic potential.

Relative Infant Dose:

Adult Dose: 100–150 mg per day.

Alternatives:

References:
1. Pharmaceutical manufacturer prescribing information, 2008.

ERTAPENEM   L3

Trade: Invanz

Other Trades: Invanz

Category: Carbapenem antibiotic

Ertapenem is an antibiotic indicated for treatment of complicated infections of the skin/subcutaneous tissues, urinary tract and respiratory tract. The manufacturer reports the concentration of ertapenem in breast milk from 5 lactating women with pelvic infections (5 to 14 days postpartum) was measured at random time points daily for 5 consecutive days following the last 1 gm dose of intravenous therapy (3–10 days of therapy). The concentration of ertapenem in breast milk within 24 hours of the last dose of therapy in all 5 women ranged from <0.13 (lower limit of quantitation) to 0.38 mg/L; peak concentrations were not assessed unfortunately. By day 5 after discontinuation of therapy, the level of ertapenem was undetectable in the breast milk of 4 women and below the lower limit of quantitation (<0.13 µg/mL) in 1 woman.[1]

The above data does not report C_{max} concentrations in milk nor the time samples were collected, so it is virtually worthless for determining infant exposure to the medication during the day and following the administration.

Using the above data and an assumed average weight of 70 kg, the mothers received about 14.28 mg/kg/day. After 24 hours, the infant would ingest about 57 µg/kg/day. The relative infant dose would be 0.4% of the maternal dose at this time. Without good data it is not possible to estimate clinical dose to the infant, but it is likely small and its oral bioavailability is poor. Almost all the penicillins and the carbapenems are safe to use in breastfeeding mothers.

Pregnancy Risk	B	Lactation Risk	L3
T ½	= 4 hours	M/P	=
Vd	= 0.11 l/kg	PB	= 95%
Tmax	= 2 hours	Oral	= Poor
MW	= 497	pKa	= 4.05

Adult Concerns: Diarrhea, infused vein complications, nausea, headache, vaginitis in females, thrombophlebitis, vomiting, fever, abdominal pain. Do not use if penicillin allergic. Seizures, altered mental status.

Pediatric Concerns: None reported via milk. However diarrhea, and perhaps less common pseudomembranous colitis could occur.

Drug Interactions: Increased levels when administered with probenecid.

Relative Infant Dose: 0.1%–0.4%

Adult Dose: 1 gm IV/IM daily.

Alternatives: Imipenem

References:

1. Pharmaceutical manufacturer prescribing information, 2003.

ERYTHROMYCIN   L3

Trade: E-Mycin, Ery-Tab, Eryc, Ilosone

Other Trades: EMU-V, Ilosone, EES, Erythrocin, E-mycin, Eryc, Erythromide, Novo-Rythro, PCE, Ilotyc, Ceplac, Erycen

Category: Macrolide antibiotic

Erythromycin is an older, narrow-spectrum antibiotic. In one study of patients receiving 400 mg three times daily, milk levels varied from 0.4 to 1.6 mg/L.[1] Doses as high as 2 gm per day produced milk levels of 1.6 to 3.2 mg/L. One case of hypertrophic pyloric stenosis apparently linked to erythromycin administration has been reported.[2] In a study of 2–3 patients who received a single 500 oral dose, milk levels at 4 hours ranged from 0.9 to 1.4 mg/L with a milk/plasma ratio of 0.92.[3] Newer macrolide-like antibiotics (azithromycin) may preclude the use of erythromycin. A recent and large study now suggests a strong positive correlation between the use of erythromycin in breastfeeding mothers and infantile hypertrophic pyloric stenosis in newborns.[4]

Pregnancy Risk	B	Lactation Risk	L3
T ½	= 1.5–2 hours	M/P	= 0.92
Vd	=	PB	= 84%
Tmax	= 2–4 hours	Oral	= Variable
MW	= 734	pKa	= 12.91

Adult Concerns: Abdominal cramping, nausea, vomiting, hepatitis, ototoxicity, and hypersensitivity.

Pediatric Concerns: Pyloric stenosis has been reported associated with the use of erythromycin early postpartum.

Drug Interactions: Erythromycin may decrease clearance of carbamazepine, cyclosporin, triazolam. Erythromycin may decrease theophylline clearance by as much as 60%. May increase terfenadine plasma levels and increase Q/T intervals. May potentiate anticoagulant effect of warfarin.

Relative Infant Dose: 1.4%–1.7%

Adult Dose: 500–800 mg QID

Alternatives: Azithromycin, clarithromycin

References:

1. Knowles JA. Drugs in milk. Pediatr Currents 1972; 1: 28–32.
2. Stang H. Pyloric stenosis associated with erythromycin ingested through breastmilk. Minn Med 1986; 69(11): 669–70, 682.
3. Matsuda S. Transfer of antibiotics into maternal milk. Biol Res Pregnancy Perinatol 1984; 5(2): 57–60.
4. Sorensen HT, Skriver MV, Pedersen L, Larsen H, Ebbesen F, Schonheyder HC. Risk of infantile hypertrophic pyloric stenosis after maternal postnatal use of macrolides. Scand J Infect Dis 2003; 35(2): 104–106.

ESCITALOPRAM   L2

Trade: Lexapro

Other Trades:

Category: Antidepressant

Escitalopram is a selective serotonin reuptake inhibitor (SSRI) used in the treatment of depression. It is the active S(+)-enantiomer of citalopram (Celexa). While this agent is very specific for the serotonin receptor site, it does apparently have a number of other side effects which may be related to activities at other receptors. Antagonism of muscarinic, histaminergic, and adrenergic receptors has been hypothesized to be associated with various anticholinergic, sedative and cardiovascular side effects.

In a case report of a 32-year-old mother taking escitalopram (5 mg/day) while breastfeeding her newborn, the reported milk level was 24.9 ng/mL at one week postpartum. The infant's daily dose was estimated to be 3.74 µg/kg. At 7.5 weeks of age, the mother was taking 10 mg/day and the milk concentration level was 76.1 ng/mL. The infant daily dose was 11.4 µg/kg. There were no adverse events reported in the infant.[1]

In a recent study of eight breastfeeding women taking an average of 10 mg/day, the total relative infant dose of escitalopram and its metabolite was reported to be 5.3% of the mothers dose.[2] The mean M/P ratio (AUC) was 2.2 for escitalopram and 2.2 for demethylescitalopram. Absolute infant doses were 7.6 µg/kg/day for escitalopram and 3.0 µg/kg/day for demethylescitalopram. The drug and its metabolite were undetectable in most of the infants tested. No adverse events in the infants were reported. Because the absolute infant dose of escitalopram is less than an equivalent antidepressant dose of racemic citalopram (Celexa), it's use is preferred over citalopram in treating depression in lactating women.

Pregnancy Risk	C	Lactation Risk	L2
T ½	= 27–32 hours	M/P	= 2.2
Vd	= 12 l/kg	PB	= 56%
Tmax	= 5 hours	Oral	= 80%
MW	= 414	pKa	= 9.5

Adult Concerns: Adverse events include nausea, sweating, dizziness, insomnia, somnolence, ejaculation disorder, diaphoresis, anorexia, and fatigue.

Pediatric Concerns: Recent data concerning the use of this product in breastfeeding mothers suggests the relative infant dose is low and levels in breastfed infant's plasma are largely undetectable.

Drug Interactions: Increased citalopram levels when used with macrolide antibiotics (erythromycin), cimetidine, and azole antifungals such as fluconazole, itraconazole, ketoconazole, etc. Carbamazepine may reduce plasma levels of citalopram. Serious reactions may occur if escitalopram is administered too soon after MAO use. Beta blocker (metoprolol) levels may increase by 2 fold when admixed with escitalopram. The combined used of escitalopram and sumatriptan (Imitrex) have been reported to produce weakness, hyperreflexia and incoordination. Escitalopram may increase levels of desipramine.

Relative Infant Dose: 5.2%–7.9%

Adult Dose: 10–40 mg daily

Alternatives: Sertraline, fluoxetine

References:
1. Castberg I, Spigset O. Excretion of Escitalopram in Breast Milk. J Clin Psychopharm 2006; 26(5): 536–538.
2. Rampono J, Hackett LP, Kristensen JH, Kohan R, Page-Sharp M, Ilett KF. Transfer of escitalopram and its metabolite demethylescitalopram into breastmilk. Br J Clin Pharmacol 2006; 62(3): 316–322.

ESMOLOL   L3

Trade: Brevibloc

Other Trades: Brevibloc

Category: Beta blocker antiarrhythmic

Esmolol is an ultra short-acting beta blocker agent (T½= 9 minutes) with low lipid solubility. It is of the same family as propranolol. It is primarily used for treatment of supraventricular tachycardia. It is only used IV and has an extremely short half-life. It is almost completely hydrolyzed in 30 minutes.[1,2] No data are available on its use in breastfeeding mothers.

Pregnancy Risk	C	Lactation Risk	L3
T ½	= 9 minutes	M/P	=
Vd	=	PB	= 55%
Tmax	= 15 minutes	Oral	= Poor
MW	= 295	pKa	= 9.5

Adult Concerns: Hypotension, bradycardia, dizziness, somnolence.

Pediatric Concerns: None reported.

Drug Interactions: Caution while coadministering esmolol with other hypotensive drugs such as reserpine, clonidine as the additive effect could cause severe hypotension, bradycardia, syncope, vertigo. Do not use esmolol with other medications that depress cardiac contractility such as verapamil, dronedarone, amiodarone, diltiazem to avoid the increased risk of fatal cardiac arrest.

Relative Infant Dose:

Adult Dose: 100 µg/kg/minute

Alternatives: Propranolol, metoprolol

References:
1.   McEvoy GE. (ed): AFHS Drug Information. New York, NY: 2003.
2.   Lacy C. Drug information handbook. Lexi-Comp Inc. Cleveland, OH, 1996.

ESOMEPRAZOLE   L2

Trade: Nexium

Other Trades: Nexium

Category: Reduces gastric acid secretion

Esomeprazole is the S-isomer of omeprazole (Prilosec) and is essentially identical to omeprazole.[1] Omeprazole is a potent inhibitor of gastric acid secretion. In a study of one patient receiving 20 mg omeprazole daily, the maternal serum concentration was negligible until 90 minutes after ingestion and then reached 950 nM at 240 min.[2] The breastmilk concentration of omeprazole began to rise minimally at 90 minutes after ingestion and peaked after 180 minutes at only 58 nM, or less than 7% of the highest serum level. This would indicate a maximum dose of 3 µg/kg/day in a breastfed infant. Omeprazole milk levels were essentially flat over 4 hours of observation. Omeprazole is extremely acid labile with a half-life of 10 minutes at pH values below 4.[3] Virtually all omeprazole ingested via milk would probably be destroyed in the stomach of the infant prior to absorption. Esomeprazole is probably compatible with breastfeeding.

Pregnancy Risk	C	Lactation Risk	L2
T ½	= 1–1.5 hours	M/P	=
Vd	= 0.23 l/kg	PB	= 97%
Tmax	= 1.5 hours	Oral	= 90%
MW	= 767.2	pKa	= 18.29

Adult Concerns: Headache, dry mouth, dizziness, diarrhea, flatulence, abdominal pain, nausea, hypertension, urinary tract infection, arthralgia, respiratory infection.

Pediatric Concerns:

Drug Interactions: Administration of esomeprazole and clarithromycin may result in increased plasma levels of esomeprazole. Omeprazole produced a 130% increase in the half-life of diazepam, reduced the plasma clearance of phenytoin by 15%, and increased phenytoin half-life by 27%. May prolong the elimination of warfarin.

Relative Infant Dose:

Adult Dose: 20–40 mg daily

Alternatives:

References:
1.   Pharmaceutical manufacturer prescribing information, 2010.

2. Marshall JK, Thompson AB, Armstrong D. Omeprazole for refractory gastroesophageal reflux disease during pregnancy and lactation. Can J Gastroenterol 1998; 12(3): 225–227.
3. Pilbrant A, Cederberg C. Development of an oral formulation of omeprazole. Scand J Gastroenterol Suppl 1985; 108: 113–120.

ESOMEPRAZOLE + NAPROXEN | L3

Trade: Vimovo

Other Trades:

Category: NSAID + Proton pump inhibitor

Esomeprazole magnesium and Naproxen is a drug combination indicated for the relief of signs and symptoms of osteoarthritis, rheumatoid arthritis and ankylosing spondylitis in patients at risk of NSAID associated gastric ulcers.[1] This product is not recommended for initial treatment of acute pain because the absorption of naproxen is delayed compared to absorption from other naproxen-containing products. Controlled studies do not extend beyond 6 months.

The excretion of esomeprazole in milk has not been studied. It is not known whether this drug is excreted in human milk. Esomeprazole is the S-isomer of omeprazole (Prilosec) and is essentially identical to omeprazole. In a study of one patient receiving 20 mg omeprazole daily, the maternal serum concentration was negligible until 90 minutes after ingestion and then reached 950 nM at 240 min.[2] The breastmilk concentration of omeprazole began to rise minimally at 90 minutes after ingestion and peaked after 180 minutes at only 58 nM, or less than 7% of the highest serum level. This would indicate a maximum dose of 3 µg/kg/day in a breastfed infant. Omeprazole milk levels were essentially flat over 4 hours of observation. Omeprazole is extremely acid labile with a half-life of 10 minutes at pH values below 4.[3] Virtually all omeprazole ingested via milk would probably be destroyed in the stomach of the infant prior to absorption.

Naproxen is a popular NSAID analgesic. It does excrete into the breastmilk, but it does not appear in quantities that would result in untoward effects in a breastfed infant. NSAIDs in general are usually compatible with breastfeeding, with some, such as ibuprofen, being completely undetectable in breastmilk.[4] In a study done at steady state in one mother consuming 375 mg of naproxen twice daily, milk levels ranged from 1.76–2.37 mg/L at 4 hours.[5,6] Total naproxen excretion in the infant's urine was only 0.26% of the maternal dose. One case of prolonged bleeding, hemorrhage, and acute anemia has been reported in a seven-day-old infant.[7] The relative infant dose on a weight-adjusted maternal daily dose would probably be less than 3.3%. Other studies have confirmed naproxen's low transfer into breastmilk, showing a 1% concentration compared to the mother's plasma levels.[8,9] Despite very low transfer into milk, there have been some reports of adverse effects in infants whose mothers were administered naproxen. In a study of twenty mothers given this medication, two reported drowsiness in their infants, while one reported vomiting.[10] Although the amount of naproxen transferred via milk is minimal, one should use with caution in nursing mothers because of its long half-life and its effect on infant cardiovascular system, kidneys, and gastrointestinal tract. However, its short term use postpartum or infrequent or occasional use would not necessarily be incompatible with breastfeeding.

Therefore, the use of esomeprazole + naproxen is probably compatible with breastfeeding for short-term use, but extra caution is urged for prolonged/long-term/chronic use.

Pregnancy Risk	C/D in 3rd trimester	Lactation Risk	L3
T ½	= Esomeprazole/naproxen: 1–1.5 hours/12–15 hours	M/P	= Esomeprazole/naproxen: /0.01
Vd	= Esomeprazole/naproxen: 0.23/0.09 l/kg	PB	= Esomeprazole/naproxen: 97%/99.7%
Tmax	= Esomeprazole/naproxen: 1.5 hours/2–4 hours	Oral	= Esomeprazole/naproxen: 90%/74–99%
MW	= Esomeprazole/naproxen: 767.2/230	pKa	= Esomeprazole/naproxen: 18.29/5.0

Adult Concerns: Hives, facial swelling, asthma (wheezing), shock, rash, stomach bleeding, gut cramps, diarrhea have been reported.

Pediatric Concerns: Watery diarrhea has been reported in one infant after several weeks of maternal use. Temporary use is OK, avoid long-term exposure while breastfeeding. One reported case of prolonged bleeding, hemorrhage, and acute anemia in a seven-day-old infant exposed to naproxen.

Drug Interactions: May potentiate efficacy and toxicity of following co-administered drugs: cyclosporine, tacrolimus, lithium, methotrexate, anticoagulants, warfarin. May decrease efficacy of following co-administered drugs: ACE inhibitors, furosemide, beta-blockers. Concomitant use with the following drugs may cause increase plasma levels of esomeprazole + naproxen: probenecid. Concomitant use with the following may decrease plasma levels and efficacy of esomeprazole + naproxen: cholestyramine. Do not use concomitantly with aspirin, selective serotonin reuptake inhibitors (SSRIs).

Relative Infant Dose:

Adult Dose: 20 mg/375–500 mg Esomeprazole/naproxen

Alternatives:

References:
1. Pharmaceutical manufacturer prescribing information, 2012.
2. Marshall JK, Thompson AB, Armstrong D. Omeprazole for refractory gastroesophageal reflux disease during pregnancy and lactation. Can J Gastroenterol 1998; 12(3): 225–227.
3. Pilbrant A, Cederberg C. Development of an oral formulation of omeprazole. Scand J Gastroenterol Suppl 1985; 108: 113–120.
4. Anon: Committee on Drugs and American Academy of Pediatrics: The transfer of drugs and other chemicals into human milk. Pediatrics 1994; 93: 137–150.
5. Jamali F, Stevens DR. Naproxen excretion in milk and its uptake by the infant. Drug Intell Clin Pharm 1983; 17(12): 910–911.
6. Jamali F. et. al. Naproxen excretion in breast milk and its uptake by sucking infant. Drug Intell Clin Pharm 1982; 16: 475 (Abstr).
7. Figalgo I. et. al. Anemia aguda, rectaorragia y hematuria asociadas a la ingestion de naproxen. Anales Espanoles de Pediatrica 1989; 30: 317–319.
8. Product Information: Prevacid(R) NapraPAC(TM), lansoprazole delayed-release capsules and naproxen tablets kit. TAP Pharmaceuticals, Lake Forest, IL, 2003a.

9. Brogden RN: Naproxen: A reveiw of its pharmacological properties and therapeutic efficacy and use. Drugs 1975; 9: 326.
10. Ito S, Blajchman A, Stephenson M, et al: Prospective follow-up of adverse reactions in breast-fed infants exposed to maternal medication. Am J Obstet Gynecol 1993; 168(5): 1393–1399.

ESTAZOLAM   L3

Trade: Prosom

Other Trades:

Category: Benzodiazepine sedative

Estazolam is a benzodiazepine sedative hypnotic that belongs to the Valium family. Estazolam, like other benzodiazepines, is secreted into rodent milk although the levels are unpublished.[1] No data are available on human milk levels. It is likely that some is secreted into human milk as well.

Pregnancy Risk	X	Lactation Risk	L3
T ½	= 10–24 hours	M/P	=
Vd	=	PB	= 93%
Tmax	= 0.5–3 hours	Oral	= Complete
MW	= 295	pKa	= 9

Adult Concerns: Sedation.

Pediatric Concerns: None reported via milk, but observe for sedation, apnea.

Drug Interactions: Certain enzyme inducers such as barbiturates may increase the metabolism of estazolam. CNS depressants may increase adverse effects of estazolam. Cimetidine may decrease metabolism of estazolam.

Relative Infant Dose:

Adult Dose: 1–2 mg daily

Alternatives: Lorazepam, midazolam, alprazolam

References:
1. Pharmaceutical manufacturer prescribing information, 1995.

ESTRADIOL + MEDROXYPROGESTERONE L3

Trade: Lunelle

Other Trades:

Category: Once-a-month birth control injection

Estradiol cypionate and Medroxyprogesterone is a drug combination indicated for use as an injectable contraceptive agent. This drug product is a once-a-month injectable birth control product. It contains medroxyprogesterone acetate (25 mg), and also contains 5 mg estradiol cypionate, which is a repository form of estrogen that is slowly released from the injection site over 30 days.

Because this injection contains estrogen, it may potentially reduce the production of milk and caution is recommended.[1] Although small amounts of estradiol may pass into breastmilk, the effects of estrogens on the infant appear minimal.

Early postpartum use of estrogens may reduce volume of milk produced and the protein content, but it is variable and depends on dose and the individual.[2,3,4,5] Breastfeeding mothers should attempt to wait until lactation is firmly established (6–8 weeks) prior to use of estrogen-containing oral contraceptives.

The effect of progestins (in this case, medroxyprogesterone), on milk production is poorly studied. Early postpartum, while progestin receptors are still present in the breast, administering progestins may actually suppress milk production just as it does in the pregnant women. This has been seen occasionally in patients early postpartum. Several days to a week later, most progestin receptors disappear from the lactocyte and breast tissues become relatively immune to the effects of progestins. Thus it is advisable to wait as long as possible postpartum prior to instituting therapy with progesterone to avoid reducing the milk supply.

Mothers should attempt to delay use of these products for as long as possible postpartum (at least 6–8 weeks), if at all. Because of the estrogen content and the prolonged release formula, caution is recommended in breastfeeding mothers.

Pregnancy Risk	X	Lactation Risk	L3
T ½	= estradiol/ MP: 60 min/14.5 hours	M/P	= estradiol/ MP: 0.08/
Vd	=	PB	= estradiol/ MP: 98%
Tmax	= estradiol/ MP: rapid	Oral	= estradiol/ MP: complete/0.6–10%
MW	= estradiol/ MP: 272/344	pKa	= estradiol/ MP:

Adult Concerns: Side effects include thromboembolism, cerebral hemorrhage, hypertension, infarction, cerebral ischemia, gallbladder disease, pulmonary embolism, thrombophlebitis. Abdominal pain, acne, etc. See package insert for numerous others.

Pediatric Concerns: Possibility of reduce milk supply. Long term follow-up of infants has shown no untoward effects.

Drug Interactions: Aminoglutethimide may decrease effectiveness and serum concentration of medroxyprogesterone. Rifampin may increase metabolism of estrogens/progestins. Anticonvulsants such as phenobarbital, phenytoin, and carbamazepine have been shown to increase metabolism of some estrogens and progestins and could reduce contraceptive effectiveness. Some antibiotics (ampicillin, tetracycline and griseofulvin) may reduce contraceptive effectiveness. St. Johns wort may also reduce contraceptive effectiveness by enhancing metabolism of numerous drugs.

Relative Infant Dose:

Adult Dose: Estradiol/medroxyprogesterone: 5 mg/25 mg injected once monthly

Alternatives: Micronor, Ovrette

References:
1. Booker DE, Pahl IR. Control of postpartum breast engorgement with oral contraceptives. Am J Obstet Gynecol 1967; 98(8): 1099–1101.
2. Booker DE, Pahl IR. Control of postpartum breast engorgement with oral contraceptives. Am J Obstet Gynecol 1967; 98(8): 1099–1101.

3. Kamal I, Hefnawi F, Ghoneim M, Abdallah M, Abdel RS. Clinical, biochemical, and experimental studies on lactation. V. Clinical effects of steroids on the initiation of lactation. Am J Obstet Gynecol 1970; 108(4): 655–658.
4. Kora SJ. Effect of oral contraceptives on lactation. Fertil Steril 1969; 20(3): 419–423.
5. Koetsawang S, Bhiraleus P, Chiemprajert T. Effects of oral contraceptives on lactation. Fertil Steril 1972; 23(1): 24–28.

ESTRADIOL, ESTRADIOL VALERATE, ESTRADIOL CYPIONATE   L3

Trade: Alora, Climara, Esclim, Estrace, Estraderm, Estrasorb, Estring, EstroGel, Femring

Other Trades: Femtrace, Depo-Estradiol, Depogen, Valergen, Delestrogen

Category: Estrogenic substances

Estradiol is an estrogenic agent available in topical, oral, vaginal, transdermal and injectable forms. Estradiol acetate, valerate and cypionate are different forms of estradiol with essentially similar pharmacological effects. Estradiol valerate and cypionate are injectable forms.

When possible, advise the nursing mother to use other forms of contraception until she has weaned her child. Although small amounts may pass into breastmilk, the effects of estrogens on the infant appear minimal. Early postpartum use of estrogens may reduce volume of milk produced and the protein content, but it is variable and depends on dose and the individual.[1,2,3,4] Breastfeeding mothers should attempt to wait until lactation is firmly established (6–8 weeks) prior to use of estrogen-containing oral contraceptives. In one study of six lactating women who received 50 or 100 mg vaginal suppositories of estradiol, the plasma levels peaked at 3 hours.[5] These doses were extremely large and are not used clinically. In another study of 11 women, the mean concentration of estradiol in breastmilk was found to be 113 pg/mL.[6] This is very close to that seen when the woman begins ovulating during lactation. If oral contraceptives are used during lactation, the transfer of estradiol to human milk will be low and will not exceed the transfer during physiologic conditions when the mother has resumed ovulation. However, suppression of lactation is still the major concern with the use of these products in breastfeeding mothers. If at all possible, do not use in breastfeeding mothers.

Pregnancy Risk	X	Lactation Risk	L3
T ½	= 21.4 hours–25.9 hours	M/P	=
Vd	=	PB	=
Tmax	= 0.5–1 hour	Oral	=
MW	= 272.39	pKa	=

Adult Concerns: Changes in vaginal bleeding patterns, breast tenderness, deep and superficial venous thrombosis, myocardial infarction, stroke, increase in blood pressure, nausea, vomiting, abdominal cramps, rash, retinal vascular thrombosis, headache, dizziness, depression, mood disturbances, increased and decreased weight, and decreased carbohydrate tolerance.

Pediatric Concerns:

Drug Interactions: Dose adjustment of thyroid hormones required for those on thyroid replacement therapy. Concomitant use with rifampin, anticonvulsants such as phenobarbital, phenytoin, carbamazepine, antibiotics such as ampicillin, tetracycline and griseofulvin, may reduce its efficacy and result in unwanted pregnancies.

Relative Infant Dose:

Adult Dose:

Alternatives:

References:
1. Booker DE, Pahl IR. Control of postpartum breast engorgement with oral contraceptives. Am J Obstet Gynecol 1967; 98(8): 1099–1101.
2. Kamal I, Hefnawi F, Ghoneim M, Abdallah M, Abdel RS. Clinical, biochemical, and experimental studies on lactation. V. Clinical effects of steroids on the initiation of lactation. Am J Obstet Gynecol 1970; 108(4): 655–658.
3. Kora SJ. Effect of oral contraceptives on lactation. Fertil Steril 1969; 20(3): 419–423.
4. Koetsawang S, Bhiraleus P, Chiemprajert T. Effects of oral contraceptives on lactation. Fertil Steril 1972; 23(1): 24–28.
5. Laukaran VH. The effects of contraceptive use on the initiation and duration of lactation. Int J Gynaecol Obstet 1987; 25 Suppl: 129–142.
6. Nilsson S, Nygren KG, Johansson ED. Transfer of estradiol to human milk. Am J Obstet Gynecol 1978; 132(6): 653–657.

ESTRIOL   L3

Trade: Ovestin, Oestriol

Other Trades:

Category: Estrogen

Estriol is a naturally secreted estrogen, typically during pregnancy in large quantities. It is not commercially available but may be used in compounded prescriptions. Conjugated estrogens comprise more than 90% of the total estrogen content of human milk and plasma.[1] Estriol glucosiduronates were the predominant estrogen metabolites (63%) in plasma. Vaginal administration of estriol is highly bioavailability and is similar to or greater than oral administration; estriol vaginal delivery may interfere with milk production as well.[2]

Pregnancy Risk	X	Lactation Risk	L3
T ½	=	M/P	=
Vd	=	PB	= 90%
Tmax	= 1–2 hours	Oral	= vaginal greater than oral
MW	=	pKa	= 13.62

Adult Concerns: Application site irritation and pruritus, breast discomfort and pain, endometrial hyperplasia, breast cancer.

Pediatric Concerns:

Drug Interactions: Dose adjustment of thyroid hormones required for those on thyroid replacement therapy. Concomitant use with rifampin, anticonvulsants such as phenobarbital, phenytoin, carbamazepine, antibiotics such as ampicillin, tetracycline and griseofulvin, may reduce its efficacy and result in unwanted pregnancies.

Relative Infant Dose:

Adult Dose:

Alternatives:

References:
1. McGarrigle HH, Lachelin GC. Oestrone, oestradiol and oestriol glucosiduronates and sulfhates in human puerperal plasma and milk. J Steroid Biochem. 1983May; 18(5): 607–11.
2. Chollet, J. A., G. Carter, et al. (2009). "Efficacy and safety of vaginal estriol and progesterone in postmenopausal women with atrophic vaginitis. " Menopause 16(5): 978–983.

ESZOPICLONE   L3

Trade: Lunesta

Other Trades:

Category: Hypnotic, sedative

Eszopiclone is a non-benzodiazepine hypnotic-sedative drug, although they both interact at the same GABA receptor.[1] Used as a night time sedative, its transfer into human milk has not yet been reported. However, a derivative which is virtually identical, zopiclone, has been studied (see zopiclone) and 1.5% of the maternal dose transferred into milk. Therefore, due to the structural similarly, one should expect about 1.5% of eszopiclone to transfer into human milk as well. The use of eszopiclone in mothers with premature infants or newborns, and particularly those with infants subject to apnea, should be avoided. Use in healthy older infants is probably less risky.

Pregnancy Risk	C	Lactation Risk	L3
T ½	= 6 hours	M/P	=
Vd	=	PB	= 59%
Tmax	= 1 hour	Oral	= >75%
MW	= 388	pKa	= 5.35

Adult Concerns: Sedation, rebound insomnia and other symptoms of withdrawal have been reported following discontinuation of eszopiclone. Headache, dry mouth, nausea, vomiting, unpleasant taste, brief memory loss, somnolence have been reported.

Pediatric Concerns: None reported. Observe closely for sedation in the infant.

Drug Interactions: Eszopiclone and lorazepam decrease each others C_{max} by 22%. Eszopiclone is metabolized by CYP3A4 and CYP2E1. Ketoconazole administration increased by 2.2 fold the exposure to eszopiclone. Additive effect with eszopiclone when mixed with alcohol. Levels of eszopiclone may be reduced by coadministration with rifampicin, a potent inducer of CYP3A4.

Relative Infant Dose:

Adult Dose: 2–3 mg at bedtime.

Alternatives: Zopiclone

References:
1. Pharmaceutical manufacturer package insert. 2005.

ETANERCEPT	L2

Trade: Enbrel
Other Trades: Enbrel
Category: Anti-arthritic

Etanercept is a dimeric fusion protein consisting of the extracellular ligand-binding portion of tumor necrosis factor bound to human IgG1. Etanercept binds specifically to tumor necrosis factor (TNF) and blocks its inflammatory and immune activity in rheumatoid arthritis patients.[1] Elevated levels of TNF are found in the synovial fluid of arthritis patients.

In a recent study of a non-breastfeeding mother who received 25 mg twice weekly, etanercept was measured in the milk retained in the breast.[2] This mother was not breastfeeding but retained some milk in the breast after 30 days. The author reported milk levels of 75 ng/mL on the day after injection. While this data is interesting, measuring drug transfer in residual breast milk following involution of alveolar tissues is simply not clinically relevant. After involution, the alveolar system would be totally open to drug transfer due to the breakdown of the tight intercellular junctions between lactocytes.

In a study of a single patient receiving etanercept first 25 mg twice weekly, then 50 mg once weekly at 3 months postpartum, levels ranged from 4.48 ng/mL at 24 hours following a 25 mg dose, to 7.50 ng/mL (0.750 µg/L) at 72 hours following a 50 mg dose. No etanercept was found in the infant's plasma compartment.[3] In another study, one patient received 25 mg twice weekly during pregnancy. Following delivery, the infant plasma levels dropped quickly. Breast milk levels at 12 weeks postpartum were only 3.5 ng/mL while the maternal plasma levels were 2872 ng/mL. None was detectable in the infant's plasma compartment.[4]

Due to its enormous molecular weight (150,000 daltons), it is extremely unlikely that clinically relevant amounts would transfer into milk in actively breastfeeding mothers. In addition, due to its protein structure, it would not be orally bioavailable in an infant. Infliximab is somewhat similar and is apparently not secreted into human milk (see infliximab).

Pregnancy Risk	B	Lactation Risk	L2
T ½	= 115 hours	M/P	=
Vd	= 0.24 l/kg	PB	=
Tmax	= 72 hours	Oral	= Nil
MW	= 150000	pKa	=

Adult Concerns: Etanercept may suppress the immune system and increase the risk of infections significantly. Incidence of infections is 38%. Headache, dizziness, cough, and rhinitis have been reported.

Pediatric Concerns: None reported via milk.

Drug Interactions: Do not administer live vaccines concurrent with etanercept.

Relative Infant Dose: 0.07%–0.2%

Adult Dose: 25 mg twice weekly

Alternatives: Infliximab

References:
1. Pharmaceutical manufacturer prescribing information, 1999.
2. Ostensen M, Eigenmann GO. Etanercept in breast milk. J Rheumatol 2004 May; 31(5): 1017–8.
3. Keeling S, Wolbink GJ. Measuring multiple etanercept levels in the breast milk of a nursing mother with rheumatoid arthritis. J Rheumatol. 2010 Jul; 37(7): 1551.
4. Murashima A, Watanabe N, Ozawa N, Saito H, Yamaguchi K. Etanercept during pregnancy and lactation in a patient with rheumatoid arthritis: drug levels in maternal serum, cord blood, breast milk and the infant's serum. Ann Rheum Dis. 2009 Nov; 68(11): 1793–4.

ETHACRYNIC ACID   L3

Trade: Edecrin

Other Trades: Edecrin

Category: Powerful loop diuretic

Ethacrynic acid is a potent, short-acting loop diuretic similar to Lasix. A significant decrease in maternal blood pressure or blood volume may reduce milk production although this is speculative. No data on transfer into human milk are available.[1,2]

Pregnancy Risk	B	Lactation Risk	L3
T ½	= 2–4 hours	M/P	=
Vd	=	PB	= 90%
Tmax	= 2 hours (oral)	Oral	= 100%
MW	= 303	pKa	= 3.5

Adult Concerns: Diuresis, hypotension, diarrhea.

Pediatric Concerns: None reported.

Drug Interactions: Increased toxicity when used with antihypertensives, other diuretics, aminoglycosides. Increased risk of arrhythmias when used with digoxin. Probenecid reduces diuresis of this product.

Relative Infant Dose:

Adult Dose: 50–200 mg daily.

Alternatives: Furosemide

References:
1. Pharmaceutical manufacturer prescribing information, 1996.
2. Lacy C. Drug information handbook. Lexi-Comp Inc. Cleveland, OH, 1996.

ETHAMBUTOL   L2

Trade: Ethambutol, Myambutol
Other Trades: Etibi, Myambutol
Category: Antitubercular drug

Ethambutol is an antimicrobial used for tuberculosis. Small amounts are secreted in milk although no studies are available which clearly document levels. In one unpublished study, the mother had an ethambutol plasma level of 1.5 mg/L three hours after a dose of 15 mg/kg daily. Following a similar dose in the same patient, the concentration in milk was 1.4 mg/L.[1] In another patient, the maternal plasma level was 4.62 mg/L and the corresponding milk concentration was 4.6 mg/L (no dose available).[1]

Pregnancy Risk	B	Lactation Risk	L2
T ½	= 3.1 hours	M/P	= 1.0
Vd	=	PB	= 8–22%
Tmax	= 2–4 hours	Oral	= 80%
MW	= 204	pKa	= 6.6, 9.5

Adult Concerns: Optic neuritis, dizziness, confusion, nausea, vomiting, anorexia.

Pediatric Concerns: None reported, but caution is recommended.

Drug Interactions: Aluminum salts may decrease oral absorption.

Relative Infant Dose: 1.5%

Adult Dose: 15–25 mg/kg daily.

Alternatives:

References:
1. Snider DE, Jr., Powell KE. Should women taking antituberculosis drugs breast-feed? Arch Intern Med 1984; 144(3): 589–590.

ETHANOL   L3

Trade: Alcohol
Other Trades:
Category: Depressant

Alcohol transfer into human milk readily, with an average milk/plasma ratio of about 1.0. This does not necessarily mean that the dose of alcohol in milk is high, only that the levels in plasma correspond closely with those in milk. The absolute amount (dose) of alcohol transferred into milk is generally low and is a function of the maternal level. Older studies, some in animals, suggested that beer (or more likely, barley) may stimulate prolactin levels.[1-4] While this may be true, we now know clearly that alcohol is a profound inhibitor of oxytocin release, and inevitably reduces milk letdown and the amount of milk delivered to the infant. Thus beer should not be considered a galactogogue.

In a study of twelve breastfeeding mothers who ingested 0.3 gm/kg of ethanol in orange juice (equivalent to 1 can of beer for the average sized woman), the mean maximum concentration of ethanol in milk was 320 mg/L.[5] This report suggests a 23% reduction (156 to 120 mL) in breastmilk production following ingestion of beer and an increase in milk odor as a function of ethanol content. In another group of 5 women, who consumed 0.4 gm/kg at one setting, milk and maternal plasma levels were similar. Levels of alcohol in milk averaged 0.44 gm/L at peak and fell to 0.09 gm/L at 180 minutes.[6] In an interesting study of the effect of alcohol on milk ingestion by infants, the rate of milk consumption by infants during the 4 hours immediately after exposure to alcohol (0.3 gm/kg) in 12 mothers was significantly less.[7] Compensatory increases in intake were then observed during the 8–16 hours after exposure when mothers refrained from drinking. Excess levels may lead to drowsiness, deep sleep, weakness, and decreased linear growth in infant. Maternal blood alcohol levels must attain 300 mg/dL before significant side effects are reported in the infant. Reduction of letdown is apparently dose-dependent and requires alcohol consumption of 1.5 to 1.9 gm/kg.[8] Other studies have suggested psychomotor delay in infants of moderate drinkers (2+ drinks daily). Avoid breastfeeding during and for at least 2 hours after drinking alcohol (moderate). Heavy drinkers should wait longer.

A new study suggests that the state of lactation metabolically changes the rate of alcohol bioavailability.[9] In this study, blood alcohol levels were significantly lower in lactating women as compared to non-lactating women. The reduced AUC levels for alcohol suggest that the metabolism of ethanol is higher in lactating women. However, the subjective effects of alcohol were still similar. Another study reported one infant that developed pseudo-Cushing syndrome as a result of exposure to alcohol in breast milk. The mother consumed at least fifty 12 ounce beers weekly in addition to other concentrated alcoholic beverages. She had stopped drinking while pregnant, and resumed postpartum. The infant showed signs of Cushing syndrome at age 8 weeks. When the mother stopped drinking while breastfeeding, the baby's appearance gradually returned to normal.[10]

Adult metabolism of alcohol is approximately 1 oz in 3 hours, so mothers who ingest alcohol in moderate amounts can generally return to breastfeeding as soon as they feel neurologically normal. A good rule is 2 hours for each drink consumed. Chronic or heavy consumers of alcohol should not breastfeed. Readers are urged to consult Koren's excellent nomogram on counseling women concerning alcohol consumption.[11] Remember, this nomogram calculates, as a function of body weight and amount of alcohol consumed, the time to "zero" plasma levels in the mother.

Pregnancy Risk	D	Lactation Risk	L3
T ½	= 0.24 hours	M/P	= 1.0
Vd	= 0.53 l/kg	PB	=
Tmax	= 30–90 minutes (oral)	Oral	= 100%
MW	= 46	pKa	= 15.9

Adult Concerns: Sedation, decreased milk supply, altered milk taste.

Pediatric Concerns: One infant developed pseudo-Cushing syndrome as a result of exposure to alcohol in breast milk. The mother consumed at least 50– 12 ounce beers weekly in addition to other concentrated alcoholic beverages. She had stopped drinking while pregnant, and resumed postpartum. The infant showed signs of Cushing syndrome at age 8 weeks. When the mother stopped drinking while breastfeeding, the baby's appearance gradually returned to normal.[10] In another case report of a heavy user, the infant was restless and insomnic for several days then exhibited violent fits and tonic-clonic seizures.[12] After removal from this mothers breast, the infant calmed. Other studies suggest changes in behavioral state such as shorter periods of sleep, cried more often, and had heightened startling reflexes after exposure to alcohol.

Drug Interactions: Increased CNS depression when used with barbiturates, benzodiazepines, chloral hydrate, and other CNS depressants. A disulfiram-like reaction (flushing, weakness, sweating, tachycardia, etc.) may occur when used with cephalosporins, chlorpropamide, disulfiram, furazolidone, metronidazole, procarbazine. Increased hypoglycemia when used with sulfonylureas and other hypoglycemic agents. Intolerance of bromocriptine.

Relative Infant Dose: 16%

Adult Dose:

Alternatives:

References:
1. Marks V, Wright JW. Endocrinological and metabolic effects of alcohol. Proc R Soc Med 1977; 70(5): 337–344.
2. De Rosa G, Corsello SM, Ruffilli MP, Della CS, Pasargiklian E. Prolactin secretion after beer. Lancet 1981; 2(8252): 934.
3. Carlson HE, Wasser HL, Reidelberger RD. Beer-induced prolactin secretion: a clinical and laboratory study of the role of salsolinol. J Clin Endocrinol Metab 1985; 60(4): 673–677.
4. Koletzko B, Lehner F. Beer and breastfeeding. Adv Exp Med Biol 2000; 478: 23–28.
5. Mennella JA, Beauchamp GK. The transfer of alcohol to human milk. Effects on flavor and the infant's behavior. N Engl J Med 1991; 325(14): 981–985.
6. da-Silva VA, Malheiros LR, Moraes-Santos AR, Barzano MA, McLean AE. Ethanol pharmacokinetics in lactating women. Braz J Med Biol Res. Oct 1993; 26(10): 1097–1103.
7. Mennella JA. Regulation of milk intake after exposure to alcohol in mothers' milk. Alcohol Clin Exp Res 2001; 25(4): 590–593.
8. Cobo E. Effect of different doses of ethanol on the milk-ejecting reflex in lactating women. Am J Obstet Gynecol 1973; 115(6): 817–821.
9. Pepino MY, Steinmeyer AL, Mennella JA. Lactational state modifies alcohol pharmacokinetics in women. Alcohol Clin Exp Res. Jun 2007; 31(6): 909–918.
10. Binkiewicz A, Robinson MJ, Senior B. Pseudo-Cushing syndrome caused by alcohol in breast milk. J Pediatr 1978 Dec; 93(6): 965–7.
11. Ho E, Collantes A, Kapur BM, Moretti M, Koren G. Alcohol and breast feeding: calculation of time to zero level in milk. Biol Neonate. 2001; 80(3): 219–222.
12. Budin P. Lecture VI. In, The nursling: the feeding and hygiene of premature and full-term infants. London. Caxton Publishing Company. 1907; 85–101.

ETHINYL ESTRADIOL   L3

Trade:

Other Trades: Activelle, Adgyn Estro, Aerodiol

Category: Estrogen

Ethinyl estradiol is an estrogenic agent. Although small amounts of estrogens may pass into breastmilk, the effects of estrogens on the infant appear minimal. In one study, ethinyl estradiol was not detected in breastmilk after administration of 50 µg/day.[1] After administration of 500 µg/day, the level in breastmilk was approximately 300 pg/mL.[1]

Early postpartum use of estrogens may reduce volume of milk produced and the protein content, but it is variable, controversial, and depends on dose and the individual.[2,3,4,5] Breastfeeding mothers should attempt to wait until lactation is firmly established (6–8 weeks) prior to use of estrogen-containing oral contraceptives. Progestin-only birth control products are preferred in breastfeeding mothers.

Pregnancy Risk	X	Lactation Risk	L3
T ½	= 36 hours	M/P	= 1: 4
Vd	=	PB	= 97%
Tmax	=	Oral	= Complete
MW	= 296	pKa	= 17.6

Adult Concerns: Observe for reduced milk production. Breakthrough bleeding is more common with this product. Fluid retention has been reported.

Pediatric Concerns: Reduced milk supply is possible. Do not use early postpartum.

Drug Interactions: Concomitant use with rifampin, anticonvulsants such as phenobarbital, phenytoin, carbamazepine, antibiotics such as ampicillin, tetracycline and griseofulvin, may reduce its efficacy and result in unwanted pregnancies.

Relative Infant Dose:

Adult Dose:

Alternatives:

References:
1. Nilsson S, Nygren KG, Johansson ED. Ethinyl estradiol in human milk and plasma after oral administration. Contraception. 1978 Feb; 17(2): 131–9.
2. Booker DE, Pahl IR. Control of postpartum breast engorgement with oral contraceptives. Am J Obstet Gynecol 1967; 98(8): 1099–1101.
3. Kamal I, Hefnawi F, Ghoneim M, Abdallah M, Abdel RS. Clinical, biochemical, and experimental studies on lactation. V. Clinical effects of steroids on the initiation of lactation. Am J Obstet Gynecol 1970; 108(4): 655–658.
3. Kora SJ. Effect of oral contraceptives on lactation. Fertil Steril 1969; 20(3): 419–423.
5. Koetsawang S, Bhiraleus P, Chiemprajert T. Effects of oral contraceptives on lactation. Fertil Steril 1972; 23(1): 24–28.

ETHINYL ESTRADIOL + ETONOGESTREL   L3

Trade: NuvaRing

Other Trades:

Category: Slow release vaginal ring contraceptive

Ethinyl estradiol and Etonogestrel is a combination product indicated for use as a contraceptive agent. This vaginal ring is a slow release product which releases on average 0.120 mg/day of etonogestrel and 0.015 mg/day of ethinyl estradiol over a

3 week period of use. Etonogestrel is the biologically active metabolite of desogestrel and has both high progestational activity with low intrinsic androgenicity.[1]

The bioavailability of ethinyl estradiol when administered intravaginally is approximately 55.6%, which is comparable to that when it is administered orally. Small amounts of estrogens and progestins are known to pass into milk, but long-term follow-up of children whose mothers used combination hormonal contraceptives while breastfeeding has shown no deleterious effects on infants. Estrogen-containing contraceptives may interfere with milk production by decreasing the quantity and quality of milk production.

The effect of progestins on milk production is poorly studied and controversial. Early postpartum, while progestin receptors are still present in the breast, administering progestins may actually suppress milk production. This has been seen occasionally in patients early postpartum. Several days to a week later, most progestin receptors disappear from the lactocytes and breast tissues become relatively immune to the effects of progestins. Thus it is advisable to wait as long as possible postpartum prior to instituting therapy with progesterone to avoid reducing the milk supply. The direct effect of progesterone therapy on the nursing infant is generally unknown, but it is believed minimal to none as natural progesterone is poorly bioavailable to the infant via milk. Several cases of gynecomastia in infants have been reported but are extremely rare.[2–6]

Pregnancy Risk	X	Lactation Risk	L3
T ½	= ethinyl estradiol/ etonogestrel: 36 hours/25 hours	M/P	=
Vd	=	PB	= ethinyl estradiol/ etonogestrel: 98.5%/66%
Tmax	=	Oral	= ethinyl estradiol/ etonogestrel: complete/ complete
MW	= ethinyl estradiol/ etonogestrel: 296/324	pKa	= ethinyl estradiol/ etonogestrel: 17.6/19.14

Adult Concerns: Do not use in patients with thrombophlebitis or thromboembolic disorders, cerebral vascular or coronary artery disease, severe hypertension. Numerous other contraindications exist, check the package insert.

Pediatric Concerns: This is an estrogen-containing contraceptive device. Estrogens in some patients may inhibit milk production significantly and change the quality of milk components. Caution patient to observe for suppression of milk production.

Drug Interactions: Concomitant use with rifampin, anticonvulsants such as phenobarbital, phenytoin, carbamazepine, antibiotics such as ampicillin, tetracycline and griseofulvin, may reduce its efficacy and result in unwanted pregnancies.

Relative Infant Dose:

Adult Dose: Ethinyl estradiol/etonogestrel: 0.015 mg/0.12 mg delivered each day for 3 weeks.

Alternatives: Progestin-only oral contraceptives.

References:

1. Pharmaceutical manufacturer Package Insert, 2003.
2. Rodriguez-Palmero M, Koletzko B, Kunz C, Jensen R. Nutritional and biochemical properties of human milk: II. Lipids, micronutrients, and bioactive factors. Clin Perinatol 1999; 26(2): 335–359.
3. Costa TH, Dorea JG. Concentration of fat, protein, lactose and energy in milk of mothers using hormonal contraceptives. Ann Trop Paediatr 1992; 12(2): 203–209.
4. Sas M, Gellen JJ, Dusitsin N, Tunkeyoon M, Chalapati S, Crawford MA, Drury PJ, Lenihan T, Ayeni O, Pinol A. An investigation on the influence of steroidal contraceptives on milk lipid and fatty acids in Hungary and Thailand. WHO Special Programme of Research, Development and Research Training in Human Reproduction. Task Force on oral contraceptives. Contracep 1986; 33(2): 159–178.
5. Shaaban MM. Contraception with progestogens and progesterone during lactation. J Steroid Biochem Mol Biol 1991; 40(4–6): 705–710.
6. Massai R, Quinteros E, Reyes MV, Caviedes R, Zepeda A, Montero JC, et al. Extended use of a progesterone-releasing vaginal ring in nursing women: a phase II clinical trial. Contracep 2005 Nov; 72(5): 352–7.

ETHINYL ESTRADIOL + LEVONORGESTREL   L3

Trade: Preven, Tri-Levlen, Nordette, Levlen, Levlite, Alesse, Seasonale, Preven Emergency Contraceptive, Trivora

Other Trades: Ovral, Triquilar

Category: Emergency contraceptive

Levonorgestrel and ethinyl estradiol can be used as an emergency contraceptive.[1] It is believed to act by preventing ovulation or fertilization by altering tubal transportation of sperm and/or ova. It may as well partially inhibit implantation by altering the endometrium. Levonorgestrel + ethinyl estradiol is an emergency contraceptive that can be used to prevent pregnancy following unprotected intercourse or a known or suspected contraceptive failure. It is not effective if the woman is already pregnant, or once the process of implantation has begun. Each tablet contains 0.25 mg levonorgestrel and 0.05 mg ethinyl estradiol. They should not be used in known or suspected pregnancy, in patients with pulmonary edema, ischemic heart disease, deep vein thrombosis, etc. The initial treatment of 2 tablets should be administered as soon as possible but within 72 hours of unprotected intercourse. This is followed by the second dose of 2 tablets 12 hours later.

Although small amounts of ethinyl estradiol may pass into breastmilk, the effects of estrogens on the infant appear minimal. Early postpartum use of estrogens may reduce volume of milk produced and the protein content, but it is variable and depends on dose and the individual.[2,3,4,5] Breastfeeding mothers should attempt to wait until lactation is firmly established (6–8 weeks) prior to use of estrogen-containing oral contraceptives.

The effect of progestins (in this case, levonorgestrel) on milk production is poorly studied. Early postpartum, while progestin receptors are still present in the breast, administering progestins may actually suppress milk production just as it does in the pregnant women. This has been seen occasionally in patients early postpartum. Several days to a week later, most progestin receptors disappear from the lactocyte and breast tissues become relatively immune to the effects of progestins. Thus it is advisable to wait as long as possible postpartum prior to instituting therapy with progesterone to avoid reducing the milk supply.

Pregnancy Risk	X	Lactation Risk	L3
T ½	= Ethinyl estradiol/ levonorgestrel: 36 hours/24 hours	M/P	= Ethinyl estradiol/ levonorgestrel: 0.25/
Vd	=	PB	= Ethinyl estradiol/ levonorgestrel: 97%/97%
Tmax	= Ethinyl estradiol/ levonorgestrel: /1–2 hours	Oral	= Ethinyl estradiol/ levonorgestrel: Complete/ complete
MW	= Ethinyl estradiol/ levonorgestrel: 296/312	pKa	= Ethinyl estradiol/ levonorgestrel: 17.6/19.8

Adult Concerns: Adverse events include nausea, vomiting, menstrual cycle disturbances, breast tenderness, headaches, abdominal pain, and dizziness.

Pediatric Concerns: None reported in infants via milk. However estrogens and even progestins may in some patients suppress milk production. Caution is recommended.

Drug Interactions: Concomitant use with rifampin, anticonvulsants such as phenobarbital, phenytoin, carbamazepine, antibiotics such as ampicillin, tetracycline and griseofulvin, may reduce its efficacy and result in unwanted pregnancies.

Relative Infant Dose:

Adult Dose: 2 tablets followed in 12 hours by 2 additional tablets.

Alternatives: Plan B

References:
1. Pharmaceutical manufacturer prescribing information, 2003.
2. Booker DE, Pahl IR. Control of postpartum breast engorgement with oral contraceptives. Am J Obstet Gynecol 1967; 98(8): 1099–1101.
3. Kamal I, Hefnawi F, Ghoneim M, Abdallah M, Abdel RS. Clinical, biochemical, and experimental studies on lactation. V. Clinical effects of steroids on the initiation of lactation. Am J Obstet Gynecol 1970; 108(4): 655–658.
4. Kora SJ. Effect of oral contraceptives on lactation. Fertil Steril 1969; 20(3): 419–423.
5. Koetsawang S, Bhiraleus P, Chiemprajert T. Effects of oral contraceptives on lactation. Fertil Steril 1972; 23(1): 24–28.

ETHINYL ESTRADIOL + NORELGESTROMIN   L3

Trade: Ortho Evra

Other Trades:

Category: Patch combination contraceptive

Ethinyl Estradiol and Norelgestromin is a combination drug indicated for use as a contraceptive agent. This is a new combination progestin and estrogen containing patch. It delivers approximately 150 µg/day norelgestromin and 20 µg/day ethinyl estradiol to the plasma compartment of the user.

Although small amounts of ethinyl estradiol may pass into breastmilk, the effects of estrogens on the infant, directly, appear minimal. However, early postpartum use of estrogens may reduce volume of milk produced and the protein content, but it is variable and depends on dose and the individual.[2,3,4,5] Breastfeeding mothers should attempt to wait until lactation is firmly established (6–8 weeks) prior to use of estrogen-containing oral contraceptives.

The effect of progestins (in this case, norelgestromin) on milk production is poorly studied. Early postpartum, while progestin receptors are still present in the breast, administering progestins may actually suppress milk production. This has been seen occasionally in patients early postpartum. Several days to a week later, most progestin receptors disappear from the lactocyte and breast tissues become relatively immune to the effects of progestins. Thus it is advisable to wait as long as possible postpartum prior to instituting therapy with progesterone to avoid reducing the milk supply.

Pregnancy Risk	X		Lactation Risk	L3
T ½	= ethinyl estradiol/ norelgestromin: 17 hours/28 hours	M/P	= ethinyl estradiol/ norelgestromin: 0.25/	
Vd	=	PB	= ethinyl estradiol/ norelgestromin: 98.5%/>97%	
Tmax	=	Oral	= ethinyl estradiol/ norelgestromin: Complete/ rapid	
MW	= ethinyl estradiol/ norelgestromin: 296/327	pKa	= ethinyl estradiol/ norelgestromin: 17.6/17.91	

Adult Concerns: Side effects include breast tenderness and enlargement headache, nausea menstrual changes, abdominal cramps and bloating ,vaginal discharge and irritation at the site of application.

Pediatric Concerns: Potential reduction of daily milk production due to estrogen content.

Drug Interactions: Same as with all combination oral contraceptives. Effectiveness may be reduced if co-administered with certain antibiotics, antifungals, anticonvulsants, protease inhibitors, or other drugs that affect hepatic metabolism. Other drugs include St. John's Wort, barbiturates, griseofulvin, rifampin, phenytoin, and carbamazepine.

Relative Infant Dose:

Adult Dose: Ethinyl estradiol/norelgestromin transdermal patch: 0.02 mg/0.15 mg delivered each day for 3 weeks.

Alternatives: Norethindrone

References:

1. Pharmaceutical manufacturer prescribing information, 2003.
2. Rodriguez-Palmero M, Koletzko B, Kunz C, Jensen R. Nutritional and biochemical properties of human milk: II. Lipids, micronutrients, and bioactive factors. Clin Perinatol 1999; 26(2): 335-359.
3. Costa TH, Dorea JG. Concentration of fat, protein, lactose and energy in milk of mothers using hormonal contraceptives. Ann Trop Paediatr 1992; 12(2): 203-209.
4. Sas M, Gellen JJ, Dusitsin N, Tunkeyoon M, Chalapati S, Crawford MA, Drury PJ, Lenihan T, Ayeni O, Pinol A. An investigation on the influence of steroidal contraceptives on milk lipid and fatty acids in Hungary and Thailand. WHO Special Programme of Research, Development and Research Training in Human Reproduction. Task Force on oral contraceptives. Contracep 1986; 33(2): 159-178.

ETHINYL ESTRADIOL + NORETHINDRONE   L3

Trade: Loestrin, Junel, Microgestin, Femhrt, Ortho-Novum, Brevinor, Norinyl 1-35, Tri-Legest, Zorane

Other Trades: Jinteli, Estrostep, Ovcon, Necon, Modicon, Brevicon, Balziva

Category: Contraceptive, antiacne

Ethinyl estradiol and Norethindrone acetate is a combination drug product indicated for use in acne vulgaris, postmenopausal osteoporosis and as a contraceptive. Although small amounts of ethinyl estradiol may pass into breastmilk, the effects of estrogens on the infant directly appear minimal. Early postpartum use of estrogens may reduce volume of milk produced and the protein content, but it is variable and depends on dose and the individual.[1,2,3,4] Breastfeeding mothers should attempt to wait until lactation is firmly established (6–8 weeks) prior to use of estrogen-containing oral contraceptives.

Norethindrone is believed to be secreted into breastmilk in small amounts. It produces a dose-dependent suppression of lactation at higher doses, although somewhat minimal at lower doses. It may reduce lactose content and reduce overall milk volume and nitrogen/protein content, resulting in lower infant weight gain although these effects are unlikely if doses are kept low.[5–9]

Pregnancy Risk	X	Lactation Risk	L3
T ½	= Ethinyl estradiol/ norethindrone: 36 hours /4–13 hours	M/P	= Ethinyl estradiol/ norethindrone: 1: 4/
Vd	=	PB	= Ethinyl estradiol/ norethindrone: 97%/97%
Tmax	= Ethinyl estradiol/ norethindrone: /1–2 hours	Oral	= Ethinyl estradiol/ norethindrone: complete/60%
MW	= Ethinyl estradiol/ norethindrone: 296/298	pKa	= Ethinyl estradiol/ norethindrone: 17.6/

Adult Concerns: Edema, chloasma, abdominal bloating, nausea, vomiting, amenorrhea, irregular menstrual cycles, breast tenderness, thromboembolism, gall bladder disease, liver disease, venous thrombosis, stroke

Pediatric Concerns: Reduction of milk supply.

Drug Interactions: Concomitant use with rifampin, anticonvulsants such as phenobarbital, phenytoin, carbamazepine, antibiotics such as ampicillin, tetracycline and griseofulvin, may reduce its efficacy and result in unwanted pregnancies.

Relative Infant Dose:

Adult Dose: 1 tablet orally daily for 21 days.

Alternatives:

References:
1. Booker DE, Pahl IR. Control of postpartum breast engorgement with oral contraceptives. Am J Obstet Gynecol 1967; 98(8): 1099–1101.
2. Kamal I, Hefnawi F, Ghoneim M, Abdallah M, Abdel RS. Clinical, biochemical, and experimental studies on lactation. V. Clinical effects of steroids on the initiation of lactation. Am J Obstet Gynecol 1970; 108(4): 655–658.
3. Kora SJ. Effect of oral contraceptives on lactation. Fertil Steril 1969; 20(3): 419–423.
4. Koetsawang S, Bhiraleus P, Chiemprajert T. Effects of oral contraceptives on lactation. Fertil Steril 1972; 23(1): 24–28.
5. Kora SJ. Effect of oral contraceptives on lactation. Fertil Steril 1969; 20(3): 419–423.
6. Miller GH, Hughes LR. Lactation and genital involution effects of a new low-dose oral contraceptive on breast-feeding mothers and their infants. Obstet Gynecol 1970; 35(1): 44–50.
7. Karim M, Ammar R, el Mahgoub S, el Ganzoury B, Fikri F, Abdou I. Injected progestogen and lactation. Br Med J 1971; 1(742): 200–203.
8. Lonnerdal B, Forsum E, Hambraeus L. Effect of oral contraceptives on composition and volume of breast milk. Am J Clin Nutr 1980; 33(4): 816–824.
9. Laukaran VH. The effects of contraceptive use on the initiation and duration of lactation. Int J Gynaecol Obstet 1987; 25 Suppl: 129–142.

ETHOSUXIMIDE   L4

Trade: Zarontin

Other Trades: Zarontin

Category: Anticonvulsant used in epilepsy

Ethosuximide is an anticonvulsant used in epilepsy. Rane's data suggest that although significant levels of ethosuximide are transferred into human milk, the plasma level in the infant is quite low.[1] A peak milk concentration of approximately 55 mg/L was reported at 1 month postpartum in a mother consuming 250 mg twice daily. Milk/plasma ratios were reported to be 1.03 on day 3 postpartum and 0.8 during the first three months of therapy. The infant's plasma reached a peak (2.9 mg/dL) at approximately 1.5 months postpartum and then declined significantly over the next 3 months suggesting increased clearance by the infant. Although these levels are considered sub-therapeutic, it is suggested that the infant's plasma levels be occasionally tested.

In another study of a women receiving 500 mg twice daily, her milk levels, as estimated from a graph, averaged 60–70 mg/L.[2] A total daily exposure to ethosuximide of 3.6–11 mg/kg as a result of nursing was predicted.

In a study by Kuhnz of 10 epileptic breastfeeding mothers (and 13 infants) receiving 3.5 to 23.6 mg/kg/day, the breastmilk concentrations were similar to those of the maternal plasma (milk/serum: 0.86) and the breastfed infants maintained serum levels between 15 and 40 μg/mL.[3] Maximum milk concentration reported was 77 mg/L although the average was 49.54 mg/L. Neonatal behavior complications such as poor suckling, sedation, and hyper-excitability occurred in 7 of the 12 infants. Interestingly, one infant who was not breastfed, exhibited severe withdrawal symptoms such as tremors, restlessness, insomnia, crying, and vomiting which lasted for 8 weeks causing a slow weight gain. Thus the question remains, is it safer to breastfeed and avoid these severe withdrawal reactions?

These studies clearly indicate that the amount of ethosuximide transferred to the infant is significant. With milk/plasma ratios of approximately 0.86–1.0 and relatively high maternal plasma levels, the maternal plasma levels are a good indication of the dose transferred to the infant. Milk levels are generally high. Caution is recommended.

Pregnancy Risk	C	Lactation Risk	L4
T ½	= 30–60 hours	M/P	= 0.94
Vd	= 0.72 l/kg	PB	=
Tmax	= 4 hours	Oral	= Complete
MW	= 141	pKa	= 9.3

Adult Concerns: Drowsiness, ataxia, nausea, vomiting, anorexia, rash.

Pediatric Concerns: Neonatal behavior complications such as poor suckling, sedation, and hyperexcitability occurred in 7 of 12 infants in one study. Milk levels are significant. Caution is recommended.

Drug Interactions: Decreased efficacy of ethosuximide when used with phenytoin, carbamazepine, primidone, phenobarbital (may reduce plasma levels). Elevated levels of ethosuximide may result when used with isoniazid.

Relative Infant Dose: 31.4%–73.5%

Adult Dose: 250–750 mg BID

Alternatives:

References:
1. Rane A, Tunell R. Ethosuximide in human milk and in plasma of a mother and her nursed infant. Br J Clin Pharmacol 1981; 12(6): 855–858.
2. Koup JR, Rose JQ, Cohen ME. Ethosuximide pharmacokinetics in a pregnant patient and her newborn. Epilepsia 1978; 19(6): 535–539.
3. Kuhnz W, Koch S, Jakob S, Hartmann A, Helge H, Nau H. Ethosuximide in epileptic women during pregnancy and lactation period. Placental transfer, serum concentrations in nursed infants and clinical status. Br J Clin Pharmacol 1984; 18(5): 671–677.

ETHOTOIN   L3

Trade: Peganone

Other Trades:

Category: Anticonvulsant

Ethotoin is a typical phenytoin-like anticonvulsant. Although no data are available on concentrations in breastmilk, its similarity to phenytoin would suggest that some is secreted via breastmilk.[1] No data are available in the literature.

Phenytoin is an old and efficient anticonvulsant. It is secreted in small amounts into breastmilk. The effect on infant is generally considered minimal if the levels in the maternal circulation are kept in low-normal range (10 µg/mL). Phenytoin levels peak in milk at 3.5 hours. In one study of 6 women receiving 200–400 mg/day of phenytoin, plasma concentrations varied from 12.8 to 78.5 µmol/L, while their milk levels ranged from 1.61 to 2.95 mg/L.[2] The milk/plasma ratios were low, ranging from 0.06 to 0.18. In only two of these infants were plasma concentrations of phenytoin detectable (0.46 and 0.72 µmol/L). No untoward effects were noted in any of these infants. Others have reported milk levels of 6 µg/mL[3], or 0.8 µg/mL.[4] Although the actual concentration in milk varies significantly between studies, the milk/plasma ratio appears relatively similar at 0.13 to 0.45. Breastmilk concentrations varied from 0.26 to 1.5 mg/L depending on the maternal dose. In a mother receiving 250 mg twice daily, milk levels were 0.26 and the milk/plasma ratio was 0.45.[5] The maternal plasma level was phenytoin was 0.58. In another study of two patients receiving 300–600 mg/d, the average milk level was 1.9 mg/L.[6] The maximum observed milk level was 2.6 mg/L.

The neonatal half-life of phenytoin is highly variable for the first week of life. Monitoring of the infants' plasma may be useful although it is not definitely required. All of the current studies indicate rather low levels of phenytoin in breastmilk and minimal plasma levels in breastfeeding infants.

Pregnancy Risk	D		Lactation Risk	L3
T ½	= 3–9 hours		M/P	=
Vd	=		PB	= 41%
Tmax	= 1–2 hours		Oral	= Complete
MW	= 204		pKa	= 16.23

Adult Concerns: Drowsiness, dizziness, insomnia, headache, blood dyscrasias.

Pediatric Concerns: None reported, but see phenytoin.

Drug Interactions: Caution is advised while administering ethotoin concomitantly with anticoagulants.

Relative Infant Dose:

Adult Dose: 1 gm per day initially, stepped up to 2–3 gm daily.

Alternatives:

References:
1. McEvoy GE. (ed): AFHS Drug Information. New York, NY: 2003.
2. Steen B, Rane A, Lonnerholm G, Falk O, Elwin CE, Sjoqvist F. Phenytoin excretion in human breast milk and plasma levels in nursed infants. Ther Drug Monit 1982; 4(4): 331–334.
3. Svenmark O, Schiller PJ, Buchthal F. 5, 5–Diphenylhydantoin (dilantin) blood levels after oral or intravenous dosage in man. Acta Pharmacol Toxicol (Copenh) 1960; 16: 331–346.
4. Kaneko S, Sato T, Suzuki K. The levels of anticonvulsants in breast milk. Br J Clin Pharmacol 1979; 7(6): 624–627.
5. Rane A, Garle M, Borga O, Sjoqvist F. Plasma disappearance of transplacentally transferred diphenylhydantoin in the newborn studied by mass fragmentography. Clin Pharmacol Ther 1974; 15(1): 39–45.
6. Mirkin BL. Diphenylhydantoin: placental transport, fetal localization, neonatal metabolism, and possible teratogenic effects. J Pediatr 1971; 78(2): 329–337.

ETIDRONATE   L3

Trade: Didronel
Other Trades: Didronel
Category: Slows bone turnover

Etidronate is a bisphosphonate that slows the dissolution of hydroxyapatite crystals in the bone, thus reducing bone calcium loss in certain syndromes such as Paget's syndrome.[1] Etidronate also reduces the remineralization of bone and can result in osteomalacia over time. It is not known how the administration of this product during active lactation would affect the maternal bone porosity. It is possible that milk calcium levels could be reduced although this has not been reported. Etidronate is poorly absorbed orally (1%) and must be administered in between meals on an empty stomach. Its penetration into milk is possible due to its small molecular weight, but it has not yet been reported. However, due to the presence of fat and calcium in milk, its oral bioavailability in infants would be exceedingly low. Whereas the plasma half-life is approximately 6 hours, the terminal elimination half-life (from bone) is >90 days.

Pregnancy Risk	C	Lactation Risk	L3
T ½	= 6 hours (plasma)	M/P	=
Vd	= 1.37 l/kg	PB	=
Tmax	= 2 hours	Oral	= 1–2.5%
MW	= 206	pKa	= 1.46

Adult Concerns: Untoward effects include loss of taste, nephrotoxicity, risk of fractures, and focal osteomalacia after prolonged use. Fever, convulsions, bone pain.

Pediatric Concerns: None reported via milk. Although unreported, it could result in reduced milk calcium levels. Oral absorption in infant would be minimal.

Drug Interactions: IV ranitidine doubles the oral absorption of alendronate (similar to etidronate). Oral products containing calcium or magnesium will significantly reduce oral bioavailability. Take on empty stomach.

Relative Infant Dose:

Adult Dose: 5–10 mg/kg daily

Alternatives:

References:
1. Drug Facts and Comparisons 1996 ed. ed. St. Louis: 1996.

ETODOLAC   L3

Trade: Etodolac, Lodine
Other Trades: Lodine, Ultradol
Category: Non-steroidal analgesic, antipyretic

Etodolac is a prototypical nonsteroidal anti-inflammatory agent (NSAID) with analgesic, antipyretic, and anti-inflammatory properties.[1] Thus far no data are available regarding its secretion into human breastmilk. Shorter half-life varieties are preferred. As with most NSAIDs, milk levels are likely minimal.

Pregnancy Risk	C/D in 3rd trimester	Lactation Risk	L3
T ½	= 7.3 hours	M/P	=
Vd	= 0.4 l/kg	PB	= 95–99%
Tmax	= 1–2 hours	Oral	= 80–100%
MW	= 287	pKa	= 4.7

Adult Concerns: Dyspepsia, nausea, diarrhea, indigestion, heartburn, abdominal pain, and gastrointestinal bleeding.

Pediatric Concerns: None reported via milk, but observe for nausea, diarrhea, indigestion. Ibuprofen probably preferred at this time.

Drug Interactions: May prolong prothrombin time when used with warfarin. Antihypertensive effects of ACE inhibitors may be blunted or completely abolished by NSAIDs. Some NSAIDs may block antihypertensive effect of beta blockers, diuretics. Used with cyclosporin, may dramatically increase renal toxicity. May increase digoxin, phenytoin, lithium levels. May increase toxicity of methotrexate. May increase bioavailability of penicillamine. Probenecid may increase NSAID levels.

Relative Infant Dose:

Adult Dose: 200–400 mg every 6–8 hours

Alternatives: Ibuprofen, Voltaren

References:
1. Pharmaceutical manufacturer prescribing information, 1995.

ETONOGESTREL IMPLANT   L3

Trade: Implanon, Nexplanon
Other Trades:
Category: Progestin

Etonogestrel is the biologically active metabolite of desogestrel and has both high progestational activity with low intrinsic androgenicity. Small amounts of progestins are known to pass into milk, but long-term follow-up of children whose mothers used hormonal contraceptives while breastfeeding has shown no deleterious effects on infants.[1] Like other progestogen-only contraceptives, the use of etonogestrel is associated with irregular menstrual bleeding and sometimes absence of bleeding. Counseling is required to ensure women make informed choices.[2] Of the contraceptives, progestin-only contraceptives are generally preferred as they produce fewer changes in milk production compared to estrogen-containing products. This product is probably quite safe for use in breastfeeding mothers, although all mothers should be counseled to observe for changes in milk production.

Pregnancy Risk	X	Lactation Risk	L3
T ½	= 25 hours	M/P	= 0.442–0.498
Vd	= 2.87 l/kg	PB	= High
Tmax	=	Oral	=
MW	= 324	pKa	= 19.14

Adult Concerns: Headache, weight gain, vaginitis, abdominal pain, irregular menstrual bleeding, acne, nausea, dizziness, depression, back pain, upper respiratory infection, sinusitis, ectopic pregnancy.

Pediatric Concerns:

Drug Interactions: Concomitant use with rifampin, anticonvulsants such as phenobarbital, phenytoin, carbamazepine, antibiotics such as ampicillin, tetracycline and griseofulvin, may reduce its efficacy and result in unwanted pregnancies.

Relative Infant Dose: 2.2%

Adult Dose:

Alternatives:

References:

1. Taneepanichskul S, Reinprayoon D, Thaithumyanon P, Praisuwanna P, Tosukhowong P, Dieben T. Effects of the etonogestrel-releasing implant Implanon and a nonmedicated intrauterine device on the growth of breast-fed infants. Contracept 2006; 73: 368–371.
2. Pharmaceutical manufacturer Package Insert, 2003.

ETOPOSIDE   L5

Trade: Toposar, Abiposid, Celltop, Eposid, Eposin, Etopofos, Etopophos, VP-16

Other Trades:

Category: Anticancer drug

Etoposide is an inhibitor of mitosis. It is commonly used to treat testicular, lung, and other cancers, and in bone marrow transplant. Oral bioavailability ranges from 50% to higher, and it is apparently associated with the dose, with lesser absorption at higher doses.[1] Etoposide is approximately 95% bound to plasma proteins. On intravenous administration, the disposition of etoposide is best described as a biphasic process, with a distribution phase half-life of about 1.5 hours and terminal elimination half-life ranging from four to eleven hours. No data are available on the transfer of etoposide into human milk; however, it is likely low. Mothers should withhold breastfeeding for at least two to three days following exposure to this agent. Withhold breastfeeding for two to three days.

Pregnancy Risk	D	Lactation Risk	L5
T ½	= 4–11 hours	M/P	=
Vd	= 0.25–0.41 l/kg	PB	= 94–97%
Tmax	= 1–1.5 hours	Oral	= 25–75%
MW	=	pKa	= 12.28

Adult Concerns: Black, tarry stools, bleeding gums, blood in the urine, chest pain, chills, cough, fever, painful or difficult urination, pale skin, pinpoint red spots on the skin, shortness of breath, sore throat, sores, ulcers, or white spots on the lips or in the mouth, swollen glands, troubled breathing with exertion, unusual bleeding or bruising, unusual tiredness or weakness, hair loss.

Pediatric Concerns:

Drug Interactions: Caution while administering with other phosphatase inhibitors such as levamisole. Co-administration with high dose cyclosporine A causes increased plasma levels and decreased clearance of etoposide.

Relative Infant Dose:

Adult Dose:

Alternatives:

References:
1. Pharmaceutical manufacturer prescribing information, 2005.

ETRAVIRINE   L5

Trade: Intelence

Other Trades:

Category: Antiretroviral agent used in HIV infections. Antiretroviral drug

Etravirine is an antiretroviral agent used for the treatment of HIV infection. There are no adequate and well-controlled studies or case reports in breastfeeding women. Breastfeeding is not recommended in mothers who have HIV.[1,2]

Pregnancy Risk	B	Lactation Risk	L5
T ½	=	M/P	=
Vd	=	PB	=
Tmax	=	Oral	=
MW	=	pKa	= <3

Adult Concerns: Nausea, rash, hyperlipidemia, hyperglycemia, elevated liver enzymes, elevated serum creatinine, peripheral neuropathy, hypersensitivity, myocardial infarction.

Pediatric Concerns:

Drug Interactions: Do not coadminister with the following: tipranavir/ritonavir, fosamprenavir/ritonavir, atazanavir/ritonavir. Do not coadminister with protease inhibitors without ritonavir. Co-administration with following drugs decreases plasma levels and efficacy of etravirine: efvirenz, nevirapine, anticonvulsants, rifabutin.

Relative Infant Dose:

Adult Dose: 200 mg twice daily

Alternatives:

References:
1.   World Health Organization: Global Programme on AIDS. Consensus statement from the WHO/UNICEF consultation on HIV transmission and breast-feeding. Geneva: WHO, 1992.
2.   Latham MC, Greiner T: Breastfeeding versus formula feeding in HIV infection. Lancet 352: 737, 1998.

ETRETINATE	L5

Trade: Tegison

Other Trades: Tigason

Category: Antipsoriatic

Etretinate is an oral Vitamin A derivative primarily used for psoriasis and sometimes acne. It is teratogenic and should not be administered to pregnant women or women about to become pregnant. Etretinate is known to transfer into animal milk although no data are available in human milk.[1,2] Etretinate is still detectable in human serum up to 2.9 years after administration has ceased due to storage at high concentrations in adipose tissue. Mothers who wish to breastfeed following therapy with this compound should be informed of its long half-life in the human. The manufacturer considers this drug to be contraindicated in breastfeeding mothers due to the potential for serious adverse effects.

Pregnancy Risk	X	Lactation Risk	L5
T ½	= 120 days (terminal)	M/P	=
Vd	= High	PB	= >99%
Tmax	= 2–6 hours	Oral	= Complete
MW	= 354	pKa	=

Adult Concerns: Dry nose, chapped lips, nose bleeds, hair loss, peeling of skin on soles, palms, sunburns, and headaches. Elevated liver enzymes, lipids. Fatigue, headache, fever.

Pediatric Concerns: None reported but great caution is urged. Premature epiphyseal closure has been reported in children treated with this product.

Drug Interactions: Milk increases absorption of oral etretinate. Exogenous vitamin A increases toxicity.

Relative Infant Dose:

Adult Dose: 0.5–0.75 mg/kg twice daily

Alternatives:

References:
1.   Pharmaceutical manufacturer prescribing information, 1995.
2.   Lacy C. Drug information handbook. Lexi-Comp Inc. Cleveland, OH, 1996.

EUCALYPTUS   L3

Trade:

Other Trades:

Category: Antimicrobial, hypoglycemic, analgesic, and anti-inflammatory.

There are many compounds contained in eucalyptus extract such as eucalyptol, cineole, and hydrocyanic acid. Antimicrobial, hypoglycemic, analgesic, and anti-inflammatory effects have been observed in animal studies.[123] Eucalyptus leaf has been traditionally used orally for treating fever, cough, infection, and dyspepsia. Eucalyptus oil also has been used topically for respiratory tract inflammation, nasal congestion, and rheumatoid arthritis.[4] There are no adequate or well-controlled studies or case reports of the use of eucalyptus in breastfeeding women. Ingestion of significant quantity may cause eucalyptus oil poisoning with depressed central nervous system and can be fatal.[4]

Pregnancy Risk	Probably Safe	Lactation Risk	L3
T ½	=	M/P	=
Vd	=	PB	=
Tmax	=	Oral	=
MW	=	pKa	=

Adult Concerns: Nausea, vomiting, hypersensitivity, contact dermatitis, diarrhea.

Pediatric Concerns:

Drug Interactions: Eucalyptus can increase hepatotoxicity of Pyrrolizidine alkaloid containing herbs such as gravel root, borage, coltsfoot, alkanna, and etc.

Relative Infant Dose:

Adult Dose:

Alternatives:

References:
1. Takahashi T, Kokubo R, Sakaino M. Antimicrobial activities of eucalyptus leaf extracts and flavonoids from Eucalyptus maculata. Lett Appl Microbiol. 2004; 39(1): 60–4.
2. Gray AM, Flatt PR. Antihyperglycemic actions of Eucalyptus globulus(Eucalyptus) are associated with pancreatic and extra-pancreatic effects in mice. J Nutr. 1998 Dec; 128(12): 2319–23.
3. Silva J, Abebe W, Sousa SM, Duarte VG, Machado MI, Matos FJ. Analgesic andanti-inflammatory effects of essential oils of Eucalyptus. J Ethnopharmacol. 2003Dec; 89(2–3): 277–83.
4. Eucalyptus. In: Natural Medicines Comprehensive Database [Internet Database]. Stockton, CA: Therapeutic Research Faculty. Date last update: 2011, May 23. Accessed on 5/24/2011.

EVEROLIMUS   L5

Trade: Zortress, Afinitor
Other Trades:
Category: Organ transplant anti-rejection

Everolimus is a macrolide immunosuppressant intended for acute rejection prophylaxis after kidney transplantation. Everolimus blocks growth factor–driven transduction signals in the T-cell response to alloantigen. It is currently used as an immunosuppressant to prevent organ transplant rejections. It has a large molecular weight and is unlikely to enter the milk compartment at high levels. However it is very fetotoxic in pregnant women and its use in breastfeeding mothers with infants should be avoided.

It is not known if everolimus is transferred into human milk. Everolimus and/or its metabolites passed into the milk of lactating rats at a concentration 3.5 times higher than in maternal serum. We recommend that the mother withhold breastfeeding for a minimum of 150 hours.

Pregnancy Risk	D	Lactation Risk	L5
T ½	= 30 hours	M/P	=
Vd	= 1.57 l/kg	PB	= 74%
Tmax	= 1–2 hours	Oral	= 30%
MW	= 958.22	pKa	= 13.43

Adult Concerns: Abdominal or stomach pain, change or loss of taste, dizziness, dry, itching skin, rash, lack or loss of strength, pain in the arms or legs, sleeplessness.

Pediatric Concerns:

Drug Interactions: Co-administration with the following increases the drug levels of everolimus: ketoconazole, itraconazole, voriconazole, clarithromycin, telithromycin, ritonavir, digoxin, cyclosporine, fluconazole, macrolide antibiotics, nicardipine, diltiazem, nelfinavir, indinavir, amprenavir. Co-administration with the following decreases drug levels and efficacy of everolimus: rifampin, rifabutin, St. John's Wort, carbamazepine, phenobarbital, phenytoin, efavirenz, nevirapine.

Relative Infant Dose:

Adult Dose: Initial dose: 0.75 mg twice daily.

Alternatives:

References:
1.   Pharmaceutical manufacturer prescribing information, 2010.

EXEMESTANE   L5

Trade: Aromasin
Other Trades:
Category: Anticancer drug

Exemestane is an irreversible, steroidal aromatase inactivator. It acts as a false substrate for the aromatase enzyme, causing its inactivation. Exemestane significantly lowers circulating estrogen concentrations in women, and it is useful in the treatment of estrogen-receptor positive breast cancer.[1] After maximum plasma concentrations are reached, levels decline polyexponentially with a mean terminal half-life of about 24 hours. It is 90% bound to plasma proteins. No data are available on its transfer into human milk. Steroids in general do not transfer significantly, so exemestane levels in milk are probably low. However, this product works irreversibly. Any present in milk could potentially suppress estrogen levels in a breastfed infant. It is not advisable to breastfeed an infant while consuming this product. A withholding period of five to seven days is recommended should the mother opt to discontinue taking this product and restart breastfeeding.

Pregnancy Risk	D	Lactation Risk	L5
T ½	= 24 hours	M/P	=
Vd	=	PB	= 90%
Tmax	= 1.2 hours	Oral	=
MW	= 296.4	pKa	=

Adult Concerns: Abdominal or stomach pain, anxiety, constipation, diarrhea, dizziness, general feeling of discomfort or illness, general feeling of tiredness or weakness, hot flashes, increased sweating, loss of appetite, nausea or vomiting, pain, trouble with sleeping.

Pediatric Concerns:

Drug Interactions: Co-administration with the following drugs may decrease drug levels and efficacy of exemestane: rifampicin, phenytoin, carbamazepine, phenobarbital, St. John's wort.

Relative Infant Dose:

Adult Dose: 25 mg once daily.

Alternatives:

References:
1. Pharmaceutical manufacturer prescribing information, 2005.

EXENATIDE   L3

Trade: Byetta
Other Trades:
Category: Improves glycemic control in diabetics

Exenatide improves glycemic control in people with Type-2 diabetes mellitus.[1] It enhances glucose-dependent insulin secretion by the pancreatic beta-cell, suppresses glucagon secretion, and slows gastric emptying. Exenatide leads to an increase in both glucose-dependent synthesis of insulin, and *in vivo* secretion of insulin from pancreatic beta cells. Exenatide therefore promotes insulin release from beta cells in the presence of elevated glucose concentrations. Exenatide is a 39-amino acid peptide and has a molecular weight of 4186 daltons which is far too large to enter milk in clinically relevant amounts. While it is reported to enter rodent milk at extremely low levels, we do not have human studies. The plasma levels of this product are extraordinarily low (picograms), and I would imagine the transfer into human milk is much lower. It would be unlikely that this product would enter milk in clinically relevant amounts, nor would it be orally bioavailable in infants. But as yet, we have no data in breastfeeding mothers and caution is recommended if this product is used.

Pregnancy Risk	C		Lactation Risk	L3
T ½	= 2.4 hours		M/P	=
Vd	= 0.4 l/kg		PB	=
Tmax	= 2.1 hours		Oral	= Nil
MW	= 4186		pKa	= 0.4

Adult Concerns: Side effects include nausea, vomiting, diarrhea, feeling jittery, dizziness, headache and dyspepsia.

Pediatric Concerns: None reported, but this product is all be unlikely to ever enter milk or be orally absorbed by an infant.

Drug Interactions: Exenatide reduced plasma levels of digoxin by 17%. Levels of lovastatin were decreased by 40%. Levels of acetaminophen were reduced by 24%.

Relative Infant Dose:

Adult Dose: Highly variable, consult prescribing information.

Alternatives:

References:
1. Pharmaceutical manufacturer prescribing information, 2010.

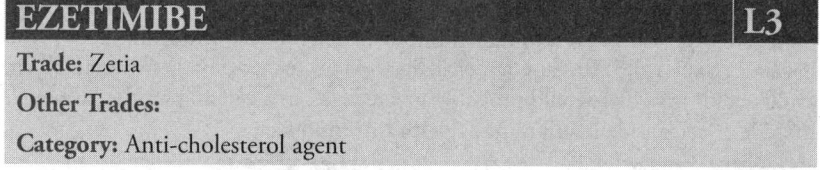

EZETIMIBE   L3

Trade: Zetia

Other Trades:

Category: Anti-cholesterol agent

Ezetimibe reduces blood cholesterol by inhibiting the absorption of cholesterol from the small intestine.[1] It appears to act at the brush border of the small intestine and inhibits the absorption of cholesterol leading to a direct reduction in delivery of cholesterol to the liver. No data are available on the transfer of this agent to milk. This is a very lipophilic agent, but has reasonably poor oral bioavailability. It is not clear at all if it would be safe for use in a breastfed infant who needs high levels of cholesterol. Some caution is recommended until data are available but it is unlikely to produce significant levels in milk.

Pregnancy Risk	C	Lactation Risk	L3
T ½	= 22 hours	M/P	=
Vd	=	PB	= >90%
Tmax	= 4–12 hours	Oral	= 35–60%
MW	= 409	pKa	= 14.44

Adult Concerns: Generally well tolerated but viral infection, headache, fatigue, and gastrointestinal symptoms such as diarrhea and abdominal pain have been reported but these symptoms are rather low in incidence.

Pediatric Concerns: No data available on transfer to human milk. Some caution is recommended.

Drug Interactions: Additive when used with statins. Ezetimibe levels increased 12-fold in a renal transplant patient receiving cyclosporine and other agents. There is an increased risk of myopathy or rhabdomyolysis when used with fibric acid products (fenofibrate).

Relative Infant Dose:

Adult Dose: 10 mg daily.

Alternatives: Cholestyramine salts

References:
1. Pharmaceutical manufacturer prescribing information, 2003.

FAMCICLOVIR   L3

Trade: Famvir
Other Trades: Famvir
Category: Antiviral for Herpes Zoster

Famciclovir is an antiviral agent used in the treatment of uncomplicated herpes zoster infection (shingles) and genital herpes. It is rapidly metabolized to the active metabolite, penciclovir. Although similar to acyclovir, no data are available on levels in human milk. Oral bioavailability of famciclovir (77%) is much better than acyclovir (15–30%). Studies with rodents suggest that the milk/plasma ratio is greater than 1.0.[1,2] Because famciclovir provides few advantages over acyclovir, at this point acyclovir would probably be preferred in a nursing mother although the side-effect profile is still minimal with this product.

Pregnancy Risk	B	Lactation Risk	L3
T ½	= 2–3 hours	M/P	= >1
Vd	= 1.13 l/kg	PB	= <20%
Tmax	= 0.9 hours	Oral	= 77%
MW	=	pKa	= 3.84

Adult Concerns: Headache, dizziness, nausea, diarrhea, fever, anorexia.
Pediatric Concerns: None reported via milk.

Drug Interactions: Cimetidine increases plasma levels of the active metabolite penciclovir. Famciclovir increases digoxin plasma levels by 19%. Probenecid significantly increases penciclovir plasma levels.

Relative Infant Dose:

Adult Dose: 125 mg twice daily.

Alternatives: Acyclovir

References:
1. Drug Facts and Comparisons 1994 ed. ed. St. Louis: 1994.
2. Pharmaceutical manufacturer prescribing information, 1995.

FAMOTIDINE   L1

Trade: Pepcid, Pepcid AC

Other Trades:

Category: Reduces gastric acid secretion

Famotidine is a typical histamine-2 receptor antagonist that reduces stomach acid secretion. In one study of 8 lactating women receiving a 40 mg/day dose, the peak concentration in breastmilk was 72 µg/L and occurred at 6 hours post-dose.[1] The milk/plasma ratios were 0.41, 1.78, and 1.33 at 2, 6, and 24 hours respectively. These levels are apparently much lower than other histamine-2 receptor antagonists (ranitidine, cimetidine) and make it a preferred choice.

Pregnancy Risk	B	Lactation Risk	L1
T ½	= 2.5–3.5 hours	M/P	= 0.41–1.78
Vd	=	PB	= 17%
Tmax	= 1–3.5 hours	Oral	= 50%
MW	= 337	pKa	= 10.5

Adult Concerns: Headache, constipation, increased liver enzymes.

Pediatric Concerns: None reported. Pediatric indications are available.

Drug Interactions: Famotidine reduces bioavailability of ketoconazole, itraconazole due to reduced oral absorption of these two products.

Relative Infant Dose: 1.9%

Adult Dose: 20–40 mg twice daily.

Alternatives: Nizatidine

References:
1. Courtney TP, Shaw RW. et. al. Excretion of famotidine in breast milk. Br J Clin Pharmacol 1988; 26: 639.

FEBUXOSTAT   L3

Trade: Uloric
Other Trades: Adenuric
Category: Xanthine oxidase inhibitor

Febuxostat is a xanthine oxidase (XO) inhibitor indicated for the chronic management of hyperuricemia in patients with gout. It is not known whether this drug is excreted in human milk. Due to its high protein binding and somewhat low oral bioavailability, minimal amounts are expected to enter breast milk. Febuxostat is transferred in the milk of rats.[1] Until more is known, caution is recommended while administering this drug in lactating women. Initially, in adults, febuxostat may increase plasma concentrations of urate and uric acid, and treatment should not be started until an acute attack of gout has completely subsided; an NSAID or colchicine should be given for at least 6 months after starting febuxostat.[1]

Pregnancy Risk	C	Lactation Risk	L3
T ½	= 5–8 hours	M/P	=
Vd	=	PB	= 99%
Tmax	= 1 hour	Oral	= 49%
MW	= 316.4	pKa	=

Adult Concerns: Side effects include liver function abnormalities, nausea, arthralgia, and rash.

Pediatric Concerns:

Drug Interactions: Febuxostat is contraindicated in patients being treated with azathioprine, mercaptopurine or theophylline.

Relative Infant Dose:

Adult Dose: 40–80 mg per day.

Alternatives:

References:
1. Pharmaceutical manufacturer prescribing information, 2010.

FELBAMATE   L4

Trade: Felbatol
Other Trades:
Category: Anticonvulsant

Felbamate is an oral antiepileptic agent for partial seizures and Lennox-Gastaut syndrome. Due to serious side effects, the FDA recommends that felbamate be given only to patients with serious seizures refractory to all other medications. Felbamate is known to be secreted in rodent milk and was detrimental to their offspring.[1] No data are available on the transfer of this drug into human milk. Due to the incidence of severe side effects, extreme caution is recommended with this medication in breastfeeding mothers.

Pregnancy Risk	C	Lactation Risk	L4
T ½	= 20–23 hours	M/P	=
Vd	= 0.7–1.0 l/kg	PB	= 25%
Tmax	= 1–4 hours	Oral	= 90%
MW	= 238	pKa	= 15.46

Adult Concerns: Aplastic anemia, weight gain, flu-like symptoms, tachycardia, nausea, vomiting, headache, insomnia.

Pediatric Concerns: None reported, but caution is urged.

Drug Interactions: Felbamate causes an increase in phenytoin plasma levels. Phenytoin produces a 45% decrease in felbamate levels. Carbamazepine levels may be decreased, whereas felbamate levels may drop by 40%. Valproic acid plasma levels may be increased.

Relative Infant Dose:

Adult Dose: 1200 mg per day in 3–4 divided doses.

Alternatives:

References:
1. Pharmaceutical manufacturer prescribing information, 1995.

FELODIPINE   L3

Trade: Plendil

Other Trades: Agon SR, Plendil ER, Plendil, Renedil

Category: Calcium channel blocker, antihypertensive

Felodipine is a calcium channel antagonist structurally related to nifedipine.[1] No data are available on the transfer of this drug into human milk. Because we have numerous studies on others in this family, it is advisable to use nifedipine or others that have breastfeeding studies available.

Pregnancy Risk	C	Lactation Risk	L3
T ½	= 11–16 hours	M/P	=
Vd	=	PB	= >99%
Tmax	= 2.5–5 hours	Oral	= 20%
MW	= 384	pKa	= <1

Adult Concerns: Headache, dizziness, edema, flushing, hypotension, constipation, cardiac arrhythmias.

Pediatric Concerns: None reported via milk, but caution is recommended.

Drug Interactions: Barbiturates may reduce bioavailability of calcium channel blockers (CCB). Calcium salts may reduce hypotensive effect. Dantrolene may increase risk of hyperkalemia and myocardial depression. Histamine-2 receptor blockers (cimetidine, ranitidine, famotidine) may increase bioavailability of certain CCBs. Hydantoins may reduce plasma levels. Quinidine increases risk of hypotension, bradycardia, tachycardia. Rifampin may reduce effects of CCBs. Vitamin D may reduce efficacy of CCBs. CCBs may increase carbamazepine, cyclosporin, encainide, prazosin levels.

Relative Infant Dose:

Adult Dose: 2.5–10 mg daily.

Alternatives: Nifedipine, Nimodipine, Verapamil

References:
1. Pharmaceutical manufacturer prescribing information, 1996.

FENDOLOPAM   L3

Trade: Corlopam

Other Trades:

Category: Dopamine Agonist

Fendolopam is a dopamine agonist used to treat severe hypertension in both adults and children.[1] It is not known whether this drug transfers into milk. Further, dopamine agonists are known to suppress prolactin release from the pituitary, so some concern exists for the use of this product in breastfeeding mothers as prolactin suppression could cause a decrease in milk production. However, its brief half-life would preclude large quantities from entering the milk compartment.

Pregnancy Risk	B	Lactation Risk	L3
T ½	= 5 minutes	M/P	=
Vd	= 0.6 l/kg	PB	=
Tmax	=	Oral	=
MW	= 305	pKa	= 9.71

Adult Concerns: Adverse effects include headache, nausea, hypotension, and dizziness.

Pediatric Concerns: In children, the most common adverse effects were hypotension and tachycardia. This medication is used in children aged <1 month to age 12 at doses of up to 0.8 µg/kg/minute for severe hypertension.

Drug Interactions: Acetaminophen use increases fendolopam levels, while beta-blockers increase the risk of hypotension.

Relative Infant Dose:

Adult Dose: Do not exceed 1.6 µg/kg/minute.

Alternatives:

References:
1. Pharmaceutical manufacturer prescribing information, 2006.

FENNEL   L3

Trade:

Other Trades:

Category: Estrogenic

Fennel is an herb native to southern Europe and Asia Minor. The oils of sweet and bitter fennel contain up to 90% trans-anethole and up to 20% fenchone and numerous other lesser oils. An acetone extract of fennel has been shown to have estrogenic effects on the genital organs of male and female rats.[1] As an herbal medicine it is reputed to increase milk secretion, promote menstruation, facilitate birth, and increased libido. The estrogenic component is believed to be a polymer of anethole such as dianethole or photoanethole.[2] Ingestion of the volatile oil may induce nausea, vomiting, seizures, pulmonary edema, and hallucinations.[3,4] An older survey of fennel samples in Italy found viable aerobic bacteria including coliforms, fecal streptococci, and salmonella species, suggesting the plant may serve as a vector for infectious gastrointestinal diseases.[5] Fennel is a popular herb that has been used since ancient times. It is primarily believed to be estrogenic. Because estrogens are known to suppress breastmilk production, its use in lactating women is questionable.

Pregnancy Risk	Possibly Hazardous	Lactation Risk	L3
T ½	=	M/P	=
Vd	=	PB	=
Tmax	=	Oral	=
MW	=	pKa	=

Adult Concerns: Allergic reactions, photodermatitis, contact dermatitis, and bacterial contamination.

Pediatric Concerns: None reported via milk. May potentially suppress milk production.

Drug Interactions:

Relative Infant Dose:

Adult Dose:

Alternatives:

References:

1. Malini T, Vanithakumari G, Megala N, Anusya S, Devi K, Elango V. Effect of Foeniculum vulgare Mill. seed extract on the genital organs of male and female rats. Indian J Physiol Pharmacol 1985; 29(1): 21–26.
2. Albert-Puleo M. Fennel and anise as estrogenic agents. J Ethnopharmacol 1980; 2(4): 337–344.
3. Marcus C, Lichtenstein EP. J. Agric Food Chem 1979; 27: 1217.
4. Duke JA. Handbook of Medicinal Herbs. Boca Raton, FL: CRC Press, 1985.
5. Ercolani GL. Bacteriological quality assessment of fresh marketed lettuce and fennel. Appl Environ Microbiol 1976; 31(6): 847–852.

FENOFIBRATE   L3

Trade: Tricor
Other Trades:
Category: Cholesterol lower agent

Fenofibrate reduces total cholesterol, LDL cholesterol, and triglycerides.[1] No data are available on its transfer into human milk however agents that reduce plasma cholesterol are not usually considered suitable for use in breastfeeding mothers. Milk levels of cholesterol are higher because the newborns need high levels of cholesterol for neurodevelopment. This and other hypocholesterolemic agents should probably not be used in breastfeeding mothers with exception of those with much older infants (>1 year).

Pregnancy Risk	C	Lactation Risk	L3
T ½	= 20 hours	M/P	=
Vd	=	PB	= 99%
Tmax	=	Oral	= 85%
MW	= 361	pKa	=

Adult Concerns: Adverse events include abdominal pain, back pain, headache, elevated liver function tests, chest pain, respiratory disorders.

Pediatric Concerns: None reported via milk, but this agent should be used with care in breastfeeding mothers due to the infants need for cholesterol.

Drug Interactions: Potentiates coumarin anticoagulants.

Relative Infant Dose:

Adult Dose: 160 mg per day.

Alternatives:

References:
1. Pharmaceutical manufacturer prescribing information, 2003.

FENOPROFEN   L2

Trade: Nalfon
Other Trades: Nalfon, Fenopron, Progesic
Category: NSAID, nonsteroidal analgesic

Fenoprofen is a typical nonsteroidal anti-inflammatory and analgesic. Following 600 mg four times daily for 4 days postpartum, the milk/plasma ratio was approximately 0.017 and fenoprofen levels in milk were too low to be accurately detected and were estimated to be approximately 1/60th of the maternal plasma level.[1] Fenoprofen was undetectable in cord blood, amniotic fluid, saliva, or washed red blood cells after multiple doses.

Pregnancy Risk	C/D in 3rd trimester	Lactation Risk	L2
T ½	= 2.5 hours	M/P	= 0.017
Vd	= 0.08–0.10 l/kg	PB	= 99%
Tmax	= 1–2 hours	Oral	= 80%
MW	= 242	pKa	= 4.5

Adult Concerns: Gastrointestinal distress and bleeding, dyspepsia, nausea, constipation, ulcers, hepatotoxicity, rash, tinnitus.

Pediatric Concerns: None reported.

Drug Interactions: May prolong prothrombin time when used with warfarin. Antihypertensive effects of ACE inhibitors may be blunted or completely abolished by NSAIDs. Some NSAIDs may block antihypertensive effect of beta blockers, diuretics. Used with cyclosporin, may dramatically increase renal toxicity. May increase digoxin, phenytoin, lithium levels. May increase toxicity of methotrexate. May increase bioavailability of penicillamine. Probenecid may increase NSAID levels.

Relative Infant Dose:

Adult Dose: 300–600 mg every 4–6 hours

Alternatives: Ibuprofen

References:
1. Rubin A. et. al. A profile of the physiological disposition and gastrointestinal effects of fenoprofen in man. Curr Med Res Opin 1974; 2: 529–544.

FENTANYL | L2

Trade: Sublimaze, Onsolis, Lazanda
Other Trades: Sublimaze, Duragesic
Category: Opiate analgesic

Fentanyl is a potent narcotic analgesic used (IV, IM, transdermally) during labor and delivery. When used parenterally, its half-life is exceedingly short.[1] The transfer of fentanyl into human milk has been documented but is low.

In a group of ten women receiving a total dose of 50 to 400 µg fentanyl IV during labor, the concentration of fentanyl in milk was generally below the level of detection (<0.05 ng/mL).[2] In a few samples, the levels were between 0.05 and 0.15 ng/mL. Using this data, an infant would ingest less than 3% of the weight-adjusted maternal dose per day. In another study of 13 women who received 2 µg/kg IV after delivery and cord clamping, fentanyl concentration in colostrum was extremely low.[3] Peak colostrum concentrations occurred at 45 minutes following intravenous administration and averaged 0.4 µg/L. Colostrum levels dropped rapidly and were undetectable after 10 hours. The authors conclude that with these small concentrations and fentanyl's low oral bioavailability, intravenous fentanyl analgesia may be used safely in breastfeeding women. The relatively low level of fentanyl found in human milk is presumably a result of the short maternal half-life, and the rather rapid redistribution out of the maternal plasma compartment. It is apparent that fentanyl transfer to milk under most clinical conditions is poor and is probably clinically unimportant. In another study of chronic exposure to fentanyl for intractable pain, the mother was receiving by transdermal patch 100 µg/hour.[4] At approximately 27 days postpartum, the infants blood was negative for both fentanyl and its metabolite norfentanyl (sensitivity 0.1 ng/mL). The mother's milk contained 6.4 ng/mL fentanyl and 6.2 ng/mL norfentanyl. The authors calculated the dose via milk at 1.3 µg/kg/day. The infant was unaffected by exposure to fentanyl.

Pregnancy Risk	C	Lactation Risk	L2
T ½	= 2–4 hours	M/P	=
Vd	= 3–8 l/kg	PB	= 80–86%
Tmax	= 7–8 minutes (IV)	Oral	= 25–75%
MW	= 336	pKa	= 8.4

Adult Concerns: Apnea, respiratory depression, muscle rigidity, hypotension, bradycardia.

Pediatric Concerns: No adverse effects reported via milk.

Drug Interactions: Increased toxicity when used with other CNS depressants, phenothiazines, tricyclic antidepressants.

Relative Infant Dose: 2.9%–5%

Adult Dose: 2–20 µg/kg injection (IV)

Alternatives: Sufentanil

References:
1. Madej TH, Strunin L. Comparison of epidural fentanyl with sufentanil. Analgesia and side effects after a single bolus dose during elective caesarean section. Anaesthesia 1987; 42(11): 1156–1161.
2. Leuschen MP, Wolf LJ, Rayburn WF. Fentanyl excretion in breast milk. Clin Pharm 1990; 9(5): 336–337.
3. Steer PL, Biddle CJ, Marley WS, Lantz RK, Sulik PL. Concentration of fentanyl in colostrum after an analgesic dose. Can J Anaesth 1992 March; 39(3): 231–5.
4. Cohen RS. Fentanyl transdermal analgesia during pregnancy and lactation. J Hum Lact. Aug 2009; 25(3): 359–361.

FENUGREEK   L3

Trade:

Other Trades:

Category: Herbal milk stimulant

Fenugreek is commonly sold as the dried, ripe seed and extracts are used as an artificial flavor for maple syrup.[1] The seeds contain from 0.1 to 0.9% diosgenin.[2] Several coumarin compounds have been noted in the seed as well as a number of alkaloids such as trigonelline, gentianin, and carpaine. The seeds also contain approximately 8% of a foul-smelling oil. Fenugreek has been noted to reduce plasma cholesterol in animals when 50% of their diet contained fenugreek seeds.[3] The high fiber content may have accounted for this change although it may be due to the steroid saponins. A hypoglycemic effect has also been noted. When added to the diet of diabetic dogs, a decrease in insulin dose and hyperglycemia was noted.[4] It is not known if these changes are due to the fiber content of the seeds or a chemical component. Fenugreek has been reported to increase the anticoagulant effect of warfarin.[5]

In a group of 10 women (non-placebo controlled) with infants born between 24 to 38 weeks gestation (mean=29 weeks) who ingested 3 fenugreek capsules 3 times daily (Nature's Way) for a week, the average milk production during the week increased significantly from a mean of 207 mL/day (range 57–1057 mL) to 464 mL/day (range 63–1140 mL).[6] No untoward effects were reported. In a study of 26 mothers of preterm infants (less than 31 weeks gestation) compared the use of fenugreek, 1725 mg (3 tablets) 3 times daily for 21 days to a placebo. Mothers initiated pumping within 12 hours of delivery and kept a daily record. Prolactin levels were drawn weekly and were not significantly changed. Data analysis revealed no statistical difference between the mothers receiving fenugreek or those receiving placebo in terms of milk volume. No adverse effects were noted in mothers or infants.[7] This study suggests that fenugreek is probably ineffective.

When dosed in moderation, fenugreek has limited toxicity and is listed in the US as a GRAS herbal (Generally Regarded As Safe). A maple syrup odor via urine and sweat is commonly reported. Higher doses may produce hypoglycemia although this is largely unsubstantiated. A stimulant effect on the isolated uterus (guinea pig) has been reported and its use in late pregnancy may not be advisable. Fenugreek's reputation as a galactagogue is widespread but undocumented. The dose commonly employed is variable but is approximately 2–3 capsules taken three times daily for a total daily dose of no more than 6 grams. The transfer of fenugreek into milk is unknown, untoward effects have only rarely been reported. Allergic reactions have been reported in patients sensitive to chickpeas and peanuts.[8]

Pregnancy Risk	Possibly Hazardous	Lactation Risk	L3
T ½	=	M/P	=
Vd	=	PB	=
Tmax	=	Oral	=
MW	=	pKa	=

Adult Concerns: Maple syrup odor in urine and sweat. Diarrhea, hypoglycemia, dyspnea (exaggeration of asthmatic symptoms). Once case of suspected gastrointestinal bleeding in a premature infant has been reported.[6] Two cases of fenugreek allergy have been reported.[7]

Pediatric Concerns: Maple syrup odor of infant urine.

Drug Interactions:

Relative Infant Dose:

Adult Dose: 6 grams per day

Alternatives: Metoclopramide, domperidone

References:
1. Review of Natural Products Facts and Comparisons, St Louis, MO 1996.
2. Sauvaire Y, Baccou JC. Extraction of diosgenin, (25R)-spirost-5-ene-3beta-ol; problems of the hydrolysis of the saponins. Lloydia 1978; 41: 247.
3. Valette G, Sauvaire Y, Baccou JC, Ribes G. Hypocholesterolaemic effect of fenugreek seeds in dogs. Atherosclerosis 1984; 50(1): 105–111.
4. Ribes G, Sauvaire Y, Baccou JC, Valette G, Chenon D, Trimble ER, Loubatieres-Mariani MM. Effects of fenugreek seeds on endocrine pancreatic secretions in dogs. Ann Nutr Metab 1984; 28(1): 37–43.
5. Lambert JP, Cormier A. Potential interaction between warfarin and boldo-fenugreek. Pharmacotherapy 2001; 21(4): 509–512.
6. Swafford S, Berens P. Effect of fenugreek on breast milk production. Abstract. ABM News and Views 2000; 6(3): 2000.
7. Reeder C, Legrand A, O'Conner-Von S., The effect of fenugreek on milk production and prolactin levels in mothers of premature infants. J Human Lact. 2011: 27: 74. Abstract.
8. Patil SP, Niphadkar PV, Bapat MM. Allergy to fenugreek (Trigonella foenum graecum). Ann Allergy Asthma Immunol 1997; 78(3): 297–300.

FERUMOXYTOL   L3

Trade: Feraheme

Other Trades:

Category: Iron replacement product.

Ferumoxytol is a uniquely formulated injectable iron replacement product. It consists of iron oxide within a carbohydrate shell.[1] This distinctive formulation allows the drug to pass through the extracellular compartment undeterred and enter the macrophages of the liver, spleen and bone marrow where eventually iron oxide is released to become a part of the storage iron pool. Iron may also be transferred from here into the plasma to be incorporated into hemoglobin. This unique design makes it effective for the treatment of iron deficiency anemia due to chronic kidney disease.

There are currently no studies on its transfer into human milk. Ferumoxytol has been successfully used for the treatment of iron-deficiency anemia in 6 pediatric patients aged 6 months to 16 years, without any reported side effects.[2] Ferumoxytol is an iron-carbohydrate complex. It is polar and non lipid-soluble. Following intravenous injection, it is primarily confined to the intravascular space. Thus, it is highly unlikely that ferumoxytol would enter breastmilk or be orally bioavailable in the infant.

Pregnancy Risk	C	Lactation Risk	L3
T ½	= 9.3–15 hours	M/P	=
Vd	= 2.3–3.16 l/kg	PB	=
Tmax	= 0.32 hour	Oral	=
MW	= 750	pKa	=

Adult Concerns: Ferumoxytol may cause nausea, dizziness, diarrhea, constipation, peripheral edema. Serious manifestations include hypotension and hypersensitivity reactions.

Pediatric Concerns: No reported complications. Can be used from 6 months to 16 years of age.

Drug Interactions: None reported.

Relative Infant Dose:

Adult Dose: 2 doses of 510 mg IV, 3–8 days apart.

Alternatives:

References:
1. Pharmaceutical manufacturer prescribing information, 2011.
2. Hassan N, Cahill J, Rajasekaran S, Kovey K. Ferumoxytol infusion in pediatric patients with gastrointestinal disorders: first case series. Ann Pharmacother. 2011 Dec; 45(12): e63. Epub 2011 Nov 24.

FESOTERODINE   L3

Trade: Toviaz

Other Trades:

Category: Anti-muscarinic

Fesoterodine is an anti-muscarinic agent used in the treatment of overactive bladder dysfunction.[1] It is rapidly metabolized *in vivo* to produce its active metabolite tolterodine. Tolterodine is a muscarinic anticholinergic agent similar in effect to atropine but is more selective for the urinary bladder. Tolterodine levels in milk have been reported in mice, where offsprings exposed to extremely high levels had slightly reduced body weight gain, but no other untoward effects. While it is more selective for the urinary bladder, preclinical trials still showed adverse effects including blurred vision, constipation, and dry mouth in adults. While we have no data on human milk, it is unlikely concentrations will be high enough to produce untoward effects in infants. However, the infant should be monitored for classic anticholinergic symptoms including dry mouth, constipation, poor tearing, etc.

Pregnancy Risk	C	Lactation Risk	L3
T ½	= 7 hours	M/P	=
Vd	= 169 l/kg	PB	= 50%
Tmax	= 5 hours	Oral	= 52%
MW	= 527.66	pKa	=

Adult Concerns: Constipation, dry eye, urinary retention, raise in intra-ocular tension, hypersensitivity reactions. Contra-indicated in patients with urinary retention and narrow-angle glaucoma.

Pediatric Concerns:

Drug Interactions: Concomitant administration with the following drugs increases the plasma levels of fesoterodine: ketoconazole, itraconazole, clarithromycin, erythromycin. Avoid coadministration with other anticholinergic agents.

Relative Infant Dose:

Adult Dose: 4–8 mg once daily.

Alternatives:

References:
1. Pharmaceutical manufacturer prescribing information, 2011.

FEXOFENADINE   L2

Trade: Allegra, Allegra Allergy 12 Hour, Allegra Allergy 24 Hour, Allegra Children's Allergy ODT, Allegra Children's Allergy, Allegra ODT

Other Trades: Allegra

Category: Antihistamine

Fexofenadine is a non-sedating histamine-1 receptor antagonist and is the active metabolite of terfenadine. It is indicated for symptoms of allergic rhinitis and other allergies. Unlike terfenadine, no cardiotoxicity has been reported with this product. In a study of 4 women receiving 60 mg/day terfenadine, no terfenadine was found in milk. However, the metabolite (fexofenadine) was present in small amounts. The average milk level of fexofenadine was 41 µg/L while the maternal plasma averaged 309 ng/mL. The time to peak for milk was 4.3 hours and the half-life in milk was 14.2 hours. The AUC (0–12) was 320 ng.hr/mL for milk and 1590 ng. hr/mL for plasma. The authors estimate that only 0.45% of the weight-adjusted maternal dose would be ingested by the infant.

Pregnancy Risk	C	Lactation Risk	L2
T ½	= 14.4 hours	M/P	= 0.21
Vd	=	PB	= 60–70%
Tmax	= 2.6 hours	Oral	= Complete
MW	= 538	pKa	= 13.2

Adult Concerns: Drowsiness, fatigue, leukopenia, nausea, dyspepsia, dry mouth, headache and throat irritation have been reported. Thus far, no cardiotoxicity has been reported .

Pediatric Concerns: None reported.

Drug Interactions: Erythromycin and ketoconazole (and potentially other azole antifungals and macrolide antibiotics) may elevate the plasma level of fexofenadine (82%) significantly.

Relative Infant Dose: 0.5%–0.7%

Adult Dose: 60 mg twice daily.

Alternatives:

References:
1. Lucas BD, Jr., Purdy CY, Scarim SK, Benjamin S, Abel SR, Hilleman DE. Terfenadine pharmacokinetics in breast milk in lactating women. Clin Pharmacol Ther 1995; 57(4): 398–402.

FIDAXOMICIN   L3

Trade: Dificid
Other Trades:
Category: Antibiotic, macrolide

Fidaxomicin is a macrolide antibiotic used for the treatment of *Clostridium difficile* infection.[1] Following oral ingestion, this antibiotic acts locally in the gastrointestinal tract against C. difficile, with minimal systemic absorption. Its active metabolite is OP-118. There are currently no studies on the transfer of this drug into human milk. But a review of its pharmacokinetic properties suggests that transfer into breastmilk would be minimal, if any transfer does occur, absorption from infant's gut should be minimal due to low oral bioavailability. However, until more established data are available, it is advisable to use this drug with caution in breastfeeding women.

Pregnancy Risk	B	Lactation Risk	L3
T ½	= 11.7 hours (11.2 hours for metabolite)	M/P	=
Vd	=	PB	=
Tmax	= 1–5 hours	Oral	= Minimal
MW	=	pKa	=

Adult Concerns: Nausea, vomiting, abdominal pain, anemia. Bowel obstruction and gastrointestinal hemorrhage are rare side-effects.

Pediatric Concerns:

Drug Interactions: When administered with cyclosporine, the plasma drug levels of fidaxomicin increased.

Relative Infant Dose:

Adult Dose: 200 mg twice daily for 10 days.

Alternatives: Metronidazole, vancomycin

References:
1. Pharmaceutical manufacturer prescribing information, 2011.

FILGRASTIM   L3

Trade: Neupogen
Other Trades: Neupogen
Category: Synthetic hematopoietic agent

Filgrastim is a large molecular weight biosynthetic protein used to stimulate neutrophil production. It is more commonly called granulocyte colony stimulating factor (G-CSF).[1] There are no data on its entry into human milk, but due to its large molecular weight (18,800 daltons) it is extremely remote that any would enter milk. Following use, the plasma levels in most individuals are often undetectable or in the picogram range. Further, due to its protein structure, it would not likely be orally bioavailable to the infant.

Pregnancy Risk	C	Lactation Risk	L3
T ½	= 3.5 hours	M/P	=
Vd	= 150 l/kg	PB	=
Tmax	= 2–8 hours	Oral	= None
MW	= 18,800	pKa	=

Adult Concerns: Transient rash, nausea and vomiting, erythema and swelling at injection site, and splenomegaly.

Pediatric Concerns: None reported via milk.

Drug Interactions: Use caution with drugs such as lithium that induce release of neutrophils.

Relative Infant Dose:

Adult Dose: 5 µg/kg daily

Alternatives:

References:
1. Pharmaceutical manufacturer prescribing information, 1999.

FINGOLIMOD   L4

Trade: Gilenya
Other Trades:
Category: Immune Modulator

Fingolimod is an immune modulator and prodrug that binds to the surface of lymphocytes and redirects them from the blood and graft sites to the lymph nodes, thus reducing the immune response in patients with Multiple Sclerosis (MS).[1] It reportedly assists in the repair of brain glial and precursor cells following injury in this syndrome. Fingolimod slows the progression of disability and reduces the frequency and severity of symptoms in patients with MS. While it decreases the heart rate, it increases the risk of infection and raises liver enzymes. Asthmatic patients may have an increase in the use of their rescue inhalers. The most common side effects include headache, flu, diarrhea, back pain, abnormal liver enzymes, and cough. It is unknown if fingolimod passes into human breast milk but it is excreted into rat milk.[2] Due to its high Vd and high protein binding, I suspect that milk levels will be low.

Pregnancy Risk	C	Lactation Risk	L4
T ½	= 6–9 days	M/P	=
Vd	= 17.4 l/kg	PB	= 99.7%
Tmax	= 12–16 hours	Oral	= 93%
MW	= 307.5	pKa	=

Adult Concerns: Headache, flu, diarrhea, back pain, abnormal liver enzymes, cough, macular edema, weakness, dizziness, bradycardia, hypertension.

Pediatric Concerns:

Drug Interactions: Ketoconazole increases fingolimod blood levels by 1.7 fold. Class Ia and III drugs can potentially cause torsades de pointes in patients who have bradycardia. Due to fingolimod's ability to cause bradycardia, patients on these medications should be monitored closely.

Relative Infant Dose:

Adult Dose: 0.5 mg daily

Alternatives:

References:
1. Kappos, L., Comi, AJ., Montalban, X., O'Connor, P., Polman, CH., Haas, T., Korn, AA., Karlsson, G., and Radue, EW. Oral fingolimod (FTY720) for relapsing multiple sclerosis. N Engl J Med. 2006 Sep 14; 355 (11): 1124–40.
2. Pharmaceutical manufacturer prescribing information, 2010.

FLAVOXATE   L3

Trade: Urispas, Apo-Flavoxate

Other Trades: Urispas

Category: Urinary tract antispasmodic

Flavoxate is used as an antispasmodic to provide relief of painful urination, urgency, nocturia, urinary frequency, or incontinence.[1] It exerts a direct smooth muscle relaxation on the bladder wall and has been used in children for enuresis. No data are available on its transfer into human milk.

Pregnancy Risk	B	Lactation Risk	L3
T ½	= <10 hours	M/P	=
Vd	=	PB	=
Tmax	= 2 hours	Oral	= Complete
MW	= 391	pKa	= 7.3

Adult Concerns: Drowsiness, dry mouth and throat, nervousness, headache, confusion, nausea, vomiting, blurred vision. Do not use with pyloric or duodenal obstruction, gastrointestinal hemorrhage, or obstructive uropathies.

Pediatric Concerns: None reported via milk.

Drug Interactions:

Relative Infant Dose:

Adult Dose: 100–200 mg three to four times daily.

Alternatives:

References:
1. Pharmaceutical manufacturer prescribing information, 1997.

FLECAINIDE ACETATE　　　　　　L3

Trade: Tambocor
Other Trades: Tambocor
Category: Antiarrhythmic agent

Flecainide is a potent antiarrhythmic used to suppress dangerous ventricular arrhythmias. In a group of 11 breastfeeding mothers receiving 100 mg oral flecainide (mean=3.2 mg/kg/day) every 12 hours for 5.5 days beginning 1 day postpartum, apparent steady-state levels of flecainide in both milk and plasma were achieved in most cases by day 4 of the study.[1] Highest daily average concentration of flecainide in milk ranged from 270 to 1529 µg/L (mean=953 µg/L) for the 11 subjects. Mean milk/plasma ratios were 3.7, 3.2, 3.5, and 2.6 on study days 2, 3, 4, and 5 respectively. After the last dose of flecainide, peak milk levels of the drug occurred at 3 to 6 hours and then declined monoexponentially. The half-life for elimination of flecainide from milk was 14.7 hours and is very similar to the plasma elimination half-life of flecainide in healthy human subjects.

Based on the pharmacokinetics of flecainide in infants, the expected average steady-state plasma concentration of flecainide in a newborn infant consuming all of the milk production of its mother (approximately 700 mL/day at the highest flecainide level of 1529 µg/L), the average daily intake by the infant would be 1.07 mg. In a normal 4 kg infant, the average plasma concentration in a breastfed infant would not be expected to exceed about 62 ng/mL. The average plasma level in infants treated with therapeutic doses is 360 ng/mL. In another study of one patient receiving 100 mg every 12 hours, milk levels of flecainide averaged 0.99 mg/L on day 4 and 5 postpartum.[2]

Levels of flecainide in milk are moderate to very low. Some caution is recommended.

Pregnancy Risk	C	Lactation Risk	L3
T ½	= 7–22 hours	M/P	= 2.6–3.7
Vd	=	PB	= 50%
Tmax	= 4.5 hours	Oral	= 90%
MW	= 414	pKa	= 9.3

Adult Concerns: Flecainide may induce arrhythmias in certain patients and congestive heart failure in approximately 2–5% of patients due to negative inotropy. Dizziness, nausea, blurred vision, dyspnea, and vomiting are reported. Flecainide should be reserved for patients with life-threatening arrhythmias. Withdrawal from flecainide therapy should be gradual due to the possibility of fatal cardiac arrest.

Pediatric Concerns: No adverse effects yet reported via milk, but observe for dizziness, faintness, dyspnea, headache, nausea, constipation.

Drug Interactions: Flecainide concentrations may be increased by digoxin and amiodarone. Arbutamine may exacerbate the arrhythmogenic effects of flecainide. Beta blockers, disopyramide, verapamil may enhance the negative inotropic effect of flecainide. Concurrent oral use of flecainide and cimetidine has been associated with a 46 to 65% increase in the elimination half-life, a 7 to 11% reduction in renal clearance, and a 15 to 32% reduction in the non-renal clearance of flecainide.

Relative Infant Dose: 4.9%–5.2%

Adult Dose: 50–100 mg twice daily.

Alternatives:

References:
1. McQuinn RL, Pisani A, Wafa S, Chang SF, Miller AM, Frappell JM, Chamberlain GV, Camm AJ. Flecainide excretion in human breast milk. Clin Pharmacol Ther 1990; 48(3): 262–267.
2. Wagner X, Jouglard J, Moulin M, Miller AM, Petitjean J, Pisapia A. Coadministration of flecainide acetate and sotalol during pregnancy: lack of teratogenic effects, passage across the placenta, and excretion in human breast milk. Am Heart J 1990; 119(3 Pt 1): 700–702.

FLOXACILLIN   L1

Trade: Flucil

Other Trades: Flucloxacillin, Flopen, Floxapen, Staphylex, Fluclox, Flu-Amp, Flu-Clomix, Magnapen

Category: Penicillin antibiotic

Floxacillin, also called flucloxacillin, is a penicillinase-resistant penicillin frequently used for resistant *staphylococcal* infections. Only trace amounts are secreted into human milk.[1] Its congener, cloxacillin, is commonly used to treat mastitis in breastfeeding mothers and has been used in thousands of breastfeeding patients without problem. Changes in gut flora are possible but unlikely.

Pregnancy Risk	B	Lactation Risk	L1
T ½	= 1.5 hours	M/P	=
Vd	= 0.11 l/kg	PB	= 94%
Tmax	= 1 hour	Oral	= 50%
MW	= 454	pKa	= 2.7

Adult Concerns: Adverse effects of floxacillin are similar to those of other penicillins, and include nausea, vomiting, diarrhea, constipation, and skin rashes, hemolytic anemia and interstitial nephritis have been reported rarely. Cases of acute hepatic cholestasis related to floxacillin therapy has been reported.

Pediatric Concerns: None reported via milk, but observe for changes in gut flora.

Drug Interactions: Concomitant penicillin and aminoglycoside therapy has been reported to result in inactivation of the aminoglycoside. Small changes in methotrexate plasma levels have been reported.

Relative Infant Dose:

Adult Dose: 250–500 mg four times daily.

Alternatives: Cloxacillin, dicloxacillin

References:
1. Pharmaceutical manufacturer prescribing information, 2010.

FLUCONAZOLE   L2

Trade: Diflucan
Other Trades: Diflucan
Category: Antifungal, particularly candida infections

Fluconazole is a synthetic triazole antifungal agent and is frequently used for vaginal, oropharyngeal, and esophageal candidiasis. Many of the triazole antifungals (itraconazole, terconazole) have similar mechanisms of action and are considered fungistatic in action. *In vivo* studies have found fluconazole to have fungistatic activity against a variety of fungal strains including *Candida albicans, Candida tropicalis, Candida glabrata*, and *Candida neoformans*. The pharmacokinetics are similar following both oral and IV administration. The drug is almost completely absorbed orally (>90%). Peak plasma levels occur in 1–2 hours after oral administration.

Fluconazole is transferred into human milk with a milk/plasma ratio of approximately 0.85.[1] Following a single 150 mg dose, milk levels at 2, 5, 24 and 48 hours were reported to be 2.93, 2.66, 1.76, and 0.98 µg/mL respectively. Maternal plasma levels at 2, 5, 24, and 48 hours were 6.4, 2.79, 2.52, and 1.19 µg/mL respectively.[1] The plasma half-life of fluconazole is 35 hours and its breastmilk half-life is 30 hours. From these data, and assuming an average milk level of 2.3 mg/L, an infant consuming 150 mL/kg/day of milk would receive an average of 0.34 mg/kg/d of fluconazole or 16% of the weight-adjusted maternal dose, and less than 5.8% of the pediatric dose (6 mg/kg/day).

In another study of one patient receiving 200 mg daily (1.5 times the above dose) for 18 days, the peak milk concentration was 4.1 mg/L at 2 hours following the dose.[2] However, the mean concentration of fluconazole in milk was not reported. Taken together, these two studies suggest a relative infant dose of 16–22% of the maternal dose.

Indication	Day 1	Daily Therapy	Minimum Duration of Therapy
Oropharyngeal candidiasis	200 mg	100 mg	14 d
Esophageal candidiasis	200 mg	100 mg	21 d
Systemic candidiasis	400 mg	200 mg	28 d
Cryptococcal meningitis acute relapse	400 mg 200 mg	200 mg 200 mg	10-12 wk after CSF culture becomes negative

Pregnancy Risk	C (D in high doses 400–800 mg/day)	Lactation Risk	L2
T ½	= 30 hours	M/P	= 0.46–0.85
Vd	=	PB	= 15%.
Tmax	= 1–2 hours	Oral	= >90%
MW	= 306	pKa	= 1.76

Adult Concerns: Adverse effects have only been reported in about 5–30% of patients, and in these, only 1–2.8% of patients have required discontinuation of the medication. Although adverse hepatic effects have been reported, they are very rare, and many occur coincident with the administration of other medications in AIDS patients. The most common complications include vomiting, diarrhea, abdominal pain, and skin rashes.

Pediatric Concerns: Pediatric complications from oral ingestion include gastrointestinal symptoms such as vomiting, nausea, diarrhea, abdominal pain. Nephrotoxicity has not been reported. No complications from exposure to breastmilk have found.

Drug Interactions: Decreased hepatic clearance of fluconazole results from use with cyclosporin, zidovudine, rifabutin, theophylline, oral hypoglycemics (glipizide and tolbutamide), warfarin, phenytoin, and terfenadine. Decreased plasma levels of fluconazole have resulted following administration with rifampin, and cimetidine.

Relative Infant Dose: 16.4%–21.5%

Adult Dose: 50–200 mg daily.

Alternatives:

References:
1. Force RW. Fluconazole concentrations in breast milk. Pediatr Infect Dis J 1995; 14(3): 235–236.
2. Schilling CG. et. al. Excretion of fluconazole in human breast milk (abstract # 130). Pharmacotherapy 1993; 13: 287.

FLUCYTOSINE   L4

Trade: Ancobon
Other Trades:
Category: Antifungal

Flucytosine is an antifungal medication used in the treatment of Candida and Cryptococcus UTI's, meningitis, pulmonary infections, and systemic infections. Flucytosine is often combined with Amphotericin B in systemic infections due to emergence of resistant strains to Flucytosine alone. There are no studies on transfer of Flucytosine into breast milk. Due to the low protein binding (2–4%), small molecular weight (129.1) and high oral bioavailability (78–89%), a moderate amount of the drug will be expected to be transferred into milk. A small amount of Flucytosine (4%) may be metabolized to 5-fluorouracil. Infant plasma drug levels should be monitored along with renal function, hepatic function, and bone marrow function if breastfeeding. Due to the side effects of Flucytosine, breastfeeding is not recommended with this drug. The half-life increases with decreasing renal function. The oral dose in neonates is 25–100 mg/kg/day; adult dose 50–150 mg/kg/day divided q 6 hours. Target trough levels are 25–50 mg/L and peak levels 50–100 mg/L. This product is probably too hazardous to use in breastfeeding women.[1-3]

Pregnancy Risk	C	Lactation Risk	L4
T ½	= 3–8 hours	M/P	=
Vd	=	PB	= 2–4%
Tmax	= 2 hours (po) faster if IV	Oral	= 78–89%
MW	= 129.1	pKa	= 2.9

Adult Concerns: Side effects include hepatotoxicity, bone marrow suppression, fatigue, hypoglycemia, hypokalemia, n/v, diarrhea, abd. pain, chest pain, and rash.

Pediatric Concerns:

Drug Interactions: Contraindicated with cytarabine. Any drugs that cause bone marrow depression, and hepatotoxicity effects such as Zidovudine should be used with caution. Aluminum hydroxide or magnesium hydroxide suspensions delay absorption and also neomycin. Drugs that impair glomerular filtration will decrease elimination of flucytosine and thus prolong T ½ and increase serum concentrations such as Amphotericin B.[4]

Relative Infant Dose:

Adult Dose: 50–150 mg/kg/day

Alternatives:

References:
1. Pharmaceutical manufacturer prescribing information, 2009.
2. Daneshmend TK, Warnock DW. Clinical pharmacokinetics of systemic antifungal drugs. Clin Pharmacokinet. 1983 Jan-Feb; 8(1): 17–42.
3. Vermes A, Guchelaar HJ, Dankert J. Flucytosine: a review of its pharmacology, clinical indications, pharmacokinetics, toxicity and drug interactions. J Antimicrob Chemother. 2000 Aug; 46(2): 171–9.

FLUDEOXYGLUCOSE F 18   L4

Trade: Fludeoxyglucose [18]F

Other Trades:

Category: PET Scanning pharmaceutical

Fludeoxyglucose [18]F (FDG) is a positron-emitting radiopharmaceutical used in conjunction with positron emission tomography (PET Scanning) to detect alterations in tissue glucose metabolism and is useful in detecting brain tumors, certain malignancies, chronic coronary artery disease, partial epilepsy, and Alzheimer's disease.[1,2,3] FDG, as a glucose analog, is taken up by high-glucose-metabolizing cells throughout the body. About 75% is sequestered within the cell until metabolized or decayed. The radioactive Fluorine-18 decays rapidly within the cell with a half-life of 110 minutes. About 20% of the dose is rapidly cleared renally by 2 hours. The urine is therefore radioactive for several hours after administration of this isotope. Thus, about 20% of the dose is rapidly cleared from the body. Only 80% remains to decay. By 24 hours (13 half-lives) only 1 part in 8200 parts of the initial radiation remains.[4] In five half-lives, about 98.5% would be decayed away. Fludeoxyglucose ^{18}F is rapidly distributed to all parts of the body that have significant glucose metabolism, including the breast. In a group of

6 lactating women, who received between 50–160 MBq FDG, amounts reported in milk were very low.[5] Decay-corrected activity measurable in breast milk ranged from 5.54 to 19.3 Bq/mL/MBq injected. Interestingly, the levels in breast tissue were quite high, but this product seems to be sequestered in lactocytes in breast tissue without penetrating into milk. The calculated maximum cumulative dose to the infant, 0.085 mSv with no interruption of breastfeeding, is well below the recommended limit of 1 mSv. Indeed, a higher radiation dose is received by the infant from close contact with the breast than from ingestion of radioactive milk. The authors suggest pumping of the milk and feeding in bottles by another individual to reduce direct exposure to radiation.

International Commission of Radiological Protection (ICRP) recommends no breastfeeding interruption; however, close contact restriction of a few hours is recommended (see radiopharmaceutical breastfeeding and close contact restriction table).[6,7] The half-life of the ^{18}F is short, only 110 minutes. Due to concentration in some tissues such as the bladder, radiation exposure could be a problem and emptying of the breast at routine intervals 'might' help reduce radiation exposure to breast tissue. The USPDI (1994) recommends interruption of breastfeeding for 12–24 hours. At 9 hours, 98.5% of the radioisotope remaining in the tissues would be decayed away.[8] It is likely that after 9 hours, almost all radioisotope would be decayed to almost background levels.

Recommend pumping and dumping of breastmilk after the procedure for at least 4 to 9 hours to minimize radiation.[6] As the infant receives more radiation from close contact with the breast, close contact should probably be avoided for about 4 hours and minimized close contact for the next 10 hours, due to release of gamma radiation from the mother.

Pregnancy Risk	C		Lactation Risk	L4
T ½	= 110 minutes		M/P	=
Vd	=		PB	= Minimal
Tmax	= 30 minutes		Oral	= Complete
MW	=		pKa	=

Adult Concerns: No untoward effects have been reported for this product.

Pediatric Concerns: None reported, but possible radiation exposure if breastfed prior to 9 hours after dose. Avoid direct contact with mothers' skin before 9 hours.

Drug Interactions:

Relative Infant Dose:

Adult Dose:

Alternatives:

References:

1. Jamieson D, Alavi A, Jolles P, Chawluk J, Reivich M. Positron emission tomography in the investigation of central nervous system disorders. Radiol Clin North Am 1988; 26(5): 1075–1088.
2. Jones SC, Alavi A, Christman D, Montanez I, Wolf AP, Reivich M. The radiation dosimetry of 2 [F-18]fluoro-2-deoxy-D-glucose in man. J Nucl Med 1982; 23(7): 613–617.

3. Som P, Atkins HL, Bandoypadhyay D, Fowler JS, MacGregor RR, Matsui K, Oster ZH, Sacker DF, Shiue CY, Turner H, Wan CN, Wolf AP, Zabinski SV. A fluorinated glucose analog, 2-fluoro-2-deoxy-D-glucose (F-18): nontoxic tracer for rapid tumor detection. J Nucl Med 1980; 21(7): 670–675.
4. Fludeoxyglucose F-18, http: //en. wikipedia. org/wiki/Fludeoxyglucose_(18F).
5. Hicks RJ, Binns D, Stabin MG. Pattern of uptake and excretion of (18)F-FDG in the lactating breast. J Nucl Med. 2001 Aug; 42(8): 1238–42.
6. Leide-Svegborn S. Radiation exposure of patients and personnel from a PET/CT procedure with 18F-FDG. Radiat Prot Dosimetry. 2010 Apr-May; 139(1–3): 208–13. Epub 2010 Feb 18.
7. ICRP, 2008. Radiation Dose to Patients from Radiopharmaceuticals–Addendum 3 to ICRP Publication 53. ICRP Publication 106. Ann. ICRP 38 (1–2).
8. Jones SC, Alavi A, Christman D, Montanez I, Wolf AP, Reivich M. The radiation dosimetry of 2 [F-18]fluoro-2-deoxy-D-glucose in man. J Nucl Med 1982; 23(7): 613–617.

FLUDROCORTISONE   L3

Trade: Florinef, Myconef

Other Trades: Florinef

Category: Mineralocorticoid

Fludrocortisone is a halogenated derivative of hydrocortisone with very potent mineralocorticoid activity and is generally used to treat Addison's disease.[1,2] Although its glucocorticoid effect is 15 times more potent than hydrocortisone, it is primarily used for its powerful ability to retain sodium in the vascular compartment (mineralocorticoid activity). It is not known if fludrocortisone penetrates into milk but if it is similar to other corticosteroids, it is very unlikely the amounts in milk will be clinically relevant until extremely high doses are used, but caution is recommended.

Pregnancy Risk	C		Lactation Risk	L3
T ½	= 3.5 hours		M/P	=
Vd	=		PB	= 42%
Tmax	= 1.7 hours		Oral	= Complete
MW	= 380		pKa	= 13.50

Adult Concerns: Hypertension, sodium retention, cardiac hypertrophy, congestive heart failure, and headache.

Pediatric Concerns: None via milk.

Drug Interactions: Excessive potassium levels may result from use with amphotericin B. Use with loop diuretics may dramatically increase potassium loss. Phenytoin, rifampin, phenobarbital, and fosphenytoin may increase hepatic metabolism of fludrocortisone and reduce its efficacy. Lithium may reduce efficacy of fludrocortisone. Tuberculin reactions may be suppressed for periods up to 6 weeks in patients receiving fludrocortisone.

Relative Infant Dose:

Adult Dose: 0.1–0.4 mg daily

Alternatives:

References:
1. Pharmaceutical manufacturer prescribing information, 1999.
2. Drug Facts and Comparisons 1999 ed. ed. St. Louis: 1999.

FLUNARIZINE   L4

Trade: Sibelium

Other Trades: Sibelium, Novo-Flunarizine

Category: Antihypertensive

Flunarizine is a calcium channel blocker primarily indicated for use in migraine headache prophylaxis and peripheral vascular disease. It has a very long half-life and a huge volume of distribution, which contributes to the long half-life.[1] No data are available on the transfer of this product into human milk. However, due to its incredibly long half-life and high volume of distribution, it is possible that this product, over time, could build up and concentrate in a breastfed infant. Other calcium channel blockers may be preferred. Use with extreme caution.

Pregnancy Risk	C	Lactation Risk	L4
T ½	= 19 days	M/P	=
Vd	= 43.2 l/kg	PB	= 99%
Tmax	= 2–4 hours	Oral	= Complete
MW	= 404	pKa	= 7.7

Adult Concerns: Extrapyramidal symptoms in elderly patients, depression, porphyria, thrombophlebitis, drowsiness, headache, dizziness.

Pediatric Concerns: None reported via milk, but caution is advised.

Drug Interactions: Prolonged bradycardia with adenosine. Sinus arrest when used with amiodarone. Hypotension and bradycardia when used with beta blockers. Increase of carbamazepine and cyclosporin plasma levels when used with flunarizine.

Relative Infant Dose:

Adult Dose: 10 mg daily

Alternatives: Nifedipine, Nimodipine, Verapamil

References:
1.   Pharmaceutical manufacturer prescribing information, 2010.

FLUNISOLIDE   L3

Trade: Nasalide, Aerobid

Other Trades: Bronalide, Rhinalar, PMS-Flunisolide, Syntaris

Category: Inhaled and intranasal steroid.

Flunisolide is a potent corticosteroid used to reduce airway hyperreactivity in asthmatics. It is also available for intranasal use for allergic rhinitis. Generally, only small levels of flunisolide are absorbed systemically (about 40%) thereby reducing systemic effects and presumably breastmilk levels as well.[1,2] After inhalation of 1 mg flunisolide, systemic availability was only 40% and plasma level was 0.4–1 ng/mL. Adrenal suppression in children has not been documented even after therapy of 2 months with 1600 μg/day. Once absorbed, flunisolide is rapidly removed from the plasma compartment by first-pass uptake in the liver. Although no data on breastmilk levels are yet available, it is unlikely that the level secreted in milk is clinically relevant.

Pregnancy Risk	C	Lactation Risk	L3
T ½	= 1.8 hours	M/P	=
Vd	= 1.8 l/kg	PB	=
Tmax	= 30 minutes	Oral	= 21% (oral)
MW	= 435	pKa	= 14.74

Adult Concerns: Most common side effect is irritation, due to vehicle, not drug itself. Loss of taste, nasal irritation, flu-like symptoms, sore throat, headache.

Pediatric Concerns: None reported. Can be used in children down to age 6.

Drug Interactions: Concurrent use with bupropion may increase the risk for seizures.

Relative Infant Dose:

Adult Dose: 1 mg daily.

Alternatives:

References:
1. Pharmaceutical manufacturer prescribing information, 1995.
2. Facts and Comparisons. St. Louis: 2010..

FLUNITRAZEPAM   L3

Trade: Rohypnol
Other Trades: Rohypnol, Hypnodorm, Raohypnol
Category: Benzodiazepine sedative

Flunitrazepam is a prototypic benzodiazepine. Frequently called the "Date Rape Pill", it induces rapid sedation and significant amnesia, particularly when mixed with alcohol.[1,2] Effects last about 8 hours. It is recommended for adult insomnia and for pediatric preanesthetic sedation. Due to its long half-life of 20 to 30 hours and being highly orally bioavailable, flunitrazepam should not be used routinely during lactation. Alternatives include lorazepam and alprazolam.

Pregnancy Risk	D	Lactation Risk	L3
T ½	= 20–30 hours	M/P	=
Vd	= 3.6 l/kg	PB	= 80%
Tmax	= 2 hours	Oral	= 80–90%
MW	= 313	pKa	= 1.8

Adult Concerns: Drowsiness, amnesia, sedation, ataxia, headache, memory impairment, tremors.

Pediatric Concerns: None reported via milk, but observe for sedation.

Drug Interactions: Clarithromycin and other macrolide antibiotics may increase plasma levels for benzodiazepines by inhibiting metabolism. May have enhanced effect when added to fentanyl, ketamine, nitrous oxide. Addition of even small amounts of alcohol may produce profound sedation, psychomotor impairment, and amnesia. Theophylline may reduce the sedative effects of benzodiazepines.

Relative Infant Dose:

Adult Dose: 2 mg daily.

Alternatives: Lorazepam, alprazolam

References:
1. Kanto J, Erkkola R, Kangas L, Pitkanen Y. Placental transfer of flunitrazepam following intramuscular administration during labour. Br J Clin Pharmacol 1987; 23(4): 491–494.
2. Kanto J, Kangas L, Leppanen T. A comparative study of the clinical effects of oral flunitrazepam, medazepam, and placebo. Int J Clin Pharmacol Ther Toxicol 1982; 20(9): 431–433.

FLUOCINOLONE   L3

Trade: Synalar, Capex Shampoo, Flucort-N, Retisert, Dermotic

Other Trades:

Category: Corticosteroid

Fluocinolone acetonide is a corticosteroid primarily used topically to reduce skin inflammation and relieve itching.[1] It is a synthetic hydrocortisone derivative. Typical dosage strength is 0.01–0.025%. Fluocinolone is a corticosteroid primarily intended for topical use. It is considered a medium-potency steroid. Following topical application to the skin, only a small amount is systemically absorbed. No data are currently available of its use in breastfeeding women. It is unlikely fluocinolone would be excreted into human milk in clinically relevant levels following topical administration.

Pregnancy Risk	C	Lactation Risk	L3
$T\frac{1}{2}$	=	M/P	=
Vd	=	PB	= >90%
Tmax	=	Oral	=
MW	=	pKa	= 14.44

Adult Concerns: Contact dermatitis, dry skin, pruritus, erythema, atrophy of skin, shiny skin, papules, hypopigmentation. May cause systemic adverse effects if used on large area, under occlusive dressing, and broken skin. Systemic side effects: HPA axis suppression, secondary infections.

Pediatric Concerns:

Drug Interactions:

Relative Infant Dose:

Adult Dose: Apply on affected areas 2–4 times daily.

Alternatives:

References:
1. Pharmaceutical manufacturer prescribing information, 2011.

FLUOCINOLONE + HYDROQUINONE + TRETINOIN   L3

Trade: Tri-Luma

Other Trades:

Category: Treatment of melasma of the face.

This combination drug product is indicated for the short-term intermittent treatment of moderate to severe melasma of the face. It is a combination drug product containing corticosteroid (fluocinolone), retinoid (tretinoin), and bleaching agent (hydroquinone).

Percutaneous absorption of unchanged tretinoin, hydroquinone and fluocinolone acetonide into the systemic circulation of two groups of healthy volunteers (total n=59) was found to be minimal following 8 weeks of daily topical application of 1 gm (Group I, n= 45) or 6 gm (Group II, n= 14) of fluocinolone + hydroquinone + tretinoin. For tretinoin, quantifiable plasma concentrations were obtained in 57.78% (26 out of 45) of Group I and 57.14% (8 out of 14) of Group II subjects. The exposure to tretinoin as reflected by the C_{max} values ranged from 2.01 to 5.34 ng/mL (Group I) and 2.0 to 4.99 ng/mL (Group II). Thus, daily topical application of this combination drug product resulted in a minimal increase of normal endogenous levels of tretinoin. The circulating tretinoin levels represent only a portion of total tretinoin-associated retinoids, which would include metabolites of tretinoin and that sequestered into peripheral tissues. For hydroquinone, quantifiable plasma concentrations were obtained in 18% (8 out of 44) of Group I subjects. The exposure to hydroquinone as reflected by the C_{max} values ranged from 25.55 to 86.52 ng/mL. All Group II subjects (6 gm dose) had post-dose plasma hydroquinone concentrations below the quantifiable limit. For fluocinolone acetonide, Groups I and II subjects had all post-dose plasma concentrations below quantifiable limits.

We do not have specific data on this combination product, but levels of the individual products are not high and milk levels will be much lower. However, caution is still recommended and a risk: benefit analysis must justify its use in breastfeeding mothers.

Pregnancy Risk	C		Lactation Risk	L3
T ½	= Fluocinolone/hydroquinone/tretinoin: / /2 hours		M/P	=
Vd	= Fluocinolone/hydroquinone/tretinoin: / /0.44 l/kg		PB	= Fluocinolone/hydroquinone/tretinoin: >90%/ /
Tmax	=		Oral	=
MW	= Fluocinolone/hydroquinone/tretinoin: 452.49/110.11/300		pKa	= Fluocinolone/hydroquinone/tretinoin: 14.44/9.96/4.79

Adult Concerns: Erythema, desquamation, burning, dryness, and pruritus at the site of topical application. The hydroquinone content may occasionally cause a blue-black pigmentation of skin at the site of application known as ochronosis.

Pediatric Concerns: No reports in the literature. Risks are moderate to low.

Drug Interactions: Avoid use with soaps or detergents with astringent, alcohol or other ingredients with drying effects on the skin. Avoid concomitant use with topical agents known to cause photosensitivity.

Relative Infant Dose:

Adult Dose:

Alternatives:

References:
1.   Pharmaceutical manufacturer prescribing information, 2005.

FLUORESCEIN   L3

Trade: AK-Fluor, Fluorescite, Funduscein-10, Ophthifluor, Fluorescein sodium, Ful-Glo, Fluorets, Fluor-I-Strip

Other Trades:

Category: Diagnostic dye in angiography

Sodium fluorescein is a yellow, water-soluble dye. A 2% fluorescein ophthalmic solution or an impregnated fluorescein strip is used topically to detect corneal abrasions, for fitting of hard contact lenses, and intravenously for fluorescein angiography. Fluorescein is used in two ways. One, in which a small amount is added directly to the eye generally by ophthalmologists and optometrists, and secondly, when much larger quantities are administered intravenously (5 mL of 10% solution). In a study of one patient who received an intravenous dose of fluorescein (5 mL of 10% fluorescein=500 mg), breastmilk levels were monitored for over 76 hours.[1] Concentrations of 372 µg/L at 6 hours and 170 µg/L at 76 hours after the dose were reported. In this patient, the half-life of fluorescein in breastmilk appeared quite long, approximating 62 hours. While the authors conclude that this is a high dose via milk, in another patient who received slightly more (910 mg IV), the patient's plasma levels of fluorescein monoglucuronide were 37,000 µg/L.[2]

Using this data, it would appear that an approximation of the milk/plasma ratio would be about 0.018, which suggests that very little of the absolute maternal dose enters milk. Nevertheless, fluorescein-induced phototoxicity remains a possibility in an infant fed breastmilk containing sodium fluorescein. One case of severe fluorescein phototoxicity has been reported in an infant receiving fluorescein intravenously.[3] If the infant is not undergoing phototherapy, it would appear that there is little risk to a breastfeeding infant.

Pregnancy Risk	C (topical), X (parenteral)	Lactation Risk	L3
T ½	= 4.4 hours (metabolite)	M/P	=
Vd	= 0.5 l/kg	PB	= 70–85%
Tmax	= 1 hour	Oral	= 50%
MW	= 376	pKa	= 9.32

Adult Concerns: Fluorescein-induced phototoxicity. Nausea, vomiting, dizziness, syncope, pruritus, seizures, following IV therapy. Severe reactions are rare. Oral fluorescein appears to elicit very few adverse reactions.

Pediatric Concerns: None reported via milk, but avoid phototherapy if used.

Drug Interactions: Interferes with numerous laboratory tests.

Relative Infant Dose: 0.8%

Adult Dose: 500 mg intravenous.

Alternatives:

References:
1. Maquire AM, Bennett J. Fluorescein elimination in human breast milk. Arch Ophthalmol 1988; 106(6): 718–719.
2. Kearns GL, Williams BJ, Timmons OD. Fluorescein phototoxicity in a premature infant. J Pediatr 1985; 107(5): 796–798.
3. Kearns GL, Williams BJ, Timmons OD. Fluorescein phototoxicity in a premature infant. J Pediatr 1985; 107(5): 796–798.

FLUORIDE   L2

Trade:

Other Trades:

Category: Hardening enamel of teeth

Fluoride is an essential element required for bone and teeth development. It is available as salts of sodium and stannic (tin). Excessive levels are known to stain teeth irreversibly. One study shows breastmilk levels of 0.024–0.172 ppm in milk (mean= 0.077 ppm) of a population exposed to fluoridated water (0.7 ppm).[1] In another study of breastfeeding women from areas low and rich in fluoride, milk fluoride levels were similar.[2] The mean fluoride concentration was 0.36 µmol/L for colostrum and 0.37 µmol/L for mature milk in the region with 1 ppm fluoride enriched water. In the region with 0.2 ppm fluoride, the mean fluoride concentration of colostrum was 0.28 µmol/L. There was no statistical difference in any of these milk fluoride levels. Fluoride probably forms calcium fluoride salts in milk which may limit the oral bioavailability of the fluoride provided by human milk. Maternal supplementation is unnecessary and not recommended in areas with high fluoride content (>0.7 ppm) in water.[3] Allergy to fluoride has been reported in one infant.[4] Younger children (2–6 years) should be instructed to use pea-sized quantities of toothpaste. Brushing should be limited to ≤ 2 times daily with fluoridated toothpaste and to spit out excess toothpaste. The American Academy of Pediatrics no longer recommends supplementing of breastfed infants with oral fluoride for the first 6 months of life. From 6 months to 3 years of age, supplement fluoride drops only if drinking water levels are less than 0.3 ppm. Bottled water may or may not contain fluoride.

Fluoride Ion and Dosing Recommendations

Fluoride Content of Drinking Water	Daily Dose, Oral (mg) In Non-Breastfed Infants
<0.3 ppm	
Birth–2 y	0.25
2–3 y	0.5
3–12 y	1
0.3-0.7 ppm	
Birth–2 y	0
2–3 y	0.25
3–12 y	0.5

Pregnancy Risk	C	Lactation Risk	L2
T ½	= 6 hours	M/P	=
Vd	= 0.5–0.7 l/kg	PB	=
Tmax	=	Oral	= 90% (Na)
MW	= 19	pKa	= 3.15

Adult Concerns: Stained enamel, allergic rash.

Pediatric Concerns: Allergy to fluoride has been reported in one infant. Do not use maternal doses >0.7 ppm.

Drug Interactions: Decreased absorption when used with magnesium, aluminum, and calcium containing products.

Relative Infant Dose:

Adult Dose: 1 mg daily.

Alternatives:

References:
1. Latifah R, Razak IA. Fluoride levels in mother's milk. J Pedod 1989; 13(2): 149–154.
2. Spak CJ, Hardell LI, De Chateau P. Fluoride in human milk. Acta Paediatr Scand 1983; 72(5): 699–701.
3. Fluoride supplementation of the breast-fed infant JAMA 1990; 263(16): 2179.
4. Shea J. et. al. Allergy to fluoride. Ann Allergy 1967; 25: 388.

FLUOROURACIL   L4

Trade: 5FU, Adrucil, Efudex, Fluoroplex, Carac, Cytosafe, Effluderm

Other Trades:

Category: Anticancer drug, actinic keratosis

Fluorouracil (5–FU) is a uracil analog used to treat a number of cancers. It is used topically for actinic keratosis, breast cancer, colorectal cancer, condyloma acuminatum, and many other cancers. Oral absorption is highly variable but averages less than 50–80%. Topical absorption through intact skin is less than 6–10%.[1] Ninety percent of the dose is accounted for during the first 24 hours, following intravenous administration. Those receiving topical therapy would not need to discontinue breastfeeding, if the surface area is minimal. If large body areas were exposed to this therapy, significant absorption could occur.

With intravenous administration of fluorouracil, the mean half-life of elimination from plasma is approximately sixteen minutes, with a range of 8–20 minutes, and is dose dependent. No intact drug can be detected in the plasma three hours after an intravenous injection. No data are available on the transfer of 5–FU to human milk. Mothers receiving injected 5–FU (IV, IM, IP) should be advised to withhold breastfeeding for a minimum of 24 hours after exposure. 5–FU is also sometimes used intraocularly following retinal surgery. Animal studies suggest that retention in the vitreous humor is long-lasting, thus the drug would be slowly released into the plasma compartment over several days. The doses here are small (5 mg) and are unlikely to produce significant plasma levels or milk levels of this drug.

Pregnancy Risk	D	Lactation Risk	L4
T ½	= 16 minutes	M/P	=
Vd	= 9 L/m²	PB	= 8–12%
Tmax	= Immediate (IV)	Oral	= 0–80%
MW	= 130	pKa	= 12.02

Adult Concerns: Nausea, vomiting, anorexia, blood dyscrasias, bone marrow suppression, myocardial toxicity, dyspnea, cardiogenic shock, rashes.

Pediatric Concerns: None reported but caution is recommended. A waiting period of 24 hours or more would largely reduce any risk.

Drug Interactions: Drug interactions are numerous and include allopurinol, cimetidine, methotrexate, leucovorin and others.

Relative Infant Dose:

Adult Dose: 6–12 mg/kg injection (IV) daily.

Alternatives:

References:
1. Pharmaceutical manufacturer prescribing information, 2005.

FLUOXETINE   L2

Trade: Prozac

Other Trades: Lovan, Zactin, Prozac, Apo-Fluoxetine, Novo-Fluoxetine

Category: Antidepressant

Fluoxetine is a very popular serotonin reuptake inhibitor (SSRI) currently used for depression and a host of other syndromes. Fluoxetine absorption is rapid and complete and the parent compound is rapidly metabolized to norfluoxetine, which is an active, long half-life metabolite (360 hours).

Both fluoxetine and norfluoxetine appear to permeate breastmilk to levels approximately ⅕ to ¼ of maternal plasma. In one patient (dose=20 mg/day), while plasma levels of fluoxetine and norfluoxetine were 100.5 µg/L and 194.5 µg/L respectively,[1] levels in milk were respectively, 28.8 µg/L and 41.6 µg/L. Milk/plasma ratios were 0.286 and 0.21 respectively. In another patient receiving 20 mg daily at bedtime, the milk concentration of fluoxetine was 67 µg/L and norfluoxetine 52 µg/L at four hours.[2] At 8 hours postdose, the concentrations fell to 17 µg/L and 13 µg/L, respectively. Using this data, the authors estimated that the total daily dose was only 15–20 µg/kg per day which represents a low exposure.

In another study of 10 breastfeeding women receiving 0.39 mg/kg/day of fluoxetine, the average breastmilk levels for fluoxetine and norfluoxetine ranged from 24.4–181.1 µg/L and 37.4–199.1 µg/L respectively.[3] Peak milk concentrations occurred within 6 hours. The milk/plasma ratios for fluoxetine and norfluoxetine were 0.88 and 0.72 respectively. Fluoxetine plasma levels in one infant were undetectable (<1 ng/mL). Using this data, an infant consuming 150 mL/kg/day would consume approximately 9.3–57 µg/kg/day total fluoxetine (and metabolite), which represents 5–9% of the maternal dose. No adverse effects were noted in the infants in this study.

In another case, severe colic, fussiness, and crying was reported.[4] The mother was receiving a dose of 20 mg fluoxetine per day. Concentrations of fluoxetine and norfluoxetine in breastmilk were 69 µg/L and 90 µg/L respectively. The plasma levels in the infant for fluoxetine and norfluoxetine were 340 ng/mL and 208 ng/mL respectively which is almost twice that of normal maternal ranges. The author does not report the maternal plasma levels but suggests they were similar to Isenberg's adult levels (100.5 ng/mL and 194.5 ng/mL for fluoxetine and norfluoxetine). In this infant, the plasma levels would approach those of a mother receiving twice the above 20 mg dose per day (40 mg/day). The symptoms resolved upon discontinuation of fluoxetine by the mother.

In a study by Brent [5], an infant exposed in utero and postpartum via milk, had moderate plasma fluoxetine levels that increased in the three weeks postpartum due to breastmilk ingestion. The infant's plasma levels of fluoxetine went from none detectable at day 13 to 61 ng/mL at day 21. The mean adult therapeutic range is 145 ng/mL. The infant in this study exhibited slight seizure activity at 3 weeks, 4 months, and 5 months.

Ilett reports that in a group of 14 women receiving 0.51 mg/kg/day fluoxetine, the mean M/P ratio was 0.67 (range 0.35 to 0.13) and 0.56 for norfluoxetine.[6] Mean total infant dose in fluoxetine equivalents was 6.81% of the weight-adjusted maternal dose. The reported infant fluoxetine and norfluoxetine plasma levels ranged from 20–252 µg/L and 17–187 µg/L respectively. Neonatal withdrawal syndrome was reported in one infant exposed in utero.[7] The mother was taking 20 mg/day, and delivered at 27 weeks. The baby was treated with nasal CPAP and phenobarbital at a dose of 5 mg/kg/day because the symptoms were interpreted as convulsions. The clinical picture was interpreted as neonatal withdrawal syndrome.[8] It is not known if these reported side effects (seizures, colic, fussiness, crying) are common, although this author has received numerous other personal communications similar to this. Indeed in one case, the infant became comatose at 11 days postpartum with high plasma levels of norfluoxetine.[9]

One case reported toxicity in a preterm infant whose mother was taking 40 mg/day. At 4 hours of age, the infant was tachypneic with a respiratory rate of 100. The infant had an erythematous rash on both cheeks and petechiae on the abdomen, chest and extremities, and scleral icterus. Plasma levels of fluoxetine and norfluoxetine at 96 hours of age were 92 and 34 ng/mL respectively, which is within the adult therapeutic range. This infant at 4 months of age had normal neurodevelopment.[10] This study suggests that seizure-like activity and toxicity can be expected in preterm infants. At present, fluoxetine is the only antidepressant cleared for use in pregnancy. This may pose an added problem in breastfed infants. Infants born of mothers receiving fluoxetine are born with full steady state plasma levels of the medication, and each time they are breastfed the level in the infant may rise further.

Several methods of reducing the risk to newborns is to reduce or eliminate the use of fluoxetine just prior to delivery, or to switch to an alternate antidepressant while breastfeeding (sertraline, paroxetine, etc.). While we do not know the real risk of side effects, they are apparently low for the population. If the patient cannot tolerate switching to another antidepressant, then fluoxetine should be continued. Age at initiation of therapy is of importance. Use in older infants (4–6 months or older) is virtually without complications because they can metabolize and excrete the medication more rapidly. Data published in 1999 also suggest that weight gain in infants breastfed from mothers who were taking fluoxetine demonstrated a growth curve significantly below that of infants who were breastfed by mothers who did not take the drug. The average deficit in measurements taken between 2 and 6 months of age was 392 grams body weight. None of these infants were noted to have unusual behavior.[11] Another report suggests that fluoxetine may induce a state of anesthesia of the vagina and nipples, although the relevance of this to breastfeeding mothers is unknown.[12] The author has had another report of a paroxetine-induced reduction of milk ejection reflex (MER). Whether or not a loss of MER is related to an anesthesia of the nipples is purely speculative.

An investigation was undertaken to study the effects of fluoxetine on the platelet 5–HT levels of the infant following lactational exposure to the drug.[13] Eleven mothers on 20–40 mg fluoxetine daily, along with their infants with ages ranging between 1 week to 6.5 months of age, were included in this study. 5–HT levels of maternal and infant plasma were assessed before taking the first fluoxetine dose, and then again at 4–12 weeks after initiation of fluoxetine therapy. It was found that although the 5–HT levels in the maternal plasma decreased significantly by 9–28% after initiation of therapy, no such difference was noted in 10 of the infants' plasma studied. However, post-exposure 5–HT levels in one infant decreased by 40%, but these levels subsequently normalized 4 months later. No untoward effects were reported in any of the infants. The authors of this study concluded that while lactational exposure to fluoxetine 20–40 mg/day causes minimal changes in platelet 5–HT levels of most infants, some caution is still recommended with its use, until more studies are done on this subject.

Current data on sertraline and escitalopram suggest these medications have difficulty entering milk, and more importantly, the infant. Therefore, they are preferred agents over fluoxetine for therapy of depression in breastfeeding mothers.[14] However, it is important to remember, that the risks of not breastfeeding far outweigh the risk of using fluoxetine. Women who can only take fluoxetine should be advised to continue breastfeeding and observe the infant for side effects. Finally, fluoxetine therapy during breastfeeding is by no means contraindicated and has been used in many thousands of women.

Pregnancy Risk	C	Lactation Risk	L2
T ½	= 2–3 days (fluoxetine)	M/P	= 0.286–0.67
Vd	= 2.6 l/kg	PB	= 94.5%
Tmax	= 1.5–12 hours	Oral	= 100%
MW	= 309	pKa	= 8.7

Adult Concerns: Nausea, tachycardia, hypotension, headache, anxiety, nervousness, insomnia, dry mouth, anorexia and visual disturbances.

Pediatric Concerns: Severe colic, fussiness, and crying have been reported in one case study.

Drug Interactions: Cimetidine may increase plasma levels 50%. Hallucinations have occurred when used with dextromethorphan. Serious fatal reactions have occurred when used after MAO inhibitors. Phenytoin may reduce plasma levels of fluoxetine by 50%. CNS toxicity may result if used with L-tryptophan. Fluoxetine may increase plasma levels of tricyclic antidepressants. Significant increase in propranolol levels have been reported. Effects of buspirone may be decreased. Serum carbamazepine levels may be increased resulting in toxicity. Bradycardia has been reported when used with diltiazem. Use with digoxin reduces digoxin levels by 15%. Lithium levels may be increased by fluoxetine with possible neurotoxicity. Sertraline did not effect lithium levels. Methadone levels have been significantly increased with SSRIs. Clearance of theophylline may be decreased by three fold. When used with warfarin, a significant increase in bleeding time has been reported.

Relative Infant Dose: 1.6%–14.6%

Adult Dose: 20–60 mg daily.

Alternatives: Sertraline, escitalopram

References:
1. Isenberg KE. Excretion of fluoxetine in human breast milk. J Clin Psychiatry 1990; 51(4): 169.
2. Burch KJ, Wells BG. Fluoxetine/norfluoxetine concentrations in human milk. Pediatrics 1992; 89(4 Pt 1): 676–677.
3. Taddio A, Ito S, Koren G. Excretion of fluoxetine and its metabolite, norfluoxetine, in human breast milk. J Clin Pharmacol 1996; 36(1): 42–47.
4. Lester BM, Cucca J, Andreozzi L, Flanagan P, Oh W. Possible association between fluoxetine hydrochloride and colic in an infant. J Am Acad Child Adolesc Psychiatry 1993; 32(6): 1253–1255.
5. Brent NB, Wisner KL. Fluoxetine and carbamazepine concentrations in a nursing mother/infant pair. Clin Pediatr (Phila) 1998; 37(1): 41–44.
6. Kristensen JH, Ilett KF, Hackett LP, Yapp P, Paech M, Begg EJ. Distribution and excretion of fluoxetine and norfluoxetine in human milk. Br J Clin Pharmacol 1999; 48(4): 521–527.
7. Hale TW, Shum S, Grossberg M. Fluoxetine toxicity in a breastfed infant. Clin Pediatr (Phila) 2001; 40(12): 681–684.
8. Nordeng H, Lindemann R, Perminov KV, Reikvam A. Neonatal withdrawl syndrome after in utero exposure to selective serotonin reuptake inhibitors. Acta Paediatr 2001; 90: 288–91.
9. Chambers CD, Anderson PO, Thomas RG, Dick LM, Felix RJ, Johnson KA, Jones KL. Weight gain in infants breastfed by mothers who take fluoxetine. Pediatrics 1999; 104(5): e61.

10. Mohan CG, Moore JJ. Fluoxetine Toxicity in a Preterm Infant. J Perinatol 2000; 20: 445–446.

11. Michael A, Mayer C. Fluoxetine-induced anaesthesia of vagina and nipples. Br J Psychiatry 2000; 176: 299.

12. Yoshida K, Smith B, Craggs M, Kumar RC. Fluoxetine in breast-milk and developmental outcome of breast-fed infants. Br J Psychiatry 1998; 172: 175–178.

13. Epperson CN, Jatlow PI, Czarkowski K, Anderson GM. Maternal fluoxetinetreatment in the postpartum period: effects on platelet serotonin and plasma druglevels in breastfeeding mother-infant pairs. Pediatrics. 2003 Nov; 112(5): e425.

14. Weissman AM, Levy BT, Hartz AJ, et. al. Pooled Analysis of Antidepressant Levels in Lactating Mothers, Breast Milk, and Nursing Infants. Am J Psychiatry 2004 June; 161(6): 1066–1078.

FLUOXETINE + OLANZAPINE   L3

Trade: Symbyax

Other Trades:

Category: Anti-depressant

Fluoxetine hydrochloride + olanzapine is a combined drug product used in the treatment of major depressive disorder and bipolar depression.[1] No data are available on the transfer of this combined drug product into human milk.

Fluoxetine is a serotonin reuptake inhibitor (SSRI). Fluoxetine absorption is rapid and complete and the parent compound rapidly yields the active metabolite, norfluoxetine. Both fluoxetine and norfluoxetine appear to permeate breastmilk to levels approximately 1/5th to ¼th of maternal plasma. In one patient (dose=20 mg/day), while plasma levels of fluoxetine and norfluoxetine were 100.5 µg/L and 194.5 µg/L respectively,[2] levels in milk were respectively, 28.8 µg/L and 41.6 µg/L. Milk/plasma ratios were 0.286 and 0.21 respectively.

In another patient receiving 20 mg daily at bedtime, the milk concentration of fluoxetine was 67 µg/L and norfluoxetine 52 µg/L at four hours.[3] At 8 hours postdose, the concentrations fell to 17 µg/L and 13 µg/L, respectively. Using this data, the authors estimated that the total daily dose was only 15–20 µg/kg per day which represents a low exposure.

In another study of 10 breastfeeding women receiving 0.39 mg/kg/day of fluoxetine, the average breastmilk levels for fluoxetine and norfluoxetine ranged from 24.4–181.1 µg/L and 37.4–199.1 µg/L respectively.[4] Peak milk concentrations occurred within 6 hours. The milk/plasma ratios for fluoxetine and norfluoxetine were 0.88 and 0.72 respectively. Fluoxetine plasma levels in one infant were undetectable (<1 ng/mL). Using this data, an infant consuming 150 mL/kg/day would consume approximately 9.3–57 µg/kg/day total fluoxetine (and metabolite), which represents 5–9% of the maternal dose. No adverse effects were noted in the infants in this study.

In another case, severe colic, fussiness, and crying was reported.[5] The mother was receiving a dose of 20 mg fluoxetine per day. Concentrations of fluoxetine and norfluoxetine in breastmilk were 69 µg/L and 90 µg/L respectively. The plasma levels in the infant for fluoxetine and norfluoxetine were 340 ng/mL and 208 ng/mL respectively which is almost twice that of normal maternal ranges. The author does not report the maternal plasma levels but suggests they were similar to Isenberg's adult levels (100.5 ng/mL and 194.5 ng/mL for fluoxetine and norfluoxetine). In this infant, the plasma levels would approach those of a mother receiving twice the above 20 mg dose per day (40 mg/day). The symptoms resolved upon discontinuation of fluoxetine by the mother.

In a study by Brent [6], an infant exposed in utero and postpartum via milk, had moderate plasma fluoxetine levels that increased in the three weeks postpartum due to breastmilk ingestion. The infant's plasma levels of fluoxetine went from none detectable at day 13 to 61 ng/mL at day 21. The mean adult therapeutic range is 145 ng/mL. The infant in this study exhibited slight seizure activity at 3 weeks, 4 months, and 5 months.

Ilett reports that in a group of 14 women receiving 0.51 mg/kg/day fluoxetine, the mean M/P ratio was 0.67 and 0.56 for norfluoxetine.[7] Mean total infant dose in fluoxetine equivalents was 6.81%. The reported infant fluoxetine and norfluoxetine plasma levels ranged from 20–252 µg/L and 17–187 µg/L respectively. Neonatal withdrawal syndrome was reported in one infant exposed in utero.[8] The mother was taking 20 mg/day, and delivered at 27 weeks. The baby was treated with nasal CPAP and phenobarbital at a dose of 5 mg/kg/day because the symptoms were interpreted as convulsions. The clinical picture was interpreted as neonatal withdrawal syndrome.[9] It is not known if these reported side effects (seizures, colic, fussiness, crying) are common, although this author has received numerous other personal communications similar to this. Indeed in one case, the infant became comatose at 11 days postpartum with high plasma levels of norfluoxetine.[10] One case reported toxicity in a preterm infant whose mother was taking 40 mg/day. At 4 hours of age, the infant was tachypneic with a respiratory rate of 100. The infant had an erythematous rash on both cheeks and petechiae on the abdomen, chest and extremities, and scleral icterus. Plasma levels of fluoxetine and norfluoxetine at 96 hours of age were 92 and 34 ng/mL respectively, which is within the adult therapeutic range. This infant at 4 months of age had normal neurodevelopment.[11] This study suggests that seizure-like activity and toxicity can be expected in preterm infants. At present, fluoxetine is the only antidepressant cleared for use in pregnancy. This may pose an added problem in breastfed infants. Infants born of mothers receiving fluoxetine are born with full steady state plasma levels of the medication, and each time they are breastfed the level in the infant may rise further.

Age at initiation of therapy is of importance. Use in older infants (4–6 months or older) is virtually without complications because they can metabolize and excrete the medication more rapidly. Data published in 1999 also suggest that weight gain in infants breastfed from mothers who were taking fluoxetine demonstrated a growth curve significantly below that of infants without exposure to the drug, the average deficit in body weight between 2 and 6 months of age being 392 grams. None of these infants were noted to have unusual behavior.[12] Finally, fluoxetine therapy during breastfeeding is by no means contraindicated and has been used in many thousands of women. Women who can only take fluoxetine should be advised to continue breastfeeding and observe the infant for side effects.

Olanzapine is an atypical antipsychotic agent.[13] It is rather unusual in that it blocks serotonin receptors rather than dopamine receptors. In a recent and excellent study of seven mother-infant nursing pairs receiving a median dose of olanzapine of 7.5 mg/day (range = 5–20 mg/day), the median infant dose ingested via milk was approximately 1.02% of the maternal dose.[14] The median milk/plasma AUC ratio was 0.38. Olanzapine was undetected in the plasma of six infants tested. All infants were healthy and experienced no observable side effects. The maximum relative infant dose was approximately 1.2%. A study of 5 mothers receiving olanzapine at a dose of 2.5–20 mg/day, reported milk/plasma ratios of 0.2 to 0.84, with an average relative infant dose of 1.6%. The authors reported no untoward effects on the infants attributable to olanzapine.[15] In a study of 37 women consuming olanzapine, early discontinuation of breastfeeding was more common in the olanzapine-exposed breastfed group (5 of 22 vs. none of 51).[13] The rate of adverse outcomes in olanzapine-exposed breastfed infants did not differ from those of the control groups. Neonatal symptoms were seen in 6 of the 30 olanzapine-exposed infants versus 2 of 51 non-exposed infants. A withdrawal syndrome was seen in three of 30 (10%) infants.[16] Breastfed infants of mothers on olanzapine did not show any significant increase in rate of adverse-effects.

Pregnancy Risk	C	Lactation Risk	L3
T ½	= Fluoxetine/olanzapine: 2–3 days/21.54 hours	M/P	= Fluoxetine/olanzapine: 0.3–0.67/0.38
Vd	= Fluoxetine/olanzapine: 2.6/14.3 l/kg	PB	= Fluoxetine/olanzapine: 94.5%/93%
Tmax	= Fluoxetine/olanzapine: 1.5–12 hours/5–8 hours	Oral	= Fluoxetine/olanzapine: 100%/>57%
MW	= Fluoxetine/olanzapine: 309/312	pKa	= Fluoxetine/olanzapine: 8.7/5.0,7.4

Adult Concerns: Commonly observed adverse effects include hypotension, peripheral edema, rise in cholesterol, blood sugar, triglycerides and prolactin levels, weight gain, sedation, somnolence, fatigue. Some of the less common and serious side-effects include seizures, diabetic ketoacidosis, strokes, suicidal ideation.

Pediatric Concerns: Severe colic, fussiness, and crying following exposure to fluoxetine has been reported in one case study.

Drug Interactions: Do not use with monoamine oxidase inhibitors, or within 2 weeks of cessation of MAO inhibitor use. Caution is advised during concurrent use with triptans, linezolid, lithium, tryptophan and tramadol. concurrent use with NSAIDs, warfarin or aspirin cold increase risk of major bleeding disorders. Avoid co-administration with benzodiazepines due to increased risk of orthostatic hypotension. Co-administration with carbamazepine decreases efficacy of olanzapine. Concomitant use with fluoxetine increases the plasma levels of olanzapine. Use with pimozide and thioridazine is contra-indicated. Concurrent use with the following drugs causes an increase in their plasma levels: clozapine, tricyclic antidepressants, haloperidol, phenytoin, antiarrhythmics.

Relative Infant Dose:

Adult Dose: Fluoxetine/olanzapine: 3–12 mg/25–50 mg once daily.

Alternatives: Sertraline, escitalopram, risperidone, haloperidol, quetiapine.

References:
1. Pharmaceutical manufacturer prescribing information, 2012.
2. Isenberg KE. Excretion of fluoxetine in human breast milk. J Clin Psychiatry 1990; 51(4): 169.

3. Burch KJ, Wells BG. Fluoxetine/norfluoxetine concentrations in human milk. Pediatrics 1992; 89(4 Pt 1): 676–677.
4. Taddio A, Ito S, Koren G. Excretion of fluoxetine and its metabolite, norfluoxetine, in human breast milk. J Clin Pharmacol 1996; 36(1): 42–47.
5. Lester BM, Cucca J, Andreozzi L, Flanagan P, Oh W. Possible association between fluoxetine hydrochloride and colic in an infant. J Am Acad Child Adolesc Psychiatry 1993; 32(6): 1253–1255.
6. Brent NB, Wisner KL. Fluoxetine and carbamazepine concentrations in a nursing mother/infant pair. Clin Pediatr (Phila) 1998; 37(1): 41–44.
7. Kristensen JH, Ilett KF, Hackett LP, Yapp P, Paech M, Begg EJ. Distribution and excretion of fluoxetine and norfluoxetine in human milk. Br J Clin Pharmacol 1999; 48(4): 521–527.
8. Hale TW, Shum S, Grossberg M. Fluoxetine toxicity in a breastfed infant. Clin Pediatr (Phila) 2001; 40(12): 681–684.
9. Nordeng H, Lindemann R, Perminov KV, Reikvam A. Neonatal withdrawl syndrome after in utero exposure to selective serotonin reuptake inhibitors. Acta Paediatr 2001; 90: 288–91.
10. Chambers CD, Anderson PO, Thomas RG, Dick LM, Felix RJ, Johnson KA, Jones KL. Weight gain in infants breastfed by mothers who take fluoxetine. Pediatrics 1999; 104(5): e61.
11. Mohan CG, Moore JJ. Fluoxetine Toxicity in a Preterm Infant. J Perinatol 2000; 20: 445–446.
12. Michael A, Mayer C. Fluoxetine-induced anaesthesia of vagina and nipples. Br J Psychiatry 2000; 176: 299.
13. Pharmaceutical manufacturer prescribing information, 1997.
14. Gardiner SJ, Kristensen JH, Begg EJ, Hackett LP,Wilson DA,Ilett KF, Kohan R and Rampono J, Transfer of olanzapine into breast milk, calculation of infant drug dose, and effect on breast-fed infants. Am J Psychiatry 2003; 160: 1428–1431.
15. Croke S, Buist A, Hackett LP, Ilett KF, Norman TR, Burrows GD. Olanzapine exretion in human breast milk: estimation of infant exposure. Int J Neuropsychoph 2002; 5: 243–247.
16. Gilad O, Merlob P, Stahl B, Klinger G. Outcome of infants exposed to olanzapine during breastfeeding. Breastfeed Med. 2011; 6(2): 55–58.

FLUPHENAZINE   L3

Trade: Prolixin, Permitil

Other Trades: Modecate, Anatensol, Apo-Fluphenazine, Moditen

Category: Psychotherapeutic agent

Fluphenazine is a phenothiazine tranquilizer and presently has the highest milligram potency of this family. Fluphenazine decanoate injections (IM) provide extremely long plasma levels with half-lives approaching 14.3 days at steady state. Members of this family generally have milk/plasma ratios ranging from 0.5 to 0.7.[1] No specific reports on fluphenazine breastmilk levels have been located. Use with caution.

Pregnancy Risk	C	Lactation Risk	L3
T ½	= 10–20 hours	M/P	=
Vd	= 220 l/kg	PB	= 91–99%
Tmax	= 1.5–2 hours	Oral	= Complete
MW	= 438	pKa	= 3.9, 8.1

Adult Concerns: Depression, seizures, appetite stimulation, blood dyscrasias, weight gain, hepatic toxicity, sedation.

Pediatric Concerns: None reported, but observe for sedation.

Drug Interactions: Increased toxicity when administered with ethanol. CNS effects may be increased when used with lithium. May stimulate the effects of narcotics including respiratory depression.

Relative Infant Dose:

Adult Dose: 1–5 mg daily.

Alternatives:

References:
1. Ayd FJ. Excretion of psychotropic drugs in breast milk. In: International Drug Therapy Newsletter. Ayd Medical Communications 8[November-December]. 1973.

FLURAZEPAM   L3

Trade: Dalmane

Other Trades: Apo-Flurazepam, Dalmane, Novo-Flupam

Category: Sedative, hypnotic

Flurazepam is a sedative, hypnotic generally used as an aid for sleep. It belongs to the benzodiazepine (Valium) family. It is rapidly and completely metabolized to several long half-life active metabolites. Because most benzodiazepines are secreted into human milk, flurazepam entry into milk should be expected.[1] However, no specific data on flurazepam breastmilk levels are available. Since flurazepam is a benzodiazepine, its kinetics should be similar to other benzodiazepines. Shorter-acting benzodiazepines (lorazepam, alprazolam) are safest during lactation provided their use is short-term or intermittent, low dose, and after the first week of life.[2] Observe for sedation in the breastfed infant. Consider usage of suitable short-acting alternatives such as lorazepam or alprazolam.

Pregnancy Risk	X	Lactation Risk	L3
T ½	= 47–100 hours	M/P	=
Vd	= 3.4–5.5 l/kg	PB	= 97%
Tmax	= 0.5–1 hours	Oral	= Complete
MW	= 388	pKa	= 1.9, 8.2

Adult Concerns: Sedation, tachycardia, jaundice, apnea.

Pediatric Concerns: None reported, but caution is recommended. Observe for sedation.

Drug Interactions: Decreased effect when used with enzyme inducers such as barbiturates. Increased toxicity when used with other CNS depressants and cimetidine.

Relative Infant Dose:

Adult Dose: 15–30 mg daily.

Alternatives: Lorazepam, alprazolam

References:
1.   Facts and Comparisons. St. Louis: 2010..
2.   Maitra R, Menkes DB. Psychotropic drugs and lactation. N Z Med J 1996; 109(1024): 217–218.

FLURBIPROFEN   L2

Trade: Ansaid, Froben, Ocufen
Other Trades: Ansaid, Froben, Ocufen
Category: Analgesic

Flurbiprofen is a nonsteroidal analgesic similar in structure to ibuprofen but used both as an ophthalmic preparation (in eyes) and orally. In one study of 12 women and following nine oral doses (50 mg/dose, 3–5 days postpartum) the milk levels of flurbiprofen in two women ranged from 0.05 to 0.07 mg/L but was <0.05 mg/L in 10 of the 12 women.[1] Concentrations in breastmilk and plasma of nursing mothers suggest that a nursing infant would receive less than 0.1 mg flurbiprofen per day, a level considered exceedingly low. In another study of 10 nursing mothers following a single 100 mg dose, the average peak concentration of flurbiprofen in breastmilk was 0.09 mg/L.[2] Both of these studies suggest that the amount of flurbiprofen transferred in human milk would be clinically insignificant to the infant.

Pregnancy Risk	B/C in 3rd trimester	Lactation Risk	L2
T ½	= 3.8–5.7 hours	M/P	= 0.008–0.013
Vd	= 0.1 l/kg	PB	= 99%
Tmax	= 1.5 hours	Oral	= Complete
MW	= 244	pKa	= 4.2

Adult Concerns: Gastrointestinal distress, diarrhea, constipation, cramping, may worsen jaundice.

Pediatric Concerns: None reported.

Drug Interactions: May prolong prothrombin time when used with warfarin. Antihypertensive effects of ACE inhibitors may be blunted or completely abolished by NSAIDs. Some NSAIDs may block antihypertensive effect of beta blockers, diuretics. Used with cyclosporin, may dramatically increase renal toxicity. May increase digoxin, phenytoin, lithium levels. May increase toxicity of methotrexate. May increase bioavailability of penicillamine. Probenecid may increase NSAID levels.

Relative Infant Dose: 0.7%–1.4%

Adult Dose: 200–300 mg daily.

Alternatives: Ibuprofen

References:
1. Smith IJ, Hinson JL, Johnson VA, Brown RD, Cook SM, Whitt RT, Wilson JT. Flurbiprofen in postpartum women: plasma and breast milk disposition. J Clin Pharmacol 1989; 29(2): 174–184.
2. Cox SR, Forbes KK. Excretion of flurbiprofen into breast milk. Pharmacotherapy 1987; 7(6): 211–215.

FLUTICASONE   L3

Trade: Flonase, Flovent, Cutivate, Veramyst
Other Trades: Flixotide, Flovent, Flonase, Flixonase
Category: Intranasal, inhaled steroid

Fluticasone is a typical steroid primarily used intranasally for allergic rhinitis and via inhalation for asthma. When instilled intranasally, the absolute bioavailability is less than 2%, so virtually none of the dose is absorbed systemically.[1] Oral absorption following inhaled fluticasone is approximately 30%, although almost instant first-pass absorption virtually eliminates plasma levels of fluticasone.[2] Peak plasma levels following inhalation of 880 µg is only 0.1 to 1.0 ng/mL. Adrenocortical suppression following oral or even systemic absorption at normal doses is extremely rare due to limited plasma levels.[3] Plasma levels are not detectable when using suggested doses. Although fluticasone is secreted into milk of rodents, the dose used was many times higher than found under normal conditions. With the above limited oral and systemic bioavailability, and rapid first-pass uptake by the liver, it is not likely that milk levels will be clinically relevant, even with rather high doses.

Pregnancy Risk	C	Lactation Risk	L3
T ½	= 7.8 hours	M/P	=
Vd	= 4.2 l/kg	PB	= 91%
Tmax	= 15–60 minutes	Oral	= Oral (1%), Inhaled (18%)
MW	= 500	pKa	= 14.48

Adult Concerns: Intranasal: pruritus, headache (1–3%), burning (3–6%), epistaxis. Adverse effects associated with inhaled fluticasone include headache, nasal congestion, and oral candidiasis.

Pediatric Concerns: When used topically on large surface areas, some adrenal suppression has been noted. No effects have been reported in breastfeeding infants. In children receiving up to 5 times the normal inhaled dose (1000 µg/day), some growth suppression was noted.

Drug Interactions: Avoid concomitant administration of fluticasone with CYP450 3A4 inhibitors such as ritonavir and ketoconazole, as this may cause increased systemic levels of fluticasone.

Relative Infant Dose:

Adult Dose: 50–110 µg inhalation daily.

Alternatives:

References:
1. Pharmaceutical manufacturer prescribing information, 1996.
2. Harding SM. The human pharmacology of fluticasone propionate. Respir Med 1990; 84 Suppl A: 25–29.
3. Todd G, Dunlop K, McNaboe J, Ryan MF, Carson D, Shields MD. Growth and adrenal suppression in asthmatic children treated with high-dose fluticasone propionate. Lancet 1996; 348(9019): 27–29.

FLUTICASONE + SALMETEROL — L3

Trade: Advair, Advair Diskus 100/50, Advair Diskus 250/50, Advair Diskus 500/50, Advair Diskus, Advair HFA

Other Trades: Seretide, Advair Inhalation Aerosol

Category: Anti-asthma, anti-inflammatory + bronchodilator

Salmeterol xinafoate and Fluticasone propionate is a combination drug product of an anti-inflammatory agent with a bronchodilator used in asthma and chronic obstructive pulmonary disease. Oral absorption following inhaled fluticasone is approximately 30%, although almost instant first-pass absorption virtually eliminates plasma levels of fluticasone.[1] Peak plasma levels following inhalation of 880 µg is only 0.1 to 1.0 nanogram/mL. Adrenocortical suppression following oral or even systemic absorption at normal doses is extremely rare due to limited plasma levels.[2] Plasma levels are not detectable when using suggested doses. Although fluticasone is secreted into milk of rodents, the dose used was many times higher than found under normal conditions. With the above limited oral and systemic bioavailability, and rapid first-pass uptake by the liver, it is not likely that milk levels will be clinically relevant, even with rather high doses.

Maternal plasma levels of salmeterol after inhaled administration are very low (85–200 pg/mL), or undetectable.[3] Studies in animals have shown that plasma and breastmilk levels are very similar. Oral absorption of both salmeterol and the xinafoate moiety are good. The terminal half-life of salmeterol is 5.5 hours, xinafoate is 11 days. No reports of use in lactating women are available. But since maternal plasma levels after inhaled administration are low to undetectable, it is highly unlikely that entry into milk should occur in clinically significant quantities.

The combined use of salmeterol and fluticasone is probably compatible with breastfeeding.

Pregnancy Risk	C	Lactation Risk	L3
T ½	= Fluticasone/salmeterol: 7.8 hours/5.5 hours	M/P	= Fluticasone/salmeterol: /1.0
Vd	= Fluticasone/salmeterol: 4.2/ l/kg	PB	= Fluticasone/salmeterol: 91%/96%
Tmax	= Fluticasone/salmeterol: 15–60 min/10–45 min	Oral	= Fluticasone/salmeterol: 1%/complete
MW	= Fluticasone/salmeterol: 500/603	pKa	= Fluticasone/salmeterol: 14.48/14.18

Adult Concerns: Headache, dizziness, pharyngitis, respiratory tract infection, throat irritation, nausea, vomiting, diarrhea, muscle pain, oral candidiasis, menstruation symptoms.

Pediatric Concerns: None reported via milk. Levels in maternal plasma too low to produce relevant levels in milk.

Drug Interactions: Increases cardiovascular risks when used concomitantly with diuretics and cytochrome P450 inhibitors. Use with caution in those on monoamine oxidase inhibitors and tricyclic antidepressants since concomitant use may potentiate effects of salmeterol. Caution advised when used concomitantly with beta-blockers due to antagonistic effect on each other.

Relative Infant Dose:

Adult Dose: Fluticasone/salmeterol: 100–500 μg/50 μg, 1–2 inhalations daily.

Alternatives:

References:
1. Harding SM. The human pharmacology of fluticasone propionate. Respir Med 1990; 84 Suppl A: 25–29.
2. Todd G, Dunlop K, McNaboe J, Ryan MF, Carson D, Shields MD. Growth and adrenal suppression in asthmatic children treated with high-dose fluticasone propionate. Lancet 1996; 348(9019): 27–29
3. Pharmaceutical manufacturer prescribing information, 1996.

FLUVASTATIN   L3

Trade: Lescol, Lescol XL

Other Trades: Vastin, Lescol

Category: Reduces blood cholesterol levels

Fluvastatin is an inhibitor of cholesterol synthesis in the liver. Fluvastatin levels in human milk are reported to be twice that of serum levels, although no exact data could be found.[1] The effect on infant is unknown but could reduce cholesterol synthesis in infant. Atherosclerosis is a chronic process and discontinuation of lipid-lowering drugs during pregnancy, and lactation should have little to no impact on the outcome of long-term therapy of primary hypercholesterolemia. Cholesterol and other products of cholesterol biosynthesis are essential components for fetal and neonatal development and the use of cholesterol-lowering drugs would not be advisable under any circumstances.

Pregnancy Risk	X	Lactation Risk	L3
T ½	= 1.2 hours	M/P	= 2.0
Vd	=	PB	= >98%
Tmax	= <1 hour	Oral	= 20–30%
MW	= 411	pKa	= 14.64

Adult Concerns: Headache, insomnia, dyspepsia, diarrhea, abdominal bloating, elevated liver enzymes.

Pediatric Concerns: None reported, but reduced plasma cholesterol levels could occur.

Drug Interactions: Anticoagulant effect of warfarin may be increased.

Relative Infant Dose:

Adult Dose: 20–40 mg daily.

Alternatives:

References:
1. Pharmaceutical manufacturer prescribing information, 1995.

FLUVOXAMINE   L2

Trade: Luvox

Other Trades: Luvox, Apo-Fluvoxamine, Alti-Fluvoxamine, Faverin, Floxyfral, Myroxim

Category: Antidepressant

Fluvoxamine is a serotonin reuptake inhibitor with antidepressant action. Although structurally dissimilar to the other serotonin reuptake inhibitors, fluvoxamine provides increased synaptic serotonin levels in the brain. It has several hepatic metabolites which are not active. Its primary indications are for the treatment of obsessive-compulsive disorders (OCD) although it also functions as an antidepressant. There are a number of significant drug-drug interactions with this product.

In a case report of one 23-year-old mother and following a dose of 100 mg twice daily for 2 weeks, the maternal plasma level of fluvoxamine base was 0.31 mg/Liter and the milk concentration was 0.09 mg/Liter.[1] The authors reported a theoretical dose to infant of 0.0104 mg/kg/day of fluvoxamine, which is only 0.5% of the maternal dose. According to the authors, the infant suffered no unwanted effects as a result of this intake and that this dose poses little risk to a nursing infant. In a study of one patient receiving 100 mg twice daily, the AUC milk/serum ratio averaged 1.32. The absolute daily dose of fluvoxamine ingested by the newborn was calculated to be 48 µg/kg/day and the relative dose was calculated to be 1.58% of the weight-adjusted maternal dose.[2] In another study of two breastfeeding women, the AUC average concentration of fluvoxamine in milk was 36 and 256 µg/L respectively.[3] The absolute infant dose was estimated at 5.4 and 38.4 µg/kg/day with a relative infant dose (% of maternal dose) of 0.8% and 1.38%. A Denver assessment on one infant indicated normal development. Fluvoxamine was not detected in the plasma of either infant (limit of detection= 2 µg/L). In a case report of a single mother receiving 25 mg three times daily, the highest milk concentration was 40 µg/L.[4] Using this data, infant would ingest approximately 6 µg/kg/day, which is 0.62% of the maternal weight-adjusted dose. Interestingly, the maternal serum concentration at 10 hours was 20 ng/mL while the infant plasma level was 9 ng/mL. Considering the clinical dose to the infant is low, this plasma level in the infant appears high. The authors suggest this may be an atypical case, or that this infant's clearance of fluvoxamine is poor. The infant showed no symptoms of adverse effects. Yoshida reported a case of a mother receiving 100 mg/day, and an infant 15 weeks postpartum.[5] In this case the concentration of fluvoxamine in maternal serum and milk was 170 µg/L and 50 µg/L respectively and a milk/plasma ratio of 0.29. The authors estimated the dose to the infant at 7.5 µg/kg/day. Developmental assessments of the infant at 4 months and 21 months suggested normal development. In a report of 2 breastfeeding women receiving 300 mg/day, Piontek was unable to detect any fluvoxamine in the plasma of two breastfed infants.[6]

In summary, the data from these all the mentioned cases suggests that only minuscule amounts of fluvoxamine are transferred to infants, that plasma levels in infants are too low to be detected, and no adverse effects have been noted.

Pregnancy Risk	C	Lactation Risk	L2
T ½	= 15.6 hours	M/P	= 1.34
Vd	=	PB	= 80%
Tmax	= 3–8 hours	Oral	= 53%
MW	= 318	pKa	= 9.4

Adult Concerns: Somnolence, insomnia, nervousness, nausea.

Pediatric Concerns: None reported several studies.

Drug Interactions: Increased toxicity may result when used with terfenadine and astemizole. Sometimes serious fatal reactions have occurred close following the use of monoamine oxidase inhibitors. Smokers have a 25% increase in the metabolism of fluvoxamine. Enhanced CNS toxicity when used with L-tryptophan. Plasma tricyclic antidepressant levels may be increased when used with fluvoxamine. Plasma levels of propranolol have been increased by five fold when used with fluvoxamine. Bradycardia has resulted when used with diltiazem. Lithium levels may be increased by fluvoxamine with possible neurotoxicity. Increased bleeding time may result when used with warfarin.

Relative Infant Dose: 0.3%–1.4%

Adult Dose: 50–300 mg daily.

Alternatives: Sertraline, paroxetine

References:
1. Wright S, Dawling S, Ashford JJ. Excretion of fluvoxamine in breast milk. Br J Clin Pharmacol 1991; 31(2): 209.
2. Hagg S, Granberg K, Carleborg L. Excretion of fluvoxamine into breast milk. Br J Clin Pharmacol 2000; 49(3): 286–288.
3. Kristensen JH, Hackett LP, Kohan R, Paech M, Ilett KF. The amount of fluvoxamine in milk is unlikely to be a cause of adverse effects in breastfed infants. J Hum Lact 2002; 18(2): 139–143.
4. Arnold LM, Suckow RF, Lichtenstein PK. Fluvoxamine concentrations in breast milk and in maternal and infant sera. J Clin Psychopharmacol 2000; 20(4): 491–493.
5. Yoshida K, Smith B, Kumar RC. Fluvoxamine in breast-milk and infant development. Br J Clin Pharmacol 1997; 44(2): 210–211.
6. Piontek CM, Wisner KL, Perel JM, Peindl KS. Serum fluvoxamine levels in breastfed infants. J Clin Psychiatry 2001; 62(2): [111]113.

FOLIC ACID   L1

Trade: Folacin, Wellcovorin

Other Trades: Bioglan Daily, Megafol, Apo-Folic, Folvite, Novo-Folacid

Category: Vitamin B_9

Folic acid is an essential vitamin. Individuals most susceptible to folic acid deficiency are pregnant women, and those receiving anticonvulsants or birth control medications. Folic acid supplementation is now strongly recommended in women prior to becoming pregnancy due to a documented reduction of spinal cord malformations. Folic acid is actively secreted into breastmilk even if mother is deficient.[1] If maternal diet is adequate, folic acid is not generally required. The infant receives all required from a normal milk supply. Cooperman determined milk folic acid content to be 15.2 ng/mL in colostrum, 16.3 ng/mL in transitional, and 33.4 ng/mL in mature milk.[2] In one study of 11 breastfeeding mothers receiving 0.8–1 mg/day of folic acid, the folic acid secreted into human milk averaged 45.6 µg/L.[3] Excessive doses (>1 mg/day) during or before pregnancy are not generally recommended. Patients on anticonvulsants often use 4 mg/day. These doses are not generally hazardous.

Pregnancy Risk	A	Lactation Risk	L1
T ½	=	M/P	=
Vd	=	PB	=
Tmax	= 30–60 minutes	Oral	= 76–93%
MW	= 441	pKa	= 4.17

Adult Concerns: Allergies, rash, nausea, anorexia, bitter taste.

Pediatric Concerns: None reported. Safe.

Drug Interactions: May increase phenytoin metabolism and reduce levels. Phenytoin, primidone, sulfasalazine, and para-aminosalicylic acid may decrease serum folate concentrations and cause deficiency. High doses of folic acid (2–4 mg/day) are recommended in young female patients consuming anticonvulsants. Oral contraceptives also impair folate metabolism producing depletion.

Relative Infant Dose:

Adult Dose: 0.4–0.8 mg daily.

Alternatives:

References:
1. Cooperman JM, Dweck HS, Newman LJ, Garbarino C, Lopez R. The folate in human milk. Am J Clin Nutr 1982; 36(4): 576–580.
2. Tamura T, Yoshimura Y, Arakawa T. Human milk folate and folate status in lactating mothers and their infants. Am J Clin Nutr 1980; 33(2): 193–197.
3. Smith AM, Picciano MF, Deering RH. Folate supplementation during lactation: maternal folate status, human milk folate content, and their relationship to infant folate status. J Pediatr Gastroenterol Nutr 1983; 2(4): 622–628.

FOLLICLE STIMULATING HORMONES   L3

Trade: Metrodin (Urofollitropin), Fertinex (Urofollitropin), FSH, Follistim (Follitropin Beta), Follitropin Alpha, Follitropin Beta, Gonal-F (Follitropin Alpha), Bravelle (Urofollitropin), Urofollitropin

Other Trades: Fertinorm HP, Metrodin

Category: FSH, follicle stimulating hormone

Follicle-stimulating hormone (FSH) is a glycoprotein gonadotropin secreted by the anterior pituitary in response to gonadotropin-releasing hormone (GnRH) from the hypothalamus.[1–3] FSH and luteinizing hormone bind to receptors in the testis and ovary and regulate gonadal function by promoting sex steroid production and gametogenesis. In the female, FSH induces growth of the graafian follicle in the ovary preparatory to the release of the ovum. Approximately 15 µg is secreted daily by the pituitary in normal individuals. Numerous forms of FSH are available and are listed below, but all work similarly. FSH is a large molecular weight peptide (34,000 daltons) and is very unlikely to enter milk or be orally bioavailable to an infant. However, it is not known if the administration of FSH, and the subsequent maternal changes in estrogen and progesterone, would alter the production of milk. It is however likely, since the onset of pregnancy is commonly followed by a decrease in milk production in most mothers.

Urofollitropin is a preparation of gonadotropin (FSH) extracted from the urine of postmenopausal women. Follitropin alpha and follitropin beta are human FSH preparations of recombinant DNA origin. Menotropins are combination products containing both FSH and luteinizing hormone (LH).

Pregnancy Risk	X	Lactation Risk	L3
T ½	= 3.9 and 70.4 hours	M/P	=
Vd	= 0.06, 1.08	PB	=
Tmax	= 6–18 hours	Oral	= None
MW	= 34,000	pKa	=

Adult Concerns: Pulmonary and vascular complications, ovarian hyperstimulation, abdominal pain, fever and chills, abdominal pain, nausea, vomiting, diarrhea, pain at injection site, bruising. Ovarian hyperstimulation.

Pediatric Concerns: None reported via milk. FSH is very unlikely to penetrate milk, and it would not be orally bioavailable. However, observe closely for reduced milk production.

Drug Interactions: Urofollitropin does not effect prolactin levels.

Relative Infant Dose:

Adult Dose: 75 units daily.

Alternatives:

References:
1. Sharma V, Riddle A, et al: Studies on folliculogenesis and in vitro fertilization outcome after the administration of follicle-stimulating hormone at different times during the menstrual cycle. Fertil Steril 1989; 51: 298–303.
2. Kjeld JM, Harsoulis P, et al: Infusions of hFSH and hLH in normal men: kinetics of human follicle stimulating hormone. Acta Endocrinologica 1976; 81: 225–233.
3. Yen SSC, Llerena LA, Pearson OH et al: Disappearance rates of endogenous follicle-stimulating hormone in serum following surgical hypophysectomy in man. J Clin Endocrinol 1970; 30: 325–329.

FONDAPARINUX SODIUM   L3

Trade: Arixtra
Other Trades: Arixtra
Category: Factor Xa inhibitor

Fondaparinux sodium is a synthetic pentasaccharide and is used for treatment and prophylaxis of deep vein thrombosis. Fondaparinux sodium causes antithrombin III-mediated inhibition of factor Xa, thus interrupting the coagulation cascade and prohibiting thrombus development.[1] As a pentasaccharide, it would neither be orally bioavailable in an infant, nor would it be likely to enter the milk compartment due to its structure. No data are available on the transmission of fondaparinux sodium to a nursing infant, but based on the kinetic profile it is highly unlikely that it would be passed to the infant.

Pregnancy Risk	B	Lactation Risk	L3
T ½	= 17–21 hours	M/P	=
Vd	= 7–11 l/kg	PB	= 94%
Tmax	= 2–3 hours	Oral	= Nil
MW	= 1728	pKa	= -2.57

Adult Concerns: Adverse reactions include bleeding, fever, nausea, and anemia.

Pediatric Concerns: No data are available, but it is neither likely to enter the milk compartment nor be orally bioavailable to the infant.

Drug Interactions: Anticoagulants, salicylates, and NSAIDs all increase the risk of bleeding when used concurrently with fondaparinux sodium.

Relative Infant Dose:

Adult Dose: 2.5–10 mg daily for 5–9 days.

Alternatives:

References:
1. Pharmaceutical manufacturer prescribing information, 2008.

FORMALDEHYDE — L4

Trade: Formaldehyde, Formalin, Methyl aldehyde
Other Trades:
Category: Preservative

Formaldehyde exposure in laboratory or embalming environments is strictly controlled by federal regulations to a permissible level of 2 ppm. At room temperature it is a colorless gas with a pungent, irritating odor detectable at 0.5 ppm. At exposure to 1–4 ppm, formaldehyde is a strong mucous membrane irritant, producing burning and lacrimation.[1] Formaldehyde is rapidly destroyed by plasma and tissue enzymes and it is very unlikely that any would enter human milk following environmental exposures. However, acute intoxications following high oral or inhaled doses could lead to significant levels of maternal plasma formic acid which could enter milk. There are no data suggesting untoward side effects in nursing infants as a result of mild to minimal environmental exposure of the mother.

Pregnancy Risk	X	Lactation Risk	L4
T ½	=	M/P	=
Vd	=	PB	=
Tmax	=	Oral	=
MW	= 30	pKa	= -4.2

Adult Concerns: Cough, mucous membrane irritation, chest pain, dyspnea, and wheezing occur in individuals exposed to 5–30 ppm.

Pediatric Concerns: None reported via milk.

Drug Interactions:

Relative Infant Dose:

Adult Dose:

Alternatives:

References:
1. Ellenhorn MJ. Medical toxicology: a primer for the medicolegal age. Clin Toxicol 1978; 13(4): 439–462.

FORMOTEROL   L3

Trade: Foradil Aerolizer, Symbicort
Other Trades:
Category: Bronchodilator

Formoterol fumarate is a long-acting selective beta-2 adrenoceptor agonist used for asthma and COPD. Following inhalation of a 120 µg dose, the maximum plasma concentration of 92 picograms/mL occurred within 5 minutes.[1] No data are available on its transfer into human milk, but the extremely low plasma levels would suggest that milk levels would be incredibly low, if even measurable. Studies of oral absorption in adults suggests that while absorption is good, plasma levels are still below detectable levels and may require large oral doses prior to attaining measurable plasma levels.[2] It is not likely the amount present in human milk would be clinically relevant to a breastfed infant.

Pregnancy Risk	C	Lactation Risk	L3
T ½	= 10 hours	M/P	=
Vd	=	PB	= 64%
Tmax	= 5 minutes	Oral	= Good
MW	= 840	pKa	=

Adult Concerns: Tremor, headache, dizziness, restlessness, palpitations, nausea, dry mouth, muscle cramps, and cough. Low serum potassium and elevated blood glucose levels can occur with high doses. Blood pressure and heart rate are minimally affected.

Pediatric Concerns: None reported via milk.

Drug Interactions: Concurrent use of xanthine derivatives, steroids, or diuretics may potentiate any hypokalemic effect. Do not use with monoamine oxidase inhibitors, tricyclic antidepressants, or drugs known to prolong QTc interval. Beta adrenergic agents may inhibit effect of formoterol.

Relative Infant Dose:

Adult Dose: 12 µg every 12 hours

Alternatives: Salmeterol, albuterol.

References:

1. Pharmaceutical manufacturer prescribing information, 2001.
2. Tattersfield AE. Long-acting beta 2-agonists. Clin Exp Allergy 1992; 22(6): 600–605.
3. Maesen FP, Smeets JJ, Gubbelmans HL, Zweers PG. Bronchodilator effect of inhaled formoterol vs salbutamol over 12 hours. Chest 1990; 97(3): 590–594.

FORMOTEROL + MOMETASONE   L3

Trade: Dulera

Other Trades:

Category: Antiasthma, anti-inflammatory/bronchodilator combination

Formoterol fumarate and Mometasone furoate is a combination of an anti-inflammatory agent with a bronchodilator. It is used via inhalation for long term control of asthma.

Formoterol is a long-acting selective beta-2 adrenoceptor agonist used for asthma and COPD. Following inhalation of a 120 µg dose, the maximum plasma concentration of 92 pg/mL occurred within 5 minutes.[1] After twice daily dosing of formoterol, 4 to 8.8 pg/mL were the steady state plasma concentrations. No data are available on its transfer into human milk, but the extremely low plasma levels would suggest that milk levels would be incredibly low, if even measurable. Studies of oral absorption in adults suggests that while absorption is good, plasma levels are still below detectable levels and may require large oral doses prior to attaining measurable plasma levels.[2,3] It is not likely the amount present in human milk would be clinically relevant to a breastfed infant.

Mometasone is a corticosteroid primarily intended for intranasal and topical use. It is considered a medium-potency steroid, similar to betamethasone and triamcinolone. It is extremely unlikely mometasone would be excreted into human milk in clinically relevant levels following topical or intranasal administration. Mometasone absolute systemic bioavailability after inhalation, given the highest dose, was 94–114 pg/mL.

Due to the low plasma concentrations and low systemic bioavailability, mometasone + formoterol should be compatible with breastfeeding.

Pregnancy Risk	C	Lactation Risk	L3
$T\frac{1}{2}$	= Formoterol/mometasone: 2.8 hours/5.8 hours	M/P	= Formoterol/mometasone: 0.5/
Vd	= Formoterol/mometasone: 4.3/ l/kg	PB	= Formoterol/mometasone: 85–90%(oral)/ 98–99%
Tmax	= Formoterol/mometasone: 32–43 min/	Oral	= Formoterol/mometasone: 0.7%/
MW	= Formoterol/mometasone: 430/427	pKa	= Formoterol/mometasone: 14.9/

Adult Concerns: Most common side effects: nasopharyngitis, sinusitis, and headache. Less common: paradoxical bronchospasm, localized infections such as *Candida albicans* of the mouth and throat. Possible side effects due to steroid content include immunosuppression, hypercorticism, adrenal suppression, decreased bone mineral density, decreased growth rate in pediatric patients, glaucoma, cataracts, hypokalemia, and hyperglycemia. Also, use caution in patients with cardiovascular disorders due to beta adrenergic effects.

Pediatric Concerns:

Drug Interactions: Concomitant administration with the following may cause increased systemic exposure to mometasone: ritonavir, atazanavir, clarithromycin, indinavir, itraconazole, nefazodone, nelfinavir, saquinavir, telithromycin. Administration of adrenergic agents such as epinephrine, dopamine should be done with caution due to possibility of additive sympathetic effects with formoterol. Potentiated hypokalemia may occur due to coadministration of formoterol with a xanthine derivative, such as aminophylline or theophylline. Potentiated hypokalemia and EKG changes are also a possibility due to concomitant use of formoterol with diuretics such as thiazides or furosemide. Use with caution with monoamine oxidase inhibitors and tricyclic antidepressants due to increased risk of cardiotoxicity. Concomitant use with beta-blockers not recommended since formoterol and beta-blockers may antagonize each other.

Relative Infant Dose:

Adult Dose: Formoterol/mometasone: 5 µg/100–200 µg, 1–2 inhalations twice daily.

Alternatives:

References:
1. Pharmaceutical manufacturer prescribing information, 2001.
2. Tattersfield AE. Long-acting beta 2-agonists. Clin Exp Allergy 1992; 22(6): 600–605.
3. Maesen FP, Smeets JJ, Gubbelmans HL, Zweers PG. Bronchodilator effect of inhaled formoterol vs salbutamol over 12 hours. Chest 1990; 97(3): 590–594.

FOSCARNET SODIUM   L4

Trade: Foscavir

Other Trades: Foscavir

Category: Antiviral for herpes, CMV infections

Foscarnet is an antiviral used to treat mucocutaneous herpes simplex manifestations and cytomegalovirus retinal infections in patients with AIDS. It is not known if foscarnet is secreted into human milk, but studies in animals indicate levels in milk were three times higher than serum levels (suggesting a milk/plasma ratio of 3.0).[1,2] Foscarnet is a potent and potentially dangerous drug that could cause significant renal toxicity, seizures, and deposition in bone and teeth. Use of this drug in breastfeeding women should be with extreme caution.

Pregnancy Risk	C	Lactation Risk	L4
T½	= 3 hours	M/P	= 3.0
Vd	=	PB	= 14–17%
Tmax	= Immediate (IV)	Oral	= 12–21%
MW	= 192	pKa	= 7.27

Adult Concerns: Fever, nausea, diarrhea, vomiting, tremor, headache, fatigue, kidney toxicity, anemia due to bone marrow suppression.

Pediatric Concerns: None reported but caution is urged.

Drug Interactions: Increased hypocalcemia with pentamidine, and increased seizures with ciprofloxacin.

Relative Infant Dose:

Adult Dose: 34–51 mg/kg injection (IV) daily.

Alternatives:

References:
1. Pharmaceutical manufacturer prescribing information, 1995.
2. Sjovall J, Karlsson A, Ogenstad S, Sandstrom E, Saarimaki M. Pharmacokinetics and absorption of foscarnet after intravenous and oral administration to patients with human immunodeficiency virus. Clin Pharmacol Ther 1988; 44(1): 65–73.

FOSFOMYCIN TROMETAMOL   L3

Trade: Monurol

Other Trades: Monuril

Category: Urinary antibiotic

Fosfomycin trometamol is a broad-spectrum antibiotic used primarily for uncomplicated urinary tract infections. It is believed safe for use in pregnancy and has been used in children less than 1 year of age. Fosfomycin absorption is largely dependent on the salt form, trometamol salts are modestly absorbed (34–58%) and calcium salts are poorly absorbed (<12%). Fosfomycin secreted into human milk would likely be in the calcium form and is unlikely to be absorbed as secreted in human milk. Foods and the acidic milieu of the stomach both significantly reduce oral absorption.[1-3] Levels secreted into human milk have been reported to be about 10% of the maternal plasma level.[4] Generally, a single 3 gm oral dose is effective treatment for many urinary tract infections in women. It is not likely that the levels present in breastmilk would produce untoward effects in a breastfeeding infant.

Pregnancy Risk	B	Lactation Risk	L3
T ½	= 4–8 hours	M/P	= 0.1
Vd	= 0.22 l/kg	PB	= <3%
Tmax	= 1.5–3 hours	Oral	= 34–58%
MW	= 138	pKa	= 7.82

Adult Concerns: Gastrointestinal symptoms include nausea, vomiting, diarrhea, epigastric discomfort, anorexia. Skin rashes and pruritus have been reported.

Pediatric Concerns: None reported via milk.

Drug Interactions: Antacids, calcium salts and foods will reduce absorption. Metoclopramide reduces serum concentration, by reducing oral bioavailability.

Relative Infant Dose:

Adult Dose: 3 gm X 1

Alternatives:

References:

1. Bergan T. Degree of absorption, pharmacokinetics of fosfomycin trometamol and duration of urinary antibacterial activity. Infection 1990; 18 Suppl 2: S65–S69.
2. Bergan T. Pharmacokinetic comparison between fosfomycin and other phosphonic acid derivatives. Chemotherapy 1990; 36 Suppl 1: 10–18.
3. Segre G, Bianchi E, Cataldi A, Zannini G. Pharmacokinetic profile of fosfomycin trometamol (Monuril). Eur Urol 1987; 13 Suppl 1: 56–63.
4. Kirby WM. Pharmacokinetics of fosfomycin. Chemotherapy 1977; 23 Suppl 1: 141–151.

FOSINOPRIL L3

Trade: Monopril

Other Trades: Monopril, Apo-Fosinopril, Jamp-Fosinopril, Mylan-Fosinopril, PMS-Fosinopril, RAN-Fosinopril, Riva-Fosinopril, Teva-Fosinopril, Staril

Category: Antihypertensive, ACE inhibitor

Fosinopril is a prodrug that is metabolized by the gut and liver upon absorption to fosinoprilat, which is an ACE inhibitor used as an antihypertensive. The manufacturer reports that the ingestion of 20 mg daily for three days resulted in barely detectable levels in human milk, although no values are provided.[1,2] Consider enalapril, benazepril, captopril as alternatives. While fosinopril is not considered incompatible with breastfeeding, the lack of data warrants caution when using this drug, particularly during the neonatal period.

Pregnancy Risk	C/D in 2nd and 3rd trimester	Lactation Risk	L3 (L4 premature)
T ½	= 11–35 hours	M/P	=
Vd	=	PB	= 95%
Tmax	= 3 hours	Oral	= 30–36%
MW	= 564	pKa	= 3.78

Adult Concerns: Anemia, dry cough, headache, dizziness, diarrhea, fatigue, nausea, vomiting, hypotension.

Pediatric Concerns: None reported via milk. Avoid using in premature infants.

Drug Interactions: Bioavailability of ACE inhibitors may be decreased when used with antacids. Capsaicin may exacerbate coughing associated with ACE inhibitor treatment. Pharmacologic effects of ACE inhibitors may be increased. Increased plasma levels of digoxin may result. Increased serum lithium levels may result when used with ACE inhibitors.

Relative Infant Dose:

Adult Dose: 20–40 mg daily.

Alternatives: Enalapril, benazepril, captopril

References:

1. Drug Facts and Comparisons 1995 ed. ed. St. Louis: 1995.
2. Pharmaceutical manufacturer prescribing information, 1995.

FOSPHENYTOIN — L2

Trade: Cerebyx

Other Trades:

Category: Anticonvulsant

Fosphenytoin is a prodrug of phenytoin. Following the parenteral injection of fosphenytoin, it is rapidly converted to the anticonvulsant phenytoin with a brief half-life of 15 minutes.[1] Thus, the active drug is phenytoin.

Phenytoin is an old and efficient anticonvulsant. It is secreted in small amounts into breastmilk. The effect on infant is generally considered minimal if the levels in the maternal circulation are kept in low-normal range (10 µg/mL). Phenytoin levels peak in milk at 3.5 hours. In one study of 6 women receiving 200–400 mg/day, plasma concentrations varied from 12.8 to 78.5 µmol/L, while their milk levels ranged from 1.61 to 2.95 mg/L.[2] The milk/plasma ratios were low, ranging from 0.06 to 0.18. In only two of these infants were plasma concentrations of phenytoin detectable (0.46 and 0.72 µmol/L). No untoward effects were noted in any of these infants. Others have reported milk levels of 6 µg/mL[3], or 0.8 µg/mL.[4] Although the actual concentration in milk varies significantly between studies, the milk/plasma ratio appears relatively similar at 0.13 to 0.45. Breastmilk concentrations varied from 0.26 to 1.5 mg/L depending on the maternal dose. In a mother receiving 250 mg twice daily, milk levels were 0.26 and the milk/plasma ratio was 0.45.[5] The maternal plasma level was phenytoin was 0.58. In another study of two patients receiving 300–600 mg/d, the average milk level was 1.9 mg/L.[6] The maximum observed milk level was 2.6 mg/L. The neonatal half-life of phenytoin is highly variable for the first week of life. Monitoring of the infants' plasma may be useful although it is not definitely required. All of the current studies indicate rather low levels of phenytoin in breastmilk and minimal plasma levels in breastfeeding infants.

Pregnancy Risk	D	Lactation Risk	L2
T ½	= 15 minutes	M/P	=
Vd	= 4–10.8 l/kg	PB	= 99%
Tmax	= 0.5 hour	Oral	=
MW	= 406	pKa	= 6.06

Adult Concerns: Side effects include headache, nausea, ecchymosis, nystagmus, tremor, etc.

Pediatric Concerns: Only one case of methemoglobinemia, drowsiness, and poor sucking has been reported with phenytoin. Most other studies suggest no problems.

Drug Interactions: Concomitant administration with following causes increased plasma drug levels of phenytoin: acute alcohol intake, amiodarone, chloramphenicol, chlordiazepoxide, cimetidine, diazepam, dicumarol, disulfiram, estrogens, ethosuximide, fluoxetine, histamine-2 receptor antagonists, halothane, isoniazid, methylphenidate, phenothiazines, phenylbutazone, salicylates, succinimides, sulfonamides, tolbutamide, trazodone. Co-administration with the following decreases plasma levels and efficacy of fosphenytoin: carbamazepine, chronic alcohol abuse, reserpine. Caution advised while co-administering with the following: phenobarbital, valproic acid, and sodium valproate. Decreased seizure threshold expected during concomitant use with tricyclic antidepressants. Concomitant administration of fosphenytoin with the following drugs may cause decreased efficacy of the following co-administered drugs: anticoagulants, corticosteroids, coumarin, digitoxin, doxycycline, estrogens, furosemide, oral contraceptives, rifampin, quinidine, theophylline, vitamin D.

Relative Infant Dose:

Adult Dose: 4–6 mg phenytoin equivalents/kg/day

Alternatives: Phenytoin

References:

1. Pharmaceutical manufacturer prescribing information, 2003.
2. Steen B, Rane A, Lonnerholm G, Falk O, Elwin CE, Sjoqvist F. Phenytoin excretion in human breast milk and plasma levels in nursed infants. Ther Drug Monit 1982; 4(4): 331–334.
3. Svensmark O, Schiller PJ, Buchthal F. 5, 5–Diphenylhydantion (dilantin) blood levels after oral or intravenous dosage in man. Acta Pharmacol Toxicol (Copenh) 1960; 16: 331–346.
4. Kaneko S, Sato T, Suzuki K. The levels of anticonvulsants in breast milk. Br J Clin Pharmacol 1979; 7(6): 624–627.
5. Rane A, Garle M, Borga O, Sjoqvist F. Plasma disappearance of transplacentally transferred diphenylhydantoin in the newborn studied by mass fragmentography. Clin Pharmacol Ther 1974; 15(1): 39–45.
6. Mirkin BL. Diphenylhydantoin: placental transport, fetal localization, neonatal metabolism, and possible teratogenic effects. J Pediatr 1971; 78(2): 329–337.

FROVATRIPTAN SUCCINATE   L3

Trade: Frova

Other Trades:

Category: Anti-migraine, 5–HT1B/1D receptor agonist

Frovatriptan is typical tryptan believed to act on intracranial arteries to prevent excessive dilation of these vessels commonly found in migraine attacks.[1] It is from the same family as sumatriptan. No data on its transfer to milk are available. Some studies suggest sumatriptan may be more effective. Sumatriptan is recommended as we have good data suggesting milk levels of sumatriptan are low and its oral bioavailability is low.

Pregnancy Risk	C	Lactation Risk	L3
T ½	= 26 hours	M/P	=
Vd	= 4.2 l/kg	PB	= 15%
Tmax	= 2–4 hours	Oral	= 30%
MW	= 379	pKa	= 10.6

Adult Concerns: May increase coronary vasoconstriction, use cautiously in patients with coronary artery disease. Events reported have included coronary artery vasospasm, transient myocardial ischemia, myocardial infarction, ventricular tachycardia and ventricular fibrillation. Commonly reported complaints include: dizziness, headache, paresthesia. Gastrointestinal symptoms include: dry mouth, dyspepsia. Fatigue, hot and cold sensations, skeletal pain, and flushing have been reported.

Pediatric Concerns: None reported via milk.

Drug Interactions: Levels of frovatriptan may increase 30% in subjects taking oral contraceptives. Frovatriptan levels may be significantly reduced (25%) by concomitant use of ergotamine. Propranolol may increase plasma levels of frovatriptan by 16–23% and half-life as well.

Relative Infant Dose:

Adult Dose: 2.5 mg initially followed by one after 2 hours if no response.

Alternatives: Sumatriptan

References:
1. Pharmaceutical manufacturer prescribing information, 2003.

FURAZOLIDONE   L2

Trade: Furoxone

Other Trades: Furoxone

Category: Gastrointestinal antibiotic

Furazolidone belongs to the nitrofurantoin family of antibiotics. It has a broad-spectrum of activity against gram-positive and gram-negative enteric organisms including cholera but is generally used for giardiasis.[1] Following an oral dose, furazolidone is poorly absorbed (<5%) and is largely inactivated in the gut. Concentrations transferred to milk are unreported, but the total amounts would be exceedingly low due to the low maternal plasma levels attained by this product. Due to poor oral absorption, systemic absorption in a breastfeeding infant would likely be minimal. Caution should be observed in early postpartum newborns due to increased risk of hyperbilirubinemia.

Pregnancy Risk	C	Lactation Risk		L2 (L4 early postpartum)
T ½	=	M/P	=	
Vd	=	PB	=	
Tmax	=	Oral	= <5%	
MW	= 225	pKa	=	

Adult Concerns: Hemolytic anemia in newborns, nausea, vomiting, diarrhea, abdominal pain. Dark yellow to brown discoloration of urine.

Pediatric Concerns: Caution is urged in neonates <1 month due to possibility of hemolytic anemia.

Drug Interactions: Increased effect when used with sympathomimetic amines, tricyclic antidepressants, monoamine oxidase inhibitors, meperidine, dextromethorphan, fluoxetine, paroxetine, sertraline, trazodone.

Relative Infant Dose:

Adult Dose: 100 mg four times daily.

Alternatives:

References:
1. Pharmaceutical manufacturer prescribing information, 2003.

FUROSEMIDE   L3

Trade: Lasix

Other Trades: Frusemide, Uremide, Apo-Furosemide, Novo-Semide, Lasix, Frusid

Category: Loop diuretic

Furosemide is a potent loop diuretic with a rather short duration of action. Furosemide has been found in breastmilk although the levels are unreported. Diuretics, by reducing blood volume, could potentially reduce breastmilk production although this is largely theoretical.[1] Furosemide is frequently used in neonates in pediatric units, so pediatric use is common. The oral bioavailability of furosemide in newborns is exceedingly poor and very high oral doses are required (1–4 mg/kg BID).[2] It is very unlikely the amount transferred into human milk would produce any effects in a nursing infant although its maternal use could suppress lactation.

Pregnancy Risk	C	Lactation Risk	L3
T ½	= 92 minutes	M/P	=
Vd	=	PB	= >98%
Tmax	= 1–2 hours	Oral	= 60–70%
MW	= 331	pKa	= 9.83

Adult Concerns: Hypotension, fluid loss, potassium loss.

Pediatric Concerns: None reported via milk.

Drug Interactions: Furosemide interferes with hypoglycemic effect of antidiabetic agents. NSAIDS may reduce diuretic effect of furosemide. Effects of antihypertensive agents may be increased. Renal clearance of lithium is decreased. Increases ototoxicity of aminoglycosides.

Relative Infant Dose:

Adult Dose: 40–80 mg twice daily.

Alternatives:

References:
1. Healy M. Suppressing lactation with oral diuretics. The Lancet 1961; 1353–1354.
2. Pharmaceutical manufacturer prescribing information, 1995.

GABAPENTIN | L2

Trade: Neurontin
Other Trades: Neurontin
Category: Anticonvulsant

Gabapentin is an older anticonvulsant used primarily for partial (focal) seizures with or without secondary generalization. It is also used for postherpetic neuralgia or neuropathic pain. Unlike many anticonvulsants, gabapentin is almost completely excreted renally without metabolism, it does not induce hepatic enzymes and is remarkably well tolerated.[1,2,3]

In a study of one breastfeeding mother who was receiving 1800 mg/day, milk levels were 11.1, 11.3, and 11.0 mg/L at 2, 4, and 8 hours respectively, following a dose of 600 mg. The milk/plasma ratio was calculated to be 0.86 and the relative infant dose was 2.34%. No adverse effects to gabapentin were noted in the infant.[4,5] In another patient receiving 2400 mg/day milk levels were 9.8, 9.0, and 7.2 mg/L at 2,4, and 8 hours respectively, after a dose of 800 mg. Using this data an infant would consume approximately 3.7% to 6.5% of the weight-adjusted maternal dose per day. No adverse events were noted in these two infants. In another study of 5 mother-infant pairs receiving 900–3200 mg gabapentin per day, the mean milk/plasma ratio ranged from 0.7 to 1.3 from 2 weeks to 3 months postpartum.[6] At 2–3 weeks, two of the five infants had detectable concentrations of gabapentin (1.3 and 1.5 µM) and one was undetectable. These levels were far below the normal plasma levels in the mothers (11–45 µM). Assuming a daily milk intake of 150 mL/day/kg, the infant dose of gabapentin was estimated to be 0.2–1.3 mg/kg/day, which is equivalent to 1.3–3.8% of the weight-normalized dose received by the mother. The plasma levels of gabapentin collected after 3 months of breastfeeding in another infant was 1.9 µM. The authors concluded that the plasma levels measured were low if at all detectable in the infants, and no adverse effects were reported in these infants.

In summary, published data reveals that the infant plasma levels following lactational exposure to gabapentin are probably too low to cause untoward effects in the breastfed infant.

Pregnancy Risk	C	Lactation Risk	L2
T ½	= 5–7 hours	M/P	= 0.7–1.3
Vd	= 0.8 l/kg	PB	= <3%
Tmax	= 1–3 hours	Oral	= 50–60%
MW	=	pKa	= 3.68, 10.70

Adult Concerns: Dizziness, somnolence, weight gain, vomiting, tremor, and CNS depression. Abrupt withdrawal may induce severe seizures.

Pediatric Concerns: None reported. Cleared for children >12 years.

Drug Interactions: Antacids reduce gabapentin absorption by 20%. Cimetidine may decrease clearance of gabapentin. No interaction has been reported with other anticonvulsants. Antacids may reduce oral absorption by 20%.

Relative Infant Dose: 6.6%

Adult Dose: 300–600 mg three times daily.

Alternatives:

References:
1. Goa KL, Sorkin EM. Gabapentin. A review of its pharmacological properties and clinical potential in epilepsy. Drugs 1993; 46(3): 409–427.
2. Ramsay RE. Clinical efficacy and safety of gabapentin. Neurology 1994; 44(6 Suppl 5): S23–S30.
3. Dichter MA, Brodie MJ. New antiepileptic drugs. N Engl J Med 1996; 334(24): 1583–1590.
4. Hale TW, Ilett KF, Hackett P. Personal communication. 2002.
5. Kristensen JH, Ilett KF, Hackett LP, Kohan R. Gabapentin and Breastfeeding: A Case Report. J Hum Lact 2006; 22(4): 426–428.
6. Ohman I, Vitols S, Tomson T. Pharmacokinetics of gabapentin during delivery, in the neonatal period, and lactation: does a fetal accumulation occur during pregnancy? Epilepsia 2005 Oct; 46(10): 1621–4.

GADOBENATE   L3

Trade: MultiHance
Other Trades:
Category: Radiological Contrast Agent

Gadobenate is a gadolinium-containing radiocontrast agent used in MRIs. Although free gadolinium is neurotoxic, it is safe when bound to the parent molecule in the contrast medium. There have been no studies on its transfer into human milk, but it is unlikely that it would accumulate in therapeutic levels.[1] The American College of Radiology concludes that it is safe for a mother-infant dyad to continue breastfeeding after the administration of a gadolinium-containing contrast medium.[2] In another review, only tiny amounts of gadolinium contrast agents reach the milk compartment and virtually none of this is absorbed orally by the infant.[3]

Pregnancy Risk	C	Lactation Risk	L3
T ½	= 1.17–2.02 hours	M/P	=
Vd	=	PB	= Low
Tmax	=	Oral	= Poor
MW	= 1058.15	pKa	= 2.39

Adult Concerns: Dizziness, nausea, vomiting, headache, taste alteration, dry mouth.

Pediatric Concerns: None reported via breast milk.

Drug Interactions: Gadobenate may compete with other drugs that use the canalicular multispecific organic anion transporter (MOAT). The coadministration of gadobenate with such drugs causes prolonged exposure to the coadministered drug. Therefore, avoid use with the following drugs: cisplatin, antracyclines (doxorubicin, daunorubicin), vinca alkaloids (vincristine, vinblastine), methotrexate, etoposide, tamoxifen, and paclitaxel. Special caution to be exercised in those with Dubin Johnson syndrome who have decreased MOAT activity.

Relative Infant Dose:

Adult Dose:

Alternatives:

References:
1. Pharmaceutical manufacturer prescribing information, 2007.
2. ACR Committee on Drugs and Contrast Media. Administration of contrast medium to breastfeeding mothers. 2004; 42–43.
3. Webb JA, Thomsen HS, Morcos SK; Members of Contrast Media Safety Committee of European Society of Urogenital Radiology (ESUR). The use of iodinated and gadolinium contrast media during pregnancy and lactation. Eur Radiol. 2005 Jun; 15(6): 1234–40. Epub 2004 Dec 18.

GADODIAMIDE   L3

Trade: Omniscan

Other Trades:

Category: Radiological Contrast Agent

Gadodiamide is a gadolinium-containing nonionic, non-iodinated water soluble contrast medium commonly used in Magnetic Resonance Imaging (MRI) scans.[1] It is quite similar to Magnevist, another gadolinium-containing agent. These agents penetrate peripheral compartments poorly, especially the brain. As such, they are extremely unlikely to enter milk as well.

Data for gadopentetate (Magnevist) support this, as its transfer into milk is negligible (<0.04%). Neither of these compounds is well absorbed orally, and neither is metabolized to any degree. It is likely that gadodiamide will penetrate milk only minimally.

The American College of Radiology concludes that it is safe for a mother-infant dyad to continue breastfeeding after the administration of a gadolinium-containing contrast medium. In another review, only tiny amounts of gadolinium contrast agents reach the milk compartment and virtually none of this is absorbed orally by the infant.[2]

Pregnancy Risk	C	Lactation Risk	L3
T ½	= 77 minutes	M/P	=
Vd	=	PB	=
Tmax	=	Oral	= Nil
MW	= 591.67	pKa	= 2.77

Adult Concerns: Nausea, headache, dizziness, fatigue, abdominal pain, diarrhea, hot flashes, myocardial infraction, nephrogenic systemic fibrosis.

Pediatric Concerns:

Drug Interactions: None reported.

Relative Infant Dose:

Adult Dose:

Alternatives:

References:
1. Pharmaceutical manufacturer prescribing information, 2007.
2. Webb JA, Thomsen HS, Morcos SK; Members of Contrast Media Safety Committee of European Society of Urogenital Radiology (ESUR). The use of iodinated andgadolinium contrast media during pregnancy and lactation. Eur Radiol. 2005 Jun; 15(6): 1234–40. Epub 2004 Dec 18.

GADOPENTETATE DIMEGLUMINE   L2

Trade: Gadolinium, Magnevist, Magnograf, Magnevistan, Viewgam

Other Trades:

Category: Contrast agent

Gadopentetate is a radiopaque agent used in magnetic resonance imaging of the kidney. It is non-ionic, non-iodinated, has low osmolarity and contains a gadolinium ion as the radiopaque entity. Following a dose of 7 mmol (6.5 gm), the amount of gadopentetate secreted in breastmilk was 3.09, 2.8, 1.08, and 0.5 and μmol/L at 2, 11, 17, and 24 hours respectively.[1] The cumulative amount excreted from both breasts in 24 hours was only 0.023% of the administered dose. Oral absorption is minimal, only 0.8% of gadopentetate is absorbed. These authors suggest that only 0.013 micromole of a gadolinium-containing compound would be absorbed by the infant in 24 hours, which is incredibly low. They further suggest that 24 hours of pumping would eliminate risks, although this seems rather extreme in view of the short (1.6 hours) half-life, poor oral bioavailability, and limited milk levels.

In another study of 19 lactating women who received 0.1 mmol/kg and one additional woman who received 0.2 mmol/kg, the cumulative amount of gadolinium excreted in breastmilk during 24 hours was 0.57 and μmol.[2] This resulted in an excreted dose of <0.04% of the IV administered maternal dose. A similar amount was noted in the patient receiving a double dose (0.2 mmol/kg). As a result, for any neonate weighing more than 1000 gm, the maximal orally ingested dose would be less than 1% of the permitted intravenous dose of 0.2 mmol/kg. According to the authors, "...that the very small amount of gadopentetate dimeglumine transferred to a nursing infant does not warrant a potentially traumatic 24-hour suspension of breastfeeding for lactating women." The American College of Radiology concludes that it is safe for a mother-infant dyad to continue breastfeeding after the administration of a gadolinium-containing contrast medium. In another review, only miniscule amounts of gadolinium contrast agents reach the milk compartment and virtually none of this is absorbed orally by the infant.[3]

Pregnancy Risk	C	Lactation Risk	L2
T ½	= 1.5–1.7 hours	M/P	=
Vd	=	PB	=
Tmax	=	Oral	= 0.8%
MW	=	pKa	=

Adult Concerns: Headache, dizziness, nausea, vomiting, pain at injection site, hypersensitivity.

Pediatric Concerns: None reported in three studies.

Drug Interactions: None reported.

Relative Infant Dose: 0.02%–0.04%

Adult Dose:

Alternatives:

References:
1. Rofsky NM, Weinreb JC, Litt AW. Quantitative analysis of gadopentetate dimeglumine excreted in breast milk. J Magn Reson Imaging 1993; 3(1): 131–132.
2. Kubik-Huch RA, Gottstein-Aalame NM, Frenzel T, Seifert B, Puchert E, Wittek S, Debatin JF. Gadopentetate dimeglumine excretion into human breast milk during lactation. Radiology 2000; 216(2): 555–558.
3. Webb JA, Thomsen HS, Morcos SK; Members of Contrast Media Safety Committee of European Society of Urogenital Radiology (ESUR). The use of iodinated andgadolinium contrast media during pregnancy and lactation. Eur Radiol. 2005 Jun; 15(6): 1234–40. Epub 2004 Dec 18.

GADOTERIDOL   L3

Trade: Prohance

Other Trades:

Category: Radiological Contrast Agent

Gadoteridol is a non-ionic, non-iodinated gadolinium chelate complex used as a radiocontrast agent in MRI scans. The metabolism of gadoteridol is unknown, but a similar gadolinium salt (gadopentetate) is not metabolized at all. The half-life is brief (1.6 hours), and the volume of distribution is very small. This suggests that gadoteridol does not penetrate tissues well and is unlikely to penetrate milk in significant quantities. A similar compound, gadopentetate, is barely detectable in breastmilk. Although not reported, the oral bioavailability is probably similar to gadopentetate, which is minimal to none. No data are available on the transfer of gadoteridol into human milk, although it is probably minimal.[1] The American College of Radiology concludes that it is safe for a mother-infant dyad to continue breastfeeding after the administration of a gadolinium-containing contrast medium. In another review, only tiny amounts of gadolinium contrast agents reach the milk compartment and virtually none of this is absorbed orally by the infant.[2]

Pregnancy Risk	C	Lactation Risk	L3
T ½	= 1.57 hours	M/P	=
Vd	=	PB	=
Tmax	=	Oral	= Poor
MW	=	pKa	=

Adult Concerns: Hypersensitivity, nausea, urticaria, taste alteration, rash, abdominal cramp, nephrogenic systemic fibrosis.

Pediatric Concerns:

Drug Interactions: None reported.

Relative Infant Dose:

Adult Dose:

Alternatives:

References:
1. Pharmaceutical manufacturer prescribing information, 2007.
2. Webb JA, Thomsen HS, Morcos SK; Members of Contrast Media Safety Committee of European Society of Urogenital Radiology (ESUR). The use of iodinated andgadolinium contrast media during pregnancy and lactation. Eur Radiol. 2005 Jun; 15(6): 1234–40. Epub 2004 Dec 18.

GADOVERSETAMIDE   L3

Trade: Optimark

Other Trades:

Category: Magnetic Resonance Imaging Agent

Gadoversetamide is a paramagnetic agent used as a contrast agent in magnetic resonance imaging (MRI). It does not enter most compartments and is confined to extracellular water with a low volume of distribution.[1] As with gadopentetate, this agent is very unlikely to penetrate milk or be orally bioavailable. However, no human data are available. Rat studies show some penetration of gadoversetamide into rat milk but rodent lactation studies do not correlate with humans. The American College of Radiology concludes that it is safe for a mother-infant dyad to continue breastfeeding after the administration of a gadolinium-containing contrast medium. In another review, only tiny amounts of gadolinium contrast agents reach the milk compartment and virtually none of this is absorbed orally by the infant.[2]

Pregnancy Risk	C	Lactation Risk	L3
T ½	= 1.7 hours	M/P	=
Vd	= 162 l/kg	PB	=
Tmax	=	Oral	= Nil
MW	= 661	pKa	=

Adult Concerns: Headache, vasodilatation, taste perversion, dizziness, nausea, and paresthesia are most commonly observed.

Pediatric Concerns:

Drug Interactions: Concurrent medications or parenteral nutrition should not be physically mixed with contrast agent and should not be administered in the same intravenous line because of the potential for chemical incompatibility.

Relative Infant Dose:

Adult Dose:

Alternatives:

References:
1. Pharmaceutical manufacturer prescribing information, 2003.
2. Webb JA, Thomsen HS, Morcos SK; Members of Contrast Media Safety Committee of European Society of Urogenital Radiology (ESUR). The use of iodinated andgadolinium contrast media during pregnancy and lactation. Eur Radiol. 2005 Jun; 15(6): 1234–40. Epub 2004 Dec 18.

GALLIUM-67 CITRATE   L4

Trade: Galliuim-67 Citrate

Other Trades:

Category: Radioactive isotope

Gallium-67 Citrate is a radioactive substance used for bone scanning. In one breastfeeding mother who received 3 mCi, the radioactive content in breastmilk was 0.15, 0.045, and 0.01 μCi/mL at 3, 7, and 14 days respectively.[1] If the infant ingested milk, the whole body exposure would have been very significant, 1.4–2.0 rad/mCi. This is significantly more than the mother's exposure of only 0.26 rad/mCi. Therefore, a significant radioactive hazard exists. Whole body scans showed intense radiation in the breast tissue of the mother. With a 14 day waiting period, the theoretical whole body dose to the infant would be 0.04 rads and 0.07 rads to the skeleton. Radioactive half-life of ^{67}Ga is 78.3 hours, while the biological half-life of the gallium ion is 9 days.

These approximations suggest that breastfeeding should be interrupted for a minimum of 1 week following a dose of 0.2 mCi, 2 weeks for 1.3 mCi, or 1 month for 4 mCi. International Commission of Radiological Protection (ICRP) recommends breastfeeding interruption of >3 weeks or cessation.[2] In one case, administration of 4.73 mCi of ^{67}Ga Citrate required 15.8 days interruption to reduce radiation exposure from breastmilk to less than 1 mSv.[3] Mountford calculated that dose of 5 mCi would probably produce radiation exposure of 1 mSv from close contact.[4] Limiting close contact to 35 minutes per hour up to a maximum 9 hours of exposure time per day for a dose of up to 2.5 mCi would reduce close contact radiation.

Recommendations: 1 month interruption for 4 mCi or more; 2 weeks interruption for 1.3 mCi; 1 week interruption for 0.2 mCi. With doses of 2.5–5.1 mCi: Avoid total contact for at least the first 4 hours. Limit close contact to 35 min every 3 hours thereafter. Estimated exposure is < 1 mSv over a month.

Pregnancy Risk	C	Lactation Risk	L4
T ½	= 78.3 hours	M/P	=
Vd	=	PB	=
Tmax	=	Oral	=
MW	=	pKa	=

Adult Concerns: Radiation hazard.

Pediatric Concerns: Significant radiation exposure. Remove from breast for 14 days.

Drug Interactions: None reported.

Relative Infant Dose:

Adult Dose: 200 mg/sq. meter IV daily

Alternatives:

References:
1. Tobin RE, Schneider PB. Uptake of ^{67}Ga in the lactating breast and its persistence in milk: case report. J Nucl Med 1976; 17(12): 1055–1056.
2. ICRP, 2008. Radiation Dose to Patients from Radiopharmaceuticals–Addendum 3 to ICRP Publication 53. ICRP Publication 106. Ann. ICRP 38 (1–2).
3. Rubow S, Klopper J, Scholtz P. Excretion of gallium 67 in human breast milk and its inadvertent ingestion by a 9-month-old child. Eur J Nucl Med. 1991; 18(10): 829–33.
4. Mountford PJ, O'Doherty MJ, Forge NI, Jeffries A, Coakley AJ. Radiation dose rates from adult patients undergoing nuclear medicine investigations. Nucl Med Commun. 1991 Sep; 12(9): 767–77.

GAMMA HYDROXYBUTYRIC ACID | L5

Trade: GBH, Gamma-OH, Somsanit, Oxybutyrate, GHB, Liquid Ecstasy

Other Trades:

Category: Illicit sedative, hallucinogen, growth stimulant

Gamma hydroxybutyrate (GHB) is a powerful, rapidly acting central nervous system depressant. GHB is indicated for the treatment of cataplexy in patients with narcolepsy, and in other countries, is sometimes used an anesthetic-hypnotic agent for general anesthesia. A natural component in the body, its function remains unknown. It is presently banned in the USA and many other countries. It is used for its ability to produce euphoric and hallucinogenic state, and for its alleged ability to release growth hormone that stimulates muscle growth. Ingestion leads to loss of muscle tone, relaxation, bradycardia to tachycardia, slowed respiration, and loss of inhibitions. Other side effects include delusions, depression, vomiting, nausea, hallucinations, seizures, delirium, agitation, amnesia, and coma. It is commonly used as a date-rape drug.[1]

It has a rather brief half-life (20–60 minutes) and <5% remains in the plasma compartment following 10 hours, and virtually none is detected in the urine after 12 hours. While these levels would depend on the dose, if the patient has returned to normal, milk levels after 12 hours would probably be low to undetectable. Although we do not have milk levels reported, but they would probably be significant during peak exposure. In patients that have dosed repeatedly for hours, a 24 hour pump and discard would be advisable. This product is strongly additive with alcohol as it is metabolized by alcohol dehydrogenase. This is a dangerous product that should never be used in breastfeeding mothers. Mothers exposed to this agent should pump and discard their milk for a minimum of 12–24 hours depending on the dose before returning the infant to the breast.

Pregnancy Risk	B	Lactation Risk	L5
T ½	= 20–60 minutes	M/P	=
Vd	= 0.4 l/kg	PB	=
Tmax	= 45 minutes	Oral	= Good
MW	= 126	pKa	= 15.98

Adult Concerns: Ingestion leads to loss of muscle tone, relaxation, bradycardia to tachycardia, slowed respiration, and loss of inhibitions. Other side effects include delusions, depression, vomiting, nausea, hallucinations, seizures, delirium, agitation, amnesia and coma.

Pediatric Concerns: No reported levels in milk, but due to its chemistry, it is likely to enter the milk compartment. Dangerous to infants.

Drug Interactions: Additive with alcohol.

Relative Infant Dose:

Adult Dose: 100 mg/kg

Alternatives:

References:
1. Baselt RC. Disposition of toxic drugs and chemicals in man. 6th ed. Foster City, CA: Chemical Toxicology Institute; 2002: 472–5.

GANCICLOVIR   L3

Trade: Zirgan, Cytovene, Valcyte, Vitracert
Other Trades:
Category: Antiviral agent

Ganciclovir is a guanosine derivative that, upon phosphorylation, inhibits DNA replication by herpes simplex viruses (HSV). It is provided as an ophthalmic gel, insert, oral tablet, or intravenous liquid. Ganciclovir ophthalmic gel is indicated for the treatment of acute herpetic keratitis (dendritic ulcers). The estimated maximum daily dose of ganciclovir administered as 1 drop, 5 times per day is 0.375 mg. Compared to maintenance doses of systemically administered ganciclovir of 900 mg (oral valganciclovir) and 5 mg/kg (IV ganciclovir), the ophthalmically administered daily dose is approximately 0.04% and 0.1% of the oral dose and IV doses, respectively, thus minimal systemic exposure is expected. It is not known whether topical ophthalmic ganciclovir administration would result in sufficient systemic absorption to produce detectable quantities in breast milk, but it is unlikely. Be aware that the oral and intravenous doses may produce much higher plasma and maternal milk levels than the ophthalmic product. Caution should be exercised when oral or intravenous products are administered to nursing or pregnant mothers.[1]

Pregnancy Risk	C	Lactation Risk	L3
T ½	= 4.8 hours	M/P	=
Vd	= 0.703 l/kg	PB	= 1–2%
Tmax	= 1.8 hours	Oral	= 60%
MW	= 255.23	pKa	=

Adult Concerns: Pain, redness, itching or inflammation. Diarrhea, nausea, vomiting. Neutropenia, anemia.

Pediatric Concerns: Maternal dose via eye drops is too low to affect infant.

Drug Interactions: Major anemia and neutropenia when used with zidovudine.

Seizures have been reported following use with imipenem. Neuropathy, diarrhea and pancreatitis have been reported when used with didanosine. Higher plasma levels of tenofovir and ganciclovir when they are used together. Increased plasma levels of ganciclovir when used with probenecid.

Relative Infant Dose:

Adult Dose: 900 mg orally once or twice daily.

Alternatives:

References:
1.   Pharmaceutical Manufacturing Prescribing Information. 2011.

GANIRELIX ACETATE   L3

Trade: Antagon (ganirelix), Cetrotide (cetrorelix), Cetrorelix
Other Trades:
Category: Synthetic gonotrophic-releasing hormone antagonist.

Ganirelix is a luteinizing hormone releasing hormone antagonist (LHRH antagonist) use in management of female infertility. Ganirelix acts by competitively inducing a rapid, reversible suppression of gonadotropin secretion.[1] This subsequently inhibits release of luteinizing hormone. The mid-cycle LH surge initiates several physiologic actions including ovulation, resumption of meiosis in the oocyte, and luteinization. This product is used to prevent the premature LH surge found in some infertile women. No data are available on the transfer of this decapeptide into human milk but it is unlikely due to its peptide structure and its larger molecular weight. In addition, it is very unlikely this decapeptide would be stable in the infants' gastrointestinal tract or orally bioavailable.

Cetrorelix acetate is also an LHRH antagonist similar in action to ganirelix.

Pregnancy Risk	X	Lactation Risk	L3
T ½	= 16.2 hours	M/P	=
Vd	= 0.62 l/kg	PB	= 82
Tmax	= 1.1 hours	Oral	= Nil
MW	= 1570	pKa	= 4.2, 9.8

Adult Concerns: Adverse events include abdominal pain, fetal death, headache, ovarian hyperstimulation syndrome, and vaginal bleeding.

Pediatric Concerns: None reported via milk, but no studies are available.

Drug Interactions:

Relative Infant Dose:

Adult Dose: 250 µg subcutaneously daily.

Alternatives:

References:
1.   Pharmaceutical manufacturer prescribing information, 2003.

GARLIC   L3

Trade:

Other Trades:

Category: Herbal antioxidant

Garlic contains a number of sulfur-containing compounds that, when ground, are metabolized to allicin, which is responsible for the pungent odor of garlic and the pharmacologic effects attributed to garlic.[1,2] Garlic has been reported to increase the levels of important plasma antioxidants, glutathione and catalase, probably due to the allicin content. Five sulfur containing compounds have been isolated that produce profound inhibition of lipid peroxidation in liver cells. A number of studies have found hypolipidemic effects of garlic oil, reducing plasma cholesterol, triglyceride levels, and elevating HDL levels significantly. Garlic oil also inhibits platelet aggregation, thus reducing risk of thrombosis. Taken together, there is significant evidence to suggest that garlic oil may reduce the risks of cardiovascular disease, reducing plasma lipids and reducing the risk of clot formation. Garlic is known to be modestly antimicrobial, having about 1% of the antimicrobial potency of penicillin. Interestingly, the hypolipidemic and antimicrobial properties appear to reside in the odorous constituents and may not be present in the deodorized oils. Although garlic oil is commonly used, the safety for long term use is still unresolved. The extract has caused a reduction in liver and kidney protein in animal studies and a potential interaction with other anticoagulants (warfarin) should be expected. Transfer of the odorous components in human milk has been documented.[3,4]

Pregnancy Risk	C		Lactation Risk	L3
T ½	=		M/P	=
Vd	=		PB	=
Tmax	=		Oral	=
MW	=		pKa	=

Adult Concerns: Few reported, but observe for excessive bleeding.

Pediatric Concerns: No studies available.

Drug Interactions: May enhance anticoagulant effects of warfarin.

Relative Infant Dose:

Adult Dose:

Alternatives:

References:
1. Bissett NG. In: Herbal Drugs and Phytopharmaceuticals. Medpharm Scientific Publishers, CRC Press, Boca Raton, 1994.
2. Review of Natural Products Facts and Comparisons, St Louis, MO 1996.
3. Mennella JA, Beauchamp GK. Maternal diet alters the sensory qualities of human milk and the nursling's behavior. Pediatrics 1991; 88(4): 737–744.
4. Mennella JA, Beauchamp GK. The effects of repeated exposure to garlic-flavored milk on the nursling's behavior. Pediatr Res 1993; 34(6): 805–808.

GATIFLOXACIN   L3

Trade: Tequin, Zymar, Zymaxid
Other Trades:
Category: Fluoroquinolone anti-injective antibiotic

Gatifloxacin is a fluoroquinolone antibiotic similar to ofloxacin, levofloxacin, and ciprofloxacin. As such, its use in pediatric age patients is not generally recommended although newer data suggest this family is safe in pediatric patients. While the manufacturer reports that gatifloxacin is secreted into animal milk, no data are available on humans. Of the numerous fluoroquinolone antibiotics, ofloxacin[1] and levofloxacin are probably preferred in breastfeeding patients due to lower milk levels. The only major risk to an infant is a change in gut flora and the possibility of overgrowth of C. Difficile (pseudomembranous colitis). If used, observe for bloody diarrhea.

Gatifloxacin ophthalmic solution: No data on its transfer into human milk is available, but the maximum plasma levels reported in one set of users was only 2.7 ng/mL. The mean C_{max} and estimated daily exposure values were 1600 and 1000 times lower than the C_{max} and AUC reported after therapeutic 400 mg oral does of moxifloxacin.[1] Thus ophthalmic exposure is extremely unlikely to produce clinically relevant levels in milk. Following the administration of a gatifloxacin ophthalmic solution (0.3% or 0.5%) to one eye of 6 healthy male subjects each in an escalated dosing regimen starting with a single 2 drop dose, then 2 drops 4 times daily for 7 days and finally 2 drops 8 times daily for 3 days, serum gatifloxacin levels were below the lower limit of quantification (5 ng/mL) in all subjects.[2] Due to the very low plasma gatifloxacin levels achieved after ophthalmic use, it is highly unlikely that infant plasma levels following breastmilk exposure would be significant enough to cause clinical effects.

Pregnancy Risk	C	Lactation Risk	L3
T ½	= 7.1 hours	M/P	=
Vd	= 1.5 l/kg	PB	= 20%
Tmax	= 1–2 hours	Oral	= 96%
MW	= 402	pKa	= 5.94, 9.21

Adult Concerns: Diarrhea, nausea, vaginitis, headache, dizziness, allergic reaction, chills, fever, palpitations, abdominal pain and other symptoms have been reported. CNS agitation, nervousness, insomnia, and paranoia have been reported. Hypoglycemia and hyperglycemia have been reported in diabetic patients.

Pediatric Concerns: None reported via milk, but no studies yet.

Drug Interactions: Probenecid may increase plasma levels of gatifloxacin by 42%. Absorption of gatifloxacin is reduced by concomitant administration with ferrous sulfate, or antacids containing aluminum and magnesium salts. A minor increase in digoxin plasma levels has been reported.

Relative Infant Dose:

Adult Dose: 400 mg daily

Alternatives: Ofloxacin, levofloxacin

References:

1. Giamarellou H, Kolokythas E, Petrikkos G, Gazis J, Aravantinos D, Sfikakis P. Pharmacokinetics of three newer quinolones in pregnant and lactating women. Am J Med 1989; 87(5A): 49S-51S.
2. Pharmaceutical manufacturer prescribing information, 2006.

GEMCITABINE   L4

Trade: Gemzar

Other Trades:

Category: Anticancer drug

Gemcitabine is a nucleoside analogue used for the treatment of metastatic breast cancer, non-small cell lung cancer, and pancreatic cancer. Gemcitabine elimination follows a two phase elimination curve. The terminal elimination half-life is reported to be 49 minutes in females but can range to as high as 638 minutes following long infusions.[1] The volume of distribution following short infusions (<70 min.) was 50 L/m^2, indicating that gemcitabine, after short infusions, is not extensively distributed into tissues. For long infusions, the volume of distribution rose to 370 L/m^2, reflecting slow equilibration of gemcitabine within the tissue compartment. Gemcitabine is metabolized to an active metabolite, gemcitabine triphosphate, which can be extracted from peripheral blood mononuclear cells. The half-life of the terminal phase for gemcitabine triphosphate from mononuclear cells ranges from 1.7 to 19.4 hours. Within one week, 92% to 98% of the dose was recovered, almost entirely in the urine. No data are available on its transfer to milk, but gemcitabine levels in milk are probably quite low, due to its low pKa (3.6). Women should be advised to withhold breastfeeding for a minimum of seven days.

Pregnancy Risk	D	Lactation Risk	L4
T ½	= 49 to 638 minutes	M/P	=
Vd	= (short infusions) 50 L/m^2; (long infusions) 370 L/m^2	PB	=
Tmax	= 30 minutes	Oral	=
MW	= 299.7	pKa	= 14.68

Adult Concerns: Constipation, hair loss, pain, sleepiness or unusual drowsiness, swelling or inflammation of the mouth, thinning of hair.

Pediatric Concerns:

Drug Interactions:

Relative Infant Dose:

Adult Dose:

Alternatives:

References:

1. Pharmaceutical manufacturer prescribing information, 2005.

GEMFIBROZIL   L3

Trade: Lopid, Gemcor

Other Trades: Ausgem, Gemhexal, Apo-Gemfibrozil, Lopid

Category: Antilipemic agent

Gemfibrozil is a hypolipidemic agent primarily used to lower triglyceride levels by decreasing serum very low density lipoproteins.[1] A slight reduction in serum cholesterol may likewise occur. Following a dose of 800 mg mean peak maternal plasma levels were 33 µg/mL. There are no data on its transfer into human milk. Reproductive studies in rodents at high doses have not revealed any evidence of harm to the fetus. But the risks of using lipid lowering drugs while pregnant, and probably while breastfeeding, may be higher than the overall risks of hyperlipidemia and, therefore, are not usually justified.

Pregnancy Risk	C	Lactation Risk	L3
T ½	= 1.5 hours	M/P	=
Vd	=	PB	= 99%
Tmax	= 1–2 hours	Oral	= 97%
MW	= 250	pKa	= 4.7

Adult Concerns: Epigastric pain, dry mouth, constipation, diarrhea and flatulence. Changes in blood chemistry including hematocrit, white blood cells, hemoglobin. Elevation of liver enzymes.

Pediatric Concerns: None reported via milk, but risk vs. benefit evaluation is recommended.

Drug Interactions: Stimulation of anticoagulants including Anisidone, dicoumarol, warfarin. Increased risk of myopathy when coadministered with HMG-CoA reductase inhibitors such as atorvastatin, fluvastatin, and other statins. Increased risk of hypoglycemia when used with glyburide, and perhaps other hypoglycemics.

Relative Infant Dose:

Adult Dose: 600 mg twice daily.

Alternatives:

References:
1. McEvoy GE. (ed): AFHS Drug Information. New York, NY: 2003.

GEMIFLOXACIN MESYLATE   L3

Trade: Factive

Other Trades: Factive

Category: Antibiotic

A member of the fluoroquinolone family, gemifloxacin is used to treat a wide range of infections caused by gram-positive and gram-negative microorganisms. It acts by inhibiting bacterial DNA synthesis. Gemifloxacin is effective against those organisms that have mutated and are insusceptible to other fluoroquinolones.[1]

No data are available on the transfer of gemifloxacin into human milk. Other fluoroquinolones are suitable however, and it is unlikely this one will be that different. Some fluoroquinolones are excreted into breastmilk (ciprofloxacin) but are safe to use. This product has a high volume of distribution, so milk levels will probably be lower than with ciprofloxacin. Observe for diarrhea in the breastfed infant.

Pregnancy Risk	C	Lactation Risk	L3
T ½	= 7 hours	M/P	=
Vd	= 4.2 l/kg	PB	= 60–70%
Tmax	= 0.5–2 hours	Oral	= 71%
MW	= 485	pKa	=

Adult Concerns: Adverse reactions include headache, rash, hyperkalemia, diarrhea, nausea, and increased liver enzyme levels.

Pediatric Concerns: No data are available. Observe for changes in gut flora.

Drug Interactions: Concurrent use of corticosteroids may increase the risk of tendon rupture. Metal cations and antacids can decrease absorption of gemifloxacin. Gemifloxacin may increase the effect of glyburide and warfarin.

Relative Infant Dose:

Adult Dose: 320 mg daily

Alternatives:

References:
1.   Pharmaceutical manufacturer prescribing information, 2004.

GENTAMICIN   L2

Trade: Garamycin
Other Trades: Palacos, Septopal, Alocomicin, Garamycin, Garatec, Cidomycin
Category: Aminoglycoside antibiotic

Gentamicin is a narrow spectrum antibiotic generally used for gram negative infections. The oral absorption of gentamicin (<1%) is generally nil with the exception of premature neonates, where small amounts may be absorbed.[1] In one study of 10 women given 80 mg three times daily IM for 5 days postpartum, milk levels were measured on day 4.[2] Gentamicin levels in milk were 0.42, 0.48, 0.49, and 0.41 mg/L at 1, 3, 5, and 7 hours respectively. The milk/plasma ratios were 0.11 at one hour and 0.44 at 7 hours. Plasma gentamicin levels in neonates were small, found in only 5 of the 10 neonates, and averaged 0.41 µg/mL. The authors estimate that daily ingestion via breastmilk would be 307 µg for a 3.6 kg neonate (normal neonatal dose= 2.5 mg/kg every 12 hours). These amounts would be clinically irrelevant in most infants.

Pregnancy Risk	C	Lactation Risk	L2
T ½	= 2–3 hours	M/P	= 0.11–0.44
Vd	= 0.28 l/kg	PB	= <10–30%
Tmax	= 30–90 minutes (IM)	Oral	= <1%
MW	=	pKa	= 8.2

Adult Concerns: Changes in gastrointestinal flora, diarrhea, kidney damage, etc.

Pediatric Concerns: None reported.

Drug Interactions: Increased toxicity when used with certain penicillins, cephalosporins, amphotericin B, loop diuretics, and neuromuscular blocking agents.

Relative Infant Dose: 2.1%

Adult Dose: 1.5–2.5 mg/kg every 8 hours

Alternatives:

References:
1. Nelson JD, McCracken GH, Jr. The current status of gentamicin for tne neonate and young infant. Am J Dis Child 1972; 124(1): 13–14.
2. Celiloglu M, Celiker S, Guven H, Tuncok Y, Demir N, Erten O. Gentamicin excretion and uptake from breast milk by nursing infants. Obstet Gynecol 1994; 84(2): 263–265.

GENTIAN VIOLET   L3

Trade: Crystal Violet, Methylrosaniline chloride, Gentian Violet

Other Trades:

Category: Antifungal, antimicrobial

Gentian violet (GV) is an older product that, when used topically and orally, is an exceptionally effective antifungal and antimicrobial.[1] It is a strong purple dye that is difficult to remove. Gentian violet has been found to be equivalent to ketoconazole and far superior to nystatin in treating oral (not esophageal) candidiasis in patients with advanced AIDS. It is also useful in treating purulent infections of the ear infected with methicillin-resistant *Staphylococcus aureus*.[3] Gentian violet (GV) solutions generally come as 1–2% solutions dissolved in a 10% solution of alcohol. For use with infants, the solution should be diluted with distilled water to 0.25 to 0.5% Gentian violet. This reduces the irritant properties of GV and reduces the alcohol content as well. While the alcohol is irritating to the nipple, it is not detrimental to the infant.[2] Higher concentrations of GV are known to be very irritating, leading to oral ulceration and necrotic skin reactions in children. If used, a small swab should be soaked in the solution, and then swabbed in the infants gingivae. Apply it directly to the affected areas in the mouth no more than once or twice daily for no more than 3–7 days. Direct application to the nipple has been reported.

Pregnancy Risk	C	Lactation Risk	L3
T ½	=	M/P	=
Vd	=	PB	=
Tmax	=	Oral	=
MW	= 408	pKa	=

Adult Concerns: Oral ulceration, stomatitis, staining of skin and clothing, nausea, vomiting, diarrhea.

Pediatric Concerns: Irritation leading to buccal ulcerations and necrotic skin reactions if used excessively and in higher concentrations. Nausea, vomiting, diarrhea.

Drug Interactions:

Relative Infant Dose:

Adult Dose: N/A

Alternatives:

References:
1. McEvoy GE. (ed): AFHS Drug Information. New York, NY: 2003.
2. Newman J. Personal communication. 1997.
3. Kayama C, Goto Y, Shimoya S, Hasegawa S, Murao S, Nakajo Y, Nibu K. Effects of Gentian Violet on Refractory Discharging Ears Infected with Methicillin-Resistant *Staphylococcus aureus*. J Otolaryngol 2006; 35(6): 384–386.

GINGER   L3

Trade:
Other Trades:
Category: Herb

There are no adequate and well-controlled studies or case reports in breastfeeding women. However, this herb has been safely used in pregnant women for many years without complications and it is unlikely it would bother a breastfeeding infant.

Pregnancy Risk	C	Lactation Risk	L3
T ½	=	M/P	=
Vd	=	PB	=
Tmax	=	Oral	=
MW	=	pKa	=

Adult Concerns: Side effects: increased bleeding risk with large doses. There is a risk of increased bleeding with large doses and as with all substances taken during pregnancy should only be used if the benefit to the mother outweighs the risk to the fetus. Ginger, in large doses, has been shown to cause a decrease in platelet aggregation that may increase the risk of bleeding.

Pediatric Concerns:

Drug Interactions:

Relative Infant Dose:

Adult Dose:

Alternatives:

References:

GINKGO BILOBA   L3

Trade:

Other Trades:

Category: Herbal antioxidant

Ginkgo Biloba (GBE) is the world's oldest living tree. Extracts of the leaves (GBE) contain numerous chemical compounds including dimeric flavones and their glycosides, amino acids such as 6-hydroxyknurenic acid, and numerous other compounds. The seeds contain ginkgo toxin, which is particularly toxic, and should not be consumed. Numerous studies reviewing ginkgo have been reported, including treatments for cerebral insufficiency, asthma, dementia, and circulatory disorders. Ginkgo appears particularly efficient at increasing cerebral blood flow, with increases varying from 20–70%.[1,2] Older patients were more responsive. This supports the clinical use of GBE to treat cognitive impairment in the elderly although more recent studies do not support its use in cognitive impairment. The anxiolytic properties of GBE have been reported to be due to monoamine oxidase inhibition in animal studies. Ginkgolides inhibit platelet-activating factor and is believed responsible for the anti-allergic and anti-asthmatic properties of this extract. No data are available on the transfer of GBE into human milk. Thus far, with exception of the seeds, GBE appears relatively non-toxic.

Pregnancy Risk	C		Lactation Risk	L3
T ½	=		M/P	=
Vd	=		PB	=
Tmax	=		Oral	=
MW	=		pKa	=

Adult Concerns: Headache, dizziness, heart palpitations, gastrointestinal symptoms, dermatologic reactions.

Pediatric Concerns: None reported via human milk.

Drug Interactions:

Relative Infant Dose:

Adult Dose:

Alternatives:

References:
1. Review of Natural Products Facts and Comparisons 1998.
2. Newall C, Anderson LA, Phillipson JD. Chamomile, German. In. Herbal Medicine. A guide for the healthcare professionals. The Pharmaceutical Press, London, 1996.

GINSENG   L3

Trade: Panax

Other Trades: Red Kooga

Category: Herbal tonic

Ginseng is perhaps the most popular and widely recognized product in the herbal remedy market. It is available in many forms, but the most common is the American root called Panax quinquefolium L. The root primarily contains steroid-like saponin glycosides (ginsenosides), of which there are at least two dozen and vary as a function of species, age, location, and season when harvested.[1] Early claims have suggested that ginseng provided strengthening effects and included increased mental capacity for work. Animal studies have suggested that ginseng can increase swimming time, prevent stress-induced ulcers, stimulate certain immune cells, etc. A number of studies, mostly small and poorly controlled, have been reported and many suggest beneficial effects of ingesting ginseng with minimal side effects. Reported toxicities have included estrogen-like effects including diffuse mammary nodularity, vaginal bleeding, etc.[2] The most commonly reported event is nervousness, excitation, morning diarrhea, and inability to concentrate. In one case report, germanium, an ingredient in ginseng preparations, produced a significant diuretic resistance.[3] A few other reports have suggested decreased platelet adhesion and increased bleeding risk with its use. No data was found concerning transfer into human milk. It is recommended that it not be used for more than 6 weeks.[4]

Pregnancy Risk	B	Lactation Risk	L3
T ½	=	M/P	=
Vd	=	PB	=
Tmax	=	Oral	=
MW	=	pKa	=

Adult Concerns: Excitement, nervousness, inability to concentrate, diarrhea, skin eruptions, hypertension, hypoglycemia, mammary nodularity. Ginseng products sometimes contain germanium, which can induce a state of severe loop-diuretic resistance.

Pediatric Concerns: None reported, but caution is urged.

Drug Interactions:

Relative Infant Dose:

Adult Dose:

Alternatives:

References:
1. Review of Natural Products Facts and Comparisons, St Louis, MO 1996.

2. Bissett NG. In: Herbal Drugs and Phytopharmaceuticals. Medpharm Scientific Publishers, CRC Press, Boca Raton, 1994.
3. Becker BN, Greene J, Evanson J, Chidsey G, Stone WJ. Ginseng-induced diuretic resistance. JAMA 1996; 276(8): 606–607.
4. The Complete German Commission E Monographs. Ed. M. Blumenthal Amer Botanical Council 1998.

GLATIRAMER   L3

Trade: Copaxone

Other Trades:

Category: Relapsing multiple sclerosis

Glatiramer is a synthetic polypeptide indicated for the treatment of relapsing, remitting multiple sclerosis.[1] It is primarily indicated for those who do not respond to interferons. Glatiramer is a mixture of random polymers of four amino acids: L-alanine, L-glutamic acid, L-lysine, and L-tyrosine. Its molecular weight ranges from 4,700 to 13,000 daltons, which would reduce its ability to enter milk. It is antigenically similar to myelin basic protein, a natural component of the myelin sheath of neurons. No data are available on its transfer into human milk, but it is very unlikely. If ingested orally, it would likely be depolymerized into individual amino acids, so toxicity is unlikely.

Pregnancy Risk	B	Lactation Risk	L3
T ½	=	M/P	=
Vd	=	PB	=
Tmax	=	Oral	= Minimal
MW	= 4700+	pKa	=

Adult Concerns: Dizziness, chest pain, palpitations, anxiety, hypertonia, sweating, nausea, weakness. Rash, hives, or severe pain where the shot is given.

Pediatric Concerns: None via milk.

Drug Interactions: None reported.

Relative Infant Dose:

Adult Dose: 20 mg subcutaneously once daily.

Alternatives: Interferon beta-1a

References:
1. Pharmaceutical manufacturer prescribing information, 2008.

GLIMEPIRIDE   L4

Trade: Amaryl

Other Trades:

Category: Lowers plasma glucose

Glimepiride is a second-generation sulfonylurea used to lower plasma glucose in patients with non-insulin dependent diabetes mellitus. No data are available on the transfer of this product into human milk. However, rodent studies demonstrated significant transfer and elevated plasma levels in pups.[1,2] Caution is urged if used in breastfeeding women. Observe for hypoglycemia in the infant.

Pregnancy Risk	C	Lactation Risk	L4
T ½	= 6–9 hours	M/P	=
Vd	= 0.113 l/kg	PB	= >99.5%
Tmax	= 2–3 hours	Oral	= 100%
MW	= 490	pKa	= 14.12

Adult Concerns: Hypoglycemia, nausea, hyponatremia, dizziness, headache, elevated liver enzymes, blurred vision.

Pediatric Concerns: None reported via milk. Observe for hypoglycemia.

Drug Interactions: The hypoglycemic effect of sulfonylureas may be increased by non-steroidal analgesics, salicylates, sulfonamides, coumarins, probenecid, and other drugs with high protein binding. Numerous other interactions exist, see product information.

Relative Infant Dose:

Adult Dose: 1–4 mg daily.

Alternatives:

References:
1. Pharmaceutical manufacturer prescribing information, 2011.
2. Bressler R, Johnson DG. Pharmacological regulation of blood glucose levels in non-insulin-dependent diabetes mellitus. Arch Intern Med 1997; 157(8): 836–848.

GLIPIZIDE   L3

Trade: Glucotrol XL, Glucotrol

Other Trades: Melizide, Minidiab, Glibenese

Category: Prolonged release hypoglycemic agent

Glipizide is a potent hypoglycemic agent that belongs to sulfonylurea family. It is formulated in regular and extended release formulations, and it is used only for non insulin-dependent (Type II) diabetes. Thus the half-life and time-to-peak depends on the formulation used. It reduces glucose levels by stimulating insulin secretion from the pancreas. In a group of 5 mothers who received daily doses of glyburide (non micronized 5 mg) or glipizide (immediate-release 5 mg) neither glyburide or glipizide were detectable in milk.[1] Detection limit for glipizide was 0.08 μg/mL. Infant plasma glucose levels were normal.

Pregnancy Risk	C	Lactation Risk	L3
T ½	= 4–6 hours	M/P	=
Vd	= 0.17–0.25 l/kg	PB	= 92–99%
Tmax	= 1–3 hours	Oral	= 80–100%
MW	= 446	pKa	= 5.9

Adult Concerns: Hypoglycemia, jaundice, nausea, vomiting, diarrhea, constipation.

Pediatric Concerns: Milk levels were undetectable in one study.

Drug Interactions: The hypoglycemic effect may be enhanced by: anticoagulants, chloramphenicol, clofibrate, fenfluramine, fluconazole, histamine-2 receptor antagonists (cimetidine, ranitidine, famotidine), magnesium salts, methyldopa, monoamine oxidase inhibitors, probenecid, salicylates, tricyclic antidepressants, sulfonamides. The hypoglycemic effect may be reduced by: beta blockers, cholestyramine, diazoxide, phenytoin, rifampin, thiazide diuretics.

Relative Infant Dose:

Adult Dose: 15–40 mg daily.

Alternatives:

References:
1. Feig DS, Briggs GG, Kraemer JM et al. Transfer of glyburide and glipizide into breast milk. Diabetes Care 2005; 28: 1851–1855.

GLIPIZIDE + METFORMIN   L3

Trade: Metaglip

Other Trades:

Category: Antidiabetic

Glipizide and Metformin hydrochloride is a combination drug product used in the management of type 2 diabetes mellitus. There are currently no studies on the transfer of this combined drug product in breastmilk.

Glipizide is a potent hypoglycemic agent that belongs to sulfonylurea family. In a group of 5 mothers who received daily doses of glyburide (non micronized 5 mg) or glipizide (immediate-release 5 mg) neither glyburide or glipizide were detectable in milk.[1] Detection limit for glipizide was 0.08 µg/mL. Infant plasma glucose levels were normal.

Metformin belongs to the biguanide family. In a study of 7 women taking metformin (median dose 1500 mg/d), the mean milk-to-plasma ratio (AUC) for metformin was 0.35.[2] The mean average concentration in milk over the dose interval was 0.27 mg/L. The absolute infant dose averaged 0.04 mg/kg/day and the mean relative infant dose was 0.28%. Metformin was present in very low or undetectable concentrations in the plasma of four of the infants who were studied. No health problems were found in the six infants who were evaluated. In another study of five subjects the median milk/plasma ratio (AUC) for metformin was 0.47.[3] The median calculated infant dose was 0.2% of the weight-adjusted maternal dose. None of the infants exposed to their mothers' milk had detectable levels of metformin in their plasma, nor were any side effects noted. In a recent study of 5 women consuming an average dose of 500 mg twice daily, the mean peak and trough metformin concentrations in breast milk were 0.42 mg/L (range 0.38–0.46 mg/L) and 0.39 mg/L (range 0.31–0.52 mg/L), respectively.[4] The average milk/serum ratio was 0.63 (range 0.36–1.00) and the estimated relative infant dose was 0.65% (range 0.43–1.08%). Blood glucose concentrations in 3 infants were normal, ranging from 47–77 mg/dL. The mothers reported no side effects were noted in the breastfed infants. Metformin is also used to treat polycystic ovary syndrome. In one study of 61 nursing infants whose mothers were taking a median of 2.55 gm/day throughout pregnancy and lactation, the growth, motor, and social development of the infants was recorded to be normal. The authors concluded that metformin was safe and effective during lactation in the first 6 months of an infant's life.[5] The relative infant dose for metformin is 0.28%-0.65%.

Based on published data, it appears that the infant plasma levels of glipizide and metformin following breastmilk exposure are too low to produce any significant clinical effects in the infant. Therefore, glipizide + metformin is probably safe to use during breastfeeding.

Pregnancy Risk	C	Lactation Risk	L3
T ½	= Glipizide/metformin: 4–6 hours/6.2 hours	M/P	= Glipizide/metformin: /0.35–0.63
Vd	= Glipizide/metformin: 0.17–0.25/3.7 l/kg	PB	= Glipizide/metformin: 92–99%/minimal
Tmax	= Glipizide/metformin: 1–3 hours/2.75 hours	Oral	= Glipizide/metformin: 80–100%/50%
MW	= Glipizide/metformin: 446/129	pKa	= Glipizide/metformin: 5.9/12.4

Adult Concerns: Hypertension hypoglycemia, abdomina pain, diarrhea, nausea, vomiting, myalgia, dizziness, upper respiratory tract infection, lactic acidosis, hemolytic anemia.

Pediatric Concerns:

Drug Interactions: Administration with the following drugs may cause severe hypoglycemia: Nonsteroidal anti-inflammatory agents, fluconazole, miconazole, chloramphenicol, fluoroquinolones, probenecid, coumarins, monoamine oxidase inhibitors, and beta-blockers. Co-administration with furosemide, cimetidine or nifedipine may cause an increase in metformin plasma levels.

Relative Infant Dose:

Adult Dose: Glipizide/metformin: 2.5–5 mg/250–500 mg 1–3 times daily.

Alternatives:

References:
1. Feig DS, Briggs GG, Kraemer JM et al. Transfer of glyburide and glipizide into breast milk. Diabetes Care 2005; 28: 1851–1855.
2. Hale TW, Kristensen JH, Hackett LP, Kohan R, Ilett KF. Transfer of metformin into human milk. Diabetologia 2002; 45(11): 1509–1514.
3. Gardiner SJ, Kirkpatrick CM, Begg EJ, Zhang M, Moore MP, Saville DJ. Transfer of metformin into human milk. Clin Pharmacol Ther 2003; 73(1): 71–77.
4. Briggs GG, Ambrose PJ, Nageotte MP, Padilla G, Wan S. Excretion of metformin into breast milk and the effect on nursing infants. Obstet Gynecol 2005 Jun; 105(6): 1437–41.
5. Glueck CJ, Salehi M, Sieve L, Wang P. Growth, motor, and social developemnt in breast- and formula- fed infants of metformin-treated women with polycyctic ovary syndrome. J Pediatr 2006; 148: 628–632.

GLUCOSAMINE   L3

Trade:

Other Trades:

Category: Antiarthritic

Glucosamine is an endogenous amino monosaccharide that has been reported effective in resolving symptoms of osteoarthritis. It is one of the salt forms of the amino sugar glucosamine, which is a constituent of cartilage proteoglycans. Administered in large doses, most is sequestered in the liver with only minimal amounts reaching other tissues, thus oral bioavailability is low. Most of the oral dose is hepatically metabolized and subsequently incorporated into other plasma proteins.[1] No data are available on transfer into human milk. Because glucosamine is primarily sequestered and metabolized in the liver, and because the plasma levels are almost undetectable, it is unlikely that any would enter human milk. Further, the fact that it is so poorly bioavailable, it is unlikely that an infant would absorb clinically relevant amounts. Do not use with warfarin, as INR levels may double causing an increased risk of bleeding complications.

Pregnancy Risk	C	Lactation Risk	L3
T ½	= 0.3 hours	M/P	=
Vd	= 0.035 l/kg	PB	=
Tmax	=	Oral	= <26%
MW	= 179	pKa	= 12.97

Adult Concerns: Minimal but include nausea, dyspepsia, vomiting, drowsiness, headache and skin rash. Peripheral edema and tachycardia have been reported. Some reports of exacerbation of asthma by glucosamine.

Pediatric Concerns: None reported via milk.

Drug Interactions: Do not use with warfarin as INR may increase significantly.

Relative Infant Dose:

Adult Dose: 500 mg three times daily.

Alternatives:

References:
1. Setnikar I, Palumbo R, Canali S, Zanolo G. Pharmacokinetics of glucosamine in man. Arzneimittelforschung 1993; 43(10): 1109–1113.

GLYBURIDE   L2

Trade: Micronase, Diabeta

Other Trades: Diaformin, Diabeta, Euglucon, Gen-Glybe, Daonil

Category: Hypoglycemic, antidiabetic agent

Glyburide is a second generation sulfonylurea agent useful in the treatment of non insulin-dependent (Type II) diabetes mellitus. It belongs to the sulfonylurea family (tolbutamide, glipizide) of hypoglycemic agents of which glyburide is one of the most potent. Glyburide apparently stimulates insulin secretion, thus reducing plasma glucose. In a study of 6 mothers who received a single dose of 5 mg, and 2 mothers who received a single dose of 10 mg glyburide, all breast milk samples were below the limit of detection of 0.005 µg/mL.[1] In a group of 5 mothers who received daily doses of glyburide (non micronized 5 mg) or glipizide (immediate-release 5 mg) neither glyburide or glipizide were detectable in milk. Infant plasma glucose levels were normal.

Pregnancy Risk	B	Lactation Risk	L2
T ½	= 4–13.7 hours	M/P	=
Vd	= 0.73 l/kg	PB	= 99%
Tmax	= 2–3 hours	Oral	= Complete
MW	= 494	pKa	= 5.3

Adult Concerns: In adults, hypoglycemia, headache, anorexia, nausea, heartburn, allergic skin rashes.

Pediatric Concerns: Milk levels undetectable. Transfer to infant of clinically relevant amounts is unlikely.

Drug Interactions: Thiazide diuretics and beta blockers may decrease efficacy of glyburide. Increased toxicity may result from use with phenylbutazone, oral anticoagulants, hydantoins, salicylates, NSAIDS, sulfonamides. Alcohol increases disulfiram effect.

Relative Infant Dose:

Adult Dose: 1.25–20 mg daily

Alternatives:

References:
1. Feig DS, Briggs GG, Kraemer JM et al. Transfer of glyburide and glipizide into breast milk. Diabetes Care 2005; 28: 1851–1855.

GLYBURIDE + METFORMIN   L3

Trade: Glucovance

Other Trades:

Category: Antidiabetic

Glyburide and Metformin hydrochloride is a combined drug product used in the management of diabetes mellitus type 2. There are currently no studies available on the transfer of glyburide + metformin into breastmilk.

Glyburide is a second generation sulfonylurea agent useful in the treatment of non insulin-dependent (Type II) diabetes mellitus. In a study of 6 mothers who received a single dose (5 mg) and 2 mothers who received a single dose of 10 mg glyburide, all breast milk samples were below the limit of detection of 0.005 µg/mL.[1] In a group of 5 mothers who received daily doses of glyburide (non micronized 5 mg) or glipizide (immediate-release 5 mg) neither glyburide or glipizide were detectable in milk. Infant plasma glucose levels were normal.

Metformin belongs to the biguanide family. In a study of 7 women taking metformin (median dose 1500 mg/d), the mean milk-to-plasma ratio (AUC) for metformin was 0.35.[2] The mean average concentration in milk over the dose interval was 0.27 mg/L. The absolute infant dose averaged 0.04 mg/kg/day and the mean relative infant dose was 0.28%. Metformin was present in very low or undetectable concentrations in the plasma of four of the infants who were studied. No health problems were found in the six infants who were evaluated. In another study of five subjects the median milk/plasma ratio (AUC) for metformin was 0.47.[3] The median calculated infant dose was 0.2% of the weight-adjusted maternal dose. None of the infants exposed to their mothers' milk had detectable levels of metformin in their plasma, nor were any side effects noted. In a recent study of 5 women consuming an average dose of 500 mg twice daily, the mean peak and trough metformin concentrations in breast milk were 0.42 mg/L (range 0.38–0.46 mg/L) and 0.39 mg/L (range 0.31–0.52 mg/L), respectively.[4] The average milk/serum ratio was 0.63 (range 0.36–1.00) and the estimated relative infant dose was 0.65% (range 0.43–1.08%). Blood glucose concentrations in 3 infants were normal, ranging from 47–77 mg/dL. The mothers reported no side effects were noted in the breastfed infants. Metformin is also used to treat polycystic ovary syndrome. In one study of 61 nursing infants whose mothers were taking a median of 2.55 gm/day throughout pregnancy and lactation, the growth, motor, and social development of the infants was recorded to be normal. The authors concluded that metformin was safe and effective during lactation in the first 6 months of an infant's life.[5] The relative infant dose for metformin is 0.28%-0.65%.

Based on the published data, it appears that the infant plasma levels of glyburide and metformin following exposure to breastmilk are too low to produce any significant clinical effects in the infant. Therefore, glyburide + metformin is probably compatible with breastfeeding.

Pregnancy Risk	B	Lactation Risk	L3
T ½	= Glyburide/metformin: 4–13.7 hours/6.2 hours	M/P	= Glyburide/metformin: /0.35–0.63
Vd	= Glyburide/metformin: 0.73/3.7 l/kg	PB	= Glyburide/metformin: 99%/minimal
Tmax	= Glyburide/metformin: 2–3 hours/2.75 hours	Oral	= Glyburide/metformin: Complete/50%
MW	= Glyburide/metformin: 494/129	pKa	= Glyburide/metformin: 5.3/12.4

Adult Concerns: Vitamin B_{12} deficiency, hypoglycemia, abdominal pain, nausea, vomiting, dizziness, headache, upper respiratory tract infection, lactic acidosis.

Pediatric Concerns:

Drug Interactions: Administration with the following drugs may cause severe hypoglycemia: Nonsteroidal anti-inflammatory agents, fluconazole, miconazole, chloramphenicol, fluoroquinolones, probenecid, coumarins, monoamine oxidase inhibitors, and beta-blockers. Co-administration with furosemide, cimetidine or nifedipine may cause an increase in metformin plasma levels.

Relative Infant Dose:

Adult Dose: Glyburide/metformin: 1.25–5mg/250–500 mg 1–3 times daily.

Alternatives:

References:
1. Feig DS, Briggs GG, Kraemer JM et al. Transfer of glyburide and glipizide into breast milk. Diabetes Care 2005; 28: 1851–1855.
2. Hale TW, Kristensen JH, Hackett LP, Kohan R, Ilett KF. Transfer of metformin into human milk. Diabetologia 2002; 45(11): 1509–1514.
3. Gardiner SJ, Kirkpatrick CM, Begg EJ, Zhang M, Moore MP, Saville DJ. Transfer of metformin into human milk. Clin Pharmacol Ther 2003; 73(1): 71–77.
4. Briggs GG, Ambrose PJ, Nageotte MP, Padilla G, Wan S. Excretion of metformin into breast milk and the effect on nursing infants. Obstet Gynecol 2005 Jun; 105(6): 1437–41.
5. Glueck CJ, Salehi M, Sieve L, Wang P. Growth, motor, and social developemnt in breast- and formula- fed infants of metformin-treated women with polycyctic ovary syndrome. J Pediatr 2006; 148: 628–632.

GLYCERIN   L3

Trade:

Other Trades:

Category: Osmotic Laxative, Ophthalmic Agent

Glycerin, also called glycerol, is a simple polyol compound that is colorless, odorless, and slightly sweet in taste.[1] It is a normal constituent in all humans and is virtually non-toxic. There are no data on the use of exogenous glycerol in breastfeeding women, but it is unlikely to be hazardous. Most would be metabolized in the gut.

Pregnancy Risk	C	Lactation Risk	L3
T ½	= 30–45 minutes	M/P	=
Vd	=	PB	=
Tmax	=	Oral	=
MW	= 92.1	pKa	=

Adult Concerns: Arrhythmias, confusion, dizziness, headache, dehydration, hyperglycemia, polydipsia, cramping pain, diarrhea, dry mouth, nausea, rectal irritation, tenesmus, vomiting.

Pediatric Concerns:

Drug Interactions:

Relative Infant Dose:

Adult Dose: 3 gm rectally; 1–3 drops ophthalmic

Alternatives:

References:
1. Pharmaceutical manufacturer prescribing information, 2001.

GLYCOPYRROLATE   L3

Trade: Robinul
Other Trades: Robinul
Category: Anticholinergic

Glycopyrrolate is a quaternary ammonium anticholinergic used prior to surgery to dry secretions. After administration, its plasma half-life is exceedingly short (<5 min.) with most of the product being distributed out of the plasma compartment rapidly.[1,2] No data are available on its transfer into human milk, but due to its short plasma half-life and its quaternary structure, it is very unlikely that significant quantities would penetrate milk. Further, along with the poor oral bioavailability of this product, it is very remote that glycopyrrolate would pose a significant risk to a breastfeeding infant.

Pregnancy Risk	B	Lactation Risk	L3
T ½	= 1.7 hours	M/P	=
Vd	= 0.64 l/kg	PB	=
Tmax	= 5 hours (oral)	Oral	= 10–25%
MW	= 398	pKa	=

Adult Concerns: Blurred vision, dry mouth, tachycardia.

Pediatric Concerns: None reported via milk.

Drug Interactions: May reduce effect of levodopa. Increased toxicity when used with amantadine and cyclopropane.

Relative Infant Dose:

Adult Dose: 1–2 mg three times daily.

Alternatives:

References:
1. Lacy C. Drug information handbook. Lexi-Comp Inc. Cleveland, OH, 1996.
2. Drug Facts and Comparisons 1996 ed. ed. St. Louis: 1996.

GOLD COMPOUNDS   L5

Trade: Ridaura, Myochrysine, Solganal
Other Trades: Myochrysine, Ridaura, Myocrisin
Category: Antiarthritic

Gold salts are anti-inflammatory agents used to treat rheumatoid arthritis. Gold salts are potent and toxic. Two injectable forms exist–gold sodium thiomalate and sodium aurothioglucose. One oral form exists, auranofin. The plasma kinetics of the gold salts are highly variable and are difficult to report, but in general, their half-lives are very extended and increase as duration of treatment continues. Auranofin is the only orally available salt form and is approximately 20–25% bioavailable. They are all probably secreted into breastmilk in small quantities.

In a study by Blau [1], milk levels of gold (gold thioglucose) following a cumulative dose of 135 mg ranged from 0.86–0.99 mg/100 mL. These are quite high and exceed the data of others although this data was challenged on arithmetical grounds by others. The subsequent publication of several other studies (see below) seem to refute the transfer of high levels of gold in milk. In one study of a patient receiving aurothiomalate (Myochrysine) 50 mg/week for 7 weeks, the concentration of gold sodium thiomalate varied from 0.022 to 0.04 mg/L at 66 hours and 7 days post-dose respectively.[2] Although the infant showed no signs or symptoms of toxicity during therapy, the authors noted that 3 months after treatment the infant developed transient facial edema of unexplained origin. In two patients treated with 50 mg aurothiomalate IM, levels in milk varied from 27–153 µg/L and reached a peak at 17 hours following the injection.[3] The authors suggested approximately 10% or more of the concentration of gold measured in maternal serum appears in breastmilk. In a study of a single patient receiving chronic aurothioglucose therapy (50 mg/week) (20 weeks), the mother's steady state plasma gold was 4.05 mg/L while it was 0.041 mg/L in breast milk.[4] The average amount of gold in breastmilk per 24 hours was only 0.0255 mg. The authors calculated that only 0.178 mg gold (0.71% of the weekly dose) would appear in the breast milk over a week. Gold was undetectable (<5 X 10(-7) mg/L) in the infant's plasma or urine even following 20 weeks. The authors suggest that It is very unlikely that more than minute amounts of gold are absorbed from the mother's breast milk when breast feeding an infant. In a study of a single patient receiving 10 mg/month aurothiomalate, Bennett found milk levels of gold ranged from 10–30 µg/L.[5] Levels in the infant's plasma were 51 µg/L.

The data published thus far varies widely. While small levels of gold may be found in milk, the oral absorption of gold is quite low, probably less than 20%. However, almost any gold absorbed would be retained in the infant for long periods (months) and some accumulation could occur following chronic therapy. For this reason prolonged exposure of a nursing infant to gold therapy is probably somewhat risky.

Pregnancy Risk	C	Lactation Risk	L5
T ½	= 3–26 days	M/P	= 0.02–0.3
Vd	= 0.1 l/kg	PB	= 95%
Tmax	= 3–6 hours (IM)	Oral	= 20–25% (auranofin)
MW	=	pKa	=

Adult Concerns: Gastrointestinal distress, diarrhea, nausea, vomiting, exfoliative dermatitis, nephrotoxicity, proteinuria, and blood dyscrasias.

Pediatric Concerns: Possible facial edema 3 months after therapy. Relationship is questionable.

Drug Interactions: Decreased gold effects with penicillamine and acetylcysteine.

Relative Infant Dose: 0.6%–2.8%

Adult Dose: 25–50 mg every week.

Alternatives: NSAIDS

References:
1.   Blau SP. Letter: Metabolism of gold during lactation. Arthritis Rheum 1973; 16(6): 777–778.

2. Bell RA, Dale IM. Gold secretion in maternal milk. Arthritis Rheum 1976; 19(6): 1374.
3. Ostensen M, Skavdal K, Myklebust G, Tomassen Y, Aarbakke J. Excretion of gold into human breast milk. Eur J Clin Pharmacol 1986; 31(2): 251–252.
4. Rooney TW, Lorber A, Veng-Pedersen P, Herman RA, Meehan R, Hade J, et al. Gold pharmacokinetics in breast milk and serum of a lactating woman. J Rheumatol 1987 Dec; 14(6): 1120–2.
5. Bennett PN, Humphries SJ, Osborne JP, Clarke AK, Taylor A. Use of sodium aurothiomalate during lactation. Br J Clin Pharmacol 1990 Jun; 29(6): 777–9.

GOLIMUMAB   L3

Trade: Simponi

Other Trades:

Category: Monoclonal antibody for arthritis

Golimumab is a monoclonal antibody tumor necrosis factor inhibitor, a pro-inflammatory mediator and has actions similar to other TNF inhibitors such as infliximab. It is described as a biological disease-modifying antirheumatic drug (DMARD). It is used in the treatment of moderately to severely active rheumatoid arthritis, active psoriatic arthritis, and active ankylosing spondylitis; a dose of 50 mg is given by subcutaneous injection once a month. In monkeys, passage into breast milk was reported. There are no studies on transfer of the drug into human milk. In the pre- and post-natal development study in cynomolgus monkeys in which golimumab was administered subcutaneously during pregnancy and lactation, golimumab was detected in the breast milk at concentrations that were approximately 400-fold lower than the maternal serum concentrations.[1] This suggests levels in human milk will be similarly low. Due to its size and structure, levels in milk will be low. Oral bioavailability will be low as well. Note: this product is commonly used with methotrexate, which can be hazardous to a breastfeeding infant.

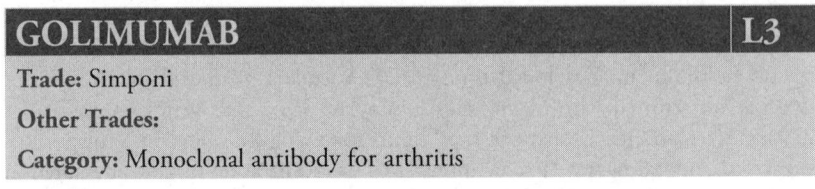

Pregnancy Risk	B	Lactation Risk	L3
T ½	= 2 weeks	M/P	=
Vd	= 58–126 ml/kg	PB	=
Tmax	= 2–6 days	Oral	= 53%
MW	= 150,000	pKa	=

Adult Concerns: Serious and sometimes fatal infections due to bacterial, mycobacterial, invasive fungal, viral, protozoal, or other opportunistic pathogens have been reported in patients receiving TNF-blocker. Observe for other infectious diseases such as tuberculosis, histoplasmosis, aspergillosis, candidiasis, coccidioidomycosis, listeriosis, and pneumocystosis.

Pediatric Concerns: None yet reported in humans, but levels in milk of monkeys was 400 fold less than plasma levels. Unlikely to enter milk or be orally bioavailable.

Drug Interactions: Methotrexate may increase the effect of this immunosuppressant.

Relative Infant Dose:

Adult Dose: 50 mg once a month.

Alternatives: Etanercept, infliximab

References:
1.   Pharmaceutical manufacturer prescribing information, 2010.

GONADORELIN   L3

Trade: Lutrepulse, Factrel

Other Trades: Wyerth-Ayerst HRF, Lutrepulse, Relisorm, Fertiral

Category: Gonadotropin-releasing hormone

Gonadorelin acetate is used for the induction of ovulation in anovulatory women with primary hypothalamic amenorrhea. Gonadorelin is a small decapeptide identical to the physiologic gonadotropin releasing hormone (GnRH) secreted by the hypothalamus which stimulates the pituitary release of luteinizing hormone (LH) and to a lesser degree follicle stimulating hormone (FSH). LH and FSH subsequently stimulate the ovary to produce follicles. Gonadorelin plasma half-life is very brief (<2–4 minutes), and it is primarily distributed to the plasma only.[1] Gonadorelin has been detected in human breastmilk at concentrations of 0.1 to 3 nanograms/mL (adult dose= 20–100 micrograms) although its oral bioavailability in the infant would be minimal to none.[2]

Pregnancy Risk	B	Lactation Risk	L3
T ½	= 2–4 minutes	M/P	=
Vd	= 0.14 l/kg	PB	=
Tmax	=	Oral	= None
MW	=	pKa	= 10.63

Adult Concerns: Ovarian hyperstimulation, bronchospasm, tachycardia, flushing, urticaria, induration at injection site.

Pediatric Concerns: None reported via milk.

Drug Interactions:

Relative Infant Dose:

Adult Dose: 1–20 µg daily.

Alternatives:

References:
1.   Reynolds JEF. (Ed): Martindale: The Extra Pharmacopoeia (electronic version). Denver, CO: Micromedex, Inc., 1990.
2.   Drug Facts and Comparisons 1996 ed. ed. St. Louis: 1996.

GOSERELIN ACETATE IMPLANT   L3

Trade: Zoladex, Histrelin, Triptorelin, Vantas (Histrelin), Supprelin (Histrelin), Trelstar (Triptorelin)

Other Trades:

Category: Inhibitor of luteinizing hormone

Goserelin acetate is a synthetic decapeptide analogue of luteinizing hormone releasing hormone (LHRH) and it acts as a potent inhibitor of pituitary gonadotropin secretion.[1] Following initial administration in males, goserelin causes an initial increase in serum luteinizing hormone (LH) and follicle stimulating hormone (FSH) levels. Chronic administration of goserelin leads to sustained suppression of these pituitary gonadotropins, and serum levels of testosterone in males. In females, a down-regulation of the pituitary gland following chronic exposure leads to suppression of gonadotropin secretion, a decrease in serum estradiol to levels consistent with the menopausal state. Serum LH and FSH are suppressed to follicular phase levels within four weeks. No data are available on its transfer into human milk but due to its structure and molecular weight it is very unlikely to enter milk, or to be orally bioavailable in the infant.

Histrelin acetate and Triptorelin pamoate are also luteinizing hormone releasing hormone (gonadotropin releasing hormone) agonists, similar to goserelin.

Pregnancy Risk	X	Lactation Risk	L3
T ½	= 2.3 hours	M/P	=
Vd	= 0.28 (females) l/kg	PB	= Low
Tmax	= 12–15 days	Oral	= Nil
MW	= 1269	pKa	= 6.2

Adult Concerns: Adverse events include hot flashes, sexual dysfunction, vaginitis, emotional lability, headache, abdominal pain, pelvic pain, depression, sweating, breast atrophy, edema, etc.

Pediatric Concerns: None reported via milk. While it is unlikely this peptide would enter milk, or be orally bioavailable to an infant, it is not known how it would affect milk production. Some caution is recommended concerning loss of milk supply.

Drug Interactions: None studied.

Relative Infant Dose:

Adult Dose: 3.6 mg subcutaneously every 28 days.

Alternatives:

References:
1. Pharmaceutical manufacturer prescribing information, 2003.

GRANISETRON   L3

Trade: Kytril
Other Trades:
Category: Antiemetic

Granisetron is an antinauseant and antiemetic agent commonly used with chemotherapy. Following a 1 mg IV dose, the peak plasma concentration was only 3.63 ng/mL.[1] No data are available on its transfer into human milk but its levels are likely to be low. Further, this family of products (see ondansetron) are not highly toxic and are commonly used in children (2+ years). It is unlikely that this product will be overtly toxic to a breastfed infant. However, when used with chemotherapeutic agents, long waiting periods should be used for elimination of the chemotherapeutic agents anyway.

Pregnancy Risk	B	Lactation Risk	L3
T ½	= 3–14 hours	M/P	=
Vd	= 2–4 l/kg	PB	= 65%
Tmax	= 1 hour	Oral	= 60%
MW	= 349	pKa	= 9

Adult Concerns: Headache, asthenia, somnolence, diarrhea, dyspepsia, abdominal pain, constipation, and fever. Rarely elevations of liver enzymes have been reported.

Pediatric Concerns: None reported via milk.

Drug Interactions: Ketoconazole may inhibit the metabolism of granisetron.

Relative Infant Dose:

Adult Dose: 2 mg orally.

Alternatives: Ondansetron

References:
1. Pharmaceutical manufacturer prescribing information, 2002.

GREPAFLOXACIN   L4

Trade: Raxar

Other Trades: Raxar

Category: Fluoroquinolone antibiotic

Grepafloxacin is a typical fluoroquinolone antibiotic similar to ciprofloxacin. The manufacturer suggests that grepafloxacin is detectable in human milk after a 400 mg dose but does not provide the exact levels.[1] Studies in rodents suggest a concentrating mechanism of about 16 times that of the plasma compartment. Because this fluoroquinolone has a rather long half-life, high volume of distribution, the ability to enter many body compartments, and is concentrated in rodent milk, it is probably advisable to use this product with extreme caution, if at all, in breastfeeding women.

Pregnancy Risk	C	Lactation Risk	L4
T ½	= 15.7 hours	M/P	=
Vd	= 5.07 l/kg	PB	= 50%
Tmax	= 2–3 hours	Oral	= 72%
MW	= 422	pKa	=

Adult Concerns: Nausea, taste perversion, dizziness, headache, diarrhea, abdominal pain.

Pediatric Concerns: None reported with this product, but diarrhea and pseudomembranous colitis has been reported with ciprofloxacin. Arthropathy has been reported following pediatric use of fluoroquinolones.

Drug Interactions: Decreased absorption with antacids. Quinolones cause increased levels of caffeine, warfarin, cyclosporine, theophylline. Cimetidine, probenecid, azlocillin increase ciprofloxacin levels and therefore may increase grepafloxacin levels in the plasma as well. Increased risk of seizures when used with foscarnet.

Relative Infant Dose:

Adult Dose: 400–600 mg daily.

Alternatives: Norfloxacin, ofloxacin, levofloxacin, ciprofloxacin.

References:
1. Pharmaceutical manufacturer prescribing information, 1999.

GRISEOFULVIN   L2

Trade: Fulvicin, Gris-PEG
Other Trades: Fulcin, Griseostatin, Grisovin, Fulvicin, Grisovin-FP
Category: Antifungal

Griseofulvin is an older class antifungal. Enhanced safety profiles with the newer families of antifungals have reduced the use of griseofulvin. The drug is primarily effective against tinea species and not *Candida albicans*.[1,2] There are no data available for humans. In one study in cows following a dose of 10 mg/kg/day for 5 days (human dose =5 mg/kg/day) milk concentrations were 0.16 mg/L. Although these data cannot be directly extrapolated to humans, they indicate transfer to milk in some species. Oral use in adults is associated with low risk of hepatic cancer. Griseofulvin is still commonly used in pediatric tinea capitis (ringworm), where it is a preferred medication.

Pregnancy Risk	C	Lactation Risk	L2
T ½	= 9–24 hours	M/P	=
Vd	=	PB	=
Tmax	= 4–8 hours	Oral	= Poor to 50%
MW	= 353	pKa	=

Adult Concerns: Headache, depression, hepatotoxicity, skin rashes, hallucinations. Symptoms of overdose include lethargy, vertigo, blurred vision, nausea, vomiting, and diarrhea.

Pediatric Concerns: None reported from breastmilk.

Drug Interactions: Barbiturates may reduce plasma levels. May inhibit warfarin activity. May reduce effectiveness of oral contraceptives. May produce increased toxicity and tachycardia when used with alcohol.

Relative Infant Dose:

Adult Dose: 500–1000 mg daily (micro) or 330–375 mg daily (ultra).

Alternatives: Fluconazole

References:

1. McEvoy GE. (ed): AFHS Drug Information. New York, NY: 2003.
2. Huddleston WA. Antifungal activity of Penicillium griseofulvin mycelium. Vet Rec 1970; 86(3): 75–76.

GUAIFENESIN   L2

Trade: Mucinex

Other Trades:

Category: Expectorant, loosens respiratory tract secretions

Guaifenesin is an expectorant used to irritate the gastric mucosa and stimulate respiratory tract secretions in order to reduce phlegm viscosity. It does not suppress coughing and should not be used in persistent cough such as with smokers. No data are available on transfer into human breastmilk. In general, clinical studies documenting the efficacy of guaifenesin are lacking, and the usefulness of this product as an expectorant is highly questionable.[1] Poor efficacy of these drugs (expectorants in general) would suggest that they do not provide enough justification for use in lactating mothers. But untoward effects have not been reported. Pediatric dose: <2 years= 12 mg/kg/day in 6 divided doses; 2–5 years= 50–100 mg every 4 hours; 6–11 years= 100–200 mg every 4 hours; Children >12 years and adults= 200–400 mg every 4 hours for a maximum of 2.4 gm/day. Always dose with large volumes of fluids.

Pregnancy Risk	C	Lactation Risk	L2
T ½	= <7 hours	M/P	=
Vd	= 1.0 l/kg	PB	=
Tmax	=	Oral	= Complete
MW	= 198	pKa	= 15.56

Adult Concerns: Vomiting, diarrhea, nausea, sedation, skin rash, gastrointestinal dyspepsia.

Pediatric Concerns: None reported.

Drug Interactions:

Relative Infant Dose:

Adult Dose: 200–400 mg every 4 hours.

Alternatives:

References:

1. Lacy C. Drug information handbook. Lexi-Comp Inc. Cleveland, OH, 1996.

GUANFACINE　　　　　　　　　　　　L3

Trade: Tenex, Intuniv

Other Trades:

Category: Antihypertensive

Guanfacine is a centrally acting antihypertensive that stimulates alpha-2 adrenergic receptors (similar to clonidine). It is now sometimes used for ADHD and other syndromes. Studies in animals indicate that guanfacine is secreted into milk (milk/plasma ratio= 0.75), but human studies are lacking.[1,2] Because this product has a low molecular weight (246), and penetrates the CNS at high levels, it is likely to penetrate milk at significant levels. Caution is urged.

Pregnancy Risk	B	Lactation Risk	L3
T ½	= 17 hours	M/P	=
Vd	= 6.3 l/kg	PB	= 20–30%
Tmax	= 2.6 hours	Oral	= 81–100%
MW	= 246	pKa	= 7.1

Adult Concerns: Bradycardia, hypotension, dry mouth, sedation, weakness, constipation.

Pediatric Concerns: None reported but observe for hypotension, sedation, weakness.

Drug Interactions: Decreased hypotensive effect when used with tricyclic antidepressants. Increased effect when used with other antihypertensive agents.

Relative Infant Dose:

Adult Dose: 1 mg daily.

Alternatives:

References:
1. Pharmaceutical manufacturer prescribing information, 1995.
2. Lacy C. Drug information handbook. Lexi-Comp Inc. Cleveland, OH, 1996.

HAEMOPHILUS B CONJUGATE VACCINE　　L3

Trade: HibTITER, Haemophilus B Vaccine, Hiberix, ProHIBiT, OmniHIB

Other Trades: PedvaxHIB, Hib Titer, Act-HIB

Category: H. influenza Vaccine

Haemophilus B conjugate (Hib) vaccine is a purified capsular polysaccharide vaccine made from Haemophilus influenza bacteria. It is non-infective. It is currently recommended for initial immunizations in children at 2 months, and at 2 month intervals, for a total of 3 injections.[1] A booster is recommended at 12–15 months. Although there are no reasons for administering to adult mothers, it would not be contraindicated in breastfeeding mothers.

Pregnancy Risk	C		Lactation Risk	L3
T ½	=		M/P	=
Vd	=		PB	=
Tmax	=		Oral	=
MW	=		pKa	=

Adult Concerns: Itching, skin rash, injection site reaction, vomiting, fever. Few anaphylactoid-type reaction.

Pediatric Concerns: Itching, skin rash, injection site reaction, vomiting, fever. Few anaphylactoid-type reaction.

Drug Interactions: Decreased immunogenicity when used with immunosuppressive agents. Immunoglobulins within 1 month may decrease antibody production.

Relative Infant Dose:

Adult Dose:

Alternatives:

References:
1. Pharmaceutical manufacturer prescribing information, 1996.

HALAZEPAM   L3

Trade: Paxipam

Other Trades:

Category: Benzodiazepine antianxiety drug

Halazepam is a benzodiazepine used to treat anxiety disorders. Halazepam is metabolized to desmethyldiazepam, which has an elimination half-life of 50–100 hours.[1] Although no information is available on halazepam levels in human milk, it should be similar to diazepam.

The benzodiazepine family, as a rule, is not ideal for breastfeeding mothers due to relatively long half-lives and the development of dependence. However, it is apparent that the shorter-acting benzodiazepines (lorazepam, alprazolam) are safest during lactation provided their use is short-term or intermittent, low dose, and after the first week of life.

Pregnancy Risk	D		Lactation Risk	L3
T ½	= 14 hours		M/P	=
Vd	= 1.0 l/kg		PB	= High
Tmax	= 1–3 hours		Oral	= Complete
MW	= 353		pKa	=

Adult Concerns: Sedation, bradycardia, euphoria, disorientation, confusion, nausea, constipation, hypotension.

Pediatric Concerns: None reported, but with diazepam some reports of lethargy, sedation, poor suckling have been found. Similar effects may be expected with halazepam.

Drug Interactions: Concurrent use of halazepam with other benzodiazepines such as zolpidem, or barbiturates such as phenobarbital, or opioid analgesics such as morphine, hydrocodone, oxycodone, hydromorphone may cause additive respiratory or CNS depression. Use with St. john's wort may decrease efficacy of halazepam.

Relative Infant Dose:

Adult Dose: 20–40 mg three to four times daily.

Alternatives: Alprazolam, lorazepam

References:
1. Pharmaceutical manufacturer prescribing information, 1995.

HALOPERIDOL   L3

Trade: Haldol

Other Trades: Serenace, Apo-Haloperidol, Haldol, Novo-Peridol, Peridol

Category: Antipsychotic

Haloperidol is a potent antipsychotic agent that is reported to increase prolactin levels in some patients. In one study of a woman treated for puerperal hypomania and receiving 5 mg twice daily, the concentration of haloperidol in milk was 0.0, 23.5, 18.0, and 3.25 µg/L on day 1, 6, 7, and 21 respectively.[1] The corresponding maternal plasma levels were 0, 40, 26, and 4 µg/L on day 1, 6, 7, and 21 respectively. The milk/plasma ratios were 0.58, 0.69, and 0.81 on days 6, 7, and 21 respectively. After 4 weeks of therapy the infant showed no symptoms of sedation and was feeding well. In another study after a mean daily dose of 29.2 mg, the concentration of haloperidol in breastmilk was 5 µg/L at 11 hours post-dose.[2]

In a study of 3 women on chronic haloperidol therapy receiving 3, 4, and 6 mg daily, milk levels were reported to be 32, 17, and 4.7 µg/L.[3] The latter levels (4.7) were taken from a patient believed to be noncompliant. Since the levels in milk are significant, some caution is recommended in breastfeeding mothers. In another study of 9 mothers receiving 1 to 40 mg/day haloperidol, breastmilk samples were randomly collected 12–15 hours after the dose. Levels in milk ranged from undetectable to 24.9 µg/L and were interestingly, not correlated with the dose.[4] In four of these infants, serum concentrations ranged from 0.8 to 2.1 µg/L.

Pregnancy Risk	C	Lactation Risk	L3
T ½	= 12–38 hours	M/P	= 0.58–0.81
Vd	= 18–30 l/kg	PB	= 92%
Tmax	= 2–6 hours	Oral	= 60%
MW	= 376	pKa	= 8.3

Adult Concerns: Extrapyramidal symptoms, sedation, anemia, tachycardia, hypotension.

Pediatric Concerns: None reported via milk. Observe for sedation, weakness.

Drug Interactions: Carbamazepine may increase metabolism and decrease effectiveness of haloperidol. CNS depressants may increase adverse effects. Epinephrine may cause hypotension. Concurrent use with lithium has caused acute encephalopathy syndromes.

Relative Infant Dose: 0.2%–12%

Adult Dose: 0.5–5 mg two to three times daily.

Alternatives: Risperidone, Olanzapine, Aripiprazole

References:
1. Whalley LJ, Blain PG, Prime JK. Haloperidol secreted in breast milk. Br Med J (Clin Res Ed) 1981; 282(6278): 1746–1747.
2. Stewart RB, Karas B, Springer PK. Haloperidol excretion in human milk. Am J Psychiatry 1980; 137(7): 849–850.
3. Ohkubo T, Shimoyama R, Sugawara K. Measurement of haloperidol in human breast milk by high-performance liquid chromatography. J Pharm Sci 1992; 81(9): 947–949.
4. Yoshida K, Smith B, Craggs M, Kumar R. Neuroleptic drugs in breast-milk: a study of pharmacokinetics and of possible adverse effects in breast-fed infants. Psychol Med. 1998 Jan; 28(1): 81–91.

HALOTHANE   L2

Trade: Fluothane

Other Trades: Fluothane

Category: Anesthetic gas

Halothane is an anesthetic gas similar to enflurane, methoxyflurane, and isoflurane. Approximately 60–80% is rapidly eliminated by exhalation the first 24 hours postoperatively, and only 15% is actually metabolized by the liver. Cote reviewed the secretion of halothane in breastmilk.[1] After a 3 hour surgery, only 2 ppm was detected in milk. At another exposure in one week, only 0.83 and 1.9 ppm were found. The authors assessed the exposure to the infant as negligible. Halothane is probably stored in the adipose tissue and eliminated for several days. There are no available data on the oral bioavailability of halothane. Pumping and dumping milk the first 4 hours postoperatively should be sufficient to eliminate any risks.

Pregnancy Risk	C	Lactation Risk	L2
T½	=	M/P	=
Vd	= 1 l/kg	PB	=
Tmax	= 10–20 minutes	Oral	=
MW	= 197	pKa	=

Adult Concerns: Nausea, vomiting, sedation, transient hepatotoxicity.

Pediatric Concerns: None reported.

Drug Interactions: When used with rifampin, or phenytoin, may have increased risk of hepatotoxicity.

Relative Infant Dose:

Adult Dose:

Alternatives:

References:

1. Cote CJ, Kenepp NB, Reed SB, Strobel GE. Trace concentrations of halothane in human breast milk. Br J Anaesth 1976; 48(6): 541–543.

HEMIN   L3

Trade: Panhematin

Other Trades: Heminevrin, Normosang

Category: Blood modifier

Intravenous hemin is used to treat acute intermittent porphyria by inhibiting delta-aminolevulinic acid synthetase, the enzyme that regulates the heme/porphyrin synthesis pathway.[1] No data are available on the levels in breast milk. However, this is a large molecular weight protein that is unlikely to enter the milk compartment, nor be orally bioavailable to an infant.

Pregnancy Risk	C		Lactation Risk	L3
T ½	=		M/P	=
Vd	=		PB	= High
Tmax	=		Oral	= Nil
MW	= 616		pKa	=

Adult Concerns: Adverse effects include pyrexia, leukocytosis, and phlebitis.

Pediatric Concerns: No data are available. Probably unable to enter milk. Would not be orally bioavailable.

Drug Interactions:

Relative Infant Dose:

Adult Dose: 1–4 mg/kg/day administered over 10–15 minutes for 3–14 days

Alternatives:

References:

1. Pharmaceutical manufacturer prescribing information, 2008.

HEPARIN   L1

Trade: Heparin

Other Trades: Hepalean, Canusal, Heplok, Pularin

Category: Anticoagulant

Heparin is an anticoagulant. It is a large protein molecule that is used subcutaneously, intramuscular, and intravenously. Due to its high molecular weight (range= 12,000–15,000 daltons),[1] it is unlikely any would transfer into breastmilk. Any present in milk would be rapidly destroyed in the gastric contents of the infant.

Pregnancy Risk	C	Lactation Risk	L1
T ½	= 1–2 hours	M/P	=
Vd	=	PB	=
Tmax	= 20 minutes	Oral	= Nil
MW	= 12–15,000	pKa	= 3.5–4.0

Adult Concerns: Hemorrhage.

Pediatric Concerns: None reported via milk.

Drug Interactions: Increased toxicity with NSAIDS, aspirin, dipyridamole, hydroxychloroquine.

Relative Infant Dose:

Adult Dose: 4,000–5,000 units every 4 hours

Alternatives:

References:
1.   McEvoy GE. (ed): AFHS Drug Information. New York, NY: 2003.

HEPATITIS A + HEPATITIS B VACCINE   L3

Trade: Twinrix
Other Trades:
Category: Vaccine

Hepatitis A + Hepatitis B vaccine combination is used for the prevention of hepatitis A and Hepatitis B infection.[1] It contains the hepatitis A vaccine as well as the recombinant Hepatitis B vaccine. It is used in those 18 years of age and older. It is administered in a 3-dose vaccine series at 0,1 and 6 months. Hepatitis A vaccine is prepared from inactivated Hepatitis A virus. There is no contraindication for receiving the vaccine during breastfeeding. Hepatitis B vaccine is an inactivated non-infectious hepatitis B surface antigen vaccine. It can be used in pediatric patients at birth. No data are available on its use in breastfeeding mothers, but it is unlikely to produce untoward effects on a breastfeeding infant since it is an inactivated virus. Hepatitis A + Hepatitis B bivalent vaccine is probably compatible with breastfeeding.

Pregnancy Risk	C	Lactation Risk	L3
T ½	=	M/P	=
Vd	=	PB	=
Tmax	=	Oral	=
MW	=	pKa	=

Adult Concerns: Redness, swelling tenderness, pain at the site of injection, headache, fatigue, diarrhea, upper respiratory tract infection, seizures, hypersensitivity reactions.

Pediatric Concerns:

Drug Interactions: Concurrent administration with corticosteroids, immunosuppressant agents, anti-cancer drugs may reduce its efficacy.

Relative Infant Dose:

Adult Dose: 1 mL intramuscular.

Alternatives:

References:
1. Pharmaceutical manufacturer prescribing information, 2011.

HEPATITIS A INFECTION   L3

Trade:

Other Trades:

Category: Syndrome

The Hepatitis A virus (HAV) belongs to the family of picornaviruses.[1] The most common mode of transmission is feco-oral. It is therefore more common in underdeveloped countries where hygiene is a regular source of concern. Other modes include transmission through contaminated food, transfusion of infected blood products, transplacental transmission,[2] and perinatal transmission.[3] In the United States the most common risk factors include ingestion of contaminated food, close contact with a child/children at a day care center, international travel, male homosexuality and use of intravenous drugs. Hepatitis A infection is an acute, self-limiting illness characterized by malaise, fever, anorexia and jaundice. It should also be noted that hepatitis A infection in children less than 6 years of age is asymptomatic 70% of the time.[1] A majority of the adult population is immune to Hepatitis A due to prior exposure. Fulminant hepatitis A infection is rare in infants and young children; chronic infection does not occur and a carrier state is unknown. Once infection occurs, viral shedding continues from onset up to 3 weeks.

No reports were found in the literature of direct transmission of hepatitis A virus in breast milk. Therefore, in view of the potential benefits of breastfeeding, it is recommended that a lactating mother with acute hepatitis A infection may continue to breastfeed. However, it is of prime importance to ensure that she take all necessary sanitary precautions to minimize feco-oral transmission to the infant. Measures such as regular handwashing before holding the baby or coming in contact with items or clothing belonging to the infant should be undertaken. Unless the mother is jaundiced and acutely ill, breastfeeding can continue without interruption.[4] Note that in infected children or infants, viral shedding can occur in their stools, despite being asymptomatic. Therefore, care givers of infected children at home and at day care centers should be cautious and maintain all hygienic and sanitary precautions to avoid exposure.

Hepatitis A vaccine and lactation: Since the hepatitis A vaccine is an inactivated vaccine, it is considered probably safe in lactating women. Therefore, lactating women travelling to endemic areas are recommended to receive the vaccine as per the general travel immunization guidelines.

Pregnancy Risk	Safer	Lactation Risk	L3
T ½	=	M/P	=
Vd	=	PB	=
Tmax	=	Oral	=
MW	=	pKa	=

Adult Concerns: Jaundice, fever, malaise.

Pediatric Concerns: None reported. Protect with gamma globulin injection.

Drug Interactions:

Relative Infant Dose:

Adult Dose:

Alternatives:

References:
1.   AAP CoID: Hepatitis A. In: Red book: 2009 Report of the committee on Infectious Diseases. Edited by Pickering LK BC, Kimberlin DW, Long SS, 29 edn; 2009: 329–337.
2.   Leikin E, Lysikiewicz A, Garry D, Tejani N: Intrauterine transmission of hepatitis A virus. Obstet Gynecol 1996, 88(4 Pt 2): 690–691.
3.   Motte A, Blanc J, Minodier P, Colson P: Acute hepatitis A in a pregnant woman at delivery. Int J Infect Dis 2009, 13(2): e49–51.
4.   Gartner L. Personal communication, 1997.

HEPATITIS A VACCINE   L3

Trade: Havrix, Vaqta

Other Trades:

Category: Vaccine

Hepatitis A vaccine is indicated for protection against hepatitis A infection. There are two hepatitis A vaccines approved by the FDA for use in the U. S., Vaqta and Havrix.[1,2] Both vaccines are made from inactivated hepatitis A virus. Both vaccine doses for adults are 1 mL initially then a booster dose of 1 mL between 6 and 12 months after the first dose. For children, Vaqta recommends an initial dose of 0.5 mL for children 2 to 17 years of age and a booster of 0.5 mL between 6 to 18 months after the initial dose. Havrix also recommends 0.5 mL for both doses but the booster should be given between 6 and 12 months of age. Seroconversion occurs within one month in 99% of cases and is expected to provide protective immunity for 20 years. Children should receive prophylaxis with the vaccine starting at 2 years of age for prevention of disease. The only contraindications to use of hepatitis A vaccine are hypersensitivity to the components. The vaccine is not approved for children under 2 years of age. Hepatitis A vaccine should not be administered with live vaccines. Travelers should be vaccinated at least one month prior to departure. For post exposure prophylaxis, the CDC recommends the patient be tested for IgM antibody to confirm Hepatitis A infection before treating any contacts of the patient. If positive, household and sexual contacts should receive immune globulin 0.02 mL/kg within two weeks of exposure. If the person received the vaccine at least one month before exposure, then they do not need the immune globulin. The vaccine should be administered the same day as the immune globulin. Common side effects of the vaccine include headache, fever, malaise, and local injection site reactions. There is no contraindication for receiving the vaccine during breastfeeding.

Pregnancy Risk	C	Lactation Risk	L3
T ½	=	M/P	=
Vd	=	PB	=
Tmax	=	Oral	=
MW	=	pKa	=

Adult Concerns: Pain at injection site, fever, headache, drowsiness, loss of appetite, fatigue, nausea, vomiting, rash, cough, otitis media, conjunctivitis, hypersensitivity.

Pediatric Concerns:

Drug Interactions:

Relative Infant Dose:

Adult Dose:

Alternatives:

References:
1. Duff B, Duff P. Hepatitis A vaccine: ready for prime time. Obstet Gynecol. 1998 Mar; 91(3): 468–71. Review.
2. Pharmaceutical manufacturer prescribing information, 2011.

HEPATITIS B IMMUNE GLOBULIN   L2

Trade: H-BIG, HEP-B-Gammagee, Hyperhep

Other Trades:

Category: Anti-Hepatitis B Immune globulins

Hepatitis B immune globulin (HBIG) is a sterile solution of immunoglobulin (10–18% protein) containing a high titer of antibodies to hepatitis B surface antigen.[1] It is most commonly used as prophylaxis therapy for infants born to hepatitis B surface antigen positive mothers. The carrier state can be prevented in about 75% of such infections in newborns given HBIG immediately after birth. HBIG is generally administered to infants born to HBsAg positive mothers who wish to breastfeed. The prophylactic dose for newborns is 0.5 mL IM (thigh) as soon after birth as possible, preferably within 1 hour.[2] The infant should also be immunized with Hepatitis B vaccine (0.5 mL IM) within 12 hours of birth (use separate site), and again at 1 and 6 months. Its use in a breastfeeding mother would not harm a breastfeeding infant.

Pregnancy Risk	C	Lactation Risk	L2
T ½	=	M/P	=
Vd	=	PB	=
Tmax	= 1–6 days	Oral	= None
MW	=	pKa	=

Adult Concerns: Pain at injection site, erythema, rash, dizziness, malaise.

Pediatric Concerns: Pain at injection site, erythema, rash.

Drug Interactions:

Relative Infant Dose:

Adult Dose: 0.06 mL/kg post-exposure X 3 over 6 weeks

Alternatives:

References:
1. Pharmaceutical manufacturer prescribing information, 1995.
2. Lawrence RA. Breastfeeding: A guide for the medical profession. St. Louis: Mosby Publishers, 1994.

HEPATITIS B INFECTION   L4

Trade: Hepatitis B Infection

Other Trades:

Category: Hepatitis B exposure

Hepatitis B virus (HBV) is a DNA virus belonging to the family hepadnaviridae.[1] Its antigenic structure is unique and is of prime diagnostic significance. Mode of transmission is mainly through blood and tissue fluids. The virus has been found to exist in human milk, serum, semen and saliva. Accordingly, various modes of transmission have been reported such as via transfusion of infected blood and blood products, use of contaminated needles, sharing of contaminated needles by illicit intravenous drug abusers, sexual contact, both heterosexual and homosexual; as well as perinatal transmission. Interestingly, transmission by sharing of razors and toothbrushes is also known.[1] HBV is one among the many carcinogenic viruses known to man, feared for its potential to cause hepatocellular carcinoma (liver cancer).[1] Hepatitis B virus (HBV) causes a wide spectrum of infections, ranging from a mild asymptomatic form to a fulminant fatal hepatitis. Chronic infection and carrier status is also known to occur.

Infants of mothers who are HBV positive (HBsAg) should be given hepatitis B immune globulin (HBIG) (preferably within 12 hours of birth) and a Hepatitis B vaccination at birth, which is believed to effectively reduce the risk of post-natal transmission, particularly via blood or body fluids from the mother.[4] While present in milk, it is not clear if HBV is infectious. These injections should be followed by the complete hepatitis B vaccine series as per the routine child immunization schedule.

Hepatitis B antigen has been detected in breastmilk.[2,3,4] Thus far, several older studies have indicated that breastfeeding poses no additional risk of transmission if these immunizations are completed, and thus far no cases of horizontal transmission of Hepatitis B via breastmilk have been reported following immunization.[5,6,7] According to the World Health Organization, The risk of transmission associated with breast milk is negligible compared to the high risk of exposure to maternal blood and body fluids at birth, and hepatitis B vaccination will substantially reduce perinatal transmission and virtually eliminate any risk of transmission through breastfeeding or breastmilk feeding.

Pregnancy Risk	Possibly Hazardous	Lactation Risk	L4
T ½	=	M/P	=
Vd	=	PB	=
Tmax	=	Oral	=
MW	=	pKa	=

Adult Concerns: Hepatitis, increased risk of liver cancer.

Pediatric Concerns: None reported if immunized with HBIG and HB vaccination.

Drug Interactions:

Relative Infant Dose:

Adult Dose:

Alternatives:

References:
1. AAP CoID: Hepatitis B. In: Red Book: 2009 Report of the Committee on Infectious Diseases. Edited by Pickering LK BC, Kimberlin DW, Long SS, 28 edn; 2009: 337–356.
2. Boxall EH, Flewett TH, Dane DS, Cameron CH, MacCallum FO, Lee TW. Letter: Hepatitis-B surface antigen in breast milk. Lancet 1974; 2(7887): 1007–1008.
3. Beasley RP, Stevens CE, Shiao IS, Meng HC. Evidence against breast-feeding as a mechanism for vertical transmission of hepatitis B. Lancet 1975; 2(7938): 740–741.
4. Woo D, Cummins M, Davies PA, Harvey DR, Hurley R, Waterson AP. Vertical transmission of hepatitis B surface antigen in carrier mothers in two west London hospitals. Arch Dis Child 1979; 54(9): 670–675.
5. Hill JB, Sheffield JS, Kim MJ, Alexander JM, Sercely B, Wendel GD: Risk of hepatitis B transmission in breast-fed infants of chronic hepatitis B carriers. Obstet Gynecol 2002, 99(6): 1049–1052.
6. Qiu L, Binns CW, Zhao Y, Zhang K, Xie X: Hepatitis B and breastfeeding in Hangzhou, Zhejiang Province, People's Republic of China. Breastfeed Med 2010, 5(3): 109–112.
7. Shi Z, Yang Y, Wang H, Ma L, Schreiber A, Li X, Sun W, Zhao X, Yang X, Zhang L et al: Breastfeeding of newborns by mothers carrying hepatitis B virus: a meta-analysis and systematic review. Arch Pediatr Adolesc Med 2011, 165(9): 837–846.

HEPATITIS B VACCINE   L2

Trade: Heptavax-B, Energix-B, Recombivax HB

Other Trades:

Category: Hepatitis B vaccination

Hepatitis B vaccine is an inactivated non-infectious hepatitis B surface antigen vaccine. It can be used in pediatric patients at birth. No data are available on its use in breastfeeding mothers, but it is unlikely to produce untoward effects on a breastfeeding infant since it is an inactivated virus. Hepatitis B vaccination is approximately 80–95% effective in preventing acute hepatitis B infections.[1,2] It requires at least 3 immunizations and the immunity lasts about 5–7 years. In infants born of HB surface antigen positive mothers, the American Academy of Pediatrics recommends that hepatitis B vaccine (along with HBIG) should be administered to the infant within 1–12 hours of birth (0.5 mL IM) and again at 1 and 6 months. If so administered, breastfeeding poses no additional risk for acquisition of HBV by the infant.

Pregnancy Risk	C		Lactation Risk	L2
T ½	=		M/P	=
Vd	=		PB	=
Tmax	=		Oral	=
MW	=		pKa	=

Adult Concerns: Pain at injection site, swelling, erythema, fever.

Pediatric Concerns: Fever, malaise, fatigue when directly injected. None reported via breastmilk.

Drug Interactions: Immunosuppressive agents would decrease effect.

Relative Infant Dose:

Adult Dose: 20 µg each for three injections over 7 months

Alternatives:

References:
1. Pharmaceutical manufacturer prescribing information, 1996.
2. American Academy of Pediatrics. Committee on Infectious Diseases. Red Book. 1997.

HEPATITIS C INFECTION   L3

Trade: Hepatitis C Infection, HCV

Other Trades:

Category: Hepatitis exposure

Hepatitis C virus (HCV) is an RNA virus belonging to the flaviviridae family.[1] The primary mode of spread is by parenteral route through exposure to HC V-contaminated blood or blood products. Besides this, sexual transmission of HCV has also been described, although rare. Infected individuals usually include illicit intravenous drug abusers and those that maintain sexual relations with multiple partners. In fact, 75% of those chronically infected with HCV are illicit drug abusers.[1] A small proportion of those infected also include health care professionals, hemophiliacs and those requiring hemodialysis. In addition, those who received blood and/or its products before 1992 are also at higher risk for acquiring the disease. Although perinatal transmission can occur, its incidence is known to be low (5–6%).[1,2,3] Symptoms of acute infection are anorexia, nausea, fatigue and jaundice. Majority of those infected become chronic asymptomatic carriers.

In one study of 17 HCV positive mothers, 11 of the 17 had HCV antibodies present in milk, but zero of the 17 had HCV-RNA in milk after birth, suggesting that the virus itself was not detected in milk.[4] However, in later studies, although HCV RNA and anti-HCV antibody have been detected in colostrum and breast milk, no greater risk of HCV transmission has been found in breastfed infants as compared to bottle-fed infants.[1,5–10] Currently a number of other studies have yet to document horizontal transmission of HCV by breastmilk.[11,12] Mothers infected with HCV should be advised that transmission of HCV by breastfeeding is possible but has not been documented. Available data seem to suggest an elevated risk of vertical transmission of HCV occurs in those co-infected with HIV and in women with elevated titers of HCV RNA. The risk of transmission of HCV via breastmilk in such cases is unknown at this time. In one study, while transmission of HCV was significantly high (21%) in HIV infected individuals, perinatal transmission of HCV was not associated with breastfeeding.[13] HCV-infected women should be counseled that transmission of HCV by breastfeeding is theoretically possible but has not yet been documented.[1,14]

The Centers for Disease Control (CDC) does not consider chronic hepatitis C infection in the mother as a contraindication to breastfeeding. The decision to breastfeed should be based largely on informed discussion between the mother and her health care provider. In view of the potential benefits of breastfeeding, a mother with HCV infection may continue to breastfeed. It may be prudent however, for mothers who are seropositive for HCV to abstain from breastfeeding if their nipples are cracked and bleeding.[1,15]

Pregnancy Risk	Possibly Hazardous	Lactation Risk	L3
T ½	=	M/P	=
Vd	=	PB	=
Tmax	=	Oral	=
MW	=	pKa	=

Adult Concerns: Cirrhosis and liver cancer

Pediatric Concerns:

Drug Interactions:

Relative Infant Dose:

Adult Dose:

Alternatives:

References:

1. AAP CoID: Hepatitis C. In: Red Book: 2009 Report of the Committee on Infectious Diseases. Edited by Pickering LK BC, Kimberlin DW, Long SS, 28 edn; 2009: 362.
2. Nagata I, Shiraki K. et. al. Mother to infant transmission of hepatitis C virus. J Pediatrics 1992; 120: 432–434.
3. Shiraki K, Ohto H, Inaba N, Fujisawa T, Tajiri H, Kanzaki S, Matsui A, Morishima T, Goto K, Kimura A et al: Guidelines for care of pregnant women carrying hepatitis C virus and their infants. Pediatr Int 2008, 50(1): 138–140.
4. Grayson ML, Braniff KM, Bowden DS, Turnidge JD. Breastfeeding and the risk of vertical transmission of hepatitis C virus. Med J Aust 1995; 163(2): 107.
5. Airoldi J, Berghella V: Hepatitis C and pregnancy. Obstet Gynecol Surv 2006, 61(10): 666–672.
6. Powell M, Bailey J, Maggio LA: Clinical inquiries. How should you manage children born to hepatitis C-positive women? J Fam Pract 2010, 59(5): 289–290.
7. Bhola K, McGuire W: Does avoidance of breast feeding reduce mother-to-infant transmission of hepatitis C virus infection? Arch Dis Child 2007, 92(4): 365–366.
8. Polywka S, Schroter M, Feucht HH, Zollner B, Laufs R: Low risk of vertical transmission of hepatitis C virus by breast milk. Clin Infect Dis 1999, 29(5): 1327–1329.
9. Ruiz-Extremera A, Salmeron J, Torres C, De Rueda PM, Gimenez F, Robles C, Miranda MT: Follow-up of transmission of hepatitis C to babies of human immunodeficiency virus-negative women: the role of breast-feeding in transmission. Pediatr Infect Dis J 2000, 19(6): 511–516.
10. Kumar RM, Shahul S. Role of breast-feeding in transmission of hepatitis C virus to infants of HCV-infected mothers. J Hepatol. 1998 Aug; 29(2): 191–7.

11. Lin HH, Kao JH, Hsu HY, Ni YH, Chang MH, Huang SC, Hwang LH, Chen PJ, Chen DS. Absence of infection in breast-fed infants born to hepatitis C virus-infected mothers. J Pediatr 1995; 126(4): 589–591.

12. Zanetti. et. al. Mother to infant transmission of hepatitis C virus. Lancet 1995; 345(8945): 289–291.

13. Paccagnini S, Principi N, Massironi E, Tanzi E, Romano L, Muggiasca ML, Ragni MC, Salvaggio L. Perinatal transmission and manifestation of hepatitis C virus infection in a high risk population. Pediatr Infect Dis J 1995; 14(3): 195–199.

14. Lawrence RA. Breastfeeding: A guide for the medical profession. St. Louis: Mosby Publishers, 1994.

15. Mast EE. Mother-to-infant hepatitis C virus transmission and breastfeeding. Adv Exp Med Biol 2004; 554: 211–6.: 211–6.

HEPATITIS E VIRUS   L4

Trade: Hepatitis E

Other Trades:

Category: Infectious disease

Hepatitis E virus (HEV) is an RNA virus belonging to the family hepeviridae.[1] Mode of transmission is mainly by feco-oral route. Therefore, this infection is largely prevalent in developing countries where maintaining food and water hygiene is an everyday challenge. However, other modes of spread such as parenteral and vertical have also been reported.[2–5] In the United States, the only reported cases are those seen in travelers returning from countries endemic for HEV. A small proportion of the cases also include those infected with the hepatitis E virus of swine origin.[1,2] Hepatitis E infection is a self-limiting illness of acute onset associated with fever, malaise, anorexia, abdominal pain, jaundice and tea-coloured urine.[6]

A study was conducted to investigate the transmission of HEV through breast milk.[7] The colostrum samples from 93 mothers who were HEV infected were studied. All 93 samples revealed the presence of anti-HEV antibody and/or HEV RNA. However, the titres in the colostrum samples were much lower as compared to the maternal serum titres. Eighty-six of these women, who were anti-HEV positive but clinically asymptomatic at the time of delivery exclusively breast-fed their infants. Although anti-HEV antibody and/or HEV RNA was found in the colostrum of these women, their infants remained healthy until 3 months of age. The infants of the remaining 6 women with acute HEV illness at the time of delivery, developed symptomatic HEV illness and became anti-HEV antibody positive within 6–8 weeks of delivery. Also, the anti-HEV antibody titres in the breast milk samples of these women also correspondingly increased. However, none of these 6 infants were breast-fed, suggesting close contact and feco-oral transmission being the most probable route of spread. Therefore, the authors of this study suggest that asymptomatic women with low anti-HEV titres may safely breast feed their infants. However, in view of possible feco-oral spread due to close contact between mother and child, mothers should be counseled to maintain all sanitary and hygienic conditions while caring for their infants. Women who are clinically ill with high anti-HEV titres or high viral RNA load are suggested to refrain from breastfeeding in view of possible transmission by either feco-oral route or via contaminated breast milk.

In conclusion, the hepatitis E virus has been isolated in breastmilk, but the extent of its infectivity to the infant is still unknown. Feco-oral transmission still appears to be the primary mode of transmission, therefore, mothers with hepatitis E infection are encouraged to take all sanitary precautions while caring for their infants. Measures such as regular handwashing before holding the baby or coming in contact with items or clothing belonging to the infant are recommended. It is advisable that mothers with active, symptomatic HEV infection temporarily refrain from breastfeeding until the symptoms subside. HEV infection is a self-limiting illness, and unlike hepatitis B and C, is not known for chronicity and does not exist in carrier state.[1] Therefore, mothers may safely continue to breastfeed once the acute illness subsides.

Pregnancy Risk	Possibly Hazardous	Lactation Risk	L4
T ½	=	M/P	=
Vd	=	PB	=
Tmax	=	Oral	=
MW	=	pKa	=

Adult Concerns: Self-limiting illness of acute onset associated with fever, malaise, anorexia, abdominal pain, jaundice and tea-coloured urine.

Pediatric Concerns:

Drug Interactions:

Relative Infant Dose:

Adult Dose:

Alternatives:

References:
1. AAP CoID: Hepatitis E. In: Red Book: 2009 Report of the Committee on Infectious Diseases. Edited by Pickering LK BC, Kimberlin DW, Long SS, 28 edn; 2009: 362.
2. Aggarwal R, Naik S: Epidemiology of hepatitis E: current status. J Gastroenterol Hepatol 2009, 24(9): 1484–1493.
3. Acharya SK, Panda SK: Hepatitis E: water, water everywhere–now a global disease. J Hepatol 2011, 54(1): 9–11.
4. Fiore S, Savasi V: Treatment of viral hepatitis in pregnancy. Expert Opin Pharmacother 2009, 10(17): 2801–2809.
5. Khuroo MS, Kamili S, Jameel S: Vertical transmission of hepatitis E virus. Lancet 1995, 345(8956): 1025–1026.
6. Bazaco MC, Albrecht SA, Malek AM: Preventing foodborne infection in pregnant women and infants. Nurs Womens Health 2008, 12(1): 46–55.
7. Chibber RM, Usmani MA, Al-Sibai MH: Should HEV infected mothers breast feed? Arch Gynecol Obstet 2004, 270(1): 15–20.

HERBAL SUPPLEMENT/TEAS   L4

Trade:

Other Trades:

Category: Herbal Remedy

Herbal supplements fall under the definition of botanicals, which are plants or plant parts that are valued for medicinal or therapeutic properties, flavor, and/or scent. Products made from botanicals that are used to maintain or improve health may be called herbal products, botanical products, or phytomedicines. Many herbal products are classified as dietary supplements, which means that they meet the definitions set forth by the FDA. Substances under this definition must be intended to supplement the diet, contain one or more dietary ingredients (including vitamins, minerals, herbs, amino acids, and other substances), be intended to be taken orally, and be labeled as being a dietary supplement. As of 2010, the FDA has enforced Good Manufacturing Processes on all dietary supplement manufacturers. These measures were put in place to ensure that manufacturers guarantee a product's identity, purity, and strength. These products are not evaluated by the FDA and are not intended to diagnose, treat, cure, or prevent any disease.[1]

It is recommended that a breastfeeding mother consult her physician or a qualified herbal specialist before beginning any herbal or homeopathic therapy. At this time there is insufficient data to determine safety regarding the wide array of products covered under this heading.

Pregnancy Risk	Possibly Hazardous	Lactation Risk	L4
T ½	=	M/P	=
Vd	=	PB	=
Tmax	=	Oral	=
MW	=	pKa	=

Adult Concerns:

Pediatric Concerns:

Drug Interactions:

Relative Infant Dose:

Adult Dose:

Alternatives:

References:

1. Dietary Supplements: Background Information. National Institutes of Health: Office of Dietary Supplements Website. Bethesda, MD. Reviewed 6/24/2011. Accessed 6/27/2011. http: //ods. od. nih. gov/factsheets/dietarysupplements/.

HEROIN   L5

Trade: Heroin

Other Trades:

Category: Narcotic analgesic

Heroin is diacetyl-morphine (diamorphine), a prodrug that is rapidly converted by plasma cholinesterases to 6-acetylmorphine and more slowly to morphine. With oral use, rapid and complete first-pass metabolism occurs in the liver. The half-life of diamorphine is only 3 minutes, with the large majority of the prodrug converted to morphine. Peak levels of morphine occur in about 30 minutes following oral doses. As an analgesic, morphine is generally considered to be an ideal choice for breastfeeding mothers when used postoperatively or for other forms of pain "in normal dosage ranges". Unfortunately, addicts and recreational users may use extraordinarily large doses of heroin, and at such doses, it is likely to be very dangerous for a breastfed infant. Heavily dependent users should probably be advised against breastfeeding and their infants converted to formula. While it could be argued that recreational users could continue to breastfeed if they avoid doing so while under the influence of the heroin or prior to its use, this still may not be advisable as it requires some understanding of the kinetics of morphine and its elimination. Heroin, as is morphine, is known to transfer into breastmilk.[1,2,3]

Pregnancy Risk	B	Lactation Risk	L5
T ½	= 1.5–2 hours	M/P	= 2.45
Vd	= 25 l/kg	PB	= 35%
Tmax	= 0.5–1 hour	Oral	= Poor
MW	= 369	pKa	= 7.6

Adult Concerns: Sedation, hypotension, euphoria, nausea, vomiting, dry mouth, respiratory depression, constipation.

Pediatric Concerns: Caution, observe for sedation. Tremors, restlessness, vomiting, poor feeding.

Drug Interactions:

Relative Infant Dose:

Adult Dose:

Alternatives:

References:
1. Feilberg VL, Rosenborg D, Broen CC, Mogensen JV. Excretion of morphine in human breast milk. Acta Anaesthesiol Scand 1989; 33(5): 426–428.
2. Wittels B, Scott DT, Sinatra RS. Exogenous opioids in human breast milk and acute neonatal neurobehavior: a preliminary study. Anesthesiology 1990; 73(5): 864–869.
3. American Academy of Pediatrics, Committee on Drugs. Transfer of drugs and other chemicals into human milk. Pediatrics 2001; 108(3): 776–89.

HERPES SIMPLEX VIRUS   L4

Trade:

Other Trades:

Category: Herpes simplex type I, II

The Herpes Simplex virus (HSV) belongs to the family of herpes viruses and consists of two distinct species, HSV-1 and HSV-2. HSV-1 is transmitted by direct contact with either the infected lesions or infected oral secretions. HSV-2 is sexually transmitted and occurs as a result of direct contact with either the infected genital lesions or infected genital secretions.

A number of cases of herpes simplex transmission via breastmilk have been reported.[1-6] In one such report, breast milk samples obtained from 34 lactating women were investigated for the presence of HSV DNA by in situ hybridization technique. Sixteen out of the thirty-four milk samples were found to be positive for HSV DNA. DNA of both HSV-1 and HSV-2 were found. This study implies that transmission of the herpes simplex virus through breast milk is a possibility and this may play a role in causing HSV infections in infants.[3] HSV-1 and HSV-2 have also been isolated from human milk, even in the absence of vesicular lesions or drainage.[4,5] In one case, a breastfed infant who was born healthy developed disseminated HSV illness postnatally.[1] It is believed that the infection was acquired via breast milk since HSV-1 was detected in the mother's milk sample. The mother however, did not give any history of herpes infection. Therefore, it is advisable that due caution be exercised in breastfeeding women with active herpes lesions of any kind, oral or genital. Lactating mothers, especially those with peri-oral herpetic lesions, should be counseled about the modes of transmission of herpes and should be warned against any direct contact between the infant and the oral lesions, such as the kind that occurs while kissing or nuzzling the infant. While holding the infant close, any active lesions anywhere should be appropriately covered to avoid direct contact with the infant.

In general, breastmilk does not appear to be a common mode of transmission of the herpes simplex virus. However, women with active lesions on one breast should avoid breast feeding from the affected breast until the lesions completely dry up, and may continue to breastfeed from the opposite breast. Other active lesions on the body should be adequately covered to avoid contact with the infant.

Pregnancy Risk	Possibly Hazardous	Lactation Risk	L4
T ½	=	M/P	=
Vd	=	PB	=
Tmax	=	Oral	=
MW	=	pKa	=

Adult Concerns: Skin eruptions, CNS changes, gingivostomatitis, skin lesions, fever.

Pediatric Concerns: Transfer of virus to infants has been reported, but may be from exposure to lesions. Cover lesions on breast.

Drug Interactions:

Relative Infant Dose:

Adult Dose: N/A

Alternatives:

References:
1. Dunkle LM, Schmidt RR, O'Connor DM. Neonatal herpes simplex infection possibly acquired via maternal breast milk. Pediatrics 1979; 63(2): 250–251.
2. Quinn PT, Lofberg JV. Maternal herpetic breast infection: another hazard of neonatal herpes simplex. Med J Aust 1978; 2(9): 411–412.
3. Kotronias D, Kapranos N: Detection of herpes simplex virus DNA in maternal breast milk by in situ hybridization with tyramide signal amplification. In Vivo 1999, 13(6): 463–466.
4. Light IJ. Postnatal acquisition of herpes simplex virus by the newborn infant: a review of the literature. Pediatrics 1979; 63(3): 480–482.
5. Sullivan-Bolyai JZ, Fife KH, Jacobs RF, Miller Z, Corey L. Disseminated neonatal herpes simplex virus type 1 from a maternal breast lesion. Pediatrics 1983; 71(3): 455–457.
6. Whitley RJ, Nahmias AJ, Visintine AM, Fleming CL, Alford CA. The natural history of herpes simplex virus infection of mother and newborn. Pediatrics 1980; 66(4): 489–494.

HEXACHLOROPHENE   L4

Trade: Septisol, Phisohex, Septi-Soft
Other Trades: Sapoderm, Dermalex
Category: Antiseptic scrub

Hexachlorophene is an antibacterial that is an effective inhibitor of gram positive organisms.[1] It is generally used topically as a surgical scrub and sometimes vaginally in mothers. Due to its lipophilic structure, it is well absorbed through intact and denuded skin producing significant levels in plasma, brain, fat, and other tissues in both adults and infants. It has been implicated in causing brain lesions (spongiform myelinopathy), blindness, and respiratory failure in both animals and humans.[2] Although there are no studies reporting concentrations of this compound in breastmilk, it is probably transferred to some degree. Transfer into breastmilk is known to occur in rodents. Topical use in infants is absolutely discouraged due to the high absorption of hexachlorophene through an infant's skin and proven toxicity.

Pregnancy Risk	C	Lactation Risk	L4
T ½	=	M/P	=
Vd	=	PB	=
Tmax	=	Oral	= Complete
MW	= 407	pKa	= 8.79

Adult Concerns: Seizures, respiratory failure, hypotension, brain lesions, blindness in overdose.

Pediatric Concerns: Following direct application, CNS injury, seizures, irritability have been reported in neonates. Toxicity via breastmilk has not been reported.

Drug Interactions:

Relative Infant Dose:

Adult Dose:

Alternatives:

References:
1. Pharmaceutical manufacturer prescribing information, 1996.
2. Tyrala EE, Hillman LS, Hillman RE, Dodson WE. Clinical pharmacology of hexachlorophene in newborn infants. J Pediatr 1977; 91(3): 481–486.

HEXYLRESORCINOL   L3

Trade:
Other Trades:
Category: Antiseptic, antihelmintic

Hexylresorcinol is an antiseptic that is commonly used in lozenge and oral spray preparations for the treatment of sore throat. It has been used as an antihelmintic in the past, though it is no longer greatly used in that capacity. This drug is absorbed both orally and through the skin. There are no reports of toxicity in humans from overdose of this medication.[1] Because its oral bioavailability is only 30%, it is unlikely that it would attain significant levels in infant's plasma or cause clinical effects in the breastfed infant.

Pregnancy Risk	Probably Safe	Lactation Risk	L3
T ½	=	M/P	=
Vd	=	PB	=
Tmax	=	Oral	= 30%
MW	= 194.3	pKa	=

Adult Concerns: Anaphylaxis, heart damage, respiratory irritation, nausea, vomiting, gastrointestinal irritation, liver damage, renal damage, skin irritation.

Pediatric Concerns: None reported.

Drug Interactions: No known drug interactions

Relative Infant Dose:

Adult Dose: 1 lozenge every 2 hours.

Alternatives:

References:
1. Hazardous Substances Data Bank Website. National Institutes of Health. U. S. National Library of Medicine. Bethesda, MD. Updated 2/4/2011. Accessed 7/25/2011. http: //toxnet. nlm. nih. gov/cgi-bin/sis/htmlgen?HSDB.

HISTAMINE   L3

Trade:

Other Trades:

Category: Diagnostic agent for asthma and gastric function

Histamine[1] is a normal substance found in the mast cells and plays a major role in the allergic response, neurotransmission, gastric acid secretion and bronchial constriction. Physiologically, it interacts at any of three different cellular receptors– H_1, H_2, and H_3. These receptors are in high concentrations in bronchi (H_1), gastric and other tissues (H_2, H_3). Histamine is primarily stored in the mast cells, which when destabilized by allergens, etc., releases histamine into the tissues and initiates the normal response to histamine. Histamine is primarily used pharmacologically as a diagnostic agent, to induce gastric acid release, or more often, stimulate bronchoconstriction in the diagnosis of asthma. Histamine is rapidly metabolized with a plasma half-life less than 3 minutes. No data are available on its transfer to human milk, but it is probably minimal. Waiting as little as 2 hours following exposure would largely eliminate all risks associated with the use of histamine in a breastfeeding mother.

Pregnancy Risk	C	Lactation Risk	L3
T ½	= <3 minutes	M/P	=
Vd	=	PB	=
Tmax	=	Oral	= Minimal
MW	= 307	pKa	= 6.9, 10.4

Adult Concerns: Side effects include flushing, vasodilation, hyper or hypotension, edema, tachycardia, headache, diarrhea, vomiting, hyperacidity, blurred vision, dizziness, bronchoconstriction, asthma symptoms.

Pediatric Concerns: None reported in breastfeeding infants. A 1–2 hour waiting period after the procedure is recommended.

Drug Interactions: Caution with use in asthmatics. Obviously, for diagnostic procedures, do not use with antihistamines.

Relative Infant Dose:

Adult Dose: Highly variable.

Alternatives:

References:
1. Pharmaceutical manufacturer prescribing information, 2005.

HIV INFECTION   L5

Trade: AIDS

Other Trades:

Category: Aids, HIV infections

The AIDS (HIV) virus has been isolated from human milk. In addition, recent reports from throughout the world have documented the transmission of HIV through human milk.[1,2,3] At least 9 or more cases in the literature currently suggest that HIV-1 is secreted and can be transmitted horizontally to the infant via breastmilk.[4,5] Although these studies clearly indicate a risk, currently no studies clearly estimate the exact risk associated with breastfeeding in HIV infected women. However, women who develop a primary HIV infection while breastfeeding may shed especially high concentrations of HIV viruses and pose a high risk of transmission to their infants. In some studies, the risk of transmission during primary infection was 29%. In various African populations, recent reports suggest the incremental risk of transmitting HIV via breastfeeding ranges from 3–12%.[6] Because the risk is now well documented, mothers infected with HIV in the USA and others countries with safe alternative sources of feeding should be advised not to breastfeed their infants.[7] Mothers at-risk for HIV should be screened and counseled prior to initiating breastfeeding.

Pregnancy Risk	Hazardous	Lactation Risk	L5 in developed countries
T ½	=	M/P	=
Vd	=	PB	=
Tmax	=	Oral	=
MW	=	pKa	=

Adult Concerns:

Pediatric Concerns: HIV transmission has been documented. HIV infected women are advised not to breastfeed.

Drug Interactions:

Relative Infant Dose:

Adult Dose:

Alternatives:

References:
1. Commitee on Pediatric AIDS. Human milk, breastfeeding, and transmission of human immunodeficiency virus in the United States. Pediatrics 1995; 96: 977–979.
2. Oxtoby MJ. Human immunodeficiency virus and other viruses in human milk: placing the issues in broader perspective. Pediatr Infect Dis J 1988; 7(12): 825–835.
3. Goldfarb J. Breastfeeding. AIDS and other infectious diseases. Clin Perinatol 1993; 20(1): 225–243.
4. Van de PP, Simonon A, Hitimana DG, Dabis F, Msellati P, Mukamabano B, Butera JB, Van Goethem C, Karita E, Lepage P. Infective and anti-infective properties of breastmilk from HIV-1-infected women. Lancet 1993; 341(8850): 914–918.
5. Dunn DT, Newell ML, Ades AE, Peckham CS. Risk of human immunodeficiency virus type 1 transmission through breastfeeding. Lancet 1992; 340(8819): 585–588.
6. St. Louis ME. et. al. The timing of HIV-1 transmission in an African setting. Presented at the First National Conference on Human Retroviruses and Related Infections. December 12–16; Washington DC. 1993.
7. Report of the committee on Infectious Diseases. American Academy of Pediatrics. 1994.

HOMATROPINE   L3

Trade: Homatromide, Novatropine, Arkitropin, Isopto Homatropine, Homatropaire

Other Trades: Acidobyl

Category: Antimuscarinic, Gastrointestinal Agent, Mydriatic-Cycloplegic

Homatropine belongs to the anti-muscarinic family of drugs, which are similar to atropine. Homatropine is rarely used today to treat duodenal or stomach ulcers or intestine problems. In rare instances, it may also be used to prevent nausea, vomiting, and motion sickness. There are no adequate and well-controlled studies or case reports of its use in breastfeeding women. However, the use of this product could produce significant drying, such as constipation, dry eyes, urinary retention, and other typical anticholinergic symptoms. It should not be used in patients with narrow angle glaucoma. The infrequent ophthalmic use of this product in breastfeeding mothers is probably not a contraindication to its use in breastfeeding women.

Pregnancy Risk	C		Lactation Risk	L3
T ½	=		M/P	=
Vd	=		PB	=
Tmax	=		Oral	=
MW	= 370		pKa	= 9.65

Adult Concerns: Observe for blurred vision, photophobia, irritation, increased ocular pressure, congestion. Do not use in patients with narrow angle glaucoma.

Pediatric Concerns: None yet reported. Systemic absorption via eyes is probably low to nil.

Drug Interactions: Avoid use with other anticholinergics such as atropine, and others. Avoid in patients with glaucoma.

Relative Infant Dose:

Adult Dose: Eye drops for refraction: instill 1 or 2 drops of homatropine 2% or 5%

Alternatives:

References:

HUMAN IMMUNE GLOBULIN IV | L2

Trade: Privigen, Flebogamma, Gammagard, Gammaplex, Carimune, Hizentra, Vivaglobin, Gammaked, Octagam

Other Trades:

Category: Treatment of primary immunodeficiency and chronic immune thrombocytopenia purpura

Intravenous Immunoglobulin (IVIG) is a blood product that is used in the treatment of immune deficiencies, inflammatory illnesses, and acute infections. Treatment is generally scheduled every three to four weeks and in autoimmune disorders, high doses (1–2 grams/kg) may used. Although there are limited data on its transfer into milk, we believe that the molecule is too large to enter into the milk compartment and therefore milk levels are low to undetectable.[1] This is a natural human immunoglobulin gm (IgG) product produced from pooled human plasma. It would not be orally bioavailable in humans.

Pregnancy Risk	C	Lactation Risk	L2
T ½	= 21–59 days	M/P	=
Vd	=	PB	=
Tmax	= Immediate (IV)	Oral	=
MW	=	pKa	=

Adult Concerns: (IVIG) For Primary Humoral Immunodeficiency: The most common adverse reactions are headache, pain, nausea, fatigue, chills, vomiting, joint swelling/effusion, pyrexia, and urticaria. Serious adverse reactions were hypersensitivity, chills, fatigue, dizziness, and increased body temperature. (IVIG) For Chronic ITP: The most common adverse reactions are headache, pyrexia/hyperthermia, positive direct antiglobulin test (DAT), anemia, vomiting, nausea, bilirubin conjugated increased, bilirubin unconjugated increased, hyperbilirubinemia, and increased blood lactate dehydrogenase. Serious adverse reactions include aseptic meningitis.

Pediatric Concerns: No major adverse reactions in breastfed infants in three studies. One case of transient rash in breastfed infant possibly caused by IVIG, following maternal administration.

Drug Interactions: Interferes with the immune response to live vaccines such as MMR vaccine, varicella vaccine, rotavirus vaccine and smallpox vaccine.

Relative Infant Dose:

Adult Dose:

Alternatives:

References:
1. Pharmaceutical Manufacturer Drug Information, 2011.

HUMAN IMMUNE GLOBULIN SC   L2

Trade: Hizentra

Other Trades:

Category: Treatment of primary immunodeficiency

Human Immune Globulin subcutaneous is indicated for the treatment of primary immunodeficiency. Treatment is generally weekly and the dose is based on previous plasma levels achieved with intravenous immune globulin (IVIG). The dose may be adjusted over time depending on clinical response and serum IgG trough levels. The serum IgG trough level should be drawn after 2 to 3 months of treatment. Although there are limited data on its transfer into milk, we believe that the molecule is too large to enter into the milk compartment and therefore milk levels are low to undetectable.[1] It would not be orally bioavailable in a human.

Pregnancy Risk	C		Lactation Risk	L2
T ½	= 21–59 days		M/P	=
Vd	=		PB	=
Tmax	= 2.9 days		Oral	=
MW	=		pKa	=

Adult Concerns: The most common adverse reactions that occur include local reactions (swelling, redness, heat, pain, and itching at the injection site), headache, vomiting, pain, and fatigue. The passive transfer of antibodies may lead to misinterpretation of the results of serological testing. The passive transfer of antibodies may also interfere with the response to live virus vaccines.

Pediatric Concerns:

Drug Interactions: Interferes with the immune response to live vaccines such as MMR vaccine, varicella vaccine, rotavirus vaccine and smallpox vaccine.

Relative Infant Dose:

Adult Dose:

Alternatives:

References:
1. Pharmaceutical manufacturer drug Information, 2011.

HUMAN PAPILLMOAVIRUS VACCINE QUADRAVALENT   L3

Trade: Gardasil (HPV4), Cervarix (HPV2)
Other Trades:
Category: HPV vaccine

This is a non-infectious recombinant vaccine prepared from the purified virus like particles from the major capsid protein of four different virus types (6,11,16, and 18). Current recommendations are to begin the series in 11– 26-year-old females, with 4 weeks between the first and second doses, and 12 weeks between the second and third doses.[1] Currently two HPV vaccines are licensed for use in the United States by the FDA. These vaccines are Gardasil and Cervarix. While both vaccines are equally effective against HPV types 16 and 18, only Gardasil has been found to be effective against HPV types 6 and 11. Gardasil is currently licensed for use in males and is also known to be effective in protecting against development of precancerous lesions of the vulva, vagina and anus. It is not known whether vaccine antigens or antibodies are excreted in human milk. One study showed an increase risk of serious adverse event, but was judged by the investigator to be non-vaccine related.[1] Also, a higher number of infants whose mothers received the vaccine had acute respiratory illnesses within 30 days after the vaccination.

Pregnancy Risk	B	Lactation Risk	L3
T ½	=	M/P	=
Vd	=	PB	=
Tmax	=	Oral	=
MW	=	pKa	=

Adult Concerns: Adverse effects included fever and injection site pain, swelling, and redness.

Pediatric Concerns: No data available.

Drug Interactions: Immunosuppressive therapies, including irradiation, antimetabolites, alkylating agents, cytotoxic drugs, and corticosteroids (used in greater than physiologic doses), may reduce the immune responses to vaccines.

Relative Infant Dose:

Adult Dose: 0.5 mL IM

Alternatives:

References:
1. Pharmaceutical manufacturer prescribing information, 2006.

HUMAN PAPILLOMAVIRUS INFECTION   L3

Trade: HPV infection
Other Trades:
Category: DNA virus infection

Human papillomaviruses (HPV) are DNA viruses and some of the most common sexually communicable diseases in the world. They are responsible not only for the presence of anogenital warts, but are also the contributing virus to the formation of flat warts, respiratory papillomatosis, and common skin warts. In addition, certain forms of papillomavirus are leading causes of cancer and dysplasia. Out of more than 100 types of this virus, more than 18 are classified as high risk, with types 16, 18, 31, and 45 being most commonly implicated in the development of cervical cancer. Types 16 and 18 are also linked to the development of oropharyngeal cancer. Types 6 and 11 are also of concern, as they most commonly result in anogenital warts, respiratory papillomatosis, and conjunctival papillomas and carcinomas.[1] Papillomaviruses are spread widely throughout the population and can reach prevalence rates of as high as 50% in school children, where cutaneous warts are common.

As a rule, close contact is required for transmission of these viruses from one individual to the next. This is evidenced by the high incidence of cutaneous warts in school children, as well as the link between public pools and plantar warts. Due to the viral nature of warts, they are often seen in immunocompromised patients. Anogenital warts most often are transferred through sexual contact and often resolve spontaneously without causing clinical effects. In the event that anogenital warts occur frequently or for prolonged periods of time, the risk for cervical cancer increases greatly.[1] It is possible to transfer HPV to an infant through the birth canal or from nongenital sites. The incubation period is varied, ranging from a few months to several years in length. It is possible that a neonate who is exposed to HPV virus will never develop clinical symptoms or may only show presence of the virus over the course of many years.[1]

HPV has been found to enter the breastmilk in one study.[2] During this study, approximately 4% of women were found to have HPV-16 DNA in breast milk samples. However, it was not established if the presence of DNA stemmed from virus in the milk or somewhere else. Another study addressed the findings of the previous one, again evaluating if HPV DNA was present within the breastmilk. This study did not find any evidence of high risk HPV within milk. At the current time, the authors of the study do not believe that evidence exists which suggests maternal to infant transfer of the virus, that would require discontinuation of breastfeeding while the mother is infected with this disease.[3]

Pregnancy Risk	Possibly Hazardous	Lactation Risk	L3
T ½	=	M/P	=
Vd	=	PB	=
Tmax	=	Oral	=
MW	=	pKa	=

Adult Concerns:

Pediatric Concerns:

Drug Interactions:

Relative Infant Dose:

Adult Dose:

Alternatives:

References:

1. American Academy of Pediatrics. Human Papillomaviruses. In: Pickering LK, Baker CJ, Kimberlin DW, Long SS, eds. Red Book: 2009 Report of the Committee on Infectious Diseases. 28th ed. Elk Grove Village, IL: American Academy of Pediatrics; 2009: 477–479
2. Sarkola, Marja MD, et. al. Human Papillomavirus DNA detected in breast milk. The Pediatric Infectious Disease Journal. 06/2010; 27(6): 557–558.
3. Mammas, Ioannis M., et al. Can "high-risk" human papillomaviruses (HPVs) be detected in human breast milk? Acta Paediatr. 2011 May; 100(5): 705–7.

HYALURONIC ACID   L3

Trade: Synvisc, Euflexxa, Healon, Hyalgan, Hylaform, Juvederm, Orthovisc, Provisc, Restylane

Other Trades: Cystistat, Durolane, Eyestil, Healon, OrthoVisc, Suplasyn

Category: Viscoelastic agent, antirheumatic, anti-wrinkle

Hyaluronic acid forms a viscoelastic solution in water, thus functioning as a joint lubricant, vitreous humor during ophthalmic surgery, and even decreasing the depth of wrinkles when injected intradermally. Sodium hyaluronate is a polysaccharide commonly found in humans in the extracellular matrix of connective tissues.[1] There are no data available on the transfer of hyaluronic acid into breastmilk, but it would be minimal to nil. The repeating chains can be quite large, and therefore size would prohibit any drug that did get absorbed from transferring into the milk compartment. A similar product is Hyalgan, which is sodium hyaluronate.

Pregnancy Risk	Probably Safe	Lactation Risk	L3
T ½	=	M/P	=
Vd	=	PB	=
Tmax	=	Oral	= Nil
MW	= Large	pKa	=

Adult Concerns: Pain at injection site. Arthralgia, bursitis, etc.

Pediatric Concerns: None reported in breastfed infants. Unlikely to enter milk.

Drug Interactions:

Relative Infant Dose:

Adult Dose:

Alternatives:

References:

1. Pharmaceutical manufacturer prescribing information, 2005.

HYDRALAZINE   L2

Trade: Apresoline
Other Trades: Alphapress, Apresoline, Novo-Hylazin, Apo-Hydralazine
Category: Antihypertensive

Hydralazine is a popular antihypertensive used for severe pre-eclampsia and gestational and postpartum hypertension. In a study of one breastfeeding mother receiving 50 mg three times daily, the concentrations of hydralazine in breastmilk at 0.5 and 2 hours after administration was 762, and 792 nmol/L respectively.[1] The respective maternal serum levels were 1525, and 580 nmol/L at the aforementioned times. From these data, an infant consuming 1000 mL of milk would consume only 0.17 mg of hydralazine, an amount too small to be clinically relevant. The published pediatric dose for hydralazine is 0.75 to 1 mg/kg/day. Since the levels in milk are far less than the clinical pediatric doses, hydralazine is probably compatible with breastfeeding.

Pregnancy Risk	C	Lactation Risk	L2
T ½	= 1.5–8 hours	M/P	= 0.49–1.36
Vd	= 1.6 l/kg	PB	= 87%
Tmax	= 2 hours	Oral	= 30–50%
MW	= 160	pKa	= 7.1

Adult Concerns: Hypotension, tachycardia, renal failure, liver toxicity, paresthesias.

Pediatric Concerns: None reported but observe for hypotension, sedation, weakness.

Drug Interactions: Increased effect with other antihypertensives, monoamine oxidase inhibitors. Decreased effect when used with indomethacin.

Relative Infant Dose: 1.2%

Adult Dose: 10–25 mg four times daily.

Alternatives:

References:
1. Liedholm H, Wahlin-Boll E, Hanson A, Ingemarsson I, Melander A. Transplacental passage and breast milk concentrations of hydralazine. Eur J Clin Pharmacol 1982; 21(5): 417–419.

HYDROCHLOROTHIAZIDE   L2

Trade: Hydrodiuril, Esidrix, Oretic, Tekturna HCT
Other Trades: Amizide, Dyazide, Modizide, Apo-Hydro, Diuchlor H, Hydrodiuril, Novo-Hydrazide, Direma, Esidrex
Category: Thiazide diuretic, antihypertensive

Hydrochlorothiazide (HCTZ) is a typical thiazide diuretic. In one study of a mother receiving a 50 mg dose each morning, milk levels were almost 25% of maternal plasma levels.[1] The dose ingested (assuming milk intake of 600 mL) would be approximately 50 µg/day, a clinically insignificant amount. The concentration of

HCTZ in the infant's serum was undetectable (<20 ng/mL). Some authors suggest that HCTZ can produce thrombocytopenia in nursing infant, although this is remote and unsubstantiated. Thiazide diuretics could potentially reduce milk production by depleting maternal blood volume although it is seldom observed. Most thiazide diuretics are considered compatible with breastfeeding if doses are kept low.

Pregnancy Risk	B	Lactation Risk	L2
T ½	= 5.6–14.8 hours	M/P	= 0.25
Vd	= 3 l/kg	PB	= 58%
Tmax	= 2 hours	Oral	= 72%
MW	= 297	pKa	= 7.9, 9.2

Adult Concerns: Fluid loss, hypotension. May reduce milk supply.

Pediatric Concerns: None reported via milk, but may reduce milk supply in mother.

Drug Interactions: May increase hypoglycemia with antidiabetic drugs. May increase hypotension associated with other antihypertensives. May increase digoxin associated arrhythmias. May increase lithium levels.

Relative Infant Dose:

Adult Dose: 25–100 mg daily.

Alternatives:

References:
1. Miller ME, Cohn RD, Burghart PH. Hydrochlorothiazide disposition in a mother and her breast-fed infant. J Pediatr 1982; 101(5): 789–791.

HYDROCHLOROTHIAZIDE + LOSARTAN   L3

Trade: Hyzaar

Other Trades:

Category: Antihypertensive agent

Hydrochlorothiazide (HCTZ) + losartan is a combined drug product of a thiazide diuretic (HCTZ) with an angiotensin II receptor blocker (losartan).[1] It is used for the management of hypertension. Currently there are no data available on the transfer of the combined drug product into breastmilk.

Hydrochlorothiazide (HCTZ) is a typical thiazide diuretic. In one study of a mother receiving a 50 mg dose each morning, milk levels were almost 25% of maternal plasma levels.[2] The dose ingested (assuming milk intake of 600 mL) would be approximately 50 µg/day, a clinically insignificant amount. The concentration of HCTZ in the infant's serum was undetectable (<20 ng/mL). Some authors suggest that HCTZ can produce thrombocytopenia in nursing infant, although this is remote and unsubstantiated. Thiazide diuretics could potentially reduce milk production by depleting maternal blood volume although it is seldom observed. Most thiazide diuretics are considered compatible with breastfeeding if doses are kept low. Losartan is an angiotensin II receptor blocker (ARB) used in the management of hypertension. No data are available on its transfer to human milk. Although it penetrates the CNS significantly, its high protein binding would probably reduce its ability to enter milk. This product is only intended for those few individuals who cannot take ACE inhibitors.

Although the likelihood of significant clinical effects in the breastfed infant with the maternal use of HCTZ + losartan is low, some caution with its use during lactation is still recommended. It should be used with caution in very premature infants.

Pregnancy Risk	C/D in 2nd and 3rd trimester	Lactation Risk	L3
T ½	= HCTZ/losartan: 5.6–14.8 hours/4–9 hours	M/P	= HCTZ/losartan: 0.25/
Vd	= HCTZ/losartan: 3/12 l/kg	PB	= HCTZ/losartan: 58%/99.8%
Tmax	= HCTZ/losartan: 2 hours/1 hour	Oral	= HCTZ/losartan: 72%/25–33%
MW	= HCTZ/losartan: 297/	pKa	= HCTZ/losartan: 7.9,9.2/14.27

Adult Concerns: Some of the more commonly reported side-effects include electrolyte imbalances, backaches, dizziness, and upper respiratory infections. More severe, and less commonly occurring adverse effects include angioedema and glaucoma.

Pediatric Concerns:

Drug Interactions: Use of this drug with dofetilide is contra-indicated due to increased risk of cardiotoxicity. Do not use concurrently with other ACE inhibitors, barbiturates, benzodiazepines, opiates or alcohol due to risk of profound hypotension and orthostatic hypotension. Concurrent use with digitalis may cause digitalis toxicity. Do not use with potassium-sparing diuretics (e. g., spironolactone, triamterene, amiloride) and potassium supplements as this may lead to hyperkalemia. Do not use concomitantly with NSAIDs in those with compromised renal function. Use with rifampin could decrease plasma levels of losartan. Use with fluconazole may increase plasma levels of losartan. Use with lithium could cause lithium toxicity.

Relative Infant Dose:

Adult Dose: HCTZ/losartan: 12.5–25 mg/50–100 mg once daily.

Alternatives:

References:
1. Pharmaceutical manufacturer prescribing information, 2011.
2. Miller ME, Cohn RD, Burghart PH. Hydrochlorothiazide disposition in a mother and her breast-fed infant. J Pediatr 1982; 101(5): 789–791.

HYDROCHLOROTHIAZIDE + OLMESARTAN   L3

Trade: Benicar HCT
Other Trades:
Category: Antihypertensive

Hydrochlorothiazide (HCTZ) + olmesartan is a combined drug product used to treat hypertension not responding to initial therapy.[1]

Hydrochlorothiazide (HCTZ) is a typical thiazide diuretic. In one study of a mother receiving a 50 mg dose each morning, milk levels were almost 25% of maternal plasma levels.[2] The dose ingested (assuming milk intake of 600 mL) would be approximately 50 µg/day, a clinically insignificant amount. The concentration of HCTZ in the infant's serum was undetectable (<20 ng/mL). Some authors suggest that HCTZ can produce thrombocytopenia in nursing infant, although this is remote and unsubstantiated. Thiazide diuretics could potentially reduce milk production by depleting maternal blood volume although it is seldom observed. Most thiazide diuretics are considered compatible with breastfeeding if doses are kept low. Olmesartan is an angiotensin II receptor antagonist used as a anti-hypertensive.[3] While it is different from the ACE inhibitors, it effectively produces the same end result, hypotension. Use in pregnancy is contraindicated. No data are available on its transfer to human milk, but its use in mothers with premature infants could be risky.

Use the drug combination of HCTZ + olmesartan with caution in those mothers with premature infants.

Pregnancy Risk	C/D in 2nd and 3rd trimester	Lactation Risk	L3
T ½	= HCTZ/olmesartan: 5.6–14.8 hours/13 hours	M/P	= HCTZ/olmesartan: 0.25/
Vd	= HCTZ/olmesartan: 3/0.24 l/kg	PB	= HCTZ/olmesartan: 58%/
Tmax	= HCTZ/olmesartan: 2 hours/1–2 hours	Oral	= HCTZ/olmesartan: 72%/26%
MW	= HCTZ/olmesartan: 297/558	pKa	= HCTZ/olmesartan: 7.9,9.2/

Adult Concerns: Nausea, vomiting, dizziness, gout, skin reactions, worsening of pre-existing renal impairment.

Pediatric Concerns:

Drug Interactions: HCTZ interactions: May increase hypoglycemia with antidiabetic drugs. May increase hypotension associated with other antihypertensives. May increase digoxin associated arrhythmias. May increase lithium levels. No major drug-drug interactions are noted with the use of olmesartan.

Relative Infant Dose:

Adult Dose: Hydrochlorothiazide/olmesartan: 12.5–50 mg/ 20–40 mg once daily

Alternatives:

References:

1. Pharmaceutical manufacturer prescribing information for Benicar-Hct, 2011.
2. Miller ME, Cohn RD, Burghart PH. Hydrochlorothiazide disposition in a mother and her breast-fed infant. J Pediatr 1982; 101(5): 789–791.
3. Pharmaceutical manufacturer prescribing information, 2003.

HYDROCHLOROTHIAZIDE + QUINAPRIL   L3

Trade: Accuretic

Other Trades:

Category: Anti-hypertensive

Hydrochlorothiazide (HCTZ) + quinapril is a combined drug product used for the management of hypertension.[1]

Hydrochlorothiazide (HCTZ) is a typical thiazide diuretic. In one study of a mother receiving a 50 mg dose each morning, milk levels were almost 25% of maternal plasma levels.[2] The dose ingested (assuming milk intake of 600 mL) would be approximately 50 µg/day, a clinically insignificant amount. The concentration of HCTZ in the infant's serum was undetectable (<20 ng/mL). Some authors suggest that HCTZ can produce thrombocytopenia in nursing infant, although this is remote and unsubstantiated. Thiazide diuretics could potentially reduce milk production by depleting maternal blood volume although it is seldom observed. Most thiazide diuretics are considered compatible with breastfeeding if doses are kept low.

Quinapril is an angiotensin converting enzyme (ACE) inhibitor used as an antihypertensive. Once in the plasma compartment, quinapril is rapidly converted to quinaprilat, the active metabolite. In a study of 6 women who received 20 mg/day, the milk/plasma ratio for quinapril was 0.12.[3] Quinapril was not detected in milk after 4 hours. No quinaprilat (metabolite) was detected in any of the milk samples. The estimated 'dose' of quinapril that would be received by the infant was 1.6% of the maternal dose, adjusted for respective weights. The authors suggest that quinapril appears to be 'safe' during breastfeeding although, as always, the risk: benefit ratio should be considered when it is to be given to a nursing mother.

The drug combination of HCTZ + quinapril is probably compatible with breastfeeding. However, this drug should be used with caution early postpartum in preterm infants.

Pregnancy Risk	D	Lactation Risk	L3
T ½	= HCTZ/quinapril: 5.6–14.8 hours/2 hours	M/P	= HCTZ/quinapril: 0.25/0.12
Vd	= HCTZ/quinapril: 3/ l/kg	PB	= HCTZ/quinapril: 58%/97%
Tmax	= HCTZ/quinapril: 2 hours/2 hours	Oral	= HCTZ/quinapril: 72%/ complete
MW	= HCTZ/quinapril: 297/474	pKa	= HCTZ/quinapril: 7.9,9.2/

Adult Concerns: The most common side effects are cough and dizziness. Some of the more serious but rare side effects include severe skin reactions, hypersensitivity reactions, gastric hemorrhage, liver impairment.

Pediatric Concerns:

Drug Interactions: HCTZ interactions: May increase hypoglycemia with antidiabetic drugs. May increase hypotension associated with other antihypertensives. May increase digoxin associated arrhythmias. May increase lithium levels. Quinapril interactions: Probenecid increases plasma levels of ACE inhibitors. ACE inhibitors and diuretics have additive hypotensive effects. Antacids reduce bioavailability of ACE inhibitors. NSAIDS reduce hypotension of ACE inhibitors. Phenothiazines increase effects of ACE inhibitors. ACE inhibitors increase digoxin and lithium plasma levels. May elevate potassium levels when potassium supplementation is added.

Relative Infant Dose:

Adult Dose: HCTZ/quinapril: 12.5–25 mg/10–20 mg once daily

Alternatives: Captopril, enalapril

References:
1. Pharmaceutical manufacturer prescribing information, 2011.
2. Miller ME, Cohn RD, Burghart PH. Hydrochlorothiazide disposition in a mother and her breast-fed infant. J Pediatr 1982; 101(5): 789–791.
3. Begg EJ, Robson RA, Gardiner SJ, Hudson LJ, Reece PA, Olson SC, Posvar EL, Sedman AJ. Quinapril and its metabolite quinaprilat in human milk. Br J Clin Pharmacol 2001; 51(5): 478–481.

HYDROCHLOROTHIAZIDE + TRIAMTERENE   L3

Trade: Dyazide, Maxzide

Other Trades: Hydrene, Apo-Triazide, Novo-Triamzide, Pro-Triazide, Riva-ZideTriamco

Category: Diuretic, anti-hypertensive

Hydrochlorothiazide (HCTZ) and Triamterene is a combination drug product indicated for use in hypertension and as a diuretic. Numerous diuretic products contain varying combinations of hydrochlorothiazide (HCTZ) and triamterene are available.

Hydrochlorothiazide (HCTZ) is a typical thiazide diuretic. In one study of a mother receiving a 50 mg dose each morning, milk levels were almost 25% of maternal plasma levels.[1] The dose ingested (assuming milk intake of 600 mL) would be approximately 50 µg/day, a clinically insignificant amount. The concentration of HCTZ in the infant's serum was undetectable (<20 ng/mL). Some authors suggest that HCTZ can produce thrombocytopenia in nursing infant, although this is remote and unsubstantiated. Thiazide diuretics could potentially reduce milk production by depleting maternal blood volume although it is seldom observed. Most thiazide diuretics are considered compatible with breastfeeding if doses are kept low.

Triamterene is a potassium sparing diuretic. Following a dose of 100–200 mg, it attains plasma levels in adults of 26–30 µg/L.[2] It is secreted in small amounts in cow's milk but no human data are available. Assuming a high milk/plasma ratio of one, an infant ingesting 125 mL/kg/day would theoretically ingest less than 4 µg/kg/day, an amount unlikely to cause clinical problems.

Since the levels of both hydrochlorothiazide and triamterene in infant's plasma are too low to produce clinical effects, it may be said that hydrochlorothiazide + triamterene is probably compatible with breastfeeding.

Pregnancy Risk	C		Lactation Risk	L3
T ½	= HCTZ/triamterene: 5.6–14.8 hours/1.5–2.5 hours	M/P	= HCTZ/triamterene: 0.25/	
Vd	= HCTZ/triamterene: 3/ l/kg	PB	= HCTZ/triamterene: 58%/55%	
Tmax	= HCTZ/triamterene: 2 hours/1.5–3 hours	Oral	= HCTZ/triamterene: 72%/30–70%	
MW	= HCTZ/triamterene: 297/253	pKa	= HCTZ/triamterene: 7.9,9.2/6.2	

Adult Concerns: Diarrhea, nausea, vomiting, hepatitis, leukopenia, hyperkalemia.

Pediatric Concerns: None reported. Hyperkalemia.

Drug Interactions: Increased risk of hyperkalemia when given with amiloride, spironolactone, and ACE inhibitors. Increased risk of toxicity with amantadine.

Relative Infant Dose: 0.2%

Adult Dose: HCTZ/triamterene: 25–50 mg/37.5–75 mg daily.

Alternatives:

References:
1. Miller ME, Cohn RD, Burghart PH. Hydrochlorothiazide disposition in a mother and her breast-fed infant. J Pediatr 1982; 101(5): 789–791.
2. Pharmaceutical manufacturer prescribing information, 2011.

HYDROCODONE   L3

Trade: Lortab, Vicodin, Maxidone, Norco

Other Trades: Hycomine, Hycodan, Robidone, Actron

Category: Analgesic for pain

Hydrocodone is a narcotic analgesic and antitussive structurally related to codeine although somewhat more potent. Its active metabolite is hydromorphone. Its use has been found to be very effective in the relief of postpartum and post-operative pain. It has also been found to very effective for the alleviation of pain associated with mastitis.[1]

Hydrocodone is commonly used in breastfeeding mothers throughout the world. In a study of two breastfeeding women taking hydrocodone for various periods,[2] patient one received a total of 63,525 µg (998.8 µg/kg) over 86.5 hours. Patient two, received 9075 µg (123.5 µg/kg) over 36 hours. In patient one, the AUC of the drug concentration in milk was 4946.1 µg/L. hr and an average milk concentration of 57.2 µg/L. The authors estimate the relative infant dose at 3.1%. In patient two, the AUC of the drug concentration in milk was 735.6 µg/L.hour and an average milk concentration of 20.4 µg/L. The authors estimate the relative infant dose at 3.7%. This paper concluded that high doses of hydrocodone in mothers who are nursing newborn or premature infants can be concerning. In another, more recent study,[3] hydrocodone and hydromorphone levels were measured in 125 breastmilk samples obtained from 30 women who were receiving 0.14–0.21 mg/kg/day (10–15 mg/day) of hydrocodone for the alleviation of postpartum pain. It was found that fully breastfed infants receive on an average of 2.4% (range: 0.2–0.9%) of the maternal hydrocodone dose. When considering total opiate exposure to both hydrocodone and hydromorphone combined, it was found that the total opiate dosage in the infants amounted to 0.7% of the therapeutic dosage commonly used in older infants. This is reassuring and suggests that when used in standard clinical dosages, the total opiate exposure to the infant is minimal and possibly clinically irrelevant. However, when calculating the hydromorphone to hydrocodone ratios in the breastmilk samples of these women, it was found that breastmilk samples from two of the women had a high hydromorphone to hydrocodone ratio of 2.8 and 3.1. These women were possibly rapid metabolizers. Although the total opiate exposure to the infants of these two women was still well below the regular pediatric therapeutic dosages, this finding raises concerns of possible untoward effects in the infants when hydrocodone is used in high doses, especially in those women who are rapid metabolizers. In conclusion, this study suggests that when used in standard postpartum dosages, hydrocodone appears to be safe in breastfeeding mothers of newborn infants. However, the authors advise against the use of high doses for prolonged periods of time, due to possible neonatal sedation and respiratory depression.

It is recommended that for treatment of postpartum pain, hydrocodone dosages should be limited to no more than 30 mg per day. If higher doses are required, then the infant should be closely monitored for possible untoward effects such as sedation and apnea. Doses more than 40 mg/day should be avoided.[3] Mothers should be advised to watch for sedation and poor weight gain in their infants.

Pregnancy Risk	C	Lactation Risk	L3
T ½	= 3.8 hours	M/P	=
Vd	= 3.3–4.7 l/kg	PB	=
Tmax	= 1.3 hours	Oral	= Complete
MW	= 299	pKa	= 8.9

Adult Concerns: Sedation, dizziness, apnea, bradycardia, nausea. Be advised that constipation can be severe.

Pediatric Concerns: Sedation observed in one infant whose mother consumed 20 mg hydrocodone + 1300 mg acetaminophen every 4 hours.[2] Neonatal sedation and apnea possible, especially with doses more than 30 mg/day.

Drug Interactions: May reduce analgesia when used with phenothiazines. May increase toxicity associated with CNS depressants and tricyclic antidepressants.

Relative Infant Dose: 2.4%–3.7%

Adult Dose: 5–10 mg every 4–6 hours

Alternatives: Codeine

References:
1. Bodley V, Powers D. Long-term treatment of a breastfeeding mother with fluconazole-resolved nipple pain caused by yeast: a case study. J Hum Lact. 1997 Dec; 13(4): 307–11.3.
2. Anderson PO et al. Hydrocodone Excretion into Breast Milk: The First Two Reported Cases. Breastfeeding Medicine Vol 2 (1) 2007; 10–14.
3. Sauberan JB, Anderson PO, Lane JR, Rafie S, Nguyen N, Rossi SS, Stellwagen LM. Breast milk hydrocodone and hydromorphone levels in mothers using hydrocodone forpostpartum pain. Obstet Gynecol. 2011 Mar; 117(3): 611–7.

HYDROCORTISONE ENEMA   L3

Trade: Colocort, Cortenema, Hycort Enema, Rectoid, Anucort, Proctosol

Other Trades:

Category: Corticosteroid

Hydrocortisone is a typical corticosteroid with weak glucocorticoid and mineralocorticoid activity.[1] The amount transferred into human milk has not been reported, but as with most steroids, is believed minimal. Hydrocortisone Rectal Suspension is absorbed from the colon, it acts both topically and systemically. Although rectal hydrocortisone has a low incidence of reported adverse reactions, prolonged use presumably may cause typical steroid systemic reactions. In a study undertaken to determine changes in concentrations of cortisol in the mammary secretion of individual women during late pregnancy, lactogenesis, established lactation and after cessation of breastfeeding, the concentration of cortisol in colostrum averaged 7.5% of that found in serum during late pregnancy. Cortisol levels in colostrum during late pregnancy was 25.5 ng/mL and fell within 2 days postpartum to 10.2 ng/mL. At 10 days, levels were 1.8 ng/mL. During established lactation, cortisol levels ranged from 0.2 to 32 ng/mL but the mean was 7.2 ng/mL.[2]

Hydrocortisone administered rectally is probably okay if used short-term. Transfer of hydrocortisone into milk is probably low, although we have no data. No adverse effects have been reported in breastfed infants.

Pregnancy Risk	C	Lactation Risk	L3
T ½	= 1–2 hours	M/P	=
Vd	= 0.48 l/kg	PB	= 90%
Tmax	=	Oral	= 96%
MW	= 362	pKa	=

Adult Concerns: Rarely local pain or burning and rectal bleeding. Sodium retention, fluid retention, congestive heart failure in susceptible patients, potassium loss, hypokalemic alkalosis, hypertension. Muscle weakness, steroid myopathy, osteoporosis, peptic ulcer, pancreatitis, ulcerative esophagitis, impaired wound healing, glaucoma, cataracts, etc.

Pediatric Concerns: None via breastfeeding have been reported.

Drug Interactions: Co-administration with the following may decrease plasma levels and efficacy of hydrocortisone: phenobarbital, phenytoin and rifampin. Concomitant administration with the following may cause increased plasma levels of hydrocortisone: troleandomycin and ketoconazole. Concomitant use of hydrocortisone with aspirin may decrease aspirin levels in blood; sudden withdrawal of hydrocortisone could cause a sudden increase in aspirin levels and could cause salicylate toxicity.

Relative Infant Dose:

Adult Dose: 100 mg nightly (60 ml) rectally.

Alternatives:

References:
1. Pharmaceutical manufacturer prescribing information, 2010.
2. Kulski JK, Hartmann PE. Changes in the concentration of cortisol in milk during different stages of human lactation. Aust J Exp Biol Med Sci. 1981 Dec; 59(Pt 6): 769–78.

HYDROCORTISONE TOPICAL   L2

Trade: Westcort, Lipsovir

Other Trades: Dermaid, Egocort, Hycor, Cortef, Cortate, Cortone, Emo-Cort, Aquacort, Dermacort

Category: Corticosteroid

Hydrocortisone is a typical corticosteroid with glucocorticoid and mineralocorticoid activity. When applied topically it suppresses inflammation and enhances healing. Initial onset of activity when applied topically is slow and may require several days for response. Absorption topically is dependent on placement; percutaneous absorption is 1% from the forearm, 2% from rectum, 4% from the scalp, 7% from the forehead, and 36% from the scrotal area.[1] The amount transferred into human milk has not been reported, but as with most steroids, is believed minimal. Applied to the nipple, only small amounts should be applied and then only after feeding; larger quantities should be removed prior to breastfeeding. 0.5 to 1% ointments, rather than creams, are generally preferred.

Pregnancy Risk	C	Lactation Risk	L2
T ½	= 1–2 hours	M/P	=
Vd	= 0.48 l/kg	PB	= 90%
Tmax	=	Oral	= 96%
MW	= 362	pKa	= 13.87

Adult Concerns: Local irritation.

Pediatric Concerns: None reported via milk.

Drug Interactions: Co-administration with the following may decrease plasma levels and efficacy of hydrocortisone: phenobarbital, phenytoin and rifampin. Concomitant administration with the following may cause increased plasma levels of hydrocortisone: troleandomycin and ketoconazole. Concomitant use of hydrocortisone with aspirin may decrease aspirin levels in blood; sudden withdrawal of hydrocortisone could cause a sudden increase in aspirin levels and could cause salicylate toxicity.

Relative Infant Dose:

Adult Dose: Apply topically four times daily.

Alternatives:

References:
1. Derendorf H, Mollmann H, Barth J, Mollmann C, Tunn S, Krieg M. Pharmacokinetics and oral bioavailability of hydrocortisone. J Clin Pharmacol 1991; 31(5): 473–476.

HYDROMORPHONE   L3

Trade: Dilaudid, Exalgo
Other Trades: Dilaudid, Hydromorph Contin, Palladone
Category: Opiate analgesic

Hydromorphone is a potent semisynthetic narcotic analgesic used to alleviate moderate to severe pain. It is approximately 7–10 times more potent that morphine, but is used in equivalently lower doses.[1] In a group of 8 women who received intranasal hydromorphone (2 mg), milk levels ranged from a high of about 6000 pg/mL at about 1 hour, to about 200 pg/mL at 24 hours, but averaged about 1.04 µg/L.[2] The observed milk/plasma ratio averaged 2.57. The half-life of hydromorphone in milk was estimated at 10.5 hours. The authors estimate a Relative Infant Dose of 0.67% of the maternal dose although I calculate it at 0.52%. Using this data an infant would consume (via milk) approximately 2.2 µg per day. This is significantly less than the clinical dose generally administered in infants and children, which is 15–30 µg/kg every 4–6 hours.

Pregnancy Risk	C	Lactation Risk	L3
T ½	= 11.1 hours	M/P	= 2.57
Vd	= 2.9 l/kg	PB	=
Tmax	= 0.27 hours	Oral	= 51%
MW	= 285	pKa	= 18.00

Adult Concerns: Hydromorphone is highly addictive. Adverse effects include dizziness, sedation, agitation, hypotension, respiratory depression, nausea, and vomiting.

Pediatric Concerns: Milk levels reported to be low. Caution recommended in weak or premature infants, or after prolonged use.

Drug Interactions: As with other opiates, barbiturates and benzodiazepines could potentiate the sedative/hypnotic properties of hydromorphone.

Relative Infant Dose: 0.7%

Adult Dose: 2–10 mg every 3–6 hours PRN

Alternatives: Codeine, hydrocodone

References:

1.   Baselt RC. Disposition of toxic drugs and chemicals in man. Foster City, CA: Chemical
     Toxicology Institute, 2000: 426–427.
2.   Edwards JE, Rudy AC, Wermeling DP, Desai N, McNamara PJ. Hydromorphone transfer into
     breast milk after intranasal administration. Pharmacotherapy 2003 February; 23(2): 153–8.

HYDROQUINONE   L3

Trade:

Other Trades:

Category: Depigmenting agent for topical applications

Hydroquinone is used for depigmentation of skin due to conditions such as
freckles, melasma, senile lentigo, and inactive chloasma.[1] Hydroquinone is rapidly
and extensively absorbed from the gut of animals. Absorption via the skin is
slower but may be more rapid with vehicles such as alcohols. The transcutaneous
absorption is reported to be about 35% which is relatively high for topical
preparations. Hydroquinone distributes rapidly and widely and is metabolized to
p-benzoquinone and other products. It is metabolized in the liver by conjugation
to monoglucuronide, monosulfate, and mercaptopuric derivatives. The excretion
of hydroquinone and its metabolites is rapid, and occurs primarily via the urine.
No data are available on its transfer into human milk. Although it is quite polar
and water soluble, it also has a rather high pKa (9.96) which could lead to some
trapping in human milk. While it does not seem to be very toxic, its chronic use in
breastfeeding mothers is probably not warranted for such benign syndromes that
could wait until the mother has weaned the infant off the breast.

Pregnancy Risk	C	Lactation Risk	L3
T ½	=	M/P	=
Vd	=	PB	=
Tmax	=	Oral	=
MW	= 110.11	pKa	= 9.96

Adult Concerns: Adverse effects include mild skin irritation and sensitivity,
dryness, and fissuring of paranasal and infraorbital areas. Cases of intoxication
and death have been reported from the oral ingestion of photographic developing
agents. Dermal applications of hydroquinone at concentration levels below 3% in
different bases caused negligible effects in male volunteers. However, there are case
reports suggesting that skin lightening creams containing 2% hydroquinone have
produced leukoderma, as well as ochronosis.

Pediatric Concerns: No reports of its use in breastfeeding mothers. While not
highly risky, its use in breastfeeding mothers may not be justified.

Drug Interactions: Combinations with corticosteroids may reduce skin irritation.

Relative Infant Dose:

Adult Dose: Apply 2–4% solutions twice daily. Limit areas treated.

Alternatives: Azelaic acid

References:
1.   Pharmaceutical manufacturer Package Insert, 2003.

HYDROXYAMPHETAMINE + TROPICAMIDE   L3

Trade: Peremyd
Other Trades:
Category: Mydriatic ophthalmic agent

An ophthalmic solution which is a combination of Hydroxyamphetamine hydrobromide and Tropicamide is currently marketed under the name of Paremyd.[1] It is indicated for use in routine diagnostic ophthalmic procedures and is recommended for topical administration in the form of eye drops. Hydroxyamphetamine is an adrenergic agent and tropicamide has anticholinergic effect. Together, they produce an additive mydriatic effect which facilitates better visualization during ophthalmic procedures. Clinically relevant mydriasis occurs within 30–60 min and lasts for 3 hours. The clinically used doses are too low to produce significant systemic levels, and therefore, the amount that enters the milk should likely be too low to produce any untoward effects in the infants. Nevertheless, it is advisable to observe the infant for possible side-effects such as dry mouth, constipation, tachycardia and restlessness. A brief with-holding period of 3–4 hours should eliminate most risk.

Pregnancy Risk	C		Lactation Risk	L3
T ½	=		M/P	=
Vd	=		PB	=
Tmax	= 30–60 min		Oral	=
MW	=		pKa	=

Adult Concerns: Dryness of eyes, blurring of vision, photophobia. A few very rare adverse effects are myocardial infarction, ventricular arrhythmias, precipitation of glaucoma.

Pediatric Concerns:

Drug Interactions:

Relative Infant Dose:

Adult Dose: 1–2 drops.

Alternatives:

References:
1. Pharmaceutical manufacturer prescribing information, 2008.

HYDROXYCHLOROQUINE   L2

Trade: Plaquenil
Other Trades: Plaquenil
Category: Antimalarial, Antirheumatic

Hydroxychloroquine (HCQ) is effective in the treatment of malaria but is also used in immune syndromes such as rheumatoid arthritis and systemic lupus erythematosus (SLE). HCQ is known to produce significant retinal damage and blindness if used over a prolonged period, and this could occur (theoretically but unlikely) in breastfed infants. Patients on this product should see an ophthalmologist routinely. It has a huge volume of distribution (Vd) which suggests milk levels will be quite low. In one study of a mother receiving 400 mg HCQ daily, the concentrations of HCQ in breastmilk were 1.46, 1.09, and 1.09 mg/L at 2.0, 9.5, and 14 hours after the dose.[1] The average milk concentration was 1.1 mg/L. The milk/plasma ratio was approximately 5.5. On a body-weight basis, the infant's dose would be 2.9% of the maternal dose. In another study of one mother receiving 200 mg twice daily, milk levels were much lower than the previous study. Only a total of 3.2 µg of hydroxychloroquine was detected in her milk over 48 hours.[2] Two breastfeeding mothers taking hydroxychloroquine were tested to determine the concentration in their breastmilk one week after delivery. The concentrations were 344 and 1424 ng/mL, which corresponded to an infant dose of 0.06 and 0.2 mg/kg/day respectively.[3] Hydroxychloroquine is mostly metabolized to chloroquine and has an incredibly long half-life. The pediatric dose for malaria prophylaxis is 5 mg/kg/week, far larger than the dose received via milk.

Due to its huge volume of distribution, milk levels are generally quite low, and therefore this drug maybe considered compatible with breastfeeding.

Pregnancy Risk	C	Lactation Risk	L2
T ½	= >40 days	M/P	= 5.5
Vd	= 580–815 l/kg	PB	= 63%
Tmax	= 1–2 hours	Oral	= 74%
MW	= 336	pKa	= 8.3, 9.7

Adult Concerns: Blood dyscrasias, nausea, vomiting, diarrhea, retinopathy, rash, aplastic anemia, psychosis, porphyria, psoriasis, corneal deposits.

Pediatric Concerns: None reported, but observe for retinal damage, blood dyscrasias.

Drug Interactions: Increased risk of blood dyscrasias when used with aurothioglucose. May increase serum digoxin levels.

Relative Infant Dose: 2.9%

Adult Dose: 400 mg every week for 10 weeks.

Alternatives:

References:
1. Nation RL, Hackett LP, Dusci LJ, Ilett KF. Excretion of hydroxychloroquine in human milk. Br J Clin Pharmacol 1984; 17(3): 368–369.
2. Ostensen M, Brown ND, Chiang PK, Aarbakke J. Hydroxychloroquine in human breast milk. Eur J Clin Pharmacol 1985; 28(3): 357.
3. Costedoat-Chalumeau N, Amoura Z, Aymard gm et al. Evidence of transplacental passage of hydroxychloroquine in humans. Arthritis Rheum 2002; 46(4): 1123–1124.

HYDROXYQUINOLINE   L3

Trade:

Other Trades:

Category: Antibacterial, antifungal

Hydroxyquinoline, also referred to as oxyquinoline, is used as an antibacterial and antifungal in individuals requiring the use of a pessary. Its derivatives have also seen use in many industries, specifically by pesticide, nylon, and dye industries. It is currently not known if this substance is present in breastmilk or if it would cause untoward effects in a breastfed child. Animal experiments indicate that small doses of ingested hydroxyquinoline may be detrimental to health. This agent was able to cause death in animal subjects with an LD-50 of 1200 mg/kg in rats.[1] Absorption may occur through the skin, potentially causing headache, nausea, nervousness, and sleeplessness. It is unlikely that this drug would cause a large number of adverse effects when used to disinfect a pessary.

Pregnancy Risk	C	Lactation Risk	L3
T ½	=	M/P	=
Vd	=	PB	=
Tmax	=	Oral	=
MW	= 145.16	pKa	= ~8.5

Adult Concerns: Headache, nausea, nervousness, sleeplessness, eye irritation, dermal irritation.

Pediatric Concerns:

Drug Interactions: No known drug interactions

Relative Infant Dose:

Adult Dose:

Alternatives:

References:
1. 8–Hydroxyquinoline Material Safety Data Sheet. Santa Cruz Biotechnology, Inc. Santa Cruz, CA. Issued May 17, 2008. Accessed July 26, 2011.

HYDROXYUREA   L3

Trade: Hydrea

Other Trades: Hydrea

Category: Antineoplastic agent

Hydroxyurea is an antineoplastic agent used to treat melanoma, leukemias, and other neoplasms. It is well absorbed orally and rapidly metabolized to urea by the liver. In one study following a dose of 500 mg three times daily for 7 days, milk samples were collected two hours after the last dose.[1] The concentration of hydroxyurea in breastmilk averaged 6.1 mg/L (range 3.8 to 8.4 mg/L). This is about 4.3% of the maternal dose which is probably too low to bother a breastfeeding infant. Approximately 80% of the dose is excreted renally within 12 hours in adults. As this product is potentially toxic, mothers receiving hydroxyurea should probably withhold breastfeeding for a minimum of 12–24 hours after the dose.

Pregnancy Risk	D	Lactation Risk	L3
T ½	= 3–4 hours	M/P	=
Vd	= 0.48 to 1.62 l/kg	PB	=
Tmax	= 2 hours	Oral	= Complete
MW	= 76	pKa	= 13.96

Adult Concerns: Bone marrow suppression, drowsiness, convulsion, hallucinations, fever, nausea, vomiting, diarrhea, constipation.

Pediatric Concerns: None reported via milk, but extreme caution is recommended due to overt toxicity of this product.

Drug Interactions: May have increased toxicity and neurotoxicity when used with fluorouracil.

Relative Infant Dose: 4.3%

Adult Dose: 80 mg/kg every 3 days

Alternatives:

References:
1.   Sylvester RK, Lobell M, Teresi ME, Brundage D, Dubowy R. Excretion of hydroxyurea into milk. Cancer 1987; 60(9): 2177–2178.

HYDROXYZINE   L1

Trade: Atarax, Vistaril

Other Trades: Apo-Hydroxyzine, Atarax, Novo-Hydroxyzin

Category: Antihistamine, antiemetic

Hydroxyzine is an antihistamine structurally similar to cyclizine and meclizine. It produces significant CNS depression, anticholinergic side effects (drying), and antiemetic side effects.[1] Hydroxyzine is largely metabolized to cetirizine. No data are available on its secretion into breastmilk, but since it is largely metabolized to cetrizine, its pharmacological behavior should be similar to cetrizine. Cetirizine is one of the preferred antihistamines during breastfeeding since it is non-sedating. Nevertheless, observe for sedation in the breastfed infant.

Pregnancy Risk	C	Lactation Risk	L1
T ½	= 3–7 hours	M/P	=
Vd	= 13–31 l/kg	PB	=
Tmax	= 2 hours	Oral	= Complete
MW	= 375	pKa	= 2.1, 7.1

Adult Concerns: Sedation, hypotension, dry mouth.

Pediatric Concerns: None reported via milk, but observe for sedation, tachycardia, dry mouth.

Drug Interactions: May reduce epinephrine vasopressor response. Increased sedation when used with CNS depressants. Increased anticholinergic side effects when admixed with other anticholinergics.

Relative Infant Dose:

Adult Dose: 50–100 mg four times daily.

Alternatives: Cetirizine, loratadine

References:
1. Paton DM, Webster DR. Clinical pharmacokinetics of H_1-receptor antagonists (the antihistamines). Clin Pharmacokinet 1985; 10(6): 477–497.

HYLAN G-F 20 — L2

Trade: Synvisc

Other Trades:

Category: Joint lubricant for arthritic pain

Hylan G-F 20 are hylan polymers made from chicken combs.[1] It is used in for treatment of osteoarthritis via intra-articular injection. Hylans are a natural complex sugar of the glycosaminoglycan similar to hyaluronic acid found in the extracellular matrix of connective tissues. Hylans are large molecular weight polymers and would not be expected to enter milk. Average molecular weight is 6 million daltons. This product would not pose a problem for a breastfeeding mother or infant.

Pregnancy Risk	Probably Safe	Lactation Risk	L2
T ½	=	M/P	=
Vd	=	PB	=
Tmax	=	Oral	= None
MW	= 6 million	pKa	=

Adult Concerns: Knee pain or swelling, rash, itching, nausea, vomiting.

Pediatric Concerns: None reported via milk. Probably too large to enter milk in clinically relevant amounts.

Drug Interactions:

Relative Infant Dose:

Adult Dose:

Alternatives:

References:
1. Pharmaceutical manufacturer prescribing information, 1999.

HYOSCYAMINE   L3

Trade: Anaspaz, Levsin, NuLev, ED-Spaz
Other Trades: Hyoscine, Levsin
Category: Anticholinergic, antisecretory agent

Hyoscyamine is an anticholinergic, antisecretory agent that belongs to the belladonna alkaloid family. Its typical effects are to dry secretions, produce constipation, dilate pupils, blur vision, and may produce urinary retention.[1,2] Although no exact amounts are listed, hyoscyamine is known to be secreted into breastmilk in trace amounts.[3] Thus far, no untoward effects from breastfeeding while using hyoscyamine have been found. Hyoscyamine drops have in the past been used directly in infants for colic although it is no longer recommended for this use. As with atropine, infants and children are especially sensitive to anticholinergics and their use is discouraged. Use with caution in breastfeeding mothers.

Pregnancy Risk	C	Lactation Risk	L3
T ½	= 3.5 hours	M/P	=
Vd	=	PB	= 50%
Tmax	= 40–90 minutes (oral)	Oral	= 81%
MW	= 289	pKa	= 9.7

Adult Concerns: Tachycardia, dry mouth, blurred vision, constipation, urinary retention.

Pediatric Concerns: Decreased heart rate, anticholinergic effects from direct use, but none reported from breastmilk ingestion. Never use directly in infants with projectile vomiting, or in infants with bilious (green) vomitus.

Drug Interactions: Decreased effect with antacids. Increased toxicity with amantadine, antimuscarinics, haloperidol, phenothiazines, tricyclic antidepressants, monoamine oxidase inhibitors.

Relative Infant Dose:

Adult Dose: 0.125–0.25 mg four times daily.

Alternatives:

References:
1. Facts and Comparisons. St. Louis: 2010.
2. Pharmaceutical manufacturer prescribing information, 2010.
3. Wilson J. Drugs in Breast Milk. New York: ADIS Press 1981.

¹²³IODINE   L5

Trade: Radioactive Iodine, Iodine-¹²³, ¹²³I, DaTscan, Ioflupane ¹²³I
Other Trades:
Category: Radioactive iodine

The normal human body contains about 9–10 mg of iodine, 90% of which resides in the thyroid gland. The thyroid gland concentrates more than 100 times the recommended daily allowance. The thyroid gland, and the cells in the lactating breast, contain a transporter (symporter) that facilitates concentration of iodine in these tissues. The normal range of iodine in human milk is reported to be 20–150 µg/L, and is a function of geography. The daily dietary requirement for lactating women is about 30% higher than for the general public.

Radioactive iodine concentrates in the thyroid gland as well as in breastmilk, and if ingested by an infant, it may suppress its thyroid function or increase the risk of future thyroid carcinomas, and produce thyroid destruction in the infant. Radioactive iodine is clinically used to ablate or destroy the thyroid (dose= 355 MBq), or in much smaller doses (7.4 MBq), to scan the thyroid for malignancies. Following ingestion, radioactive iodine concentrates in the thyroid and lactating tissues, and it is estimated 27.9% of total radioactivity is secreted via breast milk.[1] Two potential half-lives exist for radioactive iodine: one is the radioactive half-life which is solely dependent on radioactive decay of the molecule; and two, the biological half-life, which is often briefer and is the half-life of the iodine molecule itself in the human being. The latter half-life is influenced most by elimination via the kidneys and other routes. The half-life of ^{123}I is 13.2 hours. The biological or effective half-life may be shorter due to excretion in urine, feces, and milk. ^{123}I is a newer isotope that is increasing in popularity. ^{123}I has a short half-life of only 13.2 hours and is radiologically ideal for thyroid and other scans. If radioactive iodine compounds are mandatory for various "scanning" procedures, ^{123}I should be preferred.

However, the return to breastfeeding following ^{123}I therapy is dependent on the purity of this product. During manufacture of ^{123}I, ^{124}I and ^{125}I are created. If using ^{123}I, breastfeeding should be temporarily interrupted. ^{123}I is not used for ablation of the thyroid. In a study by Morita of the transfer of ^{123}I-sodium iodide, ^{123}I was excreted exponentially with an effective half-life of 5.5 hours.[2] A total of 2.5% of the total radioactivity administered was excreted in the breast milk over the 93 hours, 95% of which was excreted within the first 24 hours, and 98.2% within 36 hours. The first milk sample collected at 7 hours after administration contained 48.5% of the total radioactivity excreted. The authors estimated the potential absorption of radioactivity to an infant's thyroid in uninterrupted breast-feeding to be 30.3 mGy. With a 24-hour interruption, the absorbed radioactivity would be 1.25 mGy; with a 36-hour interruption, it would be 0.24 mGy. They recommend that breastfeeding should be curtailed for 36 hours to reduce the infant's exposure to ^{123}I radioactivity.

Ultimately, the amount of radioiodine transferred into human milk depends on the clinical dose administered to the mother and the radioisotope used. Radioiodine concentrates in milk where at least 26–45% of the dose ends up in the breast. Radiographs show major concentration in breastmilk. Low scanning doses may present an opportunity to return to breastfeeding if the counts in milk are closely monitored in the coming weeks. If one is able to measure the milk for radiation, then a return to baseline would allow a patient to re-initiate breastfeeding. Mothers exposed to radioactive iodine released from nuclear power plant disasters, should be immediately treated with potassium iodide to prevent transmission of the radioactive iodine into human milk, and the infant's thyroid. International Commission of Radiological Protection (ICRP) recommends 12 hours interruption for ^{123}I-iodohippurate, and >3 weeks interruption (or cessation) for 123-non-iodohippurate compounds.[3] See breastfeeding and close contact restriction tables in the appendix.

Breastfeeding Restrictions for thyroid imaging scans with [123]I.

[123]I SODIUM: 0.4 mCi dose: Complete cessation of breastfeeding or until counts are baseline.[4]

[123]I Hippuran: 0.5 mCi dose: 27 hours interruption.[5]

[123]I MIBG: 0.5mCi dose: 11 hours interruption 11mCi: 21 hours interruption.[5]

Note: These recommendations still permit a minimal amount of <1mSv of radiation transfer to the infant. Exposure of 1 mSv has a cancer incidence risk of 1 in 10,000 people. This amount of exposure is less than the amount an average American is exposed to from the natural environment (6.2 mSv/year). The only way to avoid all radiation exposure is to wait for 5–10 half-lives, until all of the radioisotope decays (3–6 days).

Pregnancy Risk	Hazardous		Lactation Risk	L5
T ½	= 13.2 hours		M/P	=
Vd	=		PB	=
Tmax	=		Oral	= Complete
MW	=		pKa	=

Adult Concerns: Vomiting, nausea, rash, pruritus, chest pain, tachycardia. Ablation of thyroid function. Theoretical risk of breast cancer if used in lactating women.

Pediatric Concerns:

Drug Interactions:

Relative Infant Dose:

Adult Dose:

Alternatives: Technetium-[99M]

References:
1. Robinson PS, Barker P, Campbell A, Henson P, Surveyor I, Young PR. Iodine-131 in breast milk following therapy for thyroid carcinoma. J Nucl Med 1994; 35(11): 1797–1801.
2. Morita S, Umezaki N, Ishibashi M, Kawamura S, Inada C, Hayabuchi N. Determining the breast-feeding interruption schedule after administration of ^{123}I-iodide. Ann Nucl Med 1998; 12(5): 303–306.
3. ICRP, 2008. Radiation Dose to Patients from Radiopharmaceuticals–Addendum 3 to ICRP Publication 53. ICRP Publication 106. Ann. ICRP 38 (1–2).
4. Activities of Radiopharmaceuticals from the Nuclear Regulatory Commission.
5. Montford PJ. Textbook of Radiopharmacy. Third Edition. Gordon and Breach Publishers 1999.

[125]IODINE   L5

Trade: Radioactive Iodine, Iodine-125, [125]I

Other Trades:

Category: Radioactive iodine

The normal human body contains about 9–10 mg of iodine, 90% of which resides in the thyroid gland. The thyroid gland concentrates more than 100 times the recommended daily allowance. The thyroid gland, and the cells in the lactating breast, contain a transporter (symporter) that facilitates concentration of iodine in these tissues. The normal range of iodine in human milk is reported to be 20–150 µg/L, and is a function of geography. The daily dietary requirement for lactating women is about 30% higher than for the general public.

Radioactive iodine concentrates in the thyroid gland as well as in breastmilk, and if ingested by an infant, it may suppress its thyroid function or increase the risk of future thyroid carcinomas, and produce thyroid destruction in the infant. Radioactive iodine is clinically used to ablate or destroy the thyroid (dose= 355 MBq), or in much smaller doses (7.4 MBq), to scan the thyroid for malignancies. Following ingestion, radioactive iodine concentrates in the thyroid and lactating tissues, and it is estimated 27.9% of total radioactivity is secreted via breast milk.[1] Two potential half-lives exist for radioactive iodine: one is the radioactive half-life which is solely dependent on radioactive decay of the molecule; and two, the biological half-life, which is often briefer and is the half-life of the iodine molecule itself in the human being. The latter half-life is influenced most by elimination via the kidneys and other routes. Previously published data have suggested that Iodine-125 is present in milk for at least 12 days, but these studies may be in error as they ignored the second component of the biexponential breastmilk disappearance curve.[2] The half-life of ^{125}I is 60.2 days. The biological or effective half-life may be shorter due to excretion in urine, feces, and milk.

The Nuclear Regulatory Commission has released a table of instructions to mothers concerning the use of radioisotopes. Ultimately, the amount of radioiodine transferred into human milk depends on the clinical dose administered to the mother and the radioisotope used. Radioiodine concentrates in milk where at least 26–45% of the dose ends up in the breast. Radiographs show major concentration in breastmilk. In scanning procedures where only a few microcuries are used (<14 uCi), the mother may be able to return to breastfeeding within 20 days or perhaps less depending on the dose. In cases where ablation doses are used (300–700 mCi), the risk to the breastfeeding mother (breast cancer) is significant, and the risk to the infant is major (future thyroid cancer). Low scanning doses may present an opportunity to return to breastfeeding if the counts in milk are closely monitored in the coming weeks. Using extraordinarily high ablative doses may continue to be present in milk for many weeks. If one is able to measure the milk for radiation, then a return to baseline would allow a patient to re-initiate breastfeeding. However with ablative doses, it is probably advisable to discontinue breastfeeding, dry up, and then initiate treatment to try and avoid high exposure of breast tissue. Mothers exposed to radioactive iodine released from nuclear power plant disasters, should be immediately treated with potassium iodide to prevent transmission of the radioactive iodine into human milk, and the infant's thyroid.

Breastfeeding Recommendations for ^{125}I.

^{125}I HAS: 0.2mCi dose: 277 hours (11.5 days) interruption or complete cessation.[3]

^{125}I Hippuran: 0.05 dose: 23 hours cessation.[3]

^{125}I Fibrinogen: 0.1 mCi dose: 620 hours (26 days) interruption of breastfeeding or until counts are baseline.

Note: These recommendations still permit a minimal amount of <1mSv of radiation transfer to the infant. Exposure of 1 mSv has a cancer incidence risk of 1 in 10,000 people. This amount of exposure is less than the amount an average

American is exposed to from the natural environment (6.2 mSv/year). The only way to avoid all radiation exposure is to wait for 5–10 half-lives, until all of the radioisotope decays (300–600 days).

Pregnancy Risk	Hazardous	Lactation Risk	L5
T ½	= 60.2 days	M/P	=
Vd	=	PB	=
Tmax	=	Oral	= Complete
MW	=	pKa	=

Adult Concerns: Vomiting, nausea, rash, pruritus, chest pain, tachycardia. Ablation of thyroid function. Theoretical risk of breast cancer if used in lactating women.

Pediatric Concerns: None reported, but damage to thyroid is probable if the infant is breastfed while ^{125}I levels are high.

Drug Interactions:

Relative Infant Dose:

Adult Dose:

Alternatives: Technetium-^{99M}

References:
1. Robinson PS, Barker P, Campbell A, Henson P, Surveyor I, Young PR. Iodine-131 in breast milk following therapy for thyroid carcinoma. J Nucl Med 1994; 35(11): 1797–1801.
2. Palmer KE. Excretion of ^{125}I in breast milk following administration of labelled fibrinogen. Br J Radiol 1979; 52(620): 672–673.
3. Montford PJ. Textbook of Radiopharmacy. Third Edition. Gordon and Breach Publishers 1999.

^{131}IODINE   L5

Trade: Iodine-131, ^{131}I, Radioactive Iodine, Iodotope, Hicon

Other Trades:

Category: Radioactive iodine

The normal human body contains about 9–10 mg of iodine, 90% of which resides in the thyroid gland. The thyroid gland concentrates more than 100 times the recommended daily allowance. The thyroid gland, and the cells in the lactating breast, contain a transporter (symporter) that facilitates concentration of iodine in these tissues. The normal range of iodine in human milk is reported to be 20–150 µg/L, and is a function of geography. The daily dietary requirement for lactating women is about 30% higher than for the general public.

Radioactive iodine concentrates in the thyroid gland as well as in breastmilk, and if ingested by an infant, it may suppress its thyroid function or increase the risk of future thyroid carcinomas, and produce thyroid destruction in the infant. Radioactive ^{131}I is clinically used to ablate or destroy the thyroid (dose= 355 MBq), or in much smaller doses (7.4 MBq), to scan the thyroid for malignancies. Following ingestion, radioactive iodine concentrates in the thyroid and lactating tissues, and it is estimated 27.9% of total radioactivity is secreted via breast milk.[1] Two potential half-lives exist for radioactive iodine: one is the radioactive half-life which is solely dependent on radioactive decay of the molecule; and two, the biological half-life, which is often briefer and is the half-life of the iodine molecule itself in the human being. The latter half-life is influenced most by elimination via the kidneys and other routes. Previously published data have suggested that ^{131}I is present in breastmilk for 2–14 days, but these studies may be in error as they ignored the second component of the biexponential breastmilk disappearance curve.[2] The radioactive half-life of ^{131}I is 8.1 days. The biological or effective half-life may be shorter due to excretion in urine, feces, and milk. A well done study by Dydek reviewed the transfer of both tracer and ablation doses of ^{131}I into human milk.[3] If the tracer doses are kept minimal (0.1 µCi or 3.7 kBq), breastfeeding could resume as early as the eighth day. However, if larger tracer doses (8.6 µCi or 0.317 MBq) are used, nursing could not resume until 46 days following therapy. Doses used for ablation of the maternal thyroid (111 MBq) would require an interruption of breastfeeding for a minimum of 106 days or more. However, an acceptable dose to an infant, as a result of ingestion of radioiodine, is a matter for debate although an effective dose of <1 mSv has been suggested. In another study of ^{131}I use in a mother, breastmilk levels were followed for 32 days. These authors recommend discontinuing breastfeeding for up to 50–52 days to ensure safety of the infant thyroid. Thyroid scans use either radioactive iodine or ^{99m}Technetium pertechnetate. Technetium has a very short half-life and should be preferred in breastfeeding mothers for thyroid scanning.[3] Due to the fact that significant amounts of ^{131}I are concentrated in breastmilk, women should discontinue breastfeeding prior to treatment, as the cumulative exposure to breast tissues could be excessively high. It is sometimes recommended that women discontinue breastfeeding several days to weeks before undergoing therapy or that they pump and discard milk for several weeks after exposure to iodine to reduce the overall radioactive exposure to breast tissues. The estimated dose of radioactivity to the breasts would give a "theoretical" probability of induction of breast cancer of 0.32%.[1] In addition, holding the infant close to the breast or thyroid gland for long periods may expose the infant to gamma irradiation and is not recommended. Patients should consult with the radiologist concerning exposure of the infant. One case of significant exposure was reported in a breastfed infant.[4] The mother received a 3.02 mCi dose of ^{131}I and continued to breastfeed for the next 7 days before the mother admitted breastfeeding. During this 7 day period, the infant's thyroid contained 2.7 µCi of ^{131}I, which is an effective dose equivalent of 5.5 rads. Had the mother continued to breastfeed, the dose would have been much larger and potentially dangerous. In another case report of a patient who received 14 µCi of oral ^{131}–Iodine, and then 5 mCi of ^{99m}Technetium, the mothers' milk was withdrawn and screened for radiation with a gamma counter.[5] On day 8 the measured radioactivity was 94 counts per minute (cpm). On day 13, the measured radioactivity was 30 cpm, and by day 20, the radioactivity was measured at background levels (20 cpm). This data suggests that if the ^{131}I levels administered are equal to or less than 14 µCi, then the mother could potentially return to breastfeeding after 20 days.

The Nuclear Regulatory Commission has released a table of instructions to mothers concerning the use of radioisotopes. These instructions conclude that patients should not breastfeed following the use of ^{131}I. In a study by Hammami, radioactive ^{131}I was found to transfer into breasts weeks following cessation of lactation.[6] They suggest the breast is a "radioiodine reservoir". Ultimately, the amount of radioiodine transferred into human milk depends on the clinical dose administered to the mother and the radioisotope used. Radioiodine concentrates in milk where at least 26–45% of the dose ends up in the breast. Radiographs show major concentration in breastmilk. In scanning procedures where only a few microcuries are used (< 14 uCi), the mother may be able to return to breastfeeding within 20 days or perhaps less depending on the dose. In cases where ablation doses are used (300–700 mCi), the risk to the breastfeeding mother (breast cancer) is significant, and the risk to the infant is major (future thyroid cancer). Low scanning doses may present an opportunity to return to breastfeeding if the counts in milk are closely monitored in the coming weeks. Using extraordinarily high ablative doses may continue to be present in milk for many weeks. If one is able to measure the milk for radiation, then a return to baseline would allow a patient to re-initiate breastfeeding. However with ablative doses, it is probably advisable to discontinue breastfeeding, dry up, and then initiate treatment to try and avoid high exposure of breast tissue. Mothers exposed to radioactive iodine released from nuclear power plant disasters, should be immediately treated with potassium iodide to prevent transmission of the radioactive iodine into human milk, and the infant's thyroid. International Commission of Radiological Protection (ICRP) recommends > 3 weeks breastfeeding interruption or cessation for non iodo-hippurate and 12 hours interruption for ^{131}I-iodohippurate.[7]

See extensive breastfeeding and close contract restriction tables in the appendix.

Pregnancy Risk	X		Lactation Risk	L5
T ½	= 8.1 days		M/P	=
Vd	=		PB	=
Tmax	=		Oral	= Complete
MW	=		pKa	=

Adult Concerns: Alopecia, rash, pruritus, chest pain, nausea, vomiting, tachycardia, sore throat, leukopenia, tenderness or swelling at neck, cough, hypersensitivity, anaphylaxis. Ablation of thyroid function. Theoretical risk of breast cancer if used in lactating women.

Pediatric Concerns: None reported, but damage to thyroid is probable if the infant is breastfed while ^{131}I levels are high.

Drug Interactions:

Relative Infant Dose:

Adult Dose:

Alternatives: Technetium^{99m}

References:

1. Robinson PS, Barker P, Campbell A, Henson P, Surveyor I, Young PR. Iodine-131 in breast milk following therapy for thyroid carcinoma. J Nucl Med 1994; 35(11): 1797–1801.
2. Palmer KE. Excretion of ^{125}I in breast milk following administration of labelled fibrinogen. Br J Radiol 1979; 52(620): 672–673.
3. Dydek GJ, Blue PW. Human breast milk excretion of iodine-131 following diagnostic and therapeutic administration to a lactating patient with Graves' disease. J Nucl Med 1988; 29(3): 407–410.

4. Iodine-131 dose for whole body scan administered to a breast-feeding patient. Preliminary notification of event or unusual occurrence PNO-198–038. NRC. http: //www. nrc. gov/OPA/ pn/pn19838. htm. 2004.
5. Saenz RB. Iodine-131 elimination from breast milk: a case report. J Hum Lact 2000; 16(1): 44–46.
6. Bakheet SM, Hammami MM. Patterns of radioiodine uptake by the lactating breast. Eur J Nucl Med 1994; 21(7): 604–608.
7. ICRP, 2008. Radiation Dose to Patients from Radiopharmaceuticals–Addendum 3 to ICRP Publication 53. ICRP Publication 106. Ann. ICRP 38 (1–2).
8. Activities of Radiopharmaceuticals from the Nuclear Regulatory Commission.
9. Montford PJ. Textbook of Radiopharmacy. Third Edition. Gordon and Breach Publishers 1999.
10. Adapted from American Thyroid Association Taskforce On Radioiodine Safety, Sisson JC, Freitas J, McDougall IR, Dauer LT, Hurley JR, Brierley JD, Edinboro CH, Rosenthal D, Thomas MJ, Wexler JA, Asamoah E, Avram AM, Milas M, Greenlee C. Radiation safety in the treatment of patients with thyroid diseases by radioiodine 131–I: practice recommendations of the american thyroid association. Thyroid. 2011 Apr; 21(4): 335–46. Epub 2011 Mar 18.

IBANDRONATE   L3

Trade: Boniva

Other Trades:

Category: Bisphosphonate

Ibandronate is a bisphosphonate which acts by inhibiting osteoclast-mediated bone resorption. It is therefore used in the treatment and prevention of postmenopausal osteoporosis.[1] Following oral or intravenous administration, 40 to 50% of the drug is rapidly removed from the circulation and binds to bone, thereby reducing plasma concentrations to 10% of peak plasma within 3 hours of an intravenous dose, or within 8 hours of an oral dose. It is currently not known if ibandronate is transferred into human milk. When administered in lactating rats, the concentration of ibandronate that appeared in the milk was 1.5 times the plasma concentrations.[] A review of the pharmacokinetic profile suggests that due to its relatively high protein binding and low oral bioavailability, this drug may probably not attain clinically significant plasma levels in the infant. However, until more established data are available on the transfer ibandronate into human milk, some caution is recommended when considering administration in a breastfeeding mother.

Pregnancy Risk	C	Lactation Risk	L3
T ½	= 4.6–25.5 hours	M/P	=
Vd	= 90 L l/kg	PB	= 85.7–99.5%
Tmax	= 0.5–2 hours	Oral	= 0.6%
MW	= 359.24	pKa	=

Adult Concerns: Common adverse effects include nausea, diarrhea, rise in blood pressure, abdominal pain, headache, back pain, upper respiratory infections. Some rare and serious side-effects of this drug are peptic ulcers, gastroesophageal reflux disease, esophagitis, arthralgia.

Pediatric Concerns:

Drug Interactions: Concurrent use of ibandronate with iron, calcium, magnesium and aluminum containing products may decrease the efficacy of ibandronate.

Relative Infant Dose:

Adult Dose: 3 mg IV every 3 months. 2.5 mg orally once daily or 150 mg orally once a month.

Alternatives: Alendronate, pamidronate

References:

1. Pharmaceutical manufacturer prescribing information, 2011.

IBUPROFEN   L1

Trade:

Other Trades:

Category: Analgesic, antipyretic

Ibuprofen is a nonsteroidal anti-inflammatory analgesic (NSAID). It is frequently used for fever in infants. Ibuprofen enters milk only in very low levels (less than 0.6% of maternal dose). Even large doses produce very small milk levels. In one patient receiving 400 mg twice daily, milk levels were less than 0.5 mg/L.[1] In another study of twelve women who received 400 mg doses every 6 hours for a total of 5 doses, all breastmilk levels of ibuprofen were less than 1.0 mg/L, the lower limit of the assay.[2] In another study of a single mother following the use of six 400 mg doses over 42.5 hours, ibuprofen levels at 30 minutes following the first dose were 13 mg/L.[3] The highest reported level in milk (180 µg/L) was after the third 400 mg dose at 20.5 hours. The authors suggested that an infant would receive approximately 17 µg/kg/day following maternal doses of 1.2 grams daily.

Data in these studies document that no measurable concentrations of ibuprofen are detected in breastmilk following the above doses. Ibuprofen is presently popular for therapy of fever in infants. Current recommended dose in children is 5–10 mg/kg every 6 hours. Ibuprofen is an ideal analgesic for breastfeeding mothers.

Pregnancy Risk	B/D in 3rd trimester	Lactation Risk	L1
T ½	= 1.8–2.5 hours	M/P	=
Vd	= 0.14 l/kg	PB	= >99%
Tmax	= 1–2 hours	Oral	= 80%
MW	= 206	pKa	= 4.4

Adult Concerns: Nausea, epigastric pain, dizziness, edema, gastrointestinal bleeding.

Pediatric Concerns: None reported from breastfeeding. Ideal analgesic.

Drug Interactions: Aspirin may decrease serum ibuprofen levels. May prolong prothrombin time when used with warfarin. Antihypertensive effects of ACE inhibitors may be blunted or completely abolished by NSAIDs. Some NSAIDs may block antihypertensive effect of beta blockers, diuretics. Used with cyclosporin, may dramatically increase renal toxicity. May increase digoxin, phenytoin, lithium levels. May increase toxicity of methotrexate. May increase bioavailability of penicillamine. Probenecid may increase NSAID levels.

Relative Infant Dose: 0.1%–0.7%

Adult Dose: 400 mg every 4–6 hours.

Alternatives: Acetaminophen

References:
1. Weibert RT, Townsend RJ, Kaiser DG, Naylor AJ. Lack of ibuprofen secretion into human milk. Clin Pharm 1982; 1(5): 457–458.
2. Townsend RJ, Benedetti TJ, Erickson SH, Cengiz C, Gillespie WR, Gschwend J, Albert KS. Excretion of ibuprofen into breast milk. Am J Obstet Gynecol 1984; 149(2): 184–186.
3. Walter K, Dilger C. Ibuprofen in human milk. Br J Clin Pharmacol 1997; 44: 211–2.

ICHTHAMMOL   L3

Trade: Albichthyol

Other Trades:

Category: Antiseptic, anti-inflammatory

Ichthammol is technically Ammonium bituminosulfonate and is derived from dry distillation of sulfur-rich oil shale. It has been used for the treatment of psoriasis, eczema, and other dermatologic condition for centuries. Used in 10–20% concentrations, it is still used as a "drawing salve". However, its function here is somewhat erroneous, as it only softens the skin over a lesion, permitting the formation of a pustule that is easily opened. Ichthammol is suggested to have anti-inflammatory, analgesic, antimicrobial and antifungal properties. It is well tolerated and no reports of carcinogenicity are found.[1] Pale sulfonated shale oil (4%) has been used in children to treat atopic eczema.[2] There are no studies of the topical use of ichthammol in breastfeeding women. No data are available on its use in breastfeeding mothers, however it would be largely unabsorbed transcutaneously.

Pregnancy Risk	Probably Safe	Lactation Risk	L3
T ½	=	M/P	=
Vd	=	PB	=
Tmax	=	Oral	=
MW	=	pKa	=

Adult Concerns: Staining of skin, erythema, itch.

Pediatric Concerns:

Drug Interactions:

Relative Infant Dose:

Adult Dose:

Alternatives:

References:

1. Boyd AS. Ichthammol revisited. Int J Dermatol. 2010 Jul; 49(7): 757–60. Review.
2. Korting HC, Sch√∂llmann C, Cholcha W, Wolff L; Collaborative Study Group. Efficacy and tolerability of pale sulfonated shale oil cream 4% in the treatment of mild to moderate atopic eczema in children: a multicentre, randomized vehicle-controlled trial. J Eur Acad Dermatol Venereol. 2010 Oct; 24(10): 1176–82. doi: 10.1111/j. 1468–3083.2010.03616. x.

IFOSFAMIDE   L4

Trade: Holoxan, Ifex, Ifolem, Holoxane

Other Trades:

Category: Anticancer agent

Ifosfamide (IF) is structurally similar to cyclophosphamide and is used in breast cancer. This family of drugs requires activation (metabolism) by the liver to produce the active cytotoxic agents. The oral bioavailability of IF is near 100% and reaches a peak at 1–2 hours.[1] The elimination half-life (T½ beta) ranges from 3.8 to 8.6 hours. Active metabolites stay in the plasma compartment with brief half-lives of 4–6 hours or less. Transport of IF and its metabolites into the CNS is exceedingly low (approximately 1/6th of the plasma compartment). This would suggest milk levels will probably be low when they are ultimately determined. The kinetics of this agent are highly variable depending on the renal function, creatinine clearance, liver function, etc. Waiting periods before returning to breastfeeding should be adjusted for this factor. Withhold breastfeeding for at least 72 hours.

Pregnancy Risk	D	Lactation Risk	L4
T ½	= 3.8–8.6 hours	M/P	=
Vd	= 0.72 l/kg	PB	= 20%
Tmax	= 1 hour	Oral	= 92%-100%
MW	= 261	pKa	= 3.5–4

Adult Concerns: Agitation, confusion, hallucinations, unusual tiredness.

Pediatric Concerns:

Drug Interactions: Do not administer live vaccines such as MMR, influenza, rotavirus concurrently with ifosfamide. Concurrent administration with aprepitant or fosaprepitant may cause increased plasma levels of ifosfamide. Concurrent administration with warfarin may increase risk of severe bleeding complications.

Relative Infant Dose:

Adult Dose:

Alternatives:

References:
1. Pharmaceutical manufacturer Package Insert, 2007.

ILOPERIDONE   L3

Trade: Fanapt

Other Trades:

Category: Atypical antipsychotic

Iloperidone is an atypical antipsychotic used in the treatment of schizophrenia. The dose of iloperidone must be increased slowly and administered twice daily to decrease the orthostatic hypotensive effects of the drug. Iloperidone also prolongs the QT interval and has the potential to cause leukopenia, neutropenia and agranulocytosis; therefore, ECG monitoring and monitoring of blood parameters should be done during therapy. There were no studies found on the use of iloperidone during breastfeeding although it is excreted in rat milk. The pharmaceutical information states that mothers should not breastfeed while taking iloperidone.[1] Since there is very little information on its use in breastfeeding women, other alternatives such as risperidone or quetiapine should be considered before resorting to the use of this drug.[2]

Pregnancy Risk	C	Lactation Risk	L3
T ½	= 18–33 hours	M/P	=
Vd	= 40 l/kg	PB	= 95%
Tmax	= 2–4 hours	Oral	= 96%
MW	= 426.5	pKa	=

Adult Concerns: Common side effects include weight gain, hyperprolactinemia, xerostomia, headache, dizziness, somnolence, and nasal congestion. Other side effects include fatigue, dysphagia, and suicidal intent.

Pediatric Concerns:

Drug Interactions: Concomitant administration with the following drugs increases the plasma levels of iloperidone: fluoxetine, paroxetine, ketoconazole, itraconazole, or clarithromycin. Iloperidone should not be co-administered with other drugs that could possibly prolong the QT interval such as quinidine, procainamide, amiodarone, sotalol, chlorpromazine, thioridazine, gatifloxacin, moxifloxacin, pentamidine, levomethadyl acetate, methadone.

Relative Infant Dose:

Adult Dose: 6–12 mg orally twice daily.

Alternatives: Risperidone, quetiapine, aripiprazole

References:
1. Pharmaceutical manufacturer prescribing information, 2010.
2. Howland RH. Update on newer antipsychotic drugs. J Psychosoc Nurs Ment Health Serv. 2011 Apr; 49(4): 13–5. doi: 10.3928/02793695–20110311–99.

IMATINIB MESYLATE   L5

Trade: Gleevec

Other Trades:

Category: Antineoplastic agent, tyrosine kinase inhibitor

Imatinib mesylate is a tyrosine kinase inhibitor used to treat several different types of tumors and leukemias. The metabolite half life is 40 hours, which means that 81% would be eliminated from the mother in seven days.[1] No data are available on the transfer of this medication into human milk, but due to the overt toxicity of this product, breastfeeding mothers should withhold breastfeeding for at least ten days after taking this medication. The milk should be pumped and discarded during this time. Imatinib and its active metabolite are excreted into human milk. Based on data from three breastfeeding women taking imatinib, the milk/plasma ratio is about 0.5 for imatinib and about 0.9 for the active metabolite. Considering the combined concentrations of imatinib and active metabolite, a breastfed infant could receive up to 10% of the maternal therapeutic dose based on body weight. Because of the potential for serious adverse reactions in nursing infants from imatinib, mothers should be advised against breastfeeding while taking this medication.

Pregnancy Risk	D	Lactation Risk	L5
T ½	= 18–40 hours	M/P	= 0.5/0.9 (metabolite)
Vd	=	PB	= 95%
Tmax	= 2–4 hours	Oral	= 98%
MW	= 590	pKa	= 13.45

Adult Concerns: Adverse reactions commonly seen include edema, anemia, neutropenia, thrombocytopenia, congestive heart failure, left ventricular dysfunction, hepatotoxicity, hemorrhage, gastrointestinal irritation, and dermatological reactions such as Stevens-Johnsons syndrome.

Pediatric Concerns: Strong anticancer drug. Avoid breastfeeding while taking this medication.

Drug Interactions: Warfarin, erythromycin, phenytoin, and other CYP3A4 inhibitors should not be used with imatinib.

Relative Infant Dose:

Adult Dose: 400 mg once or twice daily.

Alternatives:

References:
1. Pharmaceutical manufacturer Package Insert, 2007.

IMIPENEM + CILASTATIN   L2

Trade: Primaxin
Other Trades:
Category: Antibiotic, carbapenem

Imipenem is structurally similar to penicillins and acts similarly. Cilastatin is added to extend the half-life of imipenem. Imipenem is poorly absorbed orally and must be injected IM or IV.[1,2] Imipenem is destroyed by gastric acidity and would not be orally bioavailable. Transfer into breastmilk is probably minimal but no data are available. Changes in gastrointestinal flora could occur but is probably remote.

Pregnancy Risk	C	Lactation Risk	L2
T ½	= 0.85–1.35 hours	M/P	=
Vd	=	PB	= 20%
Tmax	= 2 hours	Oral	= Poor
MW	=	pKa	= 15

Adult Concerns: Nausea, diarrhea, vomiting, hypersensitivity reactions, superinfection, erythema multiforme, seizures.

Pediatric Concerns:

Drug Interactions: May have increased toxicity when used with other beta lactam antibiotics. Probenecid may increase toxic potential.

Relative Infant Dose:

Adult Dose:

Alternatives:

References:
1. Pharmaceutical manufacturer prescribing information, 1995.
2. McEvoy GE. (ed): AFHS Drug Information. New York, NY: 2003.

IMIPRAMINE   L2

Trade: Tofranil, Janimine

Other Trades: Melipramine, Apo-Imipramine, Impril, Novo-Pramine

Category: Tricyclic antidepressant

Imipramine is a classic tricyclic antidepressant. Imipramine is metabolized to desipramine, the active metabolite. Milk levels approximate those of maternal serum. In a patient receiving 200 mg daily at bedtime, the milk levels at 1, 9, 10, and 23 hours were 29, 24, 12, and 18 µg/L respectively.[1] However, in this study the mother was not in a therapeutic range. In another study of 4 women receiving 75–150 mg/day imipramine, levels of imipramine plus desipramine in fore milk ranged from 34–408 µg/L and in hind milk ranged from 48 to 622 µg/L.[2] In several breastfed infants, levels of imipramine plus desipramine ranged from 0.6 µg/L in one individual (maternal dose=75 mg/day) to 5.5 µg/L (maternal dose=100 mg/day).[3] Therapeutic plasma levels in older children 6–12 years are 200–225 µg/L. Two good reviews of psychotropic drugs in breastfeeding patients are available.[4,5]

The levels of imipramine in breastmilk are low and therefore, it is probably compatible with breastfeeding.

Pregnancy Risk	C	Lactation Risk	L2
T ½	= 8–16 hours	M/P	= 0.5–1.5
Vd	= 20–40 l/kg	PB	= 90%
Tmax	= 1–2 hours	Oral	= 90%
MW	= 280	pKa	= 9.5

Adult Concerns: Dry mouth, sedation, hypotension, arrhythmias, confusion, agitation, seizures.

Pediatric Concerns: None reported, but observe for sedation, dry mouth.

Drug Interactions: Barbiturates may lower serum levels of tricyclic antidepressants (TCAs). Central and respiratory depressant effects may be additive. Cimetidine has increased serum TCA concentrations. Anticholinergic symptoms may be exacerbated. Use with clonidine may produce dangerous elevations in blood pressure and hypertensive crisis. Dicumarol anticoagulant capacity may be increased when used with TCAs. Co-use with fluoxetine may increase the toxic levels and effects of TCAs. Symptoms may persist for several weeks after discontinuation of fluoxetine. Haloperidol may increase serum concentrations of TCAs. MAO inhibitors should never be given immediately after or with tricyclic antidepressants. Oral contraceptives may inhibit the metabolism of tricyclic antidepressants and may increase their plasma levels.

Relative Infant Dose: 0.1%–4.4%

Adult Dose: 75–100 mg daily.

Alternatives: Amoxapine

References:
1. Sovner R, Orsulak PJ. Excretion of imipramine and desipramine in human breast milk. Am J Psychiatry 1979; 136(4A): 451–452.
2. Yoshida K, Smith B, Kumar R. Psychotropic drugs in mothers' milk: a comprehensive review of assay methods, pharmacokinetics and of safety of breast-feeding. J Psychopharmacol. 1999; 13(1): 64–80. Review.
3. Yoshida K, Smith B, Craggs M et al. Investigation of pharmacokinetics and possible adverse effects in infants exposed to tricyclic antidepressants in breast-milk. J Affective Disord. 1997; 43: 225–37.
4. Buist A, Norman TR, Dennerstein L. Breastfeeding and the use of psychotropic medication: a review. J Affect Disord 1990; 19(3): 197–206.
5. Wisner KL, Perel JM, Findling RL. Antidepressant treatment during breast-feeding. Am J Psychiatry 1996; 153(9): 1132–1137.

IMIQUIMOD   L3

Trade: Aldara, Zyclara, Beselna, Imimor

Other Trades:

Category: Immune Modulator

Imiquimod is a toll-like receptor 7 agonist that activates immune cells to produce cytokines and helps regulate co-stimulatory molecule expression. The drug also improves the function of antigens in acquired immune cells. Imiquimod is used for the treatment of plantar warts and actinic keratoses. After topical administration of the 5% cream, serum metabolites levels have been found to be generally low and in one study, only quantifiable in 3 subjects at the end of a 21 day application.[1] The adult use of imiquimod 3.75% cream in the treatment of actinic keratoses produced similarly low serum levels when applied for 3 weeks. The amount given in this study was 18.75 mg each day for 21 days, applied to 200 sq. cm of skin. At the end of the study, mean steady state serum concentrations measured 0.323 ng/mL.[1] This concentration is much lower than the 500 ng/mL needed to elicit systemic induction of interferon alpha or interleukin 1 receptor antagonists.[2] Imiquimod has been used in young children. In a study determining the pharmacokinetics of imiquimod in children, serum levels of this drug were shown to be extremely low. After administration of 12.5–37.5 mg imiquimod each day to children aged 2–12, it was found that the median maximum concentration was ≤ 0.5 ng/mL for single doses and ≤ 1.0 ng/mL for multiple doses. One outlier was reported with concentrations as high as 9.7 ng/mL. Children in this study were all treated for molluscum contagiosum with 5% imiquimod cream. Amounts given to each child varied based on the weight of the subject and extent of disease.[3]

While there are no data on the excretion of imiquimod into human milk, milk levels will likely be far lower than 323 ng/L, which would be far too low to produce clinical effects in an infant. The manufacturer recommends that caution be used when administering imiquimod to nursing women. Infants should be observed for nausea, vomiting, and poor feeding with imiquimod use.

Pregnancy Risk	C	Lactation Risk	L3
T ½	= 23–27 hours topical, 2 hours sc, 2.5 hours oral	M/P	=
Vd	=	PB	=
Tmax	= 9 hours topical, 2.6–3.6 hours oral	Oral	= 47%
MW	= 240.3	pKa	=

Adult Concerns: Local site reactions, eczema, alopecia, rash, pruritus, infections, headache, fever, fatigue, chest pain, nausea, vomiting, diarrhea, myalgia, pharyngitis, cough, angioedema, erythema multiforme.

Pediatric Concerns:

Drug Interactions: BCG: Imiquimod may decrease the effects of this agent. Conivaptan: Do not use imiquimod within 7 days of this agent. Denosumab: This drug may increase the adverse effects of imiquimod. Echinacea: This herb may decrease the effects of imiquimod. Leflunomide: Imiquimod may increase the adverse effects of leflunomide. Do not use these drugs concurrently. Natalizumab: Imiquimod may increase the adverse effects of natalizumab. Do not use these drugs concurrently. Pimecrolimus: This drug may increase the adverse effects of imiquimod. Do not use these drugs concurrently. Roflumilast: This drug may increase the adverse effects of imiquimod. Sipuleucel-T: Imiquimod may decrease the effects of this drug. Tacrolimus: This drug may increase the adverse effects of imiquimod. Do not use these drugs concurrently. Tocilizumab: This drug may decrease the effects of imiquimod. Trastuzumab: This drug may enhance the neutropenic effects of imiquimod. Vaccines: Imiquimod may interfere with the functions of vaccines.

Relative Infant Dose:

Adult Dose: Variable topically

Alternatives:

References:

1. Kulp J, Levy S, Fein MC, Adams M, Furst J, Meng TC. Pharmacokinetics of imiquimod 3.75% cream applied daily for 3 weeks to actinic keratoses on the face and/or balding scalp. Arch Dermatol Res. 2010 Sep; 302(7): 539–44.

2. Miller RL, Gerster JF, Owens ML, Slade HB, Tomai MA (1999). Imiquimod applied topically: a novel immune response modifier and new class of drug. Int J Immunopharmacol 21: 1–14. K.
3. Myhre PE, et al. Pharmacokinetics and Safety of Imiquimod 5% Cream in the Treatment of Molluscum Contagiosum in Children. Pediatric Dermatology. Vol. 25(1); 2008.88–95.

INCOBOTULINUMTOXIN A   L3

Trade: Xeomin

Other Trades:

Category: Neuromuscular blocker

Incobotulinumtoxin A,[1] is a neurotoxin produced by *Clostridium botulinum*, spore-forming anaerobic bacillus, which appears to affect only the presynaptic membrane of the neuromuscular junction in humans, where it prevents calcium-dependent release of acetylcholine and produces a state of denervation. Muscle inactivation persists until new fibrils grow from the nerve and form junction plates on new areas of the muscle-cell walls. Intradermal injection results in temporary sweat gland denervation, reducing local sweating. No data are available on the medical use of botulin A (botulinum toxin) during breastfeeding. However, one infant was safely breastfed during maternal botulism and no botulinum toxin was detectable in the mother's milk or infant. Since the doses used medically are far lower than those that cause botulism, amounts ingested by the infant, if any, are expected to be insignificant and not cause any adverse effects in breastfed infants. Pump and discard milk for approximately 12 hours.

Pregnancy Risk	C	Lactation Risk	L3
T ½	=	M/P	=
Vd	=	PB	=
Tmax	=	Oral	= Nil
MW	= 150,000	pKa	=

Adult Concerns: Dysphagia, neck pain, muscle weakness, injection site pain, and musculoskeletal pain.

Pediatric Concerns:

Drug Interactions: No formal drug interaction studies have been conducted with Incobotulinumtoxin A. Co-administration of Incobotulinumtoxin A and aminoglycoside antibiotics, or tubocurarine-type muscle relaxants, should only be performed with caution as these agents may potentiate the effect of the toxin. Use of anticholinergic drugs after administration of Incobotulinumtoxin A may potentiate systemic anticholinergic effects.

Relative Infant Dose:

Adult Dose: For cervical dystonia = 120 Units

Alternatives:

References:
1. Pharmaceutical manufacturer prescribing information, 2010.

INDAPAMIDE   L3

Trade: Lozol

Other Trades: Dapa-Tabs, Nadide, Napamide, Natrilix, Lozide,
    Gen-Indapamide, Apo-Indapamide

Category: Antihypertensive diuretic

Indapamide is the first of a new class of indoline diuretics used to treat hypertension. No data are available on transfer of this diuretic into human milk.[1] Numerous other diuretics are available and have been studied in breastfeeding mothers. See hydrochlorothiazide, or furosemide as an alternatives.

Pregnancy Risk	B	Lactation Risk	L3
T ½	= 14 hours	M/P	=
Vd	=	PB	= 71%
Tmax	= 0.5–2 hours	Oral	= Complete
MW	= 366	pKa	= 11.69

Adult Concerns: Sodium and potassium loss, hypotension, dizziness, nausea, vomiting, constipation.

Pediatric Concerns: None reported, but observe for volume depletion.

Drug Interactions: May reduce effect of oral hypoglycemics. Cholestyramine may reduce absorption of indapamide. May increase the effect of furosemide and other diuretics. May increase toxicity and levels of lithium.

Relative Infant Dose:

Adult Dose: 2.5–5 mg daily.

Alternatives: Hydrochlorothiazide, furosemide

References:
1.   Pharmaceutical manufacturer prescribing information, 2007.

INDINAVIR   L3

Trade: Crixivan

Other Trades:

Category: Antiretroviral agent used in HIV infections.

Indinavir binds to the protease active site and inhibits the activity of the enzyme in HIV virus. This inhibition prevents cleavage of the viral polyproteins resulting in the formation of immature non-infectious viral particles. In a rodent study, indinavir milk levels were quite high[1], although usually this does not correlate closely with human milk. In a study of a single woman patient who was receiving

600 mg twice daily during the first 5 days postpartum, levels of indinavir in colostrum were 90–540% of the maternal plasma levels.[2] This should have been expected, as the milk compartment was virtually open to all plasma components the first few days postpartum. Levels of indinavir after the first week postpartum will likely be much less than above. Viral titers in milk were equivalent to those in the HAART-treated mothers, and were very low (<400 copies/mL). Because HIV may be transferred into breastmilk, breastfeeding is contraindicated in HIV infected mothers unless there are no alternative safe nutritional sources available.

Pregnancy Risk	C	Lactation Risk	L3
T ½	= 1.4–2.2 hours	M/P	=
Vd	= 195 L l/kg	PB	= 60%
Tmax	= 0.8 hours	Oral	= 30%
MW	= 711.88	pKa	= 14.21

Adult Concerns: Kidney toxicity due to stones. Asymptomatic hyperbilirubinemia, abdominal pain, nausea, diarrhea, headache.

Pediatric Concerns:

Drug Interactions: The following are drugs contra-indicated with indinavir: amiodarone, ergot derivatives, cisapride, alprazolam, triazolam, midazolam, pimozide. Concomitant use with the following causes an increase in indinavir levels: delavirdine, nelfinavir, ritonavir, itraconazole, ketoconazole. Concomitant use with the following causes a decrease in indinavir levels: efavirenz, nevirapine, carbamazepine, phenobarbitone, phenytoin, rifabutin, venlafaxine. Concomitant use of indinavir causes an increase in plasma levels of the following coadministered drugs: alfuzosin, ritonavir, saquinavir, bepridil, lidocaine, quinidine, trazodone, colchicine, felodipine, nifedipine, nicardipine, clarithromycin, bosentan, salmeterol, fluticasone, tacrolimus, cyclosporine, sirolimus. Do not use concurrently with the following drugs: rifampin, statins, St. John's wort, sildenafil, atazanavir.

Relative Infant Dose:

Adult Dose: 800 mg every 8 hours.

Alternatives:

References:
1. Lewis JS, 2nd, Terriff CM, Coulston DR, Garrison MW. Protease inhibitors: a therapeutic breakthrough for the treatment of patients with human immunodeficiency virus. Clin Ther. Mar-Apr 1997; 19(2): 187–214.
2. Colebunders R, Hodossy B, Burger D, et al. The effect of highly active antiretroviral treatment on viral load and antiretroviral drug levels in breast milk. AIDS. Nov 4 2005; 19(16): 1912–1915.

INDIUM[111]   L4

Trade: [111]Indium

Other Trades:

Category: Radioactive diagnostic agent

Indium[111] (In[111]) is a radioactive material used for imaging neuroendocrine tumors.

While the plasma half-life is extremely short (<10 minutes), with the majority of this product leaving the plasma compartment and distributing to tissue sites, the radioactive half-life is 2.8 days. In one patient receiving 12 MBq (0.32 mCi), the concentration in milk at 6 and 20 hours was 0.09 Bq/mL and 0.20 Bq/mL per MBq injected.[1] These data indicate that breastfeeding may be safe if this radiopharmaceutical is used. Assuming an ingestion of 500 cc daily, the infant would receive approximately 100 Bq per MBq given to the mother (approximately 0.1 µCi). The NRC recommends a waiting period of 1 week with doses of 20 MBq (0.5 mCi).[2] International Commission of Radiological Protection (ICRP) recommends no interruption of breastfeeding from administration of In[111] WBC and In[111] Octreotide.[3] However, close contact restriction is still warranted. Mountford estimates that a dose of 0.46 mCi will give 1 mSv radiation exposure to infant via close contact.[4] Restricting close contact to 35 minutes every 4 hours for 3 days reduces radiation exposure by 30%.[4]

Breastfeeding restrictions:

[111]In-santumomab pendetide (OncoScint): 4–6 mCi dose: 14 days interruption.

[111]In-pentetriotide (OctreoScan): 6mCi dose: 72 hours interruption.

^{111}In-DTPA (Cisternogram): 0.5–1.5 mCi dose: 14 days interruption.

^{111}In-CYT-356 (ProstaScint): 5–17 mCi dose: 14 days interruption.

^{111}In-WBC (infections): 0.5 mCi dose: 1 week interruption.[5]

[111]In-Octreotide (CSF-imaging neuroendocrine tumors): 5.3 mCi dose: <10 days interruption.

^{111}In-DTPA (CSF-cisternogram, shunt patency): 0.5 mCi dose: 1 week interruption.[5]

[111]In-Leucocytes (CSF-cisternogram, shunt patency): 0.5 mCi dose: No interruption.[6]

Close contact restrictions (6 feet separation from infant): Avoid close contact for the first 4 hours, limit close contact to 35 min per hour with maximum 9 hours per day.[4] Restricting close contact to 35 minutes every 4 hours for 3 days reduces radiation exposure by 30%.[4]

Note: These recommendations still permit a minimal amount of <1mSv of radiation transfer to the infant. Exposure of 1 mSv has a cancer incidence risk of 1 in 10,000 people. This amount of exposure is less than the amount an average American is exposed to from the natural environment (6.2 mSv/year). The only way to avoid all radiation exposure is to wait for 5–10 half-lives, until all of the radioisotope decays (14–28 days).

Pregnancy Risk	X	Lactation Risk	L4
T ½	= 2.8 days	M/P	=
Vd	=	PB	=
Tmax	= Immediate (IV)	Oral	=
MW	= 358	pKa	=

Adult Concerns: Nausea, dizziness, headache, flushing, hypotension.

Pediatric Concerns: None reported, but slight risk of radiation exposure.

Drug Interactions:

Relative Infant Dose:

Adult Dose:

Alternatives:

References:

1. Pullar M, Hartkamp A. Excretion of radioactivity in breastmilk following administration of an 113–Indium labeled chelate complex. Br J Radial 1977; 50: 846.
2. American Academy of Pediatrics, Committee on Drugs. Transfer of drugs and other chemicals into human milk. Pediatrics 2001; 108(3): 776–89.
3. ICRP, 2008. Radiation Dose to Patients from Radiopharmaceuticals–Addendum 3 to ICRP Publication 53. ICRP Publication 106. Ann. ICRP 38 (1–2).
4. Mountford PJ, O'Doherty MJ, Forge NI, Jeffries A, Coakley AJ. Radiation dose rates from adult patients undergoing nuclear medicine investigations. Nucl Med Commun. 1991 Sep; 12(9): 767–77.
5. Activities of Radiopharmaceuticals from the Nuclear Regulatory Commission.
6. Montforf PJ. Textbook of Radiopharmacy. Third edition. Gordon and Breach Publishers 1999.

INDOMETHACIN   L3

Trade: Indocin

Other Trades: Arthrexin, Hicin, Indoptol, Apo-Indomethacin, Indocid, Novo-Methacin

Category: Non-steroidal anti-inflammatory

Indomethacin is a potent, nonsteroidal anti-inflammatory agent frequently used in arthritis. It is also used in newborns in neonatal units to close a patent ductus arteriosus. There is one reported case of convulsions in an infant of a breastfeeding mother who received indomethacin early postpartum (day 7).[1] In another report of 16 women who received 75 mg to 300 mg daily (rectally). Of 20 milk samples analyzed 12 were less than 20 µg/L (limit of detection) and the median milk/plasma ratio was 0.37.[2] The eight measurable samples ranged from 23 to 115 µg/L. The authors suggest the total infant dose, assuming daily milk intake of 150 mL/kg/day, would range from 0.07% to 0.98% of the weight adjusted maternal dose. Plasma samples derived from 6 of the 7 infants were below the sensitivity of the assay (<20 µg/L) and 47 µg/L in only one infant. Dose calculations for all 16 infants showed that absolute doses ranged from <0.003 to 0.017 mg/kg/day. In six of seven infants, indomethacin levels were below detection. In one infant the plasma level was 47 µg/L. No adverse effects were noted in this study.

Based on the reported studies, indomethacin levels in breastmilk are probably too low to cause any significant adverse effects in the breastfed infant. Therefore, indomethacin use is probably compatible with breastfeeding. But since one case of convulsions has been reported with its early postpartum use, it is advisable to exercise caution in premature and newborn infants.

Pregnancy Risk	B/D in 3rd trimester	Lactation Risk	L3
T ½	= 4.5 hours	M/P	= 0.37
Vd	= 0.33–0.40 l/kg	PB	= >90%
Tmax	= 1–2: 2–4 (SR) hours	Oral	= 90%
MW	= 357	pKa	= 4.5

Adult Concerns: Renal dysfunction, gastrointestinal distress, gastric bleeding, diarrhea, clotting dysfunction.

Pediatric Concerns: One case of seizures in neonate. Additional report suggests no untoward effects. Frequently used in neonatal nurseries for patent ductus.

Drug Interactions: May prolong prothrombin time when used with warfarin. Antihypertensive effects of ACE inhibitors may be blunted or completely abolished by NSAIDs. Some NSAIDs may block antihypertensive effect of beta blockers, diuretics. Used with cyclosporin, may dramatically increase renal toxicity. May increase digoxin, phenytoin, lithium levels. May increase toxicity of methotrexate. May increase bioavailability of penicillamine. Probenecid may increase NSAID levels.

Relative Infant Dose: 1.2%

Adult Dose: 25–50 mg 2–3 times daily.

Alternatives: Ibuprofen

References:
1. Eeg-Olofsson O, Malmros I, Elwin CE, Steen B. Convulsions in a breast-fed infant after maternal indomethacin. Lancet 1978; 2(8082): 215.
2. Lebedevs TH, Wojnar-Horton RE, Yapp P, Roberts MJ, Dusci LJ, Hackett LP, Ilett KF. Excretion of indomethacin in breast milk. Br J Clin Pharmacol 1991; 32(6): 751–754.

INFLIXIMAB   L2

Trade: Remicade

Other Trades: Remicade

Category: Treatment of Crohn's, Rheumatoid arthritis

Infliximab is a monoclonal antibody to tumor necrosis factor-alpha (TNF-alpha) used to treat Crohn's disease and rheumatoid arthritis. Infliximab is a very large molecular weight IgG antibody and is largely retained in the vascular system. In a study of one breastfeeding patient who received 5 mg/kg IV, infliximab levels were determined in milk at 0, 2, 4, 8, 24, 48, 72 hours, and 4, 5, and 7 days.[1] None was detected in milk at any time (detection limit <0.1 µg/mL).

In another study, a breastfeeding mother receiving 5 infusions of 10 mg/kg during pregnancy did not have any detectable amounts of infliximab in her milk at any point.[2] The baby's serum level after delivery was 39.5 µg/mL, likely due to placental transfer. The half-life of the drug appeared to be prolonged in the newborn.[2]

Another breastfeeding mother's milk was tested 24 hours and 1 week following her first infusion of a 5 mg/kg dose. The milk levels were below the limit of quantification in both cases.[3] Infliximab is probably too large to enter milk in clinically measurable amounts. It would not be orally bioavailable. In another study of 3 patients who were at least 5 days postpartum and receiving 5 mg/kg doses, infliximab levels in milk were detectable within 12 hours of injection and peaked at 90–105 ng/mL on day 2–3 after infusion. Corresponding blood levels ranged from 18–64 µg/mL.[4] Please note, levels in milk are still $\frac{1}{200}$ th of the levels in maternal serum. Because these minuscule levels will undergo proteolysis in the infant's gastrointestinal tract, it is probably of minimal impact on the immune system of the infant. In addition, these mothers were studied early postnatally when the milk compartment is still able to leak large molecular weight proteins (i. e. IgG) into milk. Therefore, infliximab is probably compatible with breastfeeding.

Pregnancy Risk	B	Lactation Risk	L2
T ½	= 8–9.5 days	M/P	=
Vd	= 3 l/kg	PB	=
Tmax	=	Oral	= Nil
MW	= 149,100	pKa	=

Adult Concerns: Infusion-related reactions include fever, chills, pruritus, urticaria, chest pain, hypotension. A state of immunosuppression is induced thus serious infection including sepsis, disseminated tuberculosis and other infections have been reported.

Pediatric Concerns: None reported in three patients.

Drug Interactions: Concomitant use with anakinra, abatacept and tocilizumab may cause an increased risk of infections.

Relative Infant Dose: 0.3%

Adult Dose: 5 mg/kg (Crohn's)

Alternatives:

References:
1. Hale TW, Fasanmade A. Personal communication. 2002.
2. Vasiliauskas EA, Church JA, Silverman N, Barry M, Targan SR, Dubinsky MC. Case Report: Evidence for Transplacental Trasfer of Maternally Administered Infliximab to the Newborn. Clin Gastroenterol Hepatol 2006; 4: 1255–1258.
3. Peltier M, James D, Ford J, Wagner C, Davis H, Hanauer S. Infliximab levels in breast-milk of a nursing Crohn's patient. Am J Gastroenterol 2001; 96(9): S312.
4. Ben-Horin S, Yavzori M, Kopylov U, Picard O, Fudim E, Eliakim R, Chowers Y, Lang A. Detection of infliximab in breast milk of nursing mothers with inflammatory bowel disease. J Crohns Colitis. 2011 Dec; 5(6): 555–8.

INFLUENZA   L2

Trade:

Other Trades:

Category: Viral Infection

The influenza virus is an orthomyxovirus and consists of 3 types–Influenza type A, type B and type C. Most influenza epidemics are caused by type A and type

B. The influenza A virus is further classified into several subtypes, some of the most commonly known are H1N1, H1N2 and H3N2. The influenza virus is highly contagious and is transmitted from person to person through infected respiratory droplets present in the air or on surfaces. Therefore, wearing a mask to avoid inhalation of contaminated aerosol droplets and regular hand washing after contact with potentially contaminated surfaces has been recommended to decrease the risk of exposure to the virus. The incubation period is 1 to 4 days. The patient is infectious for 24 hours before the onset of symptoms. Once infected, a patient remains infectious for 3 to 7 days.[1] Influenza is characterized by moderate to high degree fever, chills, rigors, malaise, myalgia and is associated with upper respiratory tract symptoms such as cough, nasal congestion and rhinitis.

The protective benefits of breast milk in fighting respiratory illnesses in the infant has been well established. It was found that breast milk mediates an increased production of type 1 interferons in the respiratory tract of infants with influenza. Therefore, infants with influenza illness are generally encouraged to breastfeed.[2] In view of its potential benefits and since no established data on transfer of the influenza virus into breast milk exists, mothers with influenza are encouraged to continue breast feeding. It should be noted that exposure of infant to maternal illness is inevitable since the mother is contagious 24 hours prior to onset of symptoms. Lactating women with influenza can be safely treated with either oseltamivir or zanamivir, since both are compatible with breast feeding.[3] The infant should be closely monitored for any signs of respiratory illness and be treated accordingly. If, H1N1 is the virus implicated, then more restrictive breastfeeding recommendations may be recommended by the CDC.

Pregnancy Risk	Possibly Hazardous	Lactation Risk	L2
T ½	=	M/P	=
Vd	=	PB	=
Tmax	=	Oral	=
MW	=	pKa	=

Adult Concerns: Fever, sore throat, malaise, arthralgias, nausea, vomiting, diarrhea.

Pediatric Concerns:

Drug Interactions:

Relative Infant Dose:

Adult Dose:

Alternatives:

References:

1. AAP CoID: Influenza. In: Red Book: 2009 Report of the Committee on Infectious Diseases. Edited by Pickering LK BC, Kimberlin DW, Long SS, 28 edn; 2009: 400–412.
2. Melendi GA, Coviello S, Bhat N, Zea-Hernandez J, Ferolla FM, Polack FP: Breastfeeding is associated with the production of type I interferon in infants infected with influenza virus. Acta Paediatr 2010, 99(10): 1517–1521.
3. Tanaka T, Nakajima K, Murashima A, Garcia-Bournissen F, Koren G, Ito S: Safety of neuraminidase inhibitors against novel influenza A (H1N1) in pregnant and breastfeeding women. Cmaj 2009, 181(1–2): 55–58.

INFLUENZA VIRUS VACCINES | L1

Trade: Vaccine- Influenza, Flu-Imune, Fluogen, Fluzone, FluMist, Flu Vaccine, Agriflu, Fluarix, Afluria

Other Trades: Fluviral, Fluzone, FluLaval, Fluvirin

Category: Vaccine

Influenza virus vaccines come in two forms. One that is non-viable and requires injection, and the second, a live but attenuated vaccine for application in the nasal passages.

Injectable (Flu-immune, Fluogen, Fluzone, etc.): This influenza vaccine is prepared from inactivated, non-viable influenza viruses and infection of the neonate via milk would not be expected. There are no reported side effects, nor published contraindications for using influenza virus vaccine during lactation.[1,2] Influenza vaccine is now indicated for breastfeeding mothers and their infants by the American Academy of Pediatrics.

Intranasal Live Influenza Virus Vaccine (FluMist): This vaccine consists of a live but attenuated and heat unstable form of influenza virus. Virus instilled in the nasal mucosa replicate thus producing immunity in the host. Virus that escapes the nasal mucosa are unstable and die quickly. It is not known if this virus reaches the human milk compartment, but it is highly unlikely the virus could survive at this temperature in the plasma nor the milk compartment of the mother.

The CDC and the FDA recommend that all breastfeeding women be immunized. This will further protect the breastfed infant as these antibodies will pass into milk, and help protect the newborn breastfed infant from infection. Contents of influenza vaccines change from year to year. Presently, the multi-dose vials contain a small amount of mercury, but there is no evidence that this would even pass to a breastfeeding infant. Single dose vials do not contain mercury. The live attenuated vaccines, FluMist, are not recommended for breastfeeding women, although we know the risks are low. Despite misinformation, there is no squalene present in any of the influenza vaccines used in the USA.

Pregnancy Risk	C		Lactation Risk	L1	
T ½	=		M/P	=	
Vd	=		PB	=	
Tmax	=		Oral	=	
MW	=		pKa	=	

Adult Concerns: Fever, myalgia.

Pediatric Concerns: None reported in breastfeeding mothers.

Drug Interactions: Decreased effect with immunosuppressants. Influenza vaccine may be administered simultaneously (but at a separate site and with a different syringe) with other routine immunizations in children.

Relative Infant Dose:

Adult Dose: 0.5 ml injection once. FluMist is a single unit dose.

Alternatives:

References:

1. Kilbourne ED. Questions and answers. Artificial influenza immunization of nursing mothers not harmful. JAMA 1973; 226: 87.
2. Pharmaceutical manufacturer prescribing information, 2005.

INSECT STINGS   L3

Trade: Insect Stings, Spider Stings, Bee Stings

Other Trades:

Category: Insect stings, envenomations

Insect stings are primarily composed of small peptides, enzymes such as hyaluronidase, and other factors such as histamine. Because the total injection is so small, most reactions are local. In cases of systemic reactions, the secondary release of maternal reactants produces the allergic response in the injected individual. Nevertheless, the amount of injection is exceedingly small. In the case of black widow spiders, the venom is so large in molecular weight (130 kDal for alpha-toxin), it would not likely penetrate milk. In addition, most of the venoms and allergens would be destroyed in the acidic milieu of the infant's stomach. The sting of the Loxosceles spider (brown recluse, fiddleback) is primarily a local necrosis without systemic effects. No report of toxicity to nursing infants has been reported from insect stings.

Pregnancy Risk	Hazardous	Lactation Risk	L3
T ½	=	M/P	=
Vd	=	PB	=
Tmax	=	Oral	=
MW	=	pKa	=

Adult Concerns: Nausea, vomiting.

Pediatric Concerns: None reported via milk.

Drug Interactions:

Relative Infant Dose:

Adult Dose: N/A

Alternatives:

References:

INSULIN   L1

Trade: Humulin

Other Trades: Mixtard, Protaphane, Novolin, Humulin, Humalog, Iletin, Monotard

Category: Human insulin

Insulin is an anti-diabetic agent used in the management of diabetes mellitus type 1 and 2, gestational diabetes and diabetic ketoacidosis.[1] Insulin is a large peptide that is not secreted into milk. Even if secreted, it would be destroyed in the infant's gastrointestinal tract leading to minimal or no absorption.

Pregnancy Risk	B	Lactation Risk	L1
T ½	= 4–6 minutes	M/P	=
Vd	= 0.37 l/kg	PB	=
Tmax	=	Oral	=
MW	= 5808	pKa	= Varies depending on type of insulin

Adult Concerns: Hypoglycemia.

Pediatric Concerns: None reported via milk.

Drug Interactions: A decreased hypoglycemic effect may result when used with oral contraceptives, corticosteroids, diltiazem, epinephrine, thiazide diuretics, thyroid hormones and niacin. Increased hypoglycemic effects may result when used with alcohol, beta blockers, fenfluramine, monoamine oxidase inhibitors, salicylates, tetracyclines.

Relative Infant Dose:

Adult Dose: Highly Variable.

Alternatives:

References:
1. Pharmaceutical manufacturer prescribing information, 2005.

INSULIN GLARGINE   L1

Trade: Lantus

Other Trades:

Category: Long-acting recombinant insulin

Insulin glargine (rDNA origin) is a recombinant human insulin analog that is long-acting (up to 24 hours).[1] Insulin glargine differs from human insulin in that the amino acid asparagine at position A-21 is replaced by glycine and two arginines are added to the C-terminus of the B-chain. This product when administered subcutaneously precipitates and forms crystals that are slow absorbing, thus producing a sustained release formulation with a half-life of about 198 minutes. While we have no studies on its transfer into human milk, we are certain that small levels of insulin are indeed present in human milk. However, most present in milk would likely be totally destroyed in the infant's gastrointestinal tract prior to absorption. There are no contraindications to using insulin or its derivatives in breastfeeding mothers.

Pregnancy Risk	C	Lactation Risk	L1
T ½	= 5–15 minutes	M/P	=
Vd	= 0.15 l/kg	PB	= 5%
Tmax	= 6 hours	Oral	= None
MW	= 6063	pKa	=

Adult Concerns: Hypoglycemia.

Pediatric Concerns: None reported in breastfeeding infants.

Drug Interactions: A decreased hypoglycemic effect may result when used with oral contraceptives, corticosteroids, diltiazem, epinephrine, thiazide diuretics, thyroid hormones and niacin. Increased hypoglycemic effects may result when used with alcohol, beta blockers, fenfluramine, monoamine oxidase inhibitors, salicylates, tetracyclines.

Relative Infant Dose:

Adult Dose: Highly variable.

Alternatives:

References:
1. Pharmaceutical manufacturer prescribing information, 2005.

INTERFERON ALFA-2B   L3

Trade: PegIntron, Intron A
Other Trades:
Category: Antineoplastic agent

Peginterferon alfa-2b is a pegylated form of the antiviral drug interferon alfa-2b. Pegylation confers protection against enzymatic degradation systemically. It is indicated for the treatment of hepatitis C.[1] While we have no data on its use in breastfeeding mothers, other data on interferons (alfa and beta) suggest they do not readily enter the milk, and milk levels will be exceeding low. When combined with ribavirin, breastfeeding is not recommended. Ribavirin is extremely teratogenic, do not use in pregnancy.

Pregnancy Risk	C	Lactation Risk	L3
T ½	= 2–3 hours	M/P	=
Vd	= 25 to 31 L l/kg	PB	=
Tmax	= 3–12 hours	Oral	= 80–90%
MW	= 19271 daltons	pKa	=

Adult Concerns: Fever, chills, headache, fatigue, nausea, diarrhea, vomiting, dry mouth, rash, alopecia, loss of appetite, leukopenia, neutropenia, anemia, elevated liver enzymes, myalgia, flu-like symptoms, weakness, hypertension, cough.

Pediatric Concerns:

Drug Interactions:

Relative Infant Dose:

Adult Dose: 1.5 µg/kg/week.

Alternatives:

References:
1. Pharmaceutical manufacturer prescribing information, 2011.

INTERFERON ALFA-2B + RIBAVIRIN   L4

Trade: Rebetron
Other Trades:
Category: Antivirals for Hepatitis C treatment

This is a combination product containing the antiviral ribavirin and the immunomodulator drug called interferon alfa-2b. This new combination product is indicated for the long-term treatment of hepatitis C. The typical dose for an individual <75 kg consists of 1000 mg ribavirin daily in divided doses and 3 million units of interferon three times weekly.

Ribavirin is a synthetic nucleoside used as an antiviral agent and is effective in a wide variety of viral infections. It has heretofore been used acutely in respiratory syncytial virus infections in infants without major complications. However, its current use in breastfeeding patients, for treatment of Hepatitis C infections, when combined with interferon alfa (Rebetron) for periods up to one year may be more problematic as high concentrations of ribavirin could accumulate in the breastfed infant over time. No data are available on its transfer to human milk, but it is probably low and its oral bioavailability is low as well. However, ribavirin concentrates in peripheral tissues and in the red blood cells in high concentrations over time (Vd= 802).[1] Its elimination half-life at steady state averages 298 hours, which reflects slow elimination from non-plasma compartments. Red cell concentrations on average are 60 fold higher than plasma levels and may account for the occasional hemolytic anemia. It is likely the acute exposure of a breastfed infant would produce minimal side effects. However, chronic exposure over 12 months may be more risky, so caution is recommended.

Very little is known about the secretion of interferons in human milk although some interferons are known to be secreted normally and may contribute to the antiviral properties of human milk. However, interferons are large in molecular weight (16–28,000 daltons) which would limit their transfer into human milk. Following treatment with a massive dose of 30 million units IV of interferon alpha in a breastfeeding patient, the amount of interferon alpha transferred into human milk was 894, 1004, 1551, 1507, 788, 721 IU at 0 (baseline), 2, 4, 8, 12, and 24 hours respectively.[2] In a more recent study of the transfer of Interferon Beta-1a, average milk concentrations were 46.7, 97.4, 66.4, 77.5, 103.1, 108.3, 124, and 87.9 pg/mL at 0, 1, 4, 8, 12, 24, 48, and 72 hours, respectively, after dosing. Using the highest value measured (179 pg/mL), the estimated relative infant dose would be 0.006% of the maternal dose.[3] Thus interferon levels in milk are probably exceedingly low.

Interferon alfa-2B + ribavirin is extremely dangerous to a fetus and is extremely teratogenic at doses even ½₀ of the above therapeutic doses. Pregnancy must be strictly avoided if this product is used in either the male or female partner. Due to the long half-life of this product, pregnancy should be avoided for at least 6 months following use.

Pregnancy Risk	X	Lactation Risk	L4
T ½	= Interferon alfa-2B/ribavirin: 2–3 hours/298 hours	M/P	=
Vd	= Interferon alfa-2B/ribavirin: 25–31 L/2859 L l/kg	PB	= Interferon alfa-2B/ribavirin: /none
Tmax	= Interferon alfa-2B/ribavirin: 3–12 hours/1.5 hours	Oral	= Interferon alfa-2B/ribavirin: 80–90%/64%
MW	= Interferon alfa-2B/ribavirin: 19271/244	pKa	=

Adult Concerns: Anemia, insomnia, depression and irritability are common. Headache, fatigue, rigors, fever, flu-like symptoms, dizziness, nausea, myalgia, insomnia and numerous other symptoms are typical.

Pediatric Concerns: None reported via breast milk, but caution is recommended.

Drug Interactions:

Relative Infant Dose:

Adult Dose:

Alternatives:

References:
1. Lertora JJ, Rege AB, Lacour JT, Ferencz N, George WJ, VanDyke RB, Agrawal KC, Hyslop NE, Jr. Pharmacokinetics and long-term tolerance to ribavirin in asymptomatic patients infected with human immunodeficiency virus. Clin Pharmacol Ther 1991; 50(4): 442–449.
2. Kumar AR, Hale TW, Mock RE. Transfer of interferon alfa into human breast milk. J Hum Lact 2000; 16(3): 226–228.
3. Hale TW, Siddiqui AA, Baker TE. Transfer of Interferon beta -1a into Human Breastmilk. Breastfeed Med. 2011 Oct 11.

INTERFERON ALPHA-N3   L2

Trade: Alferon N, Interferon Alpha, PEG-Intron
Other Trades:
Category: Immune modulator, antiviral.

Interferon alpha is a pure clone of a single interferon subspecies with antiviral, anti-proliferative, and immunomodulatory activity. The alpha-interferons are active against various malignancies and viral syndromes such as hairy cell leukemia, melanoma, AIDS-related Kaposi's sarcoma, condyloma acuminata, and chronic hepatitis B and C infection.[1] Other forms of interferons such as the Alfa-2b (Peg-Intron) are also available. Very little is known about the secretion of interferons in human milk although some interferons are known to be secreted normally and may contribute to the antiviral properties of human milk. However, interferons are large in molecular weight (16–28,000 daltons), which would limit their transfer into human milk. Following treatment with a massive dose of 30 million units IV in one breastfeeding patient, the amount of interferon alpha transferred into human milk was 894, 1004, 1551, 1507, 788, 721 units at 0 (baseline), 2, 4, 8, 12, and 24 hours respectively.[2] Hence, even following a massive dose, no change in breastmilk levels were noted from baseline. One thousand international units is roughly equivalent to 500 nanograms of interferon.

The oral absorption of interferons is controversial and is believed to be minimal. Interferons are relatively nontoxic unless extraordinarily large doses are administered parenterally. Interferons are sometimes used in infants and children to treat idiopathic thrombocytopenia (ITP) in huge doses.

Pregnancy Risk	C	Lactation Risk	L2
T ½	= 5–7 hours	M/P	=
Vd	= 0.44 l/kg	PB	=
Tmax	= Immediate	Oral	= Low
MW	= 28,000	pKa	=

Adult Concerns: Thrombocytopenia and neutropenia. Flu-like syndrome which occurs 30 minutes after administration and persists for several hours. Fatigue, hyperglycemia, nausea and vomiting.

Pediatric Concerns: None reported via milk.

Drug Interactions: Hematologic abnormalities (granulocytopenia, thrombocytopenia) may occur when used with ACE inhibitors.

Relative Infant Dose:

Adult Dose: 0.05–0.5 mL per wart twice weekly.

Alternatives:

References:
1. Pharmaceutical manufacturer prescribing information, 1997.
2. Kumar AR, Hale TW, Mock RE. Transfer of interferon alfa into human breast milk. J Hum Lact 2000; 16(3): 226–228.

INTERFERON BETA-1A   L2

Trade: Avonex, Rebif
Other Trades: Avonex, Rebif
Category: Immune modulator

Interferon Beta-1A is a moderately large glycoprotein (166 amino acids) with antiviral, anti-proliferative, and immunomodulator activity presently used for reducing the severity and frequency of exacerbations of relapsing-remitting multiple sclerosis.[1] Interferons are large in molecular weight, generally containing 166 amino acids, which would limit their transfer into human milk. Their oral absorption is controversial but is believed to be minimal. In addition, most researchers find that plasma levels of interferons following IM injection are detectable for only a few hours, generally less than 15 hours following the dose. Thus the transfer of interferons into the plasma compartment are minimal and last only briefly. Generally they are low to undetectable.

In a recent study of the transfer of Interferon Beta-1a in six mothers receiving 30 µg per week, average milk concentrations were 46.7, 97.4, 66.4, 77.5, 103.1, 108.3, 124, and 87.9 pg/mL at 0, 1, 4, 8, 12, 24, 48, and 72 hours, respectively, after dosing. Using the highest value measured (179 pg/mL), the estimated relative infant dose would be 0.006% of the maternal dose.[2] Interferons are relatively nontoxic unless extraordinarily large doses are administered parenterally. Interferons are sometimes used in infants and children to treat idiopathic thrombocytopenia (ITP) in huge doses.

Pregnancy Risk	C	Lactation Risk	L2
T ½	= 10 hours	M/P	=
Vd	= 61.6 l/kg	PB	=
Tmax	= 3–15 hours	Oral	= Minimal
MW	= 22,500	pKa	=

Adult Concerns: Headache, myalgia, nausea, diarrhea, dyspepsia, fever, chills, malaise, sweating, depression, flu-like symptoms. These effects generally follow huge doses.

Pediatric Concerns: None reported via milk.

Drug Interactions: Do not use with live viral vaccines.

Relative Infant Dose: 0.006%

Adult Dose: 30 μg weekly I. M.

Alternatives:

References:
1. Chofflon M. Recombinant human interferon beta in relapsing-remitting multiple sclerosis: a review of the major clinical trials. Eur J Neurol 2000; 7(4): 369–380.
2. Hale TW, Siddiqui AA, Baker TE. Transfer of Interferon beta-1a into Human Breastmilk. Breastfeed Med. 2011 Oct 11.

INTERFERON BETA-1B   L2

Trade: Betaseron, Extavia
Other Trades: Betaseron, Betaferon
Category: Antiviral, immunomodulator

Interferon Beta-1B is a glycoprotein with antiviral, anti-proliferative, and immunomodulatory activity presently used for treatment of multiple sclerosis.[1,2] Very little is known about the secretion of interferons in human milk although some interferons are known to be secreted normally and may contribute to the antiviral properties of human milk. However, interferons are large in molecular weight, generally containing 165 amino acids, which would limit their transfer into human milk. In a recent study of the transfer of Interferon Beta-1a in six mothers receiving 30 μg per week, average milk concentrations were 46.7, 97.4, 66.4, 77.5, 103.1, 108.3, 124, and 87.9 pg/mL at 0, 1, 4, 8, 12, 24, 48, and 72 hours, respectively, after dosing. Using the highest value measured (179 pg/mL), the estimated relative infant dose would be 0.006% of the maternal dose.[3]

Interferons are relatively nontoxic unless extraordinarily large doses are administered parenterally. Interferons are sometimes used in infants and children to treat idiopathic thrombocytopenia (ITP) in huge doses. The transfer of interferon Beta-1a is essentially nil and it is likely the same for this product, interferon Beta-1b.

Pregnancy Risk	C	Lactation Risk	L2
T ½	= 4.3 hours	M/P	=
Vd	= 2.9 l/kg	PB	=
Tmax	= 3–15 hours (IM)	Oral	= Poor
MW	= 22,500	pKa	=

Adult Concerns: Depression, headache, myalgia, nausea, diarrhea, dyspepsia, fever, chills, malaise, sweating, depression, flu-like symptoms. These effects generally follow huge doses. Injection site necrosis has been reported in 4% of users.

Pediatric Concerns: None reported via milk. However, interferon Beta 1-a is virtually excluded from the milk compartment.

Drug Interactions: Hematologic abnormalities (granulocytopenia, thrombocytopenia) may occur when added to ACE inhibitors.

Relative Infant Dose:

Adult Dose: 0.25 mg every other day.

Alternatives: Interferon Beta 1-a

References:
1. Chiang J, Gloff CA, Yoshizawa CN, Williams GJ. Pharmacokinetics of recombinant human interferon-beta ser in healthy volunteers and its effect on serum neopterin. Pharm Res 1993; 10(4): 567–572.
2. Wills RJ. Clinical pharmacokinetics of interferons. Clin Pharmacokinet 1990; 19(5): 390–399.
3. Hale TW, Siddiqui AA, Baker TE. Transfer of Interferon beta -1a into Human Breastmilk. Breastfeed Med. 2011 Oct 11.

INULIN   L3

Trade:

Other Trades:

Category: Supplement, Diagnostic agent

Inulin is an insoluble oligosaccharide that is used as both a fiber supplement and a diagnostic agent for renal function. This agent is not metabolized, and eliminated rapidly through urine when administered intravenously. When administered orally, inulin is not broken down and is instead used as a probiotic in the gut to promote the growth of bifidobacterium. In the event of hydrolysis, the primary product of inulin is fructose. It is unlikely that this agent will be excreted into breastmilk. Inulin has been suspected of altering the absorption of several other nutrients such as calcium and glucose.[1]

Pregnancy Risk	Probably Safe	Lactation Risk	L3
T ½	=	M/P	=
Vd	=	PB	=
Tmax	=	Oral	= Nil
MW	= 6179.36	pKa	= 11.63

Adult Concerns: Bloating, flatulence, abdominal discomfort.

Pediatric Concerns:

Drug Interactions: Inulin may increase calcium absorption.

Relative Infant Dose:

Adult Dose:

Alternatives:

References:

1.   Kaur N, Gupta AK. Applications of inulin and oligofructose in health and nutrition. J Biosci. 2002 Dec; 27(7): 703–14.

IODAMIDE   L3

Trade: Isteropac, Renovue-Dip, Renovue-65

Other Trades:

Category: Radiological Contrast Agent

Iodamide is an iodinated ionic contrast medium. No data are available on the transfer into human milk; however, levels would likely be quite low due to its molecular structure and size, and due to a poor oral bioavailability, it is unlikely that it would transfer to the infant during breastfeeding.[1]

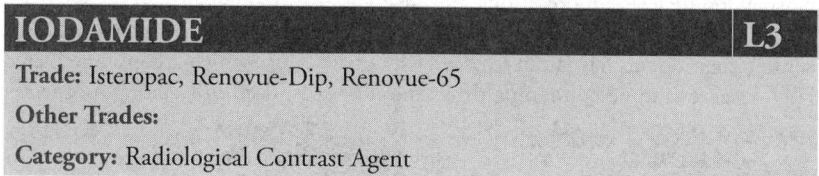

Pregnancy Risk	D	Lactation Risk	L3
T ½	= 13 hours	M/P	=
Vd	=	PB	= 5%
Tmax	=	Oral	= Poor
MW	= 627	pKa	=

Adult Concerns: Sensation of warmth, blood pressure increase or decrease, urticaria, chills, fever, pruritus, nausea, vomiting, hypersensitivity, proteinuria, headache, malaise, sneezing.

Pediatric Concerns:

Drug Interactions: Co-administration with metformin may cause lactic acidosis and acute renal failure.

Relative Infant Dose:

Adult Dose:

Alternatives:

References:

1.   Difazio LT, Singhvi SM, Heald AF, et. al. Pharmacokinetics of iodamide in normal subjects and in patients with renal impairment. J Clin Pharmacol. 1978 Jan; 18(1): 35–41.

IODINATED GLYCEROL   L4

Trade: Organidin, Iophen, R-GEN

Other Trades: Organidin

Category: Expectorant

Iodinated glycerol is a mucolytic-expectorant. This product contains 50% organically bound iodine. High levels of iodine are known to be secreted in milk.[1] Milk/plasma ratios as high as 26 have been reported. Following absorption by the infant, high levels of iodine could lead to severe thyroid depression in infants. Normal iodine levels in breastmilk are already four times higher than the RDA for infants. Expectorants, including iodine, work very poorly. Recently, many iodine containing products have been replaced with guaifenesin, which is considered safer. High levels of iodine-containing drugs should not be used in lactating mothers.

Pregnancy Risk	X	Lactation Risk	L4
T ½	=	M/P	=
Vd	=	PB	=
Tmax	=	Oral	= Complete
MW	= 258	pKa	=

Adult Concerns: Depressed thyroid function, diarrhea, nausea, vomiting, acne, dermatitis, metallic taste.

Pediatric Concerns: Iodine concentrates in milk and should not be administered to breastfeeding mothers. Infantile thyroid suppression is likely.

Drug Interactions: Increased toxicity with disulfiram, metronidazole, procarbazine, monoamine oxidase inhibitors, CNS depressants, lithium.

Relative Infant Dose:

Adult Dose:

Alternatives:

References:
1. Postellon DC, Aronow R. Iodine in mother's milk. JAMA 1982; 247(4): 463.

IODINE   L4

Trade: Iodosorb, Iodex, Iodoflex

Other Trades:

Category: Antiseptic, dietary supplement

Iodine is an essential dietary element that can be commonly found in many foods. It is most commonly used as the potassium or sodium salt. Topically Iodine is used as a topical antiseptic, although its use retards wound healing and it is no longer recommended as a topical antiseptic. Another use of iodine compound such as potassium iodide is for treatment of thyrotoxicosis, as large doses suppress thyroxine production by the thyroid gland. Foods such as seaweed, kelp, yogurt, milk, iodinated salt and fish contain higher levels of iodine. Seaweed and kelp may contain up to 20 times the recommended daily intake. Recommended dietary allowance for iodine in breastfeeding women is 290 µg/day. Excessive iodine exposure may cause thyrotoxicosis.[1] High levels of iodine are known to be pumped into human milk.[2] Milk/plasma ratios as high as 26 have been reported. Following absorption by the infant, high levels of iodine could lead to severe thyroid depression in infants. Normal iodine levels in breastmilk are already four times higher than the RDA for infants. In one study, infant subclinical hypothyroidism has been associated with excessive iodine in breastmilk (198–8484 µg/L) probably due to seaweed consumption (more than 2000 µg/day of iodine).[3] Iodine odor from a breastfed infant has been reported from a mother who used povidone-iodine vaginal gel for 6 days; however, no thyroid abnormalities were observed.[4] High levels of iodine-containing drugs should not be used in lactating mothers. Limit doses to ranges close to the RDA (290 µg/day).

Mothers who are exposed to radioactive iodine, such as from nuclear accidents, should take potassium iodide to reduce exposure of their thyroid glands to the radioactive iodine. Breastfeeding women should only take potassium iodide if they are contaminated with radioactive iodine and advised to do so by their governmental agencies. Radioactive iodine gets into breast milk avidly and therefore can transfer to the breastfed baby. Recommended Dose: 130 mg once daily for only one dose. Taking a higher dose or more frequent doses can result in adverse health effects and can even be fatal. Finally, ONLY use potassium iodide if you are advised to by your physician or government health care agency, and ONLY if you are exposed to high levels of radioactive Iodine.

Pregnancy Risk	Possibly Hazardous		Lactation Risk	L4
T ½	=		M/P	= up to 26
Vd	=		PB	=
Tmax	=		Oral	=
MW	= 127		pKa	= Completely ionized

Adult Concerns: Topical: Eczema, irritation, increase TSH, edema. Iodine intoxication: Fever, headache, hypothyroidism, metallic taste, arthralgia, pulmonary edema, rash, urticaria, lymph node enlargement.

Pediatric Concerns: Thyroid dysfunction, rash.

Drug Interactions:

Relative Infant Dose:

Adult Dose: 150 µg/day, Pregnant: 220 µg/day, Lactation: 290 µg/day.

Alternatives:

References:

1. Iodine. In: Lexi-Drugs OnlineTM Hudson, Ohio: Lexi-Comp, Inc. ; 2011. Updated periodically. Accessed 07–07–2011.
2. Postellon DC, Aronow R. Iodine in mother's milk. JAMA 1982; 247(4): 463.
3. Chung HR, Shin CH, Yang SW, Choi CW, Kim BI. Subclinical hypothyroidism in Korean preterm infants associated with high levels of iodine in breast milk. J Clin Endocrinol Metab. 2009 Nov; 94(11): 4444–7. Epub 2009 Oct 6.
4. Iodine. In: REPROTOX Database [Internet database]. Greenwood Village, Colo: Thomson Reuters (Healthcare) Inc. Updated periodically. Accessed 7–13–2011.

IODIPAMIDE   L3

Trade: Cholografin, Sinografin
Other Trades:
Category: Radiological Contrast Agent

Iodipamide is an ionic radiopaque contrast agent used to view the gallbladder and biliary tract. It is used in both adults and pediatric patients.[1] No data are available on the transfer of iodipamide into human milk; however, it is unlikely when compared to other similar agents. It has a very short half life, and it is highly protein bound. Based on kinetic data, the American College of Radiology suggests that it is safe for a mother to continue breastfeeding after receiving iodinated x-ray contrast media.[2]

Pregnancy Risk	D		Lactation Risk	L3
T ½	= 30 minutes		M/P	=
Vd	=		PB	= Very High
Tmax	=		Oral	= 10%
MW	=		pKa	= 2.63

Adult Concerns: Renal failure, hypotension, flushing, nausea, vomiting, hypersensitivity reaction. Rapid administration: warmth sensation, fever, chills, dizziness, restlessness.

Pediatric Concerns: None reported via breast milk.

Drug Interactions:

Relative Infant Dose:

Adult Dose:

Alternatives:

References:
1. Pharmaceutical manufacturer prescribing information, 2003.
2. ACR Committee on Drugs and Contrast Media. Administration of contrast medium to breastfeeding mothers. 2004; 42–43.

IODIXANOL   L3

Trade: Visipaque
Other Trades:
Category: Radiological Contrast Agent

Iodixanol is an intravenous, nonionic, water soluble radiocontrast medium with iodine concentrations of 270 and 320 mg/mL.[1] It has been studied and approved in children one year of age and older, as well as in adults. There are no studies on the transfer of iodixanol into human milk; however, it is unlikely that iodixanol would transfer into milk in any therapeutic level. Its poor oral bioavailability would further reduce any risk to an infant. Based on kinetic data, the American

College of Radiology suggests that it is safe for a mother to continue breastfeeding after receiving iodinated x-ray contrast media.[2]

Pregnancy Risk	B	Lactation Risk	L3
T ½	= 123 minutes	M/P	=
Vd	=	PB	= None
Tmax	=	Oral	= Poor
MW	= 1150.18	pKa	= 11.94

Adult Concerns: Anaphylaxis, local injection site reactions, taste perversion, headache, pruritus, nausea, rash, paresthesia, renal failure, myocardial infarction.

Pediatric Concerns:

Drug Interactions:

Relative Infant Dose:

Adult Dose:

Alternatives:

References:
1. Pharmaceutical manufacturer prescribing information, 2006
2. ACR Committee on Drugs and Contrast Media. Administration of contrast medium to breastfeeding mothers. 2004; 42–43.

IOFLUPANE [123]I   L4

Trade: DaTSCAN

Other Trades:

Category: Radiopharmaceutical agent

Ioflupane ^{123}I is a radiopharmaceutical indicated for visualization of the striatal dopamine transporter in the brain in the diagnosis of Parkinsonian syndrome.[1] It is not known if it transfers into breastmilk, but some probably does. Not all the ^{123}I is bound to this product (up to 6% is free), and any free radioactive iodine would easily transfer into milk, and to the mother's thyroid. Thyroid blocking is provided with 120 mg potassium iodide 2 hours prior to the radioactive drug. A further dose is administered 24 hour later. Infants should not breastfeed during or after the administration of potassium iodide.

Based on the physical half-life of [123]I (13.2 hours), the manufacturer recommends that breastfeeding women should consider interrupting nursing and pumping and discarding breastmilk for up to 6 days after DaTscan administration. Women should also limit their close contact with the infant during the first few half-lives to reduce exposure of the infant to gamma irradiation.

Pregnancy Risk	C		Lactation Risk	L4
T ½	= < 5 minutes		M/P	=
Vd	=		PB	=
Tmax	=		Oral	=
MW	= 427		pKa	=

Adult Concerns: Occasional hypersensitivity. Increase risk of thyroid hyperplasia if it is not blocked with prior administration of potassium iodide. Headache, nausea, vertigo, dry mouth, and dizziness have been reported.

Pediatric Concerns: Avoid breastfeeding for up to 6 days following use of this product.

Drug Interactions:

Relative Infant Dose:

Adult Dose:

Alternatives:

References:
1. Pharmaceutical manufacturer prescribing information, 2011.

IOHEXOL   L2

Trade: Accupaque, Myelo-Kit, Omnigraf, Omnipaque, Omnitrast
Other Trades:
Category: Radiological Contrast Agent

Iohexol is a nonionic radiocontrast agent. Radiopaque agents (except barium) are iodinated compounds used to visualize various organs during X-ray, CAT scans, and other radiological procedures. These compounds are highly iodinated, benzoic acid derivatives. Although under usual circumstances iodine products are contraindicated in nursing mothers (due to ion trapping in milk), these products are unique, in that they are extremely inert and are largely cleared without metabolism. The iodine is organically bound to the structure and is not biologically active.

In a study of four women who received 0.755 gm/kg (350 mg iodine/mL) of iohexol IV, the mean peak level of iohexol in milk was 35 mg/L at three hours post-injection.[1] The average concentration in milk was only 11.4 mg/L over 24 hours. Assuming a daily milk intake of 150 mL/kg body weight, the amount of iohexol transferred to an infant during the first 24 hours would be 1.7 mg/kg which corresponds to 0.23% of the maternal dose.

As a group, radiocontrast agents are virtually unabsorbed after oral administration (<0.1%).[2] Iohexol has a brief half-life of just two hours, and the estimated dose ingested by the infant is only 0.2% of the radiocontrast dose used clinically for various scanning procedures in infants. Although most company package inserts suggest that an infant be removed from the breast for 24 hours, no untoward effects have been reported with these products in breastfed infants. Because the amount of iohexol transferred into milk is so small, the authors conclude that breastfeeding is acceptable after intravenously administered iohexol. Based on kinetic data, the American College of Radiology suggests that it is safe for a mother to continue breastfeeding after receiving iodinated X-ray contrast media.[3]

Pregnancy Risk	D	Lactation Risk	L2
T ½	= 2–3.4 hours	M/P	=
Vd	=	PB	= None
Tmax	=	Oral	= Poor
MW	= 821.14	pKa	= 12.64

Adult Concerns: Local injection site reactions, nausea, vomiting, diarrhea, dizziness, headache, anxiety, arrhythmia, heart failure, renal dysfunction, hypersensitivity, cough, bronchospasm, anaphylaxis.

Pediatric Concerns: None reported in one study.

Drug Interactions:

Relative Infant Dose: 0.2%

Adult Dose:

Alternatives:

References:
1. Nielsen ST, Matheson I, Rasmussen JN, Skinnemoen K, Andrew E, Hafsahl G. Excretion of iohexol and metrizoate in human breast milk. Acta Radiol 1987; 28(5): 523–526.
2. Pharmaceutical manufacturer prescribing information, 2006.
3. ACR Committee on Drugs and Contrast Media. Administration of contrast medium to breastfeeding mothers. 2004; 42–43.

IOPAMIDOL　　　　　　　　　　　　　　　L3

Trade: Gastromiro, Iopamiro, Iopamiron, Isovue, Niopam, Pamiray, Radiomiron, Scanlux, Solutrast

Other Trades:

Category: Nonionic Radiological Contrast Agent

Iopamidol is a nonionic radiocontrast agent used for numerous radiological procedures. Although it contains significant iodine content (20–37%), the iodine is covalently bound to the parent molecule, and the bioavailability of the iodine molecule is miniscule. As with other ionic and nonionic radiocontrast agents, it is primarily extracellular and intravascular, it does not pass the blood-brain barrier, and it would be extremely unlikely that it would penetrate into human milk. However, no data are available on its transfer into human milk. As with most of these products, it is poorly absorbed from the gastrointestinal tract and rapidly excreted from the maternal circulation, due to a extremely short half-life.[1] Based on kinetic data, the American College of Radiology suggests that it is probably safe for a mother to continue breastfeeding after receiving iodinated x-ray contrast media.[2]

Pregnancy Risk	B	Lactation Risk	L3
T ½	= 2 hours	M/P	=
Vd	=	PB	= Very Low
Tmax	=	Oral	= Nil
MW	=	pKa	=

Adult Concerns: Headache, nausea, vomiting, diarrhea, pain, hot flashes, chest pain, dyspnea, rash, hives, abdominal pain, nephropathy, seizure.

Pediatric Concerns:

Drug Interactions: Iopamidol use with metformin may cause metformin-associated lactic acidosis.

Relative Infant Dose:

Adult Dose:

Alternatives:

References:
1. Pharmaceutical manufacturer prescribing information, 2004.
2. ACR Committee on Drugs and Contrast Media. Administration of contrast medium to breastfeeding mothers. 2004; 42–43.

IOPANOIC ACID   L2

Trade: Biliopaco, Cistobil, Colegraf, Colepak, Neocontrast, Telepaque

Other Trades:

Category: Radiological Contrast Agent

Iopanoic acid is a radiopaque organic iodine compound similar to dozens of other radiocontrast agents. It contains 66.7% by weight of iodine. As with all of these compounds, the iodine is organically bound to the parent molecule, and only minimal amounts are free in solution or metabolized by the body. In a group of five breastfeeding mothers who received an average of 2.77 gm of iodine (as Iopanoic acid), the amount of iopanoic acid excreted into human milk during the following 19–29 hours was 20.8 mg or about 0.08% of the maternal dose.[1] No untoward effects were noted in the infants. Since the amounts that enter breastmilk are too minimal to cause any significant adverse effects in an infant, iopanoic acid is probably compatible with breastfeeding. Based on kinetic data, the American College of Radiology suggests that it is probably safe for a mother to continue breastfeeding after receiving iodinated x-ray contrast media.[2]

Pregnancy Risk	D	Lactation Risk	L2
T ½	= 33% eliminated in 24 hours	M/P	=
Vd	=	PB	= High
Tmax	=	Oral	= Well absorbed
MW	= 570.93	pKa	= 4.8

Adult Concerns: Nausea, vomiting, diarrhea, renal failure.

Pediatric Concerns:

Drug Interactions:

Relative Infant Dose:

Adult Dose:

Alternatives:

References:
1. Holmdahl KH. Cholecystography during lactation. Acta Radiol 1956; 45(4): 305–307.
2. ACR Committee on Drugs and Contrast Media. Administration of contrast medium to breastfeeding mothers. 2004; 42–43.

IOPENTOL   L3

Trade: Imagopaque, Ivepaque

Other Trades:

Category: Radiological Contrast Agent

Iopentol is a new non-ionic contrast medium that is not yet available in the USA. There are no studies on the transfer of iopentol into human milk; however, as with virtually all of the radiocontrast agents, it is unlikely that iopentol would transfer into milk in any therapeutic level. The poor oral bioavailability further reduces risk to an infant.[1]

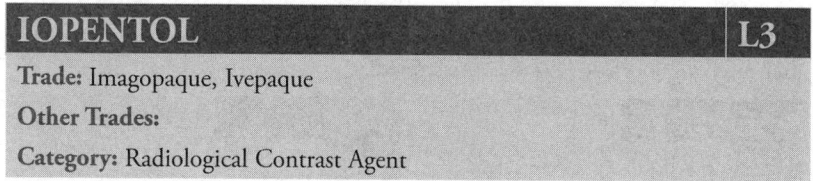

Pregnancy Risk	D	Lactation Risk	L3
T ½	= 2 hours	M/P	=
Vd	=	PB	= 3%
Tmax	=	Oral	= Poor
MW	= 835.2	pKa	=

Adult Concerns: Heat sensation, nausea.

Pediatric Concerns: Nausea, vomiting, flushing.

Drug Interactions:

Relative Infant Dose:

Adult Dose:

Alternatives:

References:
1. Pharmaceutical manufacturer prescribing information, 2006.

IOPROMIDE   L3

Trade: Clarograf, Proscope, Ultravist
Other Trades:
Category: Radiological Contrast Agent

Iopromide is a nonionic, water soluble x-ray contrast agent. Its iodine content is 48.12%, and it is available in 150, 240, 300, and 370 mg iodine/mL.[1] No data are available on the transfer of iopromide into human milk, but others in this family transfer at extraordinarily low levels, and none are orally bioavailable. Therefore, iopromide use is not likely to pose a threat to an infant and should not be a contraindication for breastfeeding. Based on kinetic data, the American College of Radiology suggests that it is probably safe for a mother to continue breastfeeding after receiving iodinated x-ray contrast media.[2]

Pregnancy Risk	D	Lactation Risk	L3
T ½	= 2 hours	M/P	=
Vd	=	PB	= 1%
Tmax	=	Oral	= Poor
MW	= 791.1	pKa	=

Adult Concerns: Headache, nausea, vomiting, headache, vasodilation, angina pectoris, local injection site hematoma, back pain, urinary urgency, nephropathy, anaphylaxis.

Pediatric Concerns:

Drug Interactions:

Relative Infant Dose:

Adult Dose:

Alternatives:

References:
1. Pharmaceutical manufacturer prescribing information, 2002.
2. ACR Committee on Drugs and Contrast Media. Administration of contrast medium to breastfeeding mothers. 2004; 42–43.

IOTHALAMATE   L3

Trade: Angio-Conray, Conray-30, Conray-43, Conray-60, Conray 325, Conray 400, Cysto-Conray, Cysto-Conray II, Vascoray
Other Trades:
Category: Radiological Contrast Agent

Iothalamate is an iodinated contrast medium, available in iodine concentrations ranging from 81 mg iodine/mL to 400 mg iodine/mL.[1] No data are available on the transfer into human milk; however, levels in milk are expected to be low to undetectable, and oral bioavailability is low. Therefore, risk to the infant would be minimal. Based on kinetic data, the American College of Radiology suggests that it is safe for a mother to continue breastfeeding after receiving iodinated x-ray contrast media.[2]

Pregnancy Risk	D	Lactation Risk	L3
T ½	= 90–92 minutes	M/P	=
Vd	=	PB	= Low
Tmax	=	Oral	=
MW	=	pKa	=

Adult Concerns: Hypersensitivity, local injection site reactions, venous thrombosis, skin necrosis.

Pediatric Concerns:

Drug Interactions: Combination with metformin may lead to lactic acidosis.

Relative Infant Dose:

Adult Dose:

Alternatives:

References:
1. Pharmaceutical manufacturer prescribing information, 2003.
2. ACR Committee on Drugs and Contrast Media. Administration of contrast medium to breastfeeding mothers. 2004; 42–43.

IOVERSOL   L3

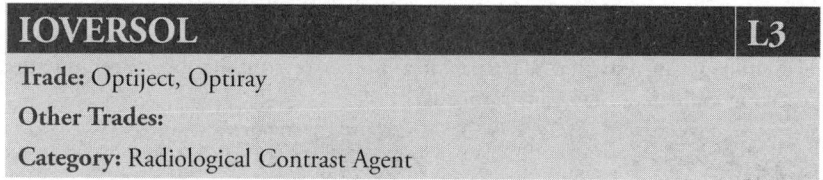

Trade: Optiject, Optiray

Other Trades:

Category: Radiological Contrast Agent

Ioversol is a typical iodinated radiocontrast agent used in computed tomographic imaging (CAT scans). The concentration of iodine varies from 16% organically bound iodine (160) to 35% iodine (350).[1] Ioversol is not metabolized, but it is excreted largely unchanged. Iodine is only minimally released; therefore, thyroid function tests remain unchanged with exception of iodine uptake studies (PBI, radioactive iodine uptake). The vascular half-life is brief, only 20 minutes. No data are available on its transfer into milk, but many others in this family have been studied and transfer to milk occur at extraordinarily low levels. Further, none of these agents are orally bioavailable. Therefore, ioversol is probably compatible with breastfeeding. Based on kinetic data, the American College of Radiology suggests that it is probably safe for a mother to continue breastfeeding after receiving iodinated x-ray contrast media.[2]

Pregnancy Risk	B	Lactation Risk	L3
T ½	= 1.5 hours	M/P	=
Vd	=	PB	= Very low
Tmax	=	Oral	= Nil
MW	= 807.12	pKa	= 11.34

Adult Concerns: Headache, chest pain, hot flashes, nausea, vomiting, back pain, rash, hives, burning sensation, nephropathy, hypersensitivity.

Pediatric Concerns:

Drug Interactions: Combination with metformin may lead to lactic acidosis.

Relative Infant Dose:

Adult Dose:

Alternatives:

References:
1. Pharmaceutical manufacturer prescribing information, 2003.
2. ACR Committee on Drugs and Contrast Media. Administration of contrast medium to breastfeeding mothers. 2004; 42–43.

IOXAGLATE   L3

Trade: Hexabrix 160, Hexabrix 200, Hexabrix 320, Hexabrix

Other Trades:

Category: Radiological Contrast Agent

Ioxaglate is an ionic dimer that offers a lower osmolarity and consequently less pain upon injection. It contains 32% iodine and is approved for both children and adults. No data are available on the transfer into human milk; however, levels are expected to be below therapeutic levels, it molecular weight is high, and oral its bioavailability is low. Based on kinetic data, the American College of Radiology suggests that it is safe for a mother to continue breastfeeding after receiving iodinated x-ray contrast media.[1]

Pregnancy Risk	B	Lactation Risk	L3
T ½	= 60–140 minutes	M/P	=
Vd	=	PB	= Low
Tmax	=	Oral	= Nil
MW	= 1268	pKa	=

Adult Concerns: Nausea, vomiting, warmth sensation, thromboembolic events, nephropathy, hypersensitivity.

Pediatric Concerns:

Drug Interactions:

Relative Infant Dose:

Adult Dose:

Alternatives:

References:
1. ACR Committee on Drugs and Contrast Media. Administration of contrast medium to breastfeeding mothers. 2004; 42–43.

IOXILAN   L3

Trade: Oxilan

Other Trades:

Category: Diagnostic Agent, Radiopharmaceutical Imaging

Ioxilan is an iodinated radio-opaque contrast agent used for diagnostic purposes. Ioxilan contains 48.1% by weight of iodine. As with all of these compounds, the iodine is organically bound to the parent molecule, and only minimal amounts are free in solution or metabolized by the body. In the case of Ioxilan, 93.7% of the original amount injected is excreted unchanged in the urine within 24 hours of administration. This suggests that very little free iodine is actually available systemically. As with other iodinated radiocontrast agents, ioxilan is excreted unchanged and little or no iodine is secreted into human milk.[1] Therefore, a brief interruption of breastfeeding for a few hours would virtually eliminate all risks. Based on kinetic data, the American College of Radiology suggests that it is probably safe for a mother to continue breastfeeding after receiving iodinated x-ray contrast media.[2]

Pregnancy Risk	B	Lactation Risk	L3
T ½	= 137 min	M/P	=
Vd	= 0.1 l/kg	PB	= Negligible
Tmax	= Immediately	Oral	= Nil
MW	= 791.12	pKa	= 6.8

Adult Concerns: Hypersensitivity to iodine may cause severe, sometimes life-threatening reactions. The risk of reaction increases with history of previous reactions to radiocontrast agents.

Pediatric Concerns: No untoward effects reported.

Drug Interactions:

Relative Infant Dose:

Adult Dose: 86 grams IV.

Alternatives:

References:
1. Holmdahl KH. Cholecystography during lactation. Acta Radiol 1956; 45(4): 305–307.
2. ACR Committee on Drugs and Contrast Media. Administration of contrast medium to breastfeeding mothers. 2004; 42–43.

IOXITALAMIC ACID   L3

Trade: Telebrix

Other Trades:

Category: Radiological Contrast Agent

Ioxitalamic acid is available in both an oral solution and an injectable solution, in concentrations ranging from 12% to 38% iodine.[1] It is used in both adults and children. There are no data available on the transfer of ioxitalamic acid into breastmilk, although levels are likely to be low. Also, oral bioavailability is extremely low. As a result, any small ingested amount would pose little threat to a breastfeeding infant. Based on kinetic data, the American College of Radiology suggests that it is safe for a mother to continue breastfeeding after receiving iodinated x-ray contrast media.[2]

Pregnancy Risk	Possibly Hazardous	Lactation Risk	L3
T ½	=	M/P	=
Vd	=	PB	=
Tmax	=	Oral	= Nil
MW	=	pKa	=

Adult Concerns: Nausea, vomiting, warmth sensation, dizziness, taste perversion.

Pediatric Concerns:

Drug Interactions:

Relative Infant Dose:

Adult Dose:

Alternatives:

References:
1. Pharmaceutical manufacturer prescribing information, 1999.
2. ACR Committee on Drugs and Contrast Media. Administration of contrast medium to breastfeeding mothers. 2004; 42–43.

IPILIMUMAB   L4

Trade: Yervoy

Other Trades:

Category: Monoclonal Antibody

Ipilimumab is an IgG1 monoclonal antibody that binds to human cytotoxic T-lymphocyte antigen 4.[1] This interaction promotes antitumor immune responses. Ipilimumab is indicated for the treatment of unresectable or metastatic melanoma.[1] This drug may cause severe immune-mediated adverse reactions such as hepatitis, enterocolitis, dermatitis, neuropathy and endocrinopathy in up to 5% of those on this medication. Therefore, occurrence of these reactions should be monitored for by evaluating laboratory chemistries, liver function tests and thyroid function tests before and after each dose.

No data exist of its transfer into breastmilk. Being of high molecular weight, it is highly unlikely that this product could transfer into breastmilk in clinically relevant amounts. However, due to the likelihood of severe immune-mediated adverse reactions in the nursing infant, a decision has to be made to either discontinue the drug or discontinue breastfeeding. Such a decision is best made after weighing the potential benefits of the drug to the mother against the potential risks to the infant. Remember that although there is no equivalent substitute to breast milk, an immune-mediated reaction in an infant could potentially be irreversible and fatal.

Pregnancy Risk	C		Lactation Risk	L4
T ½	= 14.7 days		M/P	=
Vd	= 0.1 l/kg		PB	=
Tmax	=		Oral	= Low
MW	= 148,000		pKa	=

Adult Concerns: Fatigue, diarrhea, pruritus, rash, colitis are the most common adverse effects occurring in more than 5% of those treated with this drug. Severe immune-mediated adverse reactions such as hepatitis, dermatitis, enterocolitis, neuropathy and endocrinopathy may occur in up to 5% of those on this medication. In the event of an immune-mediated reaction, this medication should be discontinued immediately and systemic high-dose corticosteroid therapy to be initiated immediately.

Pediatric Concerns:

Drug Interactions:

Relative Infant Dose:

Adult Dose: 3 mg/kg IV over 90 minutes every 3 weeks.

Alternatives:

References:
1.   Pharmaceutical manufacturer prescribing information, 2011.

IPODATE   L3

Trade: Bilivist, Biloptin, Oragrafin, Solu-Biloptin, Solubiloptine, Gastrographin
Other Trades:
Category: Radiological Contrast Agent

Not available in the USA, Ipodate is an iodine-containing oral contrast agent used for examining the gallbladder and bile ducts when gallstones are suspected. There are no studies on the transfer of ipodate into human breastmilk. However, this product releases some of its iodine content and could increase iodine levels in human milk. While it is likely that minimal drug would transfer into the milk compartment, released iodine may increase levels in milk significantly. A brief 24 hour interruption of breastfeeding is suggested. Caution should be used.[1]

Pregnancy Risk	B		Lactation Risk	L3
T ½	= 45% gone in 24 hours		M/P	=
Vd	=		PB	= High
Tmax	=		Oral	= High
MW	= 619		pKa	=

Adult Concerns: Nausea, vomiting, hypersensitivity.

Pediatric Concerns:

Drug Interactions:

Relative Infant Dose:

Adult Dose:

Alternatives:

References:
1. Pharmaceutical manufacturer prescribing information, 2008.

IPRATROPIUM BROMIDE   L2

Trade: Atrovent

Other Trades: Atrovent, Apo-Ipravent

Category: Bronchodilator in asthmatics

Ipratropium is an anticholinergic drug that is used via inhalation for dilating the bronchi of asthmatics.[1] Ipratropium is a quaternary ammonium compound, and although no data exists, it probably penetrates into breastmilk in exceedingly small levels due to its structure. It is unlikely that the infant would absorb any, due to the poor tissue distribution and oral absorption of this family of drugs.

Pregnancy Risk	B	Lactation Risk	L2
T ½	= 2 hours	M/P	=
Vd	=	PB	=
Tmax	= 1–2 hours	Oral	= 0–2%
MW	= 412	pKa	=

Adult Concerns: Nervousness, dizziness, nausea, gastrointestinal distress, dry mouth, bitter taste.

Pediatric Concerns: None reported. Commonly used in pediatric patients.

Drug Interactions: Albuterol may increase effect of ipratropium. May have increased toxicity when used with other anticholinergics.

Relative Infant Dose:

Adult Dose: 36 µg four times daily.

Alternatives:

References:
1. Pharmaceutical manufacturer prescribing information, 1996.

IRBESARTAN   L3

Trade: Avapro

Other Trades: Avapro, Avalide, Amizide

Category: Antihypertensive

Irbesartan is an angiotensin-II receptor antagonist used as an antihypertensive. Low concentrations are known to be secreted into rodent milk, but human studies are lacking.[1] Both the ACE inhibitor family and the specific AT1 inhibitors such as irbesartan are contraindicated in the 2nd and 3rd trimesters of pregnancy due to severe hypotension, neonatal skull hypoplasia, irreversible renal failure, and death in the newborn infant. However, some ACE inhibitors can be used safely in breastfeeding mothers postpartum. Some caution is recommended particularly in mothers with premature infants. Since little is known about the transfer of this drug into breastmilk, consider alternatives such as captopril or enalapril.

Pregnancy Risk	C/D in 2nd and 3rd trimester	Lactation Risk	L3
T ½	= 11–15 hours	M/P	=
Vd	= 1.3 l/kg	PB	= 90%
Tmax	= 1.5–2 hours	Oral	= 60–80%
MW	= 428	pKa	= 4.24

Adult Concerns: Headache, back pain, pharyngitis, and dizziness have been reported. The use of ACE inhibitors and angiotensin receptor blockers during pregnancy or the neonatal period is extremely dangerous and has resulted in hypotension, neonatal skull hypoplasia, anuria, renal failure and death.

Pediatric Concerns: None reported via milk, but caution is recommended.

Drug Interactions: None reported thus far.

Relative Infant Dose:

Adult Dose: 150–300 mg daily.

Alternatives: Captopril, enalapril

References:
1.   Pharmaceutical manufacturer prescribing information, 1999.

IRON   L1

Trade: Femiron, Ferate, Ferrimin 150, Proferrin ES, Spatone, Ferretts IPS
Other Trades:
Category: Metal supplement

The secretion of iron salts into breastmilk appears to be very low although the bioavailability of that present in milk is high. One recent study suggests that supplementation of infants is not generally required until the 4th month postpartum when some breastfed infants may become iron deficient although these assumptions are controversial.[1] Premature infants are more susceptible to iron deficiencies because they do not have the same hepatic stores available as full term infants. Most sources recommend iron supplementation, particularly in exclusively breastfed infants, beginning at 4th month.[1] Supplementation in pre-term infants should probably be initiated earlier. However, oral supplemental iron may block some of the antibacterial properties of human milk and lead to alternate colonization of the infants gut with non lactobacillus species. The use of relatively high doses in breastfeeding mothers is probably not contraindicated, due to the fact that iron transports very poorly to the milk compartment. Thus treatment with high maternal doses does not increase milk levels.

Pregnancy Risk	Probably Safe	Lactation Risk	L1
T ½	=	M/P	=
Vd	=	PB	=
Tmax	=	Oral	= <30%
MW	= 56	pKa	= 6.74

Adult Concerns: Constipation, nausea, gastrointestinal distress.

Pediatric Concerns: None reported via milk. Iron transports poorly into milk.

Drug Interactions: Decreased iron absorption when used with antacids, cimetidine, levodopa, penicillamine, quinolones, tetracyclines. Slightly increased absorption with ascorbic acid.

Relative Infant Dose:

Adult Dose: 50–100 mg three times daily.

Alternatives:

References:
1. Calvo EB, Galindo AC, Aspres NB. Iron status in exclusively breast-fed infants. Pediatrics 1992; 90(3): 375–379.

IRON DEXTRAN   L2

Trade: Dexferrum, Infed

Other Trades:

Category: Iron supplement

Iron dextran is a colloidal solution of ferric hydroxide in a complex with partially hydrolyzed low molecular weight dextran. It is used for severe iron deficiency anemia. Its molecular weight is approximately 180,000 daltons. Approximately 99% of the iron in iron dextran is present as a stable ferric-dextran complex. Following intramuscular (IM) injection, iron dextran is absorbed from the site principally through the lymphatic system and subsequently transferred to the reticuloendothelial system in the liver for metabolism. The initial phase of absorption lasts 3 days, which accounts for 60% of an IM dose. The other 40% requires up to 1–3 weeks to several months for complete absorption.

While there are no data available on the transfer of iron dextran into human milk, it is unlikely due to its massive molecular weight. Further, iron is transferred into human milk by a tightly controlled pumping system that first chelates the iron to a high molecular weight protein and then transfers it into the milk compartment. It is generally well known that oral dietary supplements of iron in breastfeeding mothers do not change milk levels of iron significantly.[1] Great care should be used in pregnant women. In breastfeeding mothers, supplementing with high doses is probably not contraindicated due to the poor passage of iron into milk. But some caution is still recommended.

Pregnancy Risk	C		Lactation Risk	L2
T ½	=		M/P	=
Vd	=		PB	=
Tmax	=		Oral	=
MW	=		pKa	=

Adult Concerns: Local reactions at the site of injection. Abdominal pain, dyspepsia, nausea, vomiting and diarrhea. Headache, paresthesias, weakness, changes in taste perception, faintness, syncope, folic acid deficiency, and leukocytosis. Please note: while the pregnancy risk category is only C, it has been shown to be teratogenic in other species and great care should be used in pregnant women.

Pediatric Concerns: None via breast milk.

Drug Interactions:

Relative Infant Dose:

Adult Dose:

Alternatives:

References:

1. Lawrence RA. Breastfeeding: A guide for the medical profession. St. Louis: Mosby Publishers, 1994.

IRON SUCROSE   L3

Trade: Venofer

Other Trades:

Category: Iron supplement

Iron sucrose is used in the treatment of iron-deficiency anemia in chronic renal failure. Once dissociated, the iron is incorporated into hemoglobin.[1] There have been no studies of the secretion of iron sucrose in human milk. This product is a polymerized form of polynuclear iron (III)-hydroxide in sucrose. Used intravenously, it is sequestered in the liver where it is metabolized and free iron is released into the circulation. Due to its size, iron sucrose it is unlikely to enter mature milk.

Pregnancy Risk	B		Lactation Risk	L3
T ½	= 6 hours		M/P	=
Vd	= 7.9 l/kg		PB	=
Tmax	=		Oral	= Poor
MW	= 34,000–60,000		pKa	=

Adult Concerns: Adverse reactions include hypotension, headache, nausea, and muscle cramps.

Pediatric Concerns: No data available.

Drug Interactions: Iron sucrose injection may decrease the absorption of oral iron preparations.

Relative Infant Dose:

Adult Dose: Total elemental dose of 1000 mg IV.

Alternatives:

References:
1. Pharmaceutical manufacturer prescribing information, 2005.

ISOETHARINE   L2

Trade: Bronkosol, Bronkometer

Other Trades: Numotac

Category: Bronchodilator

Isoetharine is a selective beta-2 adrenergic bronchodilator for asthmatics. There are no reports on its secretion into human milk.[1] However, plasma levels following inhalation are exceedingly low, and breastmilk levels would similarly be low. Isoetharine is rapidly metabolized in the gastrointestinal tract, so oral absorption by the infant would likely be minimal. Isoetharine is probably compatible with breastfeeding.

Pregnancy Risk	C	Lactation Risk	L2
T ½	= 1–3 hours	M/P	=
Vd	=	PB	=
Tmax	= 5–15 minutes (inhaled)	Oral	=
MW	= 239	pKa	= 12.64

Adult Concerns: Tremors and excitement, hypertension, anxiety, insomnia.

Pediatric Concerns: None reported via milk.

Drug Interactions: May have decreased effect with beta blockers and increased toxicity with other adrenergic stimulants such as epinephrine.

Relative Infant Dose:

Adult Dose:

Alternatives:

References:
1. Pharmaceutical manufacturer prescribing information, 1995.

ISOMETHEPTENE MUCATE   L3

Trade: Midrin
Other Trades: Midrin
Category: For tension and migraine headache

Isometheptene is a mild stimulate (sympathomimetic) that apparently acts by constricting dilated cranial and cerebral arterioles, thus reducing vascular headaches. It is listed as possibly effective by the FDA and is probably only marginally effective.[1] Isometheptene mucate is a component of the anti-migraine product Midrin. Midrin also contains acetaminophen and a mild sedative dichloralphenazone, of which little is known. No data are available on transfer into human milk. Due to its size and molecular composition, it is likely to attain low to moderate levels in breastmilk. Because better drugs exist for migraine therapy, this product is probably not a good choice for breastfeeding mothers. Consider sumatriptan, amitriptyline, or propranolol as alternatives.

Pregnancy Risk	C		Lactation Risk	L3
T ½	=		M/P	=
Vd	=		PB	=
Tmax	=		Oral	=
MW	= 493		pKa	=

Adult Concerns: Dizziness, skin rash, hypertension, sedation.

Pediatric Concerns: None reported. Observe for stimulation.

Drug Interactions:

Relative Infant Dose:

Adult Dose:

Alternatives: Sumatriptan, amitriptyline, propranolol

References:
1. Pharmaceutical manufacturer prescribing information, 1995.

ISONIAZID   L3

Trade: INH, Laniazid
Other Trades: Isotamine, PMS Isoniazid, Pycazide, Rimifon
Category: Antituberculosis agent

Isoniazid (INH) is an antimicrobial agent primarily used to treat tuberculosis. Following doses of 5 and 10 mg/kg, one report measured peak milk levels at 6 mg/L and 9 mg/L respectively.[1] Isoniazid was not measurable in the infant's serum but was detected in the urine of several infants. In another study, following a maternal dose of 300 mg of isoniazid, the concentration of isoniazid in milk peaked at 3 hours at 16.6 mg/L while the acetyl derivative (AcINH) was 3.76 mg/L.[2] The 24 hour excretion of INH in milk was estimated at 7 mg. The authors felt this dose was potentially hazardous to a breastfed infant.

In a recent and well-done study in seven exclusively lactating women (at 33 days or steady state) who were receiving 300 mg isoniazid daily in a single dose (and rifampin and ethambutol) the mean (AUC) of isoniazid in plasma and milk was 18.4 µg/mL/24 hours and 14.4 µg/mL/24 hours respectively.[3] The mean milk/plasma ratio (AUC) was 0.89 and the calculated relative infant dose was 1.2%. In this nicely done study, peak levels are clearly evident at 1 hour and fall rapidly at 4 hours. Caution and close monitoring of infant for liver toxicity and neuritis are suggested. Peripheral neuropathies, common in INH therapy, can be treated with 10–50 mg/day pyridoxine in adults. Suggest the mom avoid breastfeeding for 2 hours following administration of INH to avoid the peak plasma concentrations at 2 hours.

Pregnancy Risk	C	Lactation Risk	L3
T ½	= 1.1–3.1 hours	M/P	=
Vd	= 0.6 l/kg	PB	= 10–15%
Tmax	= 1–2 hours (oral)	Oral	= Complete
MW	= 137	pKa	= 1.9, 3.5

Adult Concerns: Mild hepatic dysfunction, peripheral neuritis, nausea, vomiting, dizziness.

Pediatric Concerns: None reported, but the infant should be closely monitored for toxicity including hepatitis, vision changes. Observe for fatigue, weakness, malaise, anorexia, nausea, vomiting.

Drug Interactions: Decreased effect/plasma levels of isoniazid with aluminum products. Increased toxicity/levels of oral anticoagulants, carbamazepine, cycloserine, phenytoin, certain benzodiazepines. Disulfiram reactions.

Relative Infant Dose: 1.2%–18%

Adult Dose: 5 mg/kg daily.

Alternatives:

References:
1. Snider DE, Jr., Powell KE. Should women taking antituberculosis drugs breast-feed? Arch Intern Med 1984; 144(3): 589–590.
2. Berlin CM, Lee C. Isoniazid and acetylisoniazid disposition in human milk, saliva and plasma. Fed Proc 1979; 38: 426.
3. Singh N, Golani A, Patel Z, and Maitra A. Transfer of isoniazid from circulation to breast milk in lactating women on chronic therapy for tuberculosis. BJCP 2008; 65(3): 418–422.

ISOPROTERENOL · L2

Trade: Medihaler-Iso, Isuprel

Other Trades: Isoprenaline, Isuprel, Medihaler-Iso, Saventrine

Category: Bronchodilator

Isoproterenol is an old adrenergic bronchodilator.[1] Currently it is seldom used for this purpose. There are no data available on breastmilk levels. It is probably secreted into milk in extremely small levels. Isoproterenol is rapidly metabolized in the gut, and it is unlikely a breastfeeding infant would absorb clinically significant levels.

Pregnancy Risk	C	Lactation Risk	L2
T ½	= 1–2 hours	M/P	=
Vd	= 0.5 l/kg	PB	=
Tmax	= 10 minutes (inhaled)	Oral	= Poor
MW	= 211	pKa	= 8.6

Adult Concerns: Insomnia, excitement, agitation, tachycardia.

Pediatric Concerns: None reported.

Drug Interactions: Increased toxicity when used with other adrenergic stimulants and elevation of blood pressure. When used with isoproterenol, general anesthetics may cause arrhythmias.

Relative Infant Dose:

Adult Dose: 10–30 mg four times daily.

Alternatives: Albuterol

References:
1. Drug Facts and Comparisons 1995 ed. ed. St. Louis: 1995.

ISOSORBIDE DINITRATE   L3

Trade: Angidil, Angipec, Dilatate, Isordil

Other Trades: Carvasin, Apo-ISDN, Coronex, Coradur, Apo-ISDN, Angitak, Cedocard

Category: Vasodilating agents

Isosorbide dinitrate and its mononitrate cousin are vasodilating agents used in the treatment of angina and congestive heart failure, and many other syndromes. The treatment of anal fissures with isosorbide dinitrate early postpartum may impact breastfeeding with this medication. Absorption is highly variable but once absorbed it is metabolized to a 2-mononitrate and 5-mononitrate derivatives. The 5-mononitrate has a half-life of approximately 5 hours. No data are available on the transfer of isosorbide dinitrate into human milk although small amounts may enter milk.

Pregnancy Risk	C	Lactation Risk	L3
T ½	= 5 hours (metabolite)	M/P	=
Vd	= 6.3–8.9 l/kg	PB	= Low
Tmax	= 1 hour	Oral	= 10–90%
MW	=	pKa	=

Adult Concerns: Possible side effects include heart palpitations, headache, weakness, itching and rash, nervousness, low blood pressure, and dizziness.

Pediatric Concerns: No data are available on the transfer of isosorbide dinitrate into human milk. Methemoglobinemia has been reported in pure nitrite poisoning from drinking water, but this is highly unlikely to occur with the use of this drug.

Use with some caution.

Drug Interactions: Drugs such as alcohol, aspirin and calcium channel blockers may increase the effect of isosorbide. Sildenafil may dramatically increase the effect of nitrates. Do not use with sildenafil, tadalafil, vardenafil.

Relative Infant Dose:

Adult Dose: 2.5–5 mg sublingually but highly variable. Check other resources.

Alternatives:

References:
1. Pharmaceutical manufacturer prescribing information, 2005.

ISOSORBIDE MONONITRATE — L3

Trade: Imdur
Other Trades: Duride, Corangin, Coronex, Angeze, Dynamin, Imazin, Elantan
Category: Vasodilating agent

Isosorbide mononitrate and its dinitrate cousin are vasodilating agents used in the treatment of angina and congestive heart failure, and many other syndromes. While we have no data on the transfer of isosorbide mononitrate into human milk, we know that the transfer of nitrates into human milk in general is quite poor (see nitroglycerin).

Pregnancy Risk	C	Lactation Risk	L3
T ½	= 6.2 hours	M/P	=
Vd	= 0.6 l/kg	PB	= <4%
Tmax	= 30–60 minutes	Oral	= 93%
MW	= 191	pKa	=

Adult Concerns: Cardiac dysrhythmia, edema, hypotension, dermal flushing, headache, methemoglobinemia, and other problems have been reported following the use of isosorbide mononitrate.

Pediatric Concerns: None reported. Use with some caution.

Drug Interactions: Drugs such as alcohol, aspirin and calcium channel blockers may increase the effect of isosorbides. Sildenafil may dramatically increase the effect of nitrates. Do not use with sildenafil, tadalafil, vardenafil.

Relative Infant Dose:

Adult Dose: 20 mg twice daily but highly variable. Check other resources.

Alternatives:

References:
1. Pharmaceutical manufactures prescribing information, 2005.

ISOSULFAN BLUE   L4

Trade: Lymphazurin
Other Trades:
Category: Contrast agent

Isosulfan blue is a contrast agent used for visualization of the lymphatic system drainage. Each mL of solution contains 10 mg isosulfan blue, 6.6 mg sodium monohydrogen phosphate, and 2.7 mg potassium dihydrogen phosphate.[1] Isosulfan blue has higher rate of success in detecting sentinel lymph nodes than does [99m]Technetium sulfur colloid (TSC).[2] Severe adverse reactions have been documented, such as a sudden drop in systolic arterial pressure during surgery only stabilized by continuous epinephrine infusions of 400 µg/hour.[3] Methylene blue dye has been shown to be equally effective without the chance of severe adverse side effects, and thus its use is increasing.[4] No data are available on the transfer of isosulfan blue into breast milk, and therefore caution should be used in breastfeeding mothers.

Pregnancy Risk	C	Lactation Risk	L4
T ½	=	M/P	=
Vd	=	PB	= 50%
Tmax	=	Oral	=
MW	= 566.7	pKa	=

Adult Concerns: Adverse reactions include localized swelling and itching.

Pediatric Concerns: No data were available.

Drug Interactions:

Relative Infant Dose:

Adult Dose: 0.5 ml into 3 interdigital spaces.

Alternatives:

References:
1. Pharmaceutical manufacturer prescribing information, 2006.
2. Saha S, Dan AG, Berman B et al. Lymphazurin 1% Versus [99m]mTc Sulfur Colloid for Lymphatic Mapping in Colorectal Tumors: A Comparative Analysis. Ann Surg Oncol 2003; 11(1): 21–26.
3. Stefanutto TB, Shapiro WA, Wright PMC. Anaphylactic reaction to isosulphan blue. Br J Anesth 2002; 89(3): 527–528.
4. Thevarajah S, Huston TL, Simmons RM. A comparison of the adverse reactions associated with isosulfan blue versus methylene blue dye in sentinel lymph node biopsy for breast cancer. Am J Surg 2005; 189(2): 236–239.

ISOTRETINOIN   L5

Trade: Accutane

Other Trades: Accure, Roaccutane, Accutane, Isotrex

Category: Vitamin A derivative used for acne

Isotretinoin is a synthetic derivative of the vitamin A family called retinoids. Isotretinoin is known to be incredibly teratogenic producing profound birth defects in exposed fetuses.[1] It is primarily used for cystic acne where it is extremely effective if used by skilled physicians. While only 25% reaches the plasma, the remaining is either metabolized in the gastrointestinal tract or removed first-pass by the liver. It is distributed to the liver, adrenals, ovaries, and lacrimal glands. Unlike vitamin A, isotretinoin is not stored in the liver. Secretion into milk is unknown but is likely as with other retinoids. Isotretinoin is extremely lipid soluble, and concentrations in milk may be significant. The manufacturer strongly recommends against using isotretinoin in a breastfeeding mother.

Pregnancy Risk	X	Lactation Risk	L5
T ½	= >20 hours	M/P	=
Vd	=	PB	= 99.9%
Tmax	= 3.2 hours	Oral	= 25%
MW	= 300	pKa	= 4

Adult Concerns: Cheilitis (inflammation of the lips), dry nose, pruritus, elevated serum triglycerides, arthralgia, altered blood counts, fatigue, headache, anorexia, nausea, vomiting, abnormal liver function tests, birth defects.

Pediatric Concerns: None reported, but this product poses too many risks to use in a lactating woman.

Drug Interactions: May increase clearance of carbamazepine. Avoid use of other vitamin A products.

Relative Infant Dose:

Adult Dose: 0.5–2 mg/kg daily.

Alternatives:

References:
1. Zbinden G. Investigation on the toxicity of tretinoin administered systemically to animals. Acta Derm Verereol Suppl(Stockh) 1975; 74: 36–40.

ISRADIPINE   L3

Trade: DynaCirc

Other Trades: Prescal

Category: Calcium channel blocker, antihypertensive

Isradipine is a calcium channel blocker used in the management of hypertension. It is not known if isradipine is secreted into milk. However, other calcium channel blockers are transferred only minimally (see verapamil, nifedipine).[1] Observe for lethargy, low blood pressure, and headache. Consider verapamil or nifedipine as alternatives.

Pregnancy Risk	C	Lactation Risk	L3
T ½	= 8 hours	M/P	=
Vd	=	PB	= 95%
Tmax	= 1.5 hours	Oral	= 17%
MW	= 371	pKa	= 11.44

Adult Concerns: Hypotension, headache, dizziness, fatigue, bradycardia, nausea, dyspnea.

Pediatric Concerns: None reported, but observe for hypotension, fatigue, bradycardia, apnea.

Drug Interactions: H_2 blockers may increased oral absorption of isradipine. Carbamazepine levels may be increased. Cyclosporine levels may be increased. May increase hypotension associated with fentanyl use. Digitalis levels may be increased. May increase quinidine levels including bradycardia, arrhythmias, and hypotension.

Relative Infant Dose:

Adult Dose: 2.5–10 mg twice daily.

Alternatives: Nifedipine, verapamil, nimodipine

References:

1. Pharmaceutical manufacturer prescribing information, 1996.

ITRACONAZOLE   L2

Trade: Sporanox
Other Trades: Sporanox
Category: Antifungal

Itraconazole is an antifungal agent active against a variety of fungal strains. It is extensively metabolized to hydroxyitraconazole, an active metabolite.[1] Itraconazole has an enormous volume of distribution, and large quantities (20 fold compared to plasma) concentrate in fatty tissues, liver, kidney, and skin. In a study of two women who received two oral doses of 200 mg itraconazole 12 hours apart, the average milk concentrations at 4, 24, and 48 hours after the second dose were 70, 28, and 16 µg/L respectively.[2] After 72 hours, itraconazole levels in one mother were 20 µg/L and undetectable in the other. Reported milk/plasma ratios at 4, 24, and 48 hours were 0.51, 1.61, and 1.77 respectively. However, itraconazole oral absorption in an infant is somewhat unlikely as it requires an acidic milieu for absorption, which may be unlikely in a diet high in milk. Never use with terfenadine or astemizole. Itraconazole has also been reported to induce significant bone defects in newborn animals, and it is not cleared for pediatric use. Until further studies are done, fluconazole is probably a preferred choice in breastfeeding mothers.

Pregnancy Risk	C	Lactation Risk	L2
T ½	= 64 hours	M/P	= 0.51–1.77
Vd	= 10 l/kg	PB	= 99.8%
Tmax	= 4 hours	Oral	= 55%
MW	= 706	pKa	=

Adult Concerns: Nausea, vomiting, diarrhea, epigastric pain, dizziness, rash, hypertension, abnormal liver enzymes.

Pediatric Concerns: None reported via breastmilk. Absorption via milk is unlikely.

Drug Interactions: Decreased serum levels with isoniazid, rifampin and phenytoin. Decreased absorption under alkaline conditions. Agents which increase stomach pH such as H_2 blockers (cimetidine, famotidine, nizatidine, ranitidine), omeprazole, sucralfate, and milk significantly reduce absorption. Cyclosporin levels are significantly increased by 50%. May increase phenytoin levels, inhibit warfarin metabolism, and increase digoxin levels. Significantly increases terfenadine, astemizole plasma levels.

Relative Infant Dose: 0.2%

Adult Dose: 200–400 mg daily.

Alternatives: Fluconazole

References:
1.   Pharmaceutical manufacturer prescribing information, 2011.
2.   Janssen Pharmaceuticals, personal communication. 1996.

IVACAFTOR 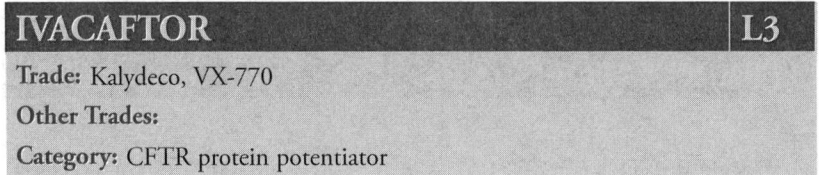 L3

Trade: Kalydeco, VX-770
Other Trades:
Category: CFTR protein potentiator

Ivacaftor is a transmembrane conductance regulator (CFTR) potentiator, indicated specifically for the treatment of cystic fibrosis due to the G551D mutation in the CFTR gene.[1] Currently there are no data available on the transfer of ivacaftor in human milk. Due to its high protein binding and high volume of distribution, it is unlikely that it would enter into milk in significant quantities. However, since so little is known about this drug, caution is urged.

Pregnancy Risk	B	Lactation Risk	L3
T ½	= 12 hours	M/P	=
Vd	= 353 L l/kg	PB	= 99%
Tmax	= 4 hours	Oral	=
MW	= 392.49	pKa	=

Adult Concerns: Nausea, diarrhea, rash, headache, pain in mouth and throat, nasal congestion are the more commonly reported side-effects. Elevation of liver enzymes may occur.

Pediatric Concerns:

Drug Interactions: Co-administration with CYP3A inhibitors (ketoconazole, fluconazole, itraconazole, clarithromycin, erythromycin, telithromycin) may increase its plasma levels and efficacy. Concomitant use with CYP3A inducers (rifampin, rifabutin, phenytoin, carbamazepine, phenobarbital, St. John's wort) decreases its efficacy and is not recommended. Avoid coadministration with grapefruit juice. Concomitant use with the following may increase plasma levels of the following coadministered drugs: midazolam, tacrolimus, digoxin, cyclosporine.

Relative Infant Dose:

Adult Dose: 150 mg every 12 hours.

Alternatives:

References:
1.   Pharmaceutical manufacturer prescribing information, 2012.

IVERMECTIN   L3

Trade: Mectizan, Stromectol, Sklice

Other Trades:

Category: Antiparasitic

Ivermectin is now widely used to treat human onchocerciasis, lymphatic filariasis, and other worms and parasites such as head lice. In a study of 4 women given 150 µg/kg orally, the maximum breastmilk concentration averaged 14.13 µg/L.[1] Milk/plasma ratios ranged from 0.39 to 0.57 with a mean of 0.51. Highest breastmilk concentration was at 4–6 hours. Average daily ingestion of ivermectin was calculated at 2.1 µg/kg which is 10 fold less than the adult dose. No adverse effects were reported in the breastfed infant. Ivermectin is probably compatible with breastfeeding.

A new topical formulation of ivermectin, Sklice, has just been introduced for head lice in infants (6 months and older). It is applied to DRY hair for 10 minutes and then washed off. Nit combing after rinsing is not necessary.

Pregnancy Risk	C	Lactation Risk	L3
T ½	= 28 hours	M/P	= 0.39–0.57
Vd	= 46.8 l/kg	PB	=
Tmax	= 4 hours	Oral	= Variable
MW	=	pKa	= 13.17

Adult Concerns: Headaches, pruritus, transient hypotension.

Pediatric Concerns: None reported.

Drug Interactions: Concurrent use of ivermectin and warfarin may cause increased plasma levels of warfarin and lead to hemorrhagic complications.

Relative Infant Dose: 1.3%

Adult Dose: 150–200 µg/kg once.

Alternatives:

References:
1.   Ogbuokiri JE, Ozumba BC, Okonkwo PO. Ivermectin levels in human breast milk. Eur J Clin Pharmacol 1994; 46(1): 89–90.

IXABEPILONE   L5

Trade: Ixempra

Other Trades:

Category: Anticancer drug

Ixabepilone is a microtubule inhibitor belonging to a class of antineoplastic agents, the epothilones and their analogs. It is approved for the treatment of aggressive metastatic or locally advanced breast cancer no longer responding to currently available chemotherapies. No data are available on its entry into human milk but small levels should be expected in milk due to its chemistry. Ixabepilone is secreted into the milk of lactating rats. After IV administration in humans of radiolabeled ixabepilone on postpartum days 7 and 9, plasma levels or radioactivity were similar to those found in milk. Withhold breastfeeding for at least 260 hours. Discard milk.

Pregnancy Risk	D	Lactation Risk	L5
T ½	= 52 hours	M/P	=
Vd	= 14.2 l/kg	PB	= 77%
Tmax	= At the end of infusion (3 hours)	Oral	=
MW	= 506	pKa	=

Adult Concerns: Unpleasant or change in taste, bone pain, cracked lips, diarrhea, constipation, discoloration of the fingernails or toenails, feeling of warmth, hair loss or thinning of the hair, heartburn, lack or loss of strength, loss of appetite, nausea, redness of the face, neck, arms, and occasionally, upper chest, stomach pain, sudden sweating, swelling or inflammation of the mouth, vomiting, weight loss.

Pediatric Concerns:

Drug Interactions: Co-administration with the following increases the plasma levels of ixabepilone: ketoconazole, erythromycin, fluconazole, or verapamil. Concomitant use with the following decreases the plasma levels of ixabepilone: rifampin, dexamethasone, phenytoin, carbamazepine, rifabutin, phenobarbital and St. John's wort. Contraindicated in patients on capecitabine with elevated liver enzymes.

Relative Infant Dose:

Adult Dose: 40 mg/m^2 IV infusion for 3 hours every 3 weeks.

Alternatives:

References:

1.   Pharmaceutical manufacturer prescribing information, 2010.

JAPANESE ENCEPHALITIS VACCINE | L3

Trade: Ixiaro

Other Trades:

Category: Vaccine

Japanese encephalitis virus (JEV) is an RNA virus belonging to the family of flaviviridae. It is an arbovirus transmitted by the bite of the Culex mosquito. This disease is prevalent in many parts of Asia. Very few cases are encountered in the United States (1 case/year), most commonly among U.S. civilians and military personnel who have travelled to endemic areas in Asia. Japanese encephalitis is characterized by a sudden onset of fever, headache, arthralgia, myalgia, followed by neurological manifestations such as headache, vomiting, rigidity and encephalitis.

Currently two Japanese encephalitis vaccines are licensed for use in the united States–the JE-VAX (inactivated mouse brain-derived vaccine) and IXIARO (inactivated vero cell culture-derived vaccine). Ixiaro is currently widely available and is licensed for those more than 17 years of age. JE-VAX is the only vaccine that can be used for children 1–16 years of age, but since the discontinuation of its manufacture in the United States since 2006, Sanofi Pasteur has reserved its remaining stock of this vaccine. When vaccination of children aged 1–16 years of age is required, healthcare providers are recommended to contact Sanofi Pasteur to order doses of JE-VAX.

Ixiaro is made from inactivated JEV proteins.[1] It is recommended in travelers who plan a prolonged stay of more than a month in an endemic area during the JEV transmission season. It is also recommended in short-term travelers who plan to spend a majority of their time in rural areas during the JEV transmission season, and in travelers travelling to an area with an ongoing JEV outbreak. It is also recommended in all laboratory workers with a potential exposure to the virus. The vaccination series should be completed 1 week prior to estimated day of travel.

There are currently no reports of transfer of the JEV vaccine in human milk. However, since it is an inactivated vaccine, it is unlikely that any exposure through breastmilk would be harmful to the infant. The Centers for Disease Control and prevention (CDC) and the ACIP states that breastfeeding is not a contra-indication to vaccination.[2] This vaccine should be administered only if the risks of acquiring the infection outweigh the risks of the vaccine itself.

Pregnancy Risk	B	Lactation Risk	L3
T ½	=	M/P	=
Vd	=	PB	=
Tmax	=	Oral	=
MW	=	pKa	=

Adult Concerns: Pain, tenderness, redness, swelling at injection site, nausea, headache, myalgia, hypersensitivity reactions. Contra-indicated in those with known hypersensitivity to protamine sulfate or thiomersal.

Pediatric Concerns:

Drug Interactions:

Relative Infant Dose:

Adult Dose: 2 doses of 0.5 mL, IM, 28 days apart.

Alternatives:

References:
1. Pharmaceutical manufacturer prescribing information, 2012.
2. Anon: Resource materials: general recommendations on immunization. Am J Prev Med 1994; 10(suppl): 60–82.

KANAMYCIN   L2

Trade: Kantrex

Other Trades: Kannasyn

Category: Antibiotic

Kanamycin is an aminoglycoside antibiotic primarily used for gram negative infections. In a study of 3 patients who received 1000 mg intravenously, milk levels at 1, 2, 4, and 6 hours were zero, 0.1 mg/L, 0.3 mg/L, 0.5 and 0.8 mg/L respectively.[1] The average milk level in this study was 0.25 mg/L although the highest milk level occurred at 1 hour following the IV infusion. The milk/plasma ratio at 6 hours was 0.045. It is probably advisable to refrain from breastfeeding for several hours following placement of the IV. This will drastically reduce the infant's exposure to kanamycin. However, poor oral absorption (only 1%) in the infant would limit amount absorbed although changes in gastrointestinal flora are possible.

Pregnancy Risk	D	Lactation Risk	L2
T ½	= 2.4 hours	M/P	= 0.045
Vd	= 0.2–0.3 l/kg	PB	= .
Tmax	= 1 hour	Oral	= 1%
MW	=	pKa	= 7.2

Adult Concerns: Diarrhea, ototoxicity, nephrotoxicity.

Pediatric Concerns: None reported, but observe for diarrhea.

Drug Interactions: May have increased toxicity when used with penicillins, cephalosporins, amphotericin B, and diuretics. May increase neuromuscular blockade when used with neuromuscular blocking agents.

Relative Infant Dose: 0.3%

Adult Dose: 5–7.5 mg/kg every 8–12 hours.

Alternatives:

References:

1. Matsuda S. Transfer of antibiotics into maternal milk. Biol Res Pregnancy Perinatol 1984; 5(2): 57–60.

KAVA-KAVA   L5

Trade:

Other Trades:

Category: Sedative and sleep enhancement

Kava is the dried rhizome and roots of Piper methysticum. While more than 20 varieties are known, the black and white grades are most popular. Kava drink is prepared from the rhizome by steeping the pulverized root in hot water. It is then filtered and consumed. It is indigenous to the islands of the South Pacific where it is used similar to alcohol to induce relaxation.[1] The activity of kava appears related to several dihydropyrones that possess CNS activity, including methysticine, kawain, dihydromethysticin, and yangonin. Studies of these agents suggest that they may induce mephenesin-like muscle relaxation in animals, similar in effect to the local anesthetics.

Masticated kava induces a local anesthetic effect in the mouth. It is not known with certainty how these agents work, but it is apparently not at the opiate receptors. However, they do induce sleep and reduce anxiety. The CNS activity of kava is due to the lipid components, not the more polar water soluble components. In humans, kava produces mild euphoria, happiness, fluent and lively speech. High doses may lead to muscle weakness, visual and auditory changes. Heavy users are underweight, have reduced plasma protein levels, facial edema, scaly rashes, elevated HDL cholesterol, blood in the urine, and abnormal CBC (elevated RBCs, reduced platelets, and lymphocytes). Discolored, flaky skin, and reddened eyes are common. Ethanol dramatically increases the toxicity of kava and should not be co-mixed. No data are available on its use in breastfeeding mothers, but care should be exercised. The German Commission E monographs state that it is contraindicated in pregnant and lactating women.[2]

Pregnancy Risk	Hazardous	Lactation Risk	L5
T ½	=	M/P	=
Vd	=	PB	=
Tmax	=	Oral	=
MW	=	pKa	=

Adult Concerns: High doses may lead to muscle weakness, visual and auditory changes. Heavy users are underweight, have reduced plasma protein levels, facial edema, scaly rashes, elevated HDL cholesterol, blood in the urine, and abnormal blood counts (elevated RBCs, reduced platelets, and lymphocytes). Discolored, flaky skin, and reddened eyes is common. Ethanol dramatically increases the toxicity of kava, and should not be co-mixed.

Pediatric Concerns: None reported but caution is recommended.

Drug Interactions: Admixing with alcohol dramatically increases toxicity of kava.

Relative Infant Dose:

Adult Dose:

Alternatives:

References:
1. Review of Natural Products Facts and Comparisons, St Louis, MO 1996.
2. The Complete German Commission E Monographs. Ed. M. Blumenthal Amer Botanical Council 1998.

KETAMINE   L3

Trade: Ketanest, Ketaset, Ketalar, Ketanest S, Ketamax, Calypsol, Brevinaze, Anesject

Other Trades:

Category: Anesthetic agent

Ketamine is a rapid acting general anesthetic agent with effects that include analgesia, anesthesia, and hallucinations. Often combined with midazolam, it is increasingly more popular, as it has fewer hemodynamic problems, and reduced postoperative depression. One interesting complication is the hallucinogenic effect commonly called a dissociative effect or emergence reaction.[1,2]

Following the use of ketamine, patients may exhibit hallucinogenic effects upon withdrawal. This is often suppressed with the addition of midazolam or other benzodiazepines. The emergent reactions are apparently age-dependent, and appear to occur more frequently in adults (30–50%) and less frequently in children (5–15%).[1] One major benefit of ketamine is the production of excellent analgesia with minimal respiratory depression. No data are available on the transfer of ketamine into human milk. It has a short half-life of 2.5 hours but its redistribution half-life out of the plasma (to muscle and tissues) is much briefer (4.68 min.), thus milk levels are likely to be low.

Pregnancy Risk	B		Lactation Risk	L3
T ½	= 2.5–3 hours		M/P	=
Vd	= 2–3 l/kg		PB	= 47%
Tmax	= 0.4 hours epidural		Oral	= 16%
MW	= 237		pKa	= 7.5

Adult Concerns: Sedation, hallucinations, normal or slightly enhanced skeletal muscle tone, cardiovascular and respiratory stimulation, and occasionally a transient and minimal respiratory depression. Diplopia and nystagmus have been reported.

Pediatric Concerns: None reported via milk. Rapid redistribution from the plasma would probably reduce levels in milk.

Drug Interactions: Prolonged recovery times may occur if used with barbiturates or narcotics. Increased neuromuscular blockade when used with atracurium and tubocurarine. Increased risk of seizures with metrizamide, and theophylline. Increased risk of cardiovascular collapse with St. John's Wort. Increased risk of respiratory depression when used with tramadol.

Relative Infant Dose:

Adult Dose: Varies but 1–2 mg/kg IV may be used for induction in adults.

Alternatives: Propfol, sufentanil.

References:

1. Bergman SA. Ketamine: review of its pharmacology and its use in pediatric anesthesia. Anesth Prog 1999; 46(1): 10–20.
2. White M, de GP, Renshof B, van KE, Dzoljic M. Pharmacokinetics of S(+) ketamine derived from target controlled infusion. Br J Anaesth 2006 March; 96(3): 330–4.
3. White PF, Ham J, Way WL, Trevor AJ. Pharmacology of ketamine isomers in surgical patients. Anesthesiology 1980 March; 52(3): 231–9.

KETOCONAZOLE   L2

Trade: Nizoral, Nizoral A-D, Xolegel, Extina

Other Trades:

Category: Antifungal, anti-dandruff

Ketoconazole is an antifungal similar in structure to miconazole and clotrimazole. It is used orally, topically, and via shampoo.[1] Ketoconazole is not detected in plasma after chronic shampooing. In a study of one patient (82 kg) receiving 200 mg daily for 10 days, milk samples were taken at 1.75, 3.25, 6.0, 8.0, and 24 hours after the tenth dose.[2] The average concentration of ketoconazole over the 24 hours was 68 µg/L while the C_{max} at 3.25 hours was 0.22 mg/L. The absorption of ketoconazole is highly variable, and could be reduced in infants due to the alkaline condition induced by milk ingestion.[3] Ketoconazole requires acidic conditions to be absorbed, and its absorption and distribution in children is not known. Regardless, ketoconazole is probably safe in breastfeeding infants.

Pregnancy Risk	C	Lactation Risk	L2
T ½	= 2–8 hours	M/P	=
Vd	=	PB	= 99%
Tmax	= 1–2 hours	Oral	= Variable (75%)
MW	= 531	pKa	= 2.94, 6.51

Adult Concerns: Nausea, vomiting, itching, dizziness, fever, chills, hypertension, hepatotoxicity.

Pediatric Concerns: None reported in one case.

Drug Interactions: Decreased ketoconazole levels occur with rifampin, isoniazid and phenytoin use. Theophylline levels may be reduced. Absorption requires acid pH, so anything increasing gastric pH will significantly reduce absorption. This includes cimetidine, ranitidine, famotidine, omeprazole, sucralfate, antacids, etc. Do not coadminister with cisapride or terfenadine (very dangerous). May increase cyclosporin levels by 50%, inhibits warfarin metabolism and prolongs coagulation.

Relative Infant Dose: 0.3%

Adult Dose: 200–400 mg daily.

Alternatives: Fluconazole

References:
1. Pharmaceutical manufacturer prescribing information, 1996.
2. Moretti ME, Ito S, Koren G. Disposition of maternal ketoconazole in breast milk. Am J Obstet Gynecol 1995; 173(5): 1625–1626.
3. Force RW, Nahata MC. Salivary concentrations of ketoconazole and fluconazole: implications for drug efficacy in oropharyngeal and esophageal candidiasis. Ann Pharmacother 1995; 29(1): 10–15.

KETOROLAC   L2

Trade: Toradol, Acular

Other Trades: Acular, Toradol

Category: Non-steroidal anti-inflammatory, analgesic

Ketorolac is a popular, nonsteroidal analgesic. Although previously used in labor and delivery, its use has subsequently been contraindicated because it is believed to adversely effect fetal circulation and inhibit uterine contractions, thus increasing the risk of hemorrhage. In a study of 10 lactating women who received 10 mg orally four times daily, milk levels of ketorolac were not detectable in 4 of the subjects.[1] In the 6 remaining patients, the concentration of ketorolac in milk 2 hours after a dose ranged from 5.2 to 7.3 µg/L on day 1 and 5.9 to 7.9 µg/L on day 2. In most patients, the breastmilk level was never above 5 µg/L. The maximum daily dose an infant could absorb (maternal dose= 40 mg/day) would range from 3.16 to 7.9 µg/day assuming a milk volume of 400 mL or 1000 mL. An infant would therefore receive less than 0.2% of the daily maternal dose (Please note, the original paper contained a misprint on the daily intake of ketorolac (mg instead of µg).

Ketorolac has been extensively studied in neonates, infants and children and is quite effective and safe. The half-life is brief and in some cases is undetectable in the infant plasma after 4 hours.[2] For a complete review of the pediatric use of ketorolac see Buck.[3] The use of ketorolac postpartum is controversial due to the risk of hemorrhage and effects on the newborn.(See FDA warnings) That said, when used after delivery when the risk of hemorrhage is minimized, ketorolac has numerous benefits over other opiate analgesics and is probably safe. The postsurgical use of ketorolac is considered safe with regard to postoperative bleeding.[4–16]

Pregnancy Risk	C/D in 3rd trimester	Lactation Risk	L2
T ½	= 2.5 hours	M/P	= 0.015–0.037
Vd	= 0.18–0.21 l/kg	PB	= 99%
Tmax	= 0.5–1 hour	Oral	= >81%
MW	= 255	pKa	= 3.5

Adult Concerns: Gastrointestinal irritability, dry mouth, nausea, vomiting, edema, or rash.

Pediatric Concerns: None reported in one study.

Drug Interactions: May prolong prothrombin time when used with warfarin. Antihypertensive effects of ACE inhibitors may be blunted or completely abolished by NSAIDs. Some NSAIDs may block antihypertensive effect of beta blockers, diuretics. Used with cyclosporin, may dramatically increase renal toxicity. May increase digoxin, phenytoin, lithium levels. May increase toxicity of methotrexate. May increase bioavailability of penicillamine. Probenecid may increase NSAID levels.

Relative Infant Dose: 0.2%

Adult Dose: 10 mg every 6 hours.

Alternatives: Ibuprofen.

References:

1. Wischnik A, Manth SM, Lloyd J, Bullingham R, Thompson JS. The excretion of ketorolac tromethamine into breast milk after multiple oral dosing. Eur J Clin Pharmacol 1989; 36(5): 521–524.
2. Cohen MN, Christians U, Henthorn T, Vu Tran Z, Moll V, Zuk J, Galinkin J. Pharmacokinetics of single-dose intravenous ketorolac in infants aged 2–11 months. Anesth Analg. 2011 Mar; 112(3): 655–60.
3. Buck ML. Use of Intravenous ketorolac for postoperative analgesia in infants. Pediatric Pharmacotherapy Newsletter, volume 17, number 8.
4. Brown CR, Mazzulla JP, Mok MS, Nussdorf RT, Rubin PD, Schwesinger WH. Comparison of repeat doses of intramuscular ketorolac tromethamine and morphine sulfate for analgesia after major surgery. Pharmacotherapy. 1990; 10(6 (Pt 2)): 45S-50S.
5. Burns JW, Aitken HA, Bullingham RE, McArdle CS, Kenny GN. Double-blind comparison of the morphine sparing effect of continuous and intermittent i.m. administration of ketorolac. British journal of anaesthesia. Sep 1991; 67(3): 235–238.
6. Cepeda MS, Vargas L, Ortegon G, Sanchez MA, Carr DB. Comparative analgesic efficacy of patient-controlled analgesia with ketorolac versus morphine after elective intraabdominal operations. Anesthesia and analgesia. Jun 1995; 80(6): 1150–1153.
7. Folsland B, Skulberg A, Halvorsen P, Helgesen KG. Placebo-controlled comparison of single intramuscular doses of ketorolac tromethamine and pethidine for post-operative analgesia. The Journal of international medical research. Jul-Aug 1990; 18(4): 305–314.
8. Gillies GW, Kenny GN, Bullingham RE, McArdle CS. The morphine sparing effect of ketorolac tromethamine. A study of a new, parenteral non-steroidal anti-inflammatory agent after abdominal surgery. Anaesthesia. Jul 1987; 42(7): 727–731.
9. Gin T, Kan AF, Lam KK, O'Meara ME. Analgesia after caesarean section with intramuscular ketorolac or pethidine. Anaesthesia and intensive care. Aug 1993; 21(4): 420–423.
10. Greer IA. Effects of ketorolac tromethamine on hemostasis. Pharmacotherapy. 1990; 10(6 (Pt 2)): 71S-76S.
11. O'Hara DA, Fanciullo G, Hubbard L, et al. Evaluation of the safety and efficacy of ketorolac versus morphine by patient-controlled analgesia for postoperative pain. Pharmacotherapy. Sep-Oct 1997; 17(5): 891–899.
12. Parker RK, Holtmann B, Smith I, White PF. Use of ketorolac after lower abdominal surgery. Effect on analgesic requirement and surgical outcome. Anesthesiology. Jan 1994; 80(1): 6–12.13.
13. Pavy TJ, Paech MJ, Evans SF. The effect of intravenous ketorolac on opioid requirement and pain after cesarean delivery. Anesthesia and analgesia. Apr 2001; 92(4): 1010–1014.
14. Stanski DR, Cherry C, Bradley R, Sarnquist FH, Yee JP. Efficacy and safety of single doses of intramuscular ketorolac tromethamine compared with meperidine for postoperative pain. Pharmacotherapy. 1990; 10(6 (Pt 2)): 40S-44S.

15. Tzeng JI, Mok MS. Combination of intramuscular Ketorolac and low dose epidural morphine for the relief of post-caesarean pain. Annals of the Academy of Medicine, Singapore. Nov 1994; 23(6 Suppl): 10–13.
16. Varrassi G, Marinangeli F, Agro F, et al. A double-blinded evaluation of propacetamol versus ketorolac in combination with patient-controlled analgesia morphine: analgesic efficacy and tolerability after gynecologic surgery. Anesthesia and analgesia. Mar 1999; 88(3): 611–616.

KETOROLAC TROMETHAMINE   L2

Trade: Sprix, Acuvail

Other Trades:

Category: Analgesic for acute moderate to severe pain

Ketorolac is a popular, nonsteroidal analgesic used in eye drops. While oral or IV ketorolac produce low levels in breastmilk, it is exceedingly unlikely that the ophthalmic product will produce high enough levels systemically in the mother to ever produce measurable levels in breastmilk.

Milk levels of ketorolac are low with the usual oral dosage,[1] but have not been measured after higher injectable dosages. Maternal use of ketorolac eye drops would not be expected to cause any adverse effects in breastfed infants. To substantially diminish the amount of drug that reaches the breastmilk after using eye drops, place pressure over the tear duct by the corner of the eye for 1 minute or more, then remove the excess solution with an absorbent tissue.

Pregnancy Risk	C/D in 3rd trimester	Lactation Risk	L2
T ½	= 4–6 hours	M/P	=
Vd	=	PB	= 99%
Tmax	= 30–60 min	Oral	= 99%
MW	= 376.41	pKa	= 3.5

Adult Concerns: Rhinalgia, nasal irritation, rhinitis, rash, bradycardia, increase liver enzymes, bradycardia, increase lacrimation.

Pediatric Concerns:

Drug Interactions: Concurrent use of ketorolac with probenecid, aspirin, pentoxifylline and other NSAIDS is contraindicated. Avoid use of ketorolac concomitantly with the following drugs: heparins, warfarin, clopidogrel, argatroban, abciximab, SSRIs, danaparoid, tacrolimus, ginkgo. For a complete list, please refer drug interactions reference.

Relative Infant Dose:

Adult Dose: One drop (0.25 mg) four times daily.

Alternatives:

References:
1. Wischnik A, Manth SM, Lloyd J, Bullingham R, Thompson JS. The excretion of ketorolac tromethamine into breast milk after multiple oral dosing. Eur J Clin Pharmacol 1989; 36(5): 521–524.

KETOTIFEN   L3

Trade: Zaditor, Zaditen, Alaway, Zyrtec Itchy-Eye Drops, Claritin Eye
Other Trades:
Category: Antihistamine

Ketotifen is a second-generation H_1-antihistamine. It is used ophthalmically to treat red eye and allergic conjunctivitis.[1] Ketotifen has been shown to enter breastmilk in animal studies, however it is not known if it is excreted into human breastmilk.[1] It is unknown if enough drug enters systemic circulation after topical administration to produce significant quantities in breastmilk. This drug has a molecular weight of 425.5, an oral bioavailability of 50%, and is distributed widely throughout the body. Based on these kinetics, it is unlikely that this drug would pose a significant risk to breastfed infants.

Pregnancy Risk	C	Lactation Risk	L3
T ½	= 21 hours	M/P	=
Vd	= 56 l/kg	PB	=
Tmax	= 2–4 hours	Oral	= 50%
MW	= 425.5	pKa	= 8.43

Adult Concerns: Syncope, rash, contact dermatitis, hyperglycemia, weight gain, xerostomia, dizziness, headache, somnolence, dyspnea, pharyngitis, rhinitis.

Pediatric Concerns:

Drug Interactions: Acetylcholinesterase Inhibitors (neostigmine, physostigmine)– may reduce the effects of ketotifen. Alcohol–may cause additional sedation along with ketotifen. Amphetamines–may reduce the sedative effect of ketotifen. Anticholinergics–may enhance the toxic effects of other anticholinergic medications. Benzylpenicylloyl polylysine–Ketotifen may diminish this agent's diagnostic ability. Betahistine–Ketotifen may diminish this agent's therapeutic effects. CNS depressants–may enhance the sedative effects of ketotifen. Droperidol–may enhance the sedative effects of ketotifen. Hydroxyzine–may enhance the sedative effects of ketotifen. Pramlintide–may enhance the effects of ketotifen. SSRI–Ketotifen may enhance this agent's toxic effects.

Relative Infant Dose:

Adult Dose: 1 drop in each eye twice daily; 1–2 mg oral twice daily.

Alternatives:

References:
1. Product Information: Zaditor(TM), ketotifen ophthalmic solution 0.025%. Novartis Ophthalmics, Duluth, GA, 2001a.

KOMBUCHA TEA   L5

Trade:
Other Trades:
Category: Herbal tea

Kombucha tea is a popular health beverage made by incubating the Kombucha mushroom in sweet black tea. During 1995, several reported cases of toxicity and one fatality was reported to the CDC.[1] Based on these reports, the Iowa Department of Health has recommended that persons refrain from drinking Kombucha tea until the role of the tea in these cases has been resolved.

Pregnancy Risk	Hazardous	Lactation Risk	L5
T ½	=	M/P	=
Vd	=	PB	=
Tmax	=	Oral	=
MW	=	pKa	=

Adult Concerns: Shortness of breath, respiratory distress, fatigue, metabolic acidosis, disseminated intravascular coagulopathy.

Pediatric Concerns: Caution is recommended.

Drug Interactions:

Relative Infant Dose:

Adult Dose: N/A

Alternatives:

References:
1. Unexplained severe illness possibly associated with consumption of Kombucha tea--Iowa, 1995 MMWR Morb Mortal Wkly Rep 1995; 44(48): 892–900.

L-METHYLFOLATE   L3

Trade: Deplin, Metafolin
Other Trades:
Category: Active folic acid metabolite

L-Methylfolate, also called Metafolin, is the active biological isomer of folate and the form of circulating folate. Approximately 10% of the population lacks the enzymes necessary to metabolize folic acid to L-methylfolate. L-Methylfolate is the form transported across cell membranes, and is bioactive. No data are available on the transport of this form of folate into human milk. However, several studies of folic acid supplementation in breastfeeding mothers clearly suggest that folate is actively transported into human milk, but most importantly, supplementing of the mother only marginally if at all, increases milk folate levels.[1,2] This suggests that even following supplementation, milk levels would be unlikely to increase, unless the mother is deficient. Thus, this product is probably not hazardous to use in a breastfeeding mother.

Pregnancy Risk	Probably Safe	Lactation Risk	L3
T ½	=	M/P	=
Vd	=	PB	=
Tmax	=	Oral	= Complete
MW	= 455	pKa	=

Adult Concerns: First-generation anticonvulsants may cause decreased serum folate levels, and high doses of folates may actually reduce plasma levels of these anticonvulsants, thereby reducing their anticonvulsant effect.

Pediatric Concerns: None reported via milk.

Drug Interactions: Do not use with anticonvulsants. First-generation anticonvulsants (carbamazepine, phenytoin, fosphenytoin, phenobarbital, primidone, valproic acid) may not only reduce plasma folate levels, but high folate administration may also reduce plasma levels of these anticonvulsants. See prescribing information.

Relative Infant Dose:

Adult Dose: 7.5 mg daily.

Alternatives: Folic acid

References:
1. Tamura T, Yoshimura Y, Arakawa T. Human milk folate and folate status in lactating mothers and their infants. Am J Clin Nutr. 1980; 33: 193–197.
2. Smith AM, Picciano MF, Deering RH. Folate supplementation during lactation: maternal folate status, human milk folate content, and their relationship to infant folate status. J Pediatr Gastroenterol Nutr. 1983; 2: 622–628.

LABETALOL   L2

Trade: Trandate, Normodyne

Other Trades: Presolol, Trandate, Labrocol

Category: Antihypertensive, beta blocker

Labetalol is a selective beta blocker with moderate lipid solubility that is used as an antihypertensive and for treating angina. In one study of 3 women receiving 600–1200 mg/day, the peak concentrations of labetalol in breastmilk were 129, 223, and 662 µg/L respectively.[1] In only one infant were measurable plasma levels found (18 µg/L) following a maternal dose of 600 mg. Therefore, only small amounts are secreted into human milk.

Pregnancy Risk	C	Lactation Risk	L2
T ½	= 6–8 hours	M/P	= 0.8–2.6
Vd	= 10 l/kg	PB	= 50%
Tmax	= 1–2 hours (oral)	Oral	= 30–40%
MW	= 328	pKa	= 7.4, 8.7

Adult Concerns: Bradycardia, hypotension, dizziness, nausea, aggravation of asthma, lethargy.

Pediatric Concerns: None reported, but observe for hypotension, bradycardia, hypoxemia, weakness.

Drug Interactions: Decreased effect when used with aluminum salts, barbiturates, calcium salts, cholestyramine, NSAIDs, ampicillin, rifampin, and salicylates. Beta blockers may reduce the effect of oral sulfonylureas (hypoglycemic agents). Increased toxicity/effect when used with other antihypertensives, contraceptives, monoamine oxidase inhibitors, cimetidine, and numerous other products. See drug interaction reference for complete listing.

Relative Infant Dose: 0.2%–0.6%

Adult Dose: 200–400 mg twice daily.

Alternatives: Propranolol, metoprolol

References:
1. Lunell NO, Kulas J, Rane A. Transfer of labetalol into amniotic fluid and breast milk in lactating women. Eur J Clin Pharmacol 1985; 28(5): 597–599.

LACOSAMIDE   L3

Trade: Vimpat
Other Trades:
Category: Anticonvulsant

Lacosamide is a new anticonvulsant used as adjunctive therapy in the treatment of partial-onset seizures in patients with epilepsy aged 17 years and older.[1] It is a functionalized amino acid that has activity in the maximal electroshock seizure test. Due to its structure, levels in milk may be significant. No data are available on its transfer into human milk, but caution is recommended until we have more data.

Pregnancy Risk	C	Lactation Risk	L3
T ½	= 13 hours	M/P	=
Vd	= 0.6 l/kg	PB	= 15%
Tmax	= 30–60 minutes	Oral	= 100%
MW	= 250	pKa	=

Adult Concerns: Lacosamide increases the risk of suicidal thoughts or behavior in patients taking these drugs for any indication. Patients treated with any anti-epileptic drug, for any indication should be monitored for the emergence or worsening of depression, suicidal thoughts or behavior, and/or any unusual changes in mood or behavior. Vertigo, eye disorders, diplopia, vision blurred, gastrointestinal disorders, nausea, vomiting, diarrhea, fatigue, gait disturbance, asthenia, contusion, dizziness, headache, ataxia, somnolence, tremor, nystagmus, depression, pruritus, impaired memory have been reported.

Pediatric Concerns: None reported yet, but caution is recommended.

Drug Interactions: None yet reported.

Relative Infant Dose:

Adult Dose: 50–600 mg per day.

Alternatives: Lamotrigine, carbamazepine

References:
1. Pharmaceutical manufacturer prescribing information, 2010.

LACTASE   L3

Trade:

Other Trades:

Category: Lactose intolerant agent

Lactase is an enzyme that metabolizes lactose (milk sugar) in the small intestine to glucose and galactose. This enzyme is naturally produced in 77% of U.S. adult populations and 100% of human infants.[1] There are no adequate and well-controlled studies or case reports in breastfeeding women, however used orally, this product is probably safe for breastfeeding women.

Pregnancy Risk	Probably Safe	Lactation Risk	L3
T ½	=	M/P	=
Vd	=	PB	=
Tmax	=	Oral	=
MW	=	pKa	=

Adult Concerns: None reported.

Pediatric Concerns:

Drug Interactions:

Relative Infant Dose:

Adult Dose: 1–2 capsules with milk

Alternatives:

References:
1. Bersaglieri T, Sabeti PC, Patterson N, Vanderploeg T, Schaffner SF, Drake JA, Rhodes M, Reich DE, Hirschhorn JN. Genetic signatures of strong recent positive selection at the lactase gene. Am J Hum Genet. 2004 Jun; 74(6): 1111–20. Epub 2004 Apr 26.

LACTIC ACID   L3

Trade:

Other Trades:

Category: Metabolite, dermatologic agent

Lactic acid is a natural product of the anaerobic branch of glucose metabolism. It is present in breast milk naturally, and may be increased during heavy exercise. Past studies have suggested that infant feeding decreased when milk contained high amounts of lactic acid.[1] Further examination of feeding habits have shown that lactic acid concentration in the milk does not appear to affect infant feeding habits or adversely affect the child.[2] When applied topically, lactic acid appears to be absorbed in amounts of no greater than 50% total dose, though absorption rates of 17–35% are more common.[3] It is unlikely that the use of topical lactic acid will produce untoward effects in infants as they already produce and consume this product naturally.

Pregnancy Risk	Probably Safe	Lactation Risk	L3
T ½	=	M/P	=
Vd	=	PB	=
Tmax	=	Oral	=
MW	= 90.09	pKa	=

Adult Concerns: Respiratory, dermal, and ocular irritation

Pediatric Concerns:

Drug Interactions: Lactic acid may promote bismuth absorption.

Relative Infant Dose:

Adult Dose: Varies depending on indication and product.

Alternatives:

References:
1. Wallace JP, Inbar G, Ernsthausen K. Infant acceptance of postexercise breast milk. Pediatrics. 1992; 89: 1245–1247.
2. Wright Kc S, Quinn TJ, Carey GB. Pediatrics. 2002; 109: 585–589.
3. Cosmetic Ingredient Review Expert Panel; International Journal of Toxicology, 17 (Suppl.1): 1–203 (1998).

LAMIVUDINE   L2

Trade: Epivir-HBV, 3TC

Other Trades: 3TC

Category: Antiviral

Lamivudine is a synthetic nucleoside analogue antiviral used for the treatment of Hepatitis B or HIV infections. It is presently in numerous other combination products (Combivir, Ziagen, etc.). In a study of 20 women receiving either 300 mg once daily or 150 mg twice daily one week postpartum, the mean breast milk concentration was 1.22 mg/L (range= 0.5–6.09) or 0.183 mg/kg/day. This is significantly less than the clinical dose normally administered to infants (4–8 mg/kg/day). The authors suggested that the amount ingested via breast milk was negligible relative to therapeutic dosing and would not provide adequate antiretroviral drug concentrations for a neonate.

In another study of 18 women receiving antiretroviral treatment for HIV infections (150 mg BID lamivudine and 200 mg BID nevirapine), median lamivudine concentrations in maternal serum, breast milk, and the infant's serum was 678 ng/mL, 1828 ng/mL and 28 ng/mL, respectively.[2] The median milk/serum ratio was 3.34 for lamivudine. The median infant concentration of lamivudine (28 ng/mL) was 5% of the inhibitory concentration (50%) which is 550 ng/mL. This data suggests that the serum levels of lamivudine attained in the infant are probably too low to produce side effects in the infant, and certainly too low to treat HIV effectively in the infant.

Pregnancy Risk	C		Lactation Risk	L2
T ½	= 5–7 hours		M/P	= 3.34
Vd	= 1.0 l/kg		PB	= <36%
Tmax	= 1–1.5 hours		Oral	= 82%
MW	= 229		pKa	=

Adult Concerns: Adverse events include lactic acidosis, severe hepatomegaly, pancreatitis, malaise, fatigue, upper respiratory infections, nausea, vomiting, headache and myalgia.

Pediatric Concerns: None reported in two studies. Dose via milk is apparently too low to produce adverse effects.

Drug Interactions: Use with co-trimoxazole (trimethoprim and sulfamethoxazole) could potentially elevate levels of lamivudine. Plasma levels of loviride were reduced by lamivudine. Do not use with ribavirin due to risk of fatal lactic acidosis.

Relative Infant Dose: 4.3%–6.4%

Adult Dose: 100 mg daily for hepatitis B infections.

Alternatives:

References:
1. Moodley J, Moodley D, Pillay K, Coovadia H, Saba J, van Leeuwen R, Goodwin C, Harrigan PR, Moore KH, Stone C, Plumb R, Johnson MA. Pharmacokinetics and antiretroviral activity of lamivudine alone or when coadministered with zidovudine in human immunodeficiency virus type 1-infected pregnant women and their offspring. J Infect Dis 1998; 178(5): 1327–1333.
2. Shapiro RL, Holland DT, Capparelli E, Lockman S, Thior I, Wester C, et al. Antiretroviral concentrations in breast-feeding infants of women in Botswana receiving antiretroviral treatment. J Infect Dis 2005 Sep 1; 192(5): 720–7.

LAMOTRIGINE   L3

Trade: Lamictal, Lamictal XR
Other Trades: Lamictal
Category: Anticonvulsant

Lamotrigine is a newer anticonvulsant primarily indicated for treatment of simple and complex partial seizures. In a study of a 24 year-old female receiving 300 mg/day lamotrigine during pregnancy, maternal serum levels and cord levels of lamotrigine at birth were 3.88 µg/mL in the mother and 3.26 µg/mL in the cord blood.[1] By day 22, the maternal serum levels were 9.61 µg/mL, the milk concentration was 6.51 mg/L, and the infant's serum level was 2.25 µg/mL. Following a reduction in dose, the prior levels decreased significantly over the next weeks. The milk/plasma ratio at the highest maternal serum level was 0.562. The estimated dose to infant would be approximately 2–5 mg per day assuming a maternal dose of 200–300 mg per day. The infant developed normally in every way. In another study of a single mother receiving 200 mg/day lamotrigine, milk levels of lamotrigine immediately prior to the next dose (trough) at steady state were 3.48 mg/L (13.6 uM).[2] The authors estimated the daily dose to infant to be 0.5 mg/kg/day. The above authors suggest that infants, while developing normally, should probably be monitored periodically for plasma levels of lamotrigine. The manufacturer reports that in a group of 5 women (no dose listed), breastmilk concentrations of lamotrigine ranged from 0.07–5.03 mg/L.[3] Breastmilk levels averaged 40–45% of maternal plasma levels. No untoward effects were noted in the infants.

In a study by Ohman of 9 breastfeeding women at 3 weeks postpartum, the median milk/plasma ratio was 0.61, and the breastfed infants maintained lamotrigine concentrations of approximately 30% of the mother's plasma levels.[4] The authors estimated the dose to the infant at 0.2–1 mg/kg/day. No adverse effects were noted in the infants. One further study of 6 breastfeeding women consuming from 175–800 (mean=400) mg/day resulted in average infant doses of 0.45 mg/kg/day, and an average infant plasma concentration of 0.6 mg/L. No adverse effects in the infants were noted.[5] In a study of four mothers with partial epilepsy on lamotrigine monotherapy, serum levels of lamotrigine in nursing newborns ranged from <1.0 to 2.0 µg/mL on day 10 of life.[6] Three babies had lamotrigine levels >1.0 µg/mL. Lamotrigine levels in newborns were on average 30% (range 20–43%) of the maternal drug level. Unfortunately, no decline was noted in two children with repeat levels at 2 months. The authors suggested significant genetic variability in the infants' ability to metabolize this drug. Close monitoring of the infant plasma levels was recommended.[6] In a recent and well-done study of thirty women under treatment with lamotrigine for seizure disorders, the average milk/plasma ratio was 0.413.[7] Infant plasma levels were 18.3% of maternal plasma levels. The theoretical daily infant dose was 0.51 mg/kg/day and the relative infant dose was 9.2% (range=3.1–21.1%). Most importantly, this study indicates that there is wide variability in milk levels that seem to be more related to the pharmacogenetic makeup of the individual than the dose. It is important to remember, that the theoretic infant dose in these studies, that ranges from 0.51 mg/kg/day to perhaps as high as 1 mg/kg/day is still significantly less than the therapeutic dose (4.4 mg/k/day) administered to 17 day-old infants with neonatal seizures.[8]

However, one case of severe apnea has been recently reported in a 16 day old breastfed infant.[9] In this case, the mother was receiving 850 mg/day, had a plasma level of 14.93 µg/mL. The plasma level of the infant was 4.87 µg/mL. Interestingly, the milk/plasma ratio was higher, 0.79 to 0.96, suggesting higher transfer into milk than in the above studies.

The use of lamotrigine in breastfeeding mothers produces significant plasma levels in some breastfed infants, although they are apparently not high enough to produce side effects in most cases. Exposure in utero is considerably higher, and levels will probably drop postnatally in newborn infants who are breastfed. Nevertheless, it is advisable to monitor the infant's plasma levels closely to ensure safety. In two recent studies by Meador et al, no untoward effects on IQ level were noted in children at age 3 years when exposed to lamotrigine during pregnancy and breastfeeding.[10,11]

Pregnancy Risk	C	Lactation Risk	L3
T ½	= 29 hours	M/P	= 0.562
Vd	= 0.9–1.3 l/kg	PB	= 55%
Tmax	= 1–4 hours	Oral	= 98%
MW	= 256	pKa	= 5.7

Adult Concerns: Rash, faintness, drowsiness, dyspepsia, fatigue, ataxia, dizziness, ataxia, somnolence, tremor, nausea, vomiting, and headache. Breast pain has been infrequently reported.

Pediatric Concerns: Breast milk levels are relatively high and relative infant dose is high as well. Reported infant plasma levels are about 30% of maternal plasma levels. One reported case of severe neonatal apnea in one infant. Closely monitor all infants exposed to lamotrigine via milk.

Drug Interactions: Acetaminophen reduces lamotrigine half-life by 15–20% and may require increased doses. Carbamazepine, phenytoin, phenobarbital, and other anticonvulsants may reduce plasma levels of lamotrigine by increasing clearance, but this is highly variable.

Relative Infant Dose: 9.2%–18.3%

Adult Dose: 150–250 mg twice daily.

Alternatives:

References:

1. Rambeck B, Kurlemann G, Stodieck SR, May TW, Jurgens U. Concentrations of lamotrigine in a mother on lamotrigine treatment and her newborn child. Eur J Clin Pharmacol 1997; 51(6): 481–484.
2. Tomson T, Ohman I, Vitols S. Lamotrigine in pregnancy and lactation: a case report. Epilepsia 1997; 38(9): 1039–1041.
3. Biddlecombe RA. Analysis of breast milk samples for lamotrigine. Internal document BDCR/93/0011. Glaxo-Wellcome 2004.
4. Ohman I, Vitols S, Tomson T. Lamotrigine in pregnancy: pharmacokinetics during delivery, in the neonate, and during lactation. Epilepsia 2000; 41(6): 709–713.
5. Page-Sharp M, Kristensen JH, Hackett LP, Beran RG, Rampono J, Hale TW, Kohan R, Ilett KF. Transfer of Lamotrigine Into Breast Milk. Ann Pharmacother 2006; 40: 1470–1471.
6. Liporace J, Kao A, D'Abreu A. Concerns regarding lamotrigine and breast-feeding. Epilepsy Behav 2004; 5(1): 102–105.
7. Newport DJ, Pennell PB, Calamaras MR, et al. Lamotrigine in breast milk and nursing infants: determination of exposure. Pediatrics. 2008; 122(1): e223-e231.
8. Barr PA, Buettiker VE, Antony JH. Efficacy of lamotrigine in refractory neonatal seizures. Pediatr Neurol. Feb 1999; 20(2): 161–163.
9. Nordmo E, Aronsen L, Wasland K, Smabrekke L, Vorren S. Severe apnea in an infant exposed to lamotrigine in breast milk. Ann Pharmacother. Nov 2009; 43(11): 1893–1897.
10. Meador KJ, Baker GA, Browning N, Clayton-Smith J, Combs-Cantrell DT, Cohen M, Kalayjian LA, Kanner A, Liporace JD, Pennell PB, Pivitera M, Loring DW. Effects of breastfeeding in children of women taking antiepileptic drugs. Neurology. Nov 30 2010; 75(22): 1954–60.
11. Meador KJ, Baker GA, Browning N, Clayton-Smith J, Combs-Cantrell DT, Cohen M, Kalayjian LA, Kanner A, Liporace JD, Pennell PB, Pivitera M, Loring DW. Cognitive function at 3 years of age after fetal exposure to antiepileptic drugs. N Eng J Med. 2009 Apr 16; 360 (16): 1597–1605.

LANSOPRAZOLE   L3

Trade: Prevacid, Prevpac, Prevacid NapraPak
Other Trades: Zoton, Prevacid
Category: Reduces stomach acid secretion

Lansoprazole is a new proton pump inhibitor that suppresses the release of acid protons from the parietal cells in the stomach, effectively raising the pH of the stomach. Structurally similar to omeprazole, it is very unstable in stomach acid and to a large degree is denatured by acidity of the infant's stomach.[1] A new study shows milk levels of omeprazole are minimal and it is likely milk levels of lansoprazole are small as well. Although there are no studies of lansoprazole in breastfeeding mothers, transfer to milk and its oral absorption (via milk) is likely to be minimal in a breastfed infant. Lansoprazole is secreted in animal milk although no data are available on the amount secreted in human milk. The only likely untoward effects would be reduced stomach acidity. This product has no current pediatric indications although it is occasionally used in severe cases of erosive gastritis.

Prevpac contains Lansoprazole, Amoxicillin, and Clarithromycin. It is primarily indicated for treatment of *Helicobacter Pylori* infections which cause stomach ulcers. Prevacid NapraPAC contains 15 mg lansoprazole and 500 mg naproxen for use in reducing the risk of NSAID-associated gastric ulcers in patients with a history of documented gastric ulcer that require the use of an NSAID for treatment of the signs and symptoms of rheumatoid arthritis, osteoarthritis, and ankylosing spondylitis.

Pregnancy Risk	B	Lactation Risk	L3
T ½	= 1.5 hours	M/P	=
Vd	= 0.5 l/kg	PB	= 97%
Tmax	= 1.7 hours	Oral	= 80% (Enteric only)
MW	= 369	pKa	= 8.85

Adult Concerns: Reduced stomach acidity. Diarrhea, nausea, elevated liver enzymes.

Pediatric Concerns: None reported via milk. It is unlikely to be absorbed while dissolved in milk due to instability in acid.

Drug Interactions: Decreased absorption of ketoconazole, itraconazole, and other drugs dependent on acid for absorption. Theophylline clearance is increased slightly. Reduced lansoprazole absorption when used with sucralfate (30%).

Relative Infant Dose:

Adult Dose: 15–30 mg three times daily.

Alternatives: Omeprazole, famotidine

References:
1.   Pharmaceutical manufacturer prescribing information, 2011.

LAPATINIB   L4

Trade: Tykerb
Other Trades:
Category: Anticancer drug

Lapatinib or lapatinib ditosylate is an orally active drug for the treatment of breast cancer (naive, ER+/EGFR+/HER2+ breast cancer patients) (triple positive) and other solid tumors. It is a dual tyrosine kinase inhibitor.[1,2] It has been approved as front-line therapy in triple positive breast cancer and as an adjuvant therapy when patients have progressed on Herceptin. There are no data available on its use in breastfeeding mothers. Due to its large molecular weight, high volume of distribution and high protein binding, milk levels will probably be exceedingly low once determined. Withhold breastfeeding for at least 120 hours. Discard milk.

Pregnancy Risk	D		Lactation Risk	L4
T ½	= 24 hours		M/P	=
Vd	= 31.4 l/kg		PB	= >99%
Tmax	= 4 hours		Oral	= Poor
MW	= 943		pKa	=

Adult Concerns: Back pain, belching, cracked lips, diarrhea, difficulty with swallowing, dry skin, heartburn, indigestion, nausea, vomiting, pain in the arms or legs, rash, redness, swelling, or painful skin, sleeplessness, sores, ulcers, or white spots on the lips, tongue, or the inside of the mouth, swelling or inflammation of the mouth, tingling of the hands and feet.

Pediatric Concerns:

Drug Interactions: Lapatinib is likely to increase exposure to drugs which are metabolized by CYP3A4 or CYP2C8, if given concurrently with lapatinib. Avoid strong CYP3A4 inhibitors. Avoid strong CYP3A4 inducers.

Relative Infant Dose:

Adult Dose: Varies according to cancer type/treatment.

Alternatives:

References:
1. Pharmaceutical manufacturer prescribing information, 2010.
2. Medina PJ, Goodin S. Lapatinib: a dual inhibitor of human epidermal growth factor receptor tyrosine kinases. Clin Ther. 2008 Aug; 30(8): 1426–47. Review.

LATANOPROST   L3

Trade: Xalatan
Other Trades: Optimol, Xalatan, Betim
Category: Prostaglandin for glaucoma

Latanoprost is a prostaglandin F2-alpha analogue used ophthalmically for the treatment of ocular hypertension and glaucoma. One drop used daily is usually effective.[1] No data are available on the transfer of this product into human milk, but it is unlikely. Prostaglandins are by nature, rapidly metabolized. Plasma levels are barely detectable and then only for 1 hour after use. Combined with the short half-life, minimal plasma levels, and poor oral bioavailability, its transfer into milk is extremely unlikely.

Pregnancy Risk	C	Lactation Risk	L3
T ½	= <30 minutes	M/P	=
Vd	= 0.16 l/kg	PB	=
Tmax	= <1 hour	Oral	= Nil
MW	= 432.59	pKa	= 15.03

Adult Concerns: Ocular irritation, headache, rash, muscle aches, joint pain.

Pediatric Concerns: None reported via milk.

Drug Interactions: Do not mix with eye drops containing thimerosal.

Relative Infant Dose:

Adult Dose: 1 drop in affected eye daily.

Alternatives:

References:
1. Pharmaceutical manufacturer prescribing information, 2011.

LEAD   L5

Trade:
Other Trades:
Category: Environmental pollutant

Lead is an environmental pollutant. It serves no useful purpose in the body and tends to accumulate in the body's bony structures based on their exposure. Due to the rapid development of the nervous system, children are particularly sensitive to elevated levels. Lead apparently transfers into human milk at a rate proportional to maternal blood levels, but the absolute degree of transfer is controversial. Studies of milk lead levels vary enormously and probably reflect the enormous difficulty in accurately measuring lead in milk. In mothers who have previously been exposed to high lead environments, the greatest chance of lead toxicity will be with her first pregnancy. Her blood levels will be highest postpartum because blood lead levels increase during lactation, and her baby's greatest chance of toxicity will be prenatal, because intestinal absorption of lead from milk is low.[1] One study evaluated lead transfer into human milk in a population of women with an average blood lead of 45 µg/dL (considered very high).[2] The average lead level in milk was 2.47 µg/dL. Using these parameters, the average intake in an infant would be 8.1 µg/kg/day. The daily permissible level by WHO is 5.0 µg/kg/day. Using these parameters, mothers contaminated with lead should not breastfeed their infants.

However, in another study of two lactating women whose blood lead levels were 29 and 33 µg/dl, the breastmilk levels were <0.005 µg/mL and <0.010 µg/mL respectively.[3] Although both infants had high lead levels (38 µg/dl and 44 µg/dl), it was probably derived from the environment or inutero. Using this data, breastfeeding would appear to be safe. In a larger study of Shanghai mothers (n=165), the transfer of lead to the fetus was highly correlated with maternal blood lead levels (maternal blood vs. cord= 13.2 µg/dL and 6.9 µg/dL).[4] Lead levels in the cord blood and breastmilk increased with the lead levels in the maternal blood, with coefficient of correlation of 0.714 and 0.353 respectively. The average concentration of lead in breastmilk for 12 occupationally exposed women (lead-exposed jobs) was 52.7 µg/L, which was almost 12 times higher than that for the occupationally non-exposed population (4.43 µg/dL). These results suggest that lead levels in milk could pose a potential health hazard to the breastfed infant but only in those mothers with high plasma lead levels.

In another rather elegant study of milk lead levels, Gulson et.al. collected samples from 21 mothers and 24 infants over a 6 month period.[5] They reported lead concentrations in milk ranging from 0.09–3.1 µg Pb/kg or ppb (mean 0.73 µg/kg) while the blood lead levels were all less than 5 µg/dL with exception of one mother. The major source of lead to the infant during this period was from maternal bone and diet. Nashashibi reports on the transfer of lead from the mother to fetus and into her breastmilk.[6] In a group of 47 women, the mean maternal blood lead concentration was 14.9 µg/dL, while in milk the mean lead level was 2.0 µg/dL. Mean lead level in cord blood was 13.1 µg/dL. These data suggest a close correlation between maternal blood and cord blood lead levels, and maternal blood and milk levels. Lead exposure to military personnel on firing ranges has been questioned. Lead levels in frequent target shooters are known to be elevated as a result of exposure to lead from unjacketed bullets and lead in primers. Breastfeeding mothers should avoid confined, unventilated ranges, but brief exposure to military firing in well-ventilated areas with jacketed bullets is probably safe. Individuals should avoid dust in such areas, sweeping, or cleaning of fire ranges.[7]

In the last decade, the permissible blood level (according to CDC) in children has dropped from 25 to less than 10 µg/dL. Lead poisoning is known to significantly alter IQ and neuropsychologic development, particularly in infants. Therefore, infants receiving breastmilk from mothers with high lead levels should be closely monitored, and both mother and infant may require chelation and the infant transferred to formula. Depending on the choice of chelator, mothers undergoing chelation therapy to remove lead may mobilize significant quantities of lead and should not breastfeed during the treatment period unless the chelator is Succimer.

Pregnancy Risk	Hazardous	Lactation Risk	L5
T ½	= 20–30 years (bone)	M/P	=
Vd	=	PB	=
Tmax	=	Oral	= 5–10%
MW	= 207	pKa	=

Adult Concerns: Constipation, abdominal pain, anemia, anorexia, vomiting, lethargy.

Pediatric Concerns: Pediatric lead poisoning, but appears unlikely via milk. More likely environmental.

Drug Interactions:

Relative Infant Dose:

Adult Dose:

Alternatives:

References:
1. Manton WI, Angle CR, Stanek KL, Kuntzelman D, Reese YR, Kuehnemann TJ. Release of lead from bone in pregnancy and lactation. Environ Res 2003; 92: 139–151.
2. Namihira D, Saldivar L, Pustilnik N, Carreon GJ, Salinas ME. Lead in human blood and milk from nursing women living near a smelter in Mexico City. J Toxicol Environ Health 1993; 38(3): 225–232.
3. Baum C, Shannon M. Lead-Poisoned lactating women have insignificant lead in breast milk. J Clin Toxicol 1995; 33(5): 540–541.
4. Li PJ, Sheng YZ, Wang QY, Gu LY, Wang YL. Transfer of lead via placenta and breast milk in human. Biomed Environ Sci 2000; 13(2): 85–89.
5. Gulson BL, Jameson CW, Mahaffey KR, Mizon KJ, Patison N, Law AJ, Korsch MJ, Salter MA. Relationships of lead in breast milk to lead in blood, urine, and diet of the infant and mother. Environ Health Perspect 1998; 106(10): 667–674.
6. Nashashibi N, Cardamakis E, Bolbos G, Tzingounis V. Investigation of kinetic of lead during pregnancy and lactation. Gynecol Obstet Invest 1999; 48(3): 158–162.
7. Gelberg KH, Depersis R. Lead exposure among target shooters. Arch Environ Occup Health. Summer 2009; 64(2): 115–120.

LEFLUNOMIDE   L4

Trade: Arava

Other Trades: Arava

Category: Antimetabolite anti-inflammatory

Leflunomide is a new anti-inflammatory agent used for arthritis. It is an immunosuppressant that reduces pyrimidine synthesis.[1] Leflunomide is metabolized to the active metabolite referred to as M1, which has a long half-life and slow elimination. This product is a potent immunosuppressant with a potential elevated risk of malignancy and teratogenicity in pregnant women. It is not known if it transfers into human milk, but use of this product while breastfeeding would be highly risky.

Pregnancy Risk	X	Lactation Risk	L4
T ½	= >15–18 hours	M/P	=
Vd	=	PB	=
Tmax	= 6–12 hours	Oral	= 80%
MW	= 270	pKa	= 10.8

Adult Concerns: Hypertension, diarrhea, respiratory infection, alopecia and rash are the most common adult side effects.

Pediatric Concerns: None via milk, but due to the danger of this product, breastfeeding is not recommended.

Drug Interactions: Cholestyramine produces a rapid reduction of plasma levels of the active metabolite. A significant increase in hepatotoxicity when admixed with other hepatotoxic drugs. Increased plasma drug levels (M1) when used with NSAIDs and rifampin May increase plasma free drug levels of tolbutamide.

Relative Infant Dose:

Adult Dose: 20 mg daily.

Alternatives:

References:
1.   Pharmaceutical manufacturer prescribing information, 1999.

LEPIRUDIN   L2

Trade: Refludan

Other Trades: Refludan

Category: Thrombin inhibitor, anticoagulant

Lepirudin is a large molecular weight polypeptide that is a direct inhibitor of thrombin.[1] It is a polypeptide that consists of 65 amino acids and has a molecular weight of 6979 daltons. Lepirudin is a recombinant hirudin. It is very unlikely this large peptide would be transported into human milk after 48 hours postnatally. Most risk would be the first 24–48 hours postnatally, when many proteins can be transported into human milk. However, it is still unlikely this agent would be stable or absorbed in the gastrointestinal tract of an infant.

One study is available on the transfer of lepirudin into breastmilk. A mother experiencing a deep vein thrombosis seven weeks postpartum was given low molecular weight heparins and developed heparin-induced thrombocytopenia. LMWH treatment was stopped and therapy with lepirudin 50 mg twice daily was started. Maternal plasma concentrations of hirudin were 0.5 to 1 mg/L 3 hours after injection. Milk samples 3 hours post-injection contained no detectable levels of hirudin. No untoward effects were noted in the infant who continued to breastfeed.[2] This product would not be orally bioavailable.

Pregnancy Risk	B	Lactation Risk	L2
T ½	= 1.3 hours	M/P	=
Vd	=	PB	=
Tmax	= 3–4 hours	Oral	= Nil
MW	= 6979	pKa	=

Adult Concerns: Hemorrhagic events, bleeding. Bronchospasm, cough, stridor, dyspnea have been reported as common.

Pediatric Concerns: None reported via milk. Levels undetectable.

Drug Interactions: Additive with other anticoagulants such as coumarin, or antithrombotic agents, etc.

Relative Infant Dose:

Adult Dose: 0.15 mg/kg/hour administered continuously.

Alternatives:

References:
1. Pharmaceutical manufacturer Prescribing Information, 2003.
2. Lindhoff-Last E, Willeke A, Thalhammer C, Nowak G, Bauersachs R. Hirudin treatment in a breastfeeding woman. Lancet 2000 Feb 5; 335: 467–68.

LETROZOLE   L4

Trade: Femara
Other Trades: Femara
Category: Aromatase inhibitor of estrogen synthesis

Letrozole is a non-competitive inhibitor of estrogen synthesis, and it is used for the treatment of estrogen-dependent tumors, particularly breast cancer. Letrozole's terminal elimination half-life is about two days and steady-state plasma concentration after daily 2.5 mg dosing is reached in two to six weeks.[1] It has a high volume of distribution and is generally used for long periods. It is well absorbed orally. No data are available on its transfer to human milk but one should expect the levels are low. However, this product works irreversibly and any present in milk could potentially suppress estrogen levels in a breastfed infant. The transfer of small amounts of this agent to an infant could seriously impair bone growth or sexual development of an infant and for this reason it is probably somewhat hazardous to use in a breastfeeding mother. It has a very long half-life which is concerning in a breastfed infant and could lead to higher plasma levels over time. It is not advisable to breastfeed an infant while consuming this product. Discontinue breastfeeding while taking this product or for a period of ten days following its discontinuation.

Pregnancy Risk	D	Lactation Risk	L4
T ½	= 48 hours	M/P	=
Vd	= 1.9 l/kg	PB	= Weak
Tmax	=	Oral	= 90%
MW	= 285	pKa	= 12.37 (pKb)

Adult Concerns: Adverse reactions include fatigue, chest pain, edema, hot flushes, hypertension, nausea, constipation, diarrhea, vomiting, bone pain, back pain, arthralgia, limb pain, dyspnea, cough, and chest wall pain.

Pediatric Concerns: None reported via milk, but this agent is probably too hazardous to use in a breastfeeding woman.

Drug Interactions: Tamoxifen may reduce letrozole plasma levels by 38%.

Relative Infant Dose:

Adult Dose: 2.5 mg daily.

Alternatives:

References:
1. Pharmaceutical manufacturer prescribing information, 2005.

LEUCOVORIN CALCIUM   L3

Trade: Leucovorin

Other Trades:

Category: Nutritive agent, methotrexate rescue

Leucovorin is an active form of folic acid, also known as the Methotrexate rescue drug. Its active component is folinic acid and its active metabolite is 5-methyltetrahydrofolate. The oral administration of leucovorin causes a significant increase in plasma folate activity. This property has been employed in the management of methotrexate toxicity as well as toxicities due to other anti-folates such as pyrimethamine and trimethoprim. Leucovorin is also used for the management of folate-deficient megaloblastic anemia, and in advanced colorectal cancer.[1] Currently there are no studies available on the transfer of leucovorin into human milk. However, considering that leucovorin is basically an active form of folic acid, which is a physiological nutrient, it is highly unlikely that leucovorin should cause any significant harm to the breastfed infant.

Pregnancy Risk	C	Lactation Risk	L3
T ½	= 3.5–5.7 hours (oral), 6.2 hours (IV or IM)	M/P	=
Vd	=	PB	=
Tmax	= 1.72–2.3 hours (oral),52 min (IM), 10 min (IV)	Oral	= 97%
MW	= 511.51	pKa	=

Adult Concerns: Diarrhea, nausea, vomiting, stomatitis, fatigue and hypersensitivity reaction.

Pediatric Concerns:

Drug Interactions: Concurrent use with fluorouracil may enhance the toxicity of fluorouracil and cause severe diarrhea, enterocolitis and even death. Concomitant use may decrease efficacy of anti-epileptics such as phenytoin, phenobarbitone, primidone and precipitate seizures.

Relative Infant Dose:

Adult Dose: Do not exceed 25 mg oral dose.

Alternatives: Folic acid

References:
1. Pharmaceutical manufacturer prescribing information, 2011.

LEUPROLIDE ACETATE   L5

Trade: Lupron, Viadur, Eligard
Other Trades: Lupron, Prostap
Category: Gonadotropin-Releasing Hormone Analog

Leuprolide is a synthetic nonapeptide analog of naturally occurring gonadotropin-releasing hormone with greater potency than the naturally occurring hormone. After initial stimulation, it inhibits gonadotropin release from the pituitary and after sustained use, suppresses ovarian and testicular hormone synthesis (2–4 weeks).[1] Almost complete suppression of estrogen, progesterone, and testosterone result.[2] Although leuprolide is contraindicated in pregnant women, no reported birth defects have been reported in humans. It is commonly used prior to fertilization but should never be used during pregnancy. It is not known whether leuprolide transfers into human milk, but due to its nonapeptide structure, it is not likely that its transfer would be extensive. In addition, animal studies have found that it has zero oral bioavailability; therefore, it is unlikely it would be orally bioavailable in the human infant if ingested via milk. Its effect on lactation is unknown, but it could suppress lactation particularly early postpartum.[3] Leuprolide would reduce estrogen and progestin levels to menopausal ranges, which may or may not suppress lactation, depending on the duration of lactation. Interestingly, several studies show no change in prolactin levels although these were not in lactating women. One study of a hyperprolactinemic patient showed significant suppression of prolactin which is the reason for my L5 risk categorization. It is of no risk to the breastfed infant, only to milk production.

Pregnancy Risk	X	Lactation Risk	L5
T ½	= 3.6 hours	M/P	=
Vd	= 0.52 l/kg	PB	= 43–49%
Tmax	= 4–6 hours	Oral	= Nil
MW	= 1400	pKa	= 9.6

Adult Concerns: Vasomotor hot flashes, gynecomastia, edema, bone pain, thrombosis, and gastrointestinal disturbances, body odor, fever, headache.

Pediatric Concerns: May suppress lactation, particularly early in lactation.

Drug Interactions:

Relative Infant Dose:

Adult Dose: 3.75 mg every month.

Alternatives:

References:
1. Sennello LT, Finley RA, Chu SY, Jagst C, Max D, Rollins DE, Tolman KG. Single-dose pharmacokinetics of leuprolide in humans following intravenous and subcutaneous administration. J Pharm Sci 1986; 75(2): 158–160.
2. Chantilis SJ, Barnett-Hamm C, Byrd WE, Carr BR. The effect of gonadotropin-releasing hormone agonist on thyroid-stimulating hormone and prolactin secretion in adult premenopausal women. Fertil Steril 1995; 64(4): 698–702.
3. Frazier SH. Personnal communication. 1997.

LEVALBUTEROL   L2

Trade: Xopenex

Other Trades:

Category: Bronchodilator

Levalbuterol is the active (R)-enantiomer of the drug substance racemic albuterol. It is a popular and new bronchodilator used in asthmatics.[1] No data are available on breastmilk levels. After inhalation, plasma levels are incredibly low averaging 1.1 ng/mL. It is very unlikely that enough would enter milk to produce clinical effects in an infant. This product is commonly used in infancy for asthma and other bronchoconstrictive illnesses.

Pregnancy Risk	C	Lactation Risk	L2
T ½	= 3.3 hours	M/P	=
Vd	=	PB	=
Tmax	= 0.2 (inhalation)	Oral	= 100%
MW	= 275	pKa	= 9.621

Adult Concerns: Tachycardia, tremors, dizziness, dyspepsia.

Pediatric Concerns: None reported via milk.

Drug Interactions: Levalbuterol effects are reduced when used with beta blockers. Cardiovascular effects are potentiated when used with monoamine oxidase inhibitors, tricyclic antidepressants, amphetamines, and inhaled anesthetics (enflurane).

Relative Infant Dose:

Adult Dose: 0.63 mg every 6–8 hours by nebulization.

Alternatives:

References:
1. Pharmaceutical manufacturer prescribing information, 2010.

LEVETIRACETAM   L3

Trade: Keppra
Other Trades: Keppra
Category: Anticonvulsant

Levetiracetam is a popular broad-spectrum antiepileptic agent. In a study of a single patient who received levetiracetam at 7 days postpartum (dose unreported), the breastmilk concentrations of levetiracetam were 99 µM three hours after administration. The corresponding plasma levels were 32 µM (milk/plasma ratio= 3.09). The mother was also ingesting phenytoin (3 x 100 mg/day) as well as valproic acid (4 x 500 mg/day). The infant was preterm (36 weeks) and unstable at birth. After the addition of levetiracetam at day 7, the infant became increasingly hypotonic and fed poorly. The infant was removed from the breast and 96 hours later the infant's plasma levetiracetam levels were 6 µM. The authors strongly advise avoidance of levetiracetam and close monitoring of the infant in breastfeeding mothers.[1] In this case, the infant was exposed to three anticonvulsants, and it is difficult to suggest that levetiracetam was solely responsible for the hypnotic condition. This is further supported by the study below.

In another study of 8 women receiving from 1500 to 3500 mg/day who were studied at birth (seven patients) and one at 10 months, the mean umbilical cord serum/maternal serum ratio was 1.14 (n= 4) at birth suggesting extensive transport of levetiracetam to the fetus.[2] The mean milk/maternal serum concentration ratio was 1.00 (range, 0.7–1.33) at 3 to 5 days after delivery (n= 7). Maternal milk levels ranged from 28 to 153 µM (4.8–26 µg/mL) but averaged 74 µM (12.6 mg/L). At 3 to 5 days after delivery, the infants had very low levetiracetam serum concentrations (<10–15 µM) (1.7–2.5 µg/mL), a finding that persisted during continued breastfeeding. One infant had a levetiracetam level of 77 uM (13 µg/mL) at day 1, but <10 µM at day 4, suggesting infants clear this product rapidly, and that breastfeeding contributes only a minimal dose. No malformations were detected at birth. No adverse effects were noted in any of the breastfeeding infants. The authors conclude that levetiracetam passes to the infant, but breastfed infants have very low serum concentrations, suggesting a rapid elimination of levetiracetam. Another study of 14 women receiving 1,000 to 3,000 mg per day had a milk-to-plasma ratio of 1.05, with an infant dose of 2.4 mg/kg/day, or 7.9% of the maternal dose. Plasma concentrations in the infants were 13% of those in the mother's plasma, ranging from 4 to 20 µmol/L. There was no evidence of accumulation of levetiracetam in this study. The authors suggest that this study should be reassuring for breastfeeding mothers taking levetiracetam.[3]

Pregnancy Risk	C	Lactation Risk	L3
T ½	= 6–8 hours	M/P	= 1.0
Vd	= 0.7 l/kg	PB	= <10%
Tmax	= 1 hour	Oral	= 100%
MW	= 170	pKa	= <-2

Adult Concerns: Somnolence, weakness, infection, headache, and dizziness.

Pediatric Concerns: None reported in one study of 8 patients.

Drug Interactions: Levetiracetam may significantly increase phenytoin plasma levels by as much as 52%.

Relative Infant Dose: 3.4%–7.8%

Adult Dose: 1000–3000 mg daily.

Alternatives: Gabapentin, lamotrigine

References:

1. Kramer G, Hosli I, et.al. Levetiracetam accumulation in human breast milk. Epilepsia 2002; 43(supplement 7): 105.
2. Johannessen SI, Helde G, Brodtkorb E. Levetiracetam concentrations in serum and in breast milk at birth and during lactation. Epilepsia. 2005; 46: 775–777.
3. Tomson T, Palm R, et.al. Pharmacokinetics of Levetiracetam during Pregnancy, Delivery, in the Neonatal Period, and Lactation. Epilepsia 2007; 48(6): 1111–1116.

LEVMETAMFETAMINE   L3

Trade: Vicks Vapor Inhaler

Other Trades:

Category: Decongestant

Levmetamfetamine is an L-isomer(R-isomer) of methamphetamine, and is used topically as a nasal decongestant.[1] Levmetamfetamine is used as a nasal decongestant for the temporary relief of nasal congestion due to a cold, hay fever, or other upper respiratory allergies. While it produces local vasoconstriction, it has little CNS effects in humans. There are no data on the use of this product in breastfeeding women. Some will probably transfer into human milk, although its oral absorption is probably low and the clinical side effects in an infant are probably minimal.

Pregnancy Risk	Probably Safe	Lactation Risk	L3
T ½	= 9–20 hours	M/P	=
Vd	=	PB	=
Tmax	=	Oral	= Low
MW	= 149.2	pKa	=

Adult Concerns: Dizziness, hypertension, tachycardia, temporary burning, stinging, sneezing, and increased nasal discharge. Increased nasal congestion with prolonged use.

Pediatric Concerns: Observe for tachycardia, and symptoms of sympathetic stimulation.

Drug Interactions:

Relative Infant Dose:

Adult Dose:

Alternatives:

References:

1. Pharmaceutical manufacturer prescribing information, 2010.

LEVOBUNOLOL   L3

Trade: Bunolol
Other Trades: Betagan, Ophtho-Bunolol
Category: Beta blocker for glaucoma

Levobunolol is a typical beta blocker used ophthalmically for treatment of glaucoma.[1] Some absorption has been reported, with resultant bradycardia in patients. No data on transfer to human milk are available. Use with caution.

Pregnancy Risk	C		Lactation Risk	L3
T ½	= 6.1 hours		M/P	=
Vd	= 5.5 l/kg		PB	=
Tmax	= 3 hours		Oral	= Complete
MW	= 291		pKa	= 16.52

Adult Concerns: Bradycardia, hypotension, headache, dizziness, fatigue, lethargy.

Pediatric Concerns: None reported via milk, but transfer of some beta blockers is reported. Observe for lethargy, hypotension, bradycardia, apnea.

Drug Interactions: May have increased toxicity when used with other systemic beta adrenergic blocking agents. May produce bradycardia following use with quinidine and verapamil.

Relative Infant Dose:

Adult Dose: 1–2 drops twice daily.

Alternatives:

References:
1. Pharmaceutical manufacturer prescribing information, 1997.

LEVOCABASTINE   L3

Trade: Livostin
Other Trades: Livostin
Category: Ophthalmic antihistamine for itching

Levocabastine is an antihistamine primarily used via nasal spray and eye drops.[1] It is used for allergic rhinitis and ophthalmic allergies.[1] After application to eye or nose, very low levels are attained in the systemic circulation (<1 ng/mL). In one nursing mother, it was calculated that the daily dose of levocabastine in the infant was about 0.5 µg, far too low to be clinically relevant.

Pregnancy Risk	C		Lactation Risk	L3
T ½	= 33–40 hours		M/P	=
Vd	=		PB	=
Tmax	= 1–2 hours		Oral	= 100%
MW	= 420.52		pKa	=

Adult Concerns: Sedation, dry mouth, fatigue, eye and nasal irritation.

Pediatric Concerns: None reported via milk.

Drug Interactions:

Relative Infant Dose:

Adult Dose: 1 drop four times daily.

Alternatives:

References:
1.   Pharmaceutical manufacturer prescribing information, 1996.

LEVOCARNITINE   L3

Trade: Carnitor, Carnitor SF

Other Trades: Carnitor

Category: Dietary Supplement

Levocarnitine supplements carnitine, a natural metabolic compound that facilitates the transfer of fatty acids into the mitochondria, thus ensuring energy production. A deficiency can be associated with excess acyl CoA esters and disruption of intermediary metabolism.[1] Supplementation has not been studied in nursing mothers but it is not likely hazardous.

Pregnancy Risk	B	Lactation Risk	L3
$T\frac{1}{2}$	= 17.4 hours	M/P	=
Vd	=	PB	= Low
Tmax	= 3.3 hours	Oral	= 10–20%
MW	= 161	pKa	= 13.52

Adult Concerns: Adverse effects include injection site pain, hypotension, diarrhea, hypervolemia, and pharyngitis.

Pediatric Concerns: No data available.

Drug Interactions:

Relative Infant Dose:

Adult Dose: 50 mg/kg every 3 hours.

Alternatives:

References:
1.   Pharmaceutical manufacturer prescribing information, 2005.

LEVOCETIRIZINE   L3

Trade: Xyzal

Other Trades:

Category: Antihistamine

Levocetirizine is a third-generation non-sedating antihistamine. It is the active metabolite (L-enantiomer) of cetirizine.[1] It has twice the binding affinity at the

H_1-receptor compared to cetirizine. No data on the transfer into human milk are available at this time. Just as with cetirizine, it is probably compatible with breastfeeding.

Pregnancy Risk	B	Lactation Risk	L3
T ½	= 8 hours	M/P	=
Vd	= 0.4 l/kg	PB	= 92%
Tmax	= 1 hour	Oral	= Complete
MW	= 389	pKa	=

Adult Concerns: Sedation, fatigue, dry mouth.

Pediatric Concerns: None reported via milk.

Drug Interactions: Increased sedation when administered with alcohol or other sedatives.

Relative Infant Dose:

Adult Dose: 5 mg daily.

Alternatives:

References:
1. Pharmaceutical manufacturer prescribing information, 2010.

LEVODOPA   L4

Trade: Dopar, Larodopa

Other Trades: Kinson, Madopar, Sinemet, Prolopa, Endo Levodopa/Carbidopa, Brocadopa, Eldopa, Weldopa

Category: Antiparkinsonian

Levodopa is a prodrug of dopamine used primarily for parkinsonian symptoms. Its use during pregnancy is extremely dangerous. In one group of 30 patients, levodopa significantly reduced prolactin plasma levels.[1] It could under certain circumstances reduce milk production as well. In a study of one mother with Parkinsonism, peak breast milk levodopa was measured to be 1.6 nmol/mL 3 hours after Sinemet CR $^{50}/_{200}$ at steady state, and returned to baseline after 6 hours. Following administration of immediate release Sinemet, milk concentrations peaked at 3.47 nmol/mL after 3 hours, and returned to baseline in 6 hours. Based on milk concentrations, the infant would have ingested a maximum of 0.023 mg/kg, much less than the dose for a 6-month-old with parkinsonism. No adverse reactions were noted in the breastfed infant, as the ingested amount was sub-therapeutic.[2]

Warning: Levodopa is known to suppress prolactin production in normal, and breastfeeding mothers.[3,4,5] In one group of 6 postpartum women (2–4 days), levodopa suppressed basal serum prolactin levels by as much as 78%.[6]

Pregnancy Risk	C	Lactation Risk	L4
T ½	= 1–3 hours	M/P	=
Vd	=	PB	= <36%
Tmax	= 1–2 hours	Oral	= 41%-70%
MW	= 197	pKa	= 9.69

Adult Concerns: Nausea, vomiting, anorexia, orthostatic hypotension. Reduces prolactin levels and may reduce milk production. Do not use in glaucoma patients with monoamine oxidase inhibitors, asthmatics, peptic ulcer disease, or parkinsonian disease.

Pediatric Concerns: None reported via milk, but reduced prolactin levels may reduce milk production.

Drug Interactions: Monoamine oxidase inhibitors may predispose to hypertensive reactions. Decreased effect when administered with phenytoin, pyridoxine, phenothiazines.

Relative Infant Dose: 1.7%

Adult Dose: 1–2 gm three times daily.

Alternatives:

References:

1. Barbieri C, Ferrari C, Caldara R, Curtarelli G. Growth hormone secretion in hypertensive patients: evidence for a derangement in central adrenergic function. Clin Sci (Lond) 1980; 58(2): 135–138.
2. Thulin PC, Woodward WR, Carter JH, Nutt JG. Levodopa in human breast milk: Clinical implications. Neurology 1998; 50: 1920–1921.
3. Ayalon D, Peyser MR et al. Effect of L-dopa on galactopoiesis and gonadotropin levels in the inappropriate lactation syndrome. Obstet Gynecol. 1974; 44: 159–70.
4. Leblanc H, Yen SS. The effect of L-dopa and chlorpromazine on prolactin and growth hormone secretion in normal women. Am J Obstet Gynecol. 1976; 126: 162–4.
5. Board JA, Fierro RJ et al. Effects of alpha- and beta-adrenergic blocking agents on serum prolactin levels in women with hyperprolactinemia and galactorrhea. Am J Obstet Gynecol. 1977; 127: 285–7.
6. Rao R, Scommegna A, Frohman LA. Integrity of central dopaminergic system in women with postpartum hyperprolactinemia. Am J Obstet Gynecol. 1982; 143: 883–7.

LEVOFLOXACIN   L3

Trade: Levaquin, Quixin

Other Trades: Levaquin

Category: Fluoroquinolone antibiotic

Levofloxacin is a pure (S) enantiomer of the racemic fluoroquinolone ofloxacin. Its kinetics, including milk levels, should be identical to ofloxacin.[1,2] The use of fluoroquinolones is increasing in pediatrics due to minimal toxicity.[3] In one case report of a mother receiving 500 mg/day, the 24 hour average milk level was reported to be approximately 5 µg/mL.[4] A peak level of 8.2 µg/mL was reported, and occurred at 5 hours after the dose. The half-life of levofloxacin in milk was estimated to be 7 hours, which would result in undetectable amounts in milk after 48 hours. The authors report the absolute infant dose would be 1.23 mg/kg/day, although this was calculated from the highest milk level of 8 samples. While the peak levels were reported to be 8.2 µg/mL, the average milk level reported was 5 µg/mL. Using this data, the relative infant dose would range from 10.5% to 17%. However, the time-to-peak interval reported in this case was 5 hours, rather than 1–1.8 hours reported following both oral and IV doses in the prescribing information. Of the 10 reported levels in this study, only 1 was above 5 µg/mL. Thus the reported average level of 5 µg/mL is probably consistent with other data. This suggests a milk/plasma ratio of approximately 0.95 which is probably correct. Thus, levofloxacin concentrations in milk peak around 1–1.8 hours and at levels close to maternal plasma levels. Observe the infant for changes in gut flora, candida overgrowth, or diarrhea.

Pregnancy Risk	C	Lactation Risk	L3
T ½	= 6–8 hours	M/P	= 0.95
Vd	= 1.27 l/kg	PB	= 24–38%
Tmax	= 1–1.8 hours	Oral	= 99%
MW	= 370	pKa	= 6.05, 8.22

Adult Concerns: Nausea, vomiting, diarrhea, abdominal cramps, gastrointestinal bleeding.

Pediatric Concerns: None reported in one case as milk levels are quite low. Observe for changes in gut flora.

Drug Interactions: Decreased absorption with antacids. Quinolones cause increased levels of caffeine, warfarin, cyclosporine, theophylline. Cimetidine, probenecid, azlocillin may increase ofloxacin levels. Increased risk of seizures when used with foscarnet.

Relative Infant Dose: 10.5%–17.2%

Adult Dose: 500 mg daily

Alternatives: Norfloxacin, ofloxacin, ciprofloxacin

References:
1. Pharmaceutical manufacturer prescribing information, 2011
2. McEvoy GE. (ed): AFHS Drug Information. New York, NY: 1997.
3. Ghaffar F, McCracken GH. Quinolones in Pediatrics. In: Hooper DC, Rubinstein E, editors. Quinolone Antimicrobial Agents. Washington, D.C.: ASM Press, 2003: 343–354.
4. Cahill JB, Bailey EM, Chien S, Johnson GM. Levofloxacin Secretion in Breast Milk: A Case Report. Pharmacother 2005; 25(1): 116–118.

LEVONORGESTREL   L3

Trade: Mirena IUD, Next Choice
Other Trades: Triquilar, Levelen, Microlut, Norplant, Microval, Norgeston
Category: Implantable, oral, and intrauterine contraceptive

Levonorgestrel (LNG) is the active progestin in Norplant and Mirena. Norplant is a contraceptive method that involves placing six match-sized, flexible capsules under the skin of a woman's upper arm. These release a low dose of synthetic progestin continuously for up to five years. Mirena is a levonorgestrel-releasing intrauterine (IUD) contraceptive that delivers 20 µg/day of levonorgestrel directly into the uterus and protects against pregnancy for up to 5 full years. The contraceptive effect of Mirena is mainly based on the local effects of levonorgestrel in the uterine cavity.

From several studies, levonorgestrel appears to produce limited, if any, effects on milk volume or quality.[1] One report of 120 women with implants at 5–6 weeks postpartum showed no change in lactation.[2] The level of progestin in the infant is approximately 10% that of maternal circulation. In a study of 9 women who were taking levonorgestrel oral mini pills (30 µg daily) and 10 women who were using the subdermal implants from 4–15 weeks postpartum, no significant differences in infant follicle stimulating hormone (FSH), luteinizing hormone (LH), or testosterone levels in urine were noted when compared to controls.[3] These results suggest that the sexual development of children exposed via milk to trace levels of lenonorgestrel is normal. The plasma concentration of levonorgestrel produced by Mirena are even lower than those produced by LNG contraceptive implants and with oral contraceptives. Because Mirena produces even lower plasma levels of this progestin, it is probably less likely to affect milk production than oral or implantable forms of progestins. In a recent study of 163 and 157 women who received Mirena intrauterine systems, or a Copper T380A intrauterine device respectively, no change in breastfeeding rate, infant growth, or infant development was noted over 12 months in either the LNG-containing insert, or the copper insert.[4] Only approximately 0.1% of the serum dose of LNG has been reported to transfer via milk to infants.[5] Increased endometrial copper concentrations have been noted in a study of 95 breastfeeding mothers with copper intrauterine devices, but no change was noted in the serum or milk copper concentrations.[6] The data from the levonorgestrel-only intrauterine devices suggests minimal to no effect on breastfeeding, but some caution is recommended as I've received numerous accounts of milk suppression following insertion of Mirena IUDs.

Pregnancy Risk	X	Lactation Risk	L3
T ½	= 24 hours	M/P	=
Vd	=	PB	= 97%
Tmax	= 1–2 hours	Oral	= Complete
MW	= 312	pKa	= 19.28

Adult Concerns: Interruption of the menstrual cycle and spotting, with headache, weight gain, and occasional depression.

Pediatric Concerns: None reported via milk. Mirena IUD has been reported to reduce milk supply. Some mothers have reported reduced milk supply with some oral, IUD, and injectable progestin-only contraceptives.

Drug Interactions: Reduced effect of carbamazepine and phenytoin.

Relative Infant Dose:

Adult Dose: Variable

Alternatives:

References:

1. Shaaban MM, Salem HT, Abdullah KA. Influence of levonorgestrel contraceptive implants, NORPLANT, initiated early postpartum upon lactation and infant growth. Contracep 1985; 32(6): 623–635.
2. Shaaban MM. Contraception with progestogens and progesterone during lactation. J Steroid Biochem Mol Biol 1991; 40(4–6): 705–710.
3. Shikary ZK, Betrabet SS, Toddywala WS, Patel DM, Datey S, Saxena BN. Pharmacodynamic effects of levonorgestrel (LNG) administered either orally or subdermally to early postpartum lactating mothers on the urinary levels of follicle stimulating hormone (FSH), luteinizing hormone (LH) and testosterone (T) in their breast-fed male infants. Contracep 1986; 34(4): 403–412.
4. Shaamash AH, Sayed GH, Hussien MM, Shaaban MM. A comparative study of the levonorgestrel-releasing intrauterine system Mirena(R) versus the Copper T380A intrauterine device during lactation: breast-feeding performance, infant growth and infant development. Contracep 2005 Nov; 72(5): 346–51.
5. Haukkamaa M, Holma P. Five year clinical performance of the new formulation of the levonorgestrel releasing intrauterine system and serum levonorgestrel concentration with the new formulation compared to that with the original one. Leiras Clinical Study Report 1996.
6. Rodrigues da Cunha AC, Dorea JG, Cantuaria AA. Intrauterine device and maternal copper metabolism during lactation. Contracep 2001; 63(1): 37–39.

LEVONORGESTREL (Plan B)   L2

Trade: Plan B, Plan B One-Step, Levonelle, NorLevo
Other Trades:
Category: Emergency contraceptive

Levonorgestrel (Plan B) is a progestin that can be used as an emergency contraceptive. It is believed to act by preventing ovulation or fertilization by altering tubal transport of sperm and/or ova.[1] It may as well partially inhibit implantation by altering the endometrium. For more details on detailed monograph on levonorgestrel. Plan B is an emergency contraceptive that can be used to prevent pregnancy following unprotected intercourse or a known or suspected contraceptive failure. It is not effective if the woman is already pregnant, or once the process of implantation has begun. To obtain maximal efficacy, the first tablet should be taken as soon as possible within 72 hours of intercourse. The second tablet should be taken 12 hour later. These agents contain a high dose of levonorgestrel (1.5 mg). In a recent study, 12 exclusively breastfeeding mothers who received a single 1.5 mg dose, levonorgestrel concentrations peaked in plasma and in milk 1–4 hours and 2–4 hours after dosing, respectively.[2] Milk/plasma ratios averaged 0.28. The estimated infant dose of levonorgestrel was only 1.6 μg during the first 24 hours. If the mother interrupts breastfeeding for 8 hours, this dose was reduced to only 1 μg. The authors recommended that to limit exposure, the mother should not breastfeed for the first 8 hours, or at most 24 hours. The amount in milk after 24 hours was only 0.09% of the total dose.

Pregnancy Risk	X		Lactation Risk	L2
T ½	= 11–45		M/P	=
Vd	=		PB	=
Tmax	= 1.6 hours		Oral	= Complete
MW	= 312		pKa	= 19.28

Adult Concerns: Adverse effects include nausea(23%), vomiting(6%), abdominal pain, fatigue, headache, heavier menstrual bleeding, dizziness, breast tenderness.

Pediatric Concerns: None reported via milk, but this progestin is unlikely to bother a breastfed infant or alter milk production in general.

Drug Interactions: Reduced effect of carbamazepine and phenytoin.

Relative Infant Dose:

Adult Dose: 0.75 mg (one tablet) initially following in 12 hours by second tablet.

Alternatives:

References:
1. Pharmaceutical manufacturer prescribing information, 2003.
2. Gainer E, Massai R, Lillo S, Reyes V, Forcelledo ML, Caviedes R, Villarroel C, Bouyer J. Levonorgestrel pharmacokinetics in plasma and milk of lactating women who take 1.5 mg for emergency contraception. Hum Reprod 2007; 22(6): 1578–1584.

LEVOTHYROXINE   L1

Trade: Synthroid, Levothroid, Unithroid, Eltroxin, Levoxyl, Thyroid, Levoxyl
Other Trades: Thyroxine, Oroxine, Eltroxin, Synthroid
Category: Thyroid supplements

Levothyroxine is also called T4. Most studies indicate that minimal levels of maternal thyroid are transferred into human milk, and further, that the amount secreted is extremely low and insufficient to protect a hypothyroid infant even while nursing.[1,2,3] The amount secreted after supplementing a breastfeeding mother is highly controversial and numerous reports conflict. Anderson[4] indicates that levothyroxine is not detectable in breast milk although others using sophisticated assay methods have shown extremely low levels (4 ng/mL). It is generally recognized that some thyroxine will transfer but the amount will be extremely low. It is important to remember that supplementation with levothyroxine is designed to bring the mother to a euthyroid state, which is equivalent to the normal breastfeeding female. Hence, the risk of using exogenous thyroxine is no different than in a normal euthyroid mother. Liothyronine (T3) appears to transfer into milk in higher concentrations than levothyroxine (T4), but liothyronine is seldom used in clinical medicine due to its short half-life (<1 day).[4]

Pregnancy Risk	A	Lactation Risk	L1
T ½	= 6–7 days	M/P	=
Vd	=	PB	= 99%
Tmax	= 2–4 hours	Oral	= 50–80%
MW	= 798	pKa	= 7.43

Adult Concerns: Nervousness, tremor, agitation, weight loss.

Pediatric Concerns: None reported via milk.

Drug Interactions: Phenytoin may decrease levothyroxine levels. Cholestyramine may decrease absorption of levothyroxine. May increase oral hypoglycemic requirements and doses. May increase effects of oral anticoagulants. Use with tricyclic antidepressants may increase toxicity.

Relative Infant Dose:

Adult Dose: 75–125 µg daily

Alternatives:

References:

1.   Mizuta H, Amino N, Ichihara K, Harada T, Nose O, Tanizawa O, Miyai K. Thyroid hormones in human milk and their influence on thyroid function of breast-fed babies. Pediatr Res 1983; 17(6): 468–471.
2.   Oberkotter LV. Thyroid function and human breast milk. Am J Dis Child 1983; 137(11): 1131.
3.   Sack J, Amado O, Lunenfeld B. Thyroxine concentration in human milk. J Clin Endocrinol Metab 1977; 45(1): 171–173.
4.   Anderson PO. Drugs and breast feeding. Semin Perinatol 1979; 3(3): 271–278.

LIDOCAINE   L2

Trade:

Other Trades:

Category: Local anesthetic

Lidocaine is an antiarrhythmic and a local anesthetic. In one study of a breastfeeding mother who received IV lidocaine for ventricular arrhythmias, the mother received approximately 965 mg over 7 hours including the bolus starting doses.[1] At seven hours, breastmilk samples were drawn and the concentration of lidocaine was 0.8 mg/L or 40% of the maternal plasma level (2.0 mg/L). Assuming that the mothers' plasma was maintained at 5 µg/mL (therapeutic=1.5–5 µg/mL), an infant consuming 1 L per day of milk would ingest approximately 2 mg/day. This amount is exceedingly low in view of the fact that the oral bioavailability of lidocaine is very poor (35%). The lidocaine dose recommended for pediatric arrhythmias is 1 mg/kg given as a bolus. Once absorbed by the liver, lidocaine is rapidly metabolized. These authors suggest that a mother could continue to breastfeed while on parenteral lidocaine. Dryden and Lo have reported the transfer of lidocaine following tumescent liposuction in a 80 kg patient.[2] The areas undergoing liposuction were infiltrated with a 52.5 mg/kg dose of lidocaine dissolved in 8400 cc of solution (total= 4200 mg). Milk samples were drawn 17 hours, and plasma levels were drawn 18 hours following the procedure because other studies show lidocaine peaks in the plasma compartment at this time postoperatively. Milk levels of lidocaine were 0.55 mg/L while plasma levels were 1.2 mg/L. Breastmilk levels were 46% of the serum level. The authors conclude that it is unlikely that toxic levels would be reached in a nursing infant. In a study of 27 parturients who received an average of 82.1 mg bupivacaine and 183.3 mg lidocaine via an epidural catheter, lidocaine milk levels at 2, 6, and 12 hours post administration were 0.86, 0.46, and 0.22 mg/L respectively.[3] Levels of bupivacaine in milk at 2, 6, and 12 hours were 0.09, 0.06, 0.04 mg/L respectively. The milk/serum ratio bases upon area under the curve values (AUC) were 1.07 and 0.34 for lidocaine and bupivacaine respectively. Based on AUC data of lidocaine and bupivacaine milk levels, the average milk concentration of these agents over 12 hours was 0.5 and 0.07 mg/L. Most of the infants had a maximal APGAR score. In a study of 7 nursing mothers who received 3.6–7.2 mL of 2% lidocaine without adrenaline, the concentration of lidocaine in milk 3 and 6 hours after injection averaged 97.5 µg/L and 52.7 µg/L respectively.[4] These authors suggest that mothers who receive local injections of lidocaine can safely breastfeed.

When administered as a local anesthetic for dental and other surgical procedures, only small quantities are used, generally less than 40 mg. However, following liposuction, the amount used via instillation in the tissues is quite high. Nevertheless, maternal plasma and milk levels do not seem to approach high concentrations and the oral bioavailability in the infant would be quite low (<35%). The topical application of lidocaine preparations to the nipple is not recommended. Oral doses as low as 100 mg have produced seizures in toddlers. Doses in infants would be much less. Two toddlers developed seizures following a dose of 15 mg/kg of 1% dibucaine ointment. For viscous lidocaine (2%) in infants and children less than 3 years of age, no more than 1.25 mL (equivalent to 25 mg) should be applied topically to the skin every 3 hours. Thus topical use to a mother's nipple is potentially hazardous.

Pregnancy Risk	B	Lactation Risk	L2
T ½	= 1.8 hours	M/P	= 0.4
Vd	= 1.3 l/kg	PB	= 70%
Tmax	= Immediate (IM, IV)	Oral	= <35%
MW	= 234	pKa	= 7.9

Adult Concerns: Bradycardia, confusion, cardiac arrest, drowsiness, seizures, bronchospasm.

Pediatric Concerns: None reported via milk. However, oral doses as low as 100 mg have produced seizures in toddlers. Doses in infants would be much less. Two toddlers developed seizures following a dose of 15 mg/kg of 1% dibucaine ointment. For viscous lidocaine (2%) in infants and children less than 3 years of age, no more than 1.25 mL (25 mg) should be applied topically to the skin every 3 hours. No data on oral use are available.

Drug Interactions: Use of local anesthetics with sulfonamides may reduce antibacterial efficacy.

Relative Infant Dose: 0.5%–3.1%

Adult Dose: 50–100 mg PRN.

Alternatives:

References:
1. Zeisler JA, Gaarder TD, De Mesquita SA. Lidocaine excretion in breast milk. Drug Intell Clin Pharm 1986; 20(9): 691–693.
2. Dryden RM, Lo MW. Breast milk lidocaine levels in tumescent liposuction. Plast Reconstr Surg 2000; 105(6): 2267–2268.
3. Ortega D, Viviand X, Lorec AM, Gamerre M, Martin C, Bruguerolle B. Excretion of lidocaine and bupivacaine in breast milk following epidural anesthesia for cesarean delivery. Acta Anaesthesiol Scand 1999; 43(4): 394–397.
4. Giuliani M, Grossi GB, Pileri M, Lajolo C, Casparrini G. Could local anesthesia while breast-feeding be harmful to infants? J Pediatr Gastroenterol Nutr 2001; 32(2): 142–144.

LINCOMYCIN   L2

Trade: Lincocin
Other Trades: Lincocin
Category: Antibiotic

Lincomycin is an effective antimicrobial used for gram positive and anaerobic infections. It is secreted into breastmilk in small but detectable levels. In a group of 9 mothers who received 500 mg every 6 hours 3 days, breastmilk concentrations ranged from 0.5 to 2.4 mg/L (mean= 1.28). In this same group, the maternal plasma levels averaged 1.37 mg/L.[1] Although effects on infant are unlikely, some modification of gut flora or diarrhea is possible.

Pregnancy Risk	B	Lactation Risk	L2
T ½	= 4.4–6.4 hours	M/P	= 0.9
Vd	=	PB	= 72%
Tmax	= 2–4 hours	Oral	= <30%
MW	= 407	pKa	= 12.97

Adult Concerns: Diarrhea, changes in gastrointestinal flora, colitis, blood dyscrasias, jaundice.

Pediatric Concerns: None reported via milk, but observe for gastrointestinal symptoms such as diarrhea.

Drug Interactions: Gastrointestinal absorption of lincomycin is decreased when used with kaolin-pectin antidiarrheals. The actions of neuromuscular blockers may be enhanced when used with lincomycin.

Relative Infant Dose: 0.7%

Adult Dose: 500 mg every 6–8 hours.

Alternatives: Clindamycin

References:
1. Medina A, Fiske N, Hjelt-Harvey I, Brown CD, Prigot A. Absorption, diffusion, and excretion of a new antibiotic lincomycin. Antimicrob Agents Chemother 1963; 161: 189–196.

LINDANE

| | L4 |

Trade: Kwell, G-well, Scabene

Other Trades: Quellada, Hexit, Kwellada, PMS-Lindane, Desitan

Category: Pediculicide, scabicide

Lindane is an older pesticide also called gamma benzene hexachloride. It is primarily indicated for treatment of pediculus capitis (head lice) and less so for scabies (crab lice).[1,2] Because of its lipophilic nature, it is significantly absorbed through the skin of neonates (up to 13%) and has produced elevated liver enzymes, seizure disorders, and hypersensitivity. It is not recommended for use in neonates or young children. Lindane is transferred into human milk although the exact amounts are unpublished. Estimates by the manufacturer indicate that the total daily dose of an infant ingesting 1 liter of milk daily (30 ng/mL) would be approximately 30 µg/day, an amount that would probably be clinically insignificant. If used in children, lindane should not be left on the skin for more than 6 hours before being washed off as peak plasma levels occur in children at about 6 hours after application. Although there are reports of some resistance, head lice and scabies should generally be treated with permethrin products (NIX, Elimite), which are much safer in pediatric patients.

Pregnancy Risk	B	Lactation Risk	L4
T ½	= 18–21 hours	M/P	=
Vd	=	PB	=
Tmax	= 6 hours	Oral	=
MW	= 290	pKa	=

Adult Concerns: Dermatitis, seizures (excess dose), nervousness, irritability, anxiety, insomnia, dizziness, aplastic anemia, thrombocytopenia, neutropenia.

Pediatric Concerns: Lindane is not recommended for children. Potential CNS toxicity includes lethargy, disorientation, restlessness, and tonic-clonic seizures.

Drug Interactions: Oil based hair dressings may enhance skin absorption.

Relative Infant Dose:

Adult Dose: Topical

Alternatives:

References:
1. Pharmaceutical manufacturer prescribing information, 1996.
2. Drug Facts and Comparisons 1996 ed. ed. St. Louis: 1996.

LINEZOLID   L3

Trade: Zyvox, Zyvoxam, Zyvoxid
Other Trades: Zyvox
Category: Antibiotic

Linezolid is a new oxazolidinone family of antibiotics primarily used for gram positive infections but has some spectrum for gram negative and anaerobic bacteria.[1] It is active against many strains, including resistant *Staphylococcus aureus* (MRSA), *Streptococcus pneumonia*, *Streptococcus pyogenes*, and others. It is indicated for use in patients with vancomycin resistant enterococcus faecium infections, staph aureus pneumonias, resistant *Streptococcus pneumonia* infections, etc. Linezolid was found in the milk of lactating rats at concentrations similar to plasma levels although the dose was not indicated (rat milk levels are always higher than humans). Using this data, with an average maternal plasma concentration of 11.5 µg/mL and a theoretical milk/plasma ratio of 1.0, an infant would ingest approximately 1.7 mg/kg/day following a maternal dose of 1200 mg/day. This amount is likely a high estimate as doses given to animals are extraordinarily high and rodent milk levels are generally many times higher than human milk.

A number of recent studies in children have found linezolid safe. The half-life is shorter in children which requires more frequent dosing. Side effects in children are the same as adults. Observe for changes in gut flora and diarrhea. High-performance liquid chromatography showed that linezolid is present in breastmilk following a single 600 mg dose. The study responsible for this test determined that linezolid reached peak concentrations of 12.36 mg/L at 2 hours after the dose was administrated. These findings in humans are consistent with those observed in animals.[2] Do not use linezolid in patients taking serotonergic agents such as paroxetine or duloxetine (SRRIs) to avoid a potential drug interaction causing a dangerous condition called serotonin syndrome.

Pregnancy Risk	C	Lactation Risk	L3
T½ = 5.2 hours		M/P =	
Vd = 0.71 l/kg		PB = 31%	
Tmax = 1.5–2.2 hours		Oral = 100%	
MW = 337		pKa = 1.7	

Adult Concerns: Thrombocytopenia has been reported in one patient. Observe for diarrhea, sometimes induced by overgrowth of C. difficile (pseudomembranous colitis). Side effects include headache, nausea, tongue discoloration, taste perversion, and vomiting. Note numerous drug-drug interactions.

Pediatric Concerns: None via milk but observe for diarrhea.

Drug Interactions: Linezolid is a reversible, nonselective inhibitor of monoamine oxidase. Therefore, it has the potential for interaction with adrenergic and serotonergic agents. This includes phenylephrine, phenylpropanolamine, pseudoephedrine, dopamine, and epinephrine. Do not use in patients taking serotonergic agents such as paroxetine or duloxetine to avoid a potential drug interaction causing a dangerous condition called serotonin syndrome.

Relative Infant Dose:

Adult Dose: 400–600 mg every 12 hours.

Alternatives: Clindamycin

References:
1. Pharmaceutical manufacturer prescribing information, 2010.
2. Sagirli et al. Determination of Linezolid in Human Breast milk by High-Performance Liquid Chromatography with Ultraviolet Detection. Journal of AOAC International. 2009; 92(6): 1658–1662.

LIOTHYRONINE — L2

Trade: Cytomel
Other Trades: Tertroxin, Cytomel
Category: Thyroid supplement

Liothyronine is also called T3. It is seldom used for thyroid replacement therapy due to its short half-life. It is generally recognized that only minimal levels of thyroid hormones are secreted in human milk although several studies have shown that hypothyroid conditions only became apparent when breastfeeding was discontinued.[1,2] Although some studies indicate that breastfeeding may briefly protect hypothyroid infants, it is apparent that the levels of T4 and T3 are too low to provide long-term protection from hypothyroid disease.[3,4,5,6] Levels of T3 reported in milk vary but, in general, are around 238 ng/dl and considerably higher than T4 levels. The maximum amount of T3 ingested daily by an infant would be 357 ng/kg/day, or approximately ⅒ the minimum requirement. From these studies, it is apparent that only exceedingly low levels of T3 are secreted into human milk and are insufficient to protect an infant from hypothyroidism.

Pregnancy Risk	A	Lactation Risk	L2
T ½	= 25 hours	M/P	=
Vd	=	PB	= Low
Tmax	= 1–2 hours	Oral	= 95%
MW	= 651	pKa	= 8.49

Adult Concerns: Tachycardia, tremor, agitation, hyperthyroidism.

Pediatric Concerns: None reported via milk.

Drug Interactions: Cholestyramine and colestipol may reduce absorption of thyroid hormones. Estrogens may decrease effectiveness of thyroid hormones. The anticoagulant effect of certain medications is increased. Serum digitalis levels are reduced in hyperthyroidism or when the hyperthyroid patient is converted to the euthyroid state. Therapeutic effects of digitalis glycosides may be reduced. A decrease in theophylline clearance can be expected.

Relative Infant Dose:

Adult Dose: 25–75 µg daily.

Alternatives:

References:
1. Bode HH, Vanjonack WJ, Crawford JD. Mitigation of cretinism by breast-feeding. Pediatrics 1978; 62(1): 13–16.
2. Rovet JF. Does breast-feeding protect the hypothyroid infant whose condition is diagnosed by newborn screening? Am J Dis Child 1990; 144(3): 319–323.
3. Varma SK, Collins M, Row A, Haller WS, Varma K. Thyroxine, tri-iodothyronine, and reverse tri-iodothyronine concentrations in human milk. J Pediatr 1978; 93(5): 803–806.
4. Hahn HB, Jr., Spiekerman AM, Otto WR, Hossalla DE. Thyroid function tests in neonates fed human milk. Am J Dis Child 1983; 137(3): 220–222.
5. Letarte J, Guyda H, Dussault JH, Glorieux J. Lack of protective effect of breast-feeding in congenital hypothyroidism: report of 12 cases. Pediatrics 1980; 65(4): 703–705.
6. Franklin R, O'Grady C, Carpenter L. Neonatal thyroid function: comparison between breast-fed and bottle-fed infants. J Pediatr 1985; 106(1): 124–126.

LIRAGLUTIDE   L3

Trade: Victoza

Other Trades:

Category: Antidiabetic, GLP-1 receptor agonist

Liraglutide is an antidiabetic medication that is used along with diet and exercise to improve glycemic control in individuals with type 2 diabetes. It is currently not known if liraglutide is excreted in human breastmilk. In rats, this drug is shown to be excreted in concentrations of approximately 50% that in the maternal plasma. There is a risk of developing thyroid C-cell tumors associated with the use of this medication. Due to a lack of data regarding the use of this drug in lactating women and the tumorigenicity shown for this agent, it is recommended that a decision to either stop breastfeeding or stop this medication should be made. Care should be taken during the first week postpartum due to a possible increased transfer of this drug into the breastmilk.[1] This drug is injected subcutaneously, and would not be orally bioavailable in a breastfed infant.

Pregnancy Risk	C	Lactation Risk	L3
T ½	= 13 hours	M/P	=
Vd	= 0.07 l/kg	PB	= >98%
Tmax	= 8–12 hours	Oral	=
MW	= 3751.2	pKa	=

Adult Concerns: Thyroid C-cell tumor, pancreatitis, hypoglycemia, nausea, diarrhea, vomiting, constipation, upper respiratory tract infection, headache, influenza.

Pediatric Concerns:

Drug Interactions: Digoxin–liraglutide may decrease the metabolism of this drug. Lisinopril–liraglutide may decrease the metabolism of this drug. Atorvastatin–liraglutide may decrease the metabolism of this drug. Acetaminophen–liraglutide may decrease the metabolism of this drug. Griseofulvin–liraglutide may increase the maximum concentration associated with this drug.

Relative Infant Dose:

Adult Dose: 0.6 mg subcutaneous once daily for one week, followed by 1.2 mg subcutaneous once daily.

Alternatives:

References:
1.   Pharmaceutical manufacturer prescribing information, 2010.

LISDEXAMFETAMINE   L3

Trade: Vyvanse
Other Trades:
Category: Stimulant for ADHD

Lisdexamfetamine dimesylate is a prodrug and is rapidly metabolized to dextroamphetamine in the gastrointestinal tract.[1] Dextroamphetamine is a potent and long-acting amphetamine. Following a 20 mg daily dose of racemic amphetamine administered at 10:00, 12:00, 14:00, and 16:00 hours each day (total= 80 mg/day) to a breastfeeding mother, amphetamine concentrations were determined in milk at 10 days and 42 days postpartum. Samples were taken at 20 minutes prior to the 10:00 hour dose and immediately prior to the 14:00 hour dose. Milk levels were 55 and 118 μg/L respectively.[2] Corresponding maternal plasma levels were 20 and 40 ng/mL at the same times. Milk/plasma ratios at these times were 2.8 and 3.0 respectively. At 42 days, breastmilk levels of amphetamine were 68 and 138 μg/L while maternal plasma levels were 9 and 21 ng/mL respectively. Milk/plasma ratios in the 42-day samples were 7.5 and 6.6 respectively. Although the milk/plasma ratios appear high, using a daily milk intake of 150mL/kg/day, the relative infant dose would be only 1.8% of the weight-normalized maternal dose, which probably accounts for the fact that the infant in this study was unaffected. In another study of 4 mothers who received 15–45 mg/day dextroamphetamine, the average absolute infant dose was 21 (11–39) μg/kg/day.[3] The authors suggest the relative infant dose was 5.7% (4–10.6). Plasma levels in the infants ranged from undetectable to 18 μg/L. No untoward effects were noted in any of the 4 infants.

The above data suggest that with normal therapeutic doses, the dose of dextroamphetamine in milk is probably subclinical. However, abusive use of this medication is common. Doses are unknown and sometimes extraordinarily high. Thus mothers should be strongly advised to withhold breastfeeding for 24 hours following the non-clinical use of dextroamphetamine.

Pregnancy Risk	C	Lactation Risk	L3
T ½	= 6.8 hours	M/P	= 2–5.2
Vd	= 3.2–5.6 l/kg	PB	= 16–20%
Tmax	= 3.5 hours	Oral	= 96%
MW	= 455	pKa	=

Adult Concerns: Nervousness, insomnia, anorexia, hyperexcitability.

Pediatric Concerns: Possible insomnia, irritability, anorexia, reduced weight gain, or poor sleeping patterns in infants. However in these studies, none of the infants were affected.

Drug Interactions: May precipitate hypertensive crisis in patients on monoamine oxidase inhibitors and arrhythmias in patients receiving general anesthetics. Increased effect/toxicity with tricyclic antidepressants, phenytoin, phenobarbital, norepinephrine, meperidine.

Relative Infant Dose: 1.8%–6.2%

Adult Dose: 30–70 mg daily

Alternatives: Methylphenidate

References:
1. Pharmaceutical manufacturer prescribing information, 2011.
2. Steiner E, Villen T, Hallberg M, Rane A. Amphetamine secretion in breast milk. Eur J Clin Pharmacol 1984; 27(1): 123–124.
3. Ilett KF, Hackett LP, Kristensen JH, Kohan R. Transfer of dexamphetamine into breast milk during treatment for attention deficit hyperactivity disorder. Br J Clin Pharmacol 2006; 63(3): 371–375.

LISINOPRIL   L3

Trade: Prinivil, Zestril

Other Trades: Prinvil, Prinivil, Zestril, Apo-Lisinopril, Carace

Category: Antihypertensive, ACE inhibitor

Lisinopril is a typical long-acting ACE inhibitor used as an antihypertensive.[1] No breastfeeding data are available on this product. ACE inhibitors in general do not transfer into human milk significantly. They should be used with caution in extremely premature infants due to renal toxicity. Consider enalapril, benazepril, captopril as alternatives.

Pregnancy Risk	C/D during third trimester		Lactation Risk	L3
T ½	= 12 hours		M/P	=
Vd	=		PB	= Low
Tmax	= 7 hours		Oral	= 29%
MW	= 442		pKa	= 3.85

Adult Concerns: Hypotension, headache, cough, gastrointestinal upset, diarrhea, nausea.

Pediatric Concerns: None reported, but observe for hypotension, weakness.

Drug Interactions: Probenecid increases plasma levels of ACE inhibitors. ACE inhibitors and diuretics have additive hypotensive effects. Antacids reduce bioavailability of ACE inhibitors. NSAIDS reduce hypotension of ACE inhibitors. Phenothiazines increase effects of ACE inhibitors. ACE inhibitors increase digoxin and lithium plasma levels. May elevate potassium levels when potassium supplementation is added.

Relative Infant Dose:

Adult Dose: 20–40 mg daily.

Alternatives: Captopril, enalapril

References:
1. McEvoy GE. (ed): AFHS Drug Information. New York, NY: 2003.

LITHIUM CARBONATE   L3

Trade: Lithobid, Eskalith

Other Trades: Lithicarb, Carbolith, Duralith, Lithane, Camcolit, Liskonum, Phasal

Category: Antimanic drug in bipolar disorders

Lithium is a potent antimanic drug used in bipolar disorder. Its use in the first trimester of pregnancy may be associated with a number of birth anomalies, particularly cardiovascular.[1] If used during pregnancy, the dose required is generally elevated due to the increased renal clearance during pregnancy. Soon after delivery, maternal lithium levels should be closely monitored as the mother's renal clearance drops to normal in the next several days. Several cases of lithium toxicity have been reported in newborns.

In a study of a 36-year-old mother who received lithium during and after pregnancy, the infant's serum lithium level was similar to the mothers at birth (maternal dose= 400 mg) but dropped to 0.03 mmol/L by the sixth day.[2] While the mother's dose increased to 800 mg/day postpartum, the infant's serum level did not rise above 10% of the maternal serum levels. At 42 days postpartum, the maternal and infant serum levels were 1.1 and 0.1 mmol/L respectively. Some toxic effects have been reported. In a mother receiving 600–1200 mg lithium daily during pregnancy, the concentration of lithium in breast milk at 3 days was 0.6 mEq/L.[3] The maternal and infant plasma levels were 1.5 mEq/L and 0.6 mEq/L respectively at 3 days. In this case the infant was floppy, unresponsive and exhibited inverted T waves which are indicative of lithium toxicity. In another study done 7 days postpartum, the milk and infant plasma levels were 0.3 mEq/L each, while the mother's plasma lithium levels were 0.9 mEq/L.[4] In a case report of a mother receiving 300 mg three times daily and breastfeeding her infant at two weeks postpartum, the mother and infant's lithium levels were 0.62 and 0.31 mmol/L respectively. The infant's neurobehavioral development and thyroid function were reported normal.[5] In a group of 11 breastfeeding mothers who received from 600 to 1500 mg/day of lithium, the authors found wide interpatient variability in lithium dose offered to the infant through breast milk which ranged from 0% to 30% of maternal weight-adjusted dose.[6]

From these studies it is apparent that lithium can permeate milk and is absorbed by the breastfed infant. If the infant continues to breastfeed, it is strongly suggested that the infant be closely monitored for serum lithium levels, and BUN/creatinine after 6 weeks or so. Levels drawn too early (7 days) may only reflect in utero exposure. Lithium does not reach steady state levels for approximately 10+ days. Clinicians may wish to wait at least this long prior to evaluating the infant's serum lithium level, or sooner if symptoms occur. In addition, lithium is known to reduce thyroxine production, and periodic thyroid evaluation should be considered. Because hydration status of the infant can alter lithium levels dramatically, the clinician should observe changes in hydration carefully. A number of studies of lithium suggest that lithium administration is not an absolute contraindication to breastfeeding, if the physician monitors the infant closely for elevated plasma lithium.[7] Current studies, as well as unpublished experience, suggest that the infant's plasma levels rise to about 30–40% of the maternal level, most often without untoward effects in the infant. Recent evidence suggests that certain anticonvulsants such as carbamazepine, valproic acid, lamotrigine, and others may be as effective as lithium in treating some forms of mania. Because these medications are probably safer to use in breastfeeding mothers, the clinician may wish to explore the use of these medications in certain breastfeeding mothers suffering from bipolar symptoms.[8]

Pregnancy Risk	D	Lactation Risk	L3 with close observation
T ½	= 17–24 hours	M/P	= 0.24–0.66
Vd	= 0.7–1.0	PB	=
Tmax	= 2–4 hours	Oral	= Complete
MW	= 74	pKa	=

Adult Concerns: Nausea, vomiting, diarrhea, frequent urination, tremor, drowsiness.

Pediatric Concerns: In one study cyanosis, T-wave abnormalities, and decreased muscle tone were reported. Other studies report no side effects. Evaluate infant lithium levels along with mothers.

Drug Interactions: Decreased lithium effect with theophylline and caffeine. Increased toxicity with alfentanil. Thiazide diuretics reduce clearance and increase toxicity. NSAIDS, haloperidol, phenothiazines, fluoxetine and ACE inhibitors may increase toxicity.

Relative Infant Dose: 12%–30.1%

Adult Dose: 600 mg three times daily.

Alternatives: Valproic acid, carbamazepine

References:

1. Schou M. Lithium treatment during pregnancy, delivery, and lactation: an update. J Clin Psychiatry 1990; 51(10): 410–413.
2. Sykes PA, Quarrie J, Alexander FW. Lithium carbonate and breast-feeding. Br Med J 1976; 2(6047): 1299.
3. Tunnessen WW, Jr., Hertz CG. Toxic effects of lithium in newborn infants: a commentary. J Pediatr 1972; 81(4): 804–807.
4. Fries H. Lithium in pregnancy. Lancet 1970; 1(7658): 1233.
5. Montgomery A. Use of lithium for treatment of bipolar disorder during pregnancy and lactation. Academy of breastfeeding Medicine News and Views 1997; 3(1): 4–5.
6. Moretti ME, Koren G, Verjee Z, Ito S. Monitoring lithium in breast milk: an individualized approach for breast-feeding mothers. Ther Drug Monit. 2003 Jun; 25(3): 364–6. Review.
7. Viguera AC, Newport, DJ, Ritchie J, Stowe Z, Whitfield T, Mogielnicki J, Baldessarini RJ, Zurick A, Cohen LS. Lithium in breast milk and nursing infants: clinical implications. Am J Psychiatry 2007; 164(2): 342–345.
8. Llewellyn A, Stowe ZN, Strader JR, Jr. The use of lithium and management of women with bipolar disorder during pregnancy and lactation. J Clin Psychiatry 1998; 59 Suppl 6: 57–64.

LOMEFLOXACIN   L3

Trade: Maxaquin
Other Trades: Okacyn
Category: Fluoroquinolone antibiotic

Lomefloxacin belongs the fluoroquinolone family of antimicrobials.[1] The fluoroquinolones in general are becoming increasingly popular in pediatric-aged patients due to the introduction of recent studies.[2] In addition, the FDA is reviewing several pediatric indications for this group. At least one case of bloody colitis (pseudomembranous colitis) has been reported in a breastfeeding infant whose mother ingested ciprofloxacin. It is reported that lomefloxacin is excreted in the milk of lactating animals although levels are low. Use with caution.

Pregnancy Risk	C	Lactation Risk	L3
T ½	= 8 hours	M/P	=
Vd	= 2 l/kg	PB	= 20.6%
Tmax	= 0.7–2.0 hours	Oral	= 92%
MW	= 351	pKa	= 6.75

Adult Concerns: Gastrointestinal distress, diarrhea, colitis, headaches, phototoxicity.

Pediatric Concerns: None reported with this drug. Pseudomembranous colitis has been reported with another member of this family. Observe closely for bloody diarrhea.

Drug Interactions: Antacids, iron salts, sucralfate, and zinc salts may interfere with the gastrointestinal absorption of the fluoroquinolones resulting in decreased serum levels. Cimetidine may interfere with the elimination of the fluoroquinolones. Nitrofurantoin may interfere with the antibacterial properties of the fluoroquinolone family. Probenecid may reduce renal clearance as much as 50%. Nephrotoxic side effects of cyclosporine may be significantly increased when used with fluoroquinolones. Phenytoin serum levels may be reduced producing a decrease in therapeutic effects. Anticoagulant effects may be increased when used with fluoroquinolones. Decreased clearance and increased plasma levels and toxicity of theophylline have been reported with the use of the fluoroquinolones.

Relative Infant Dose:

Adult Dose: 400 mg daily.

Alternatives: Norfloxacin, ofloxacin, trovafloxacin

References:
1. Pharmaceutical manufacturer prescribing information, 1996.
2. Ghaffar F, McCracken GH. Quinolones in Pediatrics. In: Hooper DC, Rubinstein E, editors. Quinolone Antimicrobial Agents. Washington, D.C.: ASM Press, 2003: 343–354.

LOPERAMIDE   L2

Trade:
Other Trades:
Category: Antidiarrheal drug

Loperamide is an antidiarrheal drug. Because it is minimally absorbed orally (0.3%), only extremely small amounts are secreted into breast milk. Following a 4 mg oral dose twice daily in 6 women (early postpartum), milk levels at 12 hours following dose averaged 0.18 µg/L, and 6 hours after the second dose were 0.27 µg/L.[1] A breastfeeding infant consuming 165 mL/kg/day of milk would ingest 2000 times less than the recommended daily dose. It is very unlikely these reported levels in milk (Relative infant dose=0.03%) would ever produce clinical effects in a breastfed infant.

Pregnancy Risk	B	Lactation Risk	L2
T ½	= 10.8 hours	M/P	= 0.5–0.36
Vd	=	PB	=
Tmax	= 4–5 hours (capsules)	Oral	= 0.3%
MW	= 477	pKa	= 8.6

Adult Concerns: Fatigue, dry mouth, respiratory depression, dry mouth, and constipation.

Pediatric Concerns: One case of mild delirium has been reported in a 4-year-old infant.

Drug Interactions: CNS depressants, phenothiazines, and tricyclic antidepressants may potentiate adverse effects.

Relative Infant Dose: 0.03%

Adult Dose: 4 mg PRN

Alternatives:

References:
1. Nikodem VC, Hofmeyr GJ. Secretion of the antidiarrhoeal agent loperamide oxide in breast milk. Eur J Clin Pharmacol 1992; 42(6): 695–696.

LOPINAVIR   L3

Trade:
Other Trades:
Category: Protease inhibitor

Lopinavir is used for treatment of HIV infection in combination with other antiretroviral agents.[1] The Centers for Disease Control and Prevention recommend that HIV-1 infected mothers not breastfeed their infants to avoid risking postnatal transmission of HIV-1. Studies in rats have demonstrated that lopinavir is secreted in milk. It is not known whether lopinavir is secreted in human milk. Because of both the potential for HIV-1 transmission and the potential for serious adverse reactions in nursing infants, mothers should be instructed not to breastfeed if they are receiving lopinavir in combination with ritonavir. Nevertheless, this drug can be used in infants down to the age of 6 months. NOTE: the oral liquid should not be used in premature babies or until 14 days after their due date, as they are unable to metabolize the propylene glycol and alcohol in the liquid preparation.

Pregnancy Risk	Probably Safe	Lactation Risk	L3
T ½	=	M/P	=
Vd	=	PB	= 98–99%
Tmax	= 2–6 hours	Oral	= poor
MW	= 629	pKa	= 13.98

Adult Concerns: Side effects of lopinavir (formulated with ritonavir) are diarrhea, pancreatitis, hepatotoxicity, headache, insomnia, and rash.

Pediatric Concerns: May be used directly in infants at age 6 months. NOTE: the oral liquid should not be used in premature babies or until 14 days after their due date, as they are unable to metabolize the propylene glycol and alcohol in the preparation.

Drug Interactions:

Relative Infant Dose:

Adult Dose: 400 mg twice daily.

Alternatives:

References:
1.   McEvoy GE. (ed): AFHS Drug Information. New York, NY: 2003.

LOPINAVIR + RITONAVIR   L3

Trade: Kaletra

Other Trades:

Category: Antiviral combination

Lopinavir + Ritonavir combined drug product is used for treatment of HIV infection in combination with other antiretroviral agents.[1] The Centers for Disease Control and Prevention (CDC) recommends that HIV-1 infected mothers not breastfeed their infants to avoid risking postnatal transmission of HIV-1. Studies in rats have demonstrated that lopinavir is secreted in milk. It is not known whether lopinavir is secreted in human milk. There are no data available on the transfer of ritonavir in breastmilk. Because of both the potential for HIV-1 transmission and the potential for serious adverse reactions in nursing infants, mothers should be instructed not to breastfeed if they are receiving lopinavir in combination with ritonavir. Nevertheless, this drug can be used in infants down to the age of 6 months. NOTE: the oral liquid should not be used in premature babies or until 14 days after their due date, as they are unable to metabolize the propylene glycol and alcohol in the liquid preparation.

Pregnancy Risk	C	Lactation Risk	L3
T ½	= 3–5 hours	M/P	=
Vd	= Lopinavir/ritonavir: 0.92–1.86/0.16–0.56 l/kg	PB	= 98%-99%
Tmax	= Lopinavir/ritonavir: 2–6 hours/2–4 hours	Oral	= Lopinavir/ritonavir: Low/80%
MW	= Lopinavir/ritonavir: 629/721	pKa	= Lopinavir/ritonavir: 13.98/

Adult Concerns: Side effects of lopinavir (formulated with ritonavir) are diarrhea, pancreatitis, hepatotoxicity, headache, insomnia, and rash.

Pediatric Concerns: May be used directly in infants at age 6 months. NOTE: the oral liquid should not be used in premature babies or until 14 days after their due date, as they are unable to metabolize the propylene glycol and alcohol in the preparation.

Drug Interactions: Numerous drug-drug interactions are known. Antihistamines (astemizole and terfenadine), ergot derivatives (dihydroergotamine, ergometrine, ergotamine, and methylergometrine), gastrointestinal prokinetics (cisapride), antipsychotics (pimozide), sedatives and hypnotics (midazolam and triazolam), and statins (simvastatin and lovastatin). Rifampicin and St. John's wort decrease the concentration of lopinavir; use with the antiretroviral is not recommended due to the possible loss of its activity and development of resistance.

Relative Infant Dose:

Adult Dose: Lopinavir/ritonavir: 400/100 mg (two 200/50 mg tablets or 5 mL oral solution) twice daily.

Alternatives:

References:
1. Pharmaceutical manufacturer prescribing information, 2010.

LORACARBEF   L3

Trade: Lorabid

Other Trades:

Category: Synthetic penicillin-like antibiotic

Loracarbef is a synthetic beta-lactam antibiotic. It is structurally similar to the cephalosporin family.[1] It is used for gram negative and gram positive infections. Pediatric indications are available for infants 6 months of age and children up to 12 years of age. No data are available on levels in breastmilk. Since so little is known about this drug, consider alternative cephalosporins.

Pregnancy Risk	B	Lactation Risk	L3
T ½	= 1 hour	M/P	=
Vd	=	PB	= 25%
Tmax	= 1.2 hours	Oral	= 90%
MW	=	pKa	= 11.45

Adult Concerns: Nausea, vomiting, diarrhea, allergic rashes.

Pediatric Concerns: None reported. Observe for gastrointestinal changes such as diarrhea.

Drug Interactions: Probenecid may increase levels of cephalosporins by reducing renal clearance.

Relative Infant Dose:

Adult Dose: 200–400 mg twice daily.

Alternatives:

References:
1. Pharmaceutical manufacturer prescribing information, 1995.

LORATADINE   L1

Trade: Alavert, Claritin, Clearatadine, Triaminic Allerchews, Children's Dimetapp ND Allergy

Other Trades:

Category: Long-acting antihistamine

Loratadine is a long-acting antihistamine with minimal sedative properties. Following 40 mg oral dose, the peak maternal plasma concentrations of loratadine and its metabolite descaboethoxyloratidine were 30.5 ng/mL and 18.6 ng/mL respectively.[1] This produced peak milk concentrations of 29.2 ng/mL and 16 ng/mL of loratadine and its metabolite respectively. Therefore the total peak milk concentrations of loratadine and its metabolite following a 40 mg maternal dose is 45.2 ng/mL. Over 48 hours, the amount of loratadine transferred via milk was 4.2 µg, which was 0.01% of the administered dose.[1] Through 48 hours, only 6.0 µg of descarboethoxyloratadine (metabolite) (7.5 µg loratadine equivalents) were excreted into breast milk. This amounts to a total of 11.7 µg or 0.029% of the administered dose of loratadine and its active metabolite were transferred via milk to the infant over 48 hours. According to the authors, a 4 kg infant would receive only 0.46% of loratadine or its metabolite on a mg/kg basis (2.9 µg/kg/day). It is very unlikely this dose would present a hazard to infants. Loratadine does not transfer into the CNS of adults, so it is unlikely to induce sedation even in infants. The half-life in neonates is not known although it is likely quite long. Pediatric formulations are available.

Pregnancy Risk	B	Lactation Risk	L1
T ½	= 8.4–28 hours	M/P	= 1.17
Vd	=	PB	= 97%
Tmax	= 1.5 hours	Oral	= Complete
MW	= 383	pKa	= 5

Adult Concerns: Sedation, dry mouth, fatigue, nausea, tachycardia, palpitations.

Pediatric Concerns: None reported, but observe for sedation, dry mouth, tachycardia.

Drug Interactions: Increased plasma levels of loratadine may result when used with ketoconazole, the macrolide antibiotics, and other products.

Relative Infant Dose: 0.3%–1.2%

Adult Dose: 10 mg daily.

Alternatives: Cetirizine

References:
1. Hilbert J, Radwanski E, Affrime MB, Perentesis G, Symchowicz S, Zampaglione N. Excretion of loratadine in human breast milk. J Clin Pharmacol 1988; 28(3): 234–239.

LORAZEPAM   L3

Trade: Ativan

Other Trades: Apo-Lorazepam, Ativan, Novo-Lorazepam, Almazine

Category: Antianxiety, sedative drug

Lorazepam is a typical benzodiazepine similar to diazepam (valium), but with a much shorter half-life. It is frequently used prenatally and pre-surgically as a sedative agent. In one prenatal study, it has been found to produce a high rate of respiratory depression, hypothermia, and feeding problems in newborns.[1] Newborns were found to secrete lorazepam for up to 11 days postpartum. In McBrides's study[2], the infants were unaffected following the prenatal use of 2.5 mg IV prior to delivery. Plasma levels of lorazepam in infants were equivalent to those of the mothers. The rate of metabolism in mother and infant appears slow but equal following delivery. In this study there were no untoward effects noted in any of the infants.

In one breastfeeding patient receiving 2.5 mg twice daily for 5 days postpartum, the breastmilk levels were 12 µg/L.[3] In another patient four hours after an oral dose of 3.5 mg, milk levels averaged 8.5 µg/L which is an RID of only 2.6%.[4] Summerfield reports an average concentration in milk of 9 µg/L and an average milk/plasma ratio of 0.22.[4] It would appear from these studies that the amount of lorazepam secreted into milk would be clinically insignificant under most conditions.

The benzodiazepine family, as a rule, is not ideal for breastfeeding mothers due to relatively long half-lives and the development of dependence. However, it is apparent that the shorter-acting benzodiazepines are safer during lactation provided their use is short-term or intermittent, low dose, and after the first week of life.[5]

Pregnancy Risk	D	Lactation Risk	L3
T ½	= 12 hours	M/P	= 0.15–0.26
Vd	= 0.9–1.3 l/kg	PB	= 85%
Tmax	= 2 hours	Oral	= 90%
MW	= 321	pKa	= 1.3, 11.5

Adult Concerns: Sedation, agitation, respiratory depression, withdrawal syndrome.

Pediatric Concerns: None reported via milk, but observe for sedation.

Drug Interactions: Increased sedation when used with morphine, alcohol, CNS depressants, monoamine oxidase inhibitors, loxapine, and tricyclic antidepressants.

Relative Infant Dose: 2.6%–2.9%

Adult Dose: 1–3 mg two-three times daily.

Alternatives: Midazolam

References:
1. Johnstone M. Effect of maternal lorazepam on the neonate. Br Med J (Clin Res Ed) 1981; 282(6280): 1973-1974.
2. McBride RJ, Dundee JW, Moore J, Toner W, Howard PJ. A study of the plasma concentrations of lorazepam in mother and neonate. Br J Anaesth 1979; 51(10): 971–978.
3. Whitelaw AG, Cummings AJ, McFadyen IR. Effect of maternal lorazepam on the neonate. Br Med J (Clin Res Ed) 1981; 282(6270): 1106–1108.
4. Summerfield RJ, Nielsen MS. Excretion of lorazepam into breast milk. Br J Anaesth 1985; 57(10): 1042–1043.
5. Maitra R, Menkes DB. Psychotropic drugs and lactation. N Z Med J 1996; 109(1024): 217–218.

LORMETAZEPAM   L3

Trade:

Other Trades: Lembrol, Noctamid, Loramet, Ergocalm

Category: Hypnotic sedative

Lormetazepam is a benzodiazepine available in the UK. It binds to the benzodiazepine receptor and enhances the GABA-a receptor. In one study of 5 breastfeeding women, delivered by cesarean section, taking 2 mg every evening for 10 days, levels of lormetazepam were below the limits of detection (below 0.2 ng/mL), except in a few milk samples.[1] At 12 and 24 h after administration, the plasma level of lormetazepam was about 3.5 ng/mL and 1.8 ng/mL in mothers, and below 0.09 ng/mL in the breastfed infants. Levels of the metabolite, Lormetazepam, were below 0.2 ng/ml. The plasma level of glucuronide varied between 24 ng/mL at 12 hours and 11 ng/mL 24 hours after administration. The milk/plasma ratio of lormetazepam was estimated to be below 0.06. The authors estimate the quantity of free and conjugated active ingredient transferred to the children via breast milk was at most 100 ng/mg, corresponding to 0.35% of the maternal dose. No free lormetazepam was found in the infants' plasma, nor were any adverse side effects noted in these infants.

Pregnancy Risk	D	Lactation Risk	L3
T ½	= 10–12 hours	M/P	= 0.06
Vd	=	PB	=
Tmax	=	Oral	= 80%
MW	= 335.2	pKa	=

Adult Concerns: Side effects are similar to other benzodiazepines and include drowsiness and sedation.

Pediatric Concerns: Milk levels are extremely low. No untoward side effects were reported in this study.

Drug Interactions: Additive respiratory depression manifested with breathing difficulty, profound sedation and coma may occur when coadministered with other sedatives/hypnotics such as phenobarbital, phenytoin, carbamazepine, alprazolam; or when administered with opiates such as morphine, codeine, hydromorphone, hydrocodone, oxycodone, fentanyl. Severe CNS depression may occur when coadministered with some herbal products such as kava, magnolia, passionflower, skull cap, tan-shen.

Relative Infant Dose: 0.4%

Adult Dose: 1mg every evening.

Alternatives: Midazolam, alprazolam

References:
1. Humpel M, Stoppelli I, Milia S, Rainer E. Pharmacokinetics and Biotransformation of the New Benzodiazepine, Lormetazepam, in Man. Eur J Clin Pharmacol 1982; 21: 421–425.

LOSARTAN   L3

Trade: Cozaar
Other Trades: Cozaar
Category: ACE-like antihypertensive

Losartan is an angiotensin II receptor blocker (ARB) used in the management of hypertension. This medication acts by selectively binding to the angiotensin II type-1 (AT1) receptors, thus preventing the attachment of angiotensin II and inhibiting the renin-angiotensin-aldosterone system (RAAS).[1,2] No data are available on its transfer to human milk. Although it penetrates the CNS significantly, its high protein binding would probably reduce its ability to enter milk significantly. This product is only intended for those few individuals who cannot tolerate ACE inhibitors.

Pregnancy Risk	C/D in 2nd and 3rd trimester	Lactation Risk	L3
T ½	= 4–9 hours	M/P	=
Vd	= 12 l/kg	PB	= 99.8%
Tmax	= 1 hour	Oral	= 25–33%
MW	=	pKa	= 14.27

Adult Concerns: Dizziness, insomnia, hypotension, anxiety, ataxia, confusion, depression. Cough or angioedema, commonly associated with ACE inhibitors does not apparently occur with losartan.

Pediatric Concerns: None reported.

Drug Interactions: Decreased effect when used with phenobarbital, ketoconazole, troleandomycin, sulfaphenazole. Increased effect when used with cimetidine, moxonidine.

Relative Infant Dose:

Adult Dose: 25–50 mg one–two times daily.

Alternatives: Captopril, enalapril

References:
1. Lacy C. Drug information handbook. Lexi-Comp Inc. Cleveland, OH, 1996.
2. Pharmaceutical manufacturer prescribing information, 1997.

LOTEPREDNOL   L3

Trade: Lotemax, Alrex

Other Trades:

Category: ophthalmic corticosteroid

Loteprednol is a corticosteroid used ophthalmically to decrease inflammation due to allergy or other inflammatory conditions. The preparation comes in 0.2% and 0.5% concentrations. The drug is mainly metabolized in the cornea. Metabolites include PJ-91, the primary metabolite, delta-1 cortienic acid etabonate, and 17-beta carboxylic acid derivative, which is inactive. Renal excretion is nil. Side effects with prolonged use include cataracts, decreased visual function, increased intra-ocular pressure, and secondary infections of the eye. No reports have been located on use during lactation.[1,2] In general, steroids, particularly ophthalmically administered steroids, would virtually never enter milk is clinically relevant amounts.

Pregnancy Risk	C	Lactation Risk	L3
T ½	= 2.8 hours	M/P	=
Vd	=	PB	= 95%
Tmax	=	Oral	= Minimal
MW	= 467.0	pKa	=

Adult Concerns: Dry eyes, blurred vision, itching, eye irritation, cataract, headache, rhinitis, increase in intraocular pressure.

Pediatric Concerns:

Drug Interactions:

Relative Infant Dose:

Adult Dose: One drop in affected eye 4 times daily.

Alternatives:

References:

1. Pharmaceutical manufacturer prescribing information, Bausch and Lomb, Inc. 2010.
2. Howes J, Novack GD. Failure to detect systemic levels, and effects of loteprednol etabonate and its metabolite, PJ-91, following chronic ocular administration. J Ocul Pharmacol Ther 1998; 14: 153–8.

LOTEPREDNOL + TOBRAMYCIN   L3

Trade: Zylet

Other Trades:

Category: Antibiotic / corticosteroid

Loteprednol etabonate and Tobramycin is a combined drug product of an antibiotic (tobramycin) with a corticosteroid (loteprednol). It is indicated for use in infections of the eye.[1] There are currently no data on the transfer of this combined drug product into breastmilk.

Loteprednol is a corticosteroid used in the eye to decrease inflammation due to allergy or other inflammatory conditions. The preparation comes in 0.2% and 0.5% concentrations. The drug is mainly metabolized in the cornea. Metabolites include PJ-91, the primary metabolite, delta-1 cortienic acid etabonate, and 17-beta carboxylic acid derivative, which is inactive. Renal excretion is 0%. Side effects with prolonged use include cataracts, decreased visual function, increased intra-ocular pressure, and secondary infections of the eye. No reports have been located on use during lactation.[2,3] In general, steroids, particularly ophthalmically administered steroids, enter milk is minimal amounts.

Tobramycin is an aminoglycoside antibiotic similar to gentamicin.[4] Although small levels of tobramycin are known to transfer into milk, they probably pose few problems. In one study of 5 patients, following an 80 mg IM dose, tobramycin levels in milk ranged from undetectable to 0.5 mg/L in only one patient.[5] In a case report of a mother receiving 150 mg three times daily for 14 days (IV), milk concentrations were determined on day four, before administration, and 60, 120, 180, 240, and 300 minutes after dosing. Tobramycin was undetectable in all samples. The limit of detection was >0.18 mg/L. No untoward effects were noted in the infant.[6] In another study of one mother who received 80 mg every 8 hours (IM), milk levels ranged from 0.6 mg/L at 1 hour to 0.58 mg/L at 8 hours post dose.[7] Levels in milk are generally low, but could produce minor changes in gut flora. As oral tobramycin is not absorbed orally, systemic levels in infant would be unexpected. The relative infant dose for tobramycin is 2.6%.

Administered ophthalmically, it is highly unlikely that either loteprednol or tobramycin would attain significant systemic levels. Therefore, amounts that enter the milk are probably minimal. Loteprednol + tobramycin eye drops are probably compatible with breastfeeding.

Pregnancy Risk	C	Lactation Risk	L3
T ½	= Loteprednol/tobramycin: 2.8 hours/2–3 hours	M/P	=
Vd	= Loteprednol/tobramycin: /0.22–0.31 l/kg	PB	= Loteprednol/tobramycin: 95%/<5%
Tmax	= Loteprednol/tobramycin: /30–90 min	Oral	= Loteprednol/tobramycin: Minimal/nil
MW	= Loteprednol/tobramycin: 467/468	pKa	= Loteprednol/tobramycin: 18.88/13.13

Adult Concerns: Headache, burning and stinging in the eye after application, glaucoma.

Pediatric Concerns: No adverse effects reported.

Drug Interactions:

Relative Infant Dose:

Adult Dose: One drop every 4–6 hours.

Alternatives:

References:

1. Pharmaceutical manufacturer prescribing information, 2011.
2. Pharmaceutical manufacturer prescribing information, Bausch and Lomb, Inc. 2010.
3. Howes J, Novack GD. Failure to detect systemic levels, and effects of loteprednol etabonate and its metabolite, PJ-91, following chronic ocular administration. J Ocul Pharmacol Ther 1998; 14: 153–8.
4. Pharmaceutical manufacturer prescribing information, 1996.
5. Takase Z. Laboratory and clinical studies on tobramycin in the field of obstetrics and gynecology. Chemotherapy (Tokyo) 1975; 23: 1402.
6. Festini F, Ciuti R, Taccetti G, Repetto T, Campana S, Martino M. Breast feeding in a woman with cystic fibrosis undergoing antibiotic intravenous treatment. J Matern Fetal Neonatal Med 2006; 19(6): 375–376.
7. Uwaydah M, Bibi S. and Salman S, Therapeutic efficacy of tobramycin--a clinical and laboratory evaluation. J Antimicrob Chemother 1975; 1: 429–437.

LOVASTATIN   L3

Trade: Mevacor

Other Trades: Mevacor, Apo-Lovastatin

Category: Hypocholesterolemic

Lovastatin is an effective inhibitor of hepatic cholesterol synthesis. It is primarily used for hypercholesterolemia. Pregnancy normally elevates maternal cholesterol and triglyceride levels. Following delivery, lipid levels gradually decline to pre-pregnancy levels within about 9 months. Small but unpublished levels are known to be secreted into human breastmilk.[1] Less than 5% of a dose reaches the maternal circulation due to extensive first-pass removal by the liver. The effect on the infant is unknown, but it could reduce hepatic cholesterol synthesis. There is little justification for using such a drug during lactation, but due to the extremely small maternal plasma levels, it is unlikely that the amount in breastmilk would be clinically active. Others in this same family of drugs include simvastatin, pravachol, atorvastatin, and fluvastatin. Atherosclerosis is a chronic process, and discontinuation of lipid-lowering drugs during pregnancy and lactation should have little to no impact on the outcome of long-term therapy of primary hypercholesterolemia. Cholesterol and other products of cholesterol biosynthesis are essential components for fetal and neonatal development, and the use of cholesterol-lowering drugs would not be advisable under most circumstances in breastfeeding mothers.

Pregnancy Risk	X	Lactation Risk	L3
T ½	= 1.1–1.7	M/P	=
Vd	=	PB	= >95%
Tmax	= 2–4 hours	Oral	= 5–30%
MW	= 405	pKa	= 13.5

Adult Concerns: Diarrhea, dyspepsia, flatulence, constipation, headache.

Pediatric Concerns: None reported but its use is not recommended.

Drug Interactions: Increased toxicity when added to gemfibrozil (myopathy, myalgia, etc), clofibrate, niacin (myopathy), erythromycin, cyclosporine, oral anticoagulants (elevated bleeding time).

Relative Infant Dose:

Adult Dose: 20–80 mg daily.

Alternatives:

References:
1. Pharmaceutical manufacturer prescribing information, 1999.

LOXAPINE   L4

Trade: Loxitane

Other Trades: Loxapac, PMS-Loxapine, Loxapac

Category: CNS tranquilizer

Loxapine is a typical antipsychotic similar to clozapine which produces pharmacologic effects similar to the phenothiazines and haloperidol family.[1] The drug does not appear to have antidepressant effects and may lower the seizure threshold. It is a powerful tranquilizer and has been found to be secreted into the milk of animals, but no data are available for human milk. This is a potent tranquilizer that could produce significant sequelae in breastfeeding infants. Numerous well studied alternatives exist, such as olanzapine, risperidone, and aripiprazole. Caution is urged.

Pregnancy Risk	C	Lactation Risk	L4
T ½	= 19 hours	M/P	=
Vd	=	PB	=
Tmax	= 1–2 hours	Oral	= 33%
MW	= 328	pKa	= 6.6

Adult Concerns: Drowsiness, tremor, rigidity, extrapyramidal symptoms.

Pediatric Concerns: None reported, but extreme caution is recommended.

Drug Interactions: Increased toxicity when used with CNS depressants, metrizamide, and monoamine oxidase inhibitors.

Relative Infant Dose:

Adult Dose: 10–50 mg two-four times daily.

Alternatives: Olanzapine, risperidone, and aripiprazole.

References:
1. McEvoy GE. (ed): AFHS Drug Information. New York, NY: 2003.

LUBIPROSTONE   L3

Trade: Amitiza

Other Trades:

Category: Gastrointestinal Agent

Lubiprostone is used for treating chronic idiopathic constipation. It is a local-acting chloride channel activator, which in turn increases chloride-rich intestinal fluid secretion without altering other serum electrolyte concentrations. Increasing the intestinal fluid secretion results in an increased motility in the intestine, and increased passage of stool.[1] No data are available on its transfer to human milk, but given that the oral absorption is nil, plasma levels in the adult are undetectable, and lubiprostone is 94% protein bound, the amount delivered to a breastfeeding infant through milk would likely be nil. Monitor baby for signs of diarrhea but this is unlikely.

Pregnancy Risk	C	Lactation Risk	L3
T ½	= 0.9–1.4 hours	M/P	=
Vd	=	PB	= 94%
Tmax	= 1.14 hours	Oral	= Nil
MW	= 390.46	pKa	= 9.68

Adult Concerns: Adverse effects include headache, nausea, and diarrhea.

Pediatric Concerns: No data are available.

Drug Interactions:

Relative Infant Dose:

Adult Dose: 24 µg twice daily.

Alternatives:

References:
1. Pharmaceutical manufacturer prescribing information, 2006.

LURASIDONE   L3

Trade: Latuda
Other Trades:
Category: Atypical antipsychotic

Lurasidone hydrochloride is an atypical antipsychotic agent used in the treatment of schizophrenia. The efficacy of lurasidone in schizophrenia is thought to be mediated through a combination of central dopamine type 2 (D_2) and serotonin type 2 (5–HT 2A) receptor antagonism. Lurasidone is present in rat milk, but there are no studies in humans. Due to its high protein binding and low oral bioavailability, lurasidone is not likely to enter breastmilk in clinically relevant amounts. Hyperglycemia and hyperprolactinemia have been reported with lurasidone use. Until more data are available in humans, caution is recommended.[1] Well studied alternatives include risperidone, olanzapine, and aripiprazole.

Pregnancy Risk	B	Lactation Risk	L3
T ½	= 18 hours	M/P	=
Vd	= 6173 l/kg	PB	= 99%
Tmax	= 1–3 hours	Oral	= 9 to 19%
MW	= 529.14	pKa	=

Adult Concerns: Most common side effects: Somnolence, akathisia, nausea, parkinsonism, and agitation. Other less common side effects: vomiting, dyspepsia, fatigue, back pain, dizziness, and anxiety.

Pediatric Concerns:

Drug Interactions: Do not use in combination with strong CYP3A4 inhibitors such as ketoconazole. Dose adjustment recommended for moderate CYP3A4 inhibitors such as diltiazem. Do not use in combination with strong CYP3A4 inducers such as rifampin or St. John's Wort.

Relative Infant Dose:

Adult Dose: 40–80 mg daily.

Alternatives: Risperidone, olanzapine, and aripiprazole.

References:
1. Pharmaceutical manufacturing prescribing information, 2011.

LUTEIN   L3

Trade: Carotenoids
Other Trades:
Category: Dietary supplement

Lutein is xantrophyll caretonoid which is the main caretonoid in retina and eye lens. Breastmilk is the main source of lutein for breastfed infant. In one study, lutein concentration in breastmilk is 159 µg/L at day 3 and 62.6 µg/L at day 30 while breastfeeding women were ingesting 1209–1258 µg of lutein daily.[1] There are no controlled studies in breastfeeding women; however, the risk of side effects to infant is probably minimal. Lutein should be given only if the potential benefit justifies the potential risk to the infant.

Pregnancy Risk	Probably Safe	Lactation Risk	L3
T ½	=	M/P	=
Vd	=	PB	=
Tmax	=	Oral	=
MW	= 569	pKa	= 18.91

Adult Concerns: None reported
Pediatric Concerns:
Drug Interactions:
Relative Infant Dose: 52.2%–138.2%
Adult Dose: 2–6 mg/day
Alternatives:

References:
1. Cena H, Castellazzi AM, Pietri A, Roggi C, Turconi G. Lutein concentration in human milk during early lactation and its relationship with dietary lutein intake. Public Health Nutr. 2009 Oct; 12(10): 1878–84. Epub 2009 Feb 16.

LUTROPIN ALFA   L3

Trade: Luveris
Other Trades:
Category: Human luteinizing hormone

Lutropin Alfa is a human luteinizing hormone (LH) of DNA recombinant origin used in the treatment of female infertility due to LH deficiency.[1] Endogenous LH promotes ovulation as well as the growth and development of the ovarian follicle. There are no studies currently on the transfer of lutropin alfa into breastmilk. However, due to its high molecular weight, transfer is unlikely. Nonetheless, some caution is recommended. It is not known if the administration of LH, and the subsequent maternal changes in estrogen and progesterone, would alter the production of milk. It is however likely, since the onset of pregnancy is commonly followed by a decrease in milk production in most mothers. Use in lactating women only if potential benefits to mother outweighs potential risks to infant.

Pregnancy Risk	X	Lactation Risk	L3
T ½	= 11–18 hours	M/P	=
Vd	= 10 l/kg	PB	=
Tmax	= 4–16 hours	Oral	= 56% (subcutaneous)
MW	= 23,390	pKa	=

Adult Concerns: Nausea, diarrhea, constipation, abdominal pain, headache. Cystic ovaries, ovarian hypertrophy and hyperstimulation.

Pediatric Concerns:

Drug Interactions:

Relative Infant Dose:

Adult Dose: 75 IU subcutaneous.

Alternatives:

References:
1. Pharmaceutical manufacturer prescribing information, 2010.

LYME DISEASE   L4

Trade: Borrelia burgdorferi infection
Other Trades:
Category: Borrelia Burgdorferi infections

Lyme disease is caused by infection with the spirochete, borrelia burgdorferi. It is a vector-borne illness transmitted by the hard Ixodes tick that generally inhabit wooded, forested areas. Lyme disease is prevalent in regions of central and eastern Europe and in eastern Asia.[1] In the United States, it is prevalent in 3 major geographical zones–southern New England, eastern mid- Atlantic and upper Midwest.[2] People of all ages may be affected. Transmission of infection is most effective 48 to 72 hours after the attachment of the infected tick.[1]

This spirochete is transferred in utero to the fetus.[3] The only evidence of possible transmission of Borrelia burgdorferi to human milk was when urine and breast milk samples from patients with skin manifestations of LD was studied using nested PCR for detection of Borrelia burgdorferi DNA. B. burgdorferi DNA was detected in breast milk samples of 2 lactating women who presented with erythema migrans–a characteristic rash associated with lyme disease. The 6-month old infant of one of them had to be hospitalized after developing fever and vomiting of unknown etiology, but the infant recovered subsequently. Therefore, although transmission of B. burgdorferi to human milk may occur, it is not known if transmission via milk is infectious.[4]

If diagnosed postpartum or in a breastfeeding mother, the mother should be treated immediately. In children (>7 years) and adults, preferred therapy is doxycycline (100 mg orally twice daily for 14–21 days), or amoxicillin (500 mg three times daily for 21 days). In breastfeeding patients, amoxicillin therapy is probably preferred but doxycycline can safely be used up to a maximum of 3 weeks. In the infant, use amoxicillin (40 mg/kg/day (max 3 gm) with probenecid (25 mg/kg/day) divided in three doses/day for a duration of 21 days.[5] Alternative therapy for adults includes clarithromycin (500 mg orally twice daily for 21 days), azithromycin (500 mg orally daily for 14–21 days), or cefuroxime axetil 500 mg orally twice daily for 21 days.[6] Although doxycycline therapy is not definitely contraindicated in breastfeeding mothers, alternates such as amoxicillin, cefuroxime, clarithromycin, or azithromycin should be preferred.

Because the spirochete antigen has been found in breast milk, breastfeeding should be withheld until treatment with an appropriate antibiotic has been initiated. Once treatment is initiated, breastfeeding may be resumed.

Pregnancy Risk	Safer	Lactation Risk	L4
T ½	=	M/P	=
Vd	=	PB	=
Tmax	=	Oral	=
MW	=	pKa	=

Adult Concerns: Acute Lyme disease: rash and influenza like symptoms

Pediatric Concerns:

Drug Interactions:

Relative Infant Dose:

Adult Dose:

Alternatives:

References:
1. Bhate C, Schwartz RA: Lyme disease: Part I. Advances and perspectives. J Am Acad Dermatol 2011, 64(4): 619–636; quiz 637–618.
2. AAP CoID: Lyme Disease (Lyme Borreliosis, Borrelia burgdorferi Infection). In: Red Book: 2009 Report of the Committee on Infectious diseases. Edited by Pickering LK BC, Kimberlin DW, Long SS, 28 edn; 2009: 430–435.
3. Stiernstedt G. Lyme borreliosis during pregnancy. Scand J Infect Dis Suppl 1990; 71: 99–100
4. Schmidt BL, Aberer E, Stockenhuber C, Klade H, Breier F, Luger A. Detection of Borrelia burgdorferi DNA by polymerase chain reaction in the urine and breast milk of patients with Lyme borreliosis. Diagn Microbiol Infect Dis 1995; 21(3): 121–128.
5. Bartlett JG. In: Pocket Book of Infectious Disease Therapy. Baltimore, USA: Williams and Wilkins, 1996.
6. Nelson JD. In: Pocket Book of Pediatric Antimicrobial Therapy. Baltimore, USA: Williams and Wilkins, 1995.

LYMPHOCYTIC CHORIOMENINGITIS VIRUS (LCMV)   L4

Trade: LCMV infection

Other Trades:

Category: Arena virus

Lymphocytic choriomeningitis, or LCMV, is a rodent-borne viral infectious disease that presents as aseptic meningitis, encephalitis, or meningoencephalitis. Its causative agent is the lymphocytic choriomeningitis virus (LCMV), a member of the family Arenaviridae. Pet mice, hamsters, guinea pigs may be infected if they have contact with wild mice or come from LCMV infected colonies. There are no adequate reports on human to human transmission of LCMV. Normally, LCMV infections are asymptomatic or mild (self-limiting disease); however, acute infections may have symptoms of fever, muscle ache, malaise, nausea, vomiting, lack of appetite, and aseptic meningitis (rare).[1]

Lymphocytic choriomeningitis virus (LCMV) has been implicated in miscarriage and congenital abnormalities.[2] LCMV is transmitted to humans via inhalation or direct contact of saliva, milk, semen, urine, nasal secretion, blood and feces of infected mice/rodents. Transmission of LCMV is more prevalent in winter months.[2] CDC estimated the prevalence of LCMV infection in human to be 2–5%. Risk of acquiring LCMV is low, mostly through contact with wild mice.[1] Pregnant women are advised to avoid contact, vacuuming, or cleaning rodent feces, urine and nesting material from wild rodents to reduce risk of LCMV infections. Proper hand washing with soap after contact with wild rodents or pets are recommended for pregnant women. Active infections of LCMV during first and second trimester have been associated with chorioretinitis, hydrocephalus, microcephaly, macrocephaly, periventricular calcification.[2] There are no treatments for LCMV currently. LCMV can be diagnosed via immunofluorescent antibody test. Previous LCMV infection does not increase risk of infant abnormalities of current and future pregnancy.[1] There are no data on viral transmission to infant from breast milk.

Pregnancy Risk	Possibly Hazardous	Lactation Risk	L4
T ½	=	M/P	=
Vd	=	PB	=
Tmax	=	Oral	=
MW	=	pKa	=

Adult Concerns: Aseptic meningitis, encephalitis

Pediatric Concerns: It is not known if LCMV is transferred into human milk, but it is likely.

Drug Interactions:

Relative Infant Dose:

Adult Dose:

Alternatives:

References:
1. Interim Guidance for Minimizing Risk for Human Lymphocytic Choriomeningitis Virus Infection Associated with Rodents. Centers for Disease Control and Prevention (2011).
2. Barton LL, Mets MB. Congenital lymphocytic choriomeningitis virus infection: decade of rediscovery. Clin Infect Dis. 2001 Aug 1; 33(3): 370–4. Epub 2001 Jul 5. Review. Erratum in: Clin Infect Dis 2001 Oct 15; 33(8): 1445.

LYSERGIC ACID DIETHYLAMIDE (LSD)   L5

Trade: LSD

Other Trades:

Category: Hallucinogen

Lysergic acid diethylamide (LSD) is a power hallucinogenic drug.[1] No data are available on transfer into breastmilk. However, due to its extreme potency and its ability to pass through the blood-brain-barrier, LSD is likely to penetrate milk and produce hallucinogenic effects in the infant. This drug is definitely CONTRAINDICATED. Maternal urine may be positive for LSD for 34–120 hours post ingestion.

Pregnancy Risk	Possibly Hazardous	Lactation Risk	L5
T ½	= 3 hours	M/P	=
Vd	=	PB	=
Tmax	= 30–60 minutes (oral)	Oral	= Complete
MW	= 268	pKa	= 7.8

Adult Concerns: Hallucinations, dilated pupils, salivation, nausea.

Pediatric Concerns: None reported via milk, but due to potency, hallucinations are likely. Contraindicated.

Drug Interactions:

Relative Infant Dose:

Adult Dose:

Alternatives:

References:
1. Ellenhorn MJ, Barceloux DG. In: Medical Toxicology. New York, NY: Elsevier, 1988.

LYSINE   L2

Trade: Lysine, L-Lysine

Other Trades:

Category: Amino acid food supplement

Lysine is a naturally occurring amino acid; the average American ingests around 6–10 grams daily. Aside from its use as a supplement in patients with poor nutrition, it is most often used for the treatment of recurrent herpes simplex infections, for which it is probably ineffective. The clinical efficacy of lysine in herpes infections is highly controversial with some advocates[1,2] and many detractors.[3] Upon absorption, most is sequestered in the liver, but blood levels do rise transiently. However, the risk of toxicity is considered quite low in both adults and infants. Rather high doses have been studied in infants as young as 4 months, with doses from 60 to 1080 mg L-lysine per 8 ounces of milk.[4] At the higher level, 5.18 grams of L-lysine was consumed. Plasma lysine levels varied only with normal limits, while urinary lysine levels were roughly proportional to the amount of supplementation. Thomas has reported an elegant study of the transfer of radiolabeled L-lysine into numerous compartments, including milk.[5,6] In a group of 5 lactating women who received L-lysine (15N-lysine and 13C-lysine (5 mg/kg/each)), milk levels of labeled lysine reached a peak at approximately 150 minutes. Labeled lysine levels in milk were slightly higher with M/P ratios ranging from 1.29 to 1.43. However, the total amount of radiolabeled lysine present in milk was still low. Only 0.54% of the administered dose of lysine was secreted into milk proteins. Further, the lysine present in milk was present as protein, not free amino acid.

Therefore supplementation of breastfeeding mothers with L-lysine will probably not result in significantly elevated levels of free lysine in milk.

Pregnancy Risk	C	Lactation Risk	L2
T ½	= 3.66 hours	M/P	=
Vd	=	PB	=
Tmax	=	Oral	= 83%
MW	= 146	pKa	= 2.18, 8.95, 10.53

Adult Concerns: Gastrointestinal distress. Lysine may cause cholesterol and triglyceride levels in the blood to rise.

Pediatric Concerns: None reported.

Drug Interactions:

Relative Infant Dose:

Adult Dose:

Alternatives:

References:
1. Griffith RS, Walsh DE, Myrmel KH, Thompson RW, Behforooz A. Success of L-lysine therapy in frequently recurrent herpes simplex infection. Treatment and prophylaxis. Dermatologica 1987; 175(4): 183–190.
2. Walsh DE, Griffith RS, Behforooz A. Subjective response to lysine in the therapy of herpes simplex. J Antimicrob Chemother 1983; 12(5): 489–496.
3. DiGiovanna JJ, Blank H. Failure of lysine in frequently recurrent herpes simplex infection. Treatment and prophylaxis. Arch Dermatol 1984; 120(1): 48–51.
4. Anderson SA, Raiten DJ. (eds): "Safety of Amino Acids in Dietary Supplements." Life Sciences Research Office, Bethesda, MD: FASEB Special Publications Office, 1999.
5. Thomas MR, Irving CS, Reeds PJ, Malphus EW, Wong WW, Boutton TW, Klein PD. Lysine and protein metabolism in the young lactating woman. Eur J Clin Nutr 1991; 45(5): 227–242.
6. Irving CS, Malphus EW, Thomas MR, Marks L, Klein PD. Infused and ingested labeled lysines: appearance in human-milk proteins. Am J Clin Nutr 1988; 47(1): 49–52.

MAGNESIUM HYDROXIDE   L1

Trade: Magnolax
Other Trades:
Category: Laxative, antacid

Magnesium hydroxide is used as an antacid and laxative. Magnesium hydroxide is poorly absorbed from maternal gastrointestinal tract. Only about 15–30% of an orally ingested magnesium product is absorbed. Magnesium rapidly deposits in bone (>50%) and is significantly distributed to tissue sites. In a comparative report of the laxative efficacy of senna vs mineral oil or magnesium hydroxide, fifty postpartum women were administered senna, the other fifty received either mineral oil or magnesium hydroxide. Doses were administered on first postpartum day, with additional doses administered on the following days. No alterations in bowel habits or abnormal stools were noted in any of the breastfed infants, indicating that magnesium hydroxide exposure through breastmilk is clinically insignificant in an infant.[1]

Pregnancy Risk	B		Lactation Risk	L1
T ½	=		M/P	=
Vd	=		PB	= 33%
Tmax	=		Oral	= 15–30%
MW	= 58		pKa	=

Adult Concerns: Hypotension, diarrhea, nausea.

Pediatric Concerns: None reported.

Drug Interactions: Decreased absorption of tetracyclines, digoxin, indomethacin, and iron salts.

Relative Infant Dose:

Adult Dose: 5–30 mL PRN

Alternatives:

References:
1. Baldwin WF. Clinical study of senna administration to nursing mothers. Can Med Assoc J 1963; 89: 566–8.

MAGNESIUM SALICYLATE   L3

Trade: Doan's Extra Strength, Doan's Regular, Keygesic-10, Momentum, Novasal
Other Trades:
Category: Topical analgesic

Magnesium salicylate is a topical analgesic most often used to treat back pain. Studies concerning the passage of magnesium salicylate into breastmilk have not been conducted, though it has been documented that salicylic acid is transferred into breastmilk.[1] As with other topical preparations, this drug does not enter the systemic circulation to the degree that an oral dosage form would. The American

Academy of Pediatrics generally deems topical preparations of salicylate derivatives to be compatible with breastfeeding.[2]

Pregnancy Risk	C	Lactation Risk	L3
T ½	= 2–3 hours (12 hours at high doses)	M/P	=
Vd	= 0.17 l/kg	PB	= 50–80%
Tmax	= 5 hours (topical)	Oral	=
MW	= 138.12	pKa	=

Adult Concerns: Burning, itching, hypermagnesemia, bleeding (less risk than aspirin), hypersensitivity reaction

Pediatric Concerns:

Drug Interactions: Alfacalcidol: This agent may increase the concentration of magnesium compounds. Bisphosphonates: Magnesium salts may decrease the concentration and effects of these agents Calcitriol: This agent may increase the concentration of magnesium compounds. Calcium channel blockers: These agents may enhance the adverse effects of magnesium salts. Magnesium salts may decrease the concentration of this agent. Mycophenolate: Magnesium salts may decrease the concentration of this agent when both drugs are administered orally. Phosphate supplements: Magnesium salts may decrease the concentration of these agents. Quinolones: Magnesium salts may decrease the absorption of these antibiotics when both are administered orally. Tetracyclines: Magnesium salts may decrease the absorption of these antibiotics when both are administered orally.Trientene: Magnesium salts may decrease the concentration of this agent.

Relative Infant Dose:

Adult Dose: 650 mg every 4 hours; use topically PRN

Alternatives:

References:
1. Gilman AG, Rall TW, Nies AS, et alGilman AG, Rall TW, Nies AS, et al (Eds): Goodman and Gilman's The Pharmacological Basis of Therapeutics, 8th. Pergamon Press, New York, NY, 1990.
2. Anon: American academy of pediatrics committee on drugs: transfer of drugs and other chemicals into human milk. Pediatrics 2001; 108(3): 776–789.

MAGNESIUM SULFATE   L1

Trade: Epsal

Other Trades:

Category: Saline laxative and anticonvulsant (IV,IM)

Magnesium is a normal plasma electrolyte. It is used pre and postnatally as an effective anticonvulsant in preeclamptic patients. In one study of 10 preeclamptic patients who received a 4 gm IV loading dose followed by 1 gm per hour IV for more than 24 hours, the average milk magnesium levels in treated subjects were 6.4 mg/dL, only slightly higher than controls (untreated) which were 4.77 mg/dL.[1] On day 2, the average milk magnesium levels in treated groups were 3.83 mg/dL, which was not significantly different from untreated controls, 3.19 mg/dL. By day 3, the treated and control groups breastmilk levels were identical (3.54 vs. 3.52 mg/dL). The mean maternal serum magnesium level on day 1 in treated groups was 3.55 mg/dL, which was significantly higher than control untreated, 1.82 mg/dL. In both treated and control subjects, levels of milk magnesium were approximately twice those of maternal serum magnesium levels, with the milk-to-serum ratio being 1.9 in treated subjects and 2.1 in control subjects. This study clearly indicates a normal concentrating mechanism for magnesium in human milk. It is well known that oral magnesium absorption is very poor, averaging only 4%.[2] Further, this study indicates that in treated groups, infants would only receive about 1.5 mg of oral magnesium more than the untreated controls. It is very unlikely that the amount of magnesium in breastmilk would be clinically relevant.

Pregnancy Risk	B	Lactation Risk	L1
T ½	= <3 hours	M/P	= 1.9
Vd	=	PB	=
Tmax	= Immediate (IV)	Oral	= 4%
MW	= 120	pKa	=

Adult Concerns: IV-hypotension, sedation, muscle weakness.

Pediatric Concerns: None reported via milk. Sedation, hypotonia following inutero exposure.

Drug Interactions: May decrease the hypertensive effect of nifedipine. May increase the depression associated with other CNS depressants, neuromuscular blocking agents, and the cardiotoxicity associated with ritodrine.

Relative Infant Dose: 0.2%

Adult Dose: 1–2 gm every 4–6 hours PRN

Alternatives:

References:
1.   Cruikshank DP, Varner MW, Pitkin RM. Breast milk magnesium and calcium concentrations following magnesium sulfate treatment. Am J Obstet Gynecol 1982; 143(6): 685–688.
2.   Morris ME, LeRoy S, Sutton SC. Absorption of magnesium from orally administered magnesium sulfate in man. J Toxicol Clin Toxicol 1987; 25: 371–82.

MALATHION   L3

Trade: Ovide, Malathion Lotion

Other Trades: A-Lices, Prioderm, Quellada M, Suleo-M

Category: Pediculicide, scabicide

Malathion is a common pesticide. It is used in lotions (0.5%) for the treatment of resistant lice and scabies.[1] It should be applied to dry hair and scalp in high enough quantities to thoroughly wet the hair and scalp. The hair should be allowed to dry naturally and shampooed 8–12 hours later. A second application at 7–9 days is required if lice are still present. It should not be used in neonates, although one case report of its use in a 7 month-old infant suggests it is relatively safe. Less than 10% of malathion is absorbed transcutaneously and is rapidly metabolized and excreted. While it belongs to the organophosphate family of insecticides, it is so rapidly metabolized and eliminated by humans (10 times) that it is relatively nontoxic under normal conditions. Since so little is absorbed systemically after its topical use, maternal levels attained will not be sufficiently high to produce significant levels in breastmilk or in the infant. Therefore, no significant clinical effects are expected in the infant following its use in breastfeeding mothers. [2,3]

Pregnancy Risk	B		Lactation Risk	L3
T ½	= 7.6 hours		M/P	=
Vd	=		PB	=
Tmax	=		Oral	= Complete
MW	=		pKa	= 18.34

Adult Concerns: Respiratory distress, excessive salivation.

Pediatric Concerns: None observed via breastfeeding.

Drug Interactions:

Relative Infant Dose:

Adult Dose:

Alternatives: Permethrin

References:
1. Pharmaceutical manufacturer prescribing information, 2010.
2. Ostrea EM Jr, Bielawski DM, Posecion NC Jr, Corrion M, Villanueva-Uy E, Jin Y, Janisse JJ, Ager JW. A comparison of infant hair, cord blood, and meconium analysis to detect fetal exposure to environmental pesticides. Environ Res. 2008 Feb; 106 (2): 277–83.
3. Lebwohl M, Clark L, and Levitt J. Therapy for head lice based on life cycle, resistance, and safety consideration. Pediatrics 207; 119: 965–74. Online access: http: //pediatrics/ aapublications.org/content/119/5/965.full.html.

MANGAFODIPIR TRISODIUM   L3

Trade: Teslascan

Other Trades:

Category: Radiological Contrast Agent

Mangafodipir is a manganese-containing radiocontrast agent used in Magnetic Resonance Imaging (MRI). It is rapidly redistributed to liver and less so to other tissues.[1] The release of manganese is significant, and whole-body stores are approximately doubled with infusion of this product. Elevated plasma manganese levels drop rapidly, with a redistribution half-life of about 25 minutes, while the terminal elimination half-life of manganese is more on the order of 10.1 hours. Manganese is effectively transported into human milk, and milk levels are apparently a function of oral intake in the mother. Consequently, manganese levels in milk could temporarily be elevated. Infants are somewhat deficient in manganese and have higher oral bioavailability of manganese, due to the relative state of deficiency.[2] For this reason, it is reasonable to assume that the use of this product in a breastfeeding woman could conceivably elevate the manganese levels of her milk significantly, although briefly. A brief interruption of breastfeeding for a few hours (four or more), followed by pumping and discarding, would significantly reduce any risk to the infant.

Pregnancy Risk	C	Lactation Risk	L3
T ½	= 10 hours	M/P	=
Vd	=	PB	= Nil
Tmax	=	Oral	= Low
MW	=	pKa	=

Adult Concerns: Local injection site reactions, nausea, vomiting, abdominal pain, warmth sensation, taste perversion, headache, hypersensitivity.

Pediatric Concerns:

Drug Interactions:

Relative Infant Dose:

Adult Dose:

Alternatives:

References:
1. Pharmaceutical manufacturer prescribing information, 2003.
2. Vuori E, Makinen SM, Kara R, Kuitunen P. The effects of the dietary intakes of copper, iron, manganese, and zinc on the trace element content of human milk. Am J Clin Nutr 1980; 33(2): 227–231.

MANNITOL   L3

Trade: Osmitrol
Other Trades:
Category: Osmotic diuretic

Mannitol is a hexahydroxy alcohol chemically related to mannose and is used as an osmotic diuretic.[1] As such, it does not readily enter the cellular compartment and remains in the extracellular compartment, thus it would not enter lactocytes. Hepatic metabolism is minimal and the drug is primarily excreted unchanged in the urine by glomerular filtration. The elimination half-life is 71–100 minutes. Mannitol does not normally enter the CNS or the eye. It is freely filtered by the kidneys with less than 10% tubular reabsorption which is the basis for its use as a diuretic. It is not known if it enters the milk compartment, but it is likely only during the first few days postpartum when the tight-junctions in the alveolar system are immature. After 48–72 hours the entry of mannitol into human milk is probably minimal. Oral absorption in infants would be minimal except early postpartum when their gastrointestinal tract is relatively porous.

Pregnancy Risk	C	Lactation Risk	L3
T ½	= 71–100 minutes	M/P	=
Vd	= Low	PB	=
Tmax	=	Oral	= 17%
MW	= 182	pKa	= 13.38

Adult Concerns: Hypernatremia, hyponatremia, elevated potassium, diarrhea, kidney failure, pulmonary edema, and congestive heart failure.

Pediatric Concerns: None reported via milk, but watery diarrhea is remotely possible. Due to its osmotic diuresis, it is possible that it could briefly reduce the production of milk.

Drug Interactions: May enhance diuresis when added with loop and other diuretics. May increase elimination of lithium.

Relative Infant Dose:

Adult Dose: Highly variable.

Alternatives:

References:
1. Pharmaceutical manufacturer prescribing information, 2003.

MAPROTILINE   L3

Trade: Ludiomil

Other Trades: Novo-Maprotilene, Ludiomil

Category: Antidepressant

Maprotiline is a unique structured (tetracyclic) antidepressant dissimilar to others but has clinical effects similar to the tricyclic antidepressants. While it has fewer anticholinergic side effects than the tricyclics, it is more sedating and has similar toxicities in overdose. In one study following an oral dose of 50 mg three times daily, milk and maternal blood levels were greater than 200 µg/L.[1] Milk/plasma ratios varied from 1.3 to 1.5. While these levels are quite low, it is not known if they are hazardous to a breastfed infant, but caution is recommended.

Pregnancy Risk	B	Lactation Risk	L3
T ½	= 27–58 hours	M/P	= 1.5
Vd	= 22.6 l/kg	PB	= 88%
Tmax	= 12 hours	Oral	= 100%
MW	= 277	pKa	= 10.5

Adult Concerns: Side effects include drowsiness, sedation, vertigo, blurred vision, dry mouth, and urinary retention. Skin rashes, seizures, myoclonus, mania and hallucinations have been reported.

Pediatric Concerns: None reported via milk, but caution is recommended.

Drug Interactions: Maprotilene levels may be decreased by barbiturates, phenytoin, and carbamazepine. Increased toxicity may result when used with CNS depressants, quinidine, monoamine oxidase inhibitors, anticholinergics, sympathomimetics, phenothiazines (seizures), benzodiazepines. Due to increased hazard of cardiotoxicity, do not admix with cisapride.

Relative Infant Dose: 1.4%

Adult Dose: 25–75 mg daily

Alternatives: Sertraline, venlafaxine, paroxetine

References:

1. Riess W. The relevance of blood level determinations during the evaluation of maprotiline in man. In: Murphy (ed): Research and Clinical Investigations in Depression. Northhampton: Cambridge Medical Publications 1976: 19–37.

MEASLES + MUMPS + RUBELLA + VARICELLA VACCINE   L3

Trade: ProQuad, MMRV vaccine

Other Trades:

Category: Vaccine

The measles + mumps + rubella + varicella (MMRV) vaccine is a combined vaccine, recommended for prevention of measles, mumps, rubella and varicella infection. As per the Advisory Commission for Immunization Practices (ACIP), it is to be administered at 12–15 months and then again at 4–6 years of age. However, if the child has a personal or family history of seizures, then the separate injections of MMR and varicella are recommended.[1]

MMR vaccine is a mixture of live, attenuated viruses from measles, mumps, and rubella strains. It is usually administered to children at 12–15 months of age. NEVER administer to a pregnant woman. Rubella, and perhaps measles and mumps virus, are undoubtedly transferred via breastmilk and have been detected in throat swabs of 56% of breastfeeding infants.[2-5] Infants exposed to the attenuated viruses via breastmilk had only mild symptoms. If medically required, MMR vaccine can be administered early postpartum.[6] A live attenuated varicella vaccine (Varivax–Merck) was recently approved for marketing by the US Food and Drug Administration. It is not known if the vaccine-acquired VZV is secreted in human milk, nor its infectiousness to infants. Interestingly, in two women with varicella-zoster infections, the virus was not culturable from milk. The antibody from the varicella zoster vaccine has been isolated in breast milk along with the DNA.[7,8] Mothers of immunodeficient infants should not breastfeed following use of this vaccine. Both the AAP[9] and the Centers for Disease Control approve the use of varicella-zoster vaccines in breastfeeding mothers, if the risk of infection is high.

The ACIP has stated that breastfeeding women may be administered both the live and killed vaccines.[10] As a general rule, vaccines are often safe to use during breastfeeding.[11]

Pregnancy Risk	C	Lactation Risk	L3
T ½	=	M/P	=
Vd	=	PB	=
Tmax	=	Oral	=
MW	=	pKa	=

Adult Concerns: Redness, pain, swelling, tenderness at site of injection, fever, skin reactions, hypersensitivity reaction. Seizures, Guillan-Barre syndrome, meningitis have rarely occurred. Contraindicated in those with ongoing acute infections, those on immunosuppressive agents or corticosteroids, those on anti-cancer drugs, those with immunodeficiency disorders, those with hypersensitivity to any of the components of the vaccine including neomycin or gelatin. Caution to be exercised in those with egg allergy.

Pediatric Concerns:

Drug Interactions: Do not administer in those on immunosuppressive agents or corticosteroids, those on anti-cancer drugs. May be administered along with other vaccines recommended at the time as per the immunization schedule.

Relative Infant Dose:

Adult Dose: 0.5 mL subcutaneous.

Alternatives:

References:

1. Product Information: PROQUAD(R) powder for solution subcutaneous injection, measles, mumps, rubella, varicella virus vaccine live solution subcutaneous injection. Merck, Whitehouse Station, NJ, 2009.
2. Buimovici-Klein E, Hite RL, Byrne T, Cooper LZ. Isolation of rubella virus in milk after postpartum immunization. J Pediatr 1977; 91(6): 939–941.
3. Losonsky GA, Fishaut JM, Strussenberg J, Ogra PL. Effect of immunization against rubella on lactation products. I. Development and characterization of specific immunologic reactivity in breast milk. J Infect Dis 1982; 145(5): 654–660.
4. Losonsky GA, Fishaut JM, Strussenberg J, Ogra PL. Effect of immunization against rubella on lactation products. II. Maternal-neonatal interactions. J Infect Dis 1982; 145(5): 661–666.
5. Landes RD, Bass JW, Millunchick EW, Oetgen WJ. Neonatal rubella following postpartum maternal immunization. J Pediatr 1980; 97(3): 465–467.
6. Lawrence RA. Breastfeeding: A guide for the medical profession. St. Louis: Mosby Publishers, 1994.
7. Frederick IB, White RJ, Braddock SW. Excretion of varicella-herpes zoster virus in breast milk. Am J Obstet Gynecol 1986; 154(5): 1116–1117.
8. Yoshida M, Yamagami N, Tezuka T, Hondo R. Case report: detection of varicella-zoster virus DNA in maternal breast milk. J Med Virol. 1992Oct; 38(2): 108–10.
9. American Academy of Pediatrics. Committee on Infectious Diseases. Red Book. 1997.
10. Anon: General recommendations on immunization; recommendations of the advisory committee on immunization practices (AICP) and the American academy of family physicians (AAFP). MMWR 2002a; 51(RR02): 1–36.
11. Schaefer CSchaefer C: Drugs During Pregnancy and Lactation, Elsevier Science B.V., Amsterdam, The Netherlands, 2001.

MEASLES + MUMPS + RUBELLA VACCINE (MMR VACCINE)   L2

Trade: MMR Vaccine, Measles–Mumps–Rubella, M-M-R II, ProQuad

Other Trades: Priorix

Category: Live attenuated triple virus vaccine

MMR vaccine is a mixture of live, attenuated viruses from measles, mumps, and rubella strains. It is usually administered to children at 12–15 months of age. NEVER administer to a pregnant woman. Rubella, and perhaps measles and mumps virus, are undoubtedly transferred via breastmilk and have been detected in throat swabs of 56% of breastfeeding infants.[1-4] Infants exposed to the attenuated viruses via breastmilk had only mild symptoms. If medically required, MMR vaccine can be administered early postpartum.[5] The American Advisory Committee on Immunization Practices has stated that breastfeeding women may be administered both the live and killed vaccines.[6] As a general rule, vaccines are often safe to use during breastfeeding.[7]

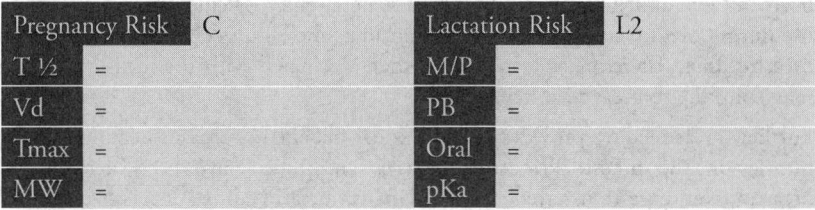

Pregnancy Risk	C		Lactation Risk	L2
T ½	=		M/P	=
Vd	=		PB	=
Tmax	=		Oral	=
MW	=		pKa	=

Adult Concerns: Mild symptoms, fever, flu-like symptoms.

Pediatric Concerns: Mild symptoms of rubella have been reported in one newborn infant.

Drug Interactions: Contraindicated in those with ongoing acute infections, those on immunosupressive agents or corticosteroids, those on anti-cancer drugs, those with immunedoficiency disorders, those with hypersensitivity to any of the components of the vaccine including neomycin or gelatin. Caution to be exercised in those with egg allergy.

Relative Infant Dose:

Adult Dose: 0.5 mL subcutaneous injection in outer aspect of upper arm.

Alternatives:

References:
1. Buimovici-Klein E, Hite RL, Byrne T, Cooper LZ. Isolation of rubella virus in milk after postpartum immunization. J Pediatr 1977; 91(6): 939–941.
2. Losonsky GA, Fishaut JM, Strussenberg J, Ogra PL. Effect of immunization against rubella on lactation products. I. Development and characterization of specific immunologic reactivity in breast milk. J Infect Dis 1982; 145(5): 654–660.
3. Losonsky GA, Fishaut JM, Strussenberg J, Ogra PL. Effect of immunization against rubella on lactation products. II. Maternal-neonatal interactions. J Infect Dis 1982; 145(5): 661–666.
4. Landes RD, Bass JW, Millunchick EW, Oetgen WJ. Neonatal rubella following postpartum maternal immunization. J Pediatr 1980; 97(3): 465–467.
5. Lawrence RA. Breastfeeding: A guide for the medical profession. St. Louis: Mosby Publishers, 1994.
6. Anon: General recommendations on immunization; recommendations of the advisory committee on immunization practices (AICP) and the American academy of family physicians (AAFP). MMWR 2002a; 51(RR02): 1–36.
7. Schaefer CSchaefer C: Drugs During Pregnancy and Lactation, Elsevier Science B.V., Amsterdam, The Netherlands, 2001.

MEASLES VIRUS VACCINE, LIVE   L2

Trade: Attenuvax

Other Trades:

Category: Vaccination for Measles

Measles vaccine is a live, attenuated vaccine indicated for the prevention of measles illness. It is administered at 12–15 months of age, as part of the routine childhood immunization schedule. This should be followed by a re-immunization at 4–6 years of age. It is usually administered along with the mumps and rubella vaccine, in the form of the MMR vaccine. There are currently no reports of transfer of the live measles virus vaccine into breastmilk. The American Advisory Committee on Immunization Practices has stated that breastfeeding women may be administered both the live and killed vaccines.[1] As a general rule, vaccines are often safe to use during breastfeeding.[2] The WHO considers measles vaccine compatible with breastfeeding. Therefore, a lactating mother vaccinated with the measles vaccine may continue to breastfeed her child.

Further, breastfeeding provides an additional benefit towards protection against measles in the infant. Protective measles antibodies have been detected in breastmilk and are transferred to the infant via breastfeeding.[3] It has been found that breastfeeding for more than 3 months is associated with a 30% decreased risk of clinical measles, and can provide protection up to the age of 10 years.[4] However, this protection is not equally as efficacious as that following measles vaccination. Therefore, while a lactating mother who has received the measles vaccine may continue to breastfeed, this does not preclude the importance of measles vaccination in the infant.

Pregnancy Risk	C		Lactation Risk	L2
T ½	=		M/P	=
Vd	=		PB	=
Tmax	=		Oral	=
MW	=		pKa	=

Adult Concerns: Headache, dizziness, rash, fever, diarrhea. Serious side effects: Anaphylaxis, encephalitis, thrombocytopenia, Steven-Johnson syndrome. Do not administer in those with hematological cancers such as leukemias, lymphomas. Do not administer in those with an acute viral illness, immunodeficiency disorders, those on corticosteroids or immunosuppressants, hypersensitivity to neomycin.

Pediatric Concerns:

Drug Interactions: Do not administer in those on cancer chemotherapy, immunosuppressants, corticosteroids.

Relative Infant Dose:

Adult Dose: 0.5 mL subcutaneous injection.

Alternatives:

References:

1. Anon: General recommendations on immunization; recommendations of the advisory committee on immunization practices (AICP) and the American academy of family physicians (AAFP). MMWR 2002a; 51(RR02): 1–36.
2. Schaefer CSchaefer C: Drugs During Pregnancy and Lactation, Elsevier Science B.V., Amsterdam, The Netherlands, 2001.
3. Adu FD, Adeniji JA. Measles antibodies in the breast milk of nursing mothers. Afr J Med Med Sci. 1995 Dec; 24(4): 385–8.
4. Silfverdal SA, Ehlin A, Montgomery SM. Breast-feeding and a subsequentdiagnosis of measles. Acta Paediatr. 2009 Apr; 98(4): 715–9. Epub 2008 Dec 24.

MEBENDAZOLE   L3

Trade: Vermox

Other Trades: Sqworm, Vermox

Category: Anthelmintic

Mebendazole is an anthelmintic used primarily for pin worms although it is active against round worms, hookworms, and a number of other nematodes. Mebendazole is poorly absorbed orally. In one patient who received 100 mg twice daily for three days, milk production was drastically reduced.[1] However in another report of four postpartum breastfeeding mothers who received 100 mg twice daily for 3 days, milk levels of mebendazole were undetectable in one patient sample. No change in milk production was noted in the latter study.[2] Considering the poor oral absorption and high protein binding, it is unlikely that mebendazole would be transmitted to the infant in clinically relevant concentrations.

Pregnancy Risk	C	Lactation Risk	L3
T ½	= 2.8–9 hours	M/P	=
Vd	=	PB	= High
Tmax	= 0.5–7.0 hours	Oral	= 2–10%
MW	= 295	pKa	= 13.92

Adult Concerns: Diarrhea, abdominal pain, nausea, vomiting, headache. Observe mother for reduced production of breast milk.

Pediatric Concerns: None reported via milk. May inhibit milk production.

Drug Interactions: Carbamazepine and phenytoin may increase metabolism of mebendazole.

Relative Infant Dose:

Adult Dose: 100 mg twice daily.

Alternatives: Pyrantel

References:
1. Rao TS. Does mebendazole inhibit lactation? N Z Med J 1983; 96(736): 589–590.
2. Kurzel RB, Toot PJ, Lambert LV, Mihelcic AS. Mebendazole and postpartum lactation. N Z Med J 1994; 107(988): 439.

MECLIZINE   L3

Trade:

Other Trades:

Category: Antiemetic, antivertigo, motion sickness

Meclizine is an antihistamine frequently used for nausea, vertigo, and motion sickness although it is inferior to scopolamine. Meclizine was previously used for nausea and vomiting of pregnancy in the USA, and still is in many countries.[1] No data are available on its secretion into breastmilk. There are no pediatric indications for this product. The use of meclizine while breastfeeding is probably safe, however monitoring for sedation in the infant is advised.

Pregnancy Risk	B	Lactation Risk	L3
T ½	= 6 hours	M/P	=
Vd	=	PB	=
Tmax	= 1–2 hours	Oral	= Complete
MW	= 391	pKa	=

Adult Concerns: Drowsiness, sedation, dry mouth, blurred vision.

Pediatric Concerns: None reported.

Drug Interactions: May have increased sedation when used with CNS depressants and other neuroleptics and anticholinergics.

Relative Infant Dose:

Adult Dose: 25–100 mg daily.

Alternatives: Dimenhydrinate, diphenhydramine, scopolamine.

References:
1. Vorherr H. Drug excretion in breast milk. Postgrad Med 1974; 56(4): 97–104.

MECLOFENAMATE   L2

Trade: Meclomen
Other Trades:
Category: Nonsteroidal anti-inflammatory agent

Meclofenamate is a nonsteroidal, anti-inflammatory agent used in the treatment of mild to moderate pain and dysmenorrhea. NSAIDS, as a class, are secreted minimally in breastmilk. Data from the manufacturer of meclofenamate reports the drug has been found in trace amounts in breastmilk.[1] Trace amounts of meclofenamate are not expected to cause clinical effects in the breastfeeding infant.

Pregnancy Risk	D	Lactation Risk	L2
T ½	= 0.8 to 2.1 hours	M/P	=
Vd	= 23 l/kg	PB	= 99%
Tmax	= 0.5–2 hours	Oral	= Complete
MW	= 336.15	pKa	=

Adult Concerns: Nausea, vomiting, diarrhea (often severe), abdominal pain, gastrointestinal bleeding, peptic ulcers, decreased hemoglobin/hematocrit, edema, rash, pruritus, headache, dizziness, and tinnitus. Contraindicated in patients that developed rhinitis, urticaria, asthma, or allergic reactions to aspirin or other anti-inflammatory agents. Caution should be used in patients on concomitant diuretic therapy, history of alchoholism, smoking, or conditions known to aggravate peptic ulcer disease, history of coagulation defects, history of gastrointestinal ulceration, bleeding, or perforation, history of liver dysfunction, hypertension or cardiac conditions aggravated by fluid retention and edema, pre-existing infection, renal dysfunction.

Pediatric Concerns:

Drug Interactions: Meclofenamate enhances the effect of warfarin. Concurrent administration of aspirin may lower meclofenamate plasma levels but doesn't affect serum salicylate levels. Greater fecal blood loss results from concomitant administration of both drugs than from either drug alone.

Relative Infant Dose:

Adult Dose: 50 mg every 4–6 hours.

Alternatives: Ibuprofen

References:
1. Pharmaceutical manufacturer prescribing information, 2010.

MEDROXYPROGESTERONE   L4

Trade: Provera, Depo-Provera, Cycrin, Sayana, DMPA

Other Trades: Farlutal, Provelle, Divina, Ralovera, Depo-Provera, Provera, Alti-MPA, Gen-Medroxy

Category: Injectable progestational agent

Medroxyprogesterone is a synthetic progestin compound. It is used orally for amenorrhea, dysmenorrhea, uterine bleeding, and infertility. It is used intramuscularly for contraception. Due to its poor oral bioavailability, it is seldom used orally. Saxena has reported that the average concentration in milk is 1.03 µg/L.[1] Koetswang reported average milk levels of 0.97 µg/L.[2]

In a series of huge studies, the World Health Organization reviewed the developmental skills of children and their weight gain following exposure to progestin-only contraceptives during lactation.[3,4] These studies documented that no adverse effects on overall development, or rate of growth, were notable. Further, they suggested there is no apparent reason to deny lactating women the use of progestin-only contraceptives, preferably after 6 weeks postpartum. There have been consistent and controversial studies suggesting that males exposed to early postnatal progestins have higher feminine scores. However, Ehrhardt's studies have provided convincing data that males exposed to early progestins were no different than controls.[5]

A number of other short and long-term studies available on development of children have found no differences with control groups.[6,7] Interestingly, an excellent study of the transfer of DMPA into breastfed infants has been published.[8] In this study of 13 breastfeeding women who received 150 mg injections of DMPA on day 43 and again on day 127 postpartum, urine and plasma collections in infants (n= 22) from day 38 to day 137 were collected. Urinary follicle stimulating hormone (FSH), luteinizing hormone (LH), unconjugated testosterone, unconjugated cortisol, medroxyprogesterone and metabolites were measured. No differences (from untreated controls) were found in LH, FSH, or unconjugated testosterone urine levels in the infants. Urine cortisol levels were not altered from those of control infants. Medroxyprogesterone or its metabolites were at no time detected in any of the infant urine samples. This data concludes that only small trace amounts of MPA are transferred to breastfeeding infants and that these amounts are not expected to have any influence on breastfeeding infants. In support of this, using calculations based on MPA levels in the blood of DMPA users and a plasma to milk MPA ratio, Benagiano and Fraser suggest that the actual amounts of MPA in the infant's system is probably at or below trace levels.[9] Koetsewant states that the small amount of MPA present in milk is unlikely to have any significant clinical adverse effects on the infant.[2] A long-term follow-up study by Jimenez found no changes in growth, development and health status in 128 breast-fed infants at 4.5 years of age.[10] DMPA mothers lactated significantly longer than controls in this study.

The use of DMPA in breastfeeding women is common but will probably always be somewhat controversial. DMPA has been documented to significantly elevate prolactin levels in breastfeeding mothers[11] and increase milk production in some mothers.[12] It is well known that estrogens suppress milk production. With progestins, it has been suggested that some women may experience a decline in milk production or arrested early production, following an injection of DMPA, particularly when the progestin is used early postpartum (12–48 hours).[13] At present there are no published data to support this, nor is the relative incidence of this untoward effect known.

Therefore, in some instances, it might be advisable to recommend treatment with oral progestin-only contraceptives postpartum rather than DMPA, so that women who experience reduced milk supply could easily withdraw from the medication without significant loss of breast milk supply. Progestins should be avoided early postnatally.[13]

Pregnancy Risk	X	Lactation Risk	L4
T ½	= 14.5 hours	M/P	=
Vd	=	PB	=
Tmax	=	Oral	= 0.6–10%
MW	= 344	pKa	= 17.61

Adult Concerns: Fluid retention, gastrointestinal distress, menstrual disorders, breakthrough bleeding, weight gain.

Pediatric Concerns: None reported via milk, although unsubstantiated reports of reduced milk supply have been made.

Drug Interactions: Aminoglutethimide may increase the hepatic clearance of medroxyprogesterone, reducing its efficacy.

Relative Infant Dose:

Adult Dose: 5–10 mg daily.

Alternatives:

References:
1.   Saxena NB. et.al. Level of contraceptive steroids in breast milk and plasma of lactating women. Contracept 1977; 16: 605–613.

2. Koetsawang S, Nukulkarn P, Fotherby K, Shrimanker K, Mangalam M, Towobola K. Transfer of contraceptive steroids in milk of women using long-acting gestagens. Contracept 1982; 25(4): 321–331.

3. Progestogen-only contraceptives during lactation: I. Infant growth. World Health Organization Task force for Epidemiological Research on Reproductive Health; Special Programme of Research, Development and Research Training in Human Reproduction. Contracept 1994; 50(1): 35–53.

4. Progestogen-only contraceptives during lactation: II. Infant development. World Health Organization, Task Force for Epidemiological Research on Reproductive Health; Special Programme of Research, Development, and Research Training in Human Reproduction. Contracep 1994; 50(1): 55–68.

5. Ehrhardt AA, Grisanti GC, Meyer-Bahlburg HF. Prenatal exposure to medroxyprogesterone acetate (MPA) in girls. Psychoneuroendocrinology 1977; 2(4): 391–398.

6. Schwallie PC. The effect of depot-medroxyprogesterone acetate on the fetus and nursing infant: a review. Contracep 1981; 23(4): 375–386.

7. Pardthaisong T, Yenchit C, Gray R. The long-term growth and development of children exposed to Depo-Provera during pregnancy or lactation. Contracep 1992; 45(4): 313–324.3.

8. Virutamasen P, Leepipatpaiboon S, Kriengsinyot R, Vichaidith P, Muia PN, Sekadde-Kigondu CB, Mati JK, Forest MG, Dikkeschei LD, Wolthers BG, d'Arcangues C. Pharmacodynamic effects of depot-medroxyprogesterone acetate (DMPA) administered to lactating women on their male infants. Contracep 1996; 54(3): 153–157.

9. Benagiano G, Fraser I. The Depo-Provera debate. Commentary on the article "Depo-Provera, a critical analysis". Contracep 1981; 24(5): 493–528.

10. Jimenez J, Ochoa M, Soler MP, Portales P. Long-term follow-up of children breast-fed by mothers receiving depot-medroxyprogesterone acetate. Contracep 1984; 30(6): 523–533.

11. Ratchanon S, Taneepanichskul S. Depot medroxyprogesterone acetate and basal serum prolactin levels in lactating women. Obstet Gynecol 2000; 96(6): 926–928.

12. Fraser IS. Long acting injectable hormonal contraceptives. Clin Reprod Fertil 1982; 1(1): 67–88.

13. Kennedy KI, Short RV, Tully MR. Premature introduction of progestin-only contraceptive methods during lactation. Contracep 1997; 55(6): 347–350.

MEFLOQUINE   L2

Trade: Lariam
Other Trades: Lariam
Category: Antimalarial

Mefloquine is an antimalarial and a structural analog of quinine. It is concentrated in red cells and therefore has a long half-life.[1] Following a single 250 mg dose in two women, the milk/plasma ratio was only 0.13 to 0.16 the first 4 days of therapy.[2] The concentration of mefloquine in milk ranged from 32 to 53 µg/L. Unfortunately, these studies were not carried out after steady state conditions, which would probably increase to some degree the amount transferred to the infant. According to the manufacturer, mefloquine is secreted in small concentrations approximately mating 3% of the maternal dose. Assuming a milk level of 53 µg/L and a daily milk intake of 150 mL/kg/day, an infant would ingest approximately 8 µg/kg/day of mefloquine, which is not sufficient to protect the infant from malaria. The therapeutic dose for malaria prophylaxis is 62 mg in a 15–19 kg infant. Thus far, no untoward effects have been reported.

Pregnancy Risk	C	Lactation Risk	L2
T ½	= 10–21 days	M/P	= 0.13–0.27
Vd	= 19 l/kg	PB	= 98%
Tmax	= 1–2 hours	Oral	= 85%
MW	= 414	pKa	= <2, 8.6

Adult Concerns: Gastrointestinal upset, dizziness, elevated liver enzymes, possible retinopathy.

Pediatric Concerns: None reported but discontinue lactation if neuropsychiatric disturbances occur.

Drug Interactions: Decreases effect of valproic acid. Increased toxicity of beta blockers, chloroquine, quinine, quinidine.

Relative Infant Dose: 0.1%–0.2%

Adult Dose: 1.25 gm once OR 250 mg every week.

Alternatives:

References:
1. Pharmaceutical manufacturer prescribing information, 1995.
2. Edstein MD, Veenendaal JR, Hyslop R. Excretion of mefloquine in human breast milk. Chemotherapy 1988; 34(3): 165–169.

MEGESTROL   L3

Trade: Megace, Megace ES
Other Trades:
Category: Progestational agent.

Megestrol is a progesterone derivative indicated in the management of advanced breast and endometrial cancer, and also used in the management of cachexia associated with AIDS.[1] Currently there are no data available of its use in breastfeeding women, or of its transfer into breastmilk. However, being a progesterone derivative, its effects are probably similar to other progestins, in that its use during lactation may suppress milk production. Early postpartum, while progestin receptors are still present in the breast, administering progestins may actually suppress milk production just as it does in the pregnant women. This has been seen occasionally in patients early postpartum. Several days to a week later, most progestin receptors disappear from the lactocyte and breast tissues become relatively immune to the effects of progestins. Thus it is advisable to wait as long as possible postpartum (at least 6–8 weeks) prior to instituting therapy with progesterone to avoid reducing the milk supply.

The direct effects of progesterone therapy on the nursing infant is generally unknown, but it is believed minimal to none as natural progesterone is poorly bioavailable to the infant via milk. Several cases of gynecomastia in infants have been reported but are extremely rare.

Pregnancy Risk	X	Lactation Risk	L3
T ½	= 34 hours	M/P	=
Vd	=	PB	=
Tmax	= 1–5 hours	Oral	=
MW	= 384.51	pKa	=

Adult Concerns: Rash, hot sweats, nausea, vomiting, diarrhea, mood swings, insomnia, impotence, rise in blood pressure, exacerbation of pre-existing diabetes are some of the more commonly reported side-effects. Severe and rare side-effects include anemia, venous thrombosis, adrenal insufficiency and pulmonary embolism.

Pediatric Concerns:

Drug Interactions: Contra-indicated with dofetilide due to increased risk of cardiac arrhythmias and cardiac arrest.

Relative Infant Dose:

Adult Dose: 400–800 mg per day.

Alternatives:

References:
1. Pharmaceutical manufacturer prescribing information, 2011.

MELATONIN   L3

Trade:

Other Trades:

Category: Hormone

Melatonin (N-acetyl-5-methoxytryptamine) is a normal hormone secreted by the pineal gland in the human brain. It is circadian in rhythm, with nighttime values considerably higher than daytime levels. It is postulated to induce a sleep-like pattern in humans. It is known to be passed into human milk and is believed responsible for entraining the newborn brain to phase shift its circadian clock to that of the mother by communicating the time of day information to the newborn.

On the average, the amount of melatonin in human milk is about 35% of the maternal plasma level but can range to as high as 80%.[1] Post feeding milk levels appear to more closely reflect the maternal plasma level than pre-feeding values, suggesting that melatonin may be transported into milk at night, during the feeding, rather than being stored in foremilk. In neonates, melatonin levels are low and progressively increase up to the age of 3 months when the characteristic diurnal rhythm is detectable.[2] Night-time melatonin levels reach a maximum at the age of 1–3 years and thereafter decline to adult values.[3,4,5] While night-time maternal serum levels average 280 pmol/L, milk levels averaged 99 pmol/L in a group of ten breastfeeding mothers.[1] The effect of orally administered melatonin on newborns is unknown, but melatonin has thus far not been associated with significant untoward effects.

Pregnancy Risk	C	Lactation Risk	L3
T ½	= 30–50 minutes	M/P	= 0.35–0.8
Vd	=	PB	=
Tmax	= 0.5–2 hours	Oral	= Complete
MW	= 232	pKa	=

Adult Concerns: Headache and confusion, drowsiness, fatigue, hypothermia, and dysphoria in depressed patients.

Pediatric Concerns: None reported.

Drug Interactions:

Relative Infant Dose:

Adult Dose:

Alternatives:

References:

1. Illnerova H, Buresova M, Presl J. Melatonin rhythm in human milk. J Clin Endocrinol Metab 1993; 77(3): 838–841.
2. Hartmann L, Roger M, Lemaitre BJ, Massias JF, Chaussain JL. Plasma and urinary melatonin in male infants during the first 12 months of life. Clin Chim Acta 1982; 121(1): 37–42.
3. Aldhous M, Franey C, Wright J, Arendt J. Plasma concentrations of melatonin in man following oral absorption of different preparations. Br J Clin Pharmacol 1985; 19(4): 517–521.
4. Attanasio A, Rager K, Gupta D. Ontogeny of circadian rhythmicity for melatonin, serotonin, and N-acetylserotonin in humans. J Pineal Res 1986; 3(3): 251–256.
5. Dollins AB, Lynch HJ, Wurtman RJ, Deng MH, Kischka KU, Gleason RE, Lieberman HR. Effect of pharmacological daytime doses of melatonin on human mood and performance. Psychopharmacology (Berl) 1993; 112(4): 490–496.

MELOXICAM   L3

Trade: Mobic

Other Trades: Mobic

Category: Nonsteroidal anti-inflammatory agent

Meloxicam is a nonsteroidal anti-inflammatory drug that appears more selective for the COX-2 receptors.[1] No data are available for transfer into human milk although it does transfer into rodent milk. Due to its long half-life and good bioavailability, another NSAID would probably be preferred.

Pregnancy Risk	C/D in 3rd trimester	Lactation Risk	L3
T ½	= 20.1 hours	M/P	=
Vd	= 0.14 l/kg	PB	= 99.4
Tmax	= 4.9 hours	Oral	= 89%
MW	= 351	pKa	= 4.2

Adult Concerns: Leukopenia, elevated liver enzymes, headache, abdominal pain, constipation, diarrhea, angina, anaphylaxis in aspirin sensitive patients.

Pediatric Concerns: None reported via milk.

Drug Interactions: May reduce coagulation in patients using anticoagulants and other platelet inhibitory drugs. NSAIDs may decrease the antihypertensive effect of ACE inhibitors. May increase blood pressure in hypertensive patients using beta blockers and other antihypertensives. May increase risk of gastric hemorrhage with calcium channel blockers. Numerous other drug-drug interactions listed, consult another text.

Relative Infant Dose:

Adult Dose: 7.5 mg/day

Alternatives: Ibuprofen, naproxen

References:
1. Pharmaceutical manufacturer prescribing information, 2002.

MELPHALAN   L5

Trade: Alkeran
Other Trades:
Category: Anticancer drug

Melphalan is an alkylating agent used in the treatment of multiple myeloma, rhabdomyosarcoma, and carcinoma of the ovary. Oral bioavailability in adults averages 61%, but it is highly variable by patient and even ranges from 9–58% in some patients.[1] Due to the wide variability, it is the most commonly used intravenously at higher doses. The terminal elimination half-life is 1.5 hours but can vary to as high as three hours. Penetration into CNS fluid is low. No data are available on its transfer to human milk, but levels are probably quite low. Mothers should be advised to withhold breastfeeding for at least 24 hours following treatment.

Pregnancy Risk	D	Lactation Risk	L5
T ½	= 1.5 hours	M/P	=
Vd	= 0.5 l/kg	PB	= 60%-90%
Tmax	=	Oral	=
MW	= 305.2	pKa	= 2.5

Adult Concerns: Nausea, vomiting, myelosuppression, secondary malignancy, hypersensitivity, thrombocytopenia, leukopenia.

Pediatric Concerns:

Drug Interactions:

Relative Infant Dose:

Adult Dose: 16 mg/m² IV.

Alternatives:

References:
1. Pharmaceutical manufacturer prescribing information, 2005.

MEMANTINE   L3

Trade: Namenda
Other Trades: Ebixa
Category: NMDA Receptor Antagonist

Memantine is used to treat moderate to severe dementia associated with Alzheimer's disease.[1] It blocks NMDA receptors, blocking glutamate from exciting the neuronal cells. The over-excitation of NMDA receptors is postulated to contribute to the disease. It binds to the magnesium binding site for longer periods of time than magnesium, causing receptor blockade under excessive stimulation. There are no data available on the transfer of memantine into human milk, but due to the large volume of distribution, it is unlikely that it would transfer to any measurable extent.

Pregnancy Risk	B	Lactation Risk	L3
T ½	= 60–80 hours	M/P	=
Vd	= 9–11 l/kg	PB	= 45%
Tmax	= 3–7 hours	Oral	= Complete
MW	= 216	pKa	= 10.27

Adult Concerns: Adverse reactions seen include hypertension, dizziness, confusion, headache, constipation, vomiting, and cough.

Pediatric Concerns: No data are available.

Drug Interactions:

Relative Infant Dose:

Adult Dose: 20 mg/day

Alternatives:

References:
1. Pharmaceutical manufacturer prescribing information, 2007.

MENINGOCOCCAL VACCINE   L1

Trade: Menomune (MPSV4), Menveo (MODC), Menactra (MCV4)
Other Trades:
Category: Vaccine

Meningococcal polysaccharide vaccine is a freeze-dried preparation of group-specific antigens from *Neisseria meningitidis*.[1] This vaccine is not infectious and is useful in preventing endemic and epidemic meningitis and meningococcemia in children and young adults. There are no contraindications for using this in breastfeeding mothers other than allergic hypersensitivity to some of the ingredients.

The vaccines currently recommended for use in USA are Menactra, Menveo and Menomune. While menveo and menomune are indicated for prevention of invasive meningococcal disease caused by *Neisseria meningitidis* in those aged 2–55 years, Menactra is used for the same indication in ages ranging from 9 months to 55 years.

Pregnancy Risk	C		Lactation Risk	L1
T ½	=		M/P	=
Vd	=		PB	=
Tmax	=		Oral	=
MW	=		pKa	=

Adult Concerns: Pain, erythema, induration at injection site. Headaches, malaise, chills and elevated temperature have been reported.

Pediatric Concerns: None via milk.

Drug Interactions:

Relative Infant Dose:

Adult Dose: 0.5 mL subcutaneously

Alternatives:

References:
1. Pharmaceutical manufacturer prescribing information, 2003.

MENOTROPINS　　　　　　　　　L3

Trade: Pergonal, Humegon, Repronex, Menopur
Other Trades: Pergonal, Humegon
Category: Produces follicle growth

Menotropins is a purified preparation of gonadotropin hormones extracted from the urine of postmenopausal women. It is a biologically standardized form containing equal activity of follicle stimulating hormone (FSH) and luteinizing hormone (LH).[1-3] Menotropins and human chorionic gonadotropins (see chorionic gonadotropins) are given sequentially to induce ovulation in the anovulatory female. FSH and LH are large molecular weight peptides and would not likely penetrate into human milk. Further, they are unstable in the gastrointestinal tract and their oral bioavailability would be minimal to zero even in an infant.

Pregnancy Risk	X	Lactation Risk	L3
T ½	= 3.9 and 70.4 hours	M/P	=
Vd	= 1.08 l/kg	PB	=
Tmax	= 6 hours	Oral	= Nil
MW	= 34,000	pKa	=

Adult Concerns: Ovarian enlargement, cysts, hemoperitoneum, fever, chills, aches, joint pains, nausea, vomiting, abdominal pain, diarrhea, bloating, rash, dizziness.

Pediatric Concerns: None reported via milk. These agents are very unlikely to enter milk. But observe closely for changes in milk production which could occur.

Drug Interactions:

Relative Infant Dose:

Adult Dose: 75–150 units each FSH and LH daily

Alternatives:

References:
1. Sharma V, Riddle A, Mason B, Whitehead M, Collins W. Studies on folliculogenesis and *in vitro* fertilization outcome after the administration of follicle-stimulating hormone at different times during the menstrual cycle. Fertil Steril 1989; 51(2): 298–303.
2. Kjeld JM, Harsoulis P, Kuku SF, Marshall JC, Kaufman B, Fraser TR. Infusions of hFSH and hLH in normal men. I. Kinetics of human follicle stimulating hormone. Acta Endocrinol (Copenh) 1976; 81(2): 225–233.
3. Yen SC, Llerena LA, Pearson OH, Littell AS. Disappearance rates of endogenous follicle-stimulating hormone in serum following surgical hypophysectomy in man. J Clin Endocrinol Metab 1970; 30(3): 325–329.

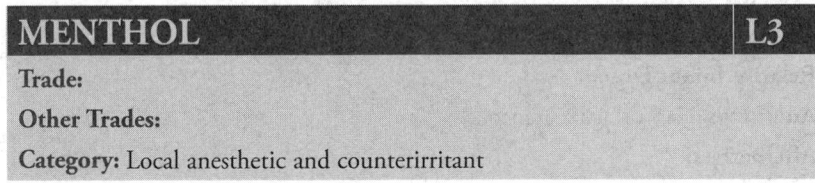

MENTHOL   L3

Trade:

Other Trades:

Category: Local anesthetic and counterirritant

Menthol is commonly used for topical analgesic and sore throat relief. Only a limited amount of menthol is absorbed systemically from topical application. Application of 300 mg of topical menthol patches produces maximum plasma concentration of 36 ng/mL.[1] Menthol is metabolized rapidly at first-pass metabolism to menthol glucuronide. Only minimal amounts of menthol would be transferred into breastmilk. According to one source, only 0.063% of the maternal dose is transferred into breastmilk.[2] Adverse effects to infant from breastfeeding are unlikely due to low relative dose and first-pass metabolism. There are no adequate and well-controlled studies in breastfeeding women.[3]

Pregnancy Risk	Probably Safe	Lactation Risk	L3
T ½	= 3–6 hours (topical)	M/P	=
Vd	=	PB	=
Tmax	= 3.4 hours (topical)	Oral	=
MW	= 156	pKa	=

Adult Concerns: Contact dermatitis. If ingested may cause nausea, vomiting, abdominal pain, drowsiness, ataxia.

Pediatric Concerns:

Drug Interactions:

Relative Infant Dose: 0.06%

Adult Dose:

Alternatives:

References:
1. Martin D, Valdez J, Boren J, Mayersohn M. Dermal absorption of camphor, menthol, and methyl salicylate in humans. J Clin Pharmacol. 2004 Oct; 44(10): 1151–7.

2. Hausner H, Bredie WL, Mⱱ∏lgaard C, Petersen MA, Mⱱ∏ller P. Differential transfer of dietary flavour compounds into human breast milk. Physiol Behav. 2008 Sep 3; 95(1–2): 118–24. Epub 2008 May 15.
3. Menthol. In: TERIS Æ Database [Internet database]. Greenwood Village, Colo: Thomson Reuters (Healthcare) Inc. Updated periodically. Accessed 07/06/2011.

MEPERIDINE   L3

Trade: Demerol
Other Trades: Pethidine, Demerol
Category: Narcotic analgesic

Meperidine is a potent opiate analgesic. It is rapidly and completely metabolized by the adult and neonatal liver to an active form, normeperidine. Significant but small amounts of meperidine are secreted into breast milk. In a study of 9 nursing mothers two hours after a 50 mg IM injection, the average concentration of meperidine in milk was 82 µg/L and a milk/plasma ratio of 1.12.[1] The highest concentration of meperidine in breastmilk at 2 hours after dose was 0.13 mg/L. In another study, the maximum concentration of meperidine in milk ranged from 134 to 244 µg/L in 5 patients at 1–2 hours after administration and 76 to 318 µg/L at 2–4 hours after administration of 25 mg intravenously (in 3 patients).[2] According to these authors, the maximum dose to an infant would be approximately 9.5 µg/kg or 1.2% to 3.5% of the weight-adjusted maternal dose. In a study of two nursing mothers who received varying amounts of meperidine following delivery (up to 1275 mg within 72 hours), the levels in milk of meperidine ranged from 36.2 to 314 µg/L with an average of 225 µg/L. Breastmilk levels of normeperidine ranged from zero to 333 µg/L with an average of 142 µg/L.[3] This study clearly shows a much longer half-life for the active metabolite, normeperidine. Normeperidine levels were detected after 56 hours post-administration in human milk (8.1 ng/mL) following a single 50 mg dose. The milk/plasma ratios varied from 0.82 to 1.59 depending on dose and timing of sampling.

In a recent study, the lactational exposure to epidural meperidine was assessed in the infants of 20 postpartum women who received a mean dose of 670 mg over 41 hours for post-cesarean pain relief.[4] Maternal plasma, infant plasma and breastmilk samples were obtained within 2 hours of cessation of meperidine administration. A second sample was obtained 6 hours later. The combined relative infant dose (RID) for both meperidine and its metabolite normeperidine at the first sampling time was 1.4%, which decreased to 0.9% within 6 hours; giving an overall mean RID of 1.65%. When meperidine and normeperidine concentrations in milk were considered independently, the mean RID for meperidine was 0.5%, while that for normeperidine was 0.65%. Therefore, at all times during the study period, the corresponding RIDs for meperidine and normeperidine remained within acceptable limits. No untoward effects were reported in the breastfed infants. Although the women in this study experienced adequate analgesia, the maternal plasma concentrations of the drug were well below the minimum effective plasma concentration required to provide clinical analgesia. This suggests that the analgesic effect of epidural meperidine is primarily local with little systemic absorption. No untoward effects were noted in the infants during the period of this study.

Published half-lives for meperidine in neonates (13 hours) and normeperidine (63 hours) are long and with time could concentrate in the plasma of a neonate. Wittels' studies[5] clearly indicate that infants from mothers treated with meperidine (post-cesarean) were neurobehaviorally depressed after three days. Infants from similar groups treated with morphine were not similarly affected.

Pregnancy Risk	C	Lactation Risk	L3
T ½	= 3.2 hours	M/P	= 0.84–1.59
Vd	= 3.7–4.2 l/kg	PB	= 65–80%
Tmax	= 30–50 minutes (IM)	Oral	= <50%
MW	= 247	pKa	= 8.6

Adult Concerns: Sedation, respiratory depression.

Pediatric Concerns: Sedation, poor suckling reflex, neurobehavioral delay.

Drug Interactions: Phenytoin may decrease analgesic effect. Meperidine may aggravate adverse effects of isoniazid. Monoamine oxidase inhibitors, fluoxetine and other SSRIs, and tricyclic antidepressants may greatly potentiate the effects of meperidine.

Relative Infant Dose: 1.1%–13.3%

Adult Dose: 50–100 mg every 3–4 hours PRN

Alternatives: Morphine, fentanyl, hydrocodone

References:
1. Peiker G, Muller B, Ihn W, Noschel H. [Excretion of pethidine in mother's milk (author's transl)]. Zentralbl Gynakol 1980; 102(10): 537–541.
2. Borgatta L, Jenny RW, Gruss L, Ong C, Barad D. Clinical significance of methohexital, meperidine, and diazepam in breast milk. J Clin Pharmacol 1997; 37(3): 186–192.
3. Quinn PG, Kuhnert BR, Kaine CJ, Syracuse CD. Measurement of meperidine and normeperidine in human breast milk by selected ion monitoring. Biomed Environ Mass Spectrom 1986; 13(3): 133–135.
4. Al-Tamimi Y, Ilett KF, Paech MJ, O'Halloran SJ, Hartmann PE. Estimation of infant dose and exposure to pethidine and norpethidine via breast milk following patient-controlled epidural pethidine for analgesia post caesarean delivery. Int J Obstet Anesth. 2011 Apr; 20(2): 128–34.
5. Wittels B, Scott DT, Sinatra RS. Exogenous opioids in human breast milk and acute neonatal neurobehavior: a preliminary study. Anesthesiology 1990; 73(5): 864–869.

MEPINDOLOL SULFATE   L2

Trade:

Other Trades: Corindolan

Category: Non-specific beta blocker

Mepindolol is a non-selective beta receptor blocking agent. In a study of 5 women (day 3 postpartum) who received 20 mg daily for 5 days, the concentrations of mepindolol in plasma and milk of five breastfeeding mothers were determined on day 1 and after 5 daily doses of mepindolol sulfate 20 mg.[1] In the newborns, plasma levels were measured once on the first and fifth days of the study. The mean maternal plasma concentration of mepindolol 2 hours after administration was 52 µg/L both after 1 and 5 doses. Average milk concentrations of mepindolol were 18 µg/L after one dose, and 22 µg/L after 5 daily doses. The average milk/plasma ratio was 0.4. Plasma levels in the newborn were below the detection limit of 1 μg/L, except for one baby in whom 2 and 5 μg/L were measured. The relative infant dose would be 1.1% of the maternal dose. No drug-related side effects were noted in these 5 infants.

Pregnancy Risk	C/D in 2nd and 3rd trimester	Lactation Risk	L2
T ½	= 3–4 hours	M/P	= <0.4
Vd	= 5.7 l/kg	PB	= 50%
Tmax	= 1–3 hours	Oral	= >95%
MW	=	pKa	=

Adult Concerns: Bradycardia, asthmatic symptoms, hypotension, sedation, weakness, hypoglycemia.

Pediatric Concerns: None reported in one study of 5 breastfed infants.

Drug Interactions: Beta blockers may reduce the effect of oral sulfonylureas (hypoglycemic agents). Increased toxicity/effect when used with other antihypertensives, contraceptives, monoamine oxidase inhibitors, cimetidine, and numerous other products. See drug interaction reference for complete listing.

Relative Infant Dose: 1%

Adult Dose: 20 mg daily.

Alternatives: Propranolol, metoprolol

References:
1. Krause W, Stoppelli I, Milia S, Rainer E. Transfer of mepindolol to newborns by breast-feeding mothers after single and repeated daily doses. Eur J Clin Pharmacol 1982; 22(1): 53–55.

MEPIVACAINE   L3

Trade: Carbocaine, Polocaine

Other Trades: Carbocaine, Polocaine

Category: Local anesthetic

Mepivacaine is a long acting local anesthetic similar to bupivacaine.[1-3] Mepivacaine is used for infiltration, peripheral nerve blocks, and central nerve blocks (epidural or caudal anesthesia). No data are available on the transfer of mepivacaine into human milk; however, its structure is practically identical to bupivacaine and one would expect its entry into human milk is similar and low. Bupivacaine enters milk in exceedingly low levels (see bupivacaine below). Due to higher fetal levels and reported toxicities, mepivacaine is never used antenatally. For use in breastfeeding patients, bupivacaine is preferred.

Bupivacaine is the most commonly employed regional anesthetic used in delivery because its concentrations in the fetus are the least of the local anesthetics. In one study of five patients, levels of bupivacaine in breastmilk were below the limits of detection (<0.02 mg/L).[4] In another study of 27 patients who received an average 82.1 mg bupivacaine via an epidural catheter,[5] the levels of bupivacaine in milk were low with a milk/serum ratio of 0.34. Most of the infants had a maximal

730   Medications and Mothers' Milk 2012

APGAR score. Bupivacaine transfer into milk is negligible. When it is used early postpartum, the minimal amount of milk secreted (30 cc/day) and the limited amount present in milk, would all but preclude any toxicity in an infant. The infant is exposed to more in utero than via milk.

Pregnancy Risk	C	Lactation Risk	L3
T ½	= 1.9–3.2 hours	M/P	=
Vd	=	PB	= 60–85%
Tmax	= 30 minutes	Oral	=
MW	= 246	pKa	= 7.6

Adult Concerns: Sedation, bradycardia, respiratory sedation, transient burning, anaphylaxis.

Pediatric Concerns: None reported via milk. Neonatal depression and convulsive seizures occurred in 7 neonates 6 hours after delivery.

Drug Interactions: Increases effect of hyaluronidase, beta blockers, monoamine oxidase inhibitors, tricyclic antidepressants, phenothiazines, and vasopressors.

Relative Infant Dose:

Adult Dose: 50–300 mg X 1

Alternatives:

References:
1. Pharmaceutical manufacturer prescribing information, 1997.
2. Hillman LS, Hillman RE, Dodson WE. Diagnosis, treatment, and follow-up of neonatal mepivacaine intoxication secondary to paracervical and pudendal blocks during labor. J Pediatr 1979; 95(3): 472–477.
3. Teramo K, Rajamaki A. Foetal and maternal plasma levels of mepivacaine and foetal acid-base balance and heart rate after paracervical block during labour. Br J Anaesth 1971; 43(4): 300–312.
4. Naulty JS. Bupivacaine in breast milk following epidural anesthesia for vaginal delivery. Regional Anesthesia 1983; 8(1): 44–45.
5. Ortega D, Viviand X, Lorec AM, Gamerre M, Martin C, Bruguerolle B. Excretion of lidocaine and bupivacaine in breast milk following epidural anesthesia for cesarean delivery. Acta Anaesthesiol Scand 1999; 43(4): 394–397.

MEPROBAMATE   L3

Trade: Equanil, Miltown

Other Trades: Equanil, Novo-Mepro, Apo-Meprobamate, Meprate

Category: Antianxiety drug

Meprobamate is an older antianxiety drug.[1] It is secreted into milk at levels 2–4 times that of the maternal plasma level.[2] It could produce some sedation in a breastfeeding infant. Avoid in lactating mothers.

Pregnancy Risk	D	Lactation Risk	L3
T ½	= 6–17 hours	M/P	= 2–4
Vd	= 0.7 l/kg	PB	= 15%
Tmax	= 1–3 hours	Oral	= Complete
MW	= 218	pKa	= 13.09

Adult Concerns: Blood dyscrasias, sedation, hypotension, withdrawal reactions.

Pediatric Concerns: None reported, but observe for sedation.

Drug Interactions: May have increased CNS depression when used with other neuroleptic depressants.

Relative Infant Dose:

Adult Dose: 300–400 mg 3 to 4 times daily.

Alternatives: Lorazepam, alprazolam

References:

1. Pharmaceutical manufacturer prescribing information, 1993.
2. Wilson JT, Brown RD, Cherek DR, Dailey JW, Hilman B, Jobe PC, Manno BR, Manno JE, Redetzki HM, Stewart JJ. Drug excretion in human breast milk: principles, pharmacokinetics and projected consequences. Clin Pharmacokinet 1980; 5(1): 1–66.

MERBROMIN   L4

Trade: Mercurochrome, Asceptichrome, Supercrome, Brocasept, Cinfacromin

Other Trades:

Category: Topical antiseptic

Merbromin is a topical antiseptic that contains mercury as a topical antiseptic. It is not available in United States due to its mercury content. There are no controlled studies in breastfeeding women and the topical absorption of mercury with this product is probably quite low. However mercury poisoning produces encephalopathy, acute renal failure, severe gastrointestinal necrosis, and numerous other systemic toxicities, particularly in infants and it is not a suitable antiseptic for use today. Mercury transfers into human milk with a milk/plasma ratio that varies according to the mercury form. Pitkin reports that in the USA, 100 unexposed women had 0.9 μg/L total mercury in their milk.[1] Mothers known to be contaminated with mercury should not breastfeed.

Pregnancy Risk	Hazardous	Lactation Risk	L4
T ½	=	M/P	=
Vd	=	PB	=
Tmax	=	Oral	=
MW	=	pKa	=

Adult Concerns: Staining of skin, contact dermatitis.

Pediatric Concerns:

Drug Interactions:

Relative Infant Dose:

Adult Dose:

Alternatives:

References:
1. Pitkin RM, Bahns JA, Filer LJ, Reynolds WA. Mercury in human maternal and cord blood, placenta, and milk. Proc Soc Exp Med 1976; 151: 65–567.

MERCAPTOPURINE   L3

Trade: Purinethol, 6–MP

Other Trades: Purinethol, Puri-Nethol

Category: Antimetabolite, immunosuppressant

6–Mercaptopurine (6–MP) is an anticancer and immunosuppressant drug that acts intracellularly as a purine antagonist, ultimately inhibiting DNA and RNA synthesis.[1] It is commonly used to treat Crohn's disease and ulcerative colitis due to its immunosuppressant effect. The drug azathioprine is metabolized to 6–Mercaptopurine, so both are essentially identical. Numerous breastfeeding studies are available with respect to azathioprine and 6–MP.

In two mothers receiving 75 mg azathioprine, the concentration of 6–MP in milk varied from 3.5–4.5 µg/L in one mother and 18 µg/L in the second mother.[2] Both levels were peak milk concentrations at 2 hours following the dose. The authors conclude that these levels would be too low to produce clinical effects in a breastfed infant. Using this data for 6–MP, an infant would absorb only 0.1% of the weight-adjusted maternal dose, which is probably too low to produce adverse effects in a breastfeeding infant. Plasma levels in treated patients is maintained at 50 ng/mL or higher. One infant continued to breastfeed during therapy and displayed no immunosuppressive effects. In another study of two infants who were breastfed by mothers receiving 75–100 mg/day azathioprine, milk levels of 6–MP were not measured. But both infants had normal blood counts, no increase in infections, and above-average growth rate.[3]

Four mothers who were receiving 1.2–2.1 mg/kg/day of azathioprine throughout pregnancy and continued postpartum were studied while breastfeeding. The mothers' blood concentrations of 6–TGN and 6–MMPN (the metabolites of azathioprine) ranged from 234–291 and 284 to 1178 pmol/100 million RBC, respectively. Neither 6–TGN nor 6–MMPN could be detected in the exposed infants. The authors suggest that breastfeeding while taking azathioprine may be safe in mothers with 'normal' TPMT enzyme activity (the enzyme responsible for metabolizing 6–TGN).[4]

Four case reports were performed with mothers taking between 50 to 100 mg/day of azathioprine. No adverse events were reported in any of the infants, and milk concentrations in two mothers proved to be undetectable.[5] Ten women at steady state on 75 to 150 mg/day azathioprine provided milk samples on days 3–4, days 7–10 and day 28 after delivery, between 3 and 18 hours after azathioprine administration. 6–MP was detected in only one case, at 1.2 and 7.6 ng/mL at 3 and 6 hours after azathioprine intake on day 28. However, 6–MP and 6–TGN were undetectable in the infants' blood. There were no signs of immunosuppression, even in three preterm neonates. The authors suggest that azathioprine therapy should not deter mothers from breastfeeding.[6] Another study of three mothers taking azathioprine while breastfeeding (doses of 100–175 mg) reported normal blood cell counts in all three infants, and only a low amount of 6–TGN in one infant on day 3. At age 3 weeks, this level decreased below the detectable range.[7] In a group of 8 lactating women who received azathioprine (75–200 mg/day), levels in milk ranged from 2–50 μg/L.[8] After 6 hours an average of 10% of the peak values were measured. The authors estimate the infants' dose to be <0.008 mg/kg/24 hours. They suggest that breastfeeding during treatment with azathioprine seems safe and should be recommended. In a 31-year-old mother with Crohn's disease being treated with 100 mg/day azathioprine, peripheral blood levels of 6–MP and 6–TGN in the infant were undetectable at day 8 or after 3 months of therapy.[9] The infant was reported to be normal after 6 months.In a recent study of the long-term follow up (median 3.3 years) of fetal and breastfeeding exposure to azathioprine (n = 11 infants), there were no differences in rates of infectious disease in azathioprine-treated groups compared to non-treated controls. The authors suggest that breastfeeding following exposure to azathioprine does not increase the risk of infections.[10]

In summary, the transport of 6-mercaptopurine into human milk is apparently quite low. However, this is a strong immunosuppressant and some caution is still recommended if it is used in a breastfeeding mother. Monitor the infant closely for signs of immunosuppression, leukopenia, thrombocytopenia, hepatotoxicity, pancreatitis, and other symptoms of 6-mercaptopurine exposure. The risks to the infant are probably low. Recent long-term data suggest that the rate of infections in treated groups is no different from non-treated controls.

Pregnancy Risk	D	Lactation Risk	L3
T ½	= 21–90 minutes	M/P	=
Vd	= 0.9 l/kg	PB	= 19%
Tmax	= 2 hours	Oral	= 50%
MW	= 170	pKa	= 7.6

Adult Concerns: Bone marrow suppression, liver toxicity, nausea, vomiting, diarrhea.

Pediatric Concerns: No data are available on 6–MP, but data on azathioprine has been published.

Drug Interactions: When used with allopurinol, reduce mercaptopurine to ⅓rd to ¼th the usual dose. When used with trimethoprim+sulfamethoxazole, may enhance bone marrow suppression. It is best to avoid the following drugs when using mercaptopurine or azathioprine: neuromuscular blocking agents (such as rocuronium, mivacurium, vercuronium, atracurium, tubocurarine), warfarin, d-penicillamine, co-trimoxazole, captopril, cimetidine, indomethacin and live vaccines.

Relative Infant Dose:

Adult Dose: 1.5–2.5 mg/kg daily

Alternatives: Infliximab

References:

1. Pharmaceutical manufacturer prescribing information, 1995.
2. Coulam CB, Moyer TP, Jiang NS, Zincke H. Breast-feeding after renal transplantation. Transplant Proc 1982; 14(3): 605–609.
3. Grekas DM, Vasiliou SS, Lazarides AN. Immunosuppressive therapy and breast-feeding after renal transplantation. Nephron 1984; 37(1): 68.
4. Gardiner SJ, Gearry RB, Roberts RL, Zhang M, Barclay ML, Begg EJ. Exposure to thiopurine drugs through breast milk is low based on metabolite concentrations in mother-infant pairs. Br J Clin Pharmacol 2006; 62(4): 453–456.
5. Moretti ME, Verjee Z, Ito S, Koren G. Breast-Feeding During Maternal Use of Azathioprine. Ann Pharmacother 2006; 40: 2269–2272.
6. Sau A, Clarke S, Bass J, Kaiser A, Marinaki A, Nelson-Piercy C. Azathioprine and breastfeeding-is it safe? BJOG 2007; 114: 498–501.
7. Bernard N, Garayt C, Chol F, Vial T, Descotes J. Prospective clinical and biological follow-up of three breastfed babies from azathioprine-treated mothers. Fundam clin Pharmacol 2007; 21 (suppl.1): 62–63. Abstract.
8. Christensen LA, Dahlerup JF, Nielsen MJ, Fallingborg JF, Schmiegelow K. Azathioprine treatment during lactation. Aliment Pharmacol Ther. 2008 Nov 15; 28(10): 1209–13. Epub 2008 Aug 30.
9. Zelinkova Z, De Boer IP, Van Dijke MJ, Kuipers EJ, Van Der Woude CJ. Azathioprine treatment during lactation. Aliment Pharmacol Ther. 2009 Jul; 30(1): 90–1;
10. Angelberger S, Reinisch W, Messerschmidt A, Miehsler W, Novacek G, Vogelsang H, Dejaco C. Long-term follow-up of babies exposed to azathioprine in utero and via breastfeeding. J Crohns Colitis. 2011 Apr; 5(2): 95–100. Epub 2010 Dec 9.

MERCURY   L5

Trade: Mercury

Other Trades:

Category: Environmental contaminate

Mercury is an environmental contaminate that is available in multiple salt forms. Elemental mercury, the form found in thermometers, is poorly absorbed orally (0.01%) but completely absorbed via inhalation (>80%).[1] Inorganic mercury causes most forms of mercury poisoning and is available in mercury disk batteries (7–15% orally bioavailable). Organic mercury (methyl mercury fungicides, phenyl mercury) is readily absorbed (90% orally). Mercury poisoning produces encephalopathy, acute renal failure, severe GI necrosis, and numerous other systemic toxicities. Mercury transfers into human milk with a milk/plasma ratio that varies according to the mercury form. Pitkin reports that in the USA that 100 unexposed women had 0.9 µg/L total mercury in their milk.[2] Concentrations of mercury in human milk are generally much higher in populations that ingest large quantities of fish. Mothers known to be contaminated with mercury should not breastfeed.

The transfer of mercury from dental amalgams has been studied to some degree. In mothers with mercury-containing amalgams, the transfer of mercury during gestation to the fetus is generally much higher than from human milk.[3,4] Mercury levels in milk are highest immediately after birth, and these are significantly correlated with the number and size of amalgam fillings present in the mother[5,6], although others disagree.[7] In this study breast milk levels of mercury dropped significantly after 2 months and are more positively associated with the amount of fish ingested, rather than the number of amalgam fillings. At birth mercury levels in milk averaged 0.9 µg/L (0.25 to 20.3 µg/L) and after two months mercury levels averaged 0.25 µg/L (0.25–11.7 µg/L). The authors suggest that the exposure to mercury of breastfed infants from maternal amalgam fillings is of minor importance compared to maternal fish consumption.

Oskarsson suggests in a study of Swedish women, that the exposure of the infant to mercury from breast milk was less than 0.3 µg/kg/d. This exposure is only approximately one-half the tolerable daily intake for adults recommended by the World Health Organization.[6]

These studies generally conclude that while mercury fillings may increase the transfer of mercury to the infant, most occurs in utero. Secondly, the transfer of mercury into human milk is transiently high at birth and then drops significantly at 2 months. Apparently the diet provides the greatest source of maternal mercury to human milk, much less is provided by older amalgam fillings. Further, the replacement of amalgam fillings should if possible be postponed until after pregnancy, and breastfeeding as the removal of amalgam fillings while breastfeeding could potentially increase the transfer of mercury to the breastfed infant and largely (this largely depends on the precautions taken by the dentist).

There are several routine precautions that the dentist could use when removing the old amalgam. Because heat during the grinding process can vaporize the mercury and enhance absorption by the mother, suggest that the dentist use copious amounts of cold water irrigation to minimize heat, use a rubber dam to isolate her mouth from the particles, and use an alternate source of air (oxygen) to minimize mercury vapor inhalation during removal of the amalgam.

While the USA has removed methylmercury from virtually all pediatric immunizations, other countries have not. In infants receiving three doses of hepatitis B vaccine and three DTP vaccines during the first 6 months of life, the exposure to ethylmercury was 25 µg Hg for each vaccine. Infant hair-Hg increased 446% during these six months, while maternal hair-Hg decreased 57%. This provides evidence that the extra mercury exposure is due to the vaccinations rather than maternal milk.[8]

The new Compact fluorescent light bulbs commonly in use today contain only 5 mg of mercury. This is 1/100 of the amount used in a single dental amalgam. Exposure to this limited amount would not be hazardous to a breastfeeding infant.

Pregnancy Risk	Hazardous	Lactation Risk	L5
T ½	= 70 days	M/P	= 0.27 -1.0
Vd	=	PB	=
Tmax	=	Oral	= Variable
MW	= 201	pKa	=

Adult Concerns: Brain damage, acute renal failure, severe GI necrosis, and numerous other systemic toxicities.

Pediatric Concerns: Mercury transfer into milk is significant. Transfer to the infant is a function of levels in the mother. Dental amalgams provide some but not significant levels of transfer. Most mercury transfers in utero, not in milk. Mercury levels in milk drop significantly after 2 months. Caution is recommended in removing amalgams while pregnant or breastfeeding.

Drug Interactions:

Relative Infant Dose:

Adult Dose:

Alternatives:

References:

1. Wofff MS. Occupationally derived chemicals in breast milk. Amer J Indust Med 1983; 4: 359–281.
2. Pickin RM, Bahns JA, Filer LJ, Reynolds WA. Mercury in human maternal and cord blood, placenta, and milk. Proc Soc Exp Med 1976; 151: 65–567.
3. Ramirez GB, Cruz MC, Pagulayan O, Ostrea E, Dalisay C. The Tagum study I: analysis and clinical correlates of mercury in maternal and cord blood, breast milk, meconium, and infants' hair. Pediatrics 2000; 106(4): 774–781.
4. Yang J, Jiang Z, Wang Y, Qureshi IA, Wu XD. Maternal-fetal transfer of metallic mercury via the placenta and milk. Ann Clin Lab Sci 1997; 27(2): 135–141
5. Drexler H, Schaller KH. The mercury concentration in breast milk resulting from amalgam fillings and dietary habits. Environ Res 1998; 77(2): 124–129.
6. Oskarsson A, Schultz A, Skerfving S, Hallen IP, Ohlin B, Lagerkvist BJ. Total and inorganic mercury in breast milk in relation to fish consumption and amalgam in lactating women. Arch Environ Health 1996; 51(3): 234–241.
7. Klemann D, Weinhold J, Strubelt O, Pentz R, Jungblut JR, Klink F. [Effects of amalgam fillings on the mercury concentrations in amniotic fluid and breast milk]. Dtsch Zahnarztl Z 1990; 45(3): 142–145.
8. Marques, RC, Dorea JG, Fonseca MF, Bastos WR, Malm O. Hair mercury in breast-fed infants exposed to thimerosal-preserved vaccines. Eur J Pediatr 2007; [Epub ahead of print].

MEROPENEM   L3

Trade: Merrem

Other Trades: Merrem, Meronem

Category: Semisynthetic carbapenem antibiotic

Meropenem is a new antibiotic similar to the older imipenem although it has greater activity against gram-negative species, but has slightly less activity against gram-positive species.[1] No data are available on its transfer into human milk but like others in this family, it is likely low. Further this agent is not orally bioavailable to any degree. Changes in gut flora could be expected in breastfed infants.

Pregnancy Risk	B	Lactation Risk	L3
T ½	= 1 hour	M/P	=
Vd	= 0.28 l/kg	PB	= 2%
Tmax	= Immediate	Oral	= Nil
MW	= 437	pKa	= 2.9, 7.8

Adult Concerns: Headache, seizures (0.5%), nausea, abdominal pain, diarrhea, and elevated liver function tests have been reported.

Pediatric Concerns: None reported via milk. Unlikely to enter milk significantly. Changes in gut flora could occur.

Drug Interactions: Increased plasma levels with probenecid.

Relative Infant Dose:

Adult Dose: 1 gm IV every 8 hours.

Alternatives: Imipenem-Cilistatin

References:
1. Pharmaceutical manufacturer prescribing information, 2003.

MESALAMINE   L3

Trade: Asacol, Pentasa, Rowasa, Canasa, Apriso, Lialda, Colazal, Balsalazide, Rowasa

Other Trades: Mesalazine, Salofalk, Mesasal, Quintasa, Asacol

Category: Anti-inflammatory in ulcerative colitis

Mesalamine or Mesalazine (UK) is an anti-inflammatory agent used in ulcerative colitis. Although it contains 5-aminosalicylic acid (5–ASA), the mechanism of action is unknown. Some 5-aminosalicylic acid can be converted into salicylic acid and absorbed, but the amount is very small. Acetyl-5-aminosalicyclic (Acetyl-5–ASA) acid is the common metabolite and has been found in breastmilk. The effect of mesalamine is primarily local on the mucosa of the colon itself. Mesalamine is poorly absorbed from the gastrointestinal tract. Only 20–30% of a dose is absorbed orally and plasma levels are exceedingly low (<2 μg/mL). Oral tablets are enteric coated for delayed absorption.

In one patient receiving 500 mg mesalamine orally three times daily, the concentration of 5–ASA in breastmilk was 0.11 mg/L, and the acetyl-5–ASA metabolite was 12.4 mg/L of milk. The milk/plasma ratio for 5–ASA was 0.27 and for acetyl-5-ASA was 5.1.[1] Using this data, the weight-adjusted relative infant dose of metabolite and active ingredient would be 8.7%. In another patient receiving 1000 mg PO three times daily, milk levels of 5-aminosalicylic acid (5–ASA) following 7 and 11 days of treatment and 5 hours following the dose were both 0.1 mg/L, and the milk/plasma ratios were 0.07 and 0.09.[2] Mesalamine is useful in patients allergic to sulfasalazine or salicylazosulfapyridine. At least one report of a watery diarrhea in an infant whose mother was using rectal 5–ASA has been reported.[3] Each time treatment was reinstated, diarrhea recurred. In a more recent study of four breastfeeding mothers ingesting mesalazine (dosage unreported), milk levels of 5–ASA ranged from 4–40 μg/L while those of its inactive metabolite, acetyl-5–ASA, were 5–14.9 mg/L. The authors did not report any complications in these breastfeeding mothers/infants.[4]

A new product, Colazal (Balsalazide), is a prodrug of mesalamine (5–ASA). Lialda is just a prolonged release formulation of mesalamine. However, its upper dosage range is 4.5 gm/day. At these newer and higher doses, some caution is recommended. Observe for gastrointestinal changes such as watery diarrhea in breastfed infants. Mesalamine administered rectally (Rowasa) is poorly absorbed systemically. About 10–30% of the administered dose can be recovered in the urine in 24 hours. However, plasma levels are exceedingly low (about 2 µg/mL or less). Breastmilk levels would be quite low as well.

Pregnancy Risk	B	Lactation Risk	L3
T ½	= 5–10 hours (metabolite)	M/P	= 0.27, 5.1
Vd	=	PB	= 55%
Tmax	= 4–12 hours	Oral	= 20–30%
MW	= 153	pKa	= 2.3, 5.69

Adult Concerns: Watery diarrhea, abdominal pain, cramps, flatulence, nausea, headache.

Pediatric Concerns: Watery diarrhea in one breastfed patient, although this appears rare.

Drug Interactions: May significantly reduce bioavailability of digoxin. Coadministration of mesalamine and azathioprine may result in an increased risk of blood disorders. Use with glyburide may increase the risk of hypoglycemia. Many more drug-drug interactions. Please check drug interaction textbook.

Relative Infant Dose: 0.1%–8.8%

Adult Dose: 800 mg three times daily.

Alternatives:

References:
1. Jenss H, Weber P, Hartmann F. 5–Aminosalicylic acid and its metabolite in breast milk during lactation. Am J Gastroenterol 1990; 85(3): 331.
2. Klotz U, Harings-Kaim A. Negligible excretion of 5-aminosalicylic acid in breast milk. Lancet 1993; 342(8871): 618–619.
3. Nelis GF. Diarrhoea due to 5-aminosalicylic acid in breast milk. Lancet 1989; 1(8634): 383.
4. Silverman DA, Ford J, Shaw I, Probert CS. Is mesalazine really safe for use in breastfeeding mothers? Gut 2005 Jan; 54(1): 170–1.

MESORIDAZINE   L4

Trade: Serentil

Other Trades: Serentil

Category: Phenothiazine antipsychotic

Mesoridazine is a typical phenothiazine antipsychotic used for treatment of schizophrenia. No data on its transfer into human milk are available.[1] However, the use of the phenothiazine family in breastfeeding mothers is risky and may increase the risk of SIDS.

Pregnancy Risk	C	Lactation Risk	L4
T ½	= 24–48 hours	M/P	=
Vd	=	PB	= 91%
Tmax	= 4 hours	Oral	= Erratic
MW	= 386	pKa	=

Adult Concerns: Adverse effects include leukopenia, eosinophilia, thrombocytopenia, anemia, aplastic anemia, hypotension, drowsiness, agitation, dystonic reactions, seizures, galactorrhea, gynecomastia, dry mouth, nausea, vomiting, constipation, priapism, incontinence, and phototoxicity.

Pediatric Concerns: None reported via milk, but use in breastfeeding mothers is discouraged due to possible sedation in infant and elevated risk of SIDS.

Drug Interactions: Decreased effect with anticonvulsants, anticholinergics. Increased toxicity when used with CNS depressants, metrizamide (increased seizures) and propranolol.

Relative Infant Dose:

Adult Dose: 25–50 mg three times daily

Alternatives: Risperidone, olanzapine, aripiprazole

References:

1. Ayd FJ. Excretion of psychotropic drugs in breast milk. In: International Drug Therapy Newsletter.Ayd Medical Communications 8[November-December]. 1973.

MESTRANOL — L3

Trade:

Other Trades:

Category: Estrogenic agent

Mestranol is a prodrug of ethinyl estradiol. Seventy percent of mestranol is converted in the liver to ethinyl estradiol. Ethinyl estradiol is an estrogenic agent. Although small amounts of estrogens may pass into breastmilk, the effects of estrogens on the infant appear minimal. In one study, ethinyl estradiol was not detected in breastmilk after administration of 50 µg/day.[1] After administration of 500 µg/day, the level in breastmilk was approximately 300 pg/mL.[1] Early postpartum use of estrogens may reduce volume of milk produced and the protein content, but it is variable, controversial, and depends on dose and the individual.[2,3,4,5] Breastfeeding mothers should attempt to wait until lactation is firmly established (6–8 weeks) prior to use of estrogen-containing oral contraceptives.

Pregnancy Risk	Hazardous	Lactation Risk	L3
T ½	=	M/P	=
Vd	=	PB	=
Tmax	=	Oral	=
MW	=	pKa	=

Adult Concerns: Observe for reduced milk production. Breakthrough bleeding is more common with this product. Fluid retention has been reported. See typical oral contraceptive contraindications.

Pediatric Concerns: Reduced milk supply is possible. Do not use early postpartum.

Drug Interactions: Concomitant use with rifampin, anticonvulsants such as phenobarbital, phenytoin, carbamazepine, antibiotics such as ampicillin, tetracycline and griseofulvin, may reduce its efficacy and result in unwanted pregnancies.

Relative Infant Dose:

Adult Dose:

Alternatives:

References:
1. Nilsson S, Nygren KG, Johansson ED. Ethinyl estradiol in human milk and plasma after oral administration. Contraception. 1978 Feb; 17(2): 131–9.
2. Booker DE, Pahl IR. Control of postpartum breast engorgement with oral contraceptives. Am J Obstet Gynecol 1967; 98(8): 1099–1101.
3. Kamal I, Hefnawi F, Ghoneim M, Abdallah M, Abdel RS. Clinical, biochemical, and experimental studies on lactation. V. Clinical effects of steroids on the initiation of lactation. Am J Obstet Gynecol 1970; 108(4): 655–658.
4. Kora SJ. Effect of oral contraceptives on lactation. Fertil Steril 1969; 20(3): 419–423.
5. Koetsawang S, Bhiraleus P, Chiemprajert T. Effects of oral contraceptives on lactation. Fertil Steril 1972; 23(1): 24–28.

MESTRANOL + NORETHYNODREL   L3

Trade: Enovid

Other Trades:

Category: Oral contraceptive agent.

Mestranol + norethynodrel is a combined oral contraceptive agent of an estrogenic agent (mestranol) with a progestin (norethynodrel).

Mestranol is an estrogenic agent and a prodrug of ethinyl estradiol. Seventy percent of it is metabolized in the liver to yield ethinyl estradiol. Ethinyl estradiol is an estrogenic agent. Although small amounts of estrogens may pass into breastmilk, the effects of estrogens on the infant appear minimal. In one study, ethinyl estradiol was not detected in breastmilk after administration of 50 μg/day.[1] After administration of 500 μg/day, the level in breastmilk was approximately 300 pg/mL.[1] Early postpartum use of estrogens may reduce volume of milk produced and the protein content, but it is variable, controversial, and depends on dose and the individual.[2,3,4,5] Breastfeeding mothers should attempt to wait until lactation is firmly established (6–8 weeks) prior to use of estrogen-containing oral contraceptives. Norethynodrel is a synthetic progestational agent used in oral contraceptives. It has limited or no effects on an infant. May decrease volume of breastmilk to some degree in some mothers if therapy initiated too soon after birth and if dose is too high.[6-8] It is advisable to wait as long as possible, preferably 6–8 weeks postpartum prior to instituting therapy with progesterone to avoid reducing the milk supply.

Breastfeeding women should be strongly advised to avoid using combination (estrogen-containing) oral contraceptives while breastfeeding because combination oral contraceptives have been shown to interfere with the production of milk and will reduce the duration of breastfeeding.[9-14] It is recommended that women wait at least 6–8 weeks postpartum to establish good milk flow, prior to beginning oral contraceptives.

Pregnancy Risk	X	Lactation Risk	L3
T ½	=	M/P	=
Vd	=	PB	=
Tmax	=	Oral	=
MW	=	pKa	=

Adult Concerns: Observe for reduced milk production. Breakthrough bleeding is more common with this product. Fluid retention has been reported. Changes in menstruation, nausea, abdominal pain, edema, breast tenderness.

Pediatric Concerns: Reduced milk supply is possible. Do not use early postpartum.

Drug Interactions: Concomitant use with rifampin, anticonvulsants such as phenobarbital, phenytoin, carbamazepine, antibiotics such as ampicillin, tetracycline and griseofulvin, may reduce its efficacy and result in unwanted pregnancies.

Relative Infant Dose:

Adult Dose: Mestranol/norethynodrel: 150 µg/9.58 mg

Alternatives:

References:

1. Nilsson S, Nygren KG, Johansson ED. Ethinyl estradiol in human milk and plasma after oral administration. Contraception. 1978 Feb; 17(2): 131–9.
2. Booker DE, Pahl IR. Control of postpartum breast engorgement with oral contraceptives. Am J Obstet Gynecol 1967; 98(8): 1099–1101.
3. Kamal I, Hefnawi F, Ghoneim M, Abdallah M, Abdel RS. Clinical, biochemical, and experimental studies on lactation. V. Clinical effects of steroids on the initiation of lactation. Am J Obstet Gynecol 1970; 108(4): 655–658.
4. Kora SJ. Effect of oral contraceptives on lactation. Fertil Steril 1969; 20(3): 419–423.
5. Koetsawang S, Bhiraleus P, Chiemprajert T. Effects of oral contraceptives on lactation. Fertil Steril 1972; 23(1): 24–28.
6. Booker DE, Pahl IR. Control of postpartum breast engorgement with oral contraceptives. Am J Obstet Gynecol 1967; 98(8): 1099–1101.
7. Laukaran VH. The effects of contraceptive use on the initiation and duration of lactation. Int J Gynaecol Obstet 1987; 25 Suppl: 129–142.
8. Kora SJ. Effect of oral contraceptives on lactation. Fertil Steril 1969; 20(3): 419–423.
9. Costa TH, Dorea JG. Concentration of fat, protein, lactose and energy in milk of mothers using hormonal contraceptives. Ann Trop Paediatr 1992; 12(2): 203–209.
10. McCann MF, Potter LS. Progestin-only oral contraception: a comprehensive review. Contraception. 1994 Dec; 50(6 Suppl 1): S1–195. Review.
11. Peralta O, D?az S, Juez G, Herreros C, Casado ME, Salvatierra AM, Miranda P, Dur?n E, Croxatto HB. Fertility regulation in nursing women: V. Long-term influence of a low-dose combined oral contraceptive initiated at day 90 postpartum upon lactation and infant growth. Contraception. 1983 Jan; 27(1): 27–38.

12. Croxatto HB, Diaz S, Peralta O, Juez G, Herreros C, Casado ME, Salvatierra AM, Miranda P, Duran E. Fertility regulation in nursing women: IV. Long-term influence of a low-dose combined oral contraceptive initiated at day 30 postpartum upon lactation and infant growth. Contraception. 1983 Jan; 27(1): 13–25.
13. Diaz S, Peralta O, Juez G, Herreros C, Casado ME, Salvatierra AM, Miranda P, Duran E, Croxatto HB. Fertility regulation in nursing women: III. Short-term influence of a low-dose combined oral contraceptive upon lactation and infant growth. Contraception. 1983 Jan; 27(1): 1–11.
14. Effects of hormonal contraceptives on breast milk composition and infant growth. World Health Organization (WHO) Task Force on Oral Contraceptives. Stud Fam Plann. 1988 Nov-Dec; 19(6 Pt 1): 361–9.

METAMIZOLE   L3

Trade: Dipyrone, Algosfar, Algozone, Analagin, Novalgin, Melubrin, Novalgina

Other Trades:

Category: Analgesic, antipyretic

Metamizole is an effective analgesic and antipyretic and was removed from the U.S. market due to serious adverse effects including agranulocytosis, aplastic anemia, thrombocytopenic purpura, and hemolytic anemia. However, it is still commonly used in many other countries. Recent analysis suggest that the risk is rather low compared to other commonly used drugs. Recent estimates suggest that the incidence rate of metamizole-induced agranulocytosis is between 0.2 and 2 cases per million person-days of use. This is lower than many commonly used drugs in the US. In one patient who took 3 doses of 500 mg orally over a 16 hour period, metamizole concentrations in mother's serum and milk and in infant's serum and urine were 3.3, 4.3 and 3.2, 3.74 µg/mL respectively.[1] Metamizole was detected in one breastfed infant's serum and urine after his mother took 1500 mg of metamizole over a 16-hour period. The infant's metamizole serum concentration was 3.2 mg/L and urine concentration was 3.74 mg/L. Two cyanotic episodes were noted in a 42 day-old infant approximately 30 minutes following the maternal dose of 1500 mg.[1] In a group of 8 women, 3–5 days postpartum, who received 1 gram doses of metamizole, milk levels of metamizole metabolites were determined between 2.5 and 5.5 hours.[2] Four metabolites were measured: 4-methylaminoantipyrine (MAA), 4-aminoantipyrine (AA), 4-formylaminoantipyrine (FAA) and 4-acetylaminoantipyrine (AAA). The sum of the mean concentrations of all four metabolites in milk was 20.37 mg/L. The mean concentration of MAA, the only active metabolite, was 11.2 µg/mL. Using the MAA data, the relative infant dose would be 1.2%. All metabolites were undetectable by 48 hours.

Because of its known complications, such as agranulocytosis and other blood dyscrasias, it is no longer recommended as an analgesic in many countries. Other safer alternatives are available. However, in severe life-threatening and refractory fever, it is a suitable antipyretic.

Pregnancy Risk	Possibly Hazardous	Lactation Risk	L3
T ½	= 2–3 hours (4–MAA)	M/P	= 1.37 (MAA)
Vd	= 0.57 l/kg	PB	= 58%
Tmax	= 1 hour	Oral	= Complete
MW	= 311	pKa	=

Adult Concerns: Metamizole was removed from the U.S. market due to serious adverse effects including agranulocytosis, aplastic anemia, thrombocytopenic purpura, and hemolytic anemia. Hypotension, skin rash, urticaria, toxic epidermal necrolysis have been reported.

Pediatric Concerns: Two cyanotic episodes were noted in a 42 day-old infant approximately 30 minutes following the maternal dose of 1500 mg.

Drug Interactions: Numerous drug-drug interactions. Reduced antihypertensive effect of beta blockers, atenolol, acebutolol, etc. Consult drug interactions text.

Relative Infant Dose: 1.2%–3%

Adult Dose: 0.5–1 gram

Alternatives: Ibuprofen, acetaminophen, ketorolac

References:

1. Rizzoni G, Furlanut M. Cyanotic crisis in a breast-fed infant from mother taking dipyrone. Hum Toxicol. 1984; 3: 505–7.
2. Zylber-Katz E, Linder N, Granit L, Levy M. Excretion of dipyrone metabolites in human breast milk. Eur J Clin Pharmacol. 1986; 30: 359–61.

METAXALONE   L3

Trade: Skelaxin

Other Trades:

Category: Sedative, skeletal muscle relaxant

Metaxalone is a centrally acting sedative used primarily as a muscle relaxant.[1] Its ability to relax skeletal muscle is weak and is probably due to its sedative properties. Hypersensitivity reactions in adults (allergic) have occurred as well as liver toxicity. No data are available on its transfer into breastmilk.

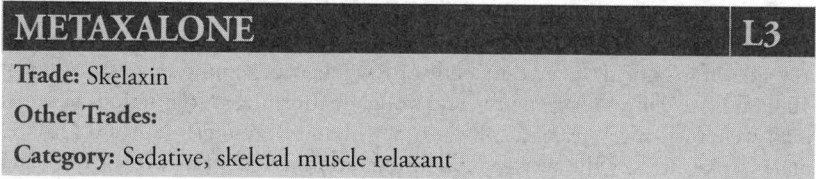

Pregnancy Risk	C	Lactation Risk	L3
T ½	= 2–3 hours	M/P	=
Vd	=	PB	=
Tmax	= 2 hours	Oral	=
MW	= 221	pKa	= 12.24

Adult Concerns: Sedation, nausea, vomiting, gastrointestinal upset, hemolytic anemia, abnormal liver function.

Pediatric Concerns: None reported. No data available.

Drug Interactions: Avoid use with other CNS depressants such as opioid analgesics, barbiturates, benzodiazepines, alcohol, chloral hydrate, kava-kava.

Relative Infant Dose:

Adult Dose: 800 mg 3–4 times daily.

Alternatives:

References:

1. Pharmaceutical manufacturer prescribing information, 1995.

METFORMIN   L1

Trade: Glucophage, Glucovance, Riomet, Glumetza

Other Trades: Diabex, Diaformin, Glucophage, Gen-Metformin, Glycon, Diguanil

Category: Oral hypoglycemic agent for diabetes

Metformin belongs to the biguanide family and is used to reduce glucose levels in non-insulin dependent diabetics. It is also used to treat polycystic ovary syndrome. Oral bioavailability is only 50%. In a study of 7 women taking metformin (median dose 1500 mg/day), the mean milk-to-plasma ratio (AUC) for metformin was 0.35.[1] The mean average concentration in milk over the dose interval was 0.27 mg/L. The absolute infant dose averaged 0.04 mg/kg/day and the mean relative infant dose was 0.28%. Metformin was present in very low or undetectable concentrations in the plasma of four of the infants who were studied. No health problems were found in the six infants who were evaluated. In another study of five subjects the median milk/plasma ratio (AUC) for metformin was 0.47.[2] The median calculated infant dose was 0.2% of the weight-adjusted maternal dose. None of the infants exposed to their mothers' milk had detectable levels of metformin in their plasma, nor were any side effects noted. In a recent study of 5 women consuming an average dose of 500 mg twice daily, the mean peak and trough metformin concentrations in breast milk were 0.42 mg/L (range 0.38–0.46 mg/L) and 0.39 mg/L (range 0.31–0.52 mg/L), respectively.[3] The average milk/serum ratio was 0.63 (range 0.36–1.00) and the estimated relative infant dose was 0.65% (range 0.43–1.08%). Blood glucose concentrations in 3 infants were normal, ranging from 47–77 mg/dL. The mothers reported no side effects were noted in the breastfed infants. In one study of 61 nursing infants whose mothers were taking a median of 2.55 gm/day throughout pregnancy and lactation, the growth, motor, and social development of the infants was recorded to be normal. The authors concluded that metformin was safe and effective during breastfeeding in the first 6 months of an infant's life.[4]

Pregnancy Risk	B	Lactation Risk	L1
T ½	= 6.2 hours (plasma)	M/P	= 0.35–0.63
Vd	= 3.7 l/kg	PB	= Minimal
Tmax	= 2.75 hours	Oral	= 50%
MW	= 129	pKa	= 12.4

Adult Concerns: Diarrhea, nausea, vomiting, bloating, lactic acidosis, hypoglycemia.

Pediatric Concerns: No side effects noted in three studies. Plasma levels undetectable.

Drug Interactions: Alcohol potentiates the effect of metformin on lactic metabolism. Cimetidine produces a 60% increase in peak metformin plasma levels. Furosemide may increase metformin plasma levels by 22%. Use of iodinated contrast material in patients receiving metformin has produced acute renal failure and been associated with lactic acidosis. Use of nifedipine increases oral bioavailability of metformin by 20%.

Relative Infant Dose: 0.3%–0.7%

Adult Dose: 500 mg twice daily.

Alternatives:

References:

1. Hale TW, Kristensen JH, Hackett LP, Kohan R, Ilett KF. Transfer of metformin into human milk. Diabetologia 2002; 45(11): 1509–1514.
2. Gardiner SJ, Kirkpatrick CM, Begg EJ, Zhang M, Moore MP, Saville DJ. Transfer of metformin into human milk. Clin Pharmacol Ther 2003; 73(1): 71–77.
3. Briggs GG, Ambrose PJ, Nageotte MP, Padilla G, Wan S. Excretion of metformin into breast milk and the effect on nursing infants. Obstet Gynecol 2005 Jun; 105(6): 1437–41.
4. Glueck CJ, Salehi M, Sieve L, Wang P. Growth, motor, and social developemnt in breast- and formula- fed infants of metformin-treated women with polycyctic ovary syndrome. J Pediatr 2006; 148: 628–632.

METFORMIN + SITAGLIPTIN   L3

Trade: Janumet

Other Trades:

Category: Anti-diabetic agent

Metformin hydrochloride and sitagliptin phosphate is a combined drug product used in the management of type 2 diabetes mellitus.[1] There are currently no studies on the transfer of this combined drug product into human milk.

Metformin belongs to the biguanide family. In a study of 7 women taking metformin (median dose 1500 mg/d), the mean milk-to-plasma ratio (AUC) for metformin was 0.35.[2] The mean average concentration in milk over the dose interval was 0.27 mg/L. The absolute infant dose averaged 0.04 mg/kg/day and the mean relative infant dose was 0.28%. Metformin was present in very low or undetectable concentrations in the plasma of four of the infants who were studied. No health problems were found in the six infants who were evaluated. In another study of five subjects the median milk/plasma ratio (AUC) for metformin was 0.47.[3] The median calculated infant dose was 0.2% of the weight-adjusted maternal dose. None of the infants exposed to their mothers' milk had detectable levels of metformin in their plasma, nor were any side effects noted.

In a recent study of 5 women consuming an average dose of 500 mg twice daily, the mean peak and trough metformin concentrations in breast milk were 0.42 mg/L (range 0.38–0.46 mg/L) and 0.39 mg/L (range 0.31–0.52 mg/L), respectively.[4] The average milk/serum ratio was 0.63 (range 0.36–1.00) and the estimated relative infant dose was 0.65% (range 0.43–1.08%). Blood glucose concentrations in 3 infants were normal, ranging from 47–77 mg/dL. The mothers reported no side effects were noted in the breastfed infants. Metformin is also used to treat polycystic ovary syndrome. In one study of 61 nursing infants whose mothers were taking a median of 2.55 gm/ day throughout pregnancy and lactation, the growth, motor, and social development of the infants was recorded to be normal. The authors concluded that metformin was safe and effective during lactation in the first 6 months of an infant's life.[5] The relative infant dose for metformin is 0.28%-0.65%.

Sitagliptin phosphate is a dipeptidyl peptidase IV inhibitor resulting in prolonged active incretin levels, thus increasing insulin release from pancreatic beta cells in type 2 diabetics and decreasing glucagon secretion from pancreatic alpha cells, and ultimately decreasing blood glucose levels.[6] It does not lower blood glucose or cause hypoglycemia in healthy subjects. There are no data available on the transfer of sitagliptin into human milk. Levels will probably be quite low due to its size and kinetics. Some caution is recommended until we have data.

Levels in milk following lactational exposure to metformin + sitagliptin are probably too low to be clinically significant. However, some caution is still recommended.

Pregnancy Risk	B	Lactation Risk	L3
T ½	= Metformin/sitagliptin: 6.2 hours/12 hours	M/P	= Metformin/sitagliptin: 0.35–0.63
Vd	= Metformin/sitagliptin: 3.7/2.8 l/kg	PB	= Metformin/sitagliptin: Minimal/38%
Tmax	= Metformin/sitagliptin: 2.75 hours/1–4 hours	Oral	= Metformin/sitagliptin: 50%/87%
MW	= Metformin/sitagliptin: 129/523	pKa	= Metformin/sitagliptin: 12.4

Adult Concerns: Headache, nasopharyngitis are more commonly encountered. Less common but serious side-effects include Stevens-Johnson syndrome, hypoglycemia, lactic acidosis, acute pancreatitis, acute renal failure, hypersensitivity reactions.

Pediatric Concerns:

Drug Interactions: Administration with the following drugs may cause severe hypoglycemia: nonsteroidal anti-inflammatory agents, fluconazole, miconazole, chloramphenicol, fluoroquinolones, probenecid, coumarins, monoamine oxidase inhibitors, and beta-blockers. Co-administration with furosemide, cimetidine or nifedipine may cause an increase in metformin plasma levels. Avoid coadministration with the following drugs: amiloride, digoxin, morphine, procainamide, quinidine, quinine, ranitidine, triamterene, trimethoprim, or vancomycin. Concomitant use with digoxin may increase blood levels of digoxin.

Relative Infant Dose:

Adult Dose: Metformin/sitagliptin: 500–1000 mg/50 mg 1–2 times daily.

Alternatives: Metformin

References:
1. Pharmaceutical manufacturer prescribing information, 2011.
2. Hale TW, Kristensen JH, Hackett LP, Kohan R, Ilett KF. Transfer of metformin into human milk. Diabetologia 2002; 45(11): 1509–1514.
3. Gardiner SJ, Kirkpatrick CM, Begg EJ, Zhang M, Moore MP, Saville DJ. Transfer of metformin into human milk. Clin Pharmacol Ther 2003; 73(1): 71–77.
4. Briggs GG, Ambrose PJ, Nageotte MP, Padilla G, Wan S. Excretion of metformin into breast milk and the effect on nursing infants. Obstet Gynecol 2005 Jun; 105(6): 1437–41.

5. Glueck CJ, Salehi M, Sieve L, Wang P. Growth, motor, and social developement in breast- and formula- fed infants of metformin-treated women with polycyctic ovary syndrome. J Pediatr 2006; 148: 628–632.
6. Pharmaceutical manufacturer prescribing information, 2008. There are no adequate and well-controlled studies in pregnant women.

METHACHOLINE CHLORIDE   L3

Trade: Arthralgen, Mecholyl, Provocholine

Other Trades:

Category: Bronchoconstrictor used for diagnosis of asthma

Methacholine is an analog of acetylcholine and is used via inhalation to diagnose asthma. When inhaled in patients prone for asthma, acute bronchoconstriction occurs, confirming the diagnosis of asthma. Although it is unlikely this product would enter milk in clinically relevant amounts, it is also unlikely to survive the gastrointestinal tract. Because this is a one-time test, a brief interruption of breastfeeding for a few hours (about 4 hours) would all but eliminate any risk.

Pregnancy Risk	C	Lactation Risk	L3
T ½	= Brief	M/P	=
Vd	=	PB	=
Tmax	= 1–4 minutes	Oral	= Low to nil
MW	= 195	pKa	=

Adult Concerns: Methacholine induces clinically apparent dyspnea, asthma and wheezing.

Pediatric Concerns: None reported via milk.

Drug Interactions: Methacholine interacts with numerous medications. Most important however are the beta blockers. Methacholine by inhalation should be avoided in patients who are receiving beta blocking agents. The use of methacholine in patients receiving beta blockers may produce exaggerated or prolonged responses that will not respond adequately to bronchodilator therapy.

Relative Infant Dose:

Adult Dose: Highly variable. Consult product information.

Alternatives:

References:
1. Pharmaceutical manufacturer prescribing information, 2005.

METHADONE   L3

Trade: Dolophine, Metadon

Other Trades: Physeptone, Biodone forte, Methex

Category: Narcotic analgesic

Methadone is a potent and very long-acting opiate analgesic. It is primarily used to prevent withdrawal in opiate addiction. In one study of 10 women receiving methadone 10–80 mg/day, the average milk/plasma ratio was 0.83.[1] Due to the variable doses used, the milk concentrations ranged from 0.05 mg/L in one patient receiving 10 mg/day, to 0.57 mg/L in a patient receiving 80 mg/day. One infant death has been reported in a breastfeeding mother receiving maintenance methadone therapy [2], although it is not clear that the only source of methadone to this infant was from breastmilk. In a more recent study of 12 breastfeeding women on methadone maintenance doses ranging from 20–80 mg/day, the mean concentration of methadone in plasma and milk was 311 (207–416) µg/L and 116 (72–160) µg/L respectively yielding a mean M/P ratio of 0.44 (0.24–0.64).[3] The mean absolute oral dose to infant was 17.4 (10.8–24) µg/kg/day. This equates to a mean of 2.79% of the maternal dose per day. In this study, 64% of the infants exhibited neonatal abstinence syndrome requiring treatment.

In two women receiving 30 mg twice daily and another who received 73 mg of methadone once daily, the average breast milk methadone concentrations was 0.169 mg/L and 0.132 mg/L respectively.[4] The milk/plasma ratios were 1.215 and 0.661 respectively. While the infant of the second mother died at 3 ½ months of SIDS, it was apparently not due to methadone, as none was present in the infant's plasma and the infant was significantly supplemented with formula. In an excellent study 8 mother/infant pairs ingesting from 40 to 105 mg/day methadone, the average (AUC) concentration of R-methadone and S-methadone enantiomers varied from 42–259 µg/L and 26–126 µg/L respectively.[5] The relative infant dose was estimated to be 2.8% of the maternal dose. Interestingly, there was little difference in methadone milk levels in immature and mature milk.

Most studies thus far show that only small amounts of methadone pass into breastmilk despite doses as high as 105 mg/day. In fact, neonatal abstinence syndromes are well known to occur in breastfeeding infants following delivery. In one study, 58% of infants developed neonatal abstinence syndrome while still breastfeeding.[3] However, some methadone is undoubtedly transferred via milk, and abrupt cessation of breastfeeding during high dose therapy has resulted in neonatal abstinence in some infants.[6]

In a recent study of eight methadone-maintained lactating women (dose= 50–105 mg/day), the concentration of methadone in milk was low (range: 2–462 ng/mL) and interestingly, were not related to maternal dose.[7] Maternal plasma levels rose over a 4 week period postpartum to reach a high at 30 days. Median milk/plasma ratios ranged from 0.22 to 0.92. The average amount of methadone ingestible by the infant was estimated to be <0.2 mg/day at day 30 postpartum. Infant plasma levels of methadone ranged from 2.2 to 8.1 ng/mL. Again, there was no correlation between maternal dose and infant plasma level. There were no significant neurobehavioral changes noted. In a recent study of 4 methadone consuming mothers whose doses ranged from 60–110 mg/day, milk levels ranged from as low as 27 ng/mL to as high as 407 ng/mL. While the dose and sampling method was high variable, the authors estimated that the average daily dose to an infant was about 330 µg/day.[8] In a group of 20 women consuming 40–200 mg/day (mean, 102 mg/day), R-methadone concentrations in milk were 1.3–3.0 times higher than S-methadone levels in all breastmilk samples studied. The average

Relative Infant Dose range of R-, S-, and total methadone were 2.7%, 1.6%, and 2.1% respectively.[9]

In summary, the dose of R plus S methadone transferred via milk is largely dose dependent but generally averages less than 2.8% of the maternal dose.[5] This is significantly less than the conventional cut-off value of 10% of the maternal dose corrected for weight. However, the amount in milk is insufficient to prevent neonatal withdrawal syndrome, although another new study suggests that it actually reduces the incidence of neonatal abstinence syndrome when infants are breastfed (OR=0.55).[10]

Pregnancy Risk	C	Lactation Risk	L3
T ½	= 13–55 hours	M/P	= 0.68 (R)
Vd	= 4–5 l/kg	PB	= 89%
Tmax	= 0.5–1 hours	Oral	= 50%
MW	= 309	pKa	= 8.6

Adult Concerns: Nausea, vomiting, constipation, respiratory depression, sedation, withdrawal syndrome.

Pediatric Concerns: Observe for sedation, respiratory depression, addiction, withdrawal syndrome. Neonatal abstinence syndrome.

Drug Interactions: Phenytoin, pentazocine, and rifampin may increase metabolism of methadone and produce withdrawal syndrome. CNS depressants, phenothiazines, tricyclic antidepressants, and monoamine oxidase inhibitors may increase adverse effects of methadone.

Relative Infant Dose: 1.9%–6.5%

Adult Dose: 2.5–10 mg every 3–4 hours PRN

Alternatives:

References:

1. Blinick G, Inturrisi CE, Jerez E, Wallach RC. Methadone assays in pregnant women and progeny. Am J Obstet Gynecol 1975; 121(5): 617–621.
2. Smialek JE, Monforte JR, Aronow R, Spitz WU. Methadone deaths in children. A continuing problem. JAMA 1977; 238(23): 2516–2517.
3. Wojnar-Horton RE, Kristensen JH, Yapp P, Ilett KF, Dusci LJ, Hackett LP. Methadone distribution and excretion into breast milk of clients in a methadone maintenance programme. Br J Clin Pharmacol 1997; 44(6): 543–547.
4. Geraghty B, Graham EA, Logan B, Weiss EL. Methadone levels in breast milk. J Hum Lact 1997; 13(3): 227–230.
5. Begg EJ, Malpas TJ, Hackett LP, Ilett KF. Distribution of R- and S-methadone into human milk during multiple, medium to high oral dosing. Br J Clin Pharmacol 2001; 52(6): 681–685.
6. Malpas TJ, Darlow BA. Neonatal abstinence syndrome following abrupt cessation of breastfeeding. N Z Med J 1999; 112(1080): 12–13.
7. Jansson LM, Choo R, Velez ML et al. Methadone maintenance and breastfeeding in the neonatal period. Pediatrics. 2008; 121: 106–114.
8. Jansson LM, Choo R, Velez ML, Lowe R, Huestis MA. Methadone maintenance and long-term lactation. Breastfeed Med. Mar 2008; 3(1): 34–37.

9. Bogen DL, Perel JM, Helsel JC, Hanusa BH, Thompson M, Wisner KL. Estimated infant exposure to enantiomer-specific methadone levels in breastmilk. Breastfeed Med. 2011 Dec; 6: 377–84.
10. Dryden C, Young D, Hepburn M, Mactier H. Maternal methadone use in pregnancy: factors associated with the development of neonatal abstinence syndrome and implications for healthcare resources. BJOG. Apr 2009; 116(5): 665–671.

METHAMPHETAMINE | L5

Trade: Desoxyephedrine, Desoxyn, Pervitin, Anadrex, Methedrine

Other Trades:

Category: CNS Stimulant

Methamphetamine is a potent CNS stimulant commonly used as a drug of abuse with a prolonged half-life. In a study of two women who were occasional recreational users of intravenous amphetamines, replicate milk samples were drawn over 24 hours.[1] The IV dose was unknown. In the 24 hours after dose, average concentrations in milk were 111 ng/mL and 281 ng/mL for methamphetamine and 4 ng/mL and 15 ng/mL for amphetamine in the two subjects. Methamphetamine is partially metabolized by N-demethylation to amphetamine. Absolute infant doses for methamphetamine plus amphetamine (as methamphetamine equivalents) were 17.5 µg/kg/day and 44.7 µg/kg/day, respectively, for subjects 1 and 2. Methamphetamine is a potent neurotoxin, known to cause dopaminergic degeneration, with loss of brain dopamine and serotonin neurons. Methamphetamine is a strong CNS stimulant that is strongly addictive. After prolonged use it is known to induce paranoid symptoms. Breastfeeding mothers should avoid using this drug, or pump and discard milk for at least 48 hours.

Pregnancy Risk	C	Lactation Risk	L5
T ½	= 4–13.6 hours	M/P	=
Vd	=	PB	=
Tmax	=	Oral	= 63%
MW	= 185.7	pKa	= 9.87

Adult Concerns: Physical effects may include anorexia, hyperactivity, mydriasis, dry mouth, headache, tachycardia, elevated blood pressure, hyperthermia, diarrhea, arrhythmia, insomnia, stroke and even death. Severe dental decay and acne are common in frequent abusers. Psychological effects include euphoria, increased libido, anxiety, grandiosity, sociability, aggressive behavior, paranoid schizophrenic symptoms, and psychosis.

Pediatric Concerns: One reported case of infant death following exposure to breast milk.[2] However, the plasma levels in the infant were reportedly too low to induce such symptoms, so the etiology of this death is in question.

Drug Interactions: Numerous. Do not use with antidepressants such as tricyclics,

SSRIs, monoamine oxidase inhibitors and numerous other CNS active medications. Consult drug interaction text.

Relative Infant Dose:

Adult Dose: 5 mg

Alternatives:

References:

1.   Bartu A, Dusci LJ, Ilett KF. Transfer of methylamphetamine and amphetamine into breast milk following recreational use of methylamphetamine. Br J Clin Pharmacol. Apr 2009; 67(4): 455–459.
2.   Ariagno R, Karch SB, Middleberg R, Stephens BG, Valdes-Dapena M. Methamphetamine ingestion by a breast-feeding mother and her infant's death: People v Henderson. JAMA. Jul 19 1995; 274(3): 215.

METHENAMINE   L3

Trade: Cystex, Hiprex, Urex

Other Trades:

Category: Antibiotic for Lower UTI

Methenamine is a polar heterocyclic organic compound that is converted into formaldehyde in urinary tract and thus acts as an anti-infective.[1] Methenamine is transferred into breastmilk in low amount. Methenamine was measured at 4.3 mg/L after 6–7 hours of taking 1 gram of methenamine hippurate.[2] Relative infant dose is calculated to be 3.62–4.52%. No adverse effect was reported from four neonates that were breastfed while mother was taking methenamine from one study.

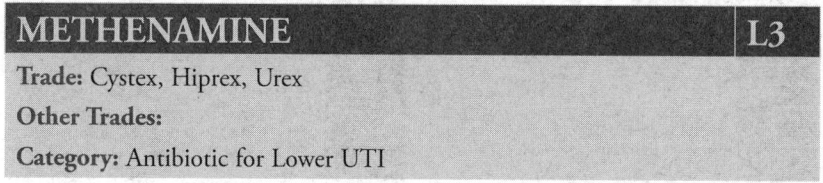

Pregnancy Risk	C		Lactation Risk	L3
T ½	= 3–6 hours		M/P	= 0.88–1.08
Vd	=		PB	=
Tmax	=		Oral	=
MW	= 140		pKa	=

Adult Concerns: Nausea, rash, vomiting, bladder irritation, pruritus, dyspepsia.

Pediatric Concerns:

Drug Interactions:

Relative Infant Dose: 3.6%–4.5%

Adult Dose: Hippurate: 1g twice daily, Mandelate 1g four times daily.

Alternatives:

References:

1.   Lexi-Comp OnlineTM, Lexi-Drugs OnlineTM, Hudson, Ohio: Lexi-Comp, Inc.; 2011; June 01, 2011.
2.   Lactmed: Drug and Lactation Database[Internet]. Bethesda, MD: National Library of Medicine. Updated 12/07/2010. [accessed 2009 Aug 4].

METHICILLIN   L3

Trade: Staphcillin, Celbenin
Other Trades: Metin, Celbenin
Category: Penicillin antibiotic

Methicillin is a penicillin antibiotic only available by IM and IV formulations.[1] It is extremely unstable at acid pH (stomach); hence, it would have only limited oral absorption in an infant or adult. No data are available on its transfer into breastmilk although it would appear to be minimal as with other penicillins. Observe for changes in gut flora and diarrhea.

Pregnancy Risk	B	Lactation Risk	L3
T ½	= 1–2 hours	M/P	=
Vd	=	PB	= 40%
Tmax	= 30–60 minutes	Oral	= Poor
MW	= 380	pKa	= 2.41

Adult Concerns: Allergic rash, thrush, diarrhea, drug fever, changes in gastrointestinal flora, renal toxicity, pseudomembranous colitis.

Pediatric Concerns: None reported via milk.

Drug Interactions: The effect of oral contraceptives may be reduced. Disulfiram and probenecid may significantly increase penicillin levels. Methicillin may increase the effect of anticoagulants.

Relative Infant Dose:

Adult Dose: 1 gm every 6 hours

Alternatives:

References:
1. Drug Facts and Comparisons 1994 ed. ed. St. Louis: 1994.

METHIMAZOLE   L2

Trade: Tapazole
Other Trades: Tapazole
Category: Antithyroid agent

Methimazole, carbimazole, and propylthiouracil (PTU) are used to inhibit the secretion of thyroxine. Carbimazole is a prodrug and is rapidly converted to methimazole.

Levels of methimazole in milk depend on the maternal dose but appear too low to produce clinical effects. In one study of a single patient receiving 2.5 mg methimazole every 12 hours, the milk/serum ratio was 1.16, and the dose per day was calculated at 16–39 µg methimazole.[1] This was equivalent to 7–16% of the maternal dose.

In another study of 35 lactating women receiving 5 to 20 mg/day of methimazole, no changes in the infant thyroid function were noted in any infant, even those at higher doses.[2] Further, studies by Lamberg in 11 women, who were treated with the methimazole derivative carbimazole (5–15 mg daily, equal to 3.3 -10 mg methimazole), found all 11 infants had normal thyroid function following maternal treatments.[3] Thus, in small maternal doses, methimazole may also be safe for the nursing mother. In a study of a woman with twins who was receiving up to 30 mg carbimazole daily, the average methimazole concentration in milk was 43 µg/L.[4] The average plasma concentrations in the twin infants were 45 and 52 ng/mL, which is below therapeutic range. Methimazole milk concentrations peaked at 2–4 hours after a carbimazole dose. No changes in thyroid function in these infants were noted. In a large study of over 134 thyrotoxic lactating mothers and their infants. Methimazole therapy was initiated at 10–30 mg/day for one month, and reduced to 5–10 mg/day subsequently. Even at methimazole doses of 20 mg/day, no changes in infant TSH, T4 or T3 were noted in over 12 months of study.[5] The authors conclude that both PTU and methimazole can safely be administered during lactation. However, during the first few months of therapy, monitoring of infant thyroid functioning is recommended.

Pregnancy Risk	D	Lactation Risk	L2
T ½	= 6–13 hours	M/P	= 1.0
Vd	=	PB	=
Tmax	= 1 hour	Oral	= 80–95%
MW	= 114	pKa	= 11.64

Adult Concerns: Hypothyroidism, hepatic dysfunction, bleeding, drowsiness, skin rash, nausea, vomiting, fever.

Pediatric Concerns: None reported in several studies, but propylthiouracil may be a preferred choice in breastfeeding women.

Drug Interactions: Use with iodinated glycerol, lithium, and potassium iodide may increase toxicity.

Relative Infant Dose: 2.3%

Adult Dose: 5–30 mg daily.

Alternatives: Propylthiouracil

References:
1. Tegler L, Lindstrom B. Antithyroid drugs in milk. Lancet 1980; 2(8194): 591.
2. Azizi F. Effect of methimazole treatment of maternal thyrotoxicosis on thyroid function in breast-feeding infants. J Pediatr 1996; 128(6): 855–858.
3. Lamberg BA, Ikonen E, Osterlund K, Teramo K, Pekonen F, Peltola J, Valimaki M. Antithyroid treatment of maternal hyperthyroidism during lactation. Clin Endocrinol (Oxf) 1984; 21(1): 81–87.
4. Rylance GW, Woods CG, Donnelly MC, Oliver JS, Alexander WD. Carbimazole and breastfeeding. Lancet 1987; 1(8538): 928.
5. Azizi F, Khoshniat M, Bahrainian M, Hedayati M. Thyroid function and intellectual development of infants nursed by mothers taking methimazole. J Clin Endocrinol Metab 2000; 85(9): 3233–3238.

METHOCARBAMOL   L3

Trade: Robaxisal, Robaxin
Other Trades: Robaxin
Category: Muscle relaxant

Methocarbamol is a centrally acting sedative and skeletal muscle relaxant. Only minimal amounts have been found in milk of dogs.[1] Observe for sedation in breastfed infant.

Pregnancy Risk	C	Lactation Risk	L3
T ½	= 0.9–1.8 hours	M/P	=
Vd	=	PB	= 46–50%
Tmax	= 1–2 hours	Oral	= Complete
MW	= 241	pKa	= 14.81

Adult Concerns: Drowsiness, nausea, metallic taste, vertigo, blurred vision, fever, headache.

Pediatric Concerns: None reported, but studies are limited.

Drug Interactions: May see increased toxicity when used with CNS depressants.

Relative Infant Dose:

Adult Dose: 4–4.5 gm every 4–6 hours

Alternatives:

References:
1. Pharmaceutical manufacturer prescribing information, 1995.

METHOHEXITAL   L3

Trade: Brevital
Other Trades: Brietal
Category: Anesthetic agent

Methohexital is an ultra short-acting barbiturate used for induction in anesthesia. The duration of action is approximately ½ that of thiopental sodium or less than 8 minutes depending on dose. Although the elimination half-life is 3.9 hours, within 30 minutes there is complete redistribution of methohexital to tissues other than the brain, primarily the liver.[1,2]

In one study of 9 women who received 120–150 mg of methohexital for induction of anesthesia, milk levels collected 1–2 hours after surgery ranged from 100 to 407 µg/L in five patients.[3] Levels in the breastmilk were found to decline rapidly within the first hour and were undetectable after 24 hours. The maximum level in milk occurred at 63 minutes after administration of anesthesia and was found to be 407 µg/L via breastmilk. The authors suggested the infant would receive a maximum of 0.04 mg of methohexital in a typical feeding (100 mL) or between 0.1 to 0.8% of the maternal weight-adjusted dosage.

Pregnancy Risk	B	Lactation Risk	L3
T ½	= 3.9 hours	M/P	= 1.1 (blood)
Vd	=	PB	= 73%
Tmax	= Instant	Oral	=
MW	= 262	pKa	= 8.3

Adult Concerns: Hypotension, lethargy, restlessness, confusion, headache, delirium and excitation

Pediatric Concerns: None reported via milk. Levels would be too low.

Drug Interactions: CNS depressants such as barbiturates, benzodiazepines, etc, may potentiate sedation with methohexital.

Relative Infant Dose: 2.8%

Adult Dose: 20–40 mg every 4–7 minutes during surgery.

Alternatives:

References:
1. Drug Facts and Comparisons 1999 ed. ed. St. Louis: 1999.
2. McEvoy GE. (ed): AFHS Drug Information. New York, NY: 2003.
3. Borgatta L, Jenny RW, Gruss L, Ong C, Barad D. Clinical Significance of Methohexital, Meperidine, and Diazepam in Breast Milk. J Clin Pharmacol 1997; 37: 186–192.

METHOTREXATE   L3

Trade: Folex, Rheumatrex

Other Trades: Ledertrexate, Methoblastin, Arthitrex

Category: Antimetabolite, anticancer, antirheumatic

Methotrexate is a potent and potentially dangerous folic acid antimetabolite used in arthritic and other immunologic syndromes. It is also used as an abortifacient in tubal pregnancies. Methotrexate is secreted into breast milk in small amounts.

Following a dose of 22.5 mg to one patient two hours post-dose, the methotrexate concentration in breastmilk was 2.6 µg/L of milk with a milk/plasma ratio of 0.08.[1] The cumulative excretion of methotrexate in the first 12 hours after oral administration was only 0.32 µg in milk. These authors conclude that methotrexate therapy in breastfeeding mothers would not pose a contraindication to breastfeeding. However, methotrexate is believed to be retained in human tissues (particularly neonatal gastrointestinal cells and ovarian cells) for long periods (months).[2]

One study has indicated a higher risk of fetal malformation in mothers who received methotrexate months prior to becoming pregnant.[3] Therefore, pregnancy should be delayed if either partner is receiving methotrexate for at least 3 months following therapy. Elimination of methotrexate is by a two-compartment model with a terminal elimination half-life of 8–15 hours.[4] Patients with poor renal function have prolonged methotrexate half-lives. It is apparent that the concentration of methotrexate in human milk is minimal, although due to the toxicity of this agent, it is probably wise to pump and discard the mother's milk for a minimum of 2–4 days. This may require extending if the dose used is quite high or frequently administered.

Methotrexate doses for ectopic pregnancy are 50 mg/m^2 per day in a single-dose regimen or two-doses regimen and 1 mg/kg/day in multidose regimen. Withhold breastfeeding for a minimum of four days.

Pregnancy Risk	X	Lactation Risk	L3
T ½	= 8–15 hours	M/P	= >0.08
Vd	= 2.6 l/kg	PB	= 34–50%
Tmax	= 1–2 hours	Oral	= 33–90%
MW	= 454	pKa	= 4.3, 5.5

Adult Concerns: Bone marrow suppression, anemia, vasculitis, vomiting, diarrhea, gastrointestinal bleeding, stomatitis, bloody diarrhea, kidney damage, seizures, etc.

Pediatric Concerns: None reported via milk, but caution is recommended.

Drug Interactions: Aminoglycosides may significantly decrease absorption of methotrexate. Etretinate has produced hepatotoxicity in several patients receiving methotrexate. The use of folic acid or its derivatives may reduce the response to MTX. The use of NSAIDs with methotrexate is contraindicated, several deaths have occurred due to elevated MTX levels. Phenytoin serum levels may be decreased. Procarbazine may increase nephrotoxicity of MTX.

Relative Infant Dose: 0.1%

Adult Dose: 10–30 mg

Alternatives:

References:
1. Johns DG, Rutherford LD, Leighton PC, Vogel CL. Secretion of methotrexate into human milk. Am J Obstet Gynecol 1972; 112(7): 978–980.
2. Fountain JR, Hutchison DJ, Waring GB, Burchenal JH. Persistence of amethopterin in normal mouse tissues. Proc Soc Exp Biol Med 1953; 83(2): 369–373.
3. Walden PA, Bagshawe KD. Pregnancies after chemotherapy for gestational trophoblastic tumours. Lancet 1979; 2(8154): 1241.
4. Grochow LB, Ames MM. A clinician's guide to chemotherapy pharmacokinetics and pharmacodynamics. 1st ed. Baltimore, MD: Williams and Wilkins; 1998.
5. American Academy of Pediatrics, Committee on Drugs. Transfer of drugs and other chemicals into human milk. Pediatrics 2001; 108(3): 776–89.

METHSCOPOLAMINE   L3

Trade: Pamine, Aerohist, AlleRx, Amdry-D

Other Trades:

Category: Anticholinergic, antispasmotic

Methscopolamine is an anticholinergic commonly used for stomach/intestinal spasms, antiemetic, antivertigo, urinary antispasmodic, to decrease salivation, to reduce stomach acid secretion and motility, and may be used for other purposes.[1] No data are available on its transfer to milk, but it is probably minimal due to its quaternary ammonium structure. Little is known about its kinetics but its effect persists for about 4–6 hours. It is commonly reported that anticholinergics suppress milk production but this data is anecdotal and has not been confirmed by this author. It is rather unlikely that this product would produce clinical levels in infants following ingestion of milk. But infants should be monitored for classic 'anticholinergic' symptoms such as drying of oral and ophthalmic secretions, constipation, and urinary retention.

Pregnancy Risk	C	Lactation Risk	L3
T ½	= <4 hours	M/P	=
Vd	=	PB	=
Tmax	=	Oral	= 10–25%
MW	= 398	pKa	=

Adult Concerns: Constipation, dry mouth, trouble urinating, nausea or dizziness, increased pulse and other anticholinergic symptoms may occur.

Pediatric Concerns: None reported via milk. Rather unlikely due to the structure of this compound.

Drug Interactions: Caution while concomitantly administering with antidepressants (tricyclic type), MAO inhibitors (e.g., phenelzine, linezolid, tranylcypromine, isocarboxazid, selegiline, furazolidone), quinidine, amantadine, antihistamines (e.g., diphenhydramine), other anticholinergics, potassium chloride supplements, antacids, absorbent-type anti-diarrhea medicines (e.g., kaolin-pectin), phenothiazines (e.g., chlorpromazine, promethazine).

Relative Infant Dose:

Adult Dose: 2.5 mg four times a day in adults.

Alternatives: Atropine

References:
1. Pharmaceutical manufacturer prescribing information, 2005.

METHYL SALICYLATE   L3

Trade:
Other Trades:
Category: Salicylate, Non-Aspirin

Methyl salicylate is a form of NSAID used to alleviate pain when applied through topical compounds and patches. The American Academy of Pediatrics recommends that salicylates be used with caution in breastfeeding women.[1] Transfer to the milk is well documented and there are concerns that rash and hypoprothrombinemia may occur in infants following salicylate administration.[2] Since methyl salicylate is similar to aspirin, methyl salicylate may have the same issue as aspirin. Aspirin is certainly implicated in Reye syndrome, but most often in older children (not infants) who have a viral illness such as flu or chickenpox. However, the amount in breastmilk is incredibly low even following the use of large therapeutic doses of methylsalicylate. Never use these products if the infant has a viral syndrome. The need for salicylates in a breastfeeding mother would require a major discussion of the risk vs benefit.

Pregnancy Risk	Probably Safe	Lactation Risk	L3
T ½	= 2–12 hours	M/P	=
Vd	=	PB	= 50–80%
Tmax	= 0.8–2.2 hours	Oral	= 15–22%
MW	= 152.1	pKa	=

Adult Concerns: Irritation, rash, gastrointestinal bleed, hypersensitivity reaction.

Pediatric Concerns:

Drug Interactions: Warfarin–Concurrent use of warfarin and methyl salicylate may result in an increased risk of bleeding.

Relative Infant Dose:

Adult Dose: Apply to affected area 3–4 times per day.

Alternatives:

References:
1. Briggs GG, Freeman RK, and Yaffe SJBriggs GG, Freeman RK, and Yaffe SJ: Drugs in Pregnancy and Lactation, 5th. Williams and Wilkins, Baltimore, MD, 1998.
2. British National Formulary, No 12, London: BMA and Pharmaceutical Society of Great Britain, 1986: 23–6.

METHYLCELLULOSE   L1

Trade:

Other Trades:

Category: Laxative agent

Methylcellulose is used as a bulk laxative for the treatment of constipation.[1] There are no data on the excretion of methylcellulose into human milk. However, it stays in the gastrointestinal tract and is totally unabsorbed. It is safe for breastfeeding mothers.

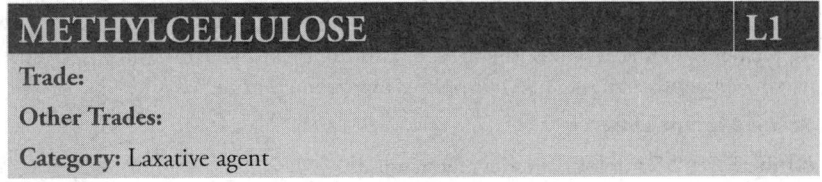

Pregnancy Risk	A	Lactation Risk	L1
T ½	=	M/P	=
Vd	=	PB	=
Tmax	=	Oral	= Nil
MW	= Very large	pKa	=

Adult Concerns: Most common: feeling of fullness. Less common: allergic reactions, chest pain, nausea and vomiting, difficulty swallowing.

Pediatric Concerns:

Drug Interactions:

Relative Infant Dose:

Adult Dose:

Alternatives:

References:
1. Pharmaceutical manufacturer prescribing information, 2011.

METHYLDOPA   L2

Trade: Aldomet

Other Trades: Aldopren, Hydopa, Nudopa, Aldomet, Apo-Methyldopa, Dopamet, Nova-Medopa

Category: Antihypertensive

Alpha-methyldopa is a centrally acting antihypertensive. It is frequently used to treat hypertension during pregnancy. In a study of 2 lactating women who received a dose of 500 mg, the maximum breastmilk concentration of methyldopa ranged from 0.2 to 0.66 mg/L.[1] In another patient who received 1000 mg dose, the maximum concentration in milk was 1.14 mg/L.[1] The milk/plasma ratios varied from 0.19 to 0.34. The authors indicated that if the infant were to ingest 750 mL of milk daily (with a maternal dose= 1000 mg), the maximum daily ingestion would be less than 855 µg or approximately 0.02% of the maternal dose. In another study of 7 women who received 0.750–2.0 gm/day of methyldopa, the free methyldopa concentrations in breastmilk ranged from zero to 0.2 mg/L while the conjugated metabolite had concentrations of 0.1 to 0.9 mg/L.[2] These studies generally indicate that the levels of methyldopa transferred to a breastfeeding infant would be too low to be clinically relevant. However, gynecomastia and galactorrhea has been reported in one full-term 2-week-old female neonate following seven days of maternal therapy with methyldopa, 250 mg three times daily.[3]

Pregnancy Risk	B	Lactation Risk	L2
T ½	= 105 minutes	M/P	= 0.19–0.34
Vd	= 0.3 l/kg	PB	= Low
Tmax	= 3–6 hours	Oral	= 25–50%
MW	= 211	pKa	= 2.2

Adult Concerns: Hemolytic anemia, hepatitis, fever, rashes, dizziness, hypotension, sleep disturbances, dry mouth, depression, colitis.

Pediatric Concerns: None reported in several studies. Gynecomastia and galactorrhea in one personal communication.

Drug Interactions: Iron supplements can interact and cause a significant increase in blood pressure. Increased toxicity with lithium has been reported.

Relative Infant Dose: 0.1%–0.4%

Adult Dose: 250–500 mg 3–4 times daily.

Alternatives:

References:

1. White WB, Andreoli JW, Cohn RD. Alpha-methyldopa disposition in mothers with hypertension and in their breast-fed infants. Clin Pharmacol Ther 1985; 37(4): 387–390.
2. Jones HM, Cummings AJ. A study of the transfer of alpha-methyldopa to the human foetus and newborn infant. Br J Clin Pharmacol 1978; 6(5): 432–434.
3. E.D.M. Personal Communication. 1997.

METHYLENE BLUE   L4

Trade: Dolsed, Atrosept, Prosed, Urimar-T
Other Trades:
Category: Diagnostic Agent

Methylene blue is a blue dye that is used in diagnostic procedures, to treat drug-induced methemoglobinemia, and to prevent ifosfamide-induced encephalopathy in oncology. No data are available on its transfer into human milk, but some should be expected. Oral absorption is considered poor.[1] The apparent half-life in humans is approximately 5.25 hours, thus interruption of breastfeeding for 24 hours is probably advisable. NEVER use in patients taking selective serotonin reuptake inhibitors (SSRIs).

Pregnancy Risk	C	Lactation Risk	L4
T ½	= 5.25	M/P	=
Vd	=	PB	=
Tmax	=	Oral	=
MW	= 319	pKa	= 3.8

Adult Concerns: Cardiac dysrhythmia and hypertension. Sweating, discoloration of skin, malignant hyperthermia, diarrhea, burning in mouth and oropharynx, nausea and vomiting

Pediatric Concerns: None reported via milk. Oral absorption is poor.

Drug Interactions: Do not use in patients taking serotonergic agents such as paroxetine or duloxetine to avoid a potential drug interaction causing a dangerous condition called serotonin syndrome.

Relative Infant Dose:

Adult Dose: 0.1–1 mg/kg

Alternatives:

References:
1. Peter C, Hongwan D, Kupfer A, Lauterburg BH. Pharmacokinetics and organ distribution of intravenous and oral methylene blue. Eur J Clin Pharmacol. 2000 Jun; 56(3): 247–50.

METHYLERGONOVINE   L2

Trade: Methergine
Other Trades: Methergine, Methylergometrine
Category: Vasoconstrictor, uterine stimulant

Methylergonovine is an amine ergot alkaloid used to control postpartum uterine bleeding. The ergot alkaloids are powerful vasoconstrictors. In a group of 8 postpartum women receiving 0.125 mg three times daily for 5 days, the concentration of methylergonovine ranged from <0.5 in 4 patients to 1.3 µg/L in one patient at one hour post dose.[1] In this study, only 5 of 16 milk samples had detectable methylergonovine levels. Using a dose of 1.3 µg/L of milk, an consume approximately 0.2 µg/kg/day, which is incredibly low compared to the usual 0.375 mg daily dose. The milk/plasma ratio averaged about 0.3.

Short-term (1 week), low-dose regimens of these agents do not apparently pose problems in nursing infants/mothers.[2] Many studies have been performed showing no difference in prolactin levels between mothers treated with methylergonovine and those receiving placebo, while some show a suppression in prolactin and thus milk production. One study suggested a 50% decrease in prolactin levels 30 to 75 minutes after a 0.2 mg intramuscular injection of methylergonovine.[3] In 30 lactating women receiving 0.6 mg orally from day 1 to day 7 postpartum, prolactin levels were significantly lower at day 7, while milk production was significantly reduced at days 3 and 7.[4] In a study of 14 postpartum women who received 0.2 mg intramuscularly, plasma prolactin concentrations were lower (141 ng/mL) as compared to the control group (266.4 ng/mL).[5] In those situations with longer therapy, milk product may be negatively affected, but it is not likely to be overly hazardous to the infant. Methylergonovine is preferred over ergonovine because it does not inhibit lactation to the same degree, and levels in milk are minimal.

Pregnancy Risk	C	Lactation Risk		L2 for acute use/ L4 for chronic use
T ½	= 3.39 hours (1.5 to 12.7 hours)	M/P	= 0.3	
Vd	=	PB	= 36%	
Tmax	= 0.5–3 hours	Oral	= 60%	
MW	= 339	pKa	= 6.7	

Adult Concerns: Nausea, vomiting, diarrhea, dizziness, rapid pulse.

Pediatric Concerns: None reported, but long term exposure is not recommended. Methylergonovine is commonly recommended early postpartum for breastfeeding mothers with bleeding.

Drug Interactions: Use caution when using with other vasoconstrictors or pressor agents.

Relative Infant Dose: 2%

Adult Dose: 0.2–0.4 mg every 6–12 hours as needed.

Alternatives:

References:
1. Erkkola R, Kanto J, Allonen H, Kleimola T, Mantyla R. Excretion of methylergometrine (methylergonovine) into the human breast milk. Int J Clin Pharmacol Biopharm 1978; 16(12): 579–580.
2. Del Pozo E, Brun DR, Hinselmann M. Lack of effect of methyl-ergonovine on postpartum lactation. Am J Obstet Gynecol 1975; 123(8): 845–846.
3. Perez-Lopez FR, Delvoye P, Denayer P, L'Hermite M, Roncero MC, Robyn C. Effectof methylergobasine maleate on serum gonadotrophin and prolactin in humans. Acta Endocrinol (Copenh) 1975; 79(4): 644–657.
4. Peters F, Lummerich M, Breckwoldt M. Inhibition of prolactin and lactation by methylergometrine hydrogenmaleate. Acta Endocrinol (Copenh) 1979; 91(2): 213–216.
5. Weiss G, Klein S, Shenkman L, Kataoka K, Hollander CS. Effect of methylergonovine on puerperal prolactin secretion. Obstet Gynecol 1975; 46(2): 209–210.

METHYLMETHACRYLATE   L3

Trade:

Other Trades:

Category: Adhesive Agent

Methylmethacrylate is a polymer used as an adhesive. In medicine, it is used for spine, hip and knee replacement surgeries. One study found undetectable levels of methyl methacrylate in milk 36 hours after a total hip arthroplasty (detection limit 0.0005 µg/mL).[1] In another study, methyl methacrylate was not detected in breast milk of surgeons after inhalation of methylmethacrylate during total joint arthroplasty.[2] Methylmethacrylate vapor starts to cause irritation once it reaches concentrations of 170–250 ppm.[3]

Pregnancy Risk	Probably Safe	Lactation Risk	L3
T ½	=	M/P	=
Vd	=	PB	=
Tmax	=	Oral	=
MW	= 100	pKa	=

Adult Concerns: Hypotension, hemorrhage, cardiac conduction irregularities, pulmonary embolism, cerebrovascular accident, new bone fracture.

Pediatric Concerns:

Drug Interactions:

Relative Infant Dose:

Adult Dose:

Alternatives:

References:
1. Hersh J, Bono JV, Padgett DE, Mancuso CA. Methyl methacrylate levels in the breast milk of a patient after total hip arthroplasty. J Arthroplasty. 1995 Feb; 10(1): 91–2.
2. Linehan CM, Gioe TJ. Serum and breast milk levels of methylmethacrylate following surgeon exposure during arthroplasty. J Bone Joint Surg Am. 2006 Sep; 88(9): 1957–61.
3. Methylmethacrylate. In: POISINDEX Æ System [Internet database]. Greenwood Village, Colo: Thomson Healthcare. Updated periodically. Accessed 06–09–2011.

METHYLPHENIDATE   L3

Trade: Ritalin, Concerta, Metadate CD, Metadate ER, Methylin, Daytrana, Focalin XR, Dexmethylphenidate

Other Trades: PMS-Methylphenidate, Riphenidate

Category: CNS stimulant, treatment of ADHD

The pharmacologic effects of methylphenidate are similar to those of amphetamines and includes CNS stimulation.[1] It is presently used for narcolepsy and attention deficit hyperactivity syndrome. In a study of 3 women receiving an average of 52 (35–80) mg/day of methylphenidate, the average drug in milk was 19 (13–28) µg/L.[2]

The milk/plasma ratio averaged 2.8 (2–3.6). The absolute infant dose averaged 2.9 (2–4.25) µg/kg/day. The average relative infant dose was 0.9% (0.7–1.1). In the one infant studied, plasma levels were <1 µg/L. These levels are probably too low to clinically relevant. Another case reported a mother taking 15 mg/day with breast milk concentrations averaging 2.5 ng/mL. The daily infant dose was estimated at 0.38 µg/kg, which corresponds to 0.16% of the maternal dose.[3] No drug was detected in breast milk 20–21 hours after the maternal dose. A mother taking 80 mg/day was determined to have a milk-to-plasma ratio of 2.7, giving an absolute infant dose of 2.3 µg/kg/day, or 0.2% of the maternal dose. Methylphenidate was not detected in the infant's plasma.[4] No adverse effects were noted in any of the infants. These levels are significantly less than for dextroamphetamine. Infants should be observed for agitation, and reduced weight gain although these are quite unlikely at these levels.

Dexmethyphenidate hydrochloride, is simply the active dextro-rotary enantiomer of methylphenidate, and therefore kinetic and breastmilk data should be similar to that of methylphenidate.

Pregnancy Risk	C	Lactation Risk	L3
T ½	= 1.4–4.2 hours	M/P	= 2.8
Vd	= 11–33 l/kg	PB	=
Tmax	= 1–3 hours	Oral	= 95%
MW	= 233	pKa	= 8.8

Adult Concerns: Nervousness, hyperactivity, insomnia, agitation, and lack of appetite.

Pediatric Concerns: None reported in 3 infants, but observe for stimulation, insomnia, anorexia, reduced weight gain.

Drug Interactions: Methylphenidate may reduce the effects of guanethidine and bretylium. May increased serum levels of tricyclic antidepressants, phenytoin, warfarin, phenobarbital, and primidone. Use with MAO inhibitors may produce significant increased effects of methylphenidate.

Relative Infant Dose: 0.2%–0.4%

Adult Dose: 10 mg 2–3 times daily. Higly variable.

Alternatives:

References:
1. Pharmaceutical manufacturer prescribing information, 1996.
2. Hackett LP, Ilett KF, Kristensen JH, Kohan R, Hale TW. Infant dose and safety of breastfeeding for dexamphetamine and methylphenidate in mothers with attention deficit hyperactivity disorder. Proceedings of the 9th International Congress of Therapeutic Drug Monitoring and Clinical Toxicology, Louisville, USA, April 23–28, 2005, Therapeutic Drug Monitoring 2005; 27: 220. (Abstract # 40).
3. Spigset O, Brede WR, Zahlsen K. Excretion of methylphenidate in Breast Milk. Am J Psychiatry 2007; 164(2): 348.
4. Hackett LP, Kristensen JH, Hale TW, Paterson R, Ilett, KF. Methylphenidate and Breast-Feeding. Ann Pharmacother 2006; 40(10): 1890–1891.

METHYLPREDNISOLONE   L2

Trade: Solu-Medrol, Depo-Medrol, Medrol
Other Trades: Neo-Medrol, Advantan, Medrol, Depo-Medrol, Solu-Medrol
Category: Corticosteroid

Methylprednisolone (MP) is the methyl derivative of prednisolone. Four milligrams of methylprednisolone is roughly equivalent to 5 mg of prednisone. Multiple dosage forms exist and include the succinate salt which is rapidly active, the methylprednisolone base which is the tablet formulation for oral use, and the methylprednisolone acetate suspension (Depo-Medrol) which is slowly absorbed over many days to weeks. Depo-Medrol is generally used intrasynovially, IM, or epidurally and is slowly absorbed from these sites. They would be very unlikely to affect a breastfed infant, but this depends on dose and duration of exposure.

For a complete description of corticosteroid use in breastfeeding mothers see the prednisone monograph. In general, the amount of methylprednisolone and other steroids transferred into human milk is minimal as long as the dose does not exceed 80 mg per day.[1] However, relating side effects of steroids administered via breastmilk and their maternal doses is rather difficult and each situation should be evaluated individually. Extended use of high doses could predispose the infant to steroid side effects including decreased linear growth rate, but these require rather high doses. Low to moderate doses are believed to have minimal effect on breastfed infants. High dose pulsed intravenous or oral administrations of methylprednisolone (MP) have become increasingly important as a treatment for acute relapses or progressively worsening of multiple sclerosis (MS).[2-6] Even though prednisolone is approved by the American Academy of Pediatrics for use in breastfeeding women, when MP is used in such high doses in patients with MS, questions concerning when mothers can return to breastfeeding have arisen. While there are extensive kinetic data on the plasma levels, metabolism and clearance of methylprednisolone from normal and MS patients[7,8], no data are available on the transfer of MP into human milk subsequent to using such high pulse IV doses in breastfeeding mothers. Simulation of MP elimination curves by the author shows a rapid and complete elimination from the maternal plasma compartment.[9] From this simulation, it would appear a brief pumping and discarding of milk for a period of 8–24 hours following the IV administration of MP (at doses up to 1 gm) would significantly reduce an infant's exposure to this corticosteroid. This simulation estimates the infant dose at 12 hours post-administration of MP to be approximately 1.24 µg/kg/day. These are only theoretical predictions as no one yet has published milk levels following IV administration of 1 gram doses.

Pregnancy Risk	C	Lactation Risk	L2
T ½	= 2.8 hours	M/P	=
Vd	= 1.5 l/kg	PB	=
Tmax	=	Oral	= Complete
MW	= 374	pKa	= 2.6, 5.0

Adult Concerns: In pediatrics, shortened stature, gastrointestinal bleeding, gastrointestinal ulceration, edema, osteoporosis.

Pediatric Concerns: None reported via breastmilk. Limit dose and length of exposure if possible. High doses and prolonged durations may inhibit epiphyseal bone growth, induce gastric ulcerations, glaucoma, etc.

Drug Interactions: Barbiturates may significantly reduce the effects of corticosteroids. Cholestyramine may reduce absorption of methylprednisolone. Oral contraceptives may reduce half-life and concentration of steroids. Ephedrine may reduce the half-life and increase clearance of certain steroids. Phenytoin may increase clearance. Corticosteroid clearance may be decreased by ketoconazole. Certain macrolide antibiotics may significantly decrease clearance of steroids. Isoniazid serum concentrations may be decreased.

Relative Infant Dose:

Adult Dose: 2–60 mg daily

Alternatives: Prednisone

References:

1. Anderson PO. Corticosteroid use by breast-feeding mothers. Clin Pharm 1987; 6(6): 445.
2. Miller DM, Weinstock-Guttman B, Bethoux F, Lee JC, Beck G, Block V, Durelli L, LaMantia L, Barnes D, Sellebjerg F, Rudick RA. A meta-analysis of methylprednisolone in recovery from multiple sclerosis exacerbations. Mult Scler 2000; 6(4): 267–273.
3. Hommes OR, Barkhof F, Jongen PJ, Frequin ST. Methylprednisolone treatment in multiple sclerosis: effect of treatment, pharmacokinetics, future. Mult Scler 1996; 1(6): 327–328.
4. Goas JY, Marion JL, Missoum A. High dose intravenous methyl prednisolone in acute exacerbations of multiple sclerosis. J Neurol Neurosurg Psychiatry 1983; 46(1): 99.
5. Sellebjerg F, Frederiksen JL, Nielsen PM, Olesen J. Double-blind, randomized, placebo-controlled study of oral, high-dose methylprednisolone in attacks of MS. Neurology 1998; 51(2): 529–534.
6. Barnes D, Hughes RA, Morris RW, Wade-Jones O, Brown P, Britton T, Francis DA, Perkin GD, Rudge P, Swash M, Katifi H, Farmer S, Frankel J. Randomised trial of oral and intravenous methylprednisolone in acute relapses of multiple sclerosis. Lancet 1997; 349(9056): 902–906.
7. Vree TB, Verwey-van Wissen CP, Lagerwerf AJ, Swolfs A, Maes RA, van Ooijen RD, Eikema Hommes OR, Jongen PJ. Isolation and identification of the C6-hydroxy and C20-hydroxy metabolites and glucuronide conjugate of methylprednisolone by preparative high-performance liquid chromatography from urine of patients receiving high-dose pulse therapy. J Chromatogr B Biomed Sci Appl 1999; 726(1–2): 157–168.
8. Vree TB, Lagerwerf AJ, Verwey-van Wissen CP, Jongen PJ. High-performance liquid chromatography analysis, preliminary pharmacokinetics, metabolism and renal excretion of methylprednisolone with its C6 and C20 hydroxy metabolites in multiple sclerosis patients receiving high-dose pulse therapy. J Chromatogr B Biomed Sci Appl 1999; 732(2): 337–348.
9. Hale TW, Ilett K. Unpublished data. 2000.

METHYLSULFONYLMETHANE   L3

Trade: MSM, Crystalline DMSO, DMSO$_2$

Other Trades:

Category: Antiarthritic

Methylsulfonylmethane (DMSO$_2$, MSM, "Crystalline DMSO") is the normal oxidation product of dimethylsulfoxide (DMSO). It is purportedly used for osteoarthritis and joint inflammations.[1] No data are available on this product, but it is probably distributed and eliminated the same as dimethylsulfoxide. MSM is well absorbed, and produces significant levels in the CNS, which would suggest it enters milk as well. It is primarily used in osteoarthritis, joint inflammation, bursitis, and allergic rhinitis, although its efficacy is questionable. It is probably somewhat safe when used briefly (up to 12 weeks), although its use in pregnant and breastfeeding women is highly questionable.

Pregnancy Risk	Probably Safe	Lactation Risk	L3
T ½	=	M/P	=
Vd	=	PB	=
Tmax	=	Oral	=
MW	= 94.1	pKa	=

Adult Concerns: Diarrhea, nausea, headache, bloating, fatigue, insomnia and difficulty with mental acuity.

Pediatric Concerns:

Drug Interactions:

Relative Infant Dose:

Adult Dose: <6 grams daily.

Alternatives:

References:
1. Pharmaceutical manufacturer prescribing information, 2011.

METOCLOPRAMIDE   L2

Trade: Reglan, Metozolv ODT

Other Trades: Maxolon, Pramin, Apo-Metoclop, Emex, Maxeran, Reglan, Gastromax, Paramid

Category: GI stimulant, prolactin stimulant

Metoclopramide, a dopamine receptor blocker, has multiple functions but is primarily used for increasing the lower esophageal sphincter tone in gastroesophageal reflux in patients with reduced gastric tone. In breastfeeding, it is sometimes used in lactating women to stimulate prolactin release from the pituitary and enhance breastmilk production.

Since 1981, a number of publications have documented major increases in breastmilk production following the use of metoclopramide, domperidone, or sulpiride. With metoclopramide, the increase in serum prolactin and breastmilk production appears dose-related up to a dose of 15 mg three times daily.[1] Many studies show 66 to 100% increases in milk production depending on the degree of breastmilk supply in the mother prior to therapy and maybe her initial prolactin levels. Doses of 15 mg/day were found ineffective, whereas doses of 30–45 mg/day were most effective. In most studies, major increases in prolactin were observed such as from 125 ng/mL to 172 ng/mL in one patient.[2] In Kauppila's study[3], the concentration of metoclopramide in milk was consistently higher than the maternal serum levels. The peak occurred at 2–3 hours after administration of the medication. During the late puerperium, the concentration of metoclopramide in the milk varied from 20 to 125 µg/L, which was less than the 28 to 157 µg/L noted during the early puerperium. The authors estimated the daily dose to infant to vary from 6 to 24 µg/kg/day during the early puerperium and from 1 to 13 µg/kg/day during the late phase. These doses are minimal compared to those used for therapy of reflux in pediatric patients (0.1 to 0.5 mg/kg/day). In these studies, only 1 of 5 infants studied had detectable blood levels of metoclopramide; hence, no accumulation or side effects were observed.

While plasma prolactin levels in the newborns were comparable to those in the mothers prior to treatment, Kauppila found slight increases in prolactin levels in 4 of 7 newborns following treatment with metoclopramide although a more recent study did not find such changes. However, prolactin levels are highly variable and subject to diurnal rhythm, thus timing is essential in measuring prolactin levels and could account for this inconsistency. In another study of 23 women with premature infants, milk production increased from 93 mL/day to 197 mL/day between the first and 7th day of therapy with 30 mg/day.[4] Prolactin levels, although varied, increased from 18.1 to 121.8 ng/mL. While basal prolactin levels were elevated significantly, metoclopramide seems to blunt the rapid rise of prolactin when milk was expressed. Nevertheless, milk production was still elevated.

Gupta studied 32 mothers with inadequate milk supply.[5] Following a dose of 10 mg three times daily, a 66–100% increase in milk supply was noted. Of twelve cases of complete lactation failure, 8 responded to treatment in an average of 3–4 days after starting therapy. In this study, 87.5% of the total 32 cases responded to metoclopramide therapy with greater milk production. No untoward effects were noted in the infants. In a study of 5 breastfeeding women who were receiving 30 mg/day, daily milk production increased significantly from 150.9 mL/day to 276.4 mL/day in this group.[6] Infant plasma prolactin levels in breastfed infants were determined as well on the 5th postnatal day and no changes were noted; thus, the amount of metoclopramide transferred in milk was not enough to change the infants' prolactin levels. In a study by Lewis in ten patients who received a single oral dose of 10 mg, the mean maternal plasma and milk levels at 2 hours was 68.5 ng/mL and 125.7 µg/L respectively.[7] Hansen's study showed that 28 women receiving 30 mg/day had no significant increase in milk production as compared to the placebo group.[8] However, this study was initiated with 96 hours of delivery, a time when virtually all mothers would have had exceedingly high plasma prolactin levels anyway. Metoclopramide should not be expected to work as a galactagogue when plasma prolactin levels are high.

It is well recognized that metoclopramide increases a mother's milk supply, but it is exceedingly dose dependent, and yet some mothers simply do not respond. In those mothers who do not respond, Kauppila's work suggests that these patients may already have elevated prolactin levels. In his study, 3 of the 5 mothers who did not respond with increased milk production, had the highest basal prolactin levels (300–400 ng/mL).[3] Thus it may be advisable to do plasma prolactin levels on under-producing mothers prior to instituting metoclopramide therapy to assess the response prior to treating. Side effects such as gastric cramping and diarrhea limit the compliance of some patients but are rare.

Withdrawing from Therapy: It is often found that upon rapid discontinuation of the medication, the supply of milk may in some instances reduce significantly. Tapering of the dose is generally recommended and one possible regimen is to decrease the dose by 10 mg per week. Long-term use of this medication (>4 weeks) may be accompanied by increased side effects such as depression in the mother although some patients have used it successfully for months. The FDA has warned that therapy longer than 3 months may be associated with tardive dyskinesis.

Two recent cases of serotonin-like reactions (agitation, dysarthria, diaphoresis and extrapyramidal movement disorder) have been reported when metoclopramide was used in patients receiving sertraline or venlafaxine.[9] Another dopamine antagonist, Domperidone, is a preferred choice but is unfortunately not available in the USA other than in compounding pharmacies.

The US FDA recently issued a black box warning concerning the association of Tardive Dyskinesia and the use of metoclopramide. But this warning is for the use more than 3 months. Use for brief periods of up to 60 days is probably safe in most instances.

Pregnancy Risk	B	Lactation Risk	L2
T ½	= 5–6 hours	M/P	= 0.5–4.06
Vd	=	PB	= 30%
Tmax	= 1–2 hours (oral)	Oral	= 30–100%
MW	= 300	pKa	= 4.5, 9.2

Adult Concerns: Diarrhea, sedation, gastric upset, nausea, extrapyramidal symptoms, severe depression.

Pediatric Concerns: None reported in infants via milk. Commonly used in pediatrics.

Drug Interactions: Anticholinergic drugs may reduce the effects of metoclopramide. Opiate analgesics may increase CNS depression. Two cases of serotonin-like syndrome have been reported when used with metoclopramide. Two recent cases of serotonin-like reactions (agitation, dysarthria, diaphoresis and extrapyramidal movement disorder) have been reported when metoclopramide was used in patients receiving sertraline or venlafaxine.

Relative Infant Dose: 4.7%–14.3%

Adult Dose: 10–15 mg three times daily.

Alternatives: Domperidone

References:
1. Kauppila A, Kivinen S, Ylikorkala O. A dose response relation between improved lactation and metoclopramide. Lancet 1981; 1(8231): 1175–1177.
2. Budd SC, Erdman SH, Long DM, Trombley SK, Udall JN, Jr. Improved lactation with metoclopramide. A case report. Clin Pediatr (Phila) 1993; 32(1): 53–57.
3. Kauppila A, Arvela P, Koivisto M, Kivinen S, Ylikorkala O, Pelkonen O. Metoclopramide and breast feeding: transfer into milk and the newborn. Eur J Clin Pharmacol 1983; 25(6): 819–823.
4. Ehrenkranz RA, Ackerman BA. Metoclopramide effect on faltering milk production by mothers of premature infants. Pediatrics 1986; 78(4): 614–620.

5. Gupta AP, Gupta PK. Metoclopramide as a lactogogue. Clin Pediatr (Phila) 1985; 24(5): 269–272.
6. Ertl T, Sulyok E, Ezer E, Sarkany I, Thurzo V, Csaba IF. The influence of metoclopramide on the composition of human breast milk. Acta Paediatr Hung 1991; 31(4): 415–422.
7. Lewis PJ, Devenish C, Kahn C. Controlled trial of metoclopramide in the initiation of breast feeding. Br J Clin Pharmacol 1980; 9(2): 217–219.
8. Hansen WF, McAndrew S, Harris K, Zimmerman MB. Metoclopramide Effect on Breastfeeding the Preterm Infant: A Randomized Trial. Obstet Gynecol 2005; 105(2): 383–389.
9. Fisher AA, Davis MW. Serotonin syndrome caused by selective serotonin reuptake-inhibitors-metoclopramide interaction. Ann Pharmacother 2002; 36: 67–71.

METOPROLOL   L3

Trade: Toprol-XL, Lopressor

Other Trades: Betaloc, Minax, Apo-Metoprolol, Betaloc, Lopressor, Novo-Metoprol

Category: Antihypertensive, beta blocker

At low doses, metoprolol is a very cardioselective beta-1 blocker, and it is used for hypertension, angina, and tachyarrhythmia. In a study of 3 women 4–6 months postpartum who received 100 mg twice daily for 4 days, the peak concentration of metoprolol ranged from 0.38 to 2.58 µmol/L, whereas the maternal plasma levels ranged from 0.1 to 0.97 µmol/L.[1] The mean milk/plasma ratio was 3.0. Assuming ingestion of 75 mL of milk at each feeding, and the maximum concentration of 2.58 µmol/L, an infant would ingest approximately 0.05 mg metoprolol at the first feeding and considerably less at subsequent feedings. In another study of 9 women receiving 50–100 mg twice daily, the maternal plasma and milk concentrations ranged from 4–556 nmol/L and 19–1690 nmol/L respectively.[2] Using this data, the authors calculated an average milk concentration throughout the day as 280 µg/L of milk. This dose is 20–40 times less than a typical clinical dose. The milk/plasma ratio in these studies averaged 3.72. Although the milk/plasma ratios for this drug are in general high, the maternal plasma levels are quite small so the absolute amount transferred to the infant are quite small. Although these levels are probably too low to be clinically relevant, clinicians should use metoprolol under close supervision.

Pregnancy Risk	C	Lactation Risk	L3
T ½	= 3–7 hours	M/P	= 3–3.72
Vd	= 2.5–5.6 l/kg	PB	= 12%
Tmax	= 2.5–3 hours	Oral	= 40–50%
MW	= 267	pKa	= 9.7

Adult Concerns: Hypotension, weakness, depression, bradycardia.

Pediatric Concerns: None reported in several studies, but close observation for hypotension, weakness, bradycardia is advised.

Drug Interactions: Decreased effect when used with aluminum salts, barbiturates, calcium salts, cholestyramine, NSAIDs, ampicillin, rifampin, and salicylates. Beta blockers may reduce the effect of oral sulfonylureas (hypoglycemic agents). Increased toxicity/effect when used with other antihypertensives, contraceptives,

MAO inhibitors, cimetidine, and numerous other products. See drug interactions reference for complete listing.

Relative Infant Dose: 1.4%

Adult Dose: 100–450 mg daily.

Alternatives: Propranolol

References:
1. Liedholm H, Melander A, Bitzen PO, Helm G, Lonnerholm G, Mattiasson I, Nilsson B, Wahlin-Boll E. Accumulation of atenolol and metoprolol in human breast milk. Eur J Clin Pharmacol 1981; 20(3): 229–231.
2. Sandstrom B, Regardh CG. Metoprolol excretion into breast milk. Br J Clin Pharmacol 1980; 9(5): 518–519.
3. Kulas J, Lunell NO, Rosing U, Steen B, Rane A. Atenolol and metoprolol. A comparison of their excretion into human breast milk. Acta Obstet Gynecol Scand Suppl 1984; 118: 65–69.

METRIZAMIDE   L2

Trade: Amipaque
Other Trades:
Category: Radiological Contrast Agent

Metrizamide is a radiographic contrast medium used mainly in myelography. It is water soluble and nonionic. Metrizamide contains 48% bound iodine by molecular weight. The iodine molecule is organically bound and is not available for uptake into breast milk due to minimal metabolism. Following subarachnoid administration of 5.06 gm the peak plasma level of 32.9 µg/mL occurred at six hours. Cumulative excretion in milk increased with time, but was extremely small with only 1.1 mg or 0.02% of the dose being recovered in milk within 44.3 hours.[1] The drug's high water solubility, nonionic characteristic, and its high molecular weight (789) also support minimal excretion into breast milk. This agent is sometimes used as an oral radiocontrast agent.[2] Only minimal oral absorption occurs (<0.4%). The authors suggest that the very small amount of metrizamide secreted in human milk is unlikely to be hazardous to the infant.

Pregnancy Risk	D	Lactation Risk	L2
T ½	= >24 hours	M/P	=
Vd	=	PB	=
Tmax	= 6 hours	Oral	= <0.4%
MW	= 789	pKa	= 10.39

Adult Concerns: Headache, irritation of meninges.

Pediatric Concerns:

Drug Interactions:

Relative Infant Dose:

Adult Dose:

Alternatives:

References:
1. Ilett KF, Hackett LP, Paterson JW, McCormick CC. Excretion of metrizamide in milk. Br J Radiol 1981; 54(642): 537–538.
2. Johansen JG. Assessment of a non-ionic contrast medium (Amipaque) in the gastrointestinal tract. Invest Radiol 1978; 13(6): 523–527.

METRIZOATE   L2

Trade: Angiocontrast, Isopaque

Other Trades:

Category: Radiological Contrast Agent

Metrizoate is an ionic radiocontrast agent. Radiopaque agents (except barium) are iodinated compounds used to visualize various organs during X-rays, CAT scans, and other radiological procedures. These compounds are highly iodinated benzoic acid derivatives. While iodine products are generally contraindicated in nursing mothers these products are unique, because they are extremely inert and are largely cleared without metabolism. In a study of four women who received metrizoate 0.58 gm/kg (350 mg Iodine/mL) IV, the peak level of metrizoate in milk was 14 mg/L at three and six hours post-injection.[1] The average milk concentration during the first 24 hours was only 11.4 mg/L. During the first 24 hours following injection, it is estimated that a total of 1.7 mg/kg would be transferred to the infant, which is only 0.3% of the maternal dose.

As a group, radiocontrast agents are virtually unabsorbed after oral administration (<0.1%). Metrizoate has a brief half-life of just two hours, and the estimated dose ingested by the infant is only 0.2% of the radiocontrast dose used clinically for various scanning procedures in infants. Although most company package inserts suggest that an infant be removed from the breast for 24 hours, no untoward effects have been reported with these products in breastfed infants. Because the amount of metrizoate transferred into milk is so small, the authors conclude that breastfeeding is acceptable after intravenously administered metrizoate.

Pregnancy Risk	D	Lactation Risk	L2
T ½	= 60–140 minutes	M/P	=
Vd	=	PB	= Very Low
Tmax	=	Oral	= Nil
MW	= 627	pKa	=

Adult Concerns: Warmth sensation, nausea, vomiting, increased blood pressure.

Pediatric Concerns:

Drug Interactions:

Relative Infant Dose:

Adult Dose:

Alternatives:

References:
1. Nielsen ST, Matheson I, Rasmussen JN, Skinnemoen K, Andrew E, Hafsahl G. Excretion of iohexol and metrizoate in human breast milk. Acta Radiol 1987; 28(5): 523–526.

METRONIDAZOLE   L2

Trade: Flagyl, Metizol, Trikacide, Protostat, Noritate, Metrocream, Metrolotion

Other Trades: Metrozine, Rozex, Apo-Metronidazole, Flagyl, NeoMetric, Novo-Nidazol

Category: Antibiotic, amebicide

Metronidazole is indicated in the treatment of vaginitis due to Trichomonas vaginalis and various anaerobic bacterial infections including giardiasis, H. pylori, B. fragilis, and *Gardnerella vaginalis*. Metronidazole has become the treatment of choice for pediatric giardiasis (AAP).

Metronidazole absorption is time and dose dependent and also depends on the route of administration (oral vs. vaginal). Following a 2 gm oral dose, milk levels were reported to peak at 50–57 mg/L at 2 hours. Milk levels after 12 hours were approximately 19 mg/L and at 24 hours were approximately 10 mg/L.[1] The average drug concentration reported in milk at 2, 8, 12, and 12–24 hours was 45.8, 27.9, 19.1, and 12.6 mg/L respectively. If breastfeeding were to continue uninterrupted, an infant would consume 21.8 mg via breastmilk. With a 12 hour discontinuation, an infant would consume only 9.8 mg.

In a group of 12 nursing mothers receiving 400 mg three times daily, the mean milk/plasma ratio was 0.91.[2] The mean milk metronidazole concentration was 15.5 mg/L. Infant plasma metronidazole levels ranged from 1.27 to 2.41 µg/mL. No adverse effects were attributable to metronidazole therapy in these infants. In another study in patients receiving 600 and 1200 mg daily, the average milk metronidazole concentration was 5.7 and 14.4 mg/L respectively.[3] The plasma levels of metronidazole (2 hours) at the 600 mg/day dose were 5 µg/mL (mother) and 0.8 µg/mL (infant). At the 1200 mg/day dose (2 hours), plasma levels were 12.5 µg/mL (mother) and 2.4 µg/mL (infant). The authors estimated the daily metronidazole dose received by the infant at 3.0 mg/kg with 500 mL milk intake per day, which is well below the advocated 10–20 mg/kg recommended therapeutic dose for infants.

For treating trichomoniasis, many physicians now recommend 2 gm single oral dose with an interruption of breastfeeding for 12–24 hours, then reinstitute breastfeeding. Thus far, no reports of untoward effects in breastfed infants have been published for the 2 gm STAT dose or the 250 mg three times daily for 10 day dosage regimen, but we suggest at least a 12 hour interruption following a 2 gram dose. In a study of 6 women receiving 400 mg three times daily for 3 days, the average milk concentration was 13.5 mg/L with a milk/plasma ratio of 0.9.[4]

For intravaginal use, metronidazole gel (MetroGel) is available. Metronidazole vaginal gel produces only 2% of the mean peak serum level concentration of a 500 mg oral metronidazole tablet. The maternal plasma level following use of each dose of vaginal gel averaged only 237 µg/L, far less than orally administered tablet formulations. Milk levels following intravaginal use would probably be exceedingly low. Milk/plasma ratios, although published for oral metronidazole, may be different for this route of administration. It is true that the relative infant dose via milk is moderately high depending on the dose and timing. Infants whose mothers ingest 1.2 gm/day will receive approximately 13.5% or less of the maternal dose or approximately 2.3 mg/kg/day. Bennett has calculated the relative infant dose from 11.7% to as high as 24% of the maternal dose.[5] Heisterberg found metronidazole levels in infant plasma to be 16% and 19% of the maternal plasma levels following doses of 600 mg/day and 1200 mg/day.[3] While these levels seem significant, it is still pertinent to remember that metronidazole is a commonly used drug in premature neonates, infants, and children, and 2.3 mg/kg/day is still much less than the therapeutic dose used in infants/children (7.5–30 mg/kg/day). Thus far, virtually no adverse effects have been reported.

INTRAVENOUS USE: Metronidazole is approximately 98% bioavailable orally and it is rapidly absorbed. In one study of intravenous kinetics, the authors found peak plasma levels of 28.9 µg/mL in adults following a 500 mg TID dose.[6] In another study of oral and intravenous kinetics, the authors used 400 mg orally, and 500 mg intravenously.[7] Following 400 mg orally, the C_{max} at 90 minutes was 17.4 µg/mL. Following 500 mg IV, the C_{max} at 90 minutes was 23.6 µg/mL. Reducing the IV dose to 400 mg would have given a plasma level of approximately 18.8 or an amount similar to the oral plasma level attained in the above group(17.4). From these two sets of data, it is apparent that the peak (C_{max}) following an intravenous dose is only slightly higher than that obtained following oral administration. In an elegant study of plasma kinetics of oral and IV metronidazole (both 500 mg and 2000 mg), Loft found that the AUC (500 mg dose) for oral and IV treatments was virtually identical (101 vs. 100 µg/mL h respectively).[8] The C_{max} (taken from graph) for oral and IV treatments were essentially the same. In another study comparing the plasma kinetics following 800 mg doses orally and IV, Bergan[9] found that plasma levels are virtually identical at 2–3 hours after the dose. Therefore, in a breastfeeding mother receiving IV metronidazole, a brief interruption of breastfeeding for perhaps 1–2 hours would expose the infant to almost identical levels as obtained from the same dose given orally.

Data from older studies with rats and mice have shown that metronidazole is potentially mutagenic/carcinogenic. Thus far, no studies in humans have found it to be mutagenic. In fact, the opposite seems to be the finding.[10,11,12] Roe suggests that metronidazole is 'essentially free of cancer risk or other serious toxic side effects'.[12] Age-gender stratified analysis did not reveal any association between short-term exposure to metronidazole and cancer in humans.[11]

Pregnancy Risk	B	Lactation Risk	L2
T ½	= 8.5 hours	M/P	= 1.15
Vd	=	PB	= 10%
Tmax	= 2–4 hours	Oral	= 100%
MW	= 171	pKa	= 2.6

Adult Concerns: Nausea, dry mouth, vomiting, diarrhea, abdominal discomfort. Drug may turn urine brown.

Pediatric Concerns: Numerous studies shown no untoward effects. One letter to the editor suggests an infant developed diarrhea, and a case of lactose intolerance. The link to metronidazole is tenuous.

Drug Interactions: Phenytoin and phenobarbital may decrease half-life of metronidazole. Alcohol may induce disulfiram-like reactions. May increase prothrombin times when used with warfarin.

Relative Infant Dose: 12.6%–13.5%

Adult Dose: 250–500 mg twice daily.

Alternatives:

References:

1. Erickson SH, Oppenheim GL, Smith GH. Metronidazole in breast milk. Obstet Gynecol 1981; 57(1): 48–50.
2. Passmore CM, McElnay JC, Rainey EA, D'Arcy PF. Metronidazole excretion in human milk and its effect on the suckling neonate. Br J Clin Pharmacol 1988; 26(1): 45–51.
3. Heisterberg L, Branebjerg PE. Blood and milk concentrations of metronidazole in mothers and infants. J Perinat Med 1983; 11(2): 114–120.
4. Amon I, Amon K. Wirkstoffkonzentrationen von metronidazol bie schwangeren und postpartal. Fortschritte der antimikrobiellen und antineoplastischen. Chemotherapie 2004; Band 2–4: 605–612.
5. Bennett PN. Use of the monographs on drugs: In: Drugs and Human Lactation. Amsterdam, Elsevier, 1996.
6. Ti TY, Lee HS, Khoo YM. Disposition of intravenous metronidazole in Asian surgical patients. Antimicrob Agents Chemother 1996; 40(10): 2248–2251.
7. Earl P, Sisson PR, Ingham HR. Twelve-hourly dosage schedule for oral and intravenous metronidazole. J Antimicrob Chemother 1989; 23(4): 619–621.
8. Loft S, Dossing M, Poulsen HE, Sonne J, Olesen KL, Simonsen K, Andreasen PB. Influence of dose and route of administration on disposition of metronidazole and its major metabolites. Eur J Clin Pharmacol 1986; 30(4): 467–473.
9. Bergan T, Leinebo O, Blom-Hagen T, Salvesen B. Pharmacokinetics and bioavailability of metronidazole after tablets, suppositories and intravenous administration. Scand J Gastroenterol Suppl 1984; 91: 45–60.
10. Falagas ME, Walker AM, Jick H, Ruthazer R, Griffith J, Snydman DR. Late incidence of cancer after metronidazole use: a matched metronidazole user/nonuser study. Clin Infect Dis 1998; 26(2): 384–388.
11. Fahrig R, Engelke M. Reinvestigation of in vivo genotoxicity studies in man. I. No induction of DNA strand breaks in peripheral lymphocytes after metronidazole therapy. Mutat Res 1997; 395(2–3): 215–221.
12. Roe FJ. Toxicologic evaluation of metronidazole with particular reference to carcinogenic, mutagenic, and teratogenic potential. Surgery 1983; 93(1 Pt 2): 158–164.

METRONIDAZOLE TOPICAL GEL   L2

Trade: MetroGel Topical

Other Trades: Metrogyl, Metro-Gel, Metrogel

Category: Topical antibacterial

Metronidazole topical gel is primarily indicated for acne and is a gel formulation containing 0.75% metronidazole. Following topical application of 1 gm of metronidazole gel to the face (equivalent to 7.5 mg metronidazole base), the maximum serum concentration was only 66 ng/mL in only one of 10 patients (In three of the ten patients, levels were undetectable).[1,2] This concentration is 100 times less than the serum concentrations achieved following the oral ingestion of just one 250 mg tablet. Therefore, the topical application of metronidazole gel provides only exceedingly low plasma levels in the mother and minimal to no levels in milk.

Pregnancy Risk	B	Lactation Risk	L2
T ½	= 8.5 hours	M/P	= 0.4–1.8
Vd	=	PB	= 10%
Tmax	=	Oral	= Complete
MW	= 171	pKa	= 2.6

Adult Concerns: Watery eyes if the gel is applied too close to eyes. Minor skin irritation, redness, milk dryness, burning.

Pediatric Concerns: None reported via milk. Milk levels would be exceedingly low to nil.

Drug Interactions: Although many known interactions with oral metronidazole are documented, due to minimal plasma levels of this preparation, they would be extremely remote.

Relative Infant Dose:

Adult Dose: Apply topically twice daily.

Alternatives:

References:
1. Drug Facts and Comparisons 1996 ed. ed. St. Louis, 1996.
2. Pharmaceutical manufacturer prescribing information, 1997.

METRONIDAZOLE VAGINAL GEL　　L2

Trade: MetroGel Vaginal
Other Trades: Metrogel
Category: Antibiotic

Metronidazole is an antibiotic used for the treatment of vaginitis. Both topical and vaginal preparations of metronidazole contain only 0.75% metronidazole. Plasma levels following administration are exceedingly low.[1] This metronidazole vaginal product produces only 2% of the mean peak serum level concentration of a 500 mg oral metronidazole tablet. The maternal plasma level following use of each dose of vaginal gel averaged 237 µg/L compared to 12,785 µg/L following an oral 500 mg tablet. Milk levels following intravaginal use would probably be exceeding low. Milk/plasma ratios, although published for oral metronidazole, may be different for this route of administration, primarily due to the low plasma levels attained with this product. Topical and intravaginal metronidazole gels are indicated for bacterial vaginosis.

Pregnancy Risk	B	Lactation Risk	L2
T ½	= 8.5 hours	M/P	=
Vd	=	PB	= 10%
Tmax	= 6–12 hours	Oral	= Complete
MW	= 171	pKa	= 2.6

Adult Concerns: Mild irritation to vaginal wall.

Pediatric Concerns: None reported.

Drug Interactions: Phenytoin and phenobarbital may decrease half-life of metronidazole. Alcohol may induce disulfiram-like reactions. May increase prothrombin times when used with warfarin.

Relative Infant Dose:

Adult Dose: 37.5 mg twice daily.

Alternatives:

References:
1. Pharmaceutical manufacturer prescribing information, 1996.

METYRAPONE   L2

Trade: Metopirone

Other Trades:

Category: Diagnostic Agent, Radiopharmaceutical Imaging

Metyrapone is an inhibitor of endogenous adrenal corticosteroid synthesis and is a diagnostic drug for diagnosis and treatment of adrenocortical hyperfunction. In a case report of a single patient who received 250 mg four times daily for almost 9 weeks, and who was 1 week postpartum, breastmilk samples were analyzed for metyrapone and its metabolite. At steady state, the average concentrations in milk and absolute and relative infant doses were 11 µg/L, 1.7 µg/kg/day, and 0.02%, respectively, for metyrapone; and 48.5 µg/L, 7.3 µg/kg/day, and 0.08%, respectively, for its metabolite, rac-metyrapol.[1] The authors suggest that maternal metyrapone use during breastfeeding is unlikely to be a significant risk to an infant.

Pregnancy Risk	C	Lactation Risk	L2
T ½	= 1.9 hours	M/P	=
Vd	=	PB	=
Tmax	= 1 hour	Oral	= Complete
MW	= 226	pKa	=

Adult Concerns: Hypertension, nausea, headache, sedation, rash, acne, alopecia and hirsutism, bone marrow depression, adrenal insufficiency have been reported.

Pediatric Concerns: None yet. Levels probably too low.

Drug Interactions: Increased risk of acetaminophen toxicity.

Relative Infant Dose: 0.06%

Adult Dose: 30 mg/kg

Alternatives:

References:
1. Hotham NJ, Ilett KF, Hackett LP, Morton MR, Muller P, Hague WM. Transfer of metyrapone and its metabolite, rac-metyrapol, into breast milk. J Hum Lact. 2009 Nov; 25(4): 451–4.

MEXILETINE   L2

Trade: Mexitil

Other Trades: Mexitil, Novo-Mexiletine

Category: Antiarrhythmic

Mexiletine hydrochloride is an antiarrhythmic agent with activity similar to lidocaine. In a study on one patient who was receiving 600 mg/day in divided doses, the milk level at steady state was 0.8 mg/L, which represented a milk/plasma ratio of 1.1.[1] Mexiletine was not detected in the infant nor were untoward effects noted. In another study on day 2 to 5 postpartum and in a patient receiving 200 mg three times daily, the mean peak concentration of mexiletine in breastmilk was 959 μg/L, and the maternal serum was 724 μg/L.[2] In this study the milk plasma ratio varied from 0.78 to 1.89 with an average of 1.45. It is unlikely this exposure would lead to untoward side effects in a breastfeeding infant.

Pregnancy Risk	C	Lactation Risk	L2
T ½	= 9.2 hours	M/P	= 1.45
Vd	= 6–12 l/kg	PB	= 63%
Tmax	= 2–3 hours (oral)	Oral	= 90%
MW	= 179	pKa	= 8.4

Adult Concerns: Arrhythmias, bradycardia, hypotension, tremors, dizziness.

Pediatric Concerns: None reported in two studies.

Drug Interactions: Aluminum, magnesium hydroxide, atropine, and narcotics may reduce the oral absorption of mexiletine. Cimetidine may increase or decrease mexiletine plasma levels. Hydantoins such as phenytoin may increase mexiletine clearance and reduce plasma levels. Rifampin may increase mexiletine clearance leading to lower levels. Mexiletine may reduce the clearance of caffeine by 50%. Serum theophylline levels may be increased significantly to toxic levels.

Relative Infant Dose: 1.4%–1.6%

Adult Dose: 200 mg every 8 hours.

Alternatives:

References:
1. Lewis AM, Patel L, Johnston A, Turner P. Mexiletine in human blood and breast milk. Postgrad Med J 1981; 57(671): 546–547.
2. Timmis AD, Jackson G, Holt DW. Mexiletine for control of ventricular dysrhythmias in pregnancy. Lancet 1980; 2(8195 pt 1): 647–648.

MICONAZOLE   L2

Trade: Oravig

Other Trades:

Category: Antifungal for candidiasis

Miconazole is an effective antifungal that is commonly used IV, topically, and intravaginally. After intravaginal application, approximately 1% of the dose is absorbed systemically.[1,2] After topical application, there is little or no absorption (0.1%). It is unlikely that the limited absorption of miconazole from vaginal application would produce significant levels in milk. Milk concentrations following oral and IV miconazole have not been reported. Oral absorption of miconazole is poor, only 25–30%. Miconazole is commonly used in pediatric patients less than 1 year of age.

Pregnancy Risk	C	Lactation Risk	L2
T ½	= 20–25 hours	M/P	=
Vd	=	PB	= 91–93%
Tmax	= Immediate (IV)	Oral	= 25–30%
MW	= 416	pKa	= 6.9

Adult Concerns: Nausea, vomiting, diarrhea, anorexia, itching, rash, local irritation.

Pediatric Concerns: None reported via milk.

Drug Interactions: May increase warfarin anticoagulant effect. May increase hypoglycemia of oral sulfonylureas. Phenytoin levels may be increased.

Relative Infant Dose:

Adult Dose: 200–1200 mg three times daily.

Alternatives:

References:
1. Facts and Comparisons. St. Louis: 2010..
2. McEvoy GE. (ed): AFHS Drug Information. New York, NY: 2003.

MICROFIBRILLAR COLLAGEN HEMOSTAT   L3

Trade: Avitene, Helistat, Hemotene
Other Trades:
Category: Hemostatic agent

Microfibrillar collagen hemostat (MCH) is an absorbable topical hemostatic agent of bovine origin. It is used to achieve hemostasis during surgical procedures when conventional methods appear to fail. Chemically it is collagen non-covalently bound to hydrochloric acid.[1,2] Collagen is an inert protein found in skin, ligaments, tendons and bones. It serves the purpose of providing cytoskeletal stability and inelasticity. Its molecular weight is 300 kDa. When MCH is applied on a bleeding surface, it attracts platelets to the surface and results in the formation of a platelet plug, which eventually helps control bleeding.[3] MCH is being used increasingly for neurosurgical procedures. This product has been known to excite local and systemic inflammatory reactions. Following its use in neurosurgical procedures, a few cases of seizures, mass occupying granulomas and encephalomyelitis have been described.[4-7] This product has the potential to pass through the circulatory system from the initial site of application, and deposit in different organs causing organ damage.[8] Its use in breastfeeding women has not been described. However, due to its high molecular weight, its transfer into breastmilk is unlikely. Being an inert protein, its systemic absorption following ingestion in milk is unlikely.

Pregnancy Risk	C	Lactation Risk	L3
T ½	=	M/P	=
Vd	=	PB	=
Tmax	=	Oral	=
MW	= 300 kDa	pKa	=

Adult Concerns: Abscess formation, hematoma, alveolitis of jaw when used in dental extraction pockets. Do not use for closure of skin incisions, on contaminated wounds and do not use on bone surfaces.

Pediatric Concerns:

Drug Interactions:

Relative Infant Dose:

Adult Dose:

Alternatives:

References:

1. Product Information: Avitene(R), microfibrillar collagen hemostat, Avicon, Inc, Ft Worth TX, 1990. Avitene(R), microfibrillar collagen hemostat, Avicon, Inc, Ft Worth TX, 1990.
2. Anon: Avitene(R)–a new topical hemostatic agent. Med Lett Drug Ther 1977; 19: 28.
3. Mason RB and Read MS: Some effects of a microcrystalline collagen preparation on blood. Haemostasis 1974; 3: 31–45.
4. Apel-Sarid L, Cochrane DD, Steinbok P, Byrne AT, Dunham C. Microfibrillarcollagen hemostat-induced necrotizing granulomatous inflammation developing aftercraniotomy: a pediatric case series. J Neurosurg Pediatr. 2010 Oct; 6(4): 385–92.
5. Sani S, Boco T, Lewis SL, Cochran E, Patel AJ, Byrne RW. Postoperative acutedisseminated encephalomyelitis after exposure to microfibrillar collagenhemostat. J Neurosurg. 2008 Jul; 109(1): 149–52.
6. O'Shaughnessy BA, Schafernak KT, DiPatri AJ Jr, Goldman S, Tomita T. Agranulomatous reaction to Avitene mimicking recurrence of a medulloblastoma. Casereport. J Neurosurg. 2006 Jan; 104(1 Suppl): 33–6.
7. Nakajima M, Kamei T, Tomimatu K, Manabe T. An intraperitoneal tumorous masscaused by granulomas of microfibrillar collagen hemostat (Avitene). Arch PatholLab Med. 1995 Dec; 119(12): 1161–3.
8. Robicsek F, Duncan GD, Born GV, Wilkinson HA, Masters TN, McClure M. Inherent dangers of simultaneous application of microfibrillar collagen hemostat andblood-saving devices. J Thorac Cardiovasc Surg. 1986 Oct; 92(4): 766–70.

MIDAZOLAM — L2

Trade: Versed

Other Trades: Hypnovel, Versed

Category: Short acting benzodiazepine sedative, hypnotic

Midazolam is a very short acting benzodiazepine primarily used as an induction or preanesthetic medication. The onset of action of midazolam is extremely rapid, its potency is greater than diazepam, and its metabolic elimination is more rapid.

With a plasma half-life of only 1.9 hours, it is preferred for rapid induction and maintenance of anesthesia.

After oral administration of 15 mg for up to 6 days postnatally in 22 women, the mean milk/plasma ratio was 0.15 and the maximum level of midazolam in breastmilk was 9 μg/L and occurred 1–2 hours after administration.[1] Midazolam and its hydroxy-metabolite were undetectable 4 hours after administration. Therefore, the amount of midazolam transferred to an infant via early milk is minimal, particularly if the baby is breastfed more than 4 hours after administration. In another study of five lactating women who received a single 2 mg IV dose, milk levels of midazolam were exceedingly low after 7 hours. The median amount of midazolam recovered within 24 hours was only 26 μg which was only 0.004% of the maternal dose of 2 mg.[2] Midazolam is so rapidly redistributed to other tissues from the plasma compartment, milk levels will invariably be exceedingly low.

Pregnancy Risk	D	Lactation Risk	L2
T ½	= 2–5 hours	M/P	= 0.15
Vd	= 1.0–2.5 l/kg	PB	= 97%
Tmax	= 20–50 minutes (oral)	Oral	= 27–44%
MW	= 326	pKa	= 6.2

Adult Concerns: Sedation, respiratory depression.

Pediatric Concerns: None reported in several studies. Milk levels exceedingly low after brief wait.

Drug Interactions: Theophylline may reduce the sedative effects of midazolam. Other CNS depressants may potentiate the depressant effects of midazolam. Cimetidine may increase plasma levels of midazolam.

Relative Infant Dose: 0.004%–0.6%

Adult Dose: 1–2.5 mg once or twice daily.

Alternatives: Lorazepam

References:
1. Matheson I, Lunde PK, Bredesen JE. Midazolam and nitrazepam in the maternity ward: milk concentrations and clinical effects. Br J Clin Pharmacol 1990; 30(6): 787–793.
2. Nitsun M, Szokol JW, Saleh HJ, Murphy GS, Vender JS, Luong L, Raikoff K, Avram MJ. Pharmacokinetics of midazolam, propofol, and fentanyl transfer to human breast milk. Clin Pharmacol Ther 2006; 79(6): 549–557.

MIDODRINE   L3

Trade: ProAmatine

Other Trades: Gutron, Amatine, Midon

Category: Vasopressor / Antihypotensive agent

Midodrine is a vasopressor used to increase blood pressure.[1] Midodrine is a prodrug that is metabolized to desglymidodrine. This metabolite is a long-acting alpha-1 agonist. It produces an increase in vascular tone and elevation of blood pressure. Desglymidodrine does not stimulate cardiac beta-1 receptors, nor does it pass the blood-brain barrier. No data are available on its transfer to human milk, but some should be expected. This product is small in molecular weight, belongs to the phenylethylamine family, is lipophilic, and is likely to penetrate milk as do the other members of this family. Some caution is recommended.

Pregnancy Risk	C	Lactation Risk	L3
T ½	= 3–4 hours (metabolite)	M/P	=
Vd	=	PB	=
Tmax	= 1–2 hours	Oral	= 93%
MW	= 290	pKa	= 7.8

Adult Concerns: Supine hypertension, pruritus, pilomotor reactions, chills, painful urination retention, and gastrointestinal symptoms have been reported. CNS reactions include headache, insomnia, stimulation, restlessness, dizziness. A vagal reflex may occur following use and produce a reflex bradycardia.

Pediatric Concerns: None reported via milk, but some caution is recommended. Observe for hypertension, insomnia, and excitement.

Drug Interactions: Additive with other adrenergic stimulants such as pseudoephedrine, ephedrine, phenylephrine or phenylpropanolamine. Digoxin may enhance or precipitate reflex bradycardia. The concurrent use of prazosin or other alpha blockers may inhibit the effects of midodrine. Use with tricyclic antidepressants may precipitate arrhythmias and tachycardia.

Relative Infant Dose:

Adult Dose: 10 mg 3 times daily at 4-hour intervals for orthostatic hypotension

Alternatives:

References:
1. Pharmaceutical manufacturer prescribing information, 2003.

MIFEPRISTONE   L3

Trade: Mifeprex
Other Trades: Mifegyn, Pencroftonum
Category: Antiprogestational agent

Mifepristone is an anti-progestational agent which competitively binds with the progesterone receptor. Based on studies with various oral doses in several animal species (mouse, rat, rabbit and monkey), the compound inhibits the activity of endogenous or exogenous progesterone.[1] Among its uses is to terminate pregnancies. Mifepristone binds to plasma protein receptors and has a biphasic elimination phase with a terminal elimination half-life of 18 hours. No data are available on its transfer into milk, but steroids transfer into human milk poorly. Interestingly, studies in monkeys[2] found increased production of colostrum and increased weight gain in infant monkeys. This correlates with the effect of progesterone receptor activation in inhibiting milk production early postnatally such as with retained placenta. In humans, mifepristone is undetectable in the milk following administration of a 200 mg dose. It may be possible to continue breastfeeding without pause when a dose of 200 mg or less is given to the mother. Levels in milk are likely to be lower than those in the serum.[3]

Pregnancy Risk	X	Lactation Risk	L3
T ½	= 18 hours	M/P	=
Vd	= 1.5 l/kg	PB	= 98%
Tmax	= 1–3 hours	Oral	= 69%
MW	= 426	pKa	= 3.7

Adult Concerns: Bleeding and cramping, abdominal pain, including uterine cramping. Other commonly reported side effects are nausea, vomiting and diarrhea. Pelvic pain, fainting, headache, dizziness, and asthenia occurred rarely.

Pediatric Concerns: No studies in humans. Studies in monkeys suggest it increases milk production early postnatally.

Drug Interactions: Do not use concurrently with clozapine as this may cause an increased risk of cardiotoxicity. Concurrent use with rifampin, phenobarbitone, phenytoin and dexamethasone decreases plasma levels and efficacy of mifepristone. Concurrent use with ketoconazole, itraconazole and erythromycin increases plasma levels of mifepristone.

Relative Infant Dose:

Adult Dose: 600 mg STAT

Alternatives:

References:
1. Pharmaceutical manufacturer prescribing information, 2005.
2. Wolf JP, Sinosich M, Anderson TL, Ulmann A, Baulieu EE, Hodgen GD. Progesterone antagonist (RU 486) for cervical dilation, labor induction, and delivery in monkeys: effectiveness in combination with oxytocin. Am J Obstet Gynecol 1989 Jan; 160(1): 45–7.
3. Saav Ingrid, Fiala Christian, Hamaleinen Jonna M, Heikinheimo Oskari,and Gemzell-Danielsson Kristina. Medical abortion in lactating women – low levels of mifepristone in breast milk. Acta Obstetricia et Gynecologica. 2010; 89: 618–622.

MIGLITOL   L2

Trade: Glyset, Diastabol

Other Trades: Glyset

Category: Anti-diabetic agent

Miglitol is an oral alpha-glycosidase inhibitor for use in non-insulin depended diabetes mellitus.[1] Miglitol delays the digestion of ingested carbohydrates thereby resulting in a small rise in blood glucose concentration following meals. Miglitol does not stimulate insulin release nor does it inhibit lactase, nor does it induce hypoglycemia. The oral absorption of miglitol is saturable in adults in doses higher than 25 mg. A dose of 100 mg is only 50–70% absorbed orally. The manufacturer reports that milk levels are very small. Total excretion into milk accounted for 0.02% of a 100 mg maternal dose. The estimated exposure to a nursing infant is approximately 0.4% of the maternal dose.[1] With such little amounts of transfer into breastmilk, it is highly unlikely that miglitol used during lactation will cause significant clinical effects in the breastfed infant. Miglitol is probably compatible with breastfeeding.

Pregnancy Risk	B	Lactation Risk	L2
T ½	= 2 hours	M/P	=
Vd	= 0.18 l/kg	PB	= <4%
Tmax	= 2–3 hours	Oral	= Variable
MW	= 207	pKa	= 5.9

Adult Concerns: Flatulence, soft stools, diarrhea, abdominal discomfort are the most commonly reported side effects.

Pediatric Concerns: No reports of use in breastfeeding mothers.

Drug Interactions: Glyburide may reduce plasma levels (17–25%) of miglitol. Only small but insignificant changes were noted when coadministered with metformin.

Relative Infant Dose: 0.4%

Adult Dose: 50 mg three times daily.

Alternatives: Metformin

References:
1.   Pharmaceutical manufacturer Prescribing Information, 2003.

MILK THISTLE   L3

Trade: Holy Thistle, Lady Thistle, Marian Thistle, Silybum, Silymarin
Other Trades:
Category: Hepatoprotectant

Milk Thistle has been used for centuries as a liver protectant.[1] Silymarin, a mixture of three isomeric flavonolignans, consists of silybin, silychristin, and silidianin.[2] Silybin is the most biologically active and is believed to be a potent antioxidant and hepatoprotective agent. Silymarin is poorly soluble in water so aqueous preparations such as teas are ineffective. The oral bioavailability is likewise poor, only 23–47% is absorbed orally. Oral forms are generally concentrated. Silymarin effects are almost exclusively on the liver and kidney and concentrates in liver cells. It is believed to inhibit oxidative damage to cells by increasing glutathione synthesis. It is believed to also stimulate the regenerative capacity of liver cells. While it has been advocated for the stimulation of milk synthesis, little evidence of efficacy exists. No data are available concerning Silymarin transfer to human milk but some probably transfers. However, it is rather devoid of reported toxicity with only brief gastrointestinal intolerance and mild allergic reactions.[3,4]

Pregnancy Risk	Probably Safe	Lactation Risk	L3
T ½	=	M/P	=
Vd	=	PB	=
Tmax	=	Oral	= 23–47%
MW	= 482	pKa	=

Adult Concerns: Mild gastrointestinal intolerance and allergic reactions.

Pediatric Concerns: None reported via milk.

Drug Interactions:

Relative Infant Dose:

Adult Dose: 200–400 mg daily via extracts.

Alternatives:

References:

1. Foster S. Milk thistle-Silybum marianum. Botanical Series No. 305. American Botanical Council, Austin, TX 1991; 3–7.
2. Leung AY. Encyclopedia of Common Natural Ingredients used in Food, Drugs and Cosmetics. J Wiley and Sons, 1980.
3. Review of Natural Products Facts and Comparisons 1999.
4. Awang D. Can Pharm J Oct 1993; 403–404.

MILNACIPRAN L3

Trade: Savella

Other Trades:

Category: Selective Serotonin and Norepinephrine Reuptake Inhibitor for fibromyalgia

Milnacipran is a selective serotonin and norepinephrine reuptake inhibitor (SSNRI) that is used in the treatment of fibromyalgia. It potentiates the serotonergic and noradrenergic activity in the brain. The drug can cause serotonin syndrome. Some of the common side effects include headache, nausea, vomiting, hypertension, tachycardia and palpitations. Milnacipran can also cause elevated liver enzymes. Animal studies show the drug is secreted into rat milk.[1] No data yet are available for its transfer into human milk, but it will probably be similar to others in this class. Milnacipran use has been known to increase the risk of suicidal tendencies. Until more is known about this drug and its transfer into breastmilk, caution is urged while using drug in lactating women.

Pregnancy Risk	C/D in 2nd and 3rd trimester	Lactation Risk	L3
T ½	= 6–8 hours	M/P	=
Vd	= 5–8 l/kg	PB	= 13%
Tmax	= 2–4 hours	Oral	= 85–90%
MW	= 282.8	pKa	= 9.6

Adult Concerns: Nausea, constipation, vomiting, headache, dizziness, flushing, and insomnia have been reported.

Pediatric Concerns: None yet via breastmilk.

Drug Interactions: As with SSRIs, use cautiously with drugs such as triptans, lithium, tryptophan, antipsychotics and dopamine antagonists. Co-administration of Milnacipran with other inhibitors of serotonin re-uptake may result in hypertension and coronary artery vasoconstriction, through additive serotonergic effects.

Relative Infant Dose:

Adult Dose: 50 mg twice daily.

Alternatives: Duloxetine, sertraline, paroxetine

References:
1. Pharmaceutical manufacturer prescribing information, 2010.

MILRINONE   L4

Trade: Primacor, Corotrop
Other Trades:
Category: Bupyridine Inotropic/Vasodilator Agent

Milrinone is a bupyridine inotropic/vasodilator agent. The drug is used in the short term treatment of heart failure (<48 hours) that is unresponsive to other modalities. There is increased mortality with long term oral use. Milrinone increases the cardiac output and decreases pulmonary capillary wedge pressure and vascular resistance with mild to moderate increases in heart rate. The drug is well absorbed after oral administration. Blood pressure, heart rate, ECG, fluid and electrolyte balance, and renal function should be monitored during therapy. The half-life is brief, 2.3 hours, therefore waiting 8 hours after last dose prior to restarting breastfeeding should eliminate risk to the infant.[1]

Pregnancy Risk	C	Lactation Risk	L4
T ½	= 0.8 to 2.3 hours	M/P	=
Vd	= 0.38 l/kg	PB	= 70%
Tmax	=	Oral	= 80%
MW	= 211.2	pKa	= 8.83

Adult Concerns: Side effects include supraventricular and ventricular arrythmias, hypotension, angina, headache, hypokalemia, tremor and thrombocytopenia.

Pediatric Concerns:

Drug Interactions:

Relative Infant Dose:

Adult Dose: 50 µg/kg over 10 min, followed by 0.59–1.13 mg/kg infusion over 24 hours.

Alternatives:

References:
1. Pharmaceutical Manufacturer Drug Insert, Baxter Healthcare Corporation, 2008.

MIMYX   L3

Trade: MimyX
Other Trades:
Category: Emollient

MimyX is an emollient hydrogel formulation used in the treatment of dermatoses. The FDA approved in July a nonsteroidal dressing for the management and relief of burning and itching associated with atopic dermatitis, allergic-contact dermatitis, radiation dermatitis, and other physician-diagnosed dermatoses in adult and pediatric patients.

The ingredients appear to be more plant based and include the following: purified water, olive oil, glycerin, pentylene glycol, palm glycerides, vegetable oil, lecithin, squalene (shark oil), betaine, palmitamide MEA, sarcosine, acetamide MEA, hydroxyethyl cellulose, sodium carbomer, carbomer, and xantham gum. No data are available on its transfer into breastmilk. This product would not likely be absorbed or bioavailable to an infant. Do not use directly on the nipple.

Pregnancy Risk	Probably Safe	Lactation Risk	L3
T ½	=	M/P	=
Vd	=	PB	=
Tmax	=	Oral	=
MW	=	pKa	=

Adult Concerns: Local site reactions such as: rash, burning, erythema, urticaria, hypersensitivity.

Pediatric Concerns:

Drug Interactions:

Relative Infant Dose:

Adult Dose: Apply on affected areas 3 times daily.

Alternatives:

References:

MINERAL OIL (PARAFFIN)   L3

Trade:
Other Trades:
Category: Laxative, Emollient

Mineral oils are a group of substances derived from petroleum with chain lengths that range in size from 15–40 carbon atoms in length. They are most often used as laxatives and emollients in topical preparations. The size of any given paraffin is indirectly related to its ability to be absorbed. Substances with greater than 34 carbons are unlikely to be absorbed due to size, while smaller molecules of less than 20 carbons are absorbed well but also broken down very quickly in the liver. Mineral hydrocarbons that are of the most concern in human subjects fall within a range of 21–28 carbons.[1,3] Rectal absorption is minimal, due to the greatest degree of absorption occurring in the small intestine.[2] As such, mineral oil is of concern only when ingested or applied topically. Ingested hydrocarbons do distribute widely throughout the body, resulting in concentrations of up to 4.5 mg/g in humans. The present molecules can include cycloalkanes, which are often found in lipogranulomas and are indicative of mineral oil presence.[1,3]

Acceptable daily intakes (ADI) vary between different mineral oils, with differences being based upon composition of any given preparation. In the case of infants less than 3 months of age, it is recommended that mineral oils be no less than 480 Da(approximately 34 carbons), and that at most 5% of the dose consist of molecules with 25 or less carbons. Total intake should not exceed 0–4 mg/kg, and substances less than 25 carbons should not exceed 0.2 mg/kg.[4] Mineral oils do transfer into breast milk, and generally appear in highest concentration towards the start of lactation. Continued breastfeeding has been shown to lower concentrations of paraffins significantly.

In one woman it was shown that n-alkanes deposited in breast milk centered around a length of 23 carbons, with a substantial amount of hydrocarbons of 22–26 carbon lengths, indicating the presence of mineral oils. Direct application of paraffins to the breast results in accumulation of mineral hydrocarbons in the milk fat. Upon administration of vaseline to the breast for 20 days, mineral hydrocarbons in the milk fat increased to 160 mg/kg.[4] In an infant who ingests 800 mL breastmilk containing 3% fat everyday, this would amount to a daily intake of 1mg/kg mineral oils. This clearly exceeds the acceptable daily intake for paraffins less than 25 carbons in length. Application of salves and ointments to the breast is only recommended after feeding, as the infant may ingest up to 40 mg/kg mineral oil from a mother who applies five daily applications of 100 mg to each breast. Based on the compositions of some body creams, this can result in a dose to the infant that measures 40 times the ADI for substances less than 25 carbons in length. Due to the fact that shorter length hydrocarbons are absorbed well by the mother, it is likely that they will also be absorbed by the infant. It should be noted that while longer chain mineral oils are not well absorbed in the gastrointestinal tract, it is possible for them to be absorbed dermally, though the rate of absorption would be very low.[4]

Toxic effects have been shown in rats when exposed to large amounts of paraffin oils, with the most significant endpoint being histiocytosis in lymph nodes.[5] It is recommended that nursing mothers avoid using paraffin containing products for breast care.[4] Mineral oil is commonly used to treat pediatric constipation, although it may prevent the absorption of oil soluble vitamins.

Pregnancy Risk	C	Lactation Risk	L3
T ½	=	M/P	=
Vd	=	PB	=
Tmax	=	Oral	= 30–60%
MW	= Varies	pKa	=

Adult Concerns: Lipid pneumonitis may occur with aspiration. Nausea, vomiting, cramps, and diarrhea may occur with oral ingestion. Anal seepage may result from rectal application. Impaired absorption of vitamins A, D, E, and K can result.

Pediatric Concerns:

Drug Interactions: Vitamin D: Paraffin may decrease absorption of cholecalciferol. Docusate: May interact with paraffin to cause inflammation of intestinal mucosa, liver, spleen, and lymph nodes. Paricalcitol: Paraffin may decrease systemic concentrations of paricalcitol. Vitamin K: Paraffin may decrease absorption of phytonadione, leading to an increased risk of bleeding.

Relative Infant Dose:

Adult Dose: Oral: 15–45 mL; Rectal: 118 mL; Topical: Apply as needed

Alternatives:

References:
1. Rose, H. G., and Liber, A. F. (1966). Accumulation of saturated hydrocarbons in human spleens. J. Lab. Clin. Med. 68, 475–483.
2. Curry CE and Butler DCurry CE and Butler D: Laxative products. In, Allen LV Jr, Berardi RR, DeSimone EM II (eds): Handbook of Nonprescription Drugs, 12th. American Pharmaceutical Association, Washington, DC, 2000a.
3. Boitnott, J. K., and Margolis, S. (1970). Saturated hydrocarbons in human tissues. III. Oil droplets in the liver and spleen. Johns Hopkins Med. J. 127, 65–78.
4. Anja Notia, Koni Grob, a, Maurus Biedermanna, Ursula Deissa and Beat J. Bruschweiler. Exposure of babies to C15–C45 mineral paraffins from human milk and breast salves. Regulatory Toxicology and Pharmacology. Volume 38, Issue 3, December 2003, Pages 317–325
5. Smith, J.H., Mallett, A.K., Priston, R.A., Brantom, P.G., Worrell, N.R., Sexsmith, C., Simpson, B.J., 1996. Ninety-day feeding study in Fischer-344 rats of highly refined petroleum-derived food-grade white oils and waxes. Toxicol. Pathol. 24, 214,-230.

MINOCYCLINE   L3/L4

Trade: Minocin, Dynacin, Arestin

Other Trades: Akamin, Minomycin, Minocin, Novo-Minocycline, Minocin, Blemix

Category: Tetracycline antibiotic

Minocycline is a broad-spectrum tetracycline antibiotic with significant side effects in pediatric patients, including dental staining and reduced bone growth.[1,2] It is probably secreted into breastmilk in small but clinically insignificant levels. Because tetracyclines, in general, bind to milk calcium they would have reduced absorption in the infant, but minocycline may be absorbed to a greater degree than the older tetracyclines. Although most tetracyclines secreted into milk are generally bound to calcium, thus inhibiting their absorption, minocycline is poorly bound and may be better absorbed in a breastfeeding infant than the older tetracyclines. While the absolute absorption of older tetracyclines may be dramatically reduced by calcium salts, the newer doxycycline and minocycline analogs bind less and their overall absorption, while slowed, may be significantly higher than earlier versions.

In a study of 2 patients receiving 200 mg orally, the concentration at peak (6 hours) was 0.8 µg/mL.[1] The authors report that the average milk level was 0.5 to 0.8 mg/L for a period of 12 hours post dose which would transfer approximately 18 µg to the infant. Thus approximately 4.2% of the maternal dose would possibly transfer to the infant via milk. Most of this would be unabsorbed orally by the infant.

Due to the risk of dental staining, and epiphyseal problems with tetracyclines in infants and children, prolonged use (more than 3 weeks) of tetracyclines should be avoided.

Pregnancy Risk	D	Lactation Risk	L3/L4 for chronic use
T ½	= 15–20 hours	M/P	=
Vd	=	PB	= 76%
Tmax	= 3 hours	Oral	= 90–100%
MW	= 457	pKa	= 2.8, 5, 7.8, 9.3

Adult Concerns: Adverse effects include gastrointestinal distress, dizziness, thyroid pigmentation, vomiting, diarrhea, nephrotoxicity, photosensitivity.

Pediatric Concerns: None via breastmilk, but pediatric side effects include decreased linear bone growth and dental staining after prolonged exposure.

Drug Interactions: Absorption may be reduced or delayed when used with dairy products, calcium, magnesium, or aluminum containing antacids, oral contraceptives, iron, zinc, sodium bicarbonate, penicillins, cimetidine. Increased toxicity may result when used with methoxyflurane anesthesia. Use with warfarin anticoagulants may increase anticoagulation.

Relative Infant Dose: 4.2%

Adult Dose: 100 mg twice daily.

Alternatives: Doxycycline

References:
1. Mizuno S, Takata M, Sano S, Ueyama T. [Minocycline]. Jpn J Antibiot. 1969 Dec; 22(6): 473–9.

MINOXIDIL   L3

Trade: Loniten, Minodyl
Other Trades: Loniten, Apo-Gain, Minox
Category: Antihypertensive

Minoxidil is a potent vasodilator and antihypertensive. It is also used for hair loss and baldness. When applied topically, only 1.4% of the dose is absorbed systemically. Following an oral dose of 7.5 mg, minoxidil was secreted into human milk in concentrations ranging from trough levels of 0.3 µg/L at 12 hours to peak levels of 41.7–55 µg/L at 1 hour following an oral dose of 7.5 mg.[1] Long-term exposure of breastfeeding infants in women ingesting oral minoxidil may not be advisable. However, in those using topical minoxidil, the limited absorption via skin would minimize systemic levels and significantly reduce risk of transfer to infant via breastmilk. It is unlikely that the amount absorbed via topical application would produce clinically relevant concentrations in breastmilk.

Pregnancy Risk	C	Lactation Risk	L3
T ½	= 3.5–4.2 hours	M/P	= 0.75–1.0
Vd	=	PB	= Low
Tmax	= 2–8 hours	Oral	= 90–95%
MW	= 209	pKa	= 4.6

Adult Concerns: Hypotension, tachycardia, headache, weight gain, skin pigmentation, rash, renal toxicity, leukopenia.

Pediatric Concerns: None reported.

Drug Interactions: Profound orthostatic hypotension when used with guanethidine. May potentiate hypotensive effect of other antihypertensives.

Relative Infant Dose: 9.1%

Adult Dose: 10–40 mg daily.

Alternatives:

References:
1.   Valdivieso A, Valdes G, Spiro TE, Westerman RL. Minoxidil in breast milk. Ann Intern Med 1985; 102(1): 135.

MIRTAZAPINE   L3

Trade: Remeron

Other Trades: Avanza, Zispin

Category: Antidepressant

Mirtazapine is a unique antidepressant structurally dissimilar to the SSRIs, tricyclic antidepressants, or the monoamine oxidase inhibitors. Mirtazapine has little or no serotonergic-like side effects, fewer anticholinergic side effects than amitriptyline, it produces less sexual dysfunction, and has not demonstrated cardiotoxic or seizure potential in a limited number of overdose cases.[1]

In a study of 3 women who received 45, 60, and 45 mg/day mirtazapine, the average concentration (AUC) in milk was 77, 75, and 47 µg/L, respectively.[2] The absolute infant dose was 10, 11.3, and 7.1 µg/kg/day, respectively. The relative infant dose was 1.9%, 1.1%, and 1.5% of the weight-normalized maternal dose, respectively. Mirtazapine was below the limit of quantitation in two of the infants and only 1.5 ng/mL in the second infant. The infants were meeting all developmental milestones and were without side effects.

Another study of 8 women taking an average of 38 mg/day showed average milk concentrations of 53 µg/L and 13 µg/L of mirtazapine and its metabolite, respectively. The average absolute infant dose was 495 µg/kg/day, indicating a relative infant dose of 1.9%. The authors of this study suggest that breastfeeding is safe during mirtazapine therapy.[3] In another mother who took 22.5 mg/day, milk levels were 130 µg/L 4 hours after dosing and 61 µg/L 10 hours after the dose (foremilk). This suggests the relative infant dose was 3.9–4.4% and 1.8–2.7%

respectively of the weight-adjusted maternal dose at these two times. At 12.5 hours post dose, infant plasma levels were undetectable.[4]

Pregnancy Risk	C	Lactation Risk	L3
T ½	= 20–40 hours	M/P	= 0.76
Vd	=	PB	= 85%
Tmax	= 2 hours	Oral	= 50%
MW	= 265	pKa	= 7.1

Adult Concerns: Drowsiness (54%), dizziness, dry mouth, constipation, increased appetite (17%), and weight gain (12%) have been reported.

Pediatric Concerns: None reported via milk but observe for sedation.

Drug Interactions: Enhanced impairment of cognitive function when administered with alcohol. Mirtazapine is a weak inhibitor of cytochrome P450 2D6 and others. Drugs metabolized by this enzyme system may have enhanced activity. Coadministration with benzodiazepines may reduce cognitive function.

Relative Infant Dose: 1.6%–6.3%

Adult Dose: 15–45 mg daily

Alternatives: Sertraline, venlafaxine, paroxetine

References:
1. Pharmaceutical manufacturer prescribing information, 1999.
2. Ilett KF, Hackett LP, Kristensen JH, Rampono J. Distribution and excretion of the novel antidepressant mirtazapine in human milk. International Lactation Consultants Meeting, Sydney, July 31– August 3, 2003.
3. Kristensen JH, Ilett KF, Rampono J, Kohan R, Hackett LP. Transfer of the antidepressant mirtazapine into breast milk. Br J Clin Pharmacol 2006; 63(3): 322–327.
4. Klier CM, Mossaheb N, Lee A, Zernig G. Mirtazapine and Breastfeeding: Maternal and Infant Plasma Levels. Am J Psychiatry 2007; 164(2): 348–349.

MISOPROSTOL   L3

Trade: Cytotec

Other Trades: Cytotec

Category: Prostaglandin hormone, gastric protectant

Misoprostol is a prostaglandin E_1 compound that is useful in treating NSAID-induced gastric ulceration. Misoprostol is absorbed orally and rapidly metabolized. Intact misoprostol is not detectable in plasma and is rapidly metabolized to misoprostol acid which is biologically active.[1]

In a study of 5 mothers receiving 200 µg, misoprostol, levels in milk rose rapidly and peaked at an average of 7.6 pg/mL at 1.1 hours, followed by a rapid decline to 0.2 pg/mL at 5 hours. The milk-to-plasma ratio was 0.05 on average. The authors suggest that misoprostol be taken immediately after a feed and the next feed be given 4 hours later, when milk levels are below 1 pg/mL.[2] Infants should be monitored for signs of diarrhea.

Pregnancy Risk	X	Lactation Risk	L3
T ½	= 20–40 minutes	M/P	= 0.05
Vd	=	PB	= 80–90%
Tmax	= 14–20 minutes (oral)	Oral	= Complete
MW	= 383	pKa	= 13.92

Adult Concerns: Diarrhea, abdominal cramps and pain, uterine bleeding and abortion.

Pediatric Concerns: None reported, but observe for diarrhea, abdominal cramps.

Drug Interactions: Levels are diminished when administered with food. Antacids reduce total bioavailability but this does not appear clinically significant.

Relative Infant Dose:

Adult Dose: 100–200 µg four times daily.

Alternatives:

References:

1. Pharmaceutical manufacturer prescribing information, 1995.
2. Vogel D, Burkhardt T, Rentsch K et al. Misoprostol versus methylergometrine: Pharmacokinetics in human milk. Am J Obstet Gynecol 2004; 191: 2168–2173.

MITOMYCIN   L5

Trade: Mutamycin, Mitomycin-C

Other Trades:

Category: Anticancer drug

Mitomycin is an antibiotic antineoplastic agent used for the treatment of cancer of the stomach, breast, pancreas, and numerous other cancers. Oral absorption is erratic due to its instability in aqueous solutions, so it is always used intravenously.[1] It is eliminated via a biexponential curve with a terminal half-life of 23–78 minutes. No data are available on its transfer into human milk. Withhold breastfeeding for a minimum of 24–48 hours.

Pregnancy Risk	D	Lactation Risk	L5
T ½	= 23–78 minutes	M/P	=
Vd	= 11–48 L/m²	PB	=
Tmax	=	Oral	=
MW	= 334	pKa	= 3.2, 6.5

Adult Concerns: Loss of appetite, nausea and vomiting, numbness or tingling in fingers and toes, purple-colored bands on nails, skin rash, unusual tiredness or weakness

Pediatric Concerns:

Drug Interactions: Do not administer concurrently with live vaccines such as MMR vaccine, influenza vaccine, varicella vaccine, rotavirus vaccine, smallpox vaccine. Co-administration with vinblastine may increase risk of pulmonary toxicity and coadministration with tamoxifen increases risk of hemolytic uremic syndrome.

Relative Infant Dose:

Adult Dose: 20 mg/m^2 IV every 6–8 weeks.

Alternatives:

References:
1. Pharmaceutical manufacturer prescribing information, 2005.

MITOXANTRONE   L5

Trade: Novantrone, Formyxan, Genefadrone, Misostol, Mitoxl, Pralifan
Other Trades: Onkotrone, Novantrone
Category: Immunosuppressant for MS

Mitoxantrone is an antineoplastic agent used in the treatment of relapsing multiple sclerosis. It is a DNA-reactive agent that intercalates into DNA via hydrogen bonding, causing cross links. It inhibits B cell, T cell, and macrophage proliferation. Terminal elimination is described by a three-compartment model. The mean alpha half-life of mitoxantrone is six to twelve minutes, the mean beta half-life is 1.1 to 3.1 hours and the mean gamma (terminal or elimination) half-life is 23 to 215 hours (median approximately 75 hours).[1]

Distribution to tissues is extensive: steady-state volume of distribution exceeds 1,000 L/m^2. Tissue concentrations of mitoxantrone appear to exceed those in the blood during the terminal elimination phase. In a study of a patient who received 3 treatments of mitoxantrone (6 mg/m^2) on days 1 to 5. Mitoxantrone levels in milk measured 120 ng/mL just after treatment (on the third day of treatment), and dropped to a stable level of 18 ng/mL for the next 28 days.[2] This agent has an enormous volume of distribution and is sequestered in at least 7 organs including the liver and bone marrow and in another study, 15% of the dose remained 35 days after exposure.[3] Assuming a mother were breastfeeding, these levels would provide about 18 µg/L of milk consumed after the first few days following exposure to the drug. In addition, it would be sequestered for long periods in the infant as well. As this is a DNA-reactive agent, and it has a huge volume of distribution leading to prolonged tissue, plasma, and milk levels, mothers should be strongly advised to not breastfeed following its use.

Pregnancy Risk	D	Lactation Risk	L5
T ½	= 23–215 hours (Median 75 hours)	M/P	=
Vd	= 14–24.7 l/kg	PB	= 78%
Tmax	=	Oral	= Poor
MW	= 517	pKa	= 5.99, 8.13

Adult Concerns: Leukopenia and thrombocytopenia are the most common adverse effects. Cardiotoxicity, nausea, vomiting, diarrhea, mucositis, hepatotoxicity, alopecia, pruritus, phlebitis have been reported. Neuropathy and paralysis of the bowel and bladder are reported.

Pediatric Concerns: None reported but extreme caution is recommended. Probably contraindicated.

Drug Interactions: Avoid vaccinations with live or attenuated vaccines (smallpox, rotavirus, etc). The half-life of mitoxantrone is increased (1.8 fold) by use with valspodar.

Relative Infant Dose: 1.8%

Adult Dose: 12 mg/m^2

Alternatives:

References:
1. Pharmaceutical manufacturer prescribing information, 2005.
2. Azuno Y, Kaku K, Fujita N, Okubo M, Kaneko T, Matsumoto N. Mitoxantrone and etoposide in breast milk. Am J Hematol 1995 Feb; 48(2): 131–2.
3. Alberts DS, Peng YM, Leigh S, Davis TP, Woodward DL. Disposition of mitoxantrone in cancer patients. Cancer Res 1985 Apr; 45(4): 1879–84.

MIVACURIUM   L3

Trade: Mivacron

Other Trades: Mivacrom

Category: Neuromuscular blocking agent

Mivacurium is a short-acting neuromuscular blocking agent used to relax skeletal muscles during surgery. Its duration is very short (6–9 minutes) and complete recovery generally occurs in 15–30 minutes.[1,2] No data are available on its transfer to breastmilk. However, it has an exceedingly short plasma half-life, a rather large molecular weight, and probably poor to no oral absorption. It is very unlikely that it would be absorbed by a breastfeeding infant.

Pregnancy Risk	C	Lactation Risk	L3
T½	= 2 minutes	M/P	=
Vd	= 147 l/kg	PB	=
Tmax	=	Oral	= Poor
MW	= 1100.18	pKa	=

Adult Concerns: Flushing, hypotension, weakness.

Pediatric Concerns: None reported.

Drug Interactions: Inhaled anesthetics, local anesthetics, calcium channel blockers, antiarrhythmic such as quinidine, and certain antibiotics such as amino glycosides, tetracyclines, vancomycin, and clindamycin may significantly prolong neuromuscular blockade with mivacurium.

Relative Infant Dose:

Adult Dose: 0.1–0.15 mg/kg every 15 minutes PRN.

Alternatives:

References:

1. McEvoy GE. (ed): AFHS Drug Information. New York, NY: 2003.
2. Pharmaceutical manufacturer prescribing information, 1995.

MOCLOBEMIDE   L3

Trade:

Other Trades: Arima, Aurorix, Apo-Moclobemide, Manerix

Category: MAO inhibitor, antidepressant.

Moclobemide is a monoamine oxidase (MAO) inhibitor. Unlike older MAO inhibitors, moclobemide is a selective and reversible inhibitor of MAO-A isozyme and thus is not plagued with the dangerous side effects of the older MAO inhibitor families. It is an effective treatment for depression.[1]

In a study by Pons in 6 lactating women, who received a single oral dose of 300 mg, the concentration of moclobemide (C_{max}) was highest at 3 hours after the dose and averaged 2.7 mg/L.[2] The average (AUC) milk concentration throughout the 12 hour period was 0.97 mg/L hour. The minimal levels of moclobemide found in milk are unlikely to produce untoward effects according to the authors. For adults, serotonergic syndrome is unlikely, but possible when admixed with SSRI antidepressants, clomipramine, fluoxetine, etc. Do not coadminister with SSRIs and tricyclic antidepressants. Do not administer with meperidine (pethidine) or dextromethorphan. Sympathomimetic hyperactivity (hypertension, headache, hyperpyrexia, arrhythmias, cerebral hemorrhage) may occur when admixed with tyramine, ephedrine, pseudoephedrine, phenylephrine, epinephrine, norepinephrine and other sympathomimetics.

Pregnancy Risk	Probably Safe	Lactation Risk	L3
T ½	= 1–2.2 hours	M/P	= 0.72
Vd	= 1–2 l/kg	PB	= 50%
Tmax	= 2 hours	Oral	= 80%
MW	= 269	pKa	= 6.3

Adult Concerns: Dry mouth, headache, dizziness, tremor, sweating, insomnia, and constipation.

Pediatric Concerns: None reported via milk.

Drug Interactions: Serotonergic syndrome is unlikely, but possible when admixed with SSRI antidepressants, clomipramine, fluoxetine, etc. Do not coadminister with SSRIs and tricyclic antidepressants. Do not administer with meperidine (pethidine) or dextromethorphan. Sympathomimetic hyperactivity (hypertension, headache, hyperpyrexia, arrhythmias, cerebral hemorrhage) may occur when admixed with tyramine, ephedrine, pseudoephedrine, phenylephrine, epinephrine, norepinephrine and other sympathomimetics.

Relative Infant Dose: 3.4%

Adult Dose: 450 mg/day

Alternatives:

References:
1. Fulton B, Benfield P. Moclobemide. An update of its pharmacological properties and therapeutic use. Drugs 1996; 52(3): 450–474.
2. Pons G, Schoerlin MP, Tam YK, Moran C, Pfefen JP, Francoual C, Pedarriosse AM, Chavinie J, Olive G. Moclobemide excretion in human breast milk. Br J Clin Pharmacol 1990; 29(1): 27–31.

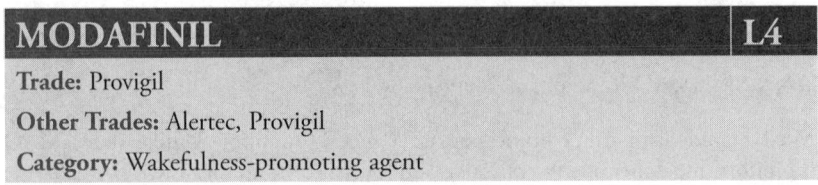

MODAFINIL   L4

Trade: Provigil

Other Trades: Alertec, Provigil

Category: Wakefulness-promoting agent

Modafinil is a wakefulness-promoting agent used for the treatment of narcolepsy.[1] Although its pharmacologic results are similar to amphetamines and methylphenidate, its method of action is unknown. No data are available on its transfer into human milk. Some caution is recommended as it is small in molecular weight and very lipid soluble, both characteristics which may ultimately lead to higher milk levels. In addition, it apparently stimulates dopamine levels. Compounds that stimulate dopamine levels in brain often reduce prolactin secretion. Milk production may suffer, but this is only a supposition.

Pregnancy Risk	C	Lactation Risk	L4
T ½	= 15 hours	M/P	=
Vd	= 0.9 l/kg	PB	= 60%
Tmax	= 2–4 hours	Oral	= Complete
MW	= 273	pKa	= 14.81

Adult Concerns: May increase incidence of headache, chest pain, palpitations, dyspnea, and transient T-wave changes on ECG. CNS changes include delusions, auditory hallucinations and sleep deprivation. Diarrhea, dry mouth, nausea, and rhinitis have been reported.

Pediatric Concerns: None reported. Observe for reduced milk supply.

Drug Interactions: May increase plasma levels of diazepam, phenytoin and propranolol. Caution when used with tricyclic and SSRI antidepressants. May induce hepatic enzymes, thus reducing circulating levels of cyclosporine, theophylline, and steroidal contraceptives.

Relative Infant Dose:

Adult Dose: 200–400 mg up to twice daily.

Alternatives:

References:
1. Pharmaceutical manufacturer prescribing information, 2001.

MOMETASONE   L3

Trade: Elocon, Nasonex, Asmanex

Other Trades:

Category: Corticosteroid

Mometasone is a corticosteroid primarily intended for intranasal and topical use. It is considered a medium-potency steroid, similar to betamethasone and triamcinolone. Following topical application to the skin, less than 0.7% is systemically absorbed over an 8 hour period.[1,2] It is extremely unlikely mometasone would be excreted into human milk in clinically relevant levels following topical or intranasal administration.

Asmanex is the inhaled version of this steroid for therapy in asthma.

Pregnancy Risk	C	Lactation Risk	L3
T ½	= 5.8 hours	M/P	=
Vd	=	PB	= 98–99%
Tmax	=	Oral	=
MW	= 427	pKa	=

Adult Concerns: Topically only minimal side effects have been reported and include irritation, burning, stinging, and dermal atrophy. After nasal administration, common adverse effects include headache, pharyngitis, epistaxis, and cough.

Pediatric Concerns: None reported via milk.

Drug Interactions: Co-administration with the following drugs increases plasma levels of mometasone: ketoconazole, indinavir, clarithromycin, itraconazole, nelfinavir, ritonavir, atazanavir, telithromycin, nefazoline, saquinavir.

Relative Infant Dose:

Adult Dose: Apply topically 2–3 times daily.

Alternatives:

References:
1. Pharmaceutical manufacturer prescribing information, 1999.
2. Drug Facts and Comparisons 1999 ed. ed. St. Louis: 1999.

MONOETHANOLAMINE OLEATE   L3

Trade: Ethamolin

Other Trades:

Category: Sclerosing Agent

Monoethanolamine is a sclerosing agent to treat varicose veins.[1] When injected intravenously, monoethanolamine oleate acts primarily by irritation of the intimal endothelium of the vein and produces an inflammatory response. This results in fibrosis and possible occlusion of the vein. There are no data on its transfer to human milk, but following injection, this product disappears from the plasma within 5 minutes. Hence a brief waiting period of perhaps an hour would significantly reduce any exposure of the milk compartment to this drug. Pump and discard all milk during this hour.

Pregnancy Risk	C	Lactation Risk	L3
T ½	= <5 minutes	M/P	=
Vd	=	PB	=
Tmax	=	Oral	=
MW	= 344	pKa	= 9.4

Adult Concerns: Pulmonary toxicity, allergic reactions, pleural effusion, edema

Pediatric Concerns:

Drug Interactions:

Relative Infant Dose:

Adult Dose:

Alternatives:

References:
1. Pharmaceutical manufacturer prescribing information, 2008.

MONTELUKAST SODIUM   L3

Trade: Singulair
Other Trades:
Category: Antiasthmatic agent

Montelukast is a leukotriene receptor inhibitor and is used as an adjunct in the treatment of asthma. The manufacturer reports that montelukast is secreted into animal milk, but no data on human milk are available.[1] This product is cleared for use in children aged 6 and above. This product does not enter the CNS nor many other tissues. Although the milk levels in humans are unreported, they are probably quite low.

Pregnancy Risk	B	Lactation Risk	L3
T ½	= 2.7–5.5 hours	M/P	=
Vd	= 0.15 l/kg	PB	= 99%
Tmax	= 2–4 hours	Oral	= 64%
MW	= 608	pKa	=

Adult Concerns: Abdominal pain, fever, dyspepsia, dental pain, dizziness, headache, cough and nasal congestion, some changes in liver enzymes.

Pediatric Concerns: None reported via milk.

Drug Interactions: Phenobarbital may reduce plasma levels by 40%. Although unreported, other inhibitors of Cytochrome P450 may affect plasma levels.

Relative Infant Dose:

Adult Dose: 10 mg daily

Alternatives: Zafirlukast

References:
1. Pharmaceutical manufacturer prescribing information, 2011.

MORINGA OLEIFERA   L3

Trade: Moringa, Mulunggay, Natalac
Other Trades:
Category: Herbal product, galactagogue

Moringa oleifera Lam (commonly known as malunggay) belongs to the plant family Moringaceae. It is widely cultivated through out the tropics and sub-tropics and has been used for centuries for various medicinal purposes. The leaves contain all essential amino acids and are rich in protein, vitamins A, B, C, and minerals. Moringa have been reported to have anti-hypertensive, hypoglycemic, anti-thyroid, hypercholesterolemic, antimicrobial and anti-tumor effects. Some of its known side-effects include hepatotoxicity, liver failure, hepatorenal syndrome. Moringa is also known for its galactagogue properties. Feeding the high protein leaves to cattle has been shown to increase weight gain by up to 32% and milk production by 43 to 65%.[1] In the Phillippines, the moringa leaves are added to chicken or shellfish soup and taken by lactating women to increase their milk supply. Malunggay capsules contain powdered moringa leaves and are available in oral formulations of 250 mg or 350 mg.

Several studies have been conducted to investigate the efficacy of malunggay as a galactagogue. In one such study, 30 hypertensive pregnant women with blood pressures of 140/90 or more were selected and administered malunggay capsules immediately post delivery.[2] The women were instructed to take the capsules every 12 hours for 4 months. The dose of malunggay administered is not mentioned. Prolactin levels were determined on three occasions: at 6 hours postpartum before capsule intake or infant suckling; at 48 hours postpartum, 30 min after infant suckling; at 4 months postpartum, 30 min after infant suckling. The infant weights were recorded at 0,1,2,4 and 16 weeks of age. Prolactin levels of the second and third extraction were significantly higher; these high prolactin levels positively correlated with earlier onset and higher breastmilk production; the infants in the treatment group showed significantly more weight gain at 4 months than those in the placebo group. The author of this study concludes that breastmilk production in hypertensive women may be enhanced with administration of malunggay capsules. Another similar study, following the same methodology, was completed with 116 women with normal pregnancies and without medical problems.[3] Similar results were obtained affirming the effectiveness of malunggay as a galactagogue. Yet another study where 68 mothers of premature babies (less than 37 weeks) were randomly selected and administered 250 mg malunggay capsules every 12 hours on postpartum days 3 to 5.[4] They were instructed to pump their milk from days 1 to 5. A significantly higher amount of breastmilk production occurred on days 4 and 5, indicating the efficacy of malunggay as galactagogues in mothers with preterm infants. This author recommends the routine use of malunggay to enhance breastmilk production in mothers of preterm infants.

Another study investigated the efficacy of antepartum malunggay capsules in promoting breastmilk production.[5] Fifty-three women at 35 weeks of gestation were randomly divided into 2 groups to either receive 2 malunggay capsules, each containing 350 mg moringa, 3 times daily, or to receive placebo. The intake of the capsules was discontinued as soon as the baby was delivered. After delivery, the postpartum mothers pumped every 4 hours for 48 hours, starting at the 6th hour postpartum. Earlier onset and higher amounts of breastmilk production was noted in the malunggay group, as compared to placebo group. After 48 hours, the total amount of breastmilk produced from the mulunggay group was 260% higher than that produced from the placebo group. The study also revealed that the amount of breastmilk produced had no correlation with the duration of antepartum intake of mulunggay capsules. Further, the increased amounts of breastmilk production in the malunggay group was not sustained past the 42nd hour. The authors of this study conclude that intake of malunngay capsule a few weeks before delivery significantly increases postpartum breastmilk production.

A comparative study was conducted to evaluate the efficacies of domperidone, metoclopramide and malunggay as galactagogues in mothers of preterm infants with lactational insufficiency.[6] Forty mothers of preterm infants with baseline milk production of <100 mL on the 2nd postpartum day were randomly selected for this study and divided into 4 groups to receive either domperidone 10 mg three times daily, or metoclopramide 10 mg three times daily, or malunggay 250 mg three times daily or milk expression using the breast pump alone. Prolactin levels were obtained before intervention and then again on days 7 and 14, 1–2 hours after oral dose or 1–2 hours after milk expression with breast pump. Milk volumes were assessed on days 7 and 14. It was noted that all the three galactagogues caused significantly higher breastmilk production as compared to milk expression with breast pump alone. Domperidone caused the highest breastmilk production, followed by metoclopramide and malunggay. There was no significant difference in the milk production caused by metoclopramide and malunggay. Further this study revealed that there is no correlation between serum prolactin levels and amount of breastmilk production, and that high serum prolactin levels is not an indicator of breastfeeding success.

In all the above mentioned studies, no adverse effects were reported. The drawbacks in all the above mentioned studies are several. Most of these studies were conducted with a small sample size which adversely affects the power of the study and does not necessarily reflect responses in a larger population. Further, these studies failed to explain the mechanism of action of malunggay as galactagogues and failed to answer if malunggay can help maintain consistently high milk production throughout the period of lactation. The safe range of dosage above which moringa toxicity is expected is also not specified. The transfer of moringa into breastmilk and its effects on the breastfed infant have also not been studied. The antepartum use of moringa is also not advised due to its known effects on uterine contraction. Until, more is known of the mechanism of action of malunggay, its transfer into breastmilk and its effectiveness as galactagogues in larger populations, it is recommended malunggay should be used in breastfeeding mothers with caution.

Pregnancy Risk	Possibly Hazardous	Lactation Risk	L3
T ½	=	M/P	=
Vd	=	PB	=
Tmax	=	Oral	=
MW	=	pKa	=

Adult Concerns: Some of its known side-effects include hepatotoxicity, liver failure, hepatorenal syndrome.

Pediatric Concerns:

Drug Interactions:

Relative Infant Dose:

Adult Dose: 250–350 mg three times a day.

Alternatives:

References:
1. "The Moringa Tree Moringa oleifera". Trees for Life International. Retrieved 2009–12–29.
2. Yabes-Almirante C., Lim C. Enhancement of breastfeeding among hypertensive mothers.
3. Yabes-Almirante C., Lim C. Effectiveness of Natalac as a galactogogue. JPMA Vol. 71/No.3 January–March 1996.
4. Estrella M.C.P., Mantaring III J.B.V., David G.Z., Taup M.A. A double-blind, randomized controlled trial on the use of malunggay (Moringa oleifera) for augmentation of the volume of breastmilk among non-nursing mothers of preterm infants. Vol.49/No.1 January-March 2000.
5. Briton-Medrano C., Perez L. The efficacy of Mulunggay (Moringa Oleifera) given to near term pregnant women in inducing early postpartum breastmilk production–a double blind randomized clinical trial.
6. Antonette M., Hernandez, Jr. E.A., Benjamin G. A comparative study on the efficacy of the different galactogogues among mothers with lactational insufficiency. The Philippine Journal of Pediatrics.

MORPHINE   L3

Trade: Duramorph, Infumorph, Embeda

Other Trades: Morphalgin, Ordine, Anamorph, Kapanol, Epimorph, Morphitec, M.O.S. MS Contin, Statex, Oramorph, Sevredol

Category: Narcotic analgesic

Morphine is a potent narcotic analgesic. In a group of 5 lactating women, the highest morphine concentration in breastmilk following two epidural doses was only 82 µg/L at 30 minutes.[1] The highest breastmilk level following 15 mg IV/IM was only 0.5 mg/L although it dropped to almost 0.01 mg/L in 4 hours. In this study and following two 4 mg epidural doses, the peak milk level was 82 µg/L or a relative infant dose of 9.1%.

In another study of women receiving morphine via PCA pumps for 12–48 hours postpartum, the concentration of morphine in breastmilk ranged from 50–60 µg/L (estimated from graph).[2] None of the infants in this study were neurobehaviorally delayed at 3 days. Because of the poor oral bioavailability of morphine (26%) it is unlikely these levels would be clinically relevant in a stable breastfeeding infant.

However, data from Robieux suggests the levels transferred to the infant are higher.[3] In this study of a single patient, plasma levels in the breastfed infant were within therapeutic range (4 ng/mL) although the infant showed no untoward signs or symptoms. However, this case was somewhat unique in that the mother received daily morphine (50 mg orally every 6 hours) during the third trimester for severe back pain. One week postpartum, the morphine was discontinued and then 5 days later reinstated due to withdrawal effects in the mother. The reported concentration in foremilk and hindmilk was 100 ng/mL and 10 ng/mL respectively and the authors suggested that the dose to the infant would be 0.8 to 12% of the maternal oral dose (0.15 to 2.41 mg/day). Although this study suggests that the amount of morphine transferred in milk can be clinically relevant, the authors calculated the infant dose from the highest milk concentration and a milk intake of 150 ml/kg/day, thus the dose of morphine to the infant would have been substantially lower (53 µg/day). This study seems flawed because the plasma levels and the doses via milk just don't correlate. That this infant showed no untoward effects, can be explained by the fact that it may have exhibited tolerance after long exposure, that the reported analgesic-therapeutic level required in neonates is actually slightly higher than in adults, or the plasma levels assayed in this infant were in error.

Infants under 1 month of age have a prolonged elimination half-life and decreased clearance of morphine relative to older infants. The clearance of morphine and its elimination begins to approach adult values by 2 months of age. In summary, morphine is probably the preferred opiate in breastfeeding mothers primarily due to its poor oral bioavailability. It is unfortunate that the clinical studies above do not necessarily suggest this. However, high doses over prolonged periods could lead to sedation and respiratory problems in newborn infants.

Pregnancy Risk	C	Lactation Risk	L3
T ½	= 1.5–2 hours	M/P	= 1.1–3.6
Vd	= 2–5 l/kg	PB	= 35%
Tmax	= 0.5–1 hour	Oral	= 26%
MW	= 285	pKa	= 8.1

Adult Concerns: Sedation, flushing, CNS depression, respiratory depression, bradycardia.

Pediatric Concerns: None reported via milk but sedation is possible with higher doses.

Drug Interactions: Barbiturates may significantly increase respiratory and CNS depressant effects of morphine. The admixture of cimetidine has produced CNS toxicity such as confusion, disorientation, respiratory depression, apnea, and seizures when used with narcotic analgesics. Diazepam may produce cardiovascular depression when used with opiates. Phenothiazines may antagonize the analgesic effect of morphine.

Relative Infant Dose: 9.1%

Adult Dose: 10–30 mg every 4 hours PRN

Alternatives: Codeine

References:

1. Feilberg VL, Rosenborg D, Broen CC, Mogensen JV. Excretion of morphine in human breast milk. Acta Anaesthesiol Scand 1989; 33(5): 426–428.
2. Wittels B, Scott DT, Sinatra RS. Exogenous opioids in human breast milk and acute neonatal neurobehavior: a preliminary study. Anesthesiology 1990; 73(5): 864–869.
3. Robieux I, Koren G, Vandenbergh H, Schneiderman J. Morphine excretion in breast milk and resultant exposure of a nursing infant. J Toxicol Clin Toxicol 1990; 28(3): 365–370.

MOXIFLOXACIN　　L3

Trade: Avelox, Vigamox

Other Trades: Avelox

Category: Fluoroquinolone antibiotic

Moxifloxacin is a quinolone antibiotic for use orally, intravenously, and in the eye.[1] It is a new-generation fluoroquinolone which exhibits improved activity against *Streptococcus pneumonia* and other species. No data are available on its transfer into human milk so until we have data, one should opt for using ofloxacin or levofloxacin for which published data are available. Moxifloxacin is known to transfer to the milk of goats and sheep, and in studies concerning those two species, the drug entered the milk to a large degree. It was believed that high concentrations in the milk compartment were achieved by way of ion trapping.[2,3] Ophthalmic use of moxifloxacin in the form of eye drops is probably OK due to low systemic levels attained. However, caution is advised with its oral or intravenous use.

Pregnancy Risk	C	Lactation Risk	L3
T ½	= 9–16 hours	M/P	=
Vd	= 1.7–3 l/kg	PB	= 50%
Tmax	= 1–3 hours	Oral	= 90%
MW	= 437	pKa	= 6.4

Adult Concerns: Nausea and diarrhea are the most common complications following oral use in adults. It should be avoided in patients with prolonged QT intervals.

Pediatric Concerns: No reports available, but changes in gut flora, and diarrhea are possible. Complications following ophthalmic use are extremely remote as the plasma levels are very low.

Drug Interactions: Moxifloxacin can be administered concurrently with food. Do not take with antacids containing magnesium, aluminum, sucralfate, metal cations such as iron or zinc. Wait a minimum of 4 hours after using these products.

Relative Infant Dose:

Adult Dose: 400 mg daily

Alternatives: Ofloxacin, levofloxacin, norfloxacin, ciprofloxacin

References:

1. Pharmaceutical manufacturer prescribing information, 2003.

2. Gouda A. Disposition kinetics of moxifloxacin in lactating ewes. The Veterinary Journal. Volume 178, Issue 2, November 2008, Pages 282–287

3. Fernandez-Varon, E., Villamayor, L., Escudero, E., Espuny, A., Carceles, C.M., 2006. Pharmacokinetics and milk penetration of moxifloxacin after intravenous and subcutaneous administration to lactating goats. The Veterinary Journal 172, 302–307.

MUMPS VIRUS VACCINE, LIVE   L3

Trade: Mumpsvax

Other Trades:

Category: Vaccination for Mumps

Mumps vaccine is a live, attenuated vaccine indicated for the prevention of mumps illness. It is administered at 12–15 months of age, as part of the routine childhood immunization schedule. This should be followed by a re-immunization at 4–6 years of age. It is usually administered along with the measles and rubella vaccine, in the form of the MMR vaccine. There are currently no reports of transfer of the live mumps virus vaccine into breastmilk. The American Advisory Committee on Immunization Practices has stated that breastfeeding women may be administered both the live and killed vaccines.[1] As a general rule, vaccines are often safe to use during breastfeeding.[2] The WHO considers mumps vaccine compatible with breastfeeding. Therefore, a lactating mother who has received the mumps vaccine may continue to breastfeed her child. Further, the antibodies present in human milk may provide some additional protection against mumps infection in the breastfed child. The breastfed infant should also receive the mumps vaccine as per the routine childhood immunization schedule.

Pregnancy Risk	X		Lactation Risk	L3
T ½	=		M/P	=
Vd	=		PB	=
Tmax	=		Oral	=
MW	=		pKa	=

Adult Concerns: Pain at injection site, fever, common cold, lymphadenopathy, rash. Serious side effects: anaphylaxis, encephalitis, thrombocytopenia, Steven-Johnson syndrome, febrile seizure. Do not administer in those with an active viral infection, or those with immunodeficiency disorders or hematologic cancers such as leukemias and lymphomas.

Pediatric Concerns:

Drug Interactions: Contraindicated in those with ongoing acute infections, those on immunosupressive agents or corticosteroids, those on anti-cancer drugs, those with immunedoficiency disorders, those with hypersensitivity to any of the components of the vaccine including neomycin or gelatin. Caution to be exercised in those with egg allergy.

Relative Infant Dose:

Adult Dose: 0.5 mL subcutaneous injection.

Alternatives:

References:
1. Anon: General recommendations on immunization; recommendations of the advisory committee on immunization practices (AICP) and the American academy of family physicians (AAFP). MMWR 2002a; 51(RR02): 1–36.
2. Schaefer CSchaefer C: Drugs During Pregnancy and Lactation, Elsevier Science B.V., Amsterdam, The Netherlands, 2001.

MUPIROCIN OINTMENT   L1

Trade: Bactroban

Other Trades: Bactroban

Category: Antibacterial ointment

Mupirocin is a topical antibiotic used for impetigo, Group A beta-hemolytic strep, *staphylococcus* infections, and Strep. pyogenes.[1] Mupirocin is only minimally absorbed following topical application. In one study, less than 0.3% of a topical dose was absorbed after 24 hours. Most remained adsorbed to the corneum layer of the skin. The drug is absorbed orally, but it is so rapidly metabolized that systemic levels are not sustained. It is quite safe for breastfeeding mothers.

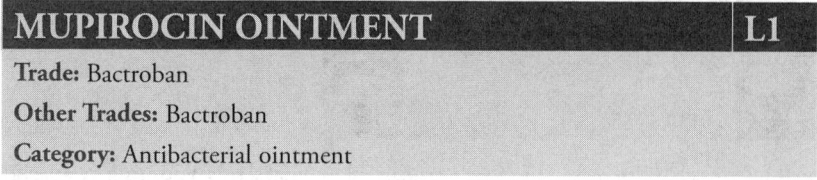

Pregnancy Risk	B	Lactation Risk	L1
T ½	= 17–36 minutes	M/P	=
Vd	=	PB	= 97%
Tmax	=	Oral	= Complete
MW	= 501	pKa	= 4.78

Adult Concerns: Rash, irritation.

Pediatric Concerns: None reported. Commonly used in pediatric patients.

Drug Interactions:

Relative Infant Dose:

Adult Dose: Apply sparingly.

Alternatives:

References:
1. Pharmaceutical manufacturer prescribing information, 2011.

MYCOPHENOLATE   L4

Trade: CellCept

Other Trades: CellCept

Category: Immunosuppressive agent

Mycophenolate is an immunosuppressive agent used to prevent rejection of allogenic transplants (kidney, heart, liver, intestine, limb, small bowel, etc.).[1] It is well absorbed and rapidly metabolized to MPA, the active metabolite. MPA glucuronide then subsequently enters the small intestine and is reabsorbed by enterohepatic recirculation. No data are available on its transfer into human milk.

The average blood level is about 63.9 µg/mL (AUC) which is relatively high. Until we have data on human breast milk levels, this agent should be considered relatively hazardous.

Pregnancy Risk	C	Lactation Risk	L4
T ½	= 17.9 hours	M/P	=
Vd	= 4 l/kg	PB	= 97%
Tmax	= 1 hour	Oral	= 94% (parent)
MW	= 433	pKa	= 5.6, 8.25

Adult Concerns: Increased risk for diarrhea, leukopenia, sepsis, vomiting, headache, tremor, insomnia, high risk of infections, lymphoma and other malignancies, bone marrow suppression.

Pediatric Concerns: This product is a high risk product for breastfeeding mothers. Great caution is recommended. See cyclosporin and others as alternatives.

Drug Interactions: Comcomitant use with azathioprine is not recommended, use cautiously with drugs that affect enterohepatic recirculation, such as cholestyramine. Avoid concurrent use of live attenuated vaccines. Numerous other drug-drug reactions occur, consult other references.

Relative Infant Dose:

Adult Dose: 1–1.5 gm orally twice daily.

Alternatives: Cyclosporine

References:
1.   Pharmaceutical manufacturer prescribing information, 2003.

NABUMETONE   L3

Trade: Relafen

Other Trades: Relafen, Relifex

Category: Anti-inflammatory agent for arthritic pain

Nabumetone is a non-steroidal anti-inflammatory agent for arthritic pain.[1] Immediately upon absorption, nabumetone is metabolized to the active metabolite. The parent drug is not detectable in plasma. It is not known if the nabumetone metabolite (6MNA) is secreted in human milk. It is known to be secreted into animal milk and has a very long half-life. Long half-life NSAIDS are not generally recommended in nursing mothers. Ketorolac and ibuprofen are ideal.

Pregnancy Risk	C/D in 3rd trimester	Lactation Risk	L3
T ½	= 22–30 hours	M/P	=
Vd	=	PB	= 99%
Tmax	= 2.5–4 hours	Oral	= 38%
MW	= 228	pKa	=

Adult Concerns: Gastrointestinal distress, nausea, vomiting, diarrhea.

Pediatric Concerns: None reported via milk. Observe for gastrointestinal distress.

Drug Interactions: May prolong prothrombin time when used with warfarin. Antihypertensive effects of ACE inhibitors may be blunted or completely abolished by NSAIDs. Some NSAIDs may block antihypertensive effect of beta blockers, diuretics. Used with cyclosporin, may dramatically increase renal toxicity. May increase digoxin, phenytoin, lithium levels. May increase toxicity of methotrexate. May increase bioavailability of penicillamine. Probenecid may increase NSAID levels.

Relative Infant Dose:

Adult Dose: 500–1000 mg 1–2 times daily.

Alternatives: Ibuprofen

References:
1. Pharmaceutical manufacturer prescribing information, 2011.

NADOLOL   L4

Trade: Corgard

Other Trades: Corgard, Syn-Nadolol, Novo-Nadolol

Category: Antihypertensive, antianginal, beta blocker

Nadolol is a long-acting beta adrenergic blocker used as an antihypertensive. It is secreted into breastmilk in moderately high concentrations. Following a maternal dose of 20 mg/day, breast milk levels at 38 hours postpartum were 146 µg/L.[1] In another study of 12 women receiving 80 mg daily the mean steady-state concentrations in milk were 357 µg/L.[2] The time to maximum concentration was 6 hours. The milk/serum ratio was reported to average 4.6. A five Kg infant would receive from 4–7% of the maternal dose. The authors recommended caution with the use of this beta blocker in breastfeeding patients. Due to its long half-life and high milk/plasma ratio, this would not be a preferred beta blocker.

Pregnancy Risk	C	Lactation Risk	L4
T ½	= 20–24 hours	M/P	= 4.6
Vd	= 1.5–3.6 l/kg	PB	= 30%
Tmax	= 2–4 hours	Oral	= 20–40%
MW	= 309	pKa	= 9.7

Adult Concerns: Hypotension, nausea, diarrhea, bradycardia, apnea, depression.

Pediatric Concerns: None reported, but due to the high M/P ratio of 4.6, this product is not recommended.

Drug Interactions: Decreased effect when used with aluminum salts, barbiturates, calcium salts, cholestyramine, NSAIDs, ampicillin, rifampin, and salicylates. Beta blockers may reduce the effect of oral sulfonylureas (hypoglycemic agents). Increased toxicity/effect when used with other antihypertensives, contraceptives, monoamine oxidase inhibitors, cimetidine, and numerous other products. See drug interaction reference for complete listing.

Relative Infant Dose: 4.4%–6.9%

Adult Dose: 40–80 mg daily.

Alternatives: Propranolol, metoprolol

References:
1. Fox RE, Marx C, Stark AR. Neonatal effects of maternal nadolol therapy. Am J Obstet Gynecol 1985; 152(8): 1045–1046.
2. Devlin RG, Duchin KL, Fleiss PM. Nadolol in human serum and breast milk. Br J Clin Pharmacol 1981; 12(3): 393–396.

NAFCILLIN   L1

Trade: Unipen, Nafcil

Other Trades: Unipen

Category: Penicillin antibiotic

Nafcillin is a penicillin antibiotic that is poorly and erratically absorbed orally.[1] The only formulations available are IV and IM. No data are available on concentration in milk, but it is likely small. Oral absorption in the infant would be minimal.

Pregnancy Risk	B	Lactation Risk	L1
T ½	= 0.5–1.5 hours	M/P	=
Vd	=	PB	= 70–90%
Tmax	= 30–60 minutes (IM).	Oral	= 50%
MW	= 436	pKa	=

Adult Concerns: Neutropenia, hypokalemia, pseudomembranous colitis, allergic rash.

Pediatric Concerns: None reported. Observe for gastrointestinal symptoms such as diarrhea. Nafcillin is frequently used in infants.

Drug Interactions: Chloramphenicol may decrease nafcillin levels. Nafcillin may inhibit efficacy of oral contraceptives. Probenecid may increase nafcillin levels. May increase anticoagulant effect of warfarin and heparin.

Relative Infant Dose:

Adult Dose: 250–1000 mg every 4–6 hours.

Alternatives:

References:
1. McEvoy GE. (ed): AFHS Drug Information. New York, NY: 2003.

NAFTIFINE   L3

Trade: Naftin
Other Trades:
Category: Antifungal

Naftifine hydrochloride is a topical allylamine medication used to treat fungal infections. Naftin is not an imidazole. The drug has anti-inflammatory and antihistaminic effects along with antifungal effects. Some degree of vasoconstriction occurs if an occulisve dressing is used which often occurs with steroid medications. No reported systemic effects have been noted with naftifine, but there have been reports of some local skin irritation. The systemic absorption of naftifine cream is between 2.5 to 6%. It is unknown if naftifine is excreted into breast milk. Theoretically, the estimate of topical absorption between 2.5 to 3.4% could suggest that 0.3 μg/kg of the drug would be excreted into milk.[1-2]

Pregnancy Risk	B	Lactation Risk	L3
T ½	= 2–3 days	M/P	=
Vd	=	PB	=
Tmax	=	Oral	=
MW	= 287	pKa	=

Adult Concerns: Stinging, burning, dry skin, skin irritation, pruritus, erythema.

Pediatric Concerns:

Drug Interactions:

Relative Infant Dose:

Adult Dose:

Alternatives: Nystatin, diflucan

References:
1. Gupta AK, Ryder JE, Cooper EA. Naftifine: a review. J Cutan Med Surg. 2008 Mar-Apr; 12(2): 51–8. Review.
2. Briggs G, Freeman, R., and Yaffe, S. A Reference Guide to Fetal and Neonatal Risk: Drugs in Pregnancy and Lactation. 2005; Seventh Edition. Vol.1 Philadelphia, PA Lippincott Williams and WIlkins.

NALBUPHINE   L2

Trade: Nubain
Other Trades: Nubain
Category: Analgesic

Nalbuphine is a potent narcotic analgesic similar in potency to morphine. Nalbuphine is both an antagonist and agonist of opiate receptors and should not be mixed with other opiates due to interference with analgesia. In a group of 20 postpartum mothers who received a single 20 mg IM nalbuphine dose, the total amount of nalbuphine excreted into human milk during a 24 hour period averaged

2.3 µg, which is equivalent to 0.012% of the maternal dosage (not weight adjusted).[1] The mean milk/plasma ratio using the AUC was 1.2. According to the authors, an oral intake of 2.3 µg nalbuphine per day by an infant would not show any measurable plasma concentrations in the neonate. In another study of 18 mothers who received 0.2 mg/kg every 4 hours over 2–3 days, the average concentration in breast milk was 42 µg/L, with a maximum of 61 µg/L. The reported infant dose was an average of 7 µg/kg/day, with a maximum of 9 µg/kg/day.[2] The authors estimate the RID = 0.59% of the weight-adjusted maternal daily dose and suggest breastfeeding is permissible.

Pregnancy Risk	B	Lactation Risk	L2
T ½	= 5 hours	M/P	= 1.2
Vd	= 2.4–7.3 l/kg	PB	=
Tmax	= 2–15 minutes (IV,IM)	Oral	= 16%
MW	= 357	pKa	=

Adult Concerns: Hypotension, sedation, withdrawal syndrome, respiratory depression.

Pediatric Concerns: Levels in milk are low. No complications reported.

Drug Interactions: May reduce efficacy of other opioid analgesics. Barbiturates may increase CNS sedation.

Relative Infant Dose: 0.5%–0.8%

Adult Dose: 10–20 mg every 3–6 hours PRN

Alternatives:

References:
1. Wischnik A, Wetzelsberger N, Lucker PW. Elimination of nalbuphine in human milk. Arzneimittelforschung 1988; 38(10): 1496–1498.
2. Jacqz-Aigrain E, Serreau R, Boissinot C, Popon M, Sobel A, Michel J, Sibony O. Excretion of Ketoprofen and Nalbuphine in Human Milk During Treatment of Maternal Pain After Delivery. Ther Drug Monit. 2007 Dec; 29(6): 815–818.

NALIDIXIC ACID   L3

Trade: NegGram

Other Trades: NegGram

Category: Urinary anti-infective

Nalidixic acid is an old urinary antiseptic and belongs to the fluoroquinolone family. In a group of 4 women receiving 1000 mg orally/day the concentration in breast milk was approximately 5 mg/L.[1] Hemolytic anemia has been reported in one infant whose mother received 1 gm nalidixic acid 4 times daily. Use with extreme caution. A number of new and less toxic choices (ofloxacin) should preclude the use of this compound.[2] A more recent study of 13 lactating women taking 2 grams of nalidixic acid, milk levels after 4 hours were 0.64 µg/mL. Levels at 10.5 hours after administration averaged 0.20 µg/mL. The maximum possible dose for a breastfeeding infant with these milk levels was 0.1 mg/kg/day, far less than the recommended dosage for children. The authors suggested that breastfeeding is not contraindicated during nalidixic acid therapy.[3] This is an old product and newer products such as ofloxacin, ciprofloxacin, or levofloxacin are preferred.

Pregnancy Risk	B	Lactation Risk	L3
T ½	= 1–2.5 hours	M/P	= 0.08–0.13
Vd	=	PB	= 93%
Tmax	= 1–2 hours	Oral	= 60%
MW	= 232	pKa	=

Adult Concerns: Hemolytic anemia, headache, drowsiness, blurred vision, nausea, vomiting.

Pediatric Concerns: Hemolytic anemia in one infant. This is an old product that should not be used currently.

Drug Interactions: Decreased efficacy/oral bioavailability when used with antacids. Increased anticoagulation with warfarin.

Relative Infant Dose: 0.4%–5.2%

Adult Dose: 1 gm 4 times daily.

Alternatives: Norfloxacin, ofloxacin, levofloxacin

References:
1. Belton EM, Jones RV. Haemolytic anaemia due to nalidixic acid. Lancet 1965; 2(7414): 691.
2. Drug Facts and Comparisons 1994 ed. ed. St. Louis: 1994.
3. Traeger A, Peiker G. Excretion of Nalidixic Acid via Mother's Milk. Arch Toxicol Suppl 1980; 4: 388–390.

NALOXONE   L3

Trade: Narcan
Other Trades: Nalone, Narcan
Category: Narcotic antagonist

Naloxone is a narcotic antagonist that when administered occupies the opiate receptor site, or when opiates are present, displaces them from the active site. It is commonly used for the treatment of opiate overdose, and now to prevent opiate abuse in patients undergoing withdrawal treatment.[1] Naloxone is poorly absorbed orally and plasma levels in adults are undetectable (<0.05 ng/mL) two hours after oral doses. Following intravenous use (0.4 mg), plasma naloxone levels averaged <0.084 µg/mL. Side effects are minimal except in narcotic-addicted patients. The AAP has advised that naloxone should not be administered (directly) to infants of narcotic-dependent mothers. Its use in breastfeeding mothers would be unlikely to cause problems as its milk levels would likely be low and its oral absorption is minimal to nil.

Pregnancy Risk	C	Lactation Risk	L3
T ½	= 64 minutes	M/P	=
Vd	= 2.6–2.8 l/kg	PB	= 45%
Tmax	=	Oral	= Nil
MW	= 399	pKa	= 7.9

Adult Concerns: Withdrawal effects in narcotic-addicted patients. Avoid direct use in infants of narcotic-addicted women. Ventricular tachycardia and fibrillation, hypertension, headache, and rarely seizures have been reported.

Pediatric Concerns: No breastfeeding studies are available. However, levels of naloxone in milk are likely to be quite low. In addition it is virtually unabsorbed orally. This product poses minimal risks to infants of women not addicted to opiates. However, even small amounts present in milk could accelerate slight withdrawal symptoms in infants of narcotic-addicted women.

Drug Interactions: Rapidly blocks the effect of most opiates precipitating withdrawal in addicts, or pain in other individuals. When used with clonidine, may reduce the hypotensive effects of this drug.

Relative Infant Dose:

Adult Dose: Highly variable but an initial dose of 0.4 to 2 mg intravenously is used for opiate withdrawal.

Alternatives:

References:
1. Pharmaceutical manufacturer prescribing information, 2005.

NALTREXONE   L1

Trade: ReVia, Vivitrol
Other Trades: ReVia, Nalorex
Category: Narcotic antagonist

Naltrexone is a long acting narcotic antagonist similar in structure to naloxone. Orally absorbed, it has been clinically used in addicts to prevent the action of injected heroin. It occupies and competes with all opioid medications for the opiate receptor. When used in addicts, it can induce rapid and long lasting withdrawal symptoms. Although the half-life appears brief, the duration of antagonism is long lasting (24–72 hours).[1-5] Naltrexone is quite lipid soluble, has a high pKa, and transfers into the brain easily (brain/plasma ratio= 0.81). It is readily metabolized to 6-beta-naltrexol (active) and two minor metabolites. The activity of naltrexone is believed to be mainly due to parent and 6-beta-naltrexol.

In a study of one patient (60 kg) receiving 50 mg/day, the average concentration of naltrexone and 6-beta-naltrexol in milk were 1.7 and 46 µg/L.[6] The milk/plasma ratios of naltrexone and 6-beta-naltrexol were 1.9 and 3.4 respectively. The absolute infant dose was 0.26 and 6.86 µg/kg/day, respectively. The authors suggest the relative infant dose is 0.06 and 1.0% (range = 0.86–1.06%). The infant was reported to have achieved all expected milestones and showed no drug-related side effects. Naltrexone was undetectable in the infants' plasma and levels of 6-beta-naltrexol were only marginally detectable, at 1.1 µg/L

Pregnancy Risk	C	Lactation Risk	L1
T ½	= 4–13 hours	M/P	= 1.9 (3.4 metabolite)
Vd	= 19 l/kg	PB	= 21%
Tmax	= 1 hour	Oral	= 96%
MW	= 341	pKa	= 7.9

Adult Concerns: Rapid opiate withdrawal symptoms. Dizziness, anorexia, rash, nausea, vomiting, and hepatocellular toxicity. Liver toxicity is common at doses approximately 5 times normal or less. A Narcan challenge test should be initiated in patients prior to therapy with naltrexone.

Pediatric Concerns: None reported in one case. Plasma levels of 6-beta-naltrexol were only marginally detectable, at 1.1 µg/L.

Drug Interactions: Suppresses narcotic analgesia and sedation.

Relative Infant Dose: 1.4%

Adult Dose: 50–150 mg daily.

Alternatives:

References:

1. Bullingham RE, McQuay HJ, Moore RA. Clinical pharmacokinetics of narcotic agonist-antagonist drugs. Clin Pharmacokinet 1983; 8(4): 332–343.
2. Crabtree BL. Review of naltrexone, a long-acting opiate antagonist. Clin Pharm 1984; 3(3): 273–280.
3. Ludden TM, Malspeis L, Baggot JD, Sokoloski TD, Frank SG, Reuning RH. Tritiated naltrexone binding in plasma from several species and tissue distribution in mice. J Pharm Sci 1976; 65(5): 712–716.
4. Verebey K, Volavka J, Mule SJ, Resnick RB. Naltrexone: disposition, metabolism, and effects after acute and chronic dosing. Clin Pharmacol Ther 1976; 20(3): 315–328.
5. Wall ME, Brine DR, Perez-Reyes M. Metabolism and disposition of naltrexone in man after oral and intravenous administration. Drug Metab Dispos 1981; 9(4): 369–375.
6. Chan CF, Page-Sharp M, Kristensen JH, O"Neil G, Ilett KF. Transfer of naltrexone and its metabolite 6,beta naltrexol into human milk. J Hum Lac 2004; 20(3): 322–326.

NAPHAZOLINE   L3

Trade: AK-Con, Albalon, Allersol, Naphcon, Ocu-Zoline, Privine, Vasoclear, Clear Eyes

Other Trades:

Category: Decongestant and vasopressor

Naphazoline is used for red eyes relief and as a nasal decongestant (spray). Over the counter products have low naphazoline concentrations (0.05%) such that systemic absorption is probably low, especially from ophthalmic preparations.[1] There are no adequate or well-controlled studies in breastfeeding women; however, the risk of side effects to a breastfed infant is probably minimal.

Pregnancy Risk	C	Lactation Risk	L3
T ½	=	M/P	=
Vd	=	PB	=
Tmax	=	Oral	=
MW	= 210	pKa	=

Adult Concerns: Irritation, blurred vision, increased intraocular pressure, dryness, rebound congestion.

Pediatric Concerns:

Drug Interactions: Combination with MOA inhibitor may increase hypertensive effect.

Relative Infant Dose:

Adult Dose: Instill 1–2 drops every 6 hours.

Alternatives:

References:
1. Pharmaceutical manufacturer prescribing information, 2011.

NAPROXEN   L3/L4

Trade: Naprosyn
Other Trades:
Category: NSAID, analgesic for arthritis

Naproxen is a popular NSAID analgesic. It does excrete into the breastmilk, but it does not appear in quantities that would result in untoward effects in a breastfed infant. NSAIDs in general are usually compatible with breastfeeding, with some, such as ibuprofen, being completely undetectable in breastmilk.[1] In a study done at steady state in one mother consuming 375 mg twice daily, milk levels ranged from 1.76–2.37 mg/L at 4 hours.[2,3] Total naproxen excretion in the infant's urine was only 0.26% of the maternal dose. Although the amount of naproxen transferred via milk is minimal, one should use with caution in nursing mothers because of its long half-life and its effects on infant cardiovascular system, kidneys, and gastrointestinal tract. However, its short term use postpartum or infrequent or occasional use would not necessarily be incompatible with breastfeeding. One case of prolonged bleeding, hemorrhage, and acute anemia has been reported in a seven-day-old infant.[4] The relative infant dose on a weight-adjusted maternal daily dose would probably be less than 3.3%. Other studies have confirmed naproxen's low transfer into breastmilk, showing a 1% concentration compared to the mother's plasma levels.[5,6] Despite very low transfer into milk, there have been some reports of adverse effects in infants whose mothers were administered naproxen. In a study of twenty mothers given this medication, two reported drowsiness in their infants, while one reported vomiting.[7]

Pregnancy Risk	C/D in 3rd trimester	Lactation Risk	L3 for acute use/ L4 for chronic use
T ½	= 12–15 hours	M/P	= 0.01
Vd	= 0.09 l/kg	PB	= 99.7%
Tmax	= 2–4 hours	Oral	= 74–99%
MW	= 230	pKa	= 5.0

Adult Concerns: Gastrointestinal distress, gastric bleeding, hemorrhage.

Pediatric Concerns: One reported case of prolonged bleeding, hemorrhage, and acute anemia in a seven-day-old infant.

Drug Interactions: May prolong prothrombin time when used with warfarin. Antihypertensive effects of ACE inhibitors may be blunted or completely abolished by NSAIDs. Some NSAIDs may block antihypertensive effect of beta blockers, diuretics. Used with cyclosporin, may dramatically increase renal toxicity. May increase digoxin, phenytoin, lithium levels. May increase toxicity of methotrexate. May increase bioavailability of penicillamine. Probenecid may increase NSAID levels.

Relative Infant Dose: 3.3%

Adult Dose: 250–500 mg twice daily.

Alternatives: Ibuprofen

References:

1. Anon: Committee on Drugs and American Academy of Pediatrics: The transfer of drugs and other chemicals into human milk. Pediatrics 1994; 93: 137–150.
2. Jamali F, Stevens DR. Naproxen excretion in milk and its uptake by the infant. Drug Intell Clin Pharm 1983; 17(12): 910–911.
3. Jamali F. et.al. Naproxen excretion in breast milk and its uptake by sucking infant. Drug Intell Clin Pharm 1982; 16: 475 (Abstr).
4. Figalgo I. et.al. Anemia aguda, rectoorragia y hematuria asociadas a la ingestion de naproxen. Anales Espanoles de Pediatrica 1989; 30: 317–319.
5. Product Information: Prevacid(R) NapraPAC(TM), lansoprazole delayed-release capsules and naproxen tablets kit. TAP Pharmaceuticals, Lake Forest, IL, 2003a.
6. Brogden RN: Naproxen: A reveiw of its pharmacological properties and therapeutic efficacy and use. Drugs 1975; 9: 326.
7. Ito S, Blajchman A, Stephenson M, et al: Prospective follow-up of adverse reactions in breast-fed infants exposed to maternal medication. Am J Obstet Gynecol 1993; 168(5): 1393–1399.

NAPROXEN + SUMATRIPTAN — L3

Trade: Treximet

Other Trades:

Category: Anti-migraine

Naproxen + sumatriptan is a combined drug product used for the treatment of migraine headaches.[1] Currently, no studies exist of the use of this combined drug product in lactating women.

Naproxen is a popular NSAID analgesic. It does excrete into the breastmilk, but it does not appear in quantities that would result in untoward effects in a breastfed infant. NSAIDs in general are usually compatible with breastfeeding, with some, such as ibuprofen, being completely undetectable in breastmilk.[2] In a study done at steady state in one mother consuming 375 mg twice daily, milk levels ranged from 1.76–2.37 mg/L at 4 hours.[3,4] Total naproxen excretion in the infant's urine was only 0.26% of the maternal dose. Although the amount of naproxen transferred via milk is minimal, one should use with caution in nursing mothers because of its long half-life and its effects on infant cardiovascular system, kidneys, and gastrointestinal tract. However, its short term use postpartum or infrequent or occasional use would not necessarily be incompatible with breastfeeding. One case of prolonged bleeding, hemorrhage, and acute anemia has been reported in a seven-day-old infant.[5] The relative infant dose would probably be less than 3.3%. Other studies have confirmed naproxen's low transfer into breastmilk, showing a 1% concentration compared to the mother's plasma levels.[6,7] Despite very low transfer into milk, there have been some reports of adverse effects in infants whose mothers were administered naproxen. In a study of twenty mothers given this medication, two reported drowsiness in their infants, while one reported vomiting.[8] Sumatriptan is a 5–HT (Serotonin) receptor agonist and a highly effective new drug for the treatment of migraine headache. It is not an analgesic, rather, it produces a rapid vasoconstriction in various regions of the brain, thus temporarily reducing the cause of migraines. In one study using 5 lactating women, each were given 6 mg subcutaneous injections and samples drawn for analysis over 8 hours.[9] The highest breastmilk levels were 87.2 µg/L at 2.6 hours post-dose and rapidly disappeared over the next 6 hours. The mean total recovery of sumatriptan in milk over the 8 hour duration was only 14.4 µg. On a weight-adjusted basis, this concentration in milk corresponded to a mean infant exposure of only 3.5% of the maternal dose. Further, assuming an oral bioavailability of only 14%, the weight-adjusted dose an infant would absorb would be approximately 0.49% of the maternal dose. The authors suggest that continued breastfeeding following sumatriptan use would not pose a significant risk to the suckling infant. The maternal plasma half-life is 1.3 hours; the milk half-life is 2.2 hours. Although the milk/plasma ratio was 4.9 (indicating significant concentrating mechanisms in milk), the absolute maternal plasma levels were small; hence, the absolute milk concentrations were low. The calculated relative infant dose for sumatripan is 3.5–15%.

The short-term or occasional use of naproxen + sumatriptan is probably compatible with breastfeeding. While very little amounts of naproxen may enter milk, higher levels of sumatriptan have been detected in milk. Observe for drowsiness, dizziness, vomiting and flushing in breastfed infants. Use with extra caution in newborn and premature infants. Consider alternatives such as acetaminophen during breastfeeding period.

Pregnancy Risk	C		Lactation Risk	L3
T ½	= Naproxen/sumatriptan: 12–15 hours/1.3 hours		M/P	= Naproxen/sumatriptan: 0.01/4.9
Vd	= Naproxen/sumatriptan: 0.09/ l/kg		PB	= Naproxen/sumatriptan: 99.7%/14–21%
Tmax	= Naproxen/sumatriptan: 2–4 hours/12 min (IM)		Oral	= Naproxen/sumatriptan: 74–99%/10–15%
MW	= Naproxen/sumatriptan: 230/413		pKa	= Naproxen/sumatriptan: 5.0/

Adult Concerns: Rare but serious side-effects include vision impairment, acute myocardial infarction, strokes.

Pediatric Concerns: Vomiting and drowsiness has been reported with naproxen use in breastfed infant. Flushing and dizziness has been reported with sumatriptan use in breastfed infant. One case of severe bleeding in a 7-day old infant with naproxen use.

Drug Interactions: The use of naproxen + sumatriptan is contra-indicated with monoamine oxidase inhibitors and ergot derivatives. Avoid coadministration with the following drugs: methotrexate, aspirin, warfarin, serotonin reuptake inhibitors, probenecid. Concomitant use decreases the plasma levels of the following coadministered drugs: ACE inhibitors, furosemide, beta-blockers such as metoprolol. Concomitant use increases plasma levels of lithium.

Relative Infant Dose:

Adult Dose: Naproxen/sumatriptan: 500 mg/85 mg once daily.

Alternatives: Zolmitriptan, acetaminophen

References:
1. Pharmaceutical manufacturer prescribing information, 2011.
2. Anon: Committee on Drugs and American Academy of Pediatrics: The transfer of drugs and other chemicals into human milk. Pediatrics 1994; 93: 137–150.
3. Jamali F, Stevens DR. Naproxen excretion in milk and its uptake by the infant. Drug Intell Clin Pharm 1983; 17(12): 910–911.
4. Jamali F. et.al. Naproxen excretion in breast milk and its uptake by sucking infant. Drug Intell Clin Pharm 1982; 16: 475 (Abstr).
5. Figalgo I. et.al. Anemia aguda, rectaorragia y hematuria asociadas a la ingestion de naproxen. Anales Espanoles de Pediatrica 1989; 30: 317–319.
6. Product Information: Prevacid(R) NapraPAC(TM), lansoprazole delayed-release capsules and naproxen tablets kit. TAP Pharmaceuticals, Lake Forest, IL, 2003a.
7. Brogden RN: Naproxen: A reveiw of its pharmacological properties and therapeutic efficacy and use. Drugs 1975; 9: 326.
8. Ito S, Blajchman A, Stephenson M, et al: Prospective follow-up of adverse reactions in breast-fed infants exposed to maternal medication. Am J Obstet Gynecol 1993; 168(5): 1393–1399.
9. Wojnar-Horton RE, Hackett LP, Yapp P, Dusci LJ, Paech M, Ilett KF. Distribution and excretion of sumatriptan in human milk. Br J Clin Pharmacol 1996; 41(3): 217–221.

NARATRIPTAN   L3

Trade: Amerge
Other Trades: Naramig
Category: Migraine headaches

Naratriptan is a serotonin receptor stimulant and is used for treatment of acute migraine headache. No data are currently available on its transfer into human milk although the manufacturer suggests it penetrates the milk of rodents.[1] Naratriptan is a close congener of sumatriptan, only slightly better absorbed orally, and may produce fewer side effects in sumatriptan-sensitive patients. Some studies suggest that sumatriptan is equal to if not more effective than naratriptan.[2] Sumatriptan has been studied in breastfeeding mothers and produces minimal milk levels.

Pregnancy Risk	C	Lactation Risk	L3
T ½	= 6 hours	M/P	=
Vd	= 2.42 l/kg	PB	= 31%
Tmax	= 2–3 hours	Oral	= 70%
MW	= 372	pKa	=

Adult Concerns: Chest discomfort including pain, pressure, heaviness, tightness has been reported. Nausea, dizziness, paresthesias are infrequently reported. Cardiovascular events are rare but include hypertension, and tachyarrhythmias.

Pediatric Concerns: None reported via milk.

Drug Interactions: Monoamine oxidase inhibitors can markedly increase naratriptan systemic effect and elimination including elevated plasma levels. Ergot containing drugs have caused prolonged vasospastic reactions, do not use within 24 hours after using an ergot-containing product. There have been rare reports of weakness, hyperreflexia, and incoordination with combined use with SSRIs such as fluoxetine, paroxetine, sertraline and fluvoxamine.

Relative Infant Dose:

Adult Dose: 1–2.5 mg every 4 hours X 2–3.

Alternatives: Sumatriptan

References:
1. Pharmaceutical manufacturer prescribing information, 1999.
2. Dahlof C, Winter P. et. al. Randomized, double-blind, placebo-controlled comparison of oral naratriptan and oral sumatriptan in the acute treatment of migraine (abstract). Neurology 1997; 48(suppl): A85–A86.

NATALIZUMAB   L3

Trade: Tysabri
Other Trades:
Category: Treatment of multiple sclerosis

Natalizumab is a recombinant humanized IgG4k monoclonal antibody used to suppress immunity in patients with multiple sclerosis. In one study of a single 28-year-old patient with an infant of 11.5 months, and who received 300 mg IV natalizumab every 4 weeks, levels in milk over a 50 day period were generally low but rising. [1] Following her first injection, levels were below the limit of quantitation for the first 13 days, and began to appear in milk slowly (Table 1). Levels in milk at 14 days were 0.333 µg/mL and rose to a peak of 0.491 µg/mL at day 28. Following another injection at day 29, levels rose from 0.491 µg/mL to 2.827 µg/mL eight days following the second infusion (day 37). The relative infant dose at day 27 (assuming a clinical dose of 600 mg total) was 4.9%. This number is quite high and concerning. However, virtually none of this IgG antibody would be orally absorbed in a 11.5 month-old infant. The infant reportedly was normal in growth and development and had no symptoms of infection.

Normally, the transfer of native IgG or similar monoclonal antibodies into human milk is low even during the colostral period, and they are easily digested prior to absorption in the GI tract of a mature infant. In the case above, levels in milk tended to rise over time (50 days). The mean average time to steady-state for natalizumab is reported to be 24 weeks following two injections (every 4 weeks). Assuming this is correct, levels in milk may continue to rise significantly over time and may reach significantly higher levels in milk at steady state. This will require further study.

At present, mothers should be advised that levels in milk may be significant although clinically unimportant due to the poor gastric absorption of this IgG monoclonal antibody.

Pregnancy Risk	C	Lactation Risk	L3
T ½	= 11 days	M/P	=
Vd	= 0.08 l/kg	PB	=
Tmax	=	Oral	= Nil
MW	= 149,000	pKa	=

Adult Concerns: Hypersensitivity reactions have been reported which include urticaria, dizziness, fever, rash, pruritus, nausea, flushing, hypotension, dyspnea and chest pain.

Pediatric Concerns: No data are available at this time.

Drug Interactions: Interferon (Avonex) reduces clearance of natalizumab by approximately 30%.

Relative Infant Dose: 4.9%

Adult Dose: 300 mg IV monthly.

Alternatives:

References:
1. Baker T, Milla M, Hale T. Transfer of natalizumab into human milk. Unpublished case report, 2012.

NEBIVOLOL   L3

Trade: Bystolic
Other Trades: Nebilet, Nebicard, Nubeta, Nodon
Category: Beta-blocker

Nebivolol is a beta-1 selective antagonist used for the treatment of hypertension.[1] No data are available on the transfer of this drug into human milk. Due to the high protein binding and very large volume of distribution, it is unlikely that nebivolol would transfer into milk in clinically relevant amounts. It is not known whether this drug is excreted in human milk. Because of the potential for beta blockers to produce serious adverse reactions in nursing infants, especially bradycardia, nebivolol is not recommended during nursing.

Pregnancy Risk	C	Lactation Risk	L3
T ½	= 10–12 hours	M/P	=
Vd	= 8–12 l/kg	PB	= 98%
Tmax	= 0.5–4 hours	Oral	= 12–96%
MW	= 442	pKa	=

Adult Concerns: Adverse reactions include edema, headache, fatigue, dizziness, insomnia, diarrhea, and nausea.

Pediatric Concerns: Neonatal hypoglycemia have been reported in breastfeeding infants during maternal use of beta blockers.

Drug Interactions:

Relative Infant Dose:

Adult Dose: 5 mg daily

Alternatives: Metoprolol

References:
1. Pharmaceutical manufacturer prescribing information, 2007.

NEDOCROMIL SODIUM   L2

Trade: Tilade
Other Trades: Tilade, Mireze
Category: Inhaled mast cell stabilizer

Nedocromil is believed to stabilize mast cells and prevent release of bronchoconstrictors in the lung following exposure to allergens. The systemic effects are minimal due to reduced plasma levels. Systemic absorption averages less than 8–17% of the total dose even after continued dosing, which is quite low.[1,2]

The poor oral bioavailability of this product and the reduced side effect profile of this family of drugs suggest that it is unlikely to produce untoward effects in a nursing infant.

Pregnancy Risk	B		Lactation Risk	L2
T ½	= 3.3 hours		M/P	=
Vd	=		PB	= 89%
Tmax	= 28 minutes		Oral	= 8–17%
MW	= 371		pKa	=

Adult Concerns: Poor taste, dizziness, headache, nausea and vomiting, sore throat, and cough.

Pediatric Concerns: None reported via milk.

Drug Interactions:

Relative Infant Dose:

Adult Dose: 3.5–4 mg four times daily.

Alternatives:

References:
1. Pharmaceutical manufacturer prescribing information, 1996.
2. Facts and Comparisons. St. Louis: 2010..

NEFAZODONE HCL   L4

Trade: Serzone

Other Trades: Serzone, Dutonin

Category: Antidepressant

Nefazodone is an antidepressant similar to trazodone but structurally dissimilar from the other serotonin reuptake inhibitors. It is rapidly metabolized to three partially active metabolites that have significantly longer half-lives (1.5 to 18 hours).[1]

In a study of one patient receiving 200 mg in the morning and 100 mg at night, the infant at 9 weeks of age (2.1 kg), was admitted for drowsiness, lethargy, failure to thrive, and poor temperature control.[2] The infant was born premature at 27 weeks. The maximum milk concentration of nefazodone was 358 µg/L while the maternal plasma C_{max} was 1270 µg/L. The concentration of the metabolites was reported to be 83 µg/L for triazoledione, 32 µg/L for HO-Nefazodone, and 18 µg/L for m-Chlorophenylpiperazine. The authors estimate the relative infant dose to be 0.45% of the weight-adjusted maternal dose. The AUC milk/plasma ratio ranged from 0.02 to 0.27.

Unfortunately, no infant plasma samples were taken for analysis. Dodd[3] recently reported a M/P ratio of only 0.1 for nefazodone in a patient receiving 200 mg twice daily. This is approximately one-third of the M/P ratio (0.27) reported by Yapp. However, the Yapp study used AUC data over many points and is probably a more accurate reflection of nefazodone transfer into milk during the day. This medication should probably not be used in breastfeeding mothers with young infants, premature infants, infants subject to apnea, or other weakened infants.

Pregnancy Risk	C	Lactation Risk	L4
T ½	= 1–4 hours	M/P	= 0.1–0.27
Vd	= 0.9 l/kg	PB	= >99%
Tmax	= 1 hour	Oral	= 20%
MW	= 507	pKa	= 6.6

Adult Concerns: Weakness, hypotension, somnolence, dizziness, dry mouth, constipation, nausea, headache.

Pediatric Concerns: Drowsiness, lethargy, failure to thrive, and poor temperature control in one infant.

Drug Interactions: Sometimes fatal reactions may occur with MAO inhibitors. Plasma levels of astemizole and terfenadine may be increased. Clinically important increases in plasma concentrations of alprazolam and triazolam have been reported. Serum concentrations of digoxin have been increased by nefazodone by 29%. Haloperidol clearance decreased by 35%. Nefazodone may decrease propranolol plasma levels by as much as 30%.

Relative Infant Dose: 1.2%

Adult Dose: 150–300 mg twice daily.

Alternatives: Sertraline, paroxetine, trazodone

References:
1. Pharmaceutical manufacturer prescribing information, 1996.
2. Yapp P, Ilett KF, Kristensen JH, Hackett LP, Paech MJ, Rampono J. Drowsiness and poor feeding in a breast-fed infant: association with nefazodone and its metabolites. Ann Pharmacother 2000; 34(11): 1269–1272.
3. Dodd S, Buist A, Burrows GD, Maguire KP, Norman TR. Determination of nefazodone and its pharmacologically active metabolites in human blood plasma and breast milk by high-performance liquid chromatography. J Chromatogr B Biomed Sci Appl 1999; 730(2): 249–255.

NEFOPAM   L3

Trade: Acupan
Other Trades:
Category: Analgesic

Nefopam hydrochloride is a non-narcotic analgesic used for post operative and musculoskeletal pain. The drug also works well for episiotomy pain.[1] The drug has also been used for shivering and intractable hiccoughs. Nefopam is structurally related to diphenhydramine and may be used as an alternative pain control method in patients who are opioid dependent. Nefopam does not appear to cause respiratory depression and is one third as potent as morphine. Nefopam is well absorbed orally and extensively metabolized by the liver. The drug is excreted largely by the kidney. In a study of five breastfeeding women who were treated with 60 mg nefopam every 4 hours for 48 hours after delivery, levels in milk were similar to plasma (M/P ratio = 1.2). Levels in milk ranged from 5.8 to 298.7 ng/mL with a mean milk level of 90.4 µg/L, and a relative infant dose of 2.6%.[2]

Pregnancy Risk	Probably Safe	Lactation Risk	L3
T ½	= 3–8 hours	M/P	= 1.2
Vd	=	PB	= 71–76%
Tmax	= Oral 1–3 hours; IM 1.5 hours	Oral	= Well absorbed
MW	= 289.8	pKa	= 9.36

Adult Concerns: Urine retention, headache, insomnia, tachycardia, diaphoresis, lightheadedness, rash, nausea, vomiting, dry mouth, and drowsiness.

Pediatric Concerns:

Drug Interactions: Increased risk of seizures when given concurrently with: amitriptyline, amoxapine, clomipramine, desipramine, dothiepin, doxepin, imipramine, lofepramine, nortriptyline, opipramol, protriptyline, and trimipramine. Increased risk of CNS excitement when given concurrently with: selegiline, toxoxatone, brofaromine, clorgyline, furazolidone, iproniazid, isocarboxazid, lazabemide, linezolid, moclobemide, rasagiline, nialamide, pargyline, phenelzine, tranylcypromine, and procarbazine.

Relative Infant Dose: 2.6%

Adult Dose: 60 mg every 4 hours.

Alternatives: Morphine, hydrocodone, oxycodone

References:
1. Bloomfield SS, Barden TP, Mitchell J. Nefopam and propoxyphene in episiotomy pain. Clin Pharmacol Ther. 1980 Apr; 27(4): 502–7.
2. Liu DT, Savage JM, Donnell D. Nefopam excretion in human milk. Br J Clin Pharmacol. 1987 Jan; 23(1): 99–101.

NEISSERIA GONORRHEAE   L2

Trade: Gonorrhea, *Gonococcal* infection
Other Trades:
Category: Infectious disease

Neisseria gonorrheae is a gram-negative bacteria, known to cause the sexually transmitted disease gonorrhea. Mode of transmission is mainly through exposure to infected genital secretions during sexual intercourse. Infection in neonates may occur due to exposure to infected secretions during vaginal delivery. *Gonococcal* infection in adults or adolescents is usually manifested by thick, purulent discharge from the cervix or urethra. Besides this burning and pain during urination, skin rash and arthritis are some of the other symptoms. Gonorrhea in women may cause infertility. In neonates, *Gonococcal* infection is manifested in the form of an eye infection called *Gonococcal* conjunctivitis or ophthalmia neonatorum. It is characterized by thick purulent conjunctival discharge. As a prophylactic measure, all neonates are routinely administered 1% tetracycline ophthalmic ointment or 0.5% erythromycin ophthalmic ointment in each eye, soon after birth. Neonates who are born to mothers with known *Gonococcal* infection are also administered a single dose of ceftriaxone.

There no studies suggesting transfer of the *Neisseria gonorrheae* bacterium into breastmilk. When a lactating mother has been diagnosed with gonorrhea, treatment should be instituted immediately with a single intramuscular dose of ceftriaxone 125 mg. Additionally, a single dose of 1 gram azithromycin should also be instituted. A lactating mother may resume breastfeeding within 24 hours of initiation of therapy. Since the mode of transmission is mainly through contact with infected secretions, it is advisable that the mother take all hygienic and sanitary precautions to avoid transmission to the infant.

Pregnancy Risk	Probably Safe	Lactation Risk	L2
T ½	=	M/P	=
Vd	=	PB	=
Tmax	=	Oral	=
MW	=	pKa	=

Adult Concerns: *Gonococcal* infection in adults or adolescents is usually manifested by thick, purulent discharge from the cervix or urethra. Besides this burning and pain during urination, skin rash and arthritis are some of the other symptoms. Gonorrhea in women may cause infertility.

Pediatric Concerns: In neonates, *Gonococcal* infection is manifested in the form of an eye infection called *Gonococcal* conjunctivitis or ophthalmia neonatorum. It is characterized by thick purulent conjunctival discharge.

Drug Interactions:

Relative Infant Dose:

Adult Dose:

Alternatives:

References:

NEOMYCIN   L3/L5

Trade: Neo-Fradin
Other Trades:
Category: Aminoglycoside antibiotic

Neomycin is an antibiotic commonly used for topical treatment of bacterial infections.[1] It is also used in preparation for bowel surgery. There are no adequate and well-controlled studies or case reports in breastfeeding women. However, contact dermatitis is a consistent problem (10% of patients) and this product should probably not be used on breastfeeding mothers, particularly on sore nipples.

Pregnancy Risk	D	Lactation Risk	L3/L5 on nipple
T ½	= 2–3 hours (12 h at high doses)	M/P	=
Vd	= 0.36 l/kg	PB	= 0%-30%
Tmax	= 1–4 hours (oral)	Oral	= 0.6–0.8%
MW	= 614.6	pKa	= 13.19

Adult Concerns: Rash, pruritus, nausea, vomiting, nephrotoxicity, ototoxicity, respiratory depression.

Pediatric Concerns:

Drug Interactions: Risk of increased respiratory depression while coadministering with non-depolarizing neuromuscular blockers such as pancuronium, atracuronium, tubocurarine. Co-administration with cyclosporine, cedofovir, tacrolimus increases risk of nephrotoxicity. Increased nephrotoxicity and ototoxicity while coadministering with furosemide, bumetanide. Increased risk of bleeding with warfarin.

Relative Infant Dose:

Adult Dose:

Alternatives:

References:
1. Pharmaceutical manufacturer prescribing information, 2011.

NEOTAME   L3

Trade: Neotame
Other Trades:
Category: Sweetener

Neotame is an artificial sweetener. It is up to 13,000 times sweeter than sugar. Neotame is rapidly metabolized and completely eliminated. There is no accumulation in the body. The major metabolic pathway is hydrolysis of the methyl ester yielding de-esterified neotame and methanol. Because only very small amounts of neotame are needed to sweeten foods, the amount of methanol derived from neotame is very small. Methanol is also found in common foods such as fruit and vegetable juices. There are no adequate and well-controlled studies or case reports in breastfeeding women.[1]

Pregnancy Risk	Probably Safe	Lactation Risk	L3
T ½	=	M/P	=
Vd	=	PB	=
Tmax	=	Oral	=
MW	= 378.5	pKa	=

Adult Concerns: No side effects listed for neotame itself but it does contain methanol. Methanol is toxic in large doses and can cause lethargy, confusion, joint aches, lower back pain, headache and asthma symptoms.

Pediatric Concerns:

Drug Interactions:

Relative Infant Dose:

Adult Dose:

Alternatives:

References:
1. www.neotame.com/pdf/neotame_science_brochure_us.pdf. Accessed Feb. 14, 2011.

NEPAFENAC   L3

Trade: Nevanac
Other Trades: Nevanac
Category: NSAID anti-inflammatory

Nepafenac is a nonsteroidal anti-inflammatory that is used ophthalmically. It is primarily used to treat the inflammation associated with extraction of cataracts and the accompanying pain. Nepafenac has been shown to be excreted in milk during animal studies, however it is not known if it is excreted in human milk.[1] Levels in human plasma are exceedingly low and levels once determined in milk, will be even lower.

Pregnancy Risk	C	Lactation Risk	L3
T ½	= 0.7–1.1 hours	M/P	=
Vd	=	PB	= 82.7–84.3%
Tmax	= 0.15–0.35 hours	Oral	= 6%
MW	= 254.28	pKa	= 19.43

Adult Concerns: Vitreous detachment, conjunctival edema, dry eye, foreign body sensation, itching of eye, ocular hyperemia, photophobia, raised intraocular pressure, reduced visual acuity, sinusitis, hypertension, headache, nausea, capsular opacity, sticky sensation.

Pediatric Concerns:

Drug Interactions: Latanoprost–Ophthalmic NSAIDs may diminish the therapeutic effect of latanoprost.

Relative Infant Dose:

Adult Dose: 1 drop three times daily.

Alternatives:

References:
1. Pharmaceutical manufacturer prescribing information, 2005.

NESIRITIDE   L3

Trade: Natrecor
Other Trades:
Category: B-type naturetic peptide

Nesiritide is a recombinant form of human B-type natriuretic peptide. It is used to treat acutely decompensated congestive heart failure.[1] No studies have been performed on the concentrations of nesiritide in human milk. However, due to the large molecular weight of this peptide (3464 Da), it is unlikely that it would pass into the milk compartment or be orally bioavailable to a breastfeeding infant.

Pregnancy Risk	C	Lactation Risk	L3
T ½	= 18 minutes	M/P	=
Vd	= 0.19 l/kg	PB	=
Tmax	= 1 hour	Oral	= Nil
MW	= 3464	pKa	=

Adult Concerns: Adverse reactions include hypotension, increased serum creatinine, ventricular tachycardia, nausea, and headache.

Pediatric Concerns: No data are available. It is unlikely to enter milk.

Drug Interactions: Increased hypotension can be seen when taken with ACE inhibitors, diuretics, and/or hypotensive agents.

Relative Infant Dose:

Adult Dose: 0.01 µg/kg/minute

Alternatives:

References:
1. Pharmaceutical manufacturer prescribing information, 2004.

NETILMICIN   L3

Trade: Netromycin
Other Trades: Netromycin, Nettilin
Category: Aminoglycoside antibiotic

Netilmicin is a typical aminoglycoside antibiotic. Poor oral absorption limits its use to IM and IV administration although some studies suggest significant oral absorption in infancy.[1,2] Only small levels are believed to be secreted into human milk although no reports exist.

Pregnancy Risk	D	Lactation Risk	L3
T ½	= 2–2.5 hours	M/P	=
Vd	=	PB	= <10%
Tmax	= 30–60 minutes (IM)	Oral	= Negligible
MW	= 476	pKa	=

Adult Concerns: Kidney damage, hearing loss, changes in gastrointestinal flora.

Pediatric Concerns: None reported, but observe for gastrointestinal symptoms such as diarrhea.

Drug Interactions: Risk of nephrotoxicity may be increased when used with cephalosporins, enflurane, methoxyflurane, and vancomycin. Auditory toxicity may increase when used with loop diuretics. The neuromuscular blocking effects of neuromuscular blocking agents may be increased when used with aminoglycosides.

Relative Infant Dose:

Adult Dose: 1.3–2.2 mg/kg every 8 hours

Alternatives:

References:
1. Pharmaceutical manufacturer prescribing information, 1995.
2. McEvoy GE. (ed): AFHS Drug Information. New York, NY: 2003.

NEUROMUSCULAR BLOCKING AGENTS | L3

Trade: Anectine, Mivacron, Tracrium, Nuromax, Pavulon, Arduan, Raplon, Zemuron, Norcuron

Other Trades:

Category: Muscle Relaxants for surgery

Neuromuscular blocking agents are similar to curare and are primarily used to relax skeletal muscle during surgery.[1,2] They typically have a three phase elimination curve. The first phase elimination is rapid, averaging about <5 minutes. The second phase half-life ranges from 7–40 minutes, and a third phase half-life is 2–3 hours. It is not known if any of these agents penetrate into human milk, but it is very unlikely. First they are large in molecular weight, have highly polar structures, and they are virtually excluded from most cells. Oral bioavailability is not reported, but it is likely small to nil. A brief waiting period (few hours) after surgery will eliminate most risks associated with the use of these products.

Pregnancy Risk	C	Lactation Risk	L3
T ½	= Variable	M/P	=
Vd	=	PB	= 50%
Tmax	=	Oral	= Nil
MW	= Large	pKa	=

Adult Concerns: Adverse effects include prolonged apnea, residual muscle weakness, and allergic reactions. Other side effects include hypotension, bronchospasms, cardiac arrhythmias. Histamine-related events include flushing, erythema, pruritus, urticaria, wheezing and bronchospasm.

Pediatric Concerns: None reported via milk. They are unlikely to penetrate into milk in significant levels.

Drug Interactions: There are literally dozens of drug-drug interactions with the neuromuscular blocking agents. Consult a more thorough text.

Relative Infant Dose:

Adult Dose: Variable depending on individual agent.

Alternatives:

References:

1. Pharmaceutical manufacturer Package Insert, 2004.
2. Baselt RC. Disposition of toxic drugs and chemicals in man. Foster City, CA: Chemical Toxicology Institute, 2000.

NEVIRAPINE   L3

Trade: Viramune

Other Trades: Viramune

Category: Antiretroviral agent used in HIV infections.

Nevirapine selectively inhibits reverse transcriptase activity and replication of HIV-1. It is commonly used concomitantly with other antiretroviral drugs to treat HIV.[1] In a study of 20 women receiving 200 mg twice daily at steady state, median nevirapine levels in maternal serum at 4 hours post dose, breast milk, and infant serum were 9534 ng/mL, 6795 ng/mL and 971 ng/mL, respectively.[2] The milk/serum ratio was 0.67. The median infant serum concentration of nevirapine (971 ng/mL) was at least 40 times the 50% inhibitory concentration and similar to peak concentrations after a single 2 mg/kg dose of nevirapine. The authors concluded that HIV-1 inhibitory concentrations of nevirapine are achieved in breastfeeding infants of mothers receiving nevirapine, exposing infants to the potential for both the beneficial as well as the adverse effects of nevirapine ingestion. Thus far, no untoward effects have been noted in the few infants studied. It is therefore apparent, that nevirapine use by the mother might significantly reduces symptoms of infection in the infant.

Infant nevirapine prophylaxis in the first 6 weeks of life is known to decrease breastfeeding HIV transmission, but the efficacy of continuation of such therapy is not known. Recently, a study was reported of the efficacy and safety of extended administration of nevirapine in a breastfeeding infant of an HIV-infected mother.[3] In this study, 1527 breastfed infants of HIV-infected mothers received 10 mg nevirapine daily for first 6 weeks of life. All the enrolled infants were HIV-negative at the time of initiation of the study. These infants were then randomized into two groups- those receiving nevirapine and those receiving placebo. All the infants were exclusively breastfed during the course of the study. The infants in the nevirapine group were administered age-appropriate increasing doses of nevirapine ranging from 10 mg daily up to 28 mg daily until 6 months of age or until cessation of breastfeeding, whichever occurred earlier. It was found that at 6 months of age, the rate of HIV-1 transmission in the nevirapine group was 1.1% as compared to 2.4% in the control group. This implies a 54% reduction in the rate of mother-to-infant transmission of HIV -1 via breastmilk. This extended nevirapine regimen was documented to be particularly effective in those mothers with CD4 cell counts of more than 350, who normally do not require antiretroviral therapy for their own health. In such mothers, there was a four-fold reduction in the rate of HIV-1 transmission via breastmilk as compared to the control group, making the rate in mothers who are not on antiretroviral therapy equivalent to those who are on antiretroviral therapy. Further, it was revealed that the rate of breastfeeding HIV transmission returns to pre-treatment levels once infant nevirapine prophylaxis is stopped. In conclusion, this study indicates that infants of mothers who do not require antiretroviral therapy for their own health may continue to exclusively breastfeed for at least 6 months of age, if the infants receive nevirapine prophylaxis during the course of breastfeeding. This allows the infant to receive the benefits of breastmilk while simultaneously avoiding the risks of HIV transmission.

Pregnancy Risk	B		Lactation Risk	L3
T ½	= 25–30 hours		M/P	= 0.67
Vd	= 1.4 l/kg		PB	= 60%
Tmax	= 4 hours		Oral	= 90%
MW	= 266		pKa	=

Adult Concerns: Reported side effects in adults are numerous and include: rash, nausea, granulocytopenia, headache, fatigue, diarrhea, abdominal pain, myalgia. Observe for liver function, CBC, routine blood chemistry.

Pediatric Concerns: None reported in several papers. Levels in milk are moderate and levels in infant plasma are supratherapeutic.

Drug Interactions: Numerous drug-drug interactions have been reported and include: didanosine, efavirenz, indinavir, lopinavir, nelfinavir, ritonavir, saquinavir, stavudine, zalcitabine, clarithromycin, ethinyl estradiol, norethindrone, fluconazole, ketoconazole, rifabutin, rifampin, St. John's Wort. Check a drug interaction reference for more.

Relative Infant Dose: 17.8%

Adult Dose: 200 mg twice daily but highly variable.

Alternatives:

References:

1. Pharmaceutical manufacturer prescribing information, 2011.
2. Shapiro RL, Holland DT, Capparelli E, Lockman S, Thior I, Wester C, et al. Antiretroviral concentrations in breast-feeding infants of women in Botswana receiving antiretroviral treatment. J Infect Dis 2005 Sep 1; 192(5): 720–7.
3. Coovadia HM, Brown ER, Fowler MG, Chipato T, Moodley D, Manji K, Musoke P,Stranix-Chibanda L, Chetty V, Fawzi W, Nakabiito C, Msweli L, Kisenge R, Guay L, Mwatha A, Lynn DJ, Eshleman SH, Richardson P, George K, Andrew P, Mofenson LM,Zwerski S, Maldonado Y; for the HPTN 046 protocol team. Efficacy and safety of an extended nevirapine regimen in infant children of breastfeeding mothers with HIV-1 infection for prevention of postnatal HIV-1 transmission (HPTN 046): a randomised, double-blind, placebo-controlled trial. Lancet. 2011 Dec 22.

NIACIN   L3

Trade: Niacin-Time, Niacor, Slo-Niacin

Other Trades: Niaspan FCT, Niodan

Category: Vitamin B₃

Niacin, also known as vitamin B_3, is an essential dietary substance, and is present in a wide variety of foods and supplements. It is a component of two coenzyme which function in oxidation-reduction reactions essential for tissue respiration. It is also used to reduce cholesterol and other fatty substances in the blood in high doses (2–6 gm/ day). Pellagra is a disease caused by niacin deficiency, and most often arises due to inadequate dietary intake. The recommended daily allowance for niacin is 14 mg/day for females, with an upper limit of 35 mg/day. In its extended release formulation, niacin has been excreted into human milk.[1] The recommended daily allowance of niacin in lactating women is 18 to 20 mg of the standard release formulation. It is currently unknown if there are clinically significant consequences when breastfeeding an infant while the mother is taking a higher dose of niacin. There is limited data concerning the use of niacin for hypercholesterolemia or hypertriglyceridemia in breastfeeding mothers. Since niacin is known to be hepatotoxic in higher doses, it is recommended that mothers control these conditions with dietary measures while breastfeeding and do not exceed the daily recommended allowance.

Pregnancy Risk	A	Lactation Risk	L3
T ½	= 45 min	M/P	=
Vd	=	PB	=
Tmax	= 45 min	Oral	= 100%
MW	= 123	pKa	= 4.85

Adult Concerns: Flushing, peripheral dilation, itching, nausea, bloating, flatulence, vomiting, abnormal liver function.

Pediatric Concerns: None reported.

Drug Interactions: Oral hypoglycemics–Niacin may produce fluctuations in blood glucose levels. Sulfinpyrazone–Niacin may inhibit uricosuric effects of this agent. Probenecid–Niacin may inhibit uricosuric effects of this agent. Lovastatin and other cholesterol lowering medications–Niacin may cause increased toxicity.

Relative Infant Dose:

Adult Dose: 10–20 mg/day.

Alternatives:

References:
1. Product Information: Niaspan(R) niacin extended release tablets. Kos Pharmaceuticals, Inc., Miami, FL, 1999.

NICARDIPINE   L2

Trade: Cardene

Other Trades: Cardene

Category: Antihypertensive, calcium channel blocker

Nicardipine is a typical calcium channel blocker structurally related to nifedipine. In a study of 11 mothers consuming 20–120 mg nicardipine daily in various dosage forms, the milk/plasma ratio at 3 hours post dose averaged 0.25 (range 0.08–0.75), and the milk concentration (C_{max}) was 7.3 µg/L (range 1.9–18.8).[1] The mean milk concentration was 4.4 µg/L (range 1.3–13.8). The authors estimate the relative infant dose to be 0.07% (range: 0.3–0.14) of the weight-adjusted maternal dose. Another study of 7 lactating women receiving a dose of 1 to 6.5 mg/hour found 82% of 34 milk samples to have undetectable levels. Six samples contained between 5.1 to 18.5 µg/L. The maximum infant exposure was calculated to be less than 300 ng/day, a level much lower than the dose used in neonates.[2]

Pregnancy Risk	C	Lactation Risk	L2
T ½	= 6–10 hours	M/P	= 0.25
Vd	= 0.6–2.0 l/kg	PB	= >95%
Tmax	= 0.5–2 hours	Oral	= 35%
MW	= 480	pKa	=

Adult Concerns: Headache, peripheral edema, flushing, hypotension, bradycardia, gingival hyperplasia.

Pediatric Concerns: None reported in one study. Levels in milk are very low.

Drug Interactions: Barbiturates may reduce bioavailability of calcium channel blockers (CCB). Calcium salts may reduce hypotensive effect. Dantrolene may increase risk of hyperkalemia and myocardial depression. H₂ blockers may increase bioavailability of certain CCBs. Hydantoins may reduce plasma levels. Quinidine increases risk of hypotension, bradycardia, tachycardia. Rifampin may reduce effects of CCBs. Vitamin D may reduce efficacy of CCBs. CCBs may increase carbamazepine, cyclosporin, encainide, prazosin levels.

Relative Infant Dose: 0.07%–0.1%

Adult Dose: 20–50 twice daily.

Alternatives: Nifedipine, nimodipine

References:
1. Jarreau P, Beller CL, Guillonneau M, Jacqz-Aigrain E. Excretion of nicardipine in human milk. 2000; 4(1): 28–30.
2. Bartels P, Hanff L, mathot R, Steegers E, Vulto A, Visser W. Nicardipine in pre-eclamptic patients: placental transfer and disposition in breast milk. BJOG 2007 Feb; 114(2): 230–3.

NICOTINE   L2

Trade: Habitrol, NicoDerm, Nicotrol, ProStep, NJOY (ENDS), Liberty Stix (ENDS), Crown Seven (ENDS), E-cigarettes, Blue Cigs (ENDS)

Other Trades: Nicabate, Habitrol, Nicoderm, Nicorette, Prostep, Nicotinell TTS

Category: Nicotine withdrawal systems

Nicotine and its metabolite cotinine are both present in milk with a milk: plasma ratio of 2.9. Fifteen lactating women (mean age, 32 years; mean weight, 72 kg) who were smokers (mean of 17 cigarettes per day) participated in a trial of the nicotine patch to assist in smoking cessation.[1] Serial milk samples were collected from the women over sequential 24-hour periods when they were smoking and when they were stabilized on the 21 mg/day, 14 mg/day, and 7 mg/day nicotine patches. Nicotine and cotinine concentrations in milk were not significantly different between smoking (mean of 17 cigarettes per day) and the 21 mg/day patch, but concentrations were significantly lower when patients were using the

14 mg/day and 7 mg/day patches than when smoking. There was also a downward trend in absolute infant dose (nicotine equivalents) from smoking or the 21 mg patch through to the 14 mg and 7 mg patches. Milk intake by the breast-fed infants was similar while their mothers were smoking (585 mL/d) and subsequently when their mothers were using the 21 mg (717 mL/d), 14 mg (731 mL/d), and 7 mg (619 mL/d) patches. The authors conclude that the absolute infant dose of nicotine and its metabolite cotinine decreases by about 70% from when subjects were smoking or using the 21 mg patch to when they were using the 7 mg patch. In addition, use of the nicotine patch had no significant influence on the milk intake by the breastfed infant. Undertaking maternal smoking cessation with the nicotine patch is, therefore, a safer option than continued smoking.

With nicotine gum, maternal serum nicotine levels average 30–60% of those found in cigarette smokers. While patches (transdermal systems) produce a sustained and lower nicotine plasma level, nicotine gum may produce large variations in peak levels when the gum is chewed rapidly, fluctuations similar to smoking itself. Mothers who choose to use nicotine gum and breastfeed should be counseled to refrain from breastfeeding for 2–3 hours after using the gum product. The nicotine inhaler only dispenses about 4 mg of nicotine following 80 inhalations, of which, only 2 mg is actually absorbed. Plasma levels slowly reach levels of about 6 ng/mL in contrast to those of a cigarette, which reach a C_{max} of approximately 49 ng/mL in only 5 minutes. These levels (6 ng/mL) are probably too low to affect a breastfeeding infant. Habitual smokeless tobacco users will receive 130–250 mg of nicotine per day compared to 180 mg per day for 1 pack of cigarettes.

E-cigarettes, also known as Electronic Nicotine Delivery Systems (ENDS) are battery-powered devices that look like conventional cigarettes and are designed to mimic and deliver the satisfying effects of a traditional cigarette without exposing the user, or the people around to the harmful compounds of tobacco smoke. E-cigarettes contain mainly 5 FDA-approved ingredients: nicotine, water, propylene glycol, glycerol and flavoring. While the nicotine content provides the gratifying effects of a regular cigarette, the propylene glycol produces vapor to mimic cigarette smoke. E-cigarettes have therefore become very popular as a safer alternative to cigarette smoking without exposure to tobacco and substances known to cause detrimental effects including lung cancer. However, these products have not been extensively studied and currently not licensed by the FDA. The amount of nicotine delivered per puff or per cartridge is also obscure. One study [2] compared the peak blood nicotine levels achieved after the use of a 16 mg e-cigarette, a nicotine inhaler and a conventional cigarette. It was reported that an e-cigarette produced peak blood nicotine levels of 1.3 ng/mL in 19.6 minutes, which is comparable to the levels obtained by a nicotine inhaler (2.1 ng/mL in 32 minutes) and much lower than those obtained by a conventional cigarette (13.4 ng/mL in 14.3 minutes). This study further revealed that the reduction in the desire to smoke is similar to that of a nicotine inhaler but that e-cigarettes are better tolerated by users.

Eissenberg,[3] later conducted a similar study and reported that the amount of nicotine delivered after 10 puffs of a 16 mg e-cigarette is little to none. Based on these findings, it can be concluded that the amount of nicotine that transfers into breastmilk after an acute inhalation of an e-cigarette is probably minimal, and comparable to that of a nicotine inhaler. But it is reported that an average e-cigarette user inhales up to 120 puffs/day.[4] This could possibly amount to significantly higher blood nicotine levels. It is too early to comment on the long-term effects of chronic use of e-cigarettes and more studies are required.

Nicotine has been suggested to cause a decrease in basal prolactin production.[5,6] One study clearly suggests that cigarette smoking significantly reduces breastmilk production at two weeks postpartum from 514 mL/day in non-smokers to 406 mL/day in smoking mothers.[7] However, Ilett's well-done study above did not detect any change in milk production at all, although the methods of these two studies were not identical. Therefore, the risk of using nicotine patches while breastfeeding is much less than the risk of formula feeding. Mothers should be advised to limit smoking as much as possible and to smoke only after they have fed their infant, or to switch to the use of nicotine patches.

Pregnancy Risk	D	Lactation Risk	L2
T ½	= 2.0 hours (non-patch)	M/P	= 2.9
Vd	=	PB	= 4.9%
Tmax	= 2–4 hours	Oral	= 30%
MW	= 162	pKa	=

Adult Concerns: Tachycardia, gastrointestinal distress, vomiting, diarrhea, rapid heart beat, and restlessness. Smoking during pregnancy has been associated with preterm births, decreased birth weight, and an increased risk of abortion and stillbirth . The use of nicotine during the last trimester has been associated with a decrease in fetal breathing movements, possibly resulting from decreased placental perfusion induced by nicotine. However, the use of nicotine patches instead of smoking is still preferred .

Pediatric Concerns: No untoward effects were noted from nicotine patch study.

Drug Interactions: Cessation of smoking may alter response to a number of medications in ex-smokers. Including are acetaminophen, caffeine, imipramine, oxazepam, pentazocine, propranolol, and theophylline. Smoking may reduce diuretic effect of furosemide. Smoking while continuing to use patches may dramatically elevate nicotine plasma levels.

Relative Infant Dose:

Adult Dose: 7–21 mg daily

Alternatives:

References:

1. Ilett KF, Hale TW, Page-Sharp M, Kristensen JH, Kohan R, Hackett LP. Use of nicotine patches in breast-feeding mothers: transfer of nicotine and cotinine into human milk. Clin Pharmacol Ther 2003; 74(6): 516–524.
2. Bullen C, McRobbie H, Thornley S, Glover M, Lin R, Laugesen M. Effect of an electronic nicotine delivery device (e cigarette) on desire to smoke and withdrawal, user preferences and nicotine delivery: randomised cross-over trial. Tob Control. 2010 Apr; 19(2): 98–103.
3. Eissenberg T. Electronic nicotine delivery devices: ineffective nicotine delivery and craving suppression after acute administration. Tob Control. 2010Feb; 19(1): 87–8.

4. Etter JF, Bullen C. Electronic cigarette: users profile, utilization,satisfaction and perceived efficacy. Addiction. 2011 Nov; 106(11): 2017–28. doi: 10.1111/j.1360–0443.2011.03505.x. Epub 2011 Jul 27.

5. Benowitz NL. Nicotine replacement therapy during pregnancy. JAMA 1991; 266(22): 3174–3177.

6. Matheson I, Rivrud GN. The effect of smoking on lactation and infantile colic. JAMA 1989; 261(1): 42–43.

7. Hopkinson JM, Schanler RJ, Fraley JK, Garza C. Milk production by mothers of premature infants: influence of cigarette smoking. Pediatrics 1992; 90(6): 934–938.

NICOTINIC ACID   L3

Trade: Nicobid, Nicolar, Niacels, Niacin, Nicotinamide, Niaspan
Other Trades:
Category: Vitamin B_3

Nicotinic acid, commonly called niacin, is a component of two coenzymes which function in oxidation-reduction reactions essential for tissue respiration. It is converted to nicotinamide *in vivo*. Although considered a vitamin, large doses (2–6 gm/day) are effective in reducing serum LDL cholesterol and triglyceride and increasing serum HDL. From numerous studies, niacin content (even when supplemented with moderately low amounts) seems to vary from about 1.1 to 3.9 mg/L under normal circumstances.[1] Supplementation apparently does increase milk niacin levels. The concentration transferred into milk as a function of dose or following high maternal doses has not been reported, but it is presumed that elevated maternal plasma levels may significantly elevate milk levels of niacin as well. Because niacin is known to be hepatotoxic in higher doses, breastfeeding mothers should not significantly exceed the RDA such as with the 2 gm/day doses used to treat hypercholesterolemia.

Pregnancy Risk	A/C in third trimester	Lactation Risk	L3
T ½	= 45 minutes	M/P	=
Vd	=	PB	=
Tmax	= 45 minutes	Oral	= Complete
MW	= 123	pKa	= 4.85

Adult Concerns: Flushing, peripheral dilation, itching, nausea, bloating, flatulence, vomiting. In high doses, some abnormal liver function tests.

Pediatric Concerns: None reported via milk, but do not exceed RDA.

Drug Interactions: Niacin may produce fluctuations in blood glucose levels and interfere with oral hypoglycemics. May inhibit uricosuric effects of sulfinpyrazone and probenecid. Increased toxicity (myopathy) when used with lovastatin and other cholesterol-lowering drugs.

Relative Infant Dose:
Adult Dose: 10–20 mg daily.

Alternatives:

References:

1. Pratt jp, Hamil BM, Moyer EZ, et.al. Metabolism of women during the reproductive cycle. XVIII. The effect of multivitamin supplements on the secretion of B vitamins in human milk. J Nutr 1951; 44(1): 141–157.

NIFEDIPINE   L2

Trade: Adalat, Procardia, Nifedical

Other Trades: Nifecard, Nyefax, Adalat, Apo-Nifed, Novo-Nifedin, Nu-Nifed, Nefensar XL

Category: Antihypertensive calcium channel blocker

Nifedipine is an effective antihypertensive. It belongs to the calcium channel blocker family of drugs. Two studies indicate that nifedipine is transferred to breastmilk in varying but generally low levels.

In one study in which the dose was varied from 10–30 mg three times daily, the highest concentration (53.35 µg/L) was measured at 1 hour after a 30 mg dose.[1] Other levels reported were 16.35 µg/L 60 minutes after a 20 mg dose and 12.89 µg/L 30 minutes after a 10 mg dose. The milk levels fell linearly with the milk half-lives estimated to be 1.4 hours for the 10 mg dose, 3.1 hours for the 20 dose, and 2.4 hours for the 30 mg dose. The milk concentration measured 8 hours following a 30 mg dose was 4.93 µg/L. In this study, using the highest concentration found and a daily intake of 150 ml/kg/day of human milk, the amount of nifedipine intake would only be 8 µg/kg/day (less than 1.8% of the therapeutic pediatric dose). The authors conclude that the amount ingested via breast milk poses little risk to an infant.

In another study, concentrations of nifedipine in human milk 1 to 8 hours after 10 mg doses varied from <1 to 10.3 µg/L (median 3.5 µg/L) in six of eleven patients.[2] In this study, milk levels three days after discontinuing medication ranged from <1 to 9.4 µg/L. The authors concluded the exposure to nifedipine through breastmilk is not significant. In a study by Penny and Lewis, following a maternal dose of 20 mg nifedipine daily for 10 days, peak breastmilk levels at 1 hour were 46 µg/L.[3] The corresponding maternal serum level was 43 µg/L. From this data the authors suggest a daily intake for an infant would be approximately 6.45 µg/kg/day. Nifedipine has been found clinically useful for nipple vasospasm. Because of the similarity to Raynaud's Phenomenon, sustained release formulations providing 30–60 mg per day are suggested.

Pregnancy Risk	C	Lactation Risk	L2
T ½	= 1.8–7 hours	M/P	= 1.0
Vd	=	PB	= 92–98%
Tmax	= 45 min-4 hours	Oral	= 50%
MW	= 346	pKa	=

Adult Concerns: Headache, peripheral edema, gingival hyperplasia, hypotension. Distortion of smell and taste.

Pediatric Concerns: None reported via milk.

Drug Interactions: Barbiturates may reduce bioavailability of calcium channel blockers (CCB). Calcium salts may reduce hypotensive effect. Dantrolene may increase risk of hyperkalemia and myocardial depression. H_2 blockers may increase bioavailability of certain CCBs. Hydantoins may reduce plasma levels. Quinidine increases risk of hypotension, bradycardia, tachycardia. Rifampin may reduce effects of CCBs. Vitamin D may reduce efficacy of CCBs. CCBs may increase carbamazepine, cyclosporin, encainide, prazosin levels.

Relative Infant Dose: 2.3%–3.4%

Adult Dose: 10–20 mg three times daily.

Alternatives: Nimodipine

References:
1. Ehrenkranz RA, Ackerman BA, Hulse JD. Nifedipine transfer into human milk. J Pediatr 1989; 114(3): 478–480.
2. Manninen AK, Juhakoski A. Nifedipine concentrations in maternal and umbilical serum, amniotic fluid, breast milk and urine of mothers and offspring. Int J Clin Pharmacol Res 1991; 11(5): 231–236.
3. Penny WJ, Lewis MJ. Nifedipine is excreted in human milk. Eur J Clin Pharmacol 1989; 36(4): 427–428.

NILOTINIB   L4

Trade: Tasigna

Other Trades:

Category: Anticancer drug

Nilotinib is used for the treatment of chronic myelogenous leukemia (CML).[1] Studies suggest it has a relatively favorable safety profile. Nilotinib is an inhibitor of the Bcr-Abl tyrosine kinase. Nilotinib was developed as a second-generation inhibitor of bcr-abl tyrosine kinase that would be effective in patients with imatinib-resistant or -intolerant CML. Nilotinib is distributed into milk in rats.[2] The drug carries a black box warning for possible heart complications. No data are available on its transfer into human milk. Due to its high protein binding, levels in milk will probably be low. Further, its oral bioavailability is poor which would reduce oral absorption in infants. This product is significantly toxic and we suggest withholding breastfeeding for 4 days.

Pregnancy Risk	D	Lactation Risk	L4
T ½	= 17 hours	M/P	=
Vd	=	PB	= 98%
Tmax	= 3 hours	Oral	= 30%
MW	= 529	pKa	= 2.1–5.4

Adult Concerns: Rash, pruritus, nausea, fatigue, headache, prolonged QT interval, and gastrointestinal disturbances. May increase bilirubin levels. Hypophosphatemia, hypokalemia, hyperkalemia, hypocalcemia, and hyponatremia have been reported.

Pediatric Concerns:

Drug Interactions: Concurrent administration with the following increases the plasma levels of nilotinib: rifampin, amiodarone, disopyramide, procainamide, quinidine and sotalol. Concomitant use with the following increases the risk of cardiotoxicity: ketokonazole, chloroquine, clarithromycin, haloperidol, methadone, moxifloxacin and pimozide. Concomitant use with midazolam increases the plasma levels of midazolam.

Relative Infant Dose:

Adult Dose: 300–400 mg twice daily.

Alternatives:

References:
1. Pharmaceutical manufacturer prescribing information, 2010.
2. Novartis Pharmaceuticals Corporation. Tasigna Æ (nilotinib) capsules prescribing information, East Hanover, NJ; 2010 Jun.

NIMODIPINE   L2

Trade: Nimotop

Other Trades: Nimotop

Category: Antihypertensive, calcium channel

Nimodipine is a calcium channel blocker although it is primarily used in preventing cerebral artery spasm and improving cerebral blood flow. Nimodipine is effective in reducing neurologic deficits following subarachnoid hemorrhage, acute stroke, and severe head trauma. It is also useful in prophylaxis of migraine.

In one study of a patient 3 days postpartum who received 60 mg every 4 hours for one week, breastmilk levels paralleled maternal serum levels with a milk/plasma ratio of approximately 0.33.[1] The highest milk concentration reported was approximately 3.5 µg/L while the maternal plasma was approximately 16 µg/L. In another study [2], a 36-year-old mother received a total dose of 46 mg IV over 24 hours. Nimodipine concentration in milk was much lower than in maternal serum, with a milk/serum ratio of 0.06 to 0.15. During IV infusion, nimodipine concentrations in milk raised initially to 2.2 µg/L and stabilized at concentrations between 0.87 and 1.6 µg/L of milk. Assuming a daily milk intake of 150 ml/kg/day, the authors estimate an infant would ingest approximately 0.063 to 0.705 µg/kg/day or 0.008 to 0.092% of the weight-adjusted dose administered to the mother. We calculate the RID at 0.001%–0.037%, which is exceedingly low.

Pregnancy Risk	C	Lactation Risk	L2
T ½	= 9 hours	M/P	= 0.06 to 0.33
Vd	= 0.94 l/kg	PB	= 95%
Tmax	= 1 hour	Oral	= 13%
MW	= 418	pKa	=

Adult Concerns: Hypotension, diarrhea, nausea, cramps.

Pediatric Concerns: None reported via milk in two studies.

Drug Interactions: When used with adenosine, prolonged bradycardia may result. Use with amiodarone may lead to sinus arrest and AV block. H_2 blockers may increase bioavailability of nimodipine. Beta blockers may increase cardiac depression. May increase carbamazepine levels when admixed. May increase cyclosporine, digoxin, quinidine plasma levels. May increase theophylline effects. Used with fentanyl, it may increase hypotension.

Relative Infant Dose: 0.001%–0.04%

Adult Dose: 60 mg every 4 hours.

Alternatives: Verapamil, nifedipine.

References:
1. Tonks AM. Nimodipine levels in breast milk. Aust N Z J Surg 1995; 65(9): 693–694.
2. Carcas AJ, Abad-Santos F, de Rosendo JM, Frias J. Nimodipine transfer into human breast milk and cerebrospinal fluid. Ann Pharmacother 1996; 30(2): 148–150.

NISOLDIPINE   L3

Trade: Sular

Other Trades: Syscor

Category: Antihypertensive

Nisoldipine is a typical calcium channel blocker antihypertensive.[1] No data are available on its transfer into human milk. For alternatives see nifedipine and verapamil. Due to its poor oral bioavailability, presence of lipids which reduce its absorption, and high protein binding, it is unlikely to penetrate milk and be absorbed by the infant (undocumented).

Pregnancy Risk	C	Lactation Risk	L3
T ½	= 7–12 hours	M/P	=
Vd	= 4 l/kg	PB	= 99%
Tmax	= 6–12 hours	Oral	= 5%
MW	= 388	pKa	=

Adult Concerns: Hypotension, bradycardia, peripheral edema.

Pediatric Concerns: None reported via milk. Observe for hypotension, sedation although unlikely.

Drug Interactions: Barbiturates may reduce bioavailability of calcium channel blockers (CCB). Calcium salts may reduce hypotensive effect. Dantrolene may increase risk of hyperkalemia and myocardial depression. H_2 blockers may increase bioavailability of certain CCBs. Hydantoins may reduce plasma levels. Quinidine increases risk of hypotension, bradycardia, tachycardia. Rifampin may reduce effects of CCBs. Vitamin D may reduce efficacy of CCBs. CCBs may increase carbamazepine, cyclosporin, encainide, prazosin levels.

Relative Infant Dose:

Adult Dose: 20–40 mg daily.

Alternatives: Nifedipine, verapamil, nimodipine

References:
1. Pharmaceutical manufacturer prescribing information, 2010.

NITAZOXANIDE   L3

Trade: Alinia

Other Trades:

Category: Antibiotic for parasitic infections

Nitazoxanide is a new thiazolide antiprotozoan agent that shows excellent *in vitro* activity against a wide variety of protozoa and helminths. It is a suitable alternative for metronidazole in many infections including *Giardia lamblia* and *Cryptosporidium parvum*. Once absorbed it is rapidly converted to the active metabolite tizoxanide.[1] No data are available on its transfer into human milk.

Pregnancy Risk	B		Lactation Risk	L3
T ½	= 1–1.6 hours		M/P	=
Vd	=		PB	= 99%
Tmax	= 4 hours		Oral	= Good
MW	= 307		pKa	=

Adult Concerns: Abdominal pain, diarrhea, headache and nausea have been reported in clinical trials.

Pediatric Concerns: None reported, but no data are available.

Drug Interactions: None reported.

Relative Infant Dose:

Adult Dose: 500 mg every 12 hours with food.

Alternatives: Metronidazole

References:
1. Pharmaceutical manufacturer package insert. 2005.

NITRAZEPAM   L2

Trade: Mogadon

Other Trades: Alodorm, Mogadon, Nitrazadon, Atempol, Nitrodos

Category: Sedative, hypnotic

Nitrazepam is a typical benzodiazepine used as a sedative. In a study of 9 women who received 5 mg nitrazepam at night, the concentration in milk increased over a period of 5 days from 30 nmol/L to 48 nmol/L.[1] The mean milk/plasma ratio after 7 hours was 0.27 in 32 paired samples and did not vary from day 1 to day 5.

The mean concentration of nitrazepam in milk was 13 μg/L and the C_{max} was 0.20 μg/L. Nitrazepam levels in a 6 day old infant were below the limits of detection. No adverse effects were noted in the infants breastfed for 5 days. Nitrazepam is probably compatible with breastfeeding but observe for sedation in the breastfed infant.

Pregnancy Risk	D	Lactation Risk	L2
T ½	= 30 hours	M/P	= 0.27
Vd	= 2–5 l/kg	PB	= 90%
Tmax	= 0.5–5 hours	Oral	= 53–94%
MW	= 281	pKa	= 3.2,10.8

Adult Concerns: Sedation, disorientation.

Pediatric Concerns: None reported, but observe for sedation.

Drug Interactions:

Relative Infant Dose: 2.9%

Adult Dose: 5–10 mg daily.

Alternatives: Alprazolam, lorazepam

References:
1. Matheson I, Lunde PK, Bredesen JE. Midazolam and nitrazepam in the maternity ward: milk concentrations and clinical effects. Br J Clin Pharmacol 1990; 30(6): 787–793.

NITRENDIPINE   L2

Trade: Baypress
Other Trades:
Category: Calcium channel blocker, antihypertensive

Nitrendipine is a typical calcium channel antihypertensive. In a group of 3 breastfeeding mothers who received 20 mg/day for 5 days, nitrendipine was excreted in breast milk at peak concentrations ranging from 4.3 to 6.5 μg/L 1–2 hours after acute dosing while its inactive pyridine metabolite ranged from 6.9 to 11.9 μg/L.[1] After 5 days of dosing, the C_{max} remained in the same range and the breast milk/plasma ratio for nitrendipine was 0.2 to 0.5. On the fourth day of continuous dosing, average concentrations of nitrendipine from 24-hour collections of the milk were 1.1 to 3.8 μg/L. Thus, nitrendipine and its metabolite are excreted in very low concentrations in human breast milk. Based on a maternal dose of 20 mg daily, a newborn infant would ingest an average of 1.7 μg/day of nitrendipine, or a relative dose of 0.095%.

Pregnancy Risk	C	Lactation Risk	L2
T ½	= 8–11 hours	M/P	= 0.2–0.5
Vd	=	PB	= 98%
Tmax	= 1–2 hours	Oral	= 16–20%
MW	= 360	pKa	=

Adult Concerns: Headache, hypotension, peripheral edema, cardiac arrhythmias, fatigue.

Pediatric Concerns: None reported via milk.

Drug Interactions: Barbiturates may reduce bioavailability of calcium channel blockers (CCB). Calcium salts may reduce hypotensive effect. Dantrolene may increase risk of hyperkalemia and myocardial depression. H_2 blockers may increase bioavailability of certain CCBs. Hydantoins may reduce plasma levels. Quinidine increases risk of hypotension, bradycardia, tachycardia. Rifampin may reduce effects of CCBs. Vitamin D may reduce efficacy of CCBs. CCBs may increase carbamazepine, cyclosporin, encainide, prazosin levels.

Relative Infant Dose: 0.1%

Adult Dose: 10–80 mg/day

Alternatives: Nifedipine, nimodipine

References:
1. White WB, Yeh SC, Krol GJ. Nitrendipine in human plasma and breast milk. Eur J Clin Pharmacol 1989; 36(5): 531–534.

NITROFURANTOIN   L2

Trade: Furadantin, Macrodantin, Furan, Macrobid

Other Trades: Apo-Nitrofurantoin, Macrodantin, Nephronex, Furadantin

Category: Urinary antibiotic

Nitrofurantoin is an old urinary tract antimicrobial. It is secreted in breastmilk but in very small amounts. In one study of 20 women receiving 100 mg four times daily, none was detected in milk.[1] In another group of 9 nursing women who received 100–200 mg every 6 hours, nitrofurantoin was undetectable in the milk of those treated with 100 mg and only trace amounts were found in those treated with 200 mg (0.3–0.5 mg/L milk).[2] In these two patients, the milk/plasma ratio ranged from 0.27 to 0.31.

In a well-done study of 4 breastfeeding mothers who ingested 100 mg nitrofurantoin with a meal, the milk/serum ratio averaged 6.21 suggesting an active transfer into milk.[3] Regardless of an active transfer, the average milk concentration throughout the day (AUC) was only 1.3 mg/L. According to the authors, the estimated dose an infant would ingest was 0.2 mg/kg/day or 6.8% of the weight-adjusted maternal dose if they consumed 200 mg/day nitrofurantoin. The therapeutic dose administered to infants is 5–7 mg/kg/day. Use with caution in infants with G6PD or in infants less than 1 month of age with hyperbilirubinemia, due to displacement of bilirubin from albumin binding sites.

Pregnancy Risk	B		Lactation Risk	L2
T ½	= 20–58 minutes		M/P	= 0.27–6.2
Vd	=		PB	= 20–60%
Tmax	= 4.9 hours		Oral	= 94%
MW	= 238		pKa	= 7.2

Adult Concerns: Nausea, vomiting, brown urine, hemolytic anemia, hepatotoxicity.

Pediatric Concerns: None reported via milk, however, do not use in infants with G6PD or in infants less than 1 month of age.

Drug Interactions: Anticholinergics increase nitrofurantoin bioavailability by delaying gastric emptying and increasing absorption. Magnesium salts may delay or decrease absorption. Uricosurics may increase nitrofurantoin levels by decreasing renal clearance.

Relative Infant Dose: 6.8%

Adult Dose: 50–100 mg four times daily.

Alternatives:

References:
1. Hosbach RH, Foster RB. Absence of nitrofurantoin from human milk. JAMA 1967; 202(11): 1057.
2. Varsano I, Fischl J, Shochet SB. The excretion of orally ingested nitrofurantoin in human milk. J Pediatr 1973; 82(5): 886–887.
3. Gerk PM, Kuhn RJ, Desai NS, McNamara PJ. Active transport of nitrofurantoin into human milk. Pharmacotherapy 2001; 21(6): 669–675.

NITROGLYCERIN, NITRATES, NITRITES | L4

Trade: Nitrostat, Nitrolingual, Nitrogard, Amyl Nitrite, Nitrong, Nitro-Bid, Nitroglyn, Minitran, Nitro-Dur

Other Trades: Anginine, Nitrolingual Spray, Nitradisc, Nitrong SR, Nitrol, Transderm-Nitro, Nitro-Dur, Deponit

Category: Vasodilator

Nitroglycerin is a rapid and short acting vasodilator used in angina and other cardiovascular problems including congestive heart failure. Nitroglycerin, as well as numerous other formulations (amyl nitrate, isosorbide dinitrate, etc.) all work by release of the nitrite and nitrate molecule. Nitrates come in numerous formulations, some for acute use (sublingual), others are more sustained (Nitro-Dur). Nitrates and Nitrites are derived from multiple sources, including medications in the form of nitroglycerin, or isosorbide dinitrate, or from food and water sources. Elevated nitrate levels in drinking water in the USA are common in rural areas. Numerous cases of nitrate-induced methemoglobinemia have been reported in infants exposed to well water with high levels of nitrates when they were fed foods/formulas prepared with contaminated water.

Only one case of a breastfed infant has been reported and it is questionable.[1] Thus far, it is less certain that the oral ingestion of nitrates can penetrate into human milk in clinically relevant amounts. Two studies suggest that while nitrates/nitrites are well absorbed orally in the mother (approximately 50%), little seems to be transported to human milk. In a study by Dusdieker[2], following a mean total nitrate intake from diet and water of 46.6, 168.1, and 272 mg/day, milk levels only averaged 4.4, 5.1, and 5.2 mg/L respectively. Thus higher maternal intake did not necessarily correlate with higher milk levels. The authors conclude that mothers who ingest nitrate of 100 mg/day or less do not produce milk with elevated nitrate levels. In a study by Green[3], milk levels were not different from maternal plasma levels. Thus it is apparent that even at relatively high rates of ingestion, nitrate levels do not concentrate in milk and may not be high enough to harm an infant. However, these studies were done using nitrates in water and may not correlate with the ingestion of high and prolonged concentrations of nitrates from medications administered orally, buccally, or transcutaneously. No studies have been found comparing milk nitrates with oral nitroglycerin or isosorbide dinitrate.

While it is apparent that milk levels are not high following the ingestion of oral nitrates, infants younger than 6 months are most at risk from nitrate intoxication because of their susceptibility to methemoglobinemia.[4] In another study of 59 women living in regions with high nitrate levels, breastmilk levels of nitrates and nitrites were 2.83 mg/L and 0.46 mg/L respectively, while those living in low nitrate regions were 2.75 mg/L and 0.32 mg/L respectively.[5] They were not significantly different. Breastfeed with caution at higher doses and with prolonged exposure. Observe the infant for methemoglobinemia.

Pregnancy Risk	C		Lactation Risk	L4
T ½	= 1–4 minutes		M/P	=
Vd	=		PB	= 60%
Tmax	= 2–20 minutes		Oral	= Complete
MW	= 227		pKa	=

Adult Concerns: Postural hypotension, flushing, headache, weakness, drug rash, exfoliative dermatitis, bradycardia, nausea, vomiting, methemoglobinemia (overdose), sweating.

Pediatric Concerns: None are reported via milk. Observe for methemoglobinemia.

Drug Interactions: IV nitroglycerin may counteract the effects of heparin. Increased toxicity when used with alcohol, beta-blockers. Calcium channel blockers may increase hypotensive effect of nitrates.

Relative Infant Dose:

Adult Dose: 1.3–6.5 mg twice daily.

Alternatives:

References:
1. Donahoe WE. Cyanosis in infants with nitrates in drinking water as a cause. Pediatrics 1949; 3: 308.
2. Dusdieker LB, Stumbo PJ, Kross BC, Dungy CI. Does increased nitrate ingestion elevate nitrate levels in human milk? Arch Pediatr Adolesc Med 1996; 150(3): 311–314.
3. Green LC, Tannenbaum SR, Fox JG. Nitrate in human and canine milk. N Engl J Med 1982; 306(22): 1367–1368.
4. Johnson CJ, Kross BC. Continuing importance of nitrate contamination of groundwater and wells in rural areas. Am J Ind Med 1990; 18(4): 449–456.
5. Paszkowski T, Sikorski R, Kozak A, Kowalski B, Jakubik J. [Contamination of human milk with nitrates and nitrites]. Pol Tyg Lek 1989; 44(46–48): 961–963.

NITROPRUSSIDE   L4

Trade: Nitropress
Other Trades: Nipride
Category: Hypotensive agent

Nitroprusside is a rapid acting hypotensive agent of short duration (1–10 minutes). Besides rapid hypotension, nitroprusside is converted metabolically to cyanogen (cyanide radical) which is potentially toxic. Although rare, significant thiocyanate toxicity can occur at higher doses (>2 µg/kg/min.) and longer durations of exposure (>1–2 days).[1] When administered orally, nitroprusside is reported to not be active although one report suggests a modest hypotensive effect. No data are available on transfer of nitroprusside nor thiocyanate into human milk. The half-life of the thiocyanate metabolite is approximately 3 days. Because the thiocyanate metabolite is orally bioavailable, some caution is advised if the mother has received nitroprusside for more than 24 hours.[2]

Pregnancy Risk	C	Lactation Risk	L4
T ½	= 3–4 minutes	M/P	=
Vd	=	PB	=
Tmax	= 1–2 minutes	Oral	= Poor
MW	=	pKa	=

Adult Concerns: Hypotension, methemoglobinemia, headache, drowsiness, cyanide toxicity, hypothyroidism, nausea, vomiting.

Pediatric Concerns: None reported but caution is urged due to thiocyanate metabolite.

Drug Interactions: Clonidine may potentiate the hypotensive effect of nitroprusside. May reduce Iodine-131 uptake and induce hypothyroidism.

Relative Infant Dose:

Adult Dose: 0.3–10 µg/kg/minute X 10 minutes

Alternatives:

References:
1. Page IH, Corcoran AC, Dustan HP, Koppanyi T. Cardiovascular actions of sodium nitroprusside in animals and hypertensive patients. Circulation 1955; 11(2): 188–198.
2. Benitz WE, Malachowski N, Cohen RS, Stevenson DK, Ariagno RL, Sunshine P. Use of sodium nitroprusside in neonates: efficacy and safety. J Pediatr 1985; 106(1): 102–110.

NITROUS OXIDE   L3

Trade:
Other Trades: Entonox
Category: Anesthetic gas

Nitrous oxide is a weak anesthetic gas. It provides good analgesia and weak anesthesia. It is rapidly eliminated from the body due to rapid exchange with nitrogen via the pulmonary alveoli (within minutes).[1] A rapid recovery generally occurs in 3–5 minutes. Due to poor lipid solubility, uptake by adipose tissue is relatively poor, and only insignificant traces of nitrous oxide circulate in blood after discontinuing inhalation of the gas. No data exists on the entry of nitrous oxide into human milk. Ingestion of nitrous oxide orally via milk is unlikely. Chronic exposure may lead to elevated risks of fetal malformations, abortions, and bone marrow toxicity (particularly in dental care workers).[2]

Pregnancy Risk	C		Lactation Risk	L3
T ½	= <3 minutes		M/P	=
Vd	=		PB	=
Tmax	= 15 minutes		Oral	= Poor
MW	= 44		pKa	=

Adult Concerns: Chronic exposure can produce bone marrow suppression, headaches, hypotension and bradycardia.

Pediatric Concerns: None reported via milk.

Drug Interactions:

Relative Infant Dose:

Adult Dose: Inhalation 30% with 70% oxygen.

Alternatives:

References:
1. General Anesthetics. In: Drug Evaluations Annual 1995 American Medical Association, 1995.
2. Adriani J. General Anesthetics. In: Clinical Management of Poisoning and Drug Overdose. W.B. Saunders and Co., 1983.

NIZATIDINE   L2

Trade: Axid

Other Trades: Tazac, Axid, Apo-Nizatidine

Category: Reduces gastric acid secretion

Nizatidine is an antisecretory, histamine-2 antagonist that reduces stomach acid secretion. In one study of 5 lactating women using a dose of 150 mg daily, milk levels of nizatidine were directly proportional to circulating maternal serum levels, yet were very low.[1] Over a 12 hour period, 96 µg (less than 0.5% of dose) was secreted into the milk. No effects on infant have been reported.

Pregnancy Risk	B		Lactation Risk	L2
T ½	= 1.5 hours		M/P	=
Vd	=		PB	= 35%
Tmax	= 0.5–3 hours		Oral	= 94%
MW	= 331		pKa	=

Adult Concerns: Headache, gastrointestinal distress.

Pediatric Concerns: None reported.

Drug Interactions: Elevated salicylate levels may occur when nizatidine is used with high doses of salicylates.

Relative Infant Dose: 0.5%

Adult Dose: 150–300 mg daily.

Alternatives: Famotidine

References:
1. Obermeyer BD, Bergstrom RF, Callaghan JT, Knadler MP, Golichowski A, Rubin A. Secretion of nizatidine into human breast milk after single and multiple doses. Clin Pharmacol Ther 1990; 47(6): 724–730.

NONOXYNOL 9 — L3

Trade: Advantage-S, Aqua Lube Plus, Conceptrol, Delfen Foam, Emko, Encare, Gynol II, Today Sponge

Other Trades:

Category: Spermicide

Nonoxynol 9 is a non-ionic surfactant used as a vaginal spermicide. In one animal study, 0.3% of nonoxynol 9 maternal dose is present in breastmilk of rats.[1] However the study could not destinguish between nonoxynol 9 or its metabolite in rodent milk. Studies in rodents are not comparable to those done in humans. There are no controlled studies in breastfeeding women reporting the level of nonoxyl 9 in breastmilk. Based on relative infant dose (RID) of 0.3%, the concentration in breasmilk would be very small.

Pregnancy Risk	C	Lactation Risk	L3
T ½	=	M/P	=
Vd	=	PB	=
Tmax	=	Oral	=
MW	= 617	pKa	=

Adult Concerns: Vaginal irritation, vaginal discomfort, vaginal pain.

Pediatric Concerns:

Drug Interactions:

Relative Infant Dose:

Adult Dose: 1 applicator 1 hour prior intercourse.

Alternatives:

References:
1. Chvapil M, Eskelson CD, Stiffel V, Owen JA, Droegemueller W. Studies on Nonoxynol-9. II. Intravaginal absorption, distribution, metabolism and excretion in rats and rabbits. Contraception. 1980 Sep; 22(3): 325–39.

NORELGESTROMIN   L3

Trade: Norelgestromin, Evra
Other Trades:
Category: Progestin

Norelgestromin is a progestational agent.[1] The effect of progestins (in this case, norelgestromin) on milk production is poorly studied. Early postpartum, while progestin receptors are still present in the breast, administering progestins may actually suppress milk production. This has been seen occasionally in patients early postpartum. Several days to a week later, most progestin receptors disappear from the lactocyte and breast tissues become relatively immune to the effects of progestins. Thus it is advisable to wait as long as possible, preferably 4–6 weeks postpartum prior to instituting therapy with progesterone to avoid reducing the milk supply.

The direct effect of progesterone therapy on the nursing infant is generally unknown, but it is believed minimal to none as natural progesterone is poorly bioavailable to the infant via milk. Several cases of gynecomastia in infants have been reported but are extremely rare.

Pregnancy Risk	X	Lactation Risk	L3
T ½	=	M/P	=
Vd	=	PB	=
Tmax	=	Oral	=
MW	= 327	pKa	= 17.91

Adult Concerns: Side effects include (in combination with ethinyl estradiol): breast tenderness and enlargement, headache, nausea, menstrual changes, abdominal cramps and bloating, vaginal discharge, and irritation at the site of application.

Pediatric Concerns:

Drug Interactions: Co-administration with the following drugs may decrease efficacy of hormonal contraceptives: barbiturates, bosentan, carbamazepine, felbamate, griseofulvin, oxcarbazine, phenytoin, rifampin, St. John's wort, topiramate. Concurrent use may increase plasma levels of the following drugs: cyclosporine, prednisone, theophyilline. Concurrent use may decrease plasma levels of the following drugs: acetaminophen, clofibric acid, lamotrigine, morphine, salicylic acid, temazepam.

Relative Infant Dose:

Adult Dose:

Alternatives:

References:
1. Pharmaceutical manufacturer prescribing information

NORETHINDRONE   L3

Trade: Aygestin, Norlutate, Micronor, NOR-Q.D., Ortho-Micronor, Errin, Camila, Jolivette, Nora-BE

Other Trades: Norethisterone, Brevinor, Micronor, Norlestrin

Category: Progestin for oral contraceptives

Norethindrone is a typical synthetic progestational agent that is used for oral contraception and other endocrine functions. It is believed to be secreted into breastmilk in small amounts. It produces a dose-dependent suppression of lactation at higher doses, although somewhat minimal at lower doses. It may reduce lactose content and reduce overall milk volume and nitrogen/protein content, resulting in lower infant weight gain although these effects are unlikely if doses are kept low.[1-5] Progestin-only mini pills are preferred oral contraceptives in breastfeeding mothers. However, recent reports claim that norethindrone can be associated with decreased breastmilk production. In a report of 13 women taking Micronor (norethindrone) who presented with poor milk production, 10 women experienced an increase in lactation upon withdrawl of Micronor.[6] While norethindrone birth control pill are considered ideal for most breastfeeding mothers, some women retain sensitivity to these products and may suffer from reduced milk production. Each and every breastfeeding mother should be individually counselled about the possible reduction in milk synthesis following the use of this product. It is advisable to wait as long as possible, preferably 6–8 weeks postpartum prior to instituting therapy with progesterone to avoid reducing the milk supply.

Pregnancy Risk	X	Lactation Risk	L3
T ½	= 4–13 hours	M/P	=
Vd	=	PB	= 97%
Tmax	= 1–2 hours	Oral	= 60%
MW	= 298	pKa	=

Adult Concerns: Changes in menstruation, breakthrough bleeding, nausea, abdominal pain, edema, breast tenderness.

Pediatric Concerns: None reported via milk. Observe for reduced milk production.

Drug Interactions: Rifampin may reduce the plasma level of norethindrone possibly decreasing its effect.

Relative Infant Dose:

Adult Dose: 0.35–5 mg daily.

Alternatives:

References:
1. Kora SJ. Effect of oral contraceptives on lactation. Fertil Steril 1969; 20(3): 419–423.
2. Miller GH, Hughes LR. Lactation and genital involution effects of a new low-dose oral contraceptive on breast-feeding mothers and their infants. Obstet Gynecol 1970; 35(1): 44–50.
3. Karim M, Ammar R, el Mahgoub S, el Ganzoury B, Fikri F, Abdou I. Injected progestogen and lactation. Br Med J 1971; 1(742): 200–203.

4. Lonnerdal B, Forsum E, Hambraeus L. Effect of oral contraceptives on composition and volume of breast milk. Am J Clin Nutr 1980; 33(4): 816–824.
5. Laukaran VH. The effects of contraceptive use on the initiation and duration of lactation. Int J Gynaecol Obstet 1987; 25 Suppl: 129–142.
6. Norethindrone (Micronor): Suspected association with decreased breast milk production. CARN 2007 July; 17(3): 4.

NORETHYNODREL   L3

Trade:

Other Trades:

Category: Progestational agent

Norethynodrel is a synthetic progestational agent used in oral contraceptives. It has limited or no effects on an infant. May decrease volume of breastmilk to some degree in some mothers if therapy initiated too soon after birth and if dose is too high.[1-3] It is advisable to wait as long as possible, preferably 4–6 weeks postpartum prior to instituting therapy with progesterone to avoid reducing the milk supply.

Pregnancy Risk	X	Lactation Risk	L3
T ½	= 8 hours	M/P	=
Vd	=	PB	=
Tmax	= 1–2 hours	Oral	=
MW	= 298	pKa	=

Adult Concerns: Changes in menstruation, breakthrough bleeding, nausea, abdominal pain, edema, breast tenderness.

Pediatric Concerns: None reported. May suppress lactation.

Drug Interactions:

Relative Infant Dose:

Adult Dose:

Alternatives:

References:

1. Booker DE, Pahl IR. Control of postpartum breast engorgement with oral contraceptives. Am J Obstet Gynecol 1967; 98(8): 1099–1101.
2. Laukaran VH. The effects of contraceptive use on the initiation and duration of lactation. Int J Gynaecol Obstet 1987; 25 Suppl: 129–142.
3. Kora SJ. Effect of oral contraceptives on lactation. Fertil Steril 1969; 20(3): 419–423.

NORFLOXACIN   L3

Trade: Noroxin

Other Trades: Noroxin

Category: Fluoroquinolone antibiotic

Norfloxacin is a fluoroquinolone antibiotic. Although other members in the fluoroquinolone family are secreted into breastmilk, only limited data are available on this drug.[1] Wise has suggested that norfloxacin is not present in breastmilk.[2] The manufacturer's product information states that doses of 200 mg do not produce detectable concentrations in milk although this was a single dose.[3] Of the fluoroquinolone family, norfloxacin, levofloxacin, or perhaps ofloxacin may be preferred over others for use in a breastfeeding mother.

Pregnancy Risk	C		Lactation Risk	L3
T ½	= 3.3 hours		M/P	=
Vd	=		PB	= 20%
Tmax	= 1–2 hours		Oral	= 30–40%
MW	= 319		pKa	=

Adult Concerns: Nausea, vomiting, gastrointestinal dyspepsia, depression, dizziness, pseudomembranous colitis in pediatric patients.

Pediatric Concerns: None reported via milk. Observe for diarrhea.

Drug Interactions: Decreased absorption with antacids. Quinolones cause increased levels of caffeine, warfarin, cyclosporine, theophylline. Cimetidine, probenecid, azlocillin increase norfloxacin levels. Increased risk of seizures when used with foscarnet.

Relative Infant Dose:

Adult Dose: 400 mg twice daily

Alternatives: Ofloxacin, levofloxacin

References:
1. Harmon T, Burkhart G, Applebaum H. Perforated pseudomembranous colitis in the breast-fed infant. J Pediatr Surg 1992; 27(6): 744–746.
2. Wise R. Norfloxacin--a review of pharmacology and tissue penetration. J Antimicrob Chemother 1984; 13 Suppl B: 59–64.
3. Pharmaceutical manufacturer prescribing information, 1999.

NORTRIPTYLINE   L2

Trade: Aventyl, Pamelor

Other Trades: Aventyl, Norventyl, Apo-Nortriptyline, Allegron

Category: Tricyclic antidepressant

Nortriptyline (NT) is a tricyclic antidepressant and is the active metabolite of amitriptyline. In one patient receiving 125 mg of nortriptyline at bedtime, milk concentrations of NT averaged 180 µg/L after 6–7 days of administration.[1] Based on these concentrations, the authors estimated the average daily infant exposure would be 27 µg/kg/day. The relative dose in milk would be 1.5% of the maternal dose. Several other authors have been unable to detect NT in maternal milk nor the serum of infants after prolonged exposure.[2,3] So far no untoward effects have been noted. A pooled analysis of 35 studies with an average dose of 78 mg/day reported a detectable level of nortriptyline in breast milk in only one patient, with a concentration of 230 ng/mL. The authors suggest that breastfeeding infants exposed to nortriptyline are unlikely to develop detectable concentrations in plasma, and therefore breastfeeding during nortriptyline therapy is not contraindicated.[4]

Pregnancy Risk	D	Lactation Risk	L2
T ½	= 16–90 hours	M/P	= 0.87–3.71
Vd	= 20–57 l/kg	PB	= 92%
Tmax	= 7–8.5 hours	Oral	= 51%
MW	= 263	pKa	= 9.7

Adult Concerns: Sedation, dry mouth, constipation, urinary retention, blurred vision.

Pediatric Concerns: None reported in several studies.

Drug Interactions: Phenobarbital may reduce effect of nortriptyline. Nortriptyline blocks the hypotensive effect of guanethidine. May increase toxicity of nortriptyline when used with clonidine. Dangerous when used with monoamine oxidase inhibitors, other CNS depressants. May increase anticoagulant effect of coumadin, warfarin. SSRIs (Prozac, Zoloft,etc) should not be used with or soon after nortriptyline or other TCAs due to serotonergic crisis.

Relative Infant Dose: 1.7%–3.1%

Adult Dose: 25 mg three to four times daily.

Alternatives: Imipramine

References:
1. Matheson I, Skjaeraasen J. Milk concentrations of flupenthixol, nortriptyline and zuclopenthixol and between-breast differences in two patients. Eur J Clin Pharmacol 1988; 35(2): 217–220.
2. Wisner KL, Perel JM. Serum nortriptyline levels in nursing mothers and their infants. Am J Psychiatry 1991; 148(9): 1234–1236.
3. Brixen-Rasmussen L, Halgrener J, Jorgensen A. Amitriptyline and nortriptyline excretion in human breast milk. Psychopharmacology (Berl) 1982; 76(1): 94–95.
4. Weissman AM, Levy BT, Hartz AJ, et.al. Pooled Analysis of Antidepressant Levels in Lactating Mothers, Breast Milk, and Nursing Infants. Am J Psychiatry 2004 June; 161(6): 1066–1078.

NYSTATIN　　　　　　　　　　　　　　L1

Trade: Mycostatin, Nilstat

Other Trades: Mycostatin, Nadostine, Nilstat, Candistatin, Nystan

Category: Antifungal

Nystatin is an antifungal primarily used for candidiasis topically and orally. The oral absorption of nystatin is extremely poor, and plasma levels are undetectable after oral administration.[1] The likelihood of secretion into milk is remote due to poor maternal absorption. It is frequently administered directly to neonates in neonatal units for candidiasis. In addition, absorption into infant circulation is equally unlikely. Current studies suggest that resistance to nystatin is growing.

Pregnancy Risk	C	Lactation Risk	L1
T ½	=	M/P	=
Vd	=	PB	=
Tmax	=	Oral	= Nil
MW	=	pKa	=

Adult Concerns: Bad taste, diarrhea, nausea, vomiting.

Pediatric Concerns: None reported. Nystatin is commonly used in infants.

Drug Interactions:

Relative Infant Dose:

Adult Dose: 500,000–1 million units three times daily.

Alternatives: Fluconazole

References:
1. Rothermel P, Faber M. Drugs in breast milk: a consumer's guide. Birth and Family J 1975; 2: 76–78.

OCTREOTIDE ACETATE   L3

Trade: SandoSTATIN, SandoSTATIN LAR

Other Trades: SandoSTATIN, SandoSTATIN LAR, Octreotide Acetate Injection, Octreotide Acetate Omega

Category: Somatostatin analog

Octreotide is a close analog of and provides activity similar to the natural hormone somatostatin.[1] Octreotide (Sandostatin LAR) is a long acting form consisting of microspheres containing octreotide. Like somatostatin, it also suppresses LH response to GnRH, decreases splanchnic blood flow, and inhibits release of serotonin, gastrin, vasoactive intestinal peptide, secretin, motilin, and pancreatic polypeptide. It is used to treat acromegaly and carcinoid tumors. Due to its molecular weight, transfer to milk is probably minimal. This product, if present in milk, would not likely be absorbed to any degree.

Pregnancy Risk	B	Lactation Risk	L3
T ½	= 1.9 hours	M/P	=
Vd	= 0.2 l/kg	PB	= 65%
Tmax	= SQ: 0.4 hour; IM: 1 hour	Oral	=
MW	= 1019	pKa	=

Adult Concerns: Nausea, diarrhea, vomiting, anorexia, abdominal discomfort, flatulence, steatorrhoea, hair loss, gallstones.

Pediatric Concerns:

Drug Interactions:

Relative Infant Dose:

Adult Dose: IM: 20 mg q 4 wk; SQ: 100–200 µg TID

Alternatives:

References:
1. Pharmaceutical manufacturer prescribing information, 2011.

OFATUMUMAB   L3

Trade: Arzerra
Other Trades:
Category: Anticancer drug

Ofatumumab is a humanized monoclonal antibody that binds specifically to both the small and large extracellular loops of the CD20 molecule. It is a cytolytic product indicated for the treatment of patients with chronic lymphocytic leukemia (CLL) refractory to fludarabine and alemtuzumab. No data are available on its use in breastfeeding mothers. However, this product does not appear overly toxic to a fetus or older individuals. The major complication is heightened rate of pneumonia or infections due to depletion of B cells. Due to its large molecular weight and the fact that it is an IgG FAB product, milk levels are likely to be quite low. Oral bioavailability will be low as well. Withhold breastfeeding for one month.

Pregnancy Risk	C	Lactation Risk	L3
T ½	= 14 days	M/P	=
Vd	= 0.07 l/kg	PB	=
Tmax	=	Oral	=
MW	= 149,000	pKa	=

Adult Concerns: Rash, diarrhea, nausea, neutropenia, anemia, fatigue, pneumonia, cough, dyspnea, upper respiratory tract infection, bronchitis, and fever.

Pediatric Concerns:

Drug Interactions:

Relative Infant Dose:

Adult Dose:

Alternatives:

References:
1. Pharmaceutical manufacturer prescribing information, 2010.

OFLOXACIN   L2

Trade: Floxin
Other Trades: Floxin, Ocuflox, Tarivid
Category: Fluoroquinolone antibiotic

Ofloxacin is a typical fluoroquinolone antimicrobial. Breastmilk concentrations are reported equal to maternal plasma levels. In one study in lactating women who received 400 mg oral doses twice daily, drug concentrations in breastmilk averaged 0.05–2.41 mg/L in milk (24 hours and 2 hours post-dose respectively).[1] The drug was still detectable in milk 24 hours after a dose. The fluoroquinolones are becoming more popular in pediatrics due to recent studies and reviews showing their safe use.[2] The only probable risk is a change in gut flora, diarrhea, and a remote risk of overgrowth of C. difficile. Ofloxacin levels in breastmilk are consistently lower

(37%) than ciprofloxacin. If a fluoroquinolone is required, ofloxacin, levofloxacin, or norfloxacin are probably the better choices for breastfeeding mothers.

Pregnancy Risk	C	Lactation Risk	L2
T ½	= 5–7 hours	M/P	= 0.98–1.66
Vd	= 1.4 l/kg	PB	= 32%
Tmax	= 0.5–2 hours	Oral	= 98%
MW	= 361	pKa	=

Adult Concerns: Nausea, vomiting, diarrhea, abdominal cramps, gastrointestinal bleeding.

Pediatric Concerns: None reported, but caution recommended. Observe for diarrhea.

Drug Interactions: Decreased absorption with antacids. Quinolones cause increased levels of caffeine, warfarin, cyclosporine, theophylline. Cimetidine, probenecid, azlocillin may increase ofloxacin levels. Increased risk of seizures when used with foscarnet.

Relative Infant Dose: 3.1%

Adult Dose: 200–400 mg twice daily.

Alternatives: Norfloxacin, trovafloxacin

References:
1. Giamarellou H, Kolokythas E, Petrikkos G, Gazis J, Aravantinos D, Sfikakis P. Pharmacokinetics of three newer quinolones in pregnant and lactating women. Am J Med 1989; 87(5A): 49S-51S.
2. Ghaffar F, McCracken GH. Quinolones in Pediatrics. In: Hooper DC, Rubinstein E, editors. Quinolone Antimicrobial Agents. Washington, D.C.: ASM Press, 2003: 343–354.

OLANZAPINE   L2

Trade: Zyprexa, Zyprexa Relprevv

Other Trades: Zyprexa

Category: Antipsychotic

Olanzapine is an atypical antipsychotic agent structurally similar to clozapine and may be used for treating schizophrenia.[1] It is rather unusual in that it blocks serotonin receptors rather than dopamine receptors.

In a recent and excellent study of seven mother-infant nursing pairs receiving a median dose of olanzapine of 7.5 mg/day (range = 5–20 mg/day), the median infant dose ingested via milk was approximately 1.02% of the maternal dose.[2] The median milk/plasma AUC ratio was 0.38. Olanzapine was undetected in the plasma of six infants tested. All infants were healthy and experienced no observable side effects. The maximum relative infant dose was approximately 1.2%.

In a case report of a mother taking 20 mg/day, the milk/plasma ratio was 0.35, giving a relative infant dose of about 4% at steady state. This milk was not fed to the infant, so infant plasma levels were not performed.[3]

In a study of 5 mothers receiving olanzapine at a dose of 2.5–20 mg/day, reported milk/plasma ratios of 0.2 to 0.84, with an average relative infant dose of 1.6%. The authors reported no untoward effects on the infants attributable to olanzapine.[4] In a study of 37 women consuming olanzapine, early discontinuation of breastfeeding was more common in the olanzapine-exposed breastfed group (5 of 22 vs. none of 51).[1] The rate of adverse outcomes in olanzapine-exposed breastfed infants did not differ from those of the control groups. Neonatal symptoms were seen in 6 of the 30 olanzapine-exposed infants versus 2 of 51 nonexposed infants. Neonatal withdrawal was seen in three of 30 (10%) infants.[5]

Pregnancy Risk	C	Lactation Risk	L2
T ½	= 21–54 hours	M/P	= 0.38
Vd	= 14.3 l/kg	PB	= 93%
Tmax	= 5–8 hours	Oral	= >57%
MW	= 312	pKa	= 5.0, 7.4

Adult Concerns: Agitation, dizziness, somnolence, constipation, weight gain, elevated liver enzymes.

Pediatric Concerns: None reported in one excellent study. Probably safe. Observe for withdrawal syndrome in some infants.

Drug Interactions: Ethanol may potentiate the effects of olanzapine. Fluvoxamine may inhibit olanzapine metabolism. Carbamazepine may increase clearance of olanzapine by 50%. Levodopa may antagonize the effect of olanzapine.

Relative Infant Dose: 0.3%–2.2%

Adult Dose: 5–10 mg daily.

Alternatives: Risperidone, haloperidol, quetiapine

References:
1. Pharmaceutical manufacturer prescribing information, 1997.
2. Gardiner SJ, Kristensen JH, Begg EJ, Hackett LP, Wilson DA,Ilett KF, Kohan R and Rampono J, Transfer of olanzapine into breast milk, calculation of infant drug dose, and effect on breast-fed infants. Am J Psychiatry 2003; 160: 1428–1431.
3. Ambresin G, Berney P, Schulz P, Bryois C. Olanzapine Excretion Into Breast Milk: A Case Report. J Clin Psychopharmacol 2004; 24(1): 93–95.
4. Croke S, Buist A, Hackett LP, Ilett KF, Norman TR, Burrows GD. Olanzapine exretion in human breast milk: estimation of infant exposure. Int J Neuropsychoph 2002; 5: 243–247.
5. Gilad O, Merlob P, Stahl B, Klinger G. Outcome of infants exposed to olanzapine during breastfeeding. Breastfeed Med.2011; 6(2): 55–58.

OLMESARTAN MEDOXOMIL   L3

Trade: Benicar

Other Trades:

Category: Antihypertensive

Olmesartan is an angiotensin II receptor antagonist used as a anti-hypertensive. Olmesartan medoxomil is a prodrug and is rapidly metabolized in the gastrointestinal tract to the active olmesartan product. It effectively blocks the angiotensin II receptor site. While it is different from the ACE inhibitors, it effectively produces the same end result, hypotension. Use in pregnancy is contraindicated. No data are available on its transfer to human milk, but its use in mothers with premature infants could be risky.

Pregnancy Risk	C/D in 2nd and 3rd trimester	Lactation Risk	L3
T ½	= 13 hours	M/P	=
Vd	= 0.24 l/kg	PB	=
Tmax	= 1–2 hours	Oral	= 26%
MW	= 558	pKa	=

Adult Concerns: Adverse effects include dizziness and low blood pressure.

Pediatric Concerns: None via milk. No data are available.

Drug Interactions: No major drug-drug interactions are noted with exception of its use with adrenergics.

Relative Infant Dose:

Adult Dose: 20–40 mg daily.

Alternatives: Captopril, enalapril

References:
1. Pharmaceutical manufacturer prescribing information, 2003.

OLOPATADINE OPHTHALMIC   L2

Trade: Patanol, Patanase, Pataday
Other Trades: Patanol, Opatanol
Category: Ophthalmic antihistamine

Olopatadine is a selective H_1-receptor antagonist and inhibitor of histamine release from mast cells. It is used topically in the eye. Kinetic studies by the manufacturer suggest that absorption is low in adults and that plasma levels are undetectable in most cases (<0.5 ng/mL).[1] Samples in which olopatadine was found in the plasma compartment were at 2 hours and were <1.3 ng/mL. Because adult plasma levels are so low, it is extremely unlikely any would be detectable in human milk. No data are available reporting levels in human milk but the risk is probably quite low.

Pregnancy Risk	C	Lactation Risk	L2
T ½	= 3 hours	M/P	=
Vd	=	PB	=
Tmax	= 2 hours	Oral	=
MW	= 373	pKa	=

Adult Concerns: Headache has been reported in 7% of patients. Asthenia, blurred vision, burning, dry eye, redness, lid edema, pruritus and rhinitis have been reported.

Pediatric Concerns: None reported via milk.

Drug Interactions:

Relative Infant Dose:

Adult Dose: One drop in affected eye twice daily.

Alternatives:

References:
1. Pharmaceutical manufacturer Prescribing Information, 2003.

OLSALAZINE   L3

Trade: Dipentum
Other Trades: Dipentum
Category: Anti-inflammatory

Olsalazine is a salicylate which is converted to 5-aminosalicylic acid (mesalamine: 5–ASA) in the gastrointestinal tract and has anti-inflammatory activity in ulcerative colitis.[1] After oral administration, only 2.4% is systemically absorbed while the majority is metabolized in the gastrointestinal tract to 5–ASA. 5–ASA is slowly and poorly absorbed. Plasma levels are exceedingly small (1.6–6.2 mmol/L), the half-life is very short, and protein binding is very high. In rodents fed up to 20 times the normal dose, olsalazine produced growth retardation in pups. In one study of a mother who received a single 500 mg dose of olsalazine, acetylated-5–ASA achieved concentrations of 0.6, 0.86, and 1.24 mmol/L in breastmilk at 10, 14, and 24 hours respectively.[2] Olsalazine, olsalazine-S, and 5–ASA were undetectable in breastmilk. While clinically significant levels in milk are remote, infants should be closely monitored for gastric changes such as diarrhea.

Pregnancy Risk	C	Lactation Risk	L3
T ½	= 0.9 hours	M/P	=
Vd	=	PB	= >99%
Tmax	= 1–2 hours	Oral	= 2.4% (olsalazine)
MW	= 346	pKa	= 3.53

Adult Concerns: Watery diarrhea, dyspepsia, diarrhea, nausea, pain/cramping, headache

Pediatric Concerns: None specifically reported with this product, but observe for diarrhea and cramping if used for longer periods.

Drug Interactions: Concurrent use with heparin, warfarin and other anticoagulants causes an increased risk of bleeding. Do not administer concurrently with varicella vaccine due to increased risk of Reye Syndrome. Concurrent administration with tamarind increases risk of salicylate toxicity.

Relative Infant Dose: 0.9%

Adult Dose: 500 mg twice daily.

Alternatives:

References:
1. Pharmaceutical manufacturer prescribing information, 2010.
2. Miller LG, Hopkinson JM, Motil KJ, Corboy JE, Andersson S. Disposition of olsalazine and metabolites in breast milk. J Clin Pharmacol 1993; 33(8): 703–706.

OMALIZUMAB   L3

Trade: Xolair
Other Trades: Xolair
Category: Monoclonal antibody

Omalizumab inhibits the binding of IgE to the high-affinity IgE receptor on the surface of mast cells and basophils. It is a large IgG monoclonal antibody used to treat persistent allergic asthma that cannot be controlled using inhaled corticosteroids. It works by inhibiting IgE binding to the receptor on mast cells and basophils, in turn decreasing the release of mediators in the allergic response.[1] The manufacturer suggests that omalizumab may be secreted into human breastmilk based on monkey studies where milk levels were only 1.5% of maternal blood levels, which would be exceedingly low. However, no studies have been performed in humans. This product would not be orally bioavailable in an infant.

Pregnancy Risk	B	Lactation Risk	L3
T ½	= 26 days	M/P	=
Vd	= 0.078 l/kg	PB	=
Tmax	= 7–8 days	Oral	= 62%
MW	= 149,000	pKa	=

Adult Concerns: Adverse reactions include headache, injection site reaction, upper respiratory tract infection, and viral infection.

Pediatric Concerns: No data are available.

Drug Interactions: No drug interactions have been noted.

Relative Infant Dose:

Adult Dose: 150–300 mg every 2–4 weeks.

Alternatives:

References:
1. Pharmaceutical manufacturer prescribing information, 2010.

OMEGA-3-ACID ETHYL ESTERS   L3

Trade: Lovaza
Other Trades:
Category: FISH OIL

Omega-3-acid ethyl esters is a lipid-regulating agent. Each 1-gram capsule contains at least 900 mg of the ethyl esters of omega-3 fatty acids sourced from fish oils.[1] These are predominantly a combination of ethyl esters of eicosapentaenoic acid (EPA–approximately 465 mg) and docosahexaenoic acid (DHA–approximately 375 mg). It is not known whether omega-3-acid ethyl esters are excreted in human milk, but we know that docosahexaenoic acid (DHA) is a common lipid in human milk. The mechanism of action of this oil is not completely understood. Potential mechanisms of action include reduction of the synthesis of triglycerides in the liver because EPA and DHA are poor substrates for the enzymes responsible for triglyceride synthesis, and EPA and DHA inhibit esterification of other fatty acids. Use caution in patients who have a known hypersensitivity to fish and/or shellfish. May prolong bleeding time. Coagulation studies should be done on patients who concurrently take anticoagulants such as warfarin or coumadin. Also, monitor bleeding time if patients are on aspirin or NSAIDS routinely.

Pregnancy Risk	C	Lactation Risk	L3
T ½	=	M/P	=
Vd	=	PB	=
Tmax	=	Oral	= Complete
MW	= DHA = 356.55 and EPA = 330.51	pKa	=

Adult Concerns: Common adverse effects: eructation, infection, flu syndrome, and dyspepsia. Monitor ALT and AST in pts with hepatic impairment. Monitor LDL's as may increase LDL in pts. Use caution in pts who have a known hypersensitivity to fish and/or shellfish. May prolong bleeding time. Coag. studies should be done on pts who concurrently take anticoagulants such as warfarin or coumadin. Also, monitor bleeding time if pts are on aspirin or NSAIDS routinely.

Pediatric Concerns:

Drug Interactions: Potential to prolong bleeding time so administer with caution in patients who take anticoagulants such as warfarin and coumadin. Also pts who take aspirin, or NSAIDs on a routine basis.

Relative Infant Dose:

Adult Dose:

Alternatives:

References:
1.   Pharmaceutical manufacturer prescribing information, 2011.

OMEPRAZOLE   L2

Trade:

Other Trades:

Category: Reduces gastric acid secretion

Omeprazole is a potent inhibitor of gastric acid secretion. In a study of one patient receiving 20 mg omeprazole daily, the maternal serum concentration was negligible until 90 minutes after ingestion and then reached 950 nM at 240 min.[1] The breastmilk concentration of omeprazole began to rise minimally at 90 minutes after ingestion and peaked after 180 minutes at only 58 nM, or less than 7% of the highest serum level. This would indicate a maximum dose of 3 µg/kg/day in a breastfed infant. Omeprazole milk levels were essentially flat over 4 hours of observation. Omeprazole is extremely acid labile with a half-life of 10 minutes at pH values below 4.[2] Virtually all omeprazole ingested via milk would probably be destroyed in the stomach of the infant prior to absorption.

Pregnancy Risk	C	Lactation Risk	L2
T ½	= 1 hour	M/P	=
Vd	=	PB	= 95%
Tmax	= 0.5–3.5 hours	Oral	= 30–40%
MW	= 345	pKa	=

Adult Concerns: Headache, diarrhea, elevated liver enzymes.

Pediatric Concerns: None reported via milk in one case.

Drug Interactions: Administration of omeprazole and clarithromycin may result in increased plasma levels of omeprazole. Omeprazole produced a 130% increase in the half-life of diazepam, reduced the plasma clearance of phenytoin by 15%, and increased phenytoin half-life by 27%. May prolong the elimination of warfarin.

Relative Infant Dose: 1.1%

Adult Dose: 20 mg twice daily.

Alternatives: Famotidine, nizatidine

References:
1. Marshall JK, Thompson AB, Armstrong D. Omeprazole for refractory gastroesophageal reflux disease during pregnancy and lactation. Can J Gastroenterol 1998; 12(3): 225–227.
2. Pilbrant A, Cederberg C. Development of an oral formulation of omeprazole. Scand J Gastroenterol Suppl 1985; 108: 113–120.

ONDANSETRON   L2

Trade: Zofran, Zuplenz

Other Trades: Zofran

Category: Antiemetic

Ondansetron is used clinically for reducing the nausea and vomiting associated with chemotherapy. It has occasionally been used during pregnancy without effect on the fetus.[1,2] It is available for oral and IV administration. Ondansetron is secreted in animal milk, but no data in humans are available. Four studies of ondansetron use in pediatric patients 4–18 years of age are available. It is commonly used in infants and children and is considered very safe.

Pregnancy Risk	B	Lactation Risk	L2
T ½	= 3.6 hours	M/P	=
Vd	=	PB	= 70–76%
Tmax	= 1.7, 3.1 (IV,PO)	Oral	= 56–66%
MW	= 293	pKa	=

Adult Concerns: Headache, drowsiness, malaise, clonic-tonic seizures, and constipation.

Pediatric Concerns: None reported via milk.

Drug Interactions: The clearance and half-life of ondansetron may be changed when used with barbiturates, carbamazepine, rifampin, phenytoin.

Relative Infant Dose:

Adult Dose: 8 mg twice daily.

Alternatives:

References:
1. Pharmaceutical manufacturer prescribing information, 1996.
2. Spratto GR. In: Nurse's Drug Reference. Albany, NY: Delmar Publishers Inc., 1995.

ORAL CONTRACEPTIVES   L3

Trade:

Other Trades: Nornyl, Cilest, Brevinor

Category: Contraceptive

Oral contraceptives are hormonal pills containing either estrogen, or progesterone, or both; used for contraceptive purposes. Oral contraceptives, particularly those containing estrogens, may decrease the volume of milk produced although this is highly controversial.[1] Quality (fat content) may similarly be reduced, although one recent study of the fat, energy, protein, and lactose concentration in milk of mothers using oral contraceptives showed no effect of contraceptives.[2] The earlier oral contraceptives are started, the greater the negative effect on lactation.[3,4] Suppression of breastmilk production with estrogen-progestin contraceptives has been suggested, but it is controversial. It seems more prevalent when they are administered early postpartum. Although it was previously believed that waiting for 6 weeks would preclude breastfeeding problems, this is apparently controversial. Numerous examples of supply problems have occurred months postpartum in some patients, but not in others. Breastfeeding women should be advised to avoid using combination (estrogen-containing) oral contraceptives while breastfeeding because combination oral contraceptives are believed to interfere with the production of milk and may reduce the duration of breastfeeding.[2,5–9]

Clinicians should suggest that the mother establish a good milk production prior to beginning oral contraceptives. Avoid combination (estrogen-progestin) contraceptives it at all possible. Use oral progestin-only preparations initially preferably after 4 weeks postpartum. Warn mothers that even progestin-only preparations may suppress milk production and to discontinue them at the first sign of low milk supply. Use medroxyprogesterone (Depo-Provera) only in those patients who have used it previously and have not experienced breastfeeding problems, or in those who have used progestin-only mini pills without problems. Attempt to wait for 4 weeks postpartum prior to using medroxyprogesterone. The transfer of progestins and estrogens into breast milk is exceedingly low, and numerous studies confirm that they have minimal or no effect on sexual development in infants.

Suggestions for OC therapy. 1) Always start with an oral progestin-only pill first, if only for a month. If milk production is sustained, then continue on the oral preparation, or a sustained release preparation like Depo medroxyprogesterone may be suitable. 2) Avoid using any form of progesterone the first week postpartum, as these may suppress early milk production. 3) Avoid estrogen-containing preparations, particularly early postpartum. While controversial, extensive clinical experience with these preparations suggest caution as signficant loss of milk supply has been frequently reported. 4) We have numerous reports of loss of milk supply following placement of Mirena IUDs. While one suggests no such loss, caution is recommended until this is clear.

Pregnancy Risk	X	Lactation Risk	L3
T ½	=	M/P	=
Vd	=	PB	=
Tmax	=	Oral	=
MW	=	pKa	=

Adult Concerns: Reduced milk production, particularly with estrogen containing preparations, but also rarely with progestin only products.

Pediatric Concerns: None reported via milk. May suppress lactation, reducing weight gain of infant.

Drug Interactions: Barbiturates, hydantoins, and rifampin, may increase the clearance of oral contraceptives resulting in decreased effectiveness of the oral contraceptives. Co-administration of griseofulvin, penicillin, or tetracyclines with oral contraceptives may decrease the efficacy of oral contraceptives possibly due to altered gut metabolism. May increase or decrease anticoagulant efficacy. Co-administration with cyclosporine, or carbamazepine may result in decreased oral contraceptive efficacy.

Relative Infant Dose:

Adult Dose:

Alternatives: Norethindrone

References:
1. Booker DE, Pahl IR. Control of postpartum breast engorgement with oral contraceptives. Am J Obstet Gynecol 1967; 98(8): 1099–1101.
2. Costa TH, Dorea JG. Concentration of fat, protein, lactose and energy in milk of mothers using hormonal contraceptives. Ann Trop Paediatr 1992; 12(2): 203–209.
3. Laukaran VH. The effects of contraceptive use on the initiation and duration of lactation. Int J Gynaecol Obstet 1987; 25 Suppl: 129–142.
4. Kora SJ. Effect of oral contraceptives on lactation. Fertil Steril 1969; 20(3): 419–423.
5. McCann MF, Potter LS. Progestin-only oral contraception: a comprehensive review. Contraception. 1994 Dec; 50(6 Suppl 1): S1–195. Review.
6. Peralta O, D?az S, Juez G, Herreros C, Casado ME, Salvatierra AM, Miranda P, Dur?n E, Croxatto HB. Fertility regulation in nursing women: V. Long-term influence of a low-dose combined oral contraceptive initiated at day 90 postpartum upon lactation and infant growth. Contraception. 1983 Jan; 27(1): 27–38.
7. Croxatto HB, D?az S, Peralta O, Juez G, Herreros C, Casado ME, Salvatierra AM, Miranda P, Dur?n E. Fertility regulation in nursing women: IV. Long-term influence of a low-dose combined oral contraceptive initiated at day 30 postpartum upon lactation and infant growth. Contraception. 1983 Jan; 27(1): 13–25.

8. Draz S, Peralta O, Juez G, Herreros C, Casado ME, Salvatierra AM, Miranda P, Duran E, Croxatto HB. Fertility regulation in nursing women: III. Short-term influence of a low-dose combined oral contraceptive upon lactation and infant growth. Contraception. 1983 Jan; 27(1): 1–11.
9. Effects of hormonal contraceptives on breast milk composition and infant growth. World Health Organization (WHO) Task Force on Oral Contraceptives. Stud Fam Plann. 1988 Nov-Dec; 19(6 Pt 1): 361–9.

ORLISTAT   L3

Trade: Xenical, Alli
Other Trades: Xenical
Category: Lipase inhibitor

Orlistat, now available over the counter as well as prescription, is used in the management of obesity. It is a reversible inhibitor of gastric and pancreatic lipases, thus it inhibits absorption of dietary fats by 30%.[1] No studies have been performed on the transmission of orlistat into the breastmilk. With high protein binding, moderately high molecular weight, and poor oral absorption, it is unlikely that orlistat would enter breastmilk in clinically relevant amounts, or affect a breastfeeding infant. However, due to orlistat's effect on the absorption of fat soluble vitamins and other fats, nutritional status of a breastfeeding mother should be closely monitored.

Pregnancy Risk	B	Lactation Risk	L3
T ½	= 1–2 hours	M/P	=
Vd	=	PB	= >99%
Tmax	= 8 hours	Oral	= Minimal
MW	= 495	pKa	=

Adult Concerns: Adverse effects include headache, oily spotting, abdominal pain, flatus with discharge, fecal urgency, fatty/oily stools, back pain, and upper respiratory infection.

Pediatric Concerns: Children aged 12–16 years experienced similar adverse effects as did the adult population.

Drug Interactions: Orlistat may decrease amiodarone and cyclosporine. Also, vitamin K absorption may be decreased leading to a change in warfarin effects. Absorption of fat soluble vitamins may be decreased with orlistat use, and thus patients should take a multivitamin containing vitamins A, D, E, and K once daily, at least 2 hours before or after orlistat.

Relative Infant Dose:

Adult Dose: 60–120 mg three times daily.

Alternatives:

References:
1. Pharmaceutical manufacturer prescribing information, 2007.

ORPHENADRINE CITRATE   L3

Trade: Norflex, Banflex, Norgesic, Flexon
Other Trades: Norgesic, Disipal, Norflex, Orfenace
Category: Muscle relaxant

Orphenadrine is an analog of diphenhydramine (Benadryl).[1] It is primarily used as a muscle relaxant although its primary effects are anticholinergic. No data are available on its secretion into breastmilk. Until more is known about the transfer of this drug into human milk, use with caution in breastfeeding mothers. Observe for sedation in the breastfed infant.

Pregnancy Risk	C	Lactation Risk	L3
T ½	= 14 hours	M/P	=
Vd	=	PB	=
Tmax	= 2–4 hours	Oral	= 95%
MW	= 269	pKa	=

Adult Concerns: Agitation, aplastic anemia, dizziness, tremor, dry mouth, nausea, constipation.

Pediatric Concerns: None reported due to limited studies.

Drug Interactions: Increased anticholinergic side effects may be noted when used with amantadine. Orphenadrine may reduce therapeutic efficacy of phenothiazine family.

Relative Infant Dose:

Adult Dose: 100 mg twice daily.

Alternatives:

References:
1. McEvoy GE. (ed): AFHS Drug Information. New York, NY: 2003.

OSELTAMIVIR PHOSPHATE   L2

Trade: Tamiflu
Other Trades: Tamiflu
Category: Anti-viral for influenza A and B

Oseltamivir is indicated for the treatment of uncomplicated acute illness due to influenza A and B infection in adults who have been symptomatic for no more than 2 days. Oseltamivir is an oral viral neuraminidase inhibitor, which blocks or prevents viral seeding or release from infected cells and prevents viral aggregation. In a recent study of one patient who was receiving 75 mg twice daily, for 5 days, the active carboxylate metabolite reached steady-state levels after 3 days and was reported to be 37–39 ng/mL.[1] Based on this data, the authors estimated the relative infant dose to be 0.5% of the maternal weight-adjusted dose. Thus, this dose is unlikely to produce clinical levels in a breastfed infant. It has recently been recommended for use in breastfeeding mothers by the CDC (Centers for Disease Control and prevention).

Pregnancy Risk	C	Lactation Risk	L2
T ½	= 6–10 hours	M/P	=
Vd	= 0.37 l/kg	PB	= 42%
Tmax	=	Oral	= 75%
MW	= 312	pKa	= 7.75

Adult Concerns: Nausea and vomiting are most common. Diarrhea, bronchitis, abdominal pain are less common.

Pediatric Concerns: None reported via milk.

Drug Interactions: None yet reported.

Relative Infant Dose: 0.5%

Adult Dose: 75 mg twice daily for 5 days.

Alternatives:

References:
1. Wentges-van HN, van EM, van der Laan JW. Oseltamivir and breastfeeding. Int J Infect Dis. 2008.

OSMOTIC LAXATIVES   L1

Trade: Milk of Magnesia, Citrate of Magnesia, Epsom Salt
Other Trades: Sorbilax, Duphalac, Acilac, Citromag
Category: Laxatives

Osmotic or saline laxatives comprise a large amount of magnesium and phosphate compounds, but all work similarly in that they osmotically pull and retain water in the gastrointestinal tract, thus functioning as laxatives. Because they are poorly absorbed, they largely stay in the gastrointestinal tract and are eliminated without significant systemic absorption.[1,2] The small amount of magnesium absorbed is rapidly cleared by the kidneys. Products considered osmotic laxatives include: Milk of Magnesia, Epsom Salts, and Citrate of Magnesia. Because milk electrolytes and ion concentrations are tightly controlled by the maternal alveolar cell, the secretion of higher than normal levels into milk is rare and unlikely. It is not known for certainty if these products enter milk in higher levels than are normally present, but it is very unlikely.

Pregnancy Risk	C	Lactation Risk	L1
T ½	=	M/P	=
Vd	=	PB	=
Tmax	=	Oral	= Poor
MW	=	pKa	=

Adult Concerns: Diarrhea, nausea, vomiting, hypocalcemia, hypermagnesemia.

Pediatric Concerns: None reported via milk.

Drug Interactions: May reduce absorption of anticoagulants such as coumarin, and dicoumarol.

Relative Infant Dose:

Adult Dose:

Alternatives:

References:
1. Drug Facts and Comparisons 1997 ed. ed. St. Louis: 1997.
2. Pharmaceutical manufacturer prescribing information, 1997.

OXALIPLATIN   L5

Trade: Eloxatin, Eloxatine, O-Plat, Oxalip

Other Trades: Eloxatin

Category: Anticancer drug

Oxaliplatin is a platinum-containing anticancer compound. Its kinetics are similar to cisplatin with a biexponential model of elimination. The decline of ultrafilterable platinum levels following oxaliplatin administration is triphasic, characterized by two relatively short distribution phases (0.43 hours and 16.8 hours) and a long terminal elimination phase (391 hours).[1,2] Check the similar drug, cisplatin, for published milk levels. Oxaliplatin is extensively bound in peripheral tissues, which accounts for its extraordinarily long elimination half-life. While breastmilk levels are unavailable, but are probably low, breastfeeding is not advisable for many days (>20–30) and should probably be discontinued for this infant, unless milk platinum levels can be measured. Two options are suggested. One, breastmilk should be tested for platinum levels and not used as long as they are measurable; two, without measuring platinum levels, breastfeeding should be permanently interrupted for this infant.

Pregnancy Risk	D	Lactation Risk	L5
T ½	= 38.7 hours	M/P	=
Vd	= Very high l/kg	PB	= >90%
Tmax	=	Oral	=
MW	= 397.3	pKa	= 1.3, 7.23

Adult Concerns: Rash, urticaria, erythema, pruritus, and, rarely, bronchospasm and hypotension.

Pediatric Concerns:

Drug Interactions: Administration of rotavirus vaccine while on oxaliplatin is contra-indicated. Concurrent use with other live vaccines such as MMR vaccine, influenza vaccine should be avoided. Use with caution while coadministering with other nephrotoxic agents.

Relative Infant Dose:

Adult Dose:

Alternatives:

References:

1. Grochow LB, Ames MM. A clinician's guide to chemotherapy pharmacokinetics and pharmacodynamics. 1st ed. Baltimore, MD: Williams and Wilkins; 1998.
2. Pharmaceutical manufacturer prescribing information, 2005.

OXAPROZIN   L3

Trade: Daypro

Other Trades: Daypro

Category: Nonsteroidal analgesic

Oxaprozin belongs to the NSAID family of analgesics and is reputed to have lesser gastrointestinal side effects than certain others.[1] Although its long half-life could prove troublesome in breastfed infants, it is probably poorly transferred to human milk. No data on transfer into human milk are available although it is known to transfer into animal milk.

Pregnancy Risk	C	Lactation Risk	L3
T ½	= 42–50 hours	M/P	=
Vd	=	PB	= 99%
Tmax	= 3–5 hours	Oral	= 95%
MW	= 293	pKa	= 4.3

Adult Concerns: Headache, nausea, abdominal pain, gastric bleeding, diarrhea, vomiting, bleeding, constipation.

Pediatric Concerns: None reported, but ibuprofen preferred in absence of data.

Drug Interactions: May prolong prothrombin time when used with warfarin. Antihypertensive effects of ACE inhibitor family may be blunted or completely abolished by NSAIDs. Some NSAIDs may block antihypertensive effect of beta blockers, diuretics. Used with cyclosporin, may dramatically increase renal toxicity. May increase digoxin, phenytoin, lithium levels. May increase toxicity of methotrexate. May increase bioavailability of penicillamine. Probenecid may increase NSAID levels.

Relative Infant Dose:

Adult Dose: 600–1200 mg daily.

Alternatives: Ibuprofen, ketorolac, naproxen

References:

1. Pharmaceutical manufacturer prescribing information, 2010.

OXAZEPAM   L3

Trade: Serax

Other Trades: Alepam, Murelax, Serepax, Apo-Oxazepam, Novoxapam, Serax, Zapex, Oxanid

Category: Benzodiazepine antianxiety drug

Oxazepam is a typical benzodiazepine and is used in anxiety disorders. Of the benzodiazepines, oxazepam is the least lipid soluble, which accounts for its low levels in milk. In one study of a patient receiving 10 mg three times daily for 3 days, the concentration of oxazepam in breastmilk was relatively constant between 24 and 30 µg/L from the evening of the first day.[1] The milk/plasma ratio ranged from 0.1 to 0.33. The authors suggest that less than 1/1000th of the maternal dose was transferred to the infant. It is unlikely that significant amounts will enter the breastmilk. In a study of a single mother who consumed 15–30 mg oxazepam daily, levels in breastmilk were approximately 10% of maternal levels at 4 hours after the dose. In 12 milk samples collected, oxazepam levels ranged from 11–26 µg/L.[2] In another study of a 22-year-old mother consuming 80 mg of diazepam and 30 mg of oxazepam, levels of diazepam and oxazepam in milk, mother's plasma and infant's plasma were reported.[3] The mean milk/plasma ratio of oxazepam was found to be 0.10, with milk concentrations ranging from 8–30 µg/L. The infant plasma concentrations on days 14 and 25 of therapy were 7.5 µg/L and 9.6 µg/L. No oxazepam was detected in milk 8 days following cessation of oxazepam. No untoward effects were noted in the infant. The authors conclude that the levels of benzodiazepines such as oxazepam in milk are minimal and are unlikely to cause untoward effects in the breastfed infant.

Pregnancy Risk	D	Lactation Risk	L3
T ½	= 12 hours	M/P	= 0.1–0.33
Vd	= 0.7–1.6 l/kg	PB	= 97%
Tmax	= 1–2 hours	Oral	= 97%
MW	= 287	pKa	= 1.7,11.6

Adult Concerns: Sedation.

Pediatric Concerns: None reported in one study.

Drug Interactions: May increase sedation when used with CNS depressants such as alcohol, barbiturates, opioids. Cimetidine may decrease metabolism and clearance of oxazepam. Cisapride can dramatically increase plasma levels of diazepam. SSRIs (fluoxetine, sertraline, paroxetine) can dramatically increase benzodiazepine levels by altering clearance, thus leading to sedation. Digoxin plasma levels may be increased.

Relative Infant Dose: 0.3%–1%

Adult Dose: 10–30 mg three-four times daily.

Alternatives:

References:

1. Wretlind M. Excretion of oxazepam in breast milk. Eur J Clin Pharmacol 1987; 33(2): 209–210.
2. Rane A, Sundwall A, Tomson G. [Oxazepam withdrawal in the neonatal period]. Lakartidningen. 1979; 76: 4416–7.
3. Dusci LJ, Good SM, Hall RW, Ilett KF. Excretion of diazepam and its metabolites in human milk during withdrawal from combination high dose diazepam and oxazepam. Br J Clin Pharmacol. 1990; 29: 123–6.

OXCARBAZEPINE   L3

Trade: Trileptal

Other Trades: Trileptal

Category: Anticonvulsant

Oxcarbazepine is a derivative of carbamazepine and is used in the treatment of partial seizures in adults and as adjunctive therapy in the treatment of partial seizures in children. It is rapidly metabolized to a longer half-life active metabolite 10-hydroxy-carbazepine (MHD). In a brief and somewhat incomplete study of a pregnant patient who received 300 mg three times daily while pregnant, plasma levels were studied in her infant for the first 5 days postpartum while the infant was breastfeeding.[1] While no breastmilk levels were reported, plasma levels of MHD in the infant were essentially the same as the mother's immediately after delivery, suggesting complete transfer transplacentally of the drug. However, while breastfeeding for the next 5 days, plasma levels of MHD in the infant declined significantly from approximately 7 µg/mL to 0.2 µg/mL on the fifth day. The decay of MHD concentrations in neonatal plasma during the first 4 days postpartum indicated first order elimination. The plasma MHD levels on day 5 amounted to 7% of those one day postpartum (93% drop in 5 days). The authors estimated the milk/plasma ratio to be 0.5. No neonatal side effects were reported by the authors.

Pregnancy Risk	C	Lactation Risk	L3
T ½	= 9 hours MHD	M/P	= 0.5
Vd	= 0.7 l/kg	PB	= 40%
Tmax	= 4.5 hours	Oral	= Complete
MW	= 252	pKa	= 10.7

Adult Concerns: Cognitive symptoms include psychomotor slowing, difficulty with concentration, speech or language problems, somnolence or fatigue, ataxia and gait disturbances. Hyponatremia has been reported.

Pediatric Concerns: None reported in one study.

Drug Interactions: Slight increases in other anticonvulsant plasma levels have been reported and include phenobarbital, phenytoin. A reduction in plasma levels of oxcarbazepine have been reported when admixed with phenobarbital, carbamazepine, phenytoin, etc. Major reductions in plasma levels of estrogens and other hormonal contraceptives has been reported and may render oral contraceptives less effective.

Relative Infant Dose:

Adult Dose: 300–600 mg twice daily.

Alternatives: Carbamazepine

References:
1. Bulau P, Paar WD, von Unruh GE. Pharmacokinetics of oxcarbazepine and 10-hydroxy-carbazepine in the newborn child of an oxcarbazepine-treated mother. Eur J Clin Pharmacol 1988; 34(3): 311–313.

OXYBUTYNIN   L3

Trade: Ditropan

Other Trades: Ditropan, Apo-Oxybutynin, Oxybutyn

Category: Anticholinergic, antispasmodic

Oxybutynin is an anticholinergic agent used to provide antispasmodic effects for conditions characterized by involuntary bladder spasms and reduces urinary urgency and frequency. It has been used in children down to 5 years of age at doses of 15 mg daily.[1] No data on transfer of this product into human milk is available. But oxybutynin is a tertiary amine which is poorly absorbed orally (only 6%). Further, the maximum plasma levels (C_{max}) generally attained are less than 31.7 ng/mL.[2] If one were to assume a theoretical M/P ratio of 1.0 (which is probably unreasonably high) and a daily ingestion of 1 L of milk, then the theoretical dose to the infant would be <2 µg/day, a dose that would be clinically irrelevant to even a neonate.

Pregnancy Risk	B	Lactation Risk	L3
T ½	= 1–2 hours	M/P	=
Vd	=	PB	=
Tmax	= 3–6 hours	Oral	= 6%
MW	= 393	pKa	= 6.96

Adult Concerns: Nausea, dry mouth, constipation, esophagitis, urinary hesitancy, flushing and urticaria. Palpitations, somnolence, hallucinations infrequently occur.

Pediatric Concerns: Suppression of lactation has been reported by the manufacturer.

Drug Interactions: May potentiate the anticholinergic effect of biperiden and other anticholinergics such as the tricyclic antidepressants. May counteract the effects of cisapride and metoclopramide.

Relative Infant Dose:

Adult Dose: 5 mg 2–4 times daily.

Alternatives:

References:
1. Pharmaceutical manufacturer prescribing information, 1997.
2. Douchamps J, Derenne F, Stockis A, Gangji D, Juvent M, Herchuelz A. The pharmacokinetics of oxybutynin in man. Eur J Clin Pharmacol 1988; 35(5): 515–520.

OXYCODONE   L3

Trade: Eth-Oxydose, Oxecta, OxyContin, Dazidox, Oxydose, Oxyfast, Oxy IR
Other Trades: Endone, Proladone, Supeudol
Category: Narcotic analgesic

Oxycodone is similar to hydrocodone and is a mild analgesic somewhat stronger than codeine. Small amounts are secreted in breastmilk. Following a dose of 5–10 mg every 4–7 hours, maternal levels peaked at 1–2 hours, and analgesia persisted for up to 4 hours.[1] Reported milk levels range from <5 to 226 µg/L. Maternal plasma levels were 14–35 µg/L. The authors suggest a milk/plasma ratio of approximately 3.4. Although active metabolites were not measured, the authors suggest that an exclusively breastfed infant would receive a maximum 8% of the maternal dosage of oxycodone. No reports of untoward effects in infants have been found although sedation is a possibility in some infants.

In another study, 50 post-cesarean women received 30 mg oxycodone rectally, and 10 mg orally up to every 2 hours as needed. The average maternal plasma levels at 0–24 hours and 24–48 hours were 18 (range 0–42) ng/mL and 12 (range 0–40) ng/mL, respectively. Average milk concentrations in samples taken during 0–24 hours and 24–48 hours were 58 (range 7–130) ng/mL and 49 (range 0–168) ng/mL, respectively. Milk/Plasma ratios were therefore calculated to be 3.2–3.4. Only one infant had a detectable level of oxycodone in their plasma, with a concentration of 6.6–7.4 ng/mL.[2] These plasma and milk levels suggest that oxycodone concentrates in the milk compartment, however, the authors suggest that at doses less than 90 mg/day for up to 3 days, maternal use of oxycodone poses only a minimal threat to breastfeeding infants. This study did not measure plasma or milk concentrations at steady state or during peak plasma concentrations, therefore, levels may have been higher at times.

In a recent retrospective study, the rate of CNS depression in breastfeeding infants was compared between 3 cohorts of breastfeeding women receiving oxycodone, codeine and acetaminophen, respectively, for alleviation of postpartum pain.[3] The mothers were receiving doses which were within the recommended adult dosages. The rates of infant CNS depression in the three groups was as follows: oxycodone group–20.1%; codeine group–16.7%; acetaminophen group–0.5%. While in the oxycodone group, symptoms appeared in mothers receiving median doses of 0.4 mg/kg/day (28 mg for a 70 kg individual), symptoms in the codeine group appeared at 1.4 mg/kg/day (98 mg/day for a 70 kg individual). Although CNS depression seemed to appear over a wide range of doses, it was found that higher doses were more likely to cause symptoms in the breastfed infant. This pattern held true for both the oxycodone as well as the codeine group. Further, maternal sedation was more likely with the use of oxycodone than with the use of codeine. Based on these findings, the authors conclude that oxycodone should not be considered a safer alternative to codeine in breastfed infants.

The data suggests that oxycodone is somewhat more risky and that the risks are dose-related. The use of doses greater than 40 mg/day should be avoided in breastfeeding mothers.

Pregnancy Risk	B	Lactation Risk	L3
T ½	= 3–6 hours	M/P	= 3.4
Vd	= 1.8–3.7 l/kg	PB	=
Tmax	= 1–2 hours	Oral	= 50%
MW	= 315	pKa	= 8.5

Adult Concerns: Drowsiness, sedation, nausea, vomiting, constipation.

Pediatric Concerns: Sedation has been reported in some infants (20.1%) at doses higher than 30 mg/day (median = 0.4 mg/kg/day).

Drug Interactions: Cigarette smoking increases effect of codeines. Increased toxicity/sedation when used with CNS depressants, phenothiazines, tricyclic antidepressants, other opiates, guanabenz, MAO inhibitors, neuromuscular blockers.

Relative Infant Dose: 1.5%–3.5%

Adult Dose: 5 mg every 6 hours.

Alternatives: Hydrocodone

References:
1. Marx CM, Pucin F, Carlson JD. et.al. Oxycodone excretion in human milk in the puerperium. Drug Intel Clin 1986; 20: 474.
2. Seaton S, Reeves M, McLean S. Oxycodone as a component of multimodal analgesia for lactating mothers after Caesarean section: Relationships between maternal plasma, breast milk and neonatal plasma levels. Aust NZ J Obstet Gyn 2007; 47: 181–85.
3. Lam J, Kelly L, Ciszkowski C, Landsmeer ML, Nauta M, Carleton BC, Hayden MR,Madadi P, Koren G. Central nervous system depression of neonates breastfed bymothers receiving oxycodone for postpartum analgesia. J Pediatr. 2012 Jan; 160(1): 33–37.e2. Epub 2011 Aug 31.

OXYMETAZOLINE   L3

Trade: Afrin, Nasacon, Sinarest Nasal, Duramist Plus, Visine L.R., Vicks Sinex 12 Hour, Neo-Synephrine 12 Hour, 4–Way Long Lasting

Other Trades:

Category: Nasal Decongestant

Oxymetazoline is a decongestant. No adequate well controlled studies exists on the use of oxymetazoline during breastfeeding; however, very little quantities of oxymetazoline are expected to reach the infant through breastmilk due to its local administration and limited absorption. Oxymetazoline has been preferred over oral systemic decongestants such as pseudoephedrine during breastfeeding.[1]

Oxymetazoline should only be used briefly, no more than 3 days. Monitor infant for insomnia, nervousness and excitation. Avoid using oxymetazoline in infants with cardiac symptoms or hypertension.

Pregnancy Risk	C	Lactation Risk	L3
T ½	= 5–8 hours	M/P	=
Vd	=	PB	=
Tmax	=	Oral	=
MW	= 260.7	pKa	= 7.67

Adult Concerns: Sneezing, rebound congestion, irritation, mucosa dryness, hypersensitivity.

Pediatric Concerns:

Drug Interactions: Atomoxetine and oxymetazoline in combination may cause tachycardia and hypertension.

Relative Infant Dose:

Adult Dose: Instill 2–3 spray in each nostril twice daily.

Alternatives:

References:
1. Anderson PO. Decongestants and milkproduction. J Hum Lact. 2000; 16: 294.Letter.

OXYMORPHONE   L3

Trade: Numorphane, Opana
Other Trades:
Category: Opiate analgesic

Oxymorphone is a potent opioid analgesic used to treat moderate to severe pain. On a weight basis, it is 8–10 times more potent than morphine, and it may produce more nausea and vomiting, but less constipation than morphine. It differs from morphine in its effects in that it generates less euphoria, sedation, itching and other histamine effects and it has no antitussive properties. It is poorly absorbed orally. Milk levels are as yet unreported. However, some caution is recommended with the prolonged use of this opioid analgesic.

Pregnancy Risk	C	Lactation Risk	L3
T ½	= 7.8 hours (oral)	M/P	=
Vd	=	PB	= 12%
Tmax	= 1.9 hours	Oral	= 10%
MW	= 337	pKa	= 8.17, 9.54

Adult Concerns: Nausea, pyrexia, somnolence, vomiting, pruritus, headache and dizziness have been reported. Tachycardia, hypotension, vomiting, constipation, dry mouth, abdominal distention, flatulence, sweating, dizziness, somnolence, headache, anxiety, sedation have been reported.

Pediatric Concerns: None yet, but observe for apnea, constipation, and sedation.

Drug Interactions: Extensive. Avoid use with other opiates, barbiturates, codeine, hydrocodone, sedatives including benzodiazepines such as diazepam, alprazolam, etc.

Relative Infant Dose:

Adult Dose: 10–20 every 4–6 hours

Alternatives: Morphine, hydrocodone, oxycodone

References:

1. Pharmaceutical manufacturer prescribing information, 2010.

OXYTOCIN   L2

Trade: Pitocin

Other Trades: Toesen, Syntocinon, Syntometrine

Category: Labor induction

Oxytocin is an endogenous nonapeptide hormone produced by the posterior pituitary and has uterine and myoepithelial muscle cell stimulant properties, as well as vasopressive and antidiuretic effects. Prepared synthetically, it is bioavailable via IV and intranasal applications. It is destroyed orally by chymotrypsin in the stomach of adults and systemically by the liver. It is known to be secreted in small amounts into human milk.

Takeda reported that mean oxytocin concentrations in human milk at postpartum day 1 to 5 were 4.5, 4.7, 4.0, 3.2, and 3.3 µIU/mL respectively.[1] The oral absorption in neonates is unknown but probably minimal. Intranasal sprays (Syntocinon) contain 40 IU/mL with a recommended typical dose being one spray (3 drops) in each nostril to induce letdown. This is roughly equivalent to 2 IU per drop or a total dose of approximately 12 IU per letdown dose. Oxytocin has been used to help mothers express milk for premature infants. The efficacy was tested in a randomized trial, where 27 mothers received intranasal oxytocin and 24 received placebo. There was no difference in total milk production between the two groups, indicating that oxytocin did not improve breast milk expression.[2] Thus this study suggests that oxytocin may not be effective in mothers 'who already have oxytocin mediated letdowns'. But it still may have some usefulness in mothers who apparently do not have letdowns. Although oxytocin is secreted in small amounts in breastmilk, no untoward effects have been noted. However, chronic use of intranasal oxytocin may lead to dependence and should be limited to the first week postpartum.

Pregnancy Risk	X	Lactation Risk	L2
T ½	= 3–5 minutes	M/P	=
Vd	=	PB	=
Tmax	=	Oral	= Minimal
MW	= >1000	pKa	= 6.56

Adult Concerns: Hypotension, hypertension, water intoxication and excessive uterine contractions, uterine hypertonicity, spasm, etc. May induce bradycardia, arrhythmias, intracranial hemorrhage, neonatal jaundice.

Pediatric Concerns: None via breast milk.

Drug Interactions: When used within 3–4 hours of cyclopropane, hypotension may result.

Relative Infant Dose:

Adult Dose: 40–80 units daily.

Alternatives:

References:
1. Takeda S, Kuwabara Y, Mizuno M. Concentrations and origin of oxytocin in breast milk. Endocrinol Jpn 1986; 33(6): 821–826.
2. Fewtrell MS, Loh KL, Blake A, Ridout DA, Hawdon J. Randomised, double blind trial of oxytocin nasal spray in mothers expressing breast milk for preterm infants. Arch Dis Child Fetal Neonatal Ed 2006; 91(3): F169–174.

PACLITAXEL   L5

Trade: Taxol, Abraxane, Abitaxel, Biotax, Paxel

Other Trades: Anzatax, Paxene, Taxol

Category: Antineoplastic agent

Paclitaxel is an antimicrotubule agent that inhibits reorganization of the microtubule network essential for mitosis in cells. It is commonly used in Kaposi's sarcoma, metastatic breast cancer and numerous other cancers. Paclitaxel is eliminated in a biphasic manner with a terminal elimination half-life of about 27 hours. It has a large molecular weight and a huge volume of distribution, which suggests extensive extravascular distribution/binding to peripheral tissues.[1]

In a study of one mother undergoing paclitaxel chemotherapy (30 mg/m^2 or 56.1 mg) for papillary thyroid cancer, milk levels were determined at 4, 28, 172, and 316 hours following infusion.[2] The AUC0–316h for paclitaxel was 247.9 mg.h/L. The Cave was 0.784 mg/L with an RID of 14.7%. Levels were below the limit of detection at 316 hours after final infusion. Because this dose was lower than normal, higher doses may require a longer duration of interruption.

This is potentially hazardous to breastfeeding infants. No data are available on the transfer of paclitaxel into human milk. Mothers should withhold breastfeeding for at least six to ten days following the use of paclitaxel.

Pregnancy Risk	D	Lactation Risk	L5
T ½	= 13–52 hours	M/P	=
Vd	= 632 L/m^2	PB	= 89–98%
Tmax	=	Oral	=
MW	= 853	pKa	=

Adult Concerns: Anaphylaxis and severe hypersensitivity reactions including fatal dyspnea and hypotension, and angioedema have been reported. Neutropenia, leukopenia, abnormal ECG, myalgia, arthralgia, nausea, vomiting, and diarrhea.

Pediatric Concerns: None reported via milk, but extreme caution is recommended.

Drug Interactions: Increased myelosuppression when admixed with cisplatin. Increased levels of doxorubicin when admixed with paclitaxel.

Relative Infant Dose: 13.9%–22.9%

Adult Dose: 135–175 mg/m^2 every 3 weeks.

Alternatives:

References:
1. Pharmaceutical manufacturer prescribing information, 2005.
2. Griffin SJ, Milla M, Baker TE, Hale TW. Transfer of carboplatin and paclitaxel into human breastmilk. Submitted, 2012.

PALIPERIDONE   L3

Trade: Invega, Invega Sustenna

Other Trades: Invega, Invega Sustenna

Category: Antipsychotic

Paliperidone, 9-hydroxyrisperidone, is an atypical antipsychotic agent used in the treatment of schizophrenia, schizoaffective disorder, and as an adjunct to mood stabilizers and/or antidepressants. It is the major metabolite of risperidone.

In a study of one patient receiving 6 mg/day of risperidone at steady state, the peak plasma level of approximately 130 µg/L occurred 4 hours after an oral dose.[1] Peak milk levels of risperidone and 9-hydroxyrisperidone were approximately 12 µg/L and 40 µg/L respectively. The estimated daily dose of risperidone and metabolite (risperidone equivalents) was 4.3% of the weight-adjusted maternal dose. The milk/plasma ratios calculated from areas under the curve over 24 hours were 0.42 and 0.24 respectively for risperidone and 6-hydroxyrisperidone. In another study, the transfer of risperidone and 9-hydroxyrisperidone into milk was studied in 2 breastfeeding women and one woman with risperidone-induced galactorrhea.[2] In case two (risperidone dose=42.1 µg/kg/day), the average concentration of risperidone and 9-hydroxyrisperidone in milk (Cav) was 2.1 and 6 µg/L respectively. The relative infant dose was 2.8% of the maternal dose. In case 3 (risperidone dose= 23.1 µg/kg/day), the average concentration of risperidone and 9-hydroxyrisperidone in milk (Cav) was 0.39 and 7.06 µg/L respectively. The milk/plasma ratio determined in 2 women was <0.5 for both risperidone compounds. The relative infant doses were 2.3%, 2.8%, and 4.7% (as risperidone equivalents) of the maternal weight-adjusted doses in these three cases. Risperidone and 9-hydroxyrisperidone were not detected in the plasma of the 2 breastfed infants studied, and no adverse effects were noted.

Paliperidone (9-hydroxyrisperidone) is known to be secreted into human milk in low levels. Paliperidone elevates prolactin levels and therefore you must monitor patients on this drug for hyperprolactinemia.

Pregnancy Risk	C		Lactation Risk	L3
T ½	= Oral: 23 hours, IM: 25–49 days		M/P	=
Vd	= 6.95 l/kg		PB	= 74%
Tmax	= Oral: 24 hours, IM: 13 days		Oral	= 28%
MW	= 427		pKa	= 2.6, 8.2

Adult Concerns: Somnolence, headache, tachycardia, tremor, weight gain, nausea, vomiting, injection site reactions, weakness, anxiety, hyperkinesia, orthostatic hypotension.

Pediatric Concerns:

Drug Interactions: Use with caution with other centrally acting drugs such as barbiturates, benzodiazepines, sedatives, tricyclic antidepressants, monoamine oxidase inhibitor, opiates and alcohol. Concomitant use with carbamazepine decreases the efficacy and plasma levels of paliperidone. The coadministration of paroxetine and divalproex increases the plasma levels of paliperidone. Contra-indicated for concomitant use with metoclopramide, mesoridazine, thioridazine, cisapride, dronedarone, pimozide.

Relative Infant Dose:

Adult Dose: 6 mg once daily.

Alternatives: Quetiapine

References:
1. Hill RC, McIvor RJ, Wojnar-Horton RE, Hackett LP, Ilett KF. Risperidone distribution and excretion into human milk: case report and estimated infant exposure during breast-feeding. J Clin Psychopharmacol 2000; 20(2): 285–286.
2. Ilett KF, Hackett LP, Kristensen JH, Vaddadi KS, Gardiner SJ, Begg EJ. Transfer of risperidone and 9-hydroxyrisperidone into human milk. Ann Pharmacother 2004; 38(2): 273–276.

PALONOSETRON   L3

Trade: Aloxi

Other Trades:

Category: Antiemetic

Palonosetron hydrochloride is a selective 5HT3 receptor antagonist, blocking serotonin binding and reducing the vomiting reflex. It is used to reduce chemotherapy induced nausea and vomiting.[1] It works similarly to ondansetron. No data are available on its transfer into human milk. Fortunately, this family of drugs is largely devoid of major side effects.

Pregnancy Risk	B		Lactation Risk	L3
T ½	= 40 hours		M/P	=
Vd	= 8.3 l/kg		PB	= 62%
Tmax	=		Oral	=
MW	= 333		pKa	=

Adult Concerns: Adverse reactions include headache, constipation, diarrhea, and dizziness.

Pediatric Concerns: No data are available.

Drug Interactions: Profound hypotension when used with apomorphine.

Relative Infant Dose:

Adult Dose: 0.25 mg 30 minutes befroe chemotherapy.

Alternatives: Ondansetron

References:
1. Pharmaceutical manufacturer prescribing information, 2004.

PAMIDRONATE   L3

Trade: Aredia

Other Trades:

Category: Bisphosphonate bone-resorption inhibitor.

Pamidronate is an inhibitor of bone-resorption. Although its mechanism of action is obscure, it possibly absorbs to the calcium phosphate crystal in bone and blocks dissolution (reabsorption) of this mineral component in bone, thus reducing turnover of bone calcium.

A 39 year-old patient presented in the first month of pregnancy with reflex sympathetic dystrophy. Because she wished to continue breastfeeding, she was treated with monthly IV doses of pamidronate (30 mg) postpartum. Following the first dose, breastmilk was assayed for pamidronate content. After infusion, breastmilk was pumped and collected into two portions: 0–24 hours and 25–48 hours. None was detected (limit of detection, 0.4 μmol/L). The authors suggested that pamidronate could be considered safe for use in lactating women. Pamidronate is poorly absorbed (0.3% to 3% of a dose) after oral administration and thus any present in milk would not likely be absorbed by the infant.

Pregnancy Risk	D	Lactation Risk	L3
T ½	= 28 hours	M/P	=
Vd	=	PB	=
Tmax	=	Oral	= 0.3% to 3%
MW	= 369	pKa	=

Adult Concerns: Adverse effects include fever and malaise, anemia (6%), leukopenia, thrombocytopenia, hypertension, hypocalcemia, abdominal pain, anorexia, constipation, nausea and vomiting. Numerous other side effects, consult package insert.

Pediatric Concerns: None reported via milk.

Drug Interactions: None reported.

Relative Infant Dose:

Adult Dose: 60 to 90 mg IV monthly

Alternatives:

References:

1. Siminoski K, Fitzgerald AA, Flesch G, Gross MS. Intravenous pamidronate for treatment of reflex sympathetic dystrophy during breast feeding. J Bone Miner Res 2000; 15(10): 2052–2055.

PANCRELIPASE   L3

Trade: Creon, Pancreaze, Zenpep, Pancrelipase, Ultracaps, Pangestyme EC, Palcaps, Panocaps, Enzymall

Other Trades: Cotazym, Cotazym S Forte, Pancrease (FM), Ultrase MT20, Cotazym (FM), Digess, Digeszyme, Pancrease (FM)

Category: Enzyme replacement

Pancrelipase is a pancreatic enzyme replacement product containing varying proportions of amylase, lipase and protease which are of porcine origin. Enzyme replacement therapy with products containing pancreatic enzymes amylase, lipase and protease are used in conditions of exocrine pancreatic insufficiency, such as that which occurs in relation with cystic fibrosis, chronic pancreatitis or after pancreatectomy.

Amylase, lipase and protease are pancreatic enzymes normally released from the pancreas into the upper gastrointestinal tract of humans to aid in the digestion of carbohydrates, fats and proteins respectively. In conditions such as cystic fibrosis or chronic pancreatitis, the pancreas lack the ability to release these enzymes, thereby hindering the digestion and consequent absorption of carbohydrates, fats and proteins. Malabsorption of these dietary nutrients eventually leads to malnutrition and ill-health. To avoid this, it is essential to supplement such patients with pancreatic enzyme replacement therapy.

There are no adequate or well-controlled studies on pancreatic enzyme replacement therapy in lactation.[1] But considering that the oral bioavailability of this product is negligible,[1] it can be presumed that none to minimal amounts get transferred into breastmilk. Further, the high molecular weight of the individual constituents of this product also makes the possibility of transfer into human milk highly unlikely. Therefore, pancreatic enzyme replacement therapy is considered compatible with breastfeeding.

Pregnancy Risk	C	Lactation Risk	L3
T ½	= Amylase/lipase/protease: 3 hours/7–13 hours	M/P	=
Vd	=	PB	=
Tmax	= 30 min	Oral	= Negligible
MW	= Amylase/lipase/protease: 50,000/47,000/43,000	pKa	=

Adult Concerns: Rash, urticaria, abdominal pain, abdominal cramping, flatulence, diarrhea, nausea, vomiting, headache, dizziness, fatigue. Contra-indicated in those with pork allergy since the product constituents are porcine-derived.[1]

Pediatric Concerns:

Drug Interactions: Co-administration with acarbose and miglitol decreases their efficacy. Concomitant use with folic acid decreases folate absorption

Relative Infant Dose:

Adult Dose: 500–2500 lipase units/kg/meal. Do not exceed 6000 lipase units/ kg/meal

Alternatives:

References:
1. Product Information: Pancreaze(Tm) delayed-release oral capsules, pancrelipase delayed-release oral capsules. McNeil Pediatrics, Titusville, NJ, 2010.

PANTOPRAZOLE   L1

Trade: Protonix

Other Trades: Pantoloc

Category: Suppresses gastric acid production

Pantoprazole is a proton-pump inhibitor similar to omeprazole. It is used primarily to suppress acid production in the stomach for treatment of gastroesophageal reflux or peptic ulcer disease. The pharmaceutical manufacturer reports 0.02% of an administered dose is excreted into milk.[1]

In a 61.6 kg patient who received a single 40 mg tablet, pantoprazole levels in milk were undetectable except at 2 hours (0.036 mg/L) and 4 hours (0.024 mg/L) after administration.[2] The pantoprazole levels in milk were estimated to be only 2.8% of the maternal plasma levels (AUC) so the M/P ratio is extraordinarily low. Using the highest concentration achieved, the relative infant dose would only be 0.95%. The daily dose would be many times lower than this as the milk levels were undetectable at 5 hours. As with all the proton-pump inhibitors, pantoprazole is completely unstable in an acid milieu and when presented in milk, it would be largely destroyed before absorption.

Pregnancy Risk	B	Lactation Risk	L1
T ½	= 1.5 hours	M/P	= 0.028
Vd	= 0.32 l/kg	PB	= 98%
Tmax	= 2–4 hours	Oral	= 77% enteric-coated
MW	= 383	pKa	= 3.8

Adult Concerns: Headache, diarrhea, flatulence, and rash.

Pediatric Concerns: None reported via milk.

Drug Interactions: None reported.

Relative Infant Dose: 1%

Adult Dose: 40–80 mg daily.

Alternatives: Omeprazole

References:
1. Pharmaceutical manufacturer prescribing information, 2003.
2. Plante L, Ferron GM, Unruh M, Mayer PR. Excretion of pantoprazole in human breast. J Reprod Med 2004 Oct; 49(10): 825–7.

PANTOTHENIC ACID   L1

Trade:

Other Trades:

Category: Vitamin B$_5$

Pantothenic acid, or vitamin B$_5$, is needed to form coenzyme-A, which is a carrier carbon within the cell. Pantothenic acid is often used in high doses in excess of 10 gm/day for the treatment of acne.[1] The recommended daily allowance for pregnant women is 6 mg/day, while breastfeeding women need 7 mg/day. The recommended dose for infants less than 6 months is 1.7 mg/day, while infants over 6 months are to receive 2 mg/day. No adverse effects from oral administration of higher oral dosages of pantothenic acid were found.[3] Concentrations found in milk are between 2 and 2.5 mg/L, with a weak correlation between maternal intake and milk levels.[2] This would correspond to a daily dose of around 0.33–0.375 mg/kg/day for breastfeeding infants.

Pregnancy Risk	A/C if dose exceeds RDA	Lactation Risk	L1
T ½	=	M/P	=
Vd	=	PB	=
Tmax	=	Oral	=
MW	= 219	pKa	= 4.4

Adult Concerns: Diarrhea at large doses. Skin rash.

Pediatric Concerns: Possible skin rash, or gastrointestinal symptoms including diarrhea if large doses are used by the mother.

Drug Interactions:

Relative Infant Dose:

Adult Dose:

Alternatives:

References:
1. Leung LH. Pantothenic acid deficiency as the pathogenesis of acne vulgaris. Med Hypotheses 1995 Jun; 44(6): 490–492.
2. Picciano MF. Handbook of milk composition. Jensen RG, ed. San Diego: Academic Press; 1995.
3. Dietary Reference Intakes for Thiamin, Riboflavin, Niacin, Vitamin B$_6$, Folate, Vitamin B$_{12}$, Pantothenic Acid, Biotin, and Choline. Food and Nutrition Board. Institude of Medicine. Washington DC: National Academy Press; 1998.

PARAMETHADIONE   L3

Trade: Paradione
Other Trades:
Category: Anticonvulsant

Paramethadione is a oxazolindinedione compound used for the treatment of seizures. It has strong sedative side effects and could induce ataxia and other sedation-related problems. There are no adequate and well-controlled studies or case reports in breastfeeding women.

Pregnancy Risk	D		Lactation Risk	L3
T ½	= 14 days		M/P	=
Vd	=		PB	=
Tmax	=		Oral	=
MW	= 157.2		pKa	=

Adult Concerns: Increase or decrease in blood pressure, rash, hair loss, nausea, vomiting, anemia, agranulocytosis, neutropenia, systemic lupus erythematosus, lymphadenopathy, myasthenia gravis, drowsiness, malaise, tonic-clonic seizure, visual disturbance, nephrotoxicity.

Pediatric Concerns:

Drug Interactions: Reduced efficacy when coadministered with evening primrose, gingko, naproxen and ketorolac.

Relative Infant Dose:

Adult Dose: 900–2400 mg 3–4 times daily

Alternatives: Valproic acid, ethosuximide, carbamazepine

References:

PARECOXIB   L3

Trade:
Other Trades: Dynastat, Rayzon, Xapit, Bextra iv/im
Category: Analgesic

Parecoxib is a parenteral cyclo-oxygenase-2 (COX-2) inhibitor indicated for the relief of post-operative pain. It is available in both intra-muscular and intra-venous formulations. Parecoxib is a prodrug for valdecoxib. Following parenteral administration, almost all of the drug is metabolized to valdecoxib, such that valdecoxib attains peak plasma concentrations with in 1 hour post-dose. Although the half-life of parecoxib lasts barely 22 minutes, the half-life of its active metabolite valdecoxib is 8–11 hours. The peak plasma concentrations of valdecoxib achieved after IM administration are similar to those following IV administration, therefore the efficacy of the drug following either administration is similar. In one reported study, 40 women were administered 40 mg IV parecoxib within 41 hours following birth for the relief of post-cesarean pain.[1] Breastmilk samples and plasma samples were obtained from these women over the subsequent 24 hours. The median milk/plasma ratios for parecoxib and its active metabolite, valdecoxib, were 0.5 and 0.14 respectively. The absolute infant doses (AID) were 0.24 µg/kg/day and 1.82 µg/kg/day for parecoxib and valdecoxib respectively, with their respective relative infant doses (RID) being 0.04% and 0.47%. The combined AID of both drugs following a single 40 mg IV dose of parecoxib was found to be approximately 2.1 µg/kg/day with a combined RID of 0.4%. The half-life of valdecoxib in milk was reported to be 8.5 hours. No untoward effects were noted in the infants. The authors of this study conclude that parecoxib administered for alleviation of post-cesarean pain is probably compatible with breastfeeding.

Therefore, although parecoxib and its active metabolite valdecoxib do transfer into breastmilk, they do so in minimal quantities. Nonetheless, since this drug has a sulfonamide group in its chemical structure, some caution is advised in the newborn and premature infants due to the increased risk of hemorrhage and kernicterus.

Pregnancy Risk	Probably Safe	Lactation Risk	L3
T ½	= 22 min (parecoxib), 8–10 hours (valdecoxib)	M/P	= 0.5
Vd	= 55 L l/kg	PB	= 98%
Tmax	= 30 min (parecoxib), 1 hour (valdecoxib)	Oral	=
MW	=	pKa	=

Adult Concerns: Peripheral edema, skin rash, abdominal pain, nausea, vomiting, upper respiratory infection. Some of the serious but rare side-effects include anaphylactic reactions, hepatitis, life-threatening skin reactions such as Stevens-Johnson syndrome, toxic epidermal necrolysis, myocardial infarction, strokes, deep vein thrombosis, pulmonary embolism. This drug is contra-indicated in those with known hypersensitivity to other sulfonamides, aspirin, NSAIDs. Contra-indicated for the relief of post-operative pain following coronary artery bypass graft (CABG).

Pediatric Concerns:

Drug Interactions: Increased risk of bleeding when used with venlafaxine, desvenlafaxine, duloxetine, milnacipran, aspirin, warfarin. Concomitant use with fluconazole and itraconazole causes increased plasma levels of valdecoxib. Co-administration with phenytoin decreases the plasma levels of valdecoxib. Concomitant use increases the plasma levels of the following drugs: warfarin, diazepam, glyburide, norethindrone, ethinyl estradiol, probably other oral contraceptives, omeprazole, dextromethorphan. Co-administration with ACE-inhibitors, furosemide, and lithium decreases their plasma concentrations and efficacy.

Relative Infant Dose: 0.4%

Adult Dose: 20–40 mg.

Alternatives:

References:

1. Paech MJ, Salman S, Ilett KF, O'Halloran SJ, Muchatuta NA. Transfer ofParecoxib and Its Primary Active Metabolite Valdecoxib via TransitionalBreastmilk Following Intravenous Parecoxib Use After Cesarean Delivery: AComparison of Naive Pooled Data Analysis and Nonlinear Mixed-Effects Modeling.Anesth Analg. 2012 Feb 17.

PAREGORIC   L3

Trade: Camphorated tincture of opium

Other Trades:

Category: Opiate analgesic used for diarrhea.

Paregoric is camphorated tincture of opium, and contains approximately 2 mg morphine per 5cc (teaspoonful) in 45% alcohol.[1] It is frequently used for diarrhea and in the past for withdrawal symptoms in neonates (Tincture of Opium is now preferred). The active ingredient in paregoric is morphine. Morphine is a potent narcotic analgesic. In a group of 5 lactating women, the highest morphine concentration in breastmilk following two epidural doses was only 82 µg/L at 30 minutes.[2] The highest breastmilk level following 15 mg IV/IM was only 0.5 mg/L although it dropped to almost 0.01 mg/L in 4 hours. In this study and following two 4 mg epidural doses, the peak milk level was 82 µg/L or a relative infant dose of 9.1%. In another study of women receiving morphine via PCA pumps for 12–48 hours postpartum, the concentration of morphine in breastmilk ranged from 50–60 µg/L.[3] None of the infants in this study were neurobehaviorally delayed at 3 days. Because of the poor oral bioavailability of morphine (26%) it is unlikely these levels would be clinically relevant in a stable breastfeeding infant. Infants under 1 month of age have a prolonged elimination half-life and decreased clearance of morphine relative to older infants. The clearance of morphine and its elimination begins to approach adult values by 2 months of age. In summary, morphine is probably the preferred opiate in breastfeeding mothers primarily due to its poor oral bioavailability. However, high doses over prolonged periods could lead to sedation and respiratory problems in newborn infants.

Due to its camphor content, the pediatric use of paregoric is discouraged but it is probably OK in breastfeeding mothers.

Pregnancy Risk	B	Lactation Risk	L3
T ½	= 1.5–2 hours	M/P	= 1.1–3.6
Vd	=	PB	= 35%
Tmax	= 0.5–1 hours	Oral	= 26%
MW	=	pKa	=

Adult Concerns: Sedation, constipation, apnea, nausea, vomiting.

Pediatric Concerns: None reported.

Drug Interactions: Do not use in combination with other CNS depressants such as other opioids (oxycodone, hydrocodone, hydromorphone, codeine), barbiturates (phenobarbital), benzodiazepines (carbamazepine, phenytoin).

Relative Infant Dose:

Adult Dose: 5–10 mL (2–4 mg morphine) 2–4 times daily.

Alternatives:

References:

1. Facts and Comparisons. St. Louis: 2010..
2. Feilberg VL, Rosenborg D, Broen CC, Mogensen JV. Excretion of morphine in human breast milk. Acta Anaesthesiol Scand 1989; 33(5): 426–428.
3. Wittels B, Scott DT, Sinatra RS. Exogenous opioids in human breast milk and acute neonatal neurobehavior: a preliminary study. Anesthesiology 1990; 73(5): 864–869.

PARICALCITOL   L3

Trade: Zemplar

Other Trades:

Category: Vitamin D analog

Paricalcitol is a vitamin D analog used in the treatment and prevention of hyperparathyroidism due to chronic kidney disease.[1] It is similar in structure to the active metabolite of vitamin D, calcitriol. There are currently no studies on the transfer of paricalcitol into human milk. It is known to be secreted in the milk of lactating rats.[2] The peak plasma concentrations attained after its oral administration in patients with chronic kidney disease was in the order of 0.06–0.11 ng/mL. Due to its very high protein binding and low plasma concentrations, it is unlikely that significant amounts would enter breastmilk. Besides this, vitamin D transfers only minimally into human milk. While levels of vitamin D are normally quite low in human milk (<20 IU/L), at least one study now suggests that supplementing a mother with extraordinarily high levels of vitamin D_2 can elevate milk levels, and subsequently lead to hypercalcemia in a breastfed infant.[3] The same may be true with the use of paricalcitol. Therefore, while this drug is probably safe if used in clinical doses, the effects of long term exposure to this drug are currently unknown. Use of excessive doses should be avoided.

Pregnancy Risk	C	Lactation Risk	L3
T ½	= 14–20 hours (in chronic kidney disease)	M/P	=
Vd	= 44–46 L l/kg	PB	= >99.8%
Tmax	= 3 hours	Oral	= 72%-86%
MW	= 416.64	pKa	=

Adult Concerns: Nausea, vomiting, diarrhea, edema, hypertension, hypercalcemia, hyperphosphatemia, hypercalciuria, gastrointestinal hemorrhage, hypersensitivity reaction. Its use is contra-indicated in the presence of hypercalcemia or vitamin D toxicity.

Pediatric Concerns:

Drug Interactions: Digitalis toxicity may occur with its use. Concomitant use of ketoconazole may cause an increase in plasma levels of paricalcitol. Use with cholestyramine or mineral oil may decrease gastrointestinal absorption of paricalcitol. Chronic concomitant us of aluminum antacids or aluminum phosphate binders may cause aluminum bone toxicity.

Relative Infant Dose:

Adult Dose: 1–2 µg daily or 2–4 µg three times a week.

Alternatives:

References:

1. Pharmaceutical manufacturer prescribing information, 2011.
2. Product Information: Zemplar(R), paricalcitol capsules. Abbott Laboratories, North Chicago, IL, 2005.
3. Greer FR, Hollis BW, Napoli JL. High concentrations of vitamin D_2 in human milk associated with pharmacologic doses of vitamin D_2. J Pediatr 1984; 105(1): 61–64.

PAROMOMYCIN   L3

Trade: Paromomycin

Other Trades: Humatin

Category: Amebicide

Paromomycin is an aminoglycoside antibiotic used to treat acute and chronic intestinal amebiasis. It interferes with bacterial protein synthesis by binding to the 30S ribosomal subunits.[1] Paromomycin is not systemically absorbed after oral ingestion and therefore poses little risk to a breastfeeding infant. It has dosing recommendations for pediatric use. It has a large molecular weight and levels in milk are likely low.

Pregnancy Risk	C		Lactation Risk	L3
T ½	=		M/P	=
Vd	=		PB	=
Tmax	=		Oral	= Nil
MW	= 615		pKa	= 5.74, 7.55

Adult Concerns: Adverse reactions include diarrhea, abdominal cramps, nausea, vomiting, and heartburn.

Pediatric Concerns: No data available.

Drug Interactions: Paromomycin decreases the effects of digoxin, vitamin A, and methotrexate. It increases the effects of anticoagulants, neuromuscular blockers, and polypeptide antibiotics.

Relative Infant Dose:

Adult Dose: 25–35 mg/kg/day in 3 divided doses for 5–10 days.

Alternatives:

References:

1. Pharmaceutical manufacturer prescribing information, 2001.

PAROXETINE   L2

Trade: Paxil

Other Trades: Aropax 20, Paxil, Seroxat

Category: Antidepressant, serotonin reuptake inhibitor

Paroxetine is a typical serotonin reuptake inhibitor. Although it undergoes hepatic metabolism, the metabolites are not active. Paroxetine is exceedingly lipophilic and distributes throughout the body with only 1% remaining in plasma. In one case report of a mother receiving 20 mg/day paroxetine at steady state[1], the breastmilk level at peak (4 hours) was 7.6 µg/L. While the maternal paroxetine dose was 333 µg/kg, the maximum daily dose to the infant was estimated at 1.14 µg/kg or 0.34% of the maternal dose.

In two studies of 6 and 4 nursing mothers respectively[2], the mean dose of paroxetine received by the infants in the first study was 1.13% (range 0.5–1.7) of the weight adjusted maternal dose. The mean M/P (AUC) was 0.39 (range 0.32–0.51) while the predicted M/P was 0.22. In the second study, the mean dose of paroxetine received by the infants was 1.25% (range 0.38–2.24%) of the weight adjusted maternal dose with a mean M/P of 0.96 (range 0.31–3.33). The drug was not detected in the plasma of 7 of the 8 infants studied and was detected (<4 mg/L) in only one infant. No adverse effects were observed in any of the infants.

In a recent study of 16 mothers by Stowe, paroxetine levels in milk were low and varied according to maternal dose.[3] Milk/plasma ratios varied from 0.056 to 1.3. Milk levels ranged from approximately 17 µg/L, 45 µg/L, 70 µg/L, 92 µg/L, and 101 µg/L in mothers receiving a dose of 10, 20, 30, 40, and 50 mg/day respectively. Levels of paroxetine were below the limit of detection (<2 ng/mL) in all 16 infants.

In a study of 6 women receiving 20–40 mg/day, the milk/plasma ratio ranged from 0.39 to 1.11 but averaged 0.69.[4] The average estimated dose to the infants ranged from 0.7 to 2.9% of the weight-adjusted maternal dose. In a seventh patient, and based on area-under-the-curve data, the milk/plasma ratio was 0.69 at a dose of 20 mg and 0.72 at a dose of 40 mg/day. The estimated dose to the infant was 1.0% and 2.0% of the weight-adjusted maternal dose at 20 and 40 mg respectively. Paroxetine levels in milk averaged 44.3 and 78.5 µg/L over 6 hours following 20 and 40 mg doses respectively. No adverse reactions or unusual behaviors were noted in any of the infants.

In another study of 24 breastfeeding mothers who received an average dose of 17.6 mg/day (range 10–40 mg/day) the average level of paroxetine in maternal serum and milk was 45.2 ng/mL and 19.2 ng/mL respectively.[5] The average milk/plasma ratio was 0.53. The authors estimated the average infant dose to be 2.88 µg/kg/day or 2.88% of the weight-adjusted maternal dose. All infant serum levels were below the limit of detection.

Yet another study of 16 mothers taking an average of 18.75 mg/day showed that paroxetine was undetectable in any of the breastfeeding infants exposed to paroxetine.[6] A pooled analysis of 68 breastfeeding mothers taking between 10–50 mg/day reported breastmilk levels between 0–153 µg/mL, with an average of 28 µg/mL. No untoward effects were noted in any of these infants exposed to paroxetine through breastmilk. One infant did experience lethargy and poor weight gain, but this infant had prenatal exposure.[7]

These studies generally conclude that paroxetine can be considered relatively 'safe' for breastfeeding infants as the absolute dose transferred is quite low. Plasma levels in the infant were generally undetectable. Recent data suggests that a neonatal withdrawal syndrome may occur in newborns exposed in utero to paroxetine[8,9] although there is significant difficulty in differentiating between withdrawal and toxicity.[10] Symptoms include jitteriness, vomiting, irritability, hypoglycemia, and necrotizing enterocolitis. Suicidal ideation and withdrawal symptoms seem worse with this product and it should not be used in adolescent patients due to the risk of suicide. In addition, the Swedish birth registries have found that pregnant women who consumed paroxetine were 1.5–2.0 times more likely to give birth to a baby with severe heart defects. Paroxetine is no longer recommended by some for use in pregnancy. While all of these complications may arise in pregnancy and in adolescents, paroxetine is still a suitable SSRI for breastfeeding women simply because the clinical dose consumed by the infant via breastmilk is exceedingly low. This said, it is still probably smart to use sertraline or another SSRI at this time.

Pregnancy Risk	D	Lactation Risk	L2
T ½	= 21 hours	M/P	= 0.056–1.3
Vd	= 3–28 l/kg	PB	= 95%
Tmax	= 5–8 hours	Oral	= Complete
MW	= 329	pKa	= 9.9

Adult Concerns: Sedation, headache, dry mouth, dizziness, nausea, insomnia, constipation, seizures. Use in children and adolescents suggests increased risk of suicide. New data may suggest an increased risk of congenital malformations if this product is used during the first trimester. Some caution is recommended.

Pediatric Concerns: Numerous studies suggest minimal to no effect on breastfed infants. A neonatal withdrawal effect (early postnatally) may occur following in utero exposure. Most studies show minimal to no plasma levels in breastfed infants. Severe heart defects have been reported in infants exposed in utero to paroxetine.

Drug Interactions: Decreased effect with phenobarbital and phenytoin. Increased toxicity with alcohol, cimetidine, MAO inhibitors (serotonergic syndrome). Increased effect with fluoxetine, tricyclic antidepressants, sertraline, phenothiazines, warfarin.

Relative Infant Dose: 1.2%–2.8%

Adult Dose: 20–50 mg daily.

Alternatives: Sertraline

References:
1. Spigset O, Carleborg L, Norstrom A, Sandlund M. Paroxetine level in breast milk. J Clin Psychiatry 1996; 57(1): 39.
2. Begg EJ, Duffull SB, Saunders DA, Buttimore RC, Ilett KF, Hackett LP, Yapp P, Wilson DA. Paroxetine in human milk. Br J Clin Pharmacol 1999; 48(2): 142–147.
3. Stowe ZN, Cohen LS, Hostetter A, Ritchie JC, Owens MJ, Nemeroff CB. Paroxetine in human breast milk and nursing infants. Am J Psychiatry 2000; 157(2): 185–189.

4. Ohman R, Hagg S, Carleborg L, Spigset O. Excretion of paroxetine into breast milk. J Clin Psychiatry 1999; 60(8): 519–523.
5. Misri S, Kim J, Riggs KW, Kostaras X. Paroxetine levels in postpartum depressed women, breast milk, and infant serum. J Clin Psychiatry 2000; 61(11): 828–832.
6. Hendrick V, Fukuchi A, Altshuler L, Widawski M, Wertheimer A, Brunhuber MV. Use of sertraline, paroxetine and fluvoxamine by nursing women. Br J Psychiatry 2001; 179: 163–166.
7. Weissman AM, Levy BT, Hartz AJ, et.al. Pooled Analysis of Antidepressant Levels in Lactating Mothers, Breast Milk, and Nursing Infants. Am J Psychiatry 2004 June; 161(6): 1066–1078.
8. Stiskal JA, Kulin N, Koren G, Ho T, Ito S. Neonatal paroxetine withdrawal syndrome. Arch Dis Child Fetal Neonatal Ed 2001; 84(2): F134–F135.
9. Nordeng H, Lindemann R, Perminov KV, Reikvam A. Neonatal withdrawl syndrome after in utero exposure to selective serotonin reuptake inhibitors. Acta Paediatr 2001; 90: 288–91.
10. Isbister GK, Dawson A, Whyte IM, Prior FH, Clancy C, Smith AJ. Neonatal paroxetine withdrawal syndrome or actually serotonin syndrome? Arch Dis Child Fetal Neonatal Ed 2001; 85(2): F147–F148.

PAZOPANIB   L5

Trade: Votrient

Other Trades:

Category: Anticancer drug

Pazopanib is a multi-tyrosine kinase inhibitor of vascular endothelial growth factor receptor. It profoundly blocks angiogenesis and could be profoundly hazardous to a newborn infant. No data are available on its transfer into human milk, but it should be expected to enter milk in low levels.[1] Withhold breastfeeding for 150 hours. Discard milk during this time.

Pregnancy Risk	D	Lactation Risk	L5
T ½	= 31 hours	M/P	=
Vd	=	PB	= >99%
Tmax	= 2–4 hours	Oral	= Good
MW	= 473	pKa	=

Adult Concerns: Diarrhea, hypertension, hair color change, nausea, fatigue, anorexia, and vomiting. Potentially serious adverse reactions include hepatotoxicity, QT prolongation and torsades de pointes, hemorrhagic events, arterial thrombotic events, and gastrointestinal perforation and fistula.

Pediatric Concerns:

Drug Interactions: Co-administration of pazopanib with the following may increase the plasma levels of pazopanib: ketoconazole, ritonavir, clarithromycin, grapefruit juice. Co-administration of pazopanib with the following decreases efficacy and plasma levels of pazopanib: rifampin.

Relative Infant Dose:

Adult Dose: 800 mg once daily.

Alternatives:

References:
1. Pharmaceutical manufacturer prescribing information, 2010.
2. Product Information: VOTRIENT(R) oral tablets, pazopanib oral tablets. GlaxoSmithKline, Research Triangle Park, NC, 2009.

PECTIN   L3

Trade:
Other Trades:
Category: Cough drop

Pectin is a purified polymerized carbohydrate obtained from citrus fruits. Pectin is used as a counter irritant in cough drops.[1] Pectin is not absorbed following oral use. It would not be orally absorbed or be transferred into human milk.

Pregnancy Risk	Probably Safe	Lactation Risk	L3
T ½	=	M/P	=
Vd	=	PB	=
Tmax	=	Oral	= Not absorbed
MW	=	pKa	=

Adult Concerns: Adverse effect in combination with fibers and guar gum: gas, diarrhea, loose stool.

Pediatric Concerns:

Drug Interactions:

Relative Infant Dose:

Adult Dose:

Alternatives:

References:
1. Pharmaceutical manufacturer prescribing information, 2010.

PEGAPTANIB SODIUM   L3

Trade: Macugen
Other Trades: Macugen
Category: Angiogenesis inhibitor

Pegaptanib is used in the treatment of neovascular age-related macular degeneration. Pegaptanib can bind to vascular endothelial growth factor inhibiting its binding with receptors and thus blocking neovascularization (inhibits intravitreal antivascular endothelial growth factor (VEGF)) and slows vision loss.[1] There have been no studies performed to measure the levels in human milk. First, the dose use for intravitreous injections is exceedingly low (0.3 mg), and levels in the plasma compartment are even lower (approximately 8 nanogram/mL). It would be exceedingly unlikely this large polymer would ever enter the milk compartment, or be orally bioavailable, or produce a clinical effect on a breastfeeding infant.

Pregnancy Risk	B		Lactation Risk	L3
T ½	= 10 days		M/P	=
Vd	=		PB	=
Tmax	=		Oral	= Nil
MW	= 50,000		pKa	=

Adult Concerns: Adverse effects include hypertension, blurred vision, corneal edema

Pediatric Concerns: No data are available.

Drug Interactions:

Relative Infant Dose:

Adult Dose: 0.3 mg every 6 weeks.

Alternatives:

References:
1. Pharmaceutical manufacturer prescribing information, 2005.

PEGFILGRASTIM   L3

Trade: Neulasta
Other Trades:
Category: Colony stimulating factor

Pegfilgrastim, the pegylated form of filgrastim, acts on hematopoietic cells stimulating production and maturation of neutrophil precursors. It is used to enhance neutrophil recovery following chemotherapy as well as to decrease infection in patients receiving myelosuppressive anti-cancer drugs.[1] There are no reported levels in human milk. Due to large molecular weight of this drug, milk levels and oral bioavailability are likely to be low. Lactation studies in rodents did not show any untoward effects on growth and development of breastfed rodents.

Pregnancy Risk	C		Lactation Risk	L3
T ½	= 15–80 hours		M/P	=
Vd	=		PB	=
Tmax	=		Oral	= Nil
MW	= 39,000		pKa	=

Adult Concerns: Adverse reactions include bone pain, alopecia, diarrhea, pyrexia, myalgia and headache. Rare cases of splenic rupture have been reported.

Pediatric Concerns: No data are available. Due to its large molecular weight, it is unlikely to enter milk in clinically relevant concentrations. No problems were noted in rodent lactation study.

Drug Interactions: Lithium may increase the expected levels of white blood cells.

Relative Infant Dose:

Adult Dose: 6 mg once per chemotherapy cycle.

Alternatives:

References:
1. Pharmaceutical manufacturer prescribing information, 2007.

PENCICLOVIR   L3

Trade: Denavir

Other Trades: Vectavir

Category: Antiviral agent

Penciclovir is an antiviral agent for the treatment of cold sores (herpes simplex labialis) of the lips and face and occasionally for herpes zoster (shingles).[1] Following topical administration, plasma levels are undetectable.[2] Because oral bioavailability is nil and maternal plasma levels are undetectable following topical therapy, it is extremely unlikely that detectable amounts would transfer into human milk or be absorbable by an infant.

Pregnancy Risk	B	Lactation Risk	L3
T ½	= 2.3 hours	M/P	=
Vd	=	PB	= <20%
Tmax	=	Oral	= 1.5%
MW	=	pKa	=

Adult Concerns: Following topical application only mild erythema was occasionally observed.

Pediatric Concerns: None reported.

Drug Interactions: None reported.

Relative Infant Dose:

Adult Dose: Topical application every 2 hours.

Alternatives:

References:
1. Hodge RA, Perkins RM. Mode of action of 9–(4-hydroxy-3-hydroxymethylbut-1-yl)guanine (BRL 39123) against herpes simplex virus in MRC-5 cells. Antimicrob Agents Chemother 1989; 33(2): 223–229.
2. Pharmaceutical manufacturer prescribing information, 2011.

PENICILLAMINE   L4

Trade: Cuprimine, Depen

Other Trades: D-Penamine, Cuprimine, Depen, Distamine, Pendramine

Category: Used in arthritis, autoimmune syndromes

Penicillamine is a potent chelating agent used to chelate copper, iron, mercury, lead, and other metals. It is also used to suppress the immune response in rheumatoid arthritis and other immunologic syndromes. It is extremely dangerous during pregnancy. Safety has not been established during lactation, but kinetics suggest it will enter milk significantly. Penicillamine is a potent drug that requires constant observation and care by attending physicians. Recommend discontinuing lactation if this drug is mandatory.[1]

Pregnancy Risk	D	Lactation Risk	L4
T ½	= 1.7–3.2 hours	M/P	=
Vd	=	PB	=
Tmax	= 1 hour	Oral	= Complete
MW	= 149	pKa	= 10.5

Adult Concerns: Anorexia, nausea, vomiting, diarrhea, alteration of taste, elevated liver enzymes, kidney damage.

Pediatric Concerns: None reported, but caution is recommended.

Drug Interactions: An increased risk of serious hematologic and renal reactions may occur if used with gold therapy, antimalarial, or other cytotoxic drugs. The absorption of penicillamine is decreased by 35% when used with iron salts. The absorption of penicillamine is decreased by 66% when used with antacids. Digoxin plasma levels may be reduced.

Relative Infant Dose:

Adult Dose: 250–500 mg four times daily.

Alternatives:

References:
1. Ostensen M, Husby G. Antirheumatic drug treatment during pregnancy and lactation. Scand J Rheumatol 1985; 14(1): 1–7.

PENICILLIN G   L1

Trade: Pfizerpen

Other Trades: Crystapen, Megacillin, Bicillin L-A, Ayercillin

Category: Antibiotic

Penicillins generally penetrate into breastmilk in small concentrations which is largely determined by class. Following IM doses of 100,000 units, the milk/plasma ratios varied between 0.03–0.13.[1,2] Milk levels varied from 7 units to 60 units/L. Possible side effects in infants would include alterations in gastrointestinal flora or allergic responses in a hypersensitive infant. Compatible with breastfeeding in non-hypersensitive infants.

Pregnancy Risk	B	Lactation Risk	L1
T ½	= <1.5 hours	M/P	= 0.03–0.13
Vd	=	PB	= 60–80%
Tmax	= 1–2 hours	Oral	= 15–30%
MW	= 372	pKa	= 2.75

Adult Concerns: Changes in gastrointestinal flora, allergic rashes.

Pediatric Concerns: None reported via milk, but observe for changes in gastrointestinal flora, diarrhea.

Drug Interactions: Probenecid may increase penicillin levels. Tetracyclines may decrease penicillin effectiveness.

Relative Infant Dose:

Adult Dose: 1.2–2.4 million units daily.

Alternatives:

References:
1. Matsuda S. Transfer of antibiotics into maternal milk. Biol Res Pregnancy Perinatol 1984; 5(2): 57–60.
2. Greene H, Burkhart B, Hobby G. Excretion of penicillin human milk following partiturition. Am J Obstet Gynecol 1946; 51: 732.

PENTAZOCINE   L3

Trade: Talwin, Talacen
Other Trades: Fortral, Talwin
Category: Analgesic

Pentazocine is a synthetic opiate and is also an opiate antagonist. Once absorbed it undergoes extensive hepatic metabolism and only small amounts achieve plasma levels.[1] It is primarily used as a mild analgesic. No data are available on transfer into breastmilk.

Pregnancy Risk	C	Lactation Risk	L3
T ½	= 2–3 hours	M/P	=
Vd	= 4.4–7.8 l/kg	PB	= 60%
Tmax	= 1–3 hours	Oral	= 18%
MW	= 285	pKa	= 9.0

Adult Concerns: Sedation, respiratory depression, nausea, vomiting, dry mouth, taste alteration.

Pediatric Concerns: None reported due to limited studies.

Drug Interactions: May reduce the analgesic effect of other opiate agonists such as morphine. Increased toxicity when used with tripelennamine can be lethal. Increased toxicity when used with CNS depressants such as phenothiazines, sedatives, hypnotics, or alcohol.

Relative Infant Dose:

Adult Dose: 50–100 mg every 3–4 hours PRN.

Alternatives:

References:
1. McEvoy GE. (ed): AFHS Drug Information. New York, NY: 2003.

PENTOBARBITAL   L3

Trade: Nembutol

Other Trades: Barbopen, Carbrital, Nembutal, Nova-Rectal, Novo-Pentobarb, Lethobarb

Category: Sedative, hypnotic.

Pentobarbital is a short acting barbiturate primarily used as a sedative. Following a dose of 100 mg for 3 days early postpartum, the concentration of pentobarbital 19 hours after the last dose was 0.17 mg/L.[1] The effect of short acting barbiturates on the breastfed infant is unknown, but significant tolerance and addiction can occur.[2-4] Use caution if used in large amounts. No reported harmful effects in breastfeeding infants.

Pregnancy Risk	D	Lactation Risk	L3
T ½	= 15–50 hours	M/P	=
Vd	= 0.5–1.0 l/kg	PB	= 35–45%
Tmax	= 30–60 minutes (oral)	Oral	= 95%
MW	= 248	pKa	= 7.9

Adult Concerns: Sedation, respiratory arrest, tachycardia, physical dependence.

Pediatric Concerns: None reported, but observe for sedation, dependence.

Drug Interactions: Barbiturates may decrease the antimicrobial activity of metronidazole. Phenobarbital may significantly reduce the serum levels and half-life of quinidine. Barbiturates decrease theophylline levels. The clearance of verapamil may be increased and its bioavailability decreased.

Relative Infant Dose: 1.8%

Adult Dose: 20–40 mg 2–4 times daily.

Alternatives:

References:

1. Wilson JT, Brown RD, Cherek DR, Dailey JW, Hilman B, Jobe PC, Manno BR, Manno JE, Redetzki HM, Stewart JJ. Drug excretion in human breast milk: principles, pharmacokinetics and projected consequences. Clin Pharmacokinet 1980; 5(1): 1–66.
2. Tyson RM, Shrader EA, Perlman HH. Drugs transmitted through breast milk. II Barbiturates. J Pediatr 1938; 14: 86–90.
3. Kaneko S, Sato T, Suzuki K. The levels of anticonvulsants in breast milk. Br J Clin Pharmacol 1979; 7(6): 624–627.
4. Horning MG. Identification and quantification of drugs and drug metabolites in human milk using GC-MS-COM methods. Mod Probl Pediatr 1975; 15: 73–79.

PENTOSAN POLYSULFATE   L2

Trade: Elmiron
Other Trades: Elmiron
Category: Urinary tract analgesic

Pentosan polysulfate is a negatively-charged synthetic sulfated polysaccharide with heparin-like properties although it is used as a urinary tract analgesic for interstitial cystitis. It is structurally related to dextran sulfate with a molecular weight of 4000–6000 daltons. Oral bioavailability is low, only 6% is absorbed systemically. Pentosan adheres to the bladder wall mucosa and may act as a buffer to control cell permeability preventing irritating solutes in the urine from reaching the cell membrane.[1,2] Although no data are available on its transfer into human milk, its large molecular weight and its poor oral bioavailability would largely preclude the transfer and absorption of clinically relevant amounts in breastfed infants.

Pregnancy Risk	B		Lactation Risk	L2
T ½	= <5 hours		M/P	=
Vd	=		PB	=
Tmax	= 3 hours		Oral	= 3%
MW	= 6000		pKa	=

Adult Concerns: Alopecia areata. Weak anticoagulant ($\frac{1}{15}$th activity of heparin). Mildly hepatotoxic. Headache, depression, insomnia, pruritus, urticaria, diarrhea, nausea, vomiting, etc. have been reported.

Pediatric Concerns: None reported via milk. Unlikely to enter milk.

Drug Interactions: May increase bleeding time when used with cisapride.

Relative Infant Dose:

Adult Dose: 100 mg three times daily.

Alternatives:

References:
1. Wagner WH. Hoe/Bay 946--a new compound with activity against the AIDS virus. Arzneimittelforschung 1989; 39(1): 112–113.
2. Asmal AC, Leary WP, Carboni J, Lockett CJ. The effects of sodium pentosan polysulphate on peripheral metabolism. S Afr Med J 1975; 49(27): 1091–1094.

PENTOSTATIN L5

Trade: Nipent
Other Trades:
Category: Anticancer drug

Pentostatin is indicated for the treatment of untreated and alpha-interferon-refractory hairy cell leukemia. It is poorly bound to proteins (<4%).[1] In humans, the mean terminal half-life is reported to be 5.7 hours, but is increased to 18 hours in patients with poor renal function. No data are available on the transfer of this agent into human milk. Mothers should withhold breastfeeding for a minimum of two days, following exposure to this agent or up to five days if renal function is poor.[1]

Pregnancy Risk	D	Lactation Risk	L5
T ½	= 3–18 hours (mean=5.7 h)	M/P	=
Vd	= 0.5 l/kg	PB	= 4%
Tmax	=	Oral	=
MW	= 268.3	pKa	=

Adult Concerns: Myelosuppression, headache, abdominal pain, fever and chills, diarrhea, nausea, vomiting, hypersensitivity reactions, and hepatotoxicity.

Pediatric Concerns:

Drug Interactions:

Relative Infant Dose:

Adult Dose: 4 mg/m^2.

Alternatives:

References:
1. Pharmaceutical manufacturer prescribing information, 2010.

PENTOXIFYLLINE L2

Trade: Trental
Other Trades: Trental, Apo-Pentoxifylline
Category: Reduces blood viscosity

Pentoxifylline and its metabolites improve the flow properties of blood by decreasing its viscosity. It is a methylxanthine derivative similar in structure to caffeine and is extensively metabolized although the metabolites do not have long half-lives. In a group of 5 breastfeeding women who received a single 400 mg dose, the mean milk/plasma ratio was 0.87 for the parent compound.[1] The milk/plasma ratios for the metabolites were lower: 0.54, 0.76, and 1.13. Average milk concentration at 2 hours following the dose was 73.9 µg/L.

Pregnancy Risk	C	Lactation Risk	L2
T ½	= 0.4–1.6 hours	M/P	=
Vd	=	PB	=
Tmax	= 1 hour	Oral	= Complete
MW	= 278	pKa	=

Adult Concerns: Bleeding, dyspepsia, bloating, diarrhea, nausea, vomiting, bad taste, dyspnea.

Pediatric Concerns: None reported.

Drug Interactions: Bleeding, and prolonged prothrombin times when used with coumarins. Use with other theophylline containing products leads to increased theophylline plasma levels.

Relative Infant Dose: 0.2%

Adult Dose: 400 mg three times a day.

Alternatives:

References:
1. Witter FR, Smith RV. The excretion of pentoxifylline and its metabolites into human breast milk. Am J Obstet Gynecol 1985; 151(8): 1094–1097.

PERFLUTREN PROTEIN TYPE A   L3

Trade: Optison, Definity
Other Trades:
Category: Diagnostic agent

Perflutren protein type A is a unique radiocontrast agent used in patients with suboptimal echocardiograms to make the left ventricular chamber opaque.[1] This product releases perflutren gas molecules that are completely eliminated in the human lung in 10 minutes. Perflutren gas is not metabolized but passes rapidly from the body. Although there are no data on levels in human milk, this product is so rapidly dissipated, that the risk to the infant would be nil. Perflutren lipid microsphere (Definity) is a new formulation of the same gas above. Again, half-life is of about 1.3 minutes.

Pregnancy Risk	C	Lactation Risk	L3
T ½	= 1.3 minutes	M/P	=
Vd	=	PB	=
Tmax	=	Oral	= Nil
MW	=	pKa	=

Adult Concerns: Adverse reactions include flushing, headache, dizziness, nausea, vomiting, and altered taste.

Pediatric Concerns: No data are available.

Drug Interactions:

Relative Infant Dose:

Adult Dose: 0.5 mL IV.

Alternatives:

References:
1.   Pharmaceutical manufacturer prescribing information, 2003.

PERINDOPRIL ERBUMINE   L3

Trade: Aceon

Other Trades: Apo-Perindopril, Coversyl

Category: ACE Inhibitor

Perindopril erbumine is an angiotensin-converting enzyme (ACE) inhibitor that is metabolized to perindoprilat. There are no known studies on perindopril and breastfeeding.[1] However, because of low reported levels in milk with similar ACE inhibitors, it is unlikely that much of the medication will be present in breastmilk. Use of another ACE inhibitor that we have more information on, such as enalapril or captopril, would be preferred.

Pregnancy Risk	D	Lactation Risk	L3
T ½	= 30–120 hours	M/P	=
Vd	= 0.16 l/kg	PB	= 10%-20%
Tmax	= 3–7 hours	Oral	= 25%
MW	= 368.47 (free acid) or 441.61 (salt form)	pKa	=

Adult Concerns: Side effects include cough, dizziness, hypotension, and impaired renal function

Pediatric Concerns:

Drug Interactions: Major drug interactions may occur with alteplase, potassium sparing diuretics, azathioprine, potassium, antacids, allopurinol, cyclosporine, lithium, and rituximab.

Relative Infant Dose:

Adult Dose: 2–8 mg/day.

Alternatives: Enalapril, captopril

References:
1.   Pharmaceutical manufacturer prescribing information, 2007.

PERMETHRIN   L2

Trade: Acticin, Elimite, Nix Creme Rinse, Pronto, A200 Lice Control

Other Trades:

Category: Insecticide, scabicide

Permethrin is a synthetic pyrethroid structure of the natural ester pyrethrum, a natural insecticide, and used to treat lice, mites, and fleas. To use, recommend that the hair be washed with detergent, and then saturated with permethrin liquid for 10 minutes before rinsing with water. One treatment is all that is required. At 14 days, a second treatment may be required if viable lice are seen. Permethrin cream is generally recommended for scabies infestations and should be applied head to toe for 8–12 hours in infants, and body (not head) only in adults. Reapplication may be needed in 7 days if live mites appear.

Permethrin absorption through the skin following application of a 5% cream is reported to be less than 2%.[1] Permethrin is rapidly metabolized by serum and tissue enzymes to inactive metabolites and rapidly excreted in the urine. Overt toxicity is very low. In spite of its rapid metabolism, some residuals are sequestered in fat tissue. In a study done in South Africa, breastmilk concentrations of permethrin was found to be between 1.1–1.6 µg/g milk fat. The source of exposure in this study was the use of indoor insecticide sprays containing permethrin or ingestion of food contaminated with permethrin. The authors suggest that the main route of exposure is probably from ingestion through diet, with some occurring due to skin contact. Inhalation is not recognized as a significant route of exposure to pyrethroids.[2] In another study in South Africa where 152 breastmilk samples were investigated, permethrin was found in 66% (101) of the samples.[3] While most samples were exceedingly low, the highest breastmilk concentration found was 14.51 µg/L. According to the authors, this suggests a daily intake of only 13.6 µg/kg, which is far lower than the set acceptable daily intake (ADI) for permethrin. The ADI for permethrin is 50 µg/kg.[3,4]Another study reported that in five infants whose mothers used permethrin during the breastfeeding period, no adverse reactions were reported.[5]

Therefore, the amounts of permethrin absorbed following topical application is far lower than the amount absorbed following oral exposure in food. Hence, the amounts ingested by the infant through milk is far lower than the acceptable daily intake for permethrin, and would therefore be unlikely to cause any significant clinical effects in the infant. The WHO considers short-term topical use of permethrin as compatible with breastfeeding.[6]

Pregnancy Risk	B		Lactation Risk	L2
T ½	=		M/P	=
Vd	=		PB	=
Tmax	=		Oral	=
MW	= 391		pKa	=

Adult Concerns: Itching, rash, skin irritation. Dyspnea has been reported in one patient.

Pediatric Concerns: None via milk.

Drug Interactions:

Relative Infant Dose:

Adult Dose:

Alternatives:

References:
1. Pharmaceutical manufacturer prescribing information, 2011.

2. Sereda B, Bouwman H, Kylin H. Comparing water, bovine milk, and indoorresidual spraying as possible sources of DDT and pyrethroid residues in breastmilk. J Toxicol Environ Health A. 2009; 72(13): 842–51.
3. Bouwman H, Sereda B, Meinhardt HM. Simultaneous presence of DDT and pyrethroidresidues in human breast milk from a malaria endemic area in South Africa.Environ Pollut. 2006 Dec; 144(3): 902–17. Epub 2006 Mar 24.
4. FAO and WHO. Joint meeting of the panel of experts on pesticide residues. 2005. http: //www.who.int/foodsafety/chem/jmpr/publications/en/index.html.
5. Ito S, Blajchman A, Stephenson M, et al: Prospective follow-up of adverse reactions in breast-fed infants exposed to maternal medication. Am J Obstet Gynecol 1993; 168(5): 1393–1399.
6. Anon: Breastfeeding and Maternal Medication. World Health Organization, Geneva, Switzerland, 2002.

PERPHENAZINE   L3

Trade:

Other Trades: Apo-Perphenazine

Category: Phenothiazine antipsychotic and antidepressant

Perphenazine is a phenothiazine derivative used as an antipsychotic or sedative. In a study of one patient receiving either 16 and 24 mg/day of perphenazine divided in two doses at 12 hour intervals, milk levels were 2.1 µg/L and 3.2 µg/L respectively.[1] The authors estimated the dose to the infant at 1.06 µg (0.3 µg/kg) or 1.59 µg (0.45 µg/kg) respective of dose. Serum perphenazine levels in the mother drawn 12 hours after doses of 16 or 24 mg/day were 2.0 and 4.9 ng/mL respectively. Hence milk/plasma ratios were approximately 1.1 and 0.7 respective of the dose. The authors estimate the dose to be approximately 0.1% of the weight-adjusted maternal dose. The authors report that during a 3 month exposure, the infant thrived and had no adverse response to the medication.

Pregnancy Risk	Probably Safe	Lactation Risk	L3
T ½	= 8–20 hours	M/P	= 0.7–1.1
Vd	=	PB	=
Tmax	=	Oral	= 40%
MW	= 404	pKa	= 7.94

Adult Concerns: Amenorrhea, galactorrhea, dreams, drowsiness, headache, lethargy, bradycardia, ECG changes, anorexia, stomach pain, nausea, hepatotoxicity, blurred vision, glycosuria, nasal congestion.

Pediatric Concerns:

Drug Interactions: The following drugs are contraindicated with perphenazine: grepafloxacin, sparfloxacin, cisapride, droperidol. Avoid the concurrent use of the following drugs: opioid analgesics such as morphine, hydromorphone, fentanyl, fluoroquinolones such as levofloxacin, moxifloxacin, pentamidine, octreotide, lithium, milnacipran. For a complete list, refer a drug interactions reference.

Relative Infant Dose: 0.1%

Adult Dose: 4–8 mg three times daily.

Alternatives:

References:
1. Olesen OV, Bartels U, Poulsen JH. Perphenazine in breast milk and serum. Am J Psychiatry. 1990 Oct; 147(10): 1378–9.

PERTUSSIS VACCINE   L2

Trade:

Other Trades:

Category: Vaccine

There are two types of pertussis vaccine, whole cell and acellular.[1] Whole cell pertussis vaccine is made form inactivated B. pertussis cells. Acellular pertussis vaccines are made from inactivated components of B. pertussis cells. Acellular pertussis vaccines only comes in combination with diphtheria and tetanus vaccines.[2] Because pertussis vaccine is an inactivated bacterial product, there is no specific contraindication in breastfeeding following injection with these vaccine. It is extremely unlikely proteins of this size would be secreted in breastmilk.

While the USA has removed methylmercury from virtually all pediatric immunizations, other countries have not. In infants receiving three doses of hepatitis B vaccine and three DTP vaccines during the first 6 months of life, the exposure to ethylmercury was 25 µg Hg for each vaccine. Infant hair-Hg increased 446% during these six months, while maternal hair-Hg decreased 57%. This provides evidence that the extra mercury exposure is due to the vaccinations rather than maternal milk.[3]

Pregnancy Risk	C	Lactation Risk	L2
T ½	=	M/P	=
Vd	=	PB	=
Tmax	=	Oral	=
MW	=	pKa	=

Adult Concerns: Local injection site reactions, irritability, fever. Rare side effects: encephalopathy, convulsions.

Pediatric Concerns:

Drug Interactions:

Relative Infant Dose:

Adult Dose:

Alternatives:

References:
1. Atkinson W, Wolfe S, Hamborsky J, eds. 2011. Pertussis. "Centers for Disease Control and Prevention. Epidemiology and Prevention of Vaccine-Preventable Diseases". 12th ed. Washington DC: Public Health Foundation.
2. Pharmaceutical manufacturer prescribing information, 2010.
3. Marques, RC, Dorea JG, Fonseca MF, Bastos WR, Malm O. Hair mercury in breast-fed infants exposed to thimerosal-preserved vaccines. Eur J Pediatr 2007; [Epub ahead of print].

PHENAZOPYRIDINE   L3

Trade:
Other Trades:
Category: Urinary tract analgesic

Phenazopyridine hydrochloride is an azo dye that is rapidly excreted in the urine, where it exerts a topical analgesic effect on urinary tract mucosa.[1] Pyridium is only moderately effective and produces a reddish-orange discoloration of the urine. It may also ruin contact lenses. It is not known if Pyridium transfers into breastmilk, but it probably does to a limited degree. This product, due to limited efficacy, should probably not be used in lactating women although it is doubtful that it would be harmful to an infant. This product is highly colored and can stain clothing. Stains can be removed by soaking in a solution of 0.25% sodium dithionite.

Pregnancy Risk	B	Lactation Risk	L3
T ½	=	M/P	=
Vd	=	PB	=
Tmax	=	Oral	= Complete
MW	= 250	pKa	= 5.1

Adult Concerns: Anemia, nausea, vomiting, diarrhea, colored urine, methemoglobinemia, hepatitis, gastrointestinal distress

Pediatric Concerns: None reported via lactation.

Drug Interactions:

Relative Infant Dose:

Adult Dose: 100–200 mg three times daily.

Alternatives:

References:
1. Drug Facts and Comparisons 1994 ed. ed. St. Louis: 1994.

PHENCYCLIDINE   L5

Trade: PCP, Angel Dust
Other Trades:
Category: Hallucinogen

Phencyclidine (PCP), also called Angel Dust, is a potent and extremely dangerous hallucinogen. High concentrations are secreted into breastmilk (>10 times plasma level) of mice.[1] Continued secretion into milk occurs over long periods of time (perhaps months). One patient who consumed PCP 41 days prior to lactating had a milk level of 3.90 µg/L.[2] PCP is extremely dangerous to a nursing infant. PCP is stored for long periods in adipose tissues. Urine samples are positive for 14–30 days in adults and probably longer in infants. The infant could test positive for PCP long after maternal exposure, particularly if breastfeeding. Definitely contraindicated.[3]

Pregnancy Risk	X	Lactation Risk	L5
T ½	= 24–51 hours	M/P	= >10
Vd	= 5.3–7.5 l/kg	PB	= 65%
Tmax	= Immediate	Oral	= Complete
MW	= 243	pKa	= 8.5

Adult Concerns: Hallucinations, psychosis.

Pediatric Concerns: Significant concentrations would likely transfer to infant. Extremely dangerous.

Drug Interactions:

Relative Infant Dose:

Adult Dose:

Alternatives:

References:
1. Nicholas JM, Lipshitz J, Schreiber EC. Phencyclidine: its transfer across the placenta as well as into breast milk. Am J Obstet Gynecol 1982; 143(2): 143–146.
2. Kaufman KR, Petrucha RA, Pitts FN, Jr., Weekes ME. PCP in amniotic fluid and breast milk: case report. J Clin Psychiatry 1983; 44(7): 269–270.
3. American Academy of Pediatrics, Committee on Drugs. Transfer of drugs and other chemicals into human milk. Pediatrics 2001; 108(3): 776–89.

PHENOBARBITAL   L3

Trade: Luminal

Other Trades: Phenobarbitone, Barbilixir, Gardenal

Category: Long acting barbiturate sedative, anticonvulsant

Phenobarbital is a long half-life barbiturate frequently used as an anticonvulsant in adults and during the neonatal period. Its long half-life in infants may lead to significant accumulation and blood levels higher than mother although this is infrequent. During the first 3–4 weeks of life, phenobarbital is poorly absorbed by the neonatal gastrointestinal tract. However, protein binding by neonatal albumin is poor, 36–43%, as compared to the adult, 51%. Thus, the volume of distribution is higher in neonates and the tissue concentrations of phenobarbital may be significantly higher. The half-life in premature infants can be extremely long (100–500 hours) and plasma levels must be closely monitored.

Although varied, milk/plasma ratios vary from 0.46 to 0.6.[1,2,3] In one study, following a dose of 30 mg four times daily, the milk concentration of phenobarbital averaged 2.74 mg/L 16 hours after the last dose.[3] The dose an infant would receive was estimated at 2–4 mg/day.[4] Phenobarbital should be administered with caution and close observation of infant is required, including plasma drug levels. One should generally expect the infant's plasma level to be approximately 30–40% of the maternal level. In some reported cases, the infant plasma levels have reached twice what the maternal plasma levels were, 2.5 hours after the maternal dose.[5] In general, the infant will receive ⅓rd of mother's dose; observe for apnea, sedation. Possibility of withdrawal symptoms such as jitteriness, irritability, crying, sweating may be expected when drug withdrawn. Baby's blood levels should be monitored if mother is on long term therapy.

Pregnancy Risk	D	Lactation Risk	L3
T ½	= 53–140 hours	M/P	= 0.4–0.6
Vd	= 0.5–0.6 l/kg	PB	= 51%
Tmax	= 8–12 hours	Oral	= 80% (Adult)
MW	= 232	pKa	= 7.2

Adult Concerns: Drowsiness, sedation, ataxia, respiratory depression, withdrawal symptoms.

Pediatric Concerns: Phenobarbital sedation has been reported, but is infrequent. Expect infant plasma levels to approximately one-third (or lower) of maternal plasma level. Withdrawal symptoms have been reported.

Drug Interactions: Barbiturates may decrease the antimicrobial activity of metronidazole. Phenobarbital may significantly reduce the serum levels and half-life of quinidine. Barbiturates decrease theophylline levels. The clearance of verapamil may be increased and its bioavailability decreased.

Relative Infant Dose: 24%

Adult Dose: 100–200 mg daily.

Alternatives:

References:
1. Tyson RM, Shrader EA, Perlman HH. Drugs transmitted through breast milk. II Barbiturates. J Pediatr 1938; 14: 86–90.
2. Kaneko S, Sato T, Suzuki K. The levels of anticonvulsants in breast milk. Br J Clin Pharmacol 1979; 7(6): 624–627.
3. Nau H, Kuhnz W, Egger HJ, Rating D, Helge H. Anticonvulsants during pregnancy and lactation. Transplacental, maternal and neonatal pharmacokinetics. Clin Pharmacokinet 1982; 7(6): 508–543.
4. Horning MG. Identification and quantification of drugs and drug metabolites in human milk using GC-MS-COM methods. Mod Probl Pediatr 1975; 15: 73–79.
5. Pote M, Kulkarni R, Agarwal M. Phenobarbital Toxic Levels in a Nursing Neonate. Indian Pediatr 2004; 41: 963–964.

PHENOL   L3

Trade:

Other Trades:

Category: Topical anesthetic

Phenol is used in oral and topical anesthetic.[1] It is caustic at concentration of 5% or greater. There are no adequate and well-controlled studies or case reports on its used topically or in breastfeeding women. Use during lactation only if potential benefit to mother outweighs the potential risks to the infant.

Pregnancy Risk	Probably Safe	Lactation Risk	L3
T ½	= 1–4.5 hours/has increased to 13.86 hours with prolonged exposure	M/P	=
Vd	=	PB	=
Tmax	= 18.8 ± 2.5 min	Oral	=
MW	= 94.11	pKa	= 9.95

Adult Concerns: Vomiting, nausea, epiglottitis, urinary symptom, arrhythmia.

Pediatric Concerns:

Drug Interactions:

Relative Infant Dose:

Adult Dose:

Alternatives:

References:
1. Phenol. In: Reprotox Æ [Internet database]. Greenwood Village, Colo: Thomson Healthcare. Updated periodically. Accessed 06/08/2011.

PHENTERMINE   L4

Trade: Fastin, Zantryl, Ionamin, Adipex-P

Other Trades: Duromine, Ionamin, Ponderax caps

Category: Appetite suppressant

Phentermine is an appetite suppressant structurally similar to the amphetamine family. As such it frequently produces CNS stimulation.[1] No data are available on its transfer to human milk. This product has a very small molecular weight (149) and would probably transfer into human milk in significant quantities and could produce stimulation, anorexia, tremors, and other CNS side effects in the newborn. The use of this product in breastfeeding mothers would be difficult to justify and is not advised.

Pregnancy Risk	C	Lactation Risk	L4
T ½	= 7–20 hours	M/P	=
Vd	=	PB	=
Tmax	= 8 hours	Oral	= Complete
MW	= 149	pKa	= 10.1

Adult Concerns: Hypertension, tachycardia, palpitations, nervousness, tremulousness, insomnia, dizziness, depression, headache, cerebral infarct, paranoid psychosis, heat stroke, nausea, vomiting, physical dependence as evidenced by withdrawal syndrome.

Pediatric Concerns: Growth impairment has been reported from direct use of phentermine in children aged 3–15 years.

Drug Interactions: Decreased effect of guanethidine, CNS depressants. Increased toxicity of MAO inhibitors, other stimulants.

Relative Infant Dose:

Adult Dose: 8 mg three times daily.

Alternatives:

References:
1. Silverstone T. Appetite suppressants. A review. Drugs 1992; 43(6): 820–836.

PHENYLEPHRINE   L3

Trade: Neo-Synephrine, Neofrin, Nostril, Prefrin Liquifilm, Ocu-Phrin, Vicks Sinex, Mydfrin, AK-Dilate

Other Trades:

Category: Decongestant

Phenylephrine is a sympathomimetic agent most commonly used as a nasal decongestant due to its vasoconstrictive properties but also for treatment of ocular uveitis, inflammation, and glaucoma as a mydriatic agent to dilate the pupil during examinations, and for cardiogenic shock.[1] Phenylephrine is a potent adrenergic stimulant and systemic effects (tachycardia, hypertension, arrhythmias), although rare, have occurred following ocular administration in some sensitive individuals. Phenylephrine is most commonly added to cold mixtures and nasal sprays for use in respiratory colds, flu, and congestion. Numerous pediatric formulations are in use and it is generally considered safe in pediatric patients.

Used ophthalmically in eye exams, the maternal dose of the medication would be very low and it is not likely to pose a problem for a breastfeeding infant. Although no data are available on its secretion into human milk, it is probable that very small amounts will be transferred into milk, but due to its poor oral bioavailability (<38%), it is not likely that it would produce clinical effects in a breastfed infant unless the maternal doses were quite high. Because of pseudoephedrine's effect on milk production, concerns that phenylephrine may suppress milk production, have not been confirmed as yet. There is no evidence that this occurs at all.

Pregnancy Risk	C	Lactation Risk	L3
T ½	= 2–3 hours	M/P	=
Vd	= 0.57 l/kg	PB	=
Tmax	= 10–60 minutes	Oral	= 38%
MW	= 203	pKa	= 9.8, 8.8

Adult Concerns: Local ocular irritation, transient tachycardia, hypertension, and sympathetic stimulation.

Pediatric Concerns: None reported via milk.

Drug Interactions: Concomitant use with other sympathomimetics may exacerbate cardiovascular effects of phenylephrine. This includes albuterol, amitriptyline, other tricyclic antidepressants, monoamine oxidase inhibitors, furazolidone, guanethidine, and others. Increased effect when used with oxytocic drugs.

Relative Infant Dose:

Adult Dose: 1–10 mg IM.

Alternatives: Oxymetazoline

References:
1. Pharmaceutical manufacturer prescribing information, 2010.

PHENYLPROPANOLAMINE   L2

Trade:

Other Trades:

Category: Adrenergic, nasal decongestant, anorexiant.

Phenylpropanolamine is an adrenergic compound frequently used in nasal decongestants and also diet pills.[1] It produces significant constriction of nasal mucosa and is a common ingredient in cold preparations. No data are available on its secretion into human milk, but due to its low molecular weight and its rapid entry past the blood-brain-barrier, it should be expected. It has recently been withdrawn from the US market.

Pregnancy Risk	C	Lactation Risk	L2
T ½	= 5.6 hours	M/P	=
Vd	= 4.5 l/kg	PB	= Low
Tmax	= 1 hour	Oral	= 100%
MW	= 188	pKa	= 9.1

Adult Concerns: Hypertension, bradycardia, AV block, arrhythmias, paranoia, seizures, psychosis, tremor, excitement, insomnia, seizures, anorexia and physical dependence.

Pediatric Concerns: None reported via milk but observe for excitement, loss of appetite, insomnia.

Drug Interactions: Hypertensive crisis when admixed with monoamine oxidase inhibitors. Increased toxicity (pressor effects) with beta blockers. Decreased effect of antihypertensives.

Relative Infant Dose:

Adult Dose: 12.5–25 mg every 4–6 hours.

Alternatives:

References:
1. Drug package insert information, 2011.

PHENYLTOLOXAMINE　　　　　　　　　　　L3

Trade: Percogesic, Dologesic, Flextra-650
Other Trades:
Category: Antihistamine/analgesic

Phenyltoloxamine is an antihistamine with analgesic properties used in over-the-counter preparations. There are no reports describing the use of phenyltoloxamine during human lactation or measuring the amount, if any, of the drug excreted into milk have been located. Similar to diphenhydramine (Benadryl), this old product should not normally be used in breastfeeding mothers, although it is probably compatible with breastfeeding.

Pregnancy Risk	C	Lactation Risk	L3
T ½	=	M/P	=
Vd	=	PB	=
Tmax	= 2–3 hours	Oral	= Well absorbed
MW	= 255	pKa	= 9.1

Adult Concerns: Tachycardia, atrioventricular block with hypertension, nausea, abdominal pain, xerostomia, drowsiness, dizziness, euphoria, faintness, blurred vision, talc embolism.

Pediatric Concerns:

Drug Interactions: Procarbazine

Relative Infant Dose:

Adult Dose:

Alternatives:

References:
1. Pharmaceutical manufacturer prescribing information, 2010.

PHENYTOIN　　　　　　　　　　　　　　L2

Trade: Dilantin
Other Trades: Dilantin, Novo-Phenytoin, Epanutin
Category: Anticonvulsant

Phenytoin is an old and efficient anticonvulsant. It is secreted in small amounts into breastmilk. The effect on infant is generally considered minimal if the levels in the maternal circulation are kept in low-normal range (10 μg/mL). Phenytoin levels peak in milk at 3.5 hours.

In one study of 6 women receiving 200–400 mg/day, plasma concentrations varied from 12.8 to 78.5 μmol/L, while their milk levels ranged from 1.61 to 2.95 mg/L.[1] The milk/plasma ratios were low, ranging from 0.06 to 0.18. In only two of these infants were plasma concentrations of phenytoin detectable (0.46 and 0.72 μmol/L). No untoward effects were noted in any of these infants. Others have reported milk levels of 6 μg/mL[2], or 0.8 μg/mL.[3] Although the actual concentration in milk varies significantly between studies, the milk/plasma ratio appears relatively similar at 0.13 to 0.45. Breastmilk concentrations varied from 0.26 to 1.5 mg/L depending on the maternal dose. In a mother receiving 250 mg twice daily, milk levels were 0.26 and the milk/plasma ratio was 0.45.[4] The maternal plasma level of phenytoin was 0.58. In another study of two patients receiving 300–600 mg/day, the average milk level was 1.9 mg/L.[5] The maximum observed milk level was 2.6 mg/L. The neonatal half-life of phenytoin is highly variable for the first week of life. Monitoring of the infants' plasma may be useful although it is not definitely required. All of the current studies indicate rather low levels of phenytoin in breastmilk and minimal plasma levels in breastfeeding infants.

Pregnancy Risk	D	Lactation Risk	L2
T ½	= 6–24 hours	M/P	= 0.18–0.45
Vd	= 0.5–0.8 l/kg	PB	= 89%
Tmax	= 4–12 hours	Oral	= 70–100%
MW	= 252	pKa	= 8.3

Adult Concerns: Sedation, hypertrophied gums, ataxia, liver toxicity.

Pediatric Concerns: Only one case of methemoglobinemia, drowsiness, and poor sucking has been reported. Most other studies suggest no problems.

Drug Interactions: Increased effects of phenytoin may occur when used with: amiodarone, benzodiazepines, chloramphenicol, cimetidine, disulfiram, ethanol, fluconazole (azoles), isoniazid, metronidazole, omeprazole, sulfonamides, valproic acid, TCAs, ibuprofen. Decreased effects of phenytoin may occur when used with: barbiturates, carbamazepine, rifampin, antacids, charcoal, sucralfate, folic acid, laxapine, nitrofurantoin, pyridoxine. Many others have been reported, please consult more complete reference.

Relative Infant Dose: 0.6%–7.7%

Adult Dose: 300 mg daily.

Alternatives:

References:
1. Steen B, Rane A, Lonnerholm G, Falk O, Elwin CE, Sjoqvist F. Phenytoin excretion in human breast milk and plasma levels in nursed infants. Ther Drug Monit 1982; 4(4): 331–334.
2. Svensmark O, Schiller PJ, Buchthal F. 5, 5–Diphenylhydantoin (dilantin) blood levels after oral or intravenous dosage in man. Acta Pharmacol Toxicol (Copenh) 1960; 16: 331–346.
3. Kaneko S, Sato T, Suzuki K. The levels of anticonvulsants in breast milk. Br J Clin Pharmacol 1979; 7(6): 624–627.
4. Rane A, Garle M, Borga O, Sjoqvist F. Plasma disappearance of transplacentally transferred diphenylhydantoin in the newborn studied by mass fragmentography. Clin Pharmacol Ther 1974; 15(1): 39–45.
5. Mirkin BL. Diphenylhydantoin: placental transport, fetal localization, neonatal metabolism, and possible teratogenic effects. J Pediatr 1971; 78(2): 329–337.

PHYTONADIONE   L1

Trade: Phytonadione, AquaMEPHYTON, Konakion, Mephyton, Vitamin K_1
Other Trades: Konakion
Category: Vitamin K_1

Vitamin K_1 is often used to reverse the effects of oral anticoagulants and to prevent hemorrhagic disease of the newborn (HDN).[1,2,3] The use of vitamin K has long been accepted primarily because it reduces the decline of the vitamin K dependent coagulation factors II, VII, IX, and X. A single IM injection of 0.5 to 1 mg or an oral dose of 1–2 mg during the neonatal period is recommended by the AAP. Although controversial, it is generally recognized that exclusive breastfeeding may not provide sufficient vitamin K_1 to provide normal clotting factors, particularly in the premature infant or those with malabsorptive disorders. Vitamin K concentration in breastmilk is normally low (<5–20 ng/mL), and most infants are born with low coagulation factors (30–60%) of normal. Although vitamin K is transferred to human milk, the amount may not be sufficient to prevent hemorrhagic disease of the newborn. Vitamin K requires the presence of bile and other factors for absorption, and neonatal absorption may be slow or delayed due to the lack of requisite gut factors.

Vitamin K_2 (menaquinones, menatetrenone) is more orally bioavailable Vitamin K. It is derived from various foods including meat, eggs, dairy, and natto. There have been some suggestions that K_2 may prevent osteoporosis.

Pregnancy Risk	C		Lactation Risk	L1
T ½	=		M/P	=
Vd	=		PB	=
Tmax	= 12 hours		Oral	= Complete
MW	= 450		pKa	=

Adult Concerns: Adverse effects include hemolytic anemia, thrombocytopenia, thrombosis, hypotension, prothrombin abnormalities, pruritus, and cutaneous reactions. Anaphylaxis.

Pediatric Concerns: Vitamin K transfer to milk is low.

Drug Interactions: Decreased effect when used with coumarin/warfarin anticoagulants.

Relative Infant Dose:

Adult Dose: 65 µg daily.

Alternatives:

References:
1. Olson JA. Recommended dietary intakes (RDI) of vitamin K in humans. Am J Clin Nutr 1987; 45(4): 687–692.
2. Lane PA, Hathaway WE. Vitamin K in infancy. J Pediatr 1985; 106(3): 351–359.
3. Vitamin and mineral supplement needs in normal children in the United States Pediatrics 1980; 66(6): 1015–1021.

PICARIDIN   L3

Trade: OFF Clean Feel, Cutter Advanced, Picaridin
Other Trades: Bayrepel
Category: Insect repellant

Picaridin, also known as Icaridin, is a newer and potentially safer alternative to the insect repellant DEET. It works by blocking the insects' ability to locate human skin. It does not cause irritation to the skin, and is odorless. Icaridin does not need to be washed off upon returning indoors. It is safe for use in children of all ages, and it will not affect plastics, synthetics, or plastic coatings. The WHO claims that icaridin is the best repellent against mosquitoes carrying Malaria.[1] The EPA suggests that icaridin has a low acute oral, inhalation, and dermal toxicity.[2]

One study concerning the absorption of picaridin in human skin attempted to show variations between formulations. In standard preparations, the average amount absorbed was 12.44% of the applied dose. In preparations containing sunscreens, the amount absorbed was shown to be lower, averaging 5.92%. Measures were also made to determine the total possible amount that could be absorbed, which resulted in 9.85% and 18.91% for the sunscreen and standard preparations respectively. It was noted that the amount of ethyl alcohol varied between the two formulations, with the standard having 60.6% alcohol content and the sunscreen formulation having 91.4%. In vivo studies showed significantly lower levels of absorption, with values ranging between 1.66% and 3.77%.[3]

Due to its lipid solubility, it is likely it would enter milk, but plasma levels are probably low. It is probably safer to use in breastfeeding mothers than DEET.

Pregnancy Risk	Probably Safe	Lactation Risk	L3
T ½	=	M/P	=
Vd	=	PB	=
Tmax	=	Oral	=
MW	= 229	pKa	=

Adult Concerns: No adverse reactions noted.

Pediatric Concerns: No adverse reactions noted.

Drug Interactions:

Relative Infant Dose:

Adult Dose:

Alternatives:

References:
1.   www.picaridin.com.
2.   www.http: //www.epa.gov/opprd001/factsheets/picaridin.pdf.
3.   Picaridin: In vitro dermal penetration study using human and rat skin. United States Environmental Protection Agency File R160418. Accessed June 27, 2011. http: //www.epa.gov/pesticides/chem_search/cleared_reviews/csr_PC-070705_26–Jun-08_a.pdf.

PILOCARPINE   L3

Trade: Isopto Carpine, Pilocar, Akarpine, Ocusert Pilo
Other Trades: Ocusert-Pilo, Minims Pilocarpine
Category: Intraocular hypotensive

Pilocarpine is a direct acting cholinergic agent used primarily in the eyes for treatment of open-angle glaucoma. The ophthalmic dose is approximately 1 mg or less per day, while the oral adult dose is approximately 15–30 mg daily.[1,2] It is not known if pilocarpine enters milk, but it probably does in low levels due to its minimal plasma levels. It is not likely that an infant would receive a clinical dose via milk, but this is presently unknown. Side effects would largely include diarrhea, gastric upset, excessive salivation, and other typical cholinergic symptoms.

Pregnancy Risk	C	Lactation Risk	L3
T ½	= 0.76–1.55 hours	M/P	=
Vd	=	PB	=
Tmax	= 1.25 hours	Oral	= Good
MW	= 208	pKa	= 7.15

Adult Concerns: Common side effects from ophthalmic use include burning or itching, blurred vision, poor night vision, headaches. Following oral use, excessive sweating may occur.

Pediatric Concerns: None reported via milk but observe for vomiting, epigastric distress, abdominal cramping and diarrhea.

Drug Interactions: A decreased response when added with anticholinergic agents. Diprivan and pilocarpine may increase myopia and increase blurred vision. Sulfacetamide ophthalmic solutions may precipitate pilocarpine prior to absorption and should not be used together.

Relative Infant Dose:

Adult Dose: 5–10 mg three times daily.

Alternatives:

References:
1. Drug Facts and Comparisons 1999 ed. ed. St. Louis: 1999.
2. Pharmaceutical manufacturer prescribing information, 1999.

PIMECROLIMUS   L2/L4

Trade: Elidel
Other Trades: Elidel
Category: Cytokine inhibitor used for atopic dermatitis

Pimecrolimus is a topical agent used as a cytokine inhibitor for atopic dermatitis. While its mechanism of action is unknown, it inhibits the release of various inflammatory cytokines for T cells and many others. Systemic absorption following topical application is minimal with reported blood concentrations consistently below 0.5 ng/mL following twice-daily application of the 1% cream.[1] Oral absorption is unreported but probably low to moderate as plasma levels of 54 ng/mL have been reported following twice daily oral doses of 30 mg.[2] Pimecrolimus is cleared for use in pediatric patients 2 years and older. No data are available on its transfer to human milk, but because the maternal plasma levels are so low, it is extremely remote that this agent would penetrate milk in clinically relevant amounts. However, its use on or around the nipples should be avoided as the clinical dose absorbed orally in the infant could be significant.

Pregnancy Risk	C	Lactation Risk	L2/L4 on nipple
T ½	=	M/P	=
Vd	=	PB	= 87%
Tmax	=	Oral	= Moderate
MW	= 810	pKa	=

Adult Concerns: Adverse reactions include excessive skin warmth and burning. Elevated risk of skin infections (varicella zoster virus infection, herpes simplex virus infection, or eczema herpeticum) and skin cancer is possible. Hives or itching, swelling of the face, tightness in the chest, and fever have been reported. The US FDA has issued a warning concerning elevated risks of skin cancers and lymphomas in patients exposed to this product. This warning is highly controversial and is not supported by many dermatologic organizations.

Pediatric Concerns: None reported via milk. It is commonly used in children 2 years old and greater. It is unlikely to penetrate milk in clinically relevant amounts. Should not be used directly on the nipple, or areola. The US FDA has issued a warning concerning elevated risks of skin cancers and lymphomas in patients exposed to this product. This warning is highly controversial and is not supported by many dermatologic organizations.

Drug Interactions:

Relative Infant Dose:

Adult Dose: Apply twice daily to skin.

Alternatives:

References:
1. Pharmaceutical manufacturer prescribing information, 2003.
2. Harper J, Green A, Scott G, Gruendl E, Dorobek B, Cardno M, Burtin P. First experience of topical SDZ ASM 981 in children with atopic dermatitis. Br J Dermatol 2001; 144(4): 781–787.

PIMOZIDE   L4

Trade: Orap

Other Trades: Orap

Category: Potent tranquilizer

Pimozide is a potent neuroleptic agent primarily used for Tourette's syndrome and chronic schizophrenia which induces a low degree of sedation.[1,2] No data are available on the secretion of pimozide into breastmilk. This is a highly risky product and numerous other antipsychotics are available. So this product is probably not worth the risk to the infant.

Pregnancy Risk	C		Lactation Risk	L4
T ½	= 55 hours		M/P	=
Vd	=		PB	=
Tmax	= 6–8 hours		Oral	= >50%
MW	= 462		pKa	= 7.32

Adult Concerns: Extrapyramidal symptoms, anorexia, weight loss, gastrointestinal distress, seizures.

Pediatric Concerns: None reported but caution is urged. No pediatric studies are found.

Drug Interactions: Increased toxicity of alfentanil, CNS depressants, guanabenz, and monoamine oxidase inhibitors. Do not use with macrolide antibiotics such as clarithromycin, erythromycin, azithromycin and dirithromycin, due to two reported deaths.

Relative Infant Dose:

Adult Dose: 7–16 mg daily.

Alternatives:

References:
1. Pharmaceutical manufacturer prescribing information, 1996.
2. Drug Facts and Comparisons 1996 ed. ed. St. Louis: 1996.

PINDOLOL   L3

Trade: Visken

Other Trades: Apio-Pindol, Gen-Pindol, Novo-Pindol, Nu-Pindol, PMS-Pindol, Visken

Category: Antihypertensive

Pindolol is a nonselective beta blocker that is used as an antihypertensives and antiarrhythmic. In one study of six hypertensive pregnant women, ages 25–35 years, with a gestational age of 37–40 weeks, patients were given 10 mg pindolol tablets every 12 hours for a minimum of 3 days during pregnancy and after delivery. A single breastmilk sample was collected on the day of delivery from 11 to 14 hours post dose. Two pindolol metabolites were measured in milk, (-)-S-pindolol whose concentration averaged 3.1 µg/L (range 1.5 to 3.9 µg/L) and (+)-R-pindolol averaging 1.9 µg/L (range 1.2 to 4.2 µg/L).[1] The authors estimate that a fully breastfed infant would receive an average of 0.36% of the weight-adjusted maternal dose. This data unfortunately was collected during the colostral phase, and probably overestimates the actual dose during regular lactation.

Pregnancy Risk	B	Lactation Risk	L3
T ½	= 3–4 hours	M/P	=
Vd	= 2 l/kg	PB	= 40%
Tmax	= 1 hour	Oral	= >95%
MW	= 248	pKa	= 9.52

Adult Concerns: Reversible mental depression progressing to catatonia, short-term memory loss, swelling of the face, fingers, feet, or lower legs.

Pediatric Concerns: None reported in one study.

Drug Interactions: While taking beta blockers, patients with a history of severe anaphylactic reaction to a variety of allergens may be more reactive to repeated challenge, either accidental, diagnostic, or therapeutic. Such patients may be unresponsive to the usual doses of epinephrine used to treat allergic reactions.

Relative Infant Dose: 0.4%

Adult Dose: 10–60 mg/day.

Alternatives:

References:
1. Gonçalves PV, Cavalli RC, da Cunha SP, Lanchote VL. Determination of pindolol enantiomers in amniotic fluid and breast milk by high-performance liquid chromatography: applications to pharmacokinetics in pregnant and lactating women. J Chromatogr B Analyt Technol Biomed Life Sci. 2007 Jun 1; 852(1–2): 640–5.

PIOGLITAZONE   L3

Trade: Actos

Other Trades:

Category: Oral antidiabetic agent

Pioglitazone is a thiazolidinedione family oral antidiabetic agent similar to troglitazone and rosiglitazone. It acts primarily by increasing insulin receptor sensitivity. In essence, the insulin receptor is activated reducing insulin resistance. This family also decreases hepatic gluconeogenesis and increases insulin-dependent muscle glucose uptake. They do not increase the release or secretion of insulin. No data are available on its entry into human milk. Due to its high plasma protein binding, transfer into milk is probably low, but there are no studies currently to confirm this. Preferably, use other anti-diabetic agents on which there are more published data.

Pregnancy Risk	C	Lactation Risk	L3
T ½	= 16–24 hours	M/P	=
Vd	= 0.63 l/kg	PB	= >99%
Tmax	= 2 hours	Oral	=
MW	= 392	pKa	= 5.2, 6.8

Adult Concerns: Hypoglycemia, upper respiratory tract infection, headache, sinusitis, myalgia, elevated liver enzymes. Elevated CPK, edema, anemia, and pharyngitis have been reported but are rare.

Pediatric Concerns: None reported via milk, but no data are available.

Drug Interactions: May reduce plasma levels of oral contraceptives, estrogens and progestins, by 30% which could lead to loss of contraception.

Relative Infant Dose:

Adult Dose: 15–30 mg once daily.

Alternatives: Metformin, glyburide, glipizide.

References:
1. Pharmaceutical manufacturer prescribing information, 2011.

## PIPERACILLIN	L2

Trade: Zosyn, Pipracil
Other Trades: Pipril, Tazocin, Pipracil
Category: Penicillin antibiotic

Piperacillin is an extended-spectrum penicillin. It is not absorbed orally and must be given IM or IV.[1] Concentrations of piperacillin secreted into milk are believed to be extremely low.[2] Its poor oral absorption would limit its absorption.

Pregnancy Risk	B		Lactation Risk	L2
T ½	= 0.6–1.3 hours		M/P	=
Vd	=		PB	= 30%
Tmax	= 30–50 minutes		Oral	= Poor
MW	= 518		pKa	= 4.14

Adult Concerns: Allergic skin rash, blood dyscrasias, diarrhea, nausea, vomiting, kidney toxicity, changes in gastrointestinal flora.

Pediatric Concerns: None reported via milk.

Drug Interactions: Tetracyclines may reduce penicillin effectiveness. Probenecid may increase penicillin levels.

Relative Infant Dose:

Adult Dose: 4–5 gm 2–3 times daily.

Alternatives:

References:
1. Pharmaceutical manufacturer prescribing information, 1996.
2. Chaplin S, Sanders GL, Smith JM. Drug excretion in human breast milk. Adv Drug React Ac Pois Rev 1982; 1: 255–287.

PIPERACILLIN + TAZOBACTAM   L2

Trade: Zosyn, Novaplus Zosyn
Other Trades: PiperTaz, Tazosin
Category: Antibiotic penicillin

Piperacillin sodium and Tazobactam sodium is a combined drug product indicated for use in pneumonias, appendicitis, pelvic inflammatory disease, peritonitis and infections of skin and subcutaneous tissues.[1]

Piperacillin is an extended-spectrum penicillin. It is not absorbed orally and must be given IM or IV. Tazobactam is a penicillin-like inhibitor of the enzyme beta lactamase and has few clinical effects. Piperacillin with tazobactam, the pharmacokinetics of piperacillin do not appear to be altered by tazobactam, but piperacillin reduces the renal clearance of tazobactam. Concentrations of piperacillin secreted into milk are believed to be extremely low[2]; tazobactam concentrations in human milk have not been studied. Studies in women suggest that this medication poses minimal risk to the infant when used during breastfeeding. Its poor oral absorption would limit its absorption.

Pregnancy Risk	B	Lactation Risk	L2
T ½	= 0.7–1.2 hours	M/P	=
Vd	= 10 to 16 L l/kg	PB	= 30%
Tmax	= Immediately	Oral	=
MW	=	pKa	= 4.14 / 2.1

Adult Concerns: Diarrhea, nausea, vomiting, headache, insomnia, rash, itching, fever, moniliasis.

Pediatric Concerns:

Drug Interactions: Avoid concurrent use with vancuronium due to increased risk of paralysis and respiratory depression. Avoid coadministration with methotrexate to avoid methotrexate toxicity. Concurrent use with probenecid may cause increased plasma levels of piperacillin.

Relative Infant Dose:

Adult Dose:

Alternatives:

References:
1. Pharmaceutical manufacturer prescribing information, 1996.
2. Chaplin S, Sanders GL, Smith JM. Drug excretion in human breast milk. Adv Drug React Ac Pois Rev 1982; 1: 255–287.

PIRBUTEROL ACETATE   L3

Trade: Maxair
Other Trades: Maxair, Evirel
Category: Bronchodilator for asthmatics

Pirbuterol is a classic beta-2 drug (similar to albuterol) for dilating pulmonary bronchi in asthmatic patients. It is administered by inhalation and, occasionally, orally.[1] Plasma levels are all but undetectable with normal inhaled doses. No data are available on levels in milk, but they would probably be minimal if administered via inhalation. Oral preparations would provide much higher plasma levels and would be associated with a higher risk for breastfeeding infants.

Pregnancy Risk	C	Lactation Risk	L3
T ½	= 2–3 hours	M/P	=
Vd	=	PB	=
Tmax	= 5 minutes (Aerosol)	Oral	= Complete
MW	= 240	pKa	= 3.0, 7.0, 10.3

Adult Concerns: Irritability, tremors, dry mouth, excitement, palpitations, and tachycardia.

Pediatric Concerns: None reported via milk, but observe for irritability, tremors.

Drug Interactions: Decreased effect when used with beta blockers. Increased toxicity with other beta agonists, monoamine oxidase inhibitors, and tricyclic antidepressants.

Relative Infant Dose:

Adult Dose: 0.2–0.4 mg every 4–6 hours.

Alternatives:

References:
1.   Pharmaceutical manufacturer prescribing information, 1993, 1994.

PIROXICAM   L2

Trade: Feldene
Other Trades: Candyl, Mobilis, Pirox, Apo-Piroxicam, Feldene, Novo-Pirocam
Category: Non-steroidal analgesic for arthritis

Piroxicam is a typical nonsteroidal anti-inflammatory commonly used in arthritics. In one patient taking 40 mg/day, breastmilk levels were 0.22 mg/L at 2.5 hours after dose.[1] In another study of long-term therapy in four lactating women receiving 20 mg/day, the mean piroxicam concentration in breastmilk was 78 µg/L which is approximately 1–3% of the maternal plasma concentration.[2] The daily dose ingested by the infant was calculated to average 3.4% of the weight-adjusted maternal dose of piroxicam. Even though piroxicam has a very long half-life, this report suggests its use to be safe in breastfeeding mothers.

Pregnancy Risk	C/D in 3rd trimester	Lactation Risk	L2
T ½	= 30–86 hours	M/P	= 0.008–0.013
Vd	= 0.31 l/kg	PB	= 99.3%
Tmax	= 3–5 hours	Oral	= Complete
MW	= 331	pKa	= 5.1

Adult Concerns: Gastric distress, gastrointestinal bleeding, constipation, vomiting, edema, dizziness, liver toxicity.

Pediatric Concerns: None reported via milk in several studies.

Drug Interactions: May prolong prothrombin time when used with warfarin. Antihypertensive effects of ACE inhibitors may be blunted or completely abolished by NSAIDs. Some NSAIDs may block antihypertensive effect of beta blockers, diuretics. Used with cyclosporin, may dramatically increase renal toxicity. May increase digoxin, phenytoin, lithium levels. May increase toxicity of methotrexate. May increase bioavailability of penicillamine. Probenecid may increase NSAID levels.

Relative Infant Dose: 3.4%–5.8%

Adult Dose: 20 mg daily.

Alternatives: Ibuprofen

References:
1. Ostensen M. Piroxicam in human breast milk. Eur J Clin Pharmacol 1983; 25(6): 829–830.
2. Ostensen M, Matheson I, Laufen H. Piroxicam in breast milk after long-term treatment. Eur J Clin Pharmacol 1988; 35(5): 567–569.

PNEUMOCOCCAL VACCINE   L1

Trade: Prevnar, Pneumovax 23 (PPSV23), Prevnar 13 (PCV13)

Other Trades: Pneuno 23, Pneumovax 23

Category: Vaccine

The pneumococcal vaccine is an inactivated product that consists of a mixture of polysaccharides from the 23 most prevalent types of *Streptococcus pneumonia*. It is non-infectious. It is available as a formulation containing 7 strains (7-valent) conjugate, and a 23 strain (valent) conjugate vaccine. The 7-valent vaccine is for use in children less than 2 years of age, and is recommended at ages 2, 4, 6 and 12–15 months. The 23-valent vaccine is for use in adults aged 65 years or older (one dose), anyone aged two years or older that is immunocompromized, or anyone who has or is getting a cochlear implant.[1] Although technically not approved for use in breastfeeding mothers, Prevnar 7 is recommended by the AAP for use in infants 2 months of age and older. The CDC also suggests Pneumovax is of minimal risk to a breastfeeding infant. Therefore it is unlikely to produce any untoward effects in a breastfed infant.

Pregnancy Risk	C	Lactation Risk	L1
T ½	=	M/P	=
Vd	=	PB	=
Tmax	=	Oral	= Nil
MW	=	pKa	=

Adult Concerns: Adverse reactions with the 23-valent conjugate vaccine include malaise, headache, nausea, vomiting, serum sickness, and fever.

Pediatric Concerns: Adverse reactions with the 7-valent pneumococcal conjugate vaccine include fever, irritability, drowsiness, erythema, decreased appetite, vomiting, diarrhea, and local tenderness.

Drug Interactions: Immunosupressants may decrease the efficacy of the vaccine.

Relative Infant Dose:

Adult Dose: 0.5 mL IM.

Alternatives:

References:
1. Pharmaceutical manufacturer prescribing information, 2007.

PODOFILOX   L3

Trade: Condylox, Podophyllotoxin
Other Trades:
Category: Antimitotic agent use topically for treatment of genital warts.

Podofilox (also called Podophyllotoxin) is an antimitotic agent used to treat genital warts and Condyloma acuminatum. Its transcutaneous absorption is minimal, plasma levels in 52 patients following use of 0.05 mL of 0.5% podofilox solution to external genitalia did not result in detectable serum levels. However, applications of 0.1 to 1.5 mL resulted in plasma levels of 1–17 ng/mL one to two hours post treatment. The drug does not accumulate after multiple treatments. No data are available on its transfer to human milk. It would be advisable to limit the dosage used in breastfeeding women, and to wait for a minimum of 4 hours following application before breastfeeding. The infant should be closely monitored for gastrointestinal distress. The use of this product in breastfeeding women should be avoided if possible.

Pregnancy Risk	C	Lactation Risk	L3
T ½	= 1–4.5 hours	M/P	=
Vd	=	PB	=
Tmax	= 1–2 hours	Oral	=
MW	= 414	pKa	= 13.42

Adult Concerns: Burning, pain, inflammation, erosion and itching at site of injection. Insomnia, bleeding, tenderness, malodor, dizziness, scaring have been reported.

Pediatric Concerns: No data are available, but extreme caution is recommended if used. A brief waiting period of 4 hours or more following application is recommended.

Drug Interactions:

Relative Infant Dose:

Adult Dose: Variable, but 0.5% solution applied topically every 12 hours is indicated for genital warts.

Alternatives:

References:
1. Pharmaceutical manufacturer prescribing information, 2005.

POLIDOCANOL   L3

Trade: Asclera

Other Trades:

Category: Sclerosing Agent

Polidocanol is a sclerosing agent used to treat varicose veins.[1] There are no adequate or well-controlled studies or case reports in breast feeding women. The adverse effects of using polidocanol are mainly local. One time treatment poses minimal harm to the infant, since the half-life is short and the effects are local. However, since the manufacturer has obtained little pharmacokinetic data, the effects are uncertain.

Pregnancy Risk	C	Lactation Risk	L3
T ½	= 1.5 hours	M/P	=
Vd	=	PB	=
Tmax	=	Oral	=
MW	= 580	pKa	= 6.5–8

Adult Concerns: Allergic reactions, injections site reactions, pain, thrombosis

Pediatric Concerns: None reported.

Drug Interactions:

Relative Infant Dose:

Adult Dose:

Alternatives: Glycerin

References:
1. Pharmaceutical manufacturer prescribing information, 2011.

POLIO VACCINE, INACTIVATED   L2

Trade: Ipol
Other Trades:
Category: Vaccine

Inactivated polio vaccine is administered for the prevention of poliomyelitis.[1] There are no adequate studies that determine the infant risk when using this medication during breastfeeding. If previously unimmunized or if traveling to an area endemic for polio, a lactating woman may receive inactivated poliovirus vaccine. Her infant should receive the inactivated polio vaccine according to the recommended childhood immunization schedule.[2]

Pregnancy Risk	C	Lactation Risk	L2
T ½	=	M/P	=
Vd	=	PB	=
Tmax	=	Oral	=
MW	=	pKa	=

Adult Concerns: Pain at site of injection, fever, fatigue, loss of appetite, vomiting, irritability.

Pediatric Concerns: None reported via breast milk. Adverse reactions via IPV administration: Local injection site reactions, fever, loss of appetite, vomiting, rash, irritability.

Drug Interactions:

Relative Infant Dose:

Adult Dose:

Alternatives:

References:
1. Pharmaceutical manufacturer prescribing information, 2009.
2. Pickering LK, Baker CJ, Long SS, McMillan JA, eds. Red Book: 2009 Report of the Committee on Infectious Diseases. 28th ed. Elk Grove Village, IL: American Academy of Pediatrics. 2009.

POLIO VACCINE, ORAL   L2

Trade: Vaccine-Live Oral Trivalent Polio
Other Trades:
Category: Vaccine

Oral polio vaccine is a mixture of three, live, attenuated oral polio viruses.[1] Human milk contains oral polio antibodies consistent with that of the maternal circulation.[2] Early exposure of the infant may reduce production of antibodies in the infant later on but this is not a major problem. Immunization of infant prior to 6 weeks of age is not recommended due to reduced antibody production. At this age, the effect of breastmilk antibodies on the infant's development of antibodies is believed minimal. Wait until infant is 6 weeks of age before immunizing mother.

Pregnancy Risk	C	Lactation Risk	L2
T ½	=	M/P	=
Vd	=	PB	=
Tmax	=	Oral	=
MW	=	pKa	=

Adult Concerns: Rash, fever.

Pediatric Concerns: None reported via milk.

Drug Interactions: May have inadequate response when used with immunosuppressants. Cholera vaccine may reduce seroconversion rate when coadministered, wait at least 30 days.

Relative Infant Dose:

Adult Dose:

Alternatives:

References:
1. Pharmaceutical manufacturer prescribing information, 1996.
2. Adcock E, Greene H. Poliovirus antibodies in breast-fed infants. Lancet 1971; 2(7725): 662–663.

POLYETHYLENE GLYCOL   L3

Trade:

Other Trades:

Category: Topical, lubricant, laxative

Polyethylene glycols are derivatives of paraffins (mineral oils) and used in a large variety of applications. They are commonly used in ointments, suppositories, lubricants, plasticizers, binders, paints, polishes, paper coatings, cosmetics, hair preparations, and food additives. These agents generally exhibit little to no toxicity, and systemic absorption is unlikely when used topically or when ingested along with electrolytes for bowel cleansing purposes. The molecular weights of these agents vary, with each preparation's molecular weight being denoted by a number after the name of the compound. For instance, polyethylene glycol 200 would consist of molecules averaging a molecular weight of 200. The weight of the chosen agent is important due to altered kinetics and incidence rates of adverse effects.[1] Although no data are available on transfer into human milk, it is highly unlikely that enough maternal absorption would occur to produce milk levels.

Pregnancy Risk	C	Lactation Risk	L3
T ½	=	M/P	=
Vd	=	PB	=
Tmax	=	Oral	= 0.2% (varies)
MW	= Variable	pKa	=

Adult Concerns: Urticaria, bloating, cramping, diarrhea, flatulence, nausea, anaphylactic shock.

Pediatric Concerns:

Drug Interactions: No known drug interactions.

Relative Infant Dose:

Adult Dose: Variable

Alternatives:

References:
1. Polyethylene Glycol. TERIS. Reprotox System. Reviewed 12/06. Accessed 7/21/11.

POLYETHYLENE GLYCOL-ELECTROLYTE SOLUTIONS   L3

Trade: GoLYTELY, Col-Lav, Colovage, Colyte, OCL, MoviPrep

Other Trades: PegLyte

Category: Bowel evacuant

Polyethylene glycol electrolyte solutions (PEG-ES) are saline laxatives.[1] It is a non-absorbable solution used as an osmotic agent to cleanse the bowel. It is completely non-absorbed from the adult gastrointestinal tract and would not likely penetrate human milk. This product is often used in children and infants prior to gastrointestinal surgery. Although no data are available on transfer into human milk, it is highly unlikely that enough maternal absorption would occur to produce milk levels.

Pregnancy Risk	C	Lactation Risk	L3
T ½	=	M/P	=
Vd	=	PB	=
Tmax	=	Oral	= Nil
MW	=	pKa	=

Adult Concerns: Diarrhea, bad taste, intestinal fullness. Do not use in gastrointestinal obstruction, gastric retention, bowel preformation, toxic colitis, megacolon or ileus.

Pediatric Concerns: None reported via milk.

Drug Interactions: Due to intense diarrhea produced, it would dramatically reduce oral absorption of any other orally administered medicine.

Relative Infant Dose:

Adult Dose: 240 mL every 10 minutes up to 4 L.

Alternatives:

References:
1. Pharmaceutical manufacturer prescribing information, 1996.

POLYMYXIN B SULFATE   L2

Trade:
Other Trades: Aerocortin
Category: Antibacterial

Polymyxin B is a commonly used topical, ophthalmic, and rarely injectable antibiotic. Most commonly used with other antibiotics, including neomycin and corticosteroids (hydrocortisone), it is commonly used to treat conjunctivitis, blepharitis, keratitis, and other topical infections.[1] It primarily covers most gram negative bacteria and some gram positive. It has been used in infants via injection (40,000 units/kg/day) but this is extremely rare. When applied ophthalmically, it is almost completely unabsorbed into surrounding tissues. No data are available on its transfer to human milk. However, when used topically it is very unlikely enough would be absorbed transcutaneously to produce plasma or milk levels. Orally, it would be largely destroyed by the gastric acid in the infant as it is very unstable in acidic milieu. When applied topically to nipples in small amounts, it is unlikely to produce problems in a breastfed infant.

Pregnancy Risk	B	Lactation Risk	L2
T ½	= 6 hours	M/P	=
Vd	=	PB	= Low
Tmax	= 2 hours	Oral	= Nil
MW	= Large	pKa	=

Adult Concerns: Plasma concentrations exceeding 5 µg/mL in adults may produce paresthesias, dizziness, weakness, drowsiness, ataxia, etc. But these are only seen following IM, IV, or intrathecal injections, not via topical application.

Pediatric Concerns: The adult observations are rarely seen in children.

Drug Interactions: Additive effects when polymyxin is added to neuromuscular blockers. Incompatible with acids, alkali solutions, amphotericin B solutions.

Relative Infant Dose:

Adult Dose: Topical: 10,000–25,000 units/mL.

Alternatives:

References:
1. Pharmaceutical manufacturer prescribing information, 2011.

POSACONAZOLE   L3

Trade: Noxafil
Other Trades:
Category: antifungal for candidiasis

Posaconazole is an antifungal medication used in the treatment of oropharyngeal candidiasis. The drug is also used in the treatment of chromoblastomycosis, invasive aspergillosis, mycetoma infections, fusariosis, and coccidioidomycosis. There is no increase in plasma concentration with daily doses above 800 mg. Steady state is reached in seven to ten days. The pharmacokinetics are linear with a high fat meal. The drug is absorbed slowly from the gastrointestinal tract. The drug also has a large volume of distribution. Elimination is 77% via feces and 14% via urine. Sixty-six percent is excreted unchanged in the feces. Posaconazole has been found to be excreted in rat milk, but no human studies have been conducted on excretion into breast milk.[1-2] This drug's kinetic parameters suggest that significant transfer into breastmilk is unlikely, however, caution is still advised due to its relatively long half-life.

Pregnancy Risk	C	Lactation Risk	L3
T ½	= 35 hours	M/P	=
Vd	= Large l/kg	PB	= 98%
Tmax	= 5 hours	Oral	=
MW	= 700.8	pKa	= 3.6, 4.6

Adult Concerns: Headache, cough, fever, bacteremia, thrombocytopenia, hypokalemia, abdominal pain, nausea, vomiting, diarrhea, hypertension, increase liver enzymes, anemia, renal failure, QT prolongation.

Pediatric Concerns:

Drug Interactions: Do not coadminister posaconazole with the following drugs: sirolimus–can result in sirolimus toxicity; pimozide, quinidine can result in cardiotoxicity, simvastatin can result in rhabdomyolysis, ergot alkaloids can result in ergotism. Posaconazole increases concentrations of cyclosporine or tacrolimus. Concomitant use with midazolam can increase its sedative/hypnotic efficacy.

Relative Infant Dose:

Adult Dose:

Alternatives:

References:
1. Moton A, Krishna G, Ma L, O'Mara F, Prasad P, McLeod J, Preston RA.Pharmacokinetics of a single dose of the antifungal posaconazole as oralsuspension in subjects with hepatic impairment. Curr Med Res Opin. 2010Jan; 26(1): 1–7.
2. Courtney R, Pai S, Laughlin M, Lim J, Batra V. Pharmacokinetics, safety, andtolerability of oral posaconazole administered in single and multiple doses inhealthy adults. Antimicrob Agents Chemother. 2003 Sep; 47(9): 2788–95.

POTASSIUM IODIDE   L4

Trade: SSKI

Other Trades:

Category: Antithyroid agent, Expectorant

Potassium iodide is frequently used to suppress thyroxine secretion in hyperthyroid patients (thyroid storm). About 30% of the oral dose administered is taken up by the thyroid gland, 20% goes to fecal excretion, the rest is cleared renally. Thus the biological half-lives are: blood, 6 hours; thyroid gland, 80 days; rest of the body, 12 days.[1] Most of a dose administered is rapidly cleared from the body via feces and urine. Part (30%) is sequestered for long periods in the thyroid gland. Because plasma iodine is the only source of iodine uptake in breastmilk, and it is cleared rapidly with a 6 hour half-life, mothers could theoretically return to breastfeeding after exposure to potassium iodide within approximately 24–48 hours. Iodide salts are known to be secreted into milk in high concentrations.[2,3] Milk/plasma ratios as high at 15–23 have been reported. Iodides are sequestered in the thyroid gland at high levels and can potentially cause severe thyroid depression in a breastfed infant.[1] Use with extreme caution if at all in breastfeeding mothers. Combined with the fact that it is a poor expectorant and that it is concentrated in breastmilk, it is not recommended in breastfeeding mothers. However, following treatment of thyroid storm, mothers should pump and discard milk for at least 24–48 hours.

Pregnancy Risk	D	Lactation Risk	L4
T ½	= 6 hours (blood)	M/P	= 23
Vd	=	PB	=
Tmax	=	Oral	= Complete
MW	= 166	pKa	=

Adult Concerns: Thyroid depression, goiter, gastrointestinal distress, rash, gastrointestinal bleeding, fever, weakness.

Pediatric Concerns: Thyroid suppression may occur. Do not use doses higher than RDA.

Drug Interactions:

Relative Infant Dose:

Adult Dose: 5–10 mg daily.

Alternatives:

References:
1. KKramer GH, Hauck BM, Chamberlain MJ. Biological half-life of iodine in adults with intact thyroid function and in athyreotic persons. Radiat Prot Dosimetry.2002; 102(2): 129–35.
2. Delange F, Chanoine JP, Abrassart C, Bourdoux P. Topical iodine, breastfeeding, and neonatal hypothyroidism. Arch Dis Child 1988; 63(1): 106–107.
3. Postellon DC, Aronow R. Iodine in mother's milk. JAMA 1982; 247(4): 463.

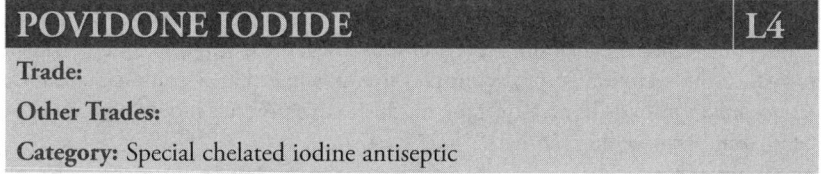

POVIDONE IODIDE   L4

Trade:

Other Trades:

Category: Special chelated iodine antiseptic

Povidone iodide is a chelated form of iodine. It is primarily used as an antiseptic and antimicrobial. When placed on the adult skin, very little is absorbed. When used intravaginally, significant and increased plasma levels of iodine have been documented. In a study of 62 pregnant women who used povidone-iodine douches, significant increases in plasma iodine were noted, and a seven fold increase in fetal thyroid iodine content was reported.[1] Topical application to infants has resulted in significant absorption through the skin. Once plasma levels are attained in the mother, iodide rapidly sequesters in human milk at high milk/plasma ratios.[2,3]

High oral iodine intake in mothers is documented to produce thyroid suppression in breastfed infants.[2] Use with extreme caution or not at all. Repeated use of povidone iodide is not recommended in nursing mothers or their infants.

Pregnancy Risk	D	Lactation Risk	L4
T ½	=	M/P	= >23
Vd	=	PB	=
Tmax	=	Oral	= Complete
MW	=	pKa	=

Adult Concerns: Iodine toxicity, hypothyroidism, goiter, neutropenia.

Pediatric Concerns: Transfer of absorbed iodine could occur leading to neonatal thyroid suppression. Avoid if possible.

Drug Interactions:

Relative Infant Dose:

Adult Dose:

Alternatives:

References:
1. Mahillon I, Peers W, Bourdoux P, Ermans AM, Delange F. Effect of vaginal douching with povidone-iodine during early pregnancy on the iodine supply to mother and fetus. Biol Neonate 1989; 56(4): 210–217.
2. Delange F, Chanoine JP, Abrassart C, Bourdoux P. Topical iodine, breastfeeding, and neonatal hypothyroidism. Arch Dis Child 1988; 63(1): 106–107.
3. Postellon DC, Aronow R. Iodine in mother's milk. JAMA 1982; 247(4): 463.

PRAMIPEXOLE   L4

Trade: Mirapex

Other Trades: Mirepexin

Category: Dopamine agonist for Parkinson's disease

Pramipexole is a non-ergot dopamine agonist for use in treating the symptoms of Parkinson's disease and restless leg syndrome.[1] While rodent studies showed rather high levels in milk, rats studies simply don't correlate with humans. No human studies are available concerning levels in milk. Regardless, pramipexole is known to reduce the secretion of prolactin, and it is possible that it could significantly reduce milk synthesis in breastfeeding mothers. This product should probably not be used in breastfeeding mothers.

Pregnancy Risk	C	Lactation Risk	L4
T ½	= 8 hours	M/P	=
Vd	= 7.14 l/kg	PB	= 15%
Tmax	= 2 hours	Oral	= >90%
MW	= 302	pKa	= 9.6

Adult Concerns: Adverse events include falling asleep during the day. Such events may occur without warning. Other adverse effects include dizziness, insomnia, extrapyramidal symptoms, headache, nausea, vomiting, constipation, dry mouth, postural hypotension and confusion.

Pediatric Concerns: None reported via milk, but inhibition of prolactin secretion could severely reduce milk production.

Drug Interactions: Cimetidine produced a 50% increase in pramipexole levels. Dopamine antagonists such as metoclopramide, domperidone, and others, may significantly interfere with the activity of pramipexole.

Relative Infant Dose:

Adult Dose: 1.5–4.5 mg/day.

Alternatives:

References:
1. Pharmaceutical manufacturer prescribing information, 2003.

PRAMLINTIDE ACETATE   L3

Trade: Symlin

Other Trades:

Category: Antihyperglycemic agent for diabetics

Pramlintide acetate is an anti hyperglycemic agent used in diabetics.[1] Pramlintide is a synthetic analog of human amylin, a naturally occurring peptide created by the pancreatic beta cells that contributes to glucose control during the postprandial period. Amylin is co-located in beta cells and is co-secreted with insulin in response to food intake. Amylin has a number of biologic functions including: slowing gastric emptying, and suppressing glucagon secretion, which reduces glucose output by the liver. It also reduces appetite by action in the CNS. In diabetics both insulin and amylin secretion are reduced in response to food. Pramlintide is a small peptide with a molecular weight of 3949 daltons and is administered subcutaneously. Although we do not have data on its transfer to milk, this product is probably far too large to enter milk in clinically relevant amounts after the first 3–7 days postpartum. Being a small peptide, it is also unlikely to be absorbed orally in infants. Even when injected subcutaneously it is only 30–40% bioavailable. It would probably not be contraindicated in breastfeeding mothers, but we have no data yet and some caution is certainly recommended.

Pregnancy Risk	C	Lactation Risk	L3
T ½	= 48 minutes	M/P	=
Vd	=	PB	=
Tmax	= 20 minutes	Oral	= 40%
MW	= 3949	pKa	=

Adult Concerns: Pramlintide in combination with insulin may lead to hypoglycemia. Nausea, headache, anorexia, vomiting, dizziness have been reported.

Pediatric Concerns: None reported via milk. Unlikely to enter milk or be orally bioavailable in the infant.

Drug Interactions: May affect the absorption of many drugs due to its affect on gastric emptying.

Relative Infant Dose:

Adult Dose: Highly variable, consult prescribing information.

Alternatives:

References:
1. Pharmaceutical manufacturer prescribing information, 2005.

PRAMOXINE   L3

Trade: Curasore, Prax, Proctofoam-NS, Tronolane, Sarna Sensitive, Proctofoam, PramoxGel

Other Trades:

Category: OTC antihistamine

Pramoxine is a topical anesthetic used to for the treatment of pruritus, and inflammation secondary to hemorrhoids, proctitis, cryptitis, and fissures.[1] Because this agent is used topically, it is not likely to be absorbed systemically. Do not use directly on the nipple. There are no adequate and well-controlled studies or case reports in breastfeeding women.

Pregnancy Risk	C	Lactation Risk	L3
T ½	=	M/P	=
Vd	=	PB	=
Tmax	= 3–5 min	Oral	=
MW	= 293	pKa	= 7.1

Adult Concerns: Contact dermatitis, stinging, eczema, angioedema.

Pediatric Concerns:

Drug Interactions:

Relative Infant Dose:

Adult Dose:

Alternatives:

References:
1. Pharmaceutical manufacturer prescribing information, 2010.

PRASUGREL   L4

Trade: Effient

Other Trades:

Category: Platelet aggregation inhibitor

Prasugrel hydrochloride binds irreversibly to platelet receptors preventing platelet aggregation. Prasugrel reduces ischemic events seen (such as stent thrombosis) in acute coronary syndrome in patients who are undergoing percutaneous coronary intervention.[1] Prasugrel is a prodrug that is metabolized to both active and inactive chemicals. Approximately 68% of the drug is excreted in urine and 27% in feces. Most patients have a 50% decrease in platelet aggregation within one hour of dosing. Steady state was reached following 3 to 5 days of a 10 mg daily dose after loading with 60 mg. Platelet aggregation was inhibited 70%. Bleeding time was prolonged when coadministered with warfarin.

No studies on the transfer of prasugrel into breast milk are available. Because prasugrel produces an irreversible inhibition of platelet aggregation, any present in milk could inhibit an infant's platelet function for a prolonged period. Because aspirin affects platelet aggregation similarly, and its milk levels are quite low, it would appear to be an ideal alternative. However, aspirin also inhibits platelet aggregation for long periods as well and may increase the risk of Reye' s syndrome in infants. Prasugrel and aspirin are often given together to prevent thrombotic complications after placement of coronary stents. Caution is urged while using this drug in lactating women.

Pregnancy Risk	B	Lactation Risk	L4
T ½	= 7 hours (range 2–15 hours)	M/P	=
Vd	= 0.62–0.97 l/kg	PB	= 98%
Tmax	= 30 minutes	Oral	= >79%
MW	= 409.9	pKa	= 5.1

Adult Concerns: Bleeding, bruising.

Pediatric Concerns: None reported, but observe for prolonged bleeding times, bruising, bleeding.

Drug Interactions: Warfarin, heparin, clopidogrel, aspirin, NSAIDS, may increase risk of bleeding.

Relative Infant Dose:

Adult Dose: 10 mg daily.

Alternatives: Aspirin (low dose)

References:
1. Pharmaceutical manufacturer prescribing information, 2010.
2. Armani AM. Prasugrel: an efficacy and safety review of a new antiplatelet therapy option. Crit Pathw Cardiol. 2010 Dec; 9(4): 199–202.

PRAVASTATIN   L3

Trade: Pravachol

Other Trades: Pravachol, Lipostat

Category: Lowers blood cholesterol

Pravastatin belongs to the HMG-CoA reductase family of cholesterol lowering drugs.[1] Small amounts are believed to be secreted into human milk but the levels were unreported. The effect on an infant is unknown, but it could reduce cholesterol synthesis. Atherosclerosis is a chronic process and discontinuation of lipid-lowering drugs during pregnancy and lactation should have little to no impact on the outcome of long-term therapy of primary hypercholesterolemia. Cholesterol and other products of cholesterol biosynthesis are essential components for fetal and neonatal development and the use of cholesterol-lowering drugs during the period of lactation and could pose some risk to a newborn. However, pravastatin is poorly absorbed orally and the risk to an infant is probably minimal.

Pregnancy Risk	X		Lactation Risk	L3
T ½	= 77 hours		M/P	=
Vd	=		PB	= 50%
Tmax	= 1–1.5 hours		Oral	= 17%
MW	= 446		pKa	= 4.7

Adult Concerns: Leukopenia, elevated liver enzymes, depression, neuropathy, etc.

Pediatric Concerns: None reported via milk but studies are limited.

Drug Interactions: The anticoagulant effect of warfarin may be increased. Use with bile acid sequestrants may reduce pravastatin bioavailability by 50%. May increase toxicities of cyclosporine. Concurrent use of niacin may increase risk of severe myopathy.

Relative Infant Dose:

Adult Dose: 10–20 mg daily.

Alternatives:

References:
1. Pharmaceutical manufacturer prescribing information, 2012.

PRAZEPAM L3

Trade: Centrax

Other Trades: Centrax

Category: Antianxiety agent

Prazepam is a typical benzodiazepine that belongs to diazepam family. It has a long half-life in adults. Peak plasma level occurs 6 hours post-dose.[1] An active metabolite with a longer half-life is produced. No data are available on transfer into human milk. Most benzodiazepines have high milk/plasma ratios and transfer into milk readily. Observe infant closely for sedation.

Pregnancy Risk	D		Lactation Risk	L3
T ½	= 30–100 hours		M/P	=
Vd	= 12–14 l/kg		PB	= >70%
Tmax	= 6 hours		Oral	= Complete
MW	= 325		pKa	= 2.7

Adult Concerns: Sedation, hypotension, depression.

Pediatric Concerns: None reported via milk, but benzodiazepines may induce sedation in breastfed infants.

Drug Interactions: May decrease effect of levodopa. May produce increased toxicity when used with other CNS depressants, disulfiram, cimetidine, anticoagulants, and digoxin.

Relative Infant Dose:

Adult Dose: 10 mg three times daily.

Alternatives: Lorazepam, alprazolam

References:
1.   Facts and Comparisons. St. Louis: 2010..

PRAZIQUANTEL	L2

Trade: Biltricide
Other Trades: Biltricide
Category: Anthelmintic

Praziquantel is a trematodicide used for treatment of schistosome infections and infestations of liver flukes. In a study of 10 women who received 1) a single dose of 50 mg/kg; or 2) 20 mg/kg three times daily, milk and plasma levels were determined at multiple time intervals over the next 32 hours.[1] In group 1, the average milk concentration was 0.19 mg/L. In group 2, the average milk concentration was 0.198 mg/L. Throughout the duration of this study, the infants in group 1 ingested 27.4 µg and those in group 2 ingested 25.6 µg of praziquantel. On average, the maternal plasma concentrations were four times higher than milk concentrations. Using this data, the relative infant dose would be approximately 0.05% of the maternal dose in both groups. These values are probably too low to harm an infant.

Pregnancy Risk	B	Lactation Risk	L2
T ½	= 0.8–1.5 hours, metabolite 4.5 hours	M/P	= 0.25%
Vd	=	PB	= 80%
Tmax	= 1–3 hours	Oral	= 80%
MW	= 312	pKa	=

Adult Concerns: Fever, dizziness, headache, abdominal pain, drowsiness and malaise.

Pediatric Concerns: None reported via milk.

Drug Interactions: May increase levels of albendazole with admixed. Carbamazepine, dexamethasone, and phenytoin may decrease praziquantel AUC significantly. Cimetidine may increase plasma levels by 300%.

Relative Infant Dose: 0.05%–0.06%

Adult Dose: 10–25 mg/kg BID-TID X 1 day

Alternatives:

References:
1.   Leopold G, Ungethum W, Groll E, Diekmann HW, Nowak H, Wegner DH. Clinical pharmacology in normal volunteers of praziquantel, a new drug against schistosomes and cestodes. An example of a complex study covering both tolerance and pharmacokinetics. Eur J Clin Pharmacol 1978; 14(4): 281–291.

PRAZOSIN   L4

Trade: Minipress
Other Trades: Pressin, Minipress, Apo-Prazo, Novo-Prazin, Hypovasl
Category: Strong antihypertensive

Prazosin is a selective alpha-1 adrenergic antagonist used to control hypertension. It is structurally similar to doxazosin and terazosin.[1,2] Others in this family (doxazosin) are known to concentrate in milk. Exercise extreme caution when administering to nursing mothers.

Pregnancy Risk	C	Lactation Risk	L4
T ½	= 2–3 hours	M/P	=
Vd	= 0.6 l/kg	PB	= 97%
Tmax	= 2–3 hours	Oral	=
MW	= 383	pKa	= 6.5

Adult Concerns: Leukopenia, tachycardia, hypotension, dizziness, fainting, headache, edema, diarrhea, urinary frequency.

Pediatric Concerns: None reported via milk, but some in this family are concentrated in milk. Observe extreme caution.

Drug Interactions: Beta blockers may enhance acute postural hypotensive reaction. The antihypertensive action of prazosin may be decreased by NSAIDs. Verapamil appears to increase serum prazosin levels. The antihypertensive effect of clonidine may be decreased when used with prazosin.

Relative Infant Dose:

Adult Dose: 3–7.5 mg twice daily.

Alternatives: Clonidine

References:
1. Drug Facts and Comparisons 1994 ed. ed. St. Louis: 1994.
2. Pharmaceutical manufacturer prescribing information, 1993, 1994.

PREDNICARBATE   L3

Trade: Dermatop
Other Trades:
Category: High potency steroid ointment

Prednicarbate is a high potency steroid ointment.[1] Its absorption via skin surfaces is exceedingly low, even in infants. Its oral absorption is not reported but would probably be equivalent to prednisolone, or high. If recommended for topical application on the nipple, other less potent steroids should be suggested, including hydrocortisone or triamcinolone. If applied to the nipple, only extremely small amounts should be applied.

Pregnancy Risk	C		Lactation Risk	L3
T ½	=		M/P	=
Vd	=		PB	=
Tmax	=		Oral	=
MW	= 488		pKa	=

Adult Concerns: Symptoms of adrenal steroid suppression, fluid retention, gastric erosions.

Pediatric Concerns: None reported via milk.

Drug Interactions:

Relative Infant Dose:

Adult Dose:

Alternatives:

References:
1. Pharmaceutical manufacturer prescribing information, 2011.

PREDNISONE-PREDNISOLONE   L2

Trade: Prednisone, Prednisolone, Desonate, Fluorometholone Ophthalmic Solution

Other Trades:

Category: Steroid, corticosteroid

Small amounts of most corticosteroids are secreted into breastmilk. Following a 10 mg oral dose of prednisone, peak milk levels of prednisolone and prednisone were 1.6 µg/L and 2.67 µg/L, respectively.[1] In a group of 10 women who received 10–80 mg/day prednisolone, the milk levels were only 5–25% of the maternal serum levels.[2] In one patient who received 80 mg/day prednisolone, the peak plasma concentration at 1 hour was 317 µg/L. The AUC average milk concentration in this mother was 156 µg/L over 6 hours.[2] This is significantly less than 2% of the weight-normalized maternal dose. Because this last estimate was only determined over 6 hours and this dose was administered once each 24 hours, the total daily estimate would be much less than the 2% estimate. In another study of a single patient who received 120 mg prednisone/day, the total combined steroid levels (prednisone + prednisolone) peaked at 2 hours.[3] The peak level of combined steroid was 627 µg/L. Assuming the infant received 120 mL of milk every 4 hours, the total possible ingestion would only be 47 µg/day. In a group of 7 women who received radioactive labeled prednisolone 5 mg, the total recovery per liter of milk during the 48 hours after the dose was 0.14%.[4]

In small doses, most steroids are certainly not contraindicated in nursing mothers. Whenever possible use low-dose alternatives such as aerosols or inhalers. Following administration, wait at least 4 hours if possible prior to feeding infant to reduce exposure. With high doses (>40 mg/day), particularly for long periods, steroids could potentially produce problems in infant growth and development, although we have absolutely no data in this area, or which doses would pose problems. Brief applications of high dose steroids are probably not contraindicated as the overall exposure is low. With prolonged high dose therapy, the infant should be closely monitored for growth and development.

Pregnancy Risk	D/C in 2nd and 3rd trimester	Lactation Risk	L2
T ½	= 2–3 hours	M/P	= 0.25
Vd	=	PB	= >90%
Tmax	= 1–2 hours (maternal plasma) 1 hour (milk)	Oral	= Complete
MW	= 358	pKa	= 13.9

Adult Concerns: Gastric distress, gastric ulceration, glaucoma, thinning of skin.

Pediatric Concerns: None reported via milk. Limit degree and duration of exposure if possible. Use inhaled or intranasal steroids to reduce exposure. Short-term use is safe.

Drug Interactions: Decreased effect when used with barbiturates, phenytoin, rifampin.

Relative Infant Dose: 1.8%–5.3%

Adult Dose: 5–120 mg/day.

Alternatives:

References:
1. Katz FH, Duncan BR. Letter: Entry of prednisone into human milk. N Engl J Med 1975; 293(22): 1154.
2. Ost L, Wettrell G, Bjorkhem I, Rane A. Prednisolone excretion in human milk. J Pediatr 1985; 106(6): 1008–1011.
3. Berlin CM, Kaiser DG, Demmers L. Excretion of prednisone and prednisolone in human milk. Pharmacologist 1979; 21: 264.
4. McKenzie SA, Selley JA, Agnew JE. Secretion of prednisolone into breast milk. Arch Dis Child 1975; 50(11): 894–896.

PREGABALIN   L3

Trade: Lyrica
Other Trades: Lyrica
Category: Analgesic

Pregabalin binds to a subunit of voltage gated calcium channels in central nervous system tissues reducing the release of several neurotransmitters. It is used in the management of neuropathic pain associated with diabetic peripheral neuropathy, and postherpetic neuralgia.[1] There are no data available on the transfer of pregabalin into human milk. However, due to the kinetics of the drug, its passage into the milk compartment is probable, and its oral bioavailability to the infant would be high. Therefore, nursing mothers should use caution taking pregabalin while nursing.

Pregnancy Risk	C		Lactation Risk	L3
T ½	= 6 hours		M/P	=
Vd	= 0.5 l/kg		PB	=
Tmax	= 1.5 hours		Oral	= 90%
MW	= 159		pKa	= 4.2 and 10.6

Adult Concerns: Adverse reactions include asthenia, dry mouth, edema, dizziness, somnolence, and constipation.

Pediatric Concerns: No data available in infants.

Drug Interactions: Pregabalin should not be used with CNS depressants or thiazolidinediones.

Relative Infant Dose:

Adult Dose: 150–600 mg/day in divided doses.

Alternatives:

References:
1. Pharmaceutical manufacturer prescribing information, 2004.

PRIMAQUINE PHOSPHATE   L3

Trade:

Other Trades: Primacin, Primaquine phosphate

Category: Antimalarial

Primaquine is a typical antimalarial medication that is primarily used as chemoprophylaxis after the patient has returned from the region of exposure with the intention of preventing relapses of plasmodium vivax and or ovale. It is used in pediatric patients at a dose of 0.3 mg/kg/day for 14 days.[1-3] No data are available on its transfer into human milk. Maternal plasma levels are rather low, only 53–107 ng/mL, suggesting that milk levels might be rather low as well.

Pregnancy Risk	C		Lactation Risk	L3
T ½	= 4–7 hours		M/P	=
Vd	=		PB	=
Tmax	= 1–2 hours		Oral	= 96%
MW	= 259		pKa	=

Adult Concerns: Blood dyscrasias including granulocytopenia, anemia, leukocytosis, methemoglobinemia. Arrhythmia, hypertension, abdominal pain, cramps, visual (ocular) disturbances.

Pediatric Concerns: None reported from milk.

Drug Interactions: Elevated risk of blood dyscrasias with aurothioglucose. May reduce plasma levels of oral contraceptives.

Relative Infant Dose:

Adult Dose: 15 mg daily.

Alternatives:

References:

1. Mihaly GW, Ward SA, Edwards G, Orme ML, Breckenridge AM. Pharmacokinetics of primaquine in man: identification of the carboxylic acid derivative as a major plasma metabolite. Br J Clin Pharmacol 1984; 17(4): 441–446.
2. Mihaly GW, Ward SA, Edwards G, Nicholl DD, Orme ML, Breckenridge AM. Pharmacokinetics of primaquine in man. I. Studies of the absolute bioavailability and effects of dose size. Br J Clin Pharmacol 1985; 19(6): 745–750.
3. Bhatia SC, Saraph YS, Revankar SN, Doshi KJ, Bharucha ED, Desai ND, Vaidya AB, Subrahmanyam D, Gupta KC, Satoskar RS. Pharmacokinetics of primaquine in patients with P. vivax malaria. Eur J Clin Pharmacol 1986; 31(2): 205–210.

PRIMIDONE   L3

Trade: Mysoline

Other Trades: Apo-Primidone, Mysoline, Sertan, Misolyne

Category: Anticonvulsant

Primidone is a barbiturate and an anticonvulsant with sedative/hypnotic properties. It is metabolized in adults to several derivatives including phenobarbital. After chronic therapy, levels of phenobarbital rise to a therapeutic range. Hence, problems for the infant would not only include primidone but, subsequently, phenobarbital. In one study of 2 women receiving primidone, the steady-state concentrations of primidone in neonatal serum via ingestion of breastmilk were 0.7 and 2.5 µg/mL.[1] The steady-state phenobarbital levels in neonatal serum were between 2.0 to 13.0 µg/mL. The calculated dose of phenobarbital per day received by each infant ranged from 1.8 to 8.9 mg/day. Some sedation has been reported, particularly during the neonatal period. In another group of 4 women receiving 7.3 mg/kg/day primidone, levels in milk averaged 4.2 mg/L.[2] In another patient receiving 750 mg/day primidone and valproic acid 2.4 gm/d, breastmilk levels of primidone averaged 6 mg/L.[3]

Pregnancy Risk	D	Lactation Risk	L3
T½	= 5–18 hours (primidone), 75–120 hours metabolite	M/P	= 0.72
Vd	= 0.5–1.0 l/kg	PB	= 25%
Tmax	= 1–2 hours	Oral	= 90%
MW	= 218	pKa	=

Adult Concerns: Sedation, apnea, reduced suckling.

Pediatric Concerns: Some sedation, during neonatal period.

Drug Interactions: Acetazolamide may decrease primidone plasma levels. Co-administration of carbamazepine may lower primidone and phenobarbital concentrations and elevate carbamazepine concentrations. Use of phenytoin may reduce primidone concentrations. Primidone concentrations may be increased when used with isoniazid. The clearance of primidone may be decreased with nicotinamide.

Relative Infant Dose: 8.4%–8.6%

Adult Dose: 250 mg three times daily.

Alternatives:

References:

1. Kuhnz W, Koch S, Helge H, Nau H. Primidone and phenobarbital during lactation period in epileptic women: total and free drug serum levels in the nursed infants and their effects on neonatal behavior. Dev Pharmacol Ther 1988; 11(3): 147–154.
2. Nau H, Rating D, Hauser I et al. Placental transfer and pharmacokinetics of primidone and its metabolites phenobarbital, PEMA, and hydroxyphenobarbital in neonates and infants of epileptic mothers. Eur J Clin Pharmacol. 1980; 18: 31–42.
3. Espir MLE, Benton P, Will E et al. Sodium valproate–some clinical and pharmacological aspects. In: Legg NJ, ed. Clinical and pharmacological aspects of sodium valproate in the treatment of epilepsy: proceedings of a symposium. 1976; 145–51.

PROBENECID   L2

Trade: Benemid, Benecid, Probanalan, Proben, Apurina, Uricosid

Other Trades:

Category: Uricosuric agent/Used in treatment of gout

Probenecid is a uricosuric agent which accelerates the urinary excretion of uric acid by inhibiting the reabsorption of uric acid in the proximal convoluted tubule in the kidney. Hence it dramatically reduces plasma uric acid. It is also used to prevent the elimination of various penicillins and cephalosporins and is used to prolong their elimination half-lives. In a study of a single patient consuming 500 mg four times daily, milk levels of probenecid averaged 964 µg/L corresponding to an absolute dose of 145 µg/kg/day and a relative infant dose of 0.7%.[1] In this case of a mother receiving both probenecid and cephalexin, the infant suffered adverse effects (diarrhea). This complication was probably due to prolonged and increased exposure to cephalexin induced by small levels of probenecid.

Pregnancy Risk	C	Lactation Risk	L2
T ½	= 6–12 hours	M/P	= 0.03
Vd	=	PB	= 75–95%
Tmax	= 2–4 hours	Oral	= Complete
MW	= 285	pKa	=

Adult Concerns: Adverse reactions include, headache, dizziness, hepatic necrosis, vomiting, nausea, anorexia and sore gums. Nephrotic syndrome may occur with presence of uric acid stones, renal colic and urinary frequency. Anaphylaxis, fever, urticaria, pruritus, aplastic anemia, leukopenia, neutropenia, and thrombocytopenia have been reported.

Pediatric Concerns: Although milk levels are quite low, the renal excretion of many drugs is significantly impeded by probenecid. Thus when used in combination with other medications, the infant may have complications from altered half-lives of other medications. Observe closely for drug-drug interactions.

Drug Interactions: Profound increases in plasma levels and prolonged half-lives of penicillin and cephalosporin products when probenecid administered. Salicylates antagonizes the uricosuric effect of probenecid. Probenecid produces a modest increase in free sulfonamide plasma concentrations but a significant increase in total sulfonamide plasma levels. Probenecid may prolong or enhance the action of oral sulfonylureas and thereby increase the risk of hypoglycemia. Probenecid has been shown to more than double the plasma levels of oseltamivir. It has been reported that patients receiving probenecid require significantly less thiopental for induction of anesthesia. In addition, ketamine and thiopental anesthesia may be prolonged. The concomitant use of probenecid increases the mean plasma half-life of a number of drugs, including: indomethacin, acetaminophen, naproxen, ketoprofen, meclofenamate, lorazepam, and rifampin. In animals, probenecid may dramatically increase plasma concentrations of methotrexate.

Relative Infant Dose: 0.7%

Adult Dose: 500 mg four times daily or less.

Alternatives:

References:
1. Ilett KF, Hackett LP, Ingle B, Bretz PJ. Transfer of probenecid and cephalexin into breast milk. Ann Pharmacother 2006 May; 40(5): 986–9.

PROBIOTICS   L3

Trade:

Other Trades:

Category: Gastrointestinal Agent, Antidiarrheal, Microflora Replacement

Probiotics are micro-organisms that are identical or similar to natural microflora that are found in the gut. They are defined as living organisms that elicit a beneficial health effect when ingested or applied to the body. While most of these products are used orally, there have been some instances of vaginal administration. Common organisms found in these products are Lactobacillus, Bifidobacterium, and Saccharomyces species.[1] When ingested or used vaginally, these products are considered safe and are usually well tolerated. There has long been a concern that, due to the activity of these preparations, the organisms could penetrate the blood stream and cause a systemic infection in the infant.[1] While there are few reports of such problems occurring, it should be noted that such infections have been noted in the past.[2] The risk does remain low, with estimated incidences being less than 1 per 1 million for Lactobacillus[3], and 1 per 5.6 million for Saccharomyces.[4] No reports of Bifidobacterium infection have been reported from probiotic use.[5] Risk factors that can determine the possibility for adverse reactions include immunosuppression, severe illness, central catheters, and injury to the gut.[3]

Due to the fact that probiotics are not often absorbed systemically, it is unlikely that they will transfer into breast milk.[1] Lactobacillus has been reported to appear in the colostrum, though the amounts reported were not clinically significant and most likely stemmed from external contamination.[6] There are currently no published data regarding adverse effects in breastfed infants whose mothers were actively taking probiotics.[1] These should probably not be used in a mother with a premature infant with a poorly developed GI tract.

Pregnancy Risk	Probably Safe	Lactation Risk	L3
T ½	=	M/P	=
Vd	=	PB	=
Tmax	=	Oral	=
MW	=	pKa	=

Adult Concerns: Chest pain, endocarditis, rash, burping, gas, constipation, vomiting, hiccups, septicemia, fungemia.

Pediatric Concerns:

Drug Interactions: The use of antibiotics may negate or hinder the effects of probiotics.

Relative Infant Dose:

Adult Dose: Dosing varies, most often taken 1–2 times daily.

Alternatives:

References:
1. Bozzo P, Einarson A, Elias J. Are probiotics safe for use during pregnancy and lactation? Canadian Family Physician. Vol 57: MARCH 2011.
2. Snydman DR. The safety of probiotics. Clin Infect Dis 2008; 46(Suppl 2): S104–11.
3. Borriello SP, Hammes WP, Holzapfel W, Marteau P, Schrezenmeir J, Vaara M,et al. Safety of probiotics that contain lactobacilli or bifidobacteria. Clin InfectDis 2003; 36(6): 775–80. Epub 2003 Mar 5.
4. Karpa KD. Probiotics for Clostridium difficile diarrhea: putting it into perspective. Ann Pharmacother 2007; 41(7): 1284–7. Epub 2007 Jun 26.
5. Boyle RJ, Robins-Browne RM, Tang ML. Probiotic use in clinical practice: what are the risks? Am J Clin Nutr 2006; 83(6): 1256–64.
6. Abrahamsson TR, Sinkiewicz G, Jakobsson T, Fredrikson M, Björkstén B. Probiotic lactobacilli in breast milk and infant stool in relation to oral intake during the first year of life. J Pediatr Gastroenterol Nutr 2009; 49(3): 349–54.

PROCAINAMIDE   L3

Trade: Pronestyl, Procan
Other Trades: Pronestyl, Procan SR, Apo-Procainamide
Category: Antiarrhythmic

Procainamide is an antiarrhythmic agent. Procainamide and its active metabolite are secreted into breastmilk in moderate concentrations. In one patient receiving 500 mg four times daily, the breast milk levels of procainamide at 0, 3, 6, 9, and 12 hours were 5.3, 3.9, 10.2, 4.8, and 2.6 mg/L respectively.[1] The milk/serum ratio varied from 1.0 at 12 hours to 7.3 at 6 hours post-dose (mean= 4.3). The milk levels averaged 5.4 mg/L for parent drug and 3.5 mg/L for metabolite. Although levels in milk are still too small to provide significant blood levels in an infant, use with caution.

Pregnancy Risk	C	Lactation Risk	L3
T ½	= 3.0 hours	M/P	= 1–7.3
Vd	= 2 l/kg	PB	= 16%
Tmax	= 0.75–2.5 hours	Oral	= 75–90%
MW	= 235	pKa	= 9.2

Adult Concerns: Nausea, vomiting, liver toxicity, blood dyscrasias, hypotension.

Pediatric Concerns: None reported via milk. Observe for liver toxicity, hypotension, but very unlikely.

Drug Interactions: Propranolol may increase procainamide serum levels. Cimetidine and ranitidine appear to increase bioavailability of procainamide. Use with lidocaine may increase cardio depressant action of procainamide.

Relative Infant Dose: 5.4%

Adult Dose: 500–1000 mg every 4–6 hours.

Alternatives:

References:
1. Pittard WB, III, Glazier H. Procainamide excretion in human milk. J Pediatr 1983; 102(4): 631–633.

PROCAINE HCL   L3

Trade: Novocain

Other Trades:

Category: Local anesthetic

Procaine is an ester-type local anesthetic with low potential for systemic toxicity and short duration of action.[1] Procaine is generally used for infiltration or local anesthesia, peripheral nerve block, or rarely, spinal anesthesia. Procaine is rapidly metabolized by plasma pseudocholinesterase to p-aminobenzoic acid.[2] No data are available on its transfer to human milk, but it is unlikely. Most other local anesthetics (see bupivacaine, lidocaine) penetrate milk only poorly and it is likely that procaine, due to its brief plasma half-life, would produce even lower milk levels. Due to its ester bond, it would be poorly bioavailable.

Pregnancy Risk	C	Lactation Risk	L3
T ½	= 7.7 minutes	M/P	=
Vd	=	PB	= 5.8%
Tmax	=	Oral	= Poor
MW	= 236	pKa	= 9.1

Adult Concerns: High plasma concentrations of procaine due to excessive dosage, or inadvertent intravascular injection may result in systemic adverse effects involving the cardiovascular and central nervous systems including nervousness, drowsiness, or blurred vision. Allergic reactions due to the p-aminobenzoic acid metabolite have been reported and may produce urticaria and edema.

Pediatric Concerns: None reported via milk.

Drug Interactions: Enhanced neuromuscular blockade which increases risk of paralysis may occur when coadministered with neuromuscular blocking agents such as succinyl chloride, cisatracurium and rapacuronium. Use with sulfonamide antibiotics such as sulfadiazine, sulfadoxine, sulfasalazine, sulfamethoxazole may antagonize antibiotic efficacy. Concurrent use with St. John's Wort increases risk of hypotension and cardiovascular collapse.

Relative Infant Dose:

Adult Dose: 350–600 mg X 1.

Alternatives:

References:
1. Drug Facts and Comparisons 1999 ed. ed. St. Louis: 1999.
2. McEvoy GE. (ed): AFHS Drug Information. New York, NY: 2003.

PROCHLORPERAZINE   L3

Trade: Compazine

Other Trades: Stemetil, Prorazin, Stemetil, Nu-Prochlor, Buccastem

Category: Antiemetic, tranquilizer-sedative

Prochlorperazine is a phenothiazine primarily used as an antiemetic in adults and pediatric patients.[1] There are no data yet concerning breastmilk levels but other phenothiazine derivatives enter milk in small amounts. Because infants are extremely hypersensitive to these compounds, I suggest caution in younger infants. This product may also increase prolactin levels.[2] Consider promethazine as a safer alternative, although neonatal apnea is a consistent problem with this family of drugs. Use with extreme caution in infants subject to apnea.

Pregnancy Risk	C	Lactation Risk	L3
T ½	= 6–10 hours (single dose), 14–22 hours (repeated dose).	M/P	=
Vd	= 20–22.1 l/kg	PB	= 90%
Tmax	= 4–8 hours	Oral	= 12.5% oral
MW	= 374	pKa	=

Adult Concerns: Sedation, extrapyramidal effects, seizures, weight gain, liver toxicity.

Pediatric Concerns: None reported via milk, but caution is recommended.

Drug Interactions: May have increased toxicity when used with other CNS depressants, anticonvulsants. Epinephrine may cause hypotension.

Relative Infant Dose:

Adult Dose: 5–10 mg 3–4 times daily.

Alternatives: Promethazine

References:
1. Facts and Comparisons. St. Louis: 2010..
2. McEvoy GE. (ed): AFHS Drug Information. New York, NY: 2003.

PROGESTERONE   L3

Trade: Crinone, Prometrium, Progesterone Vaginal Ring, Prochieve, Endometrin
Other Trades: Crinone, Gesterol, Cyclogest, Gestone
Category: Progestational agent

Progesterone is a naturally occurring steroid (progestin) that is secreted by the ovary, placenta, and adrenal gland. Oral administration is hampered by rapid and extensive intestinal and liver metabolism leading to poorly sustained serum concentrations and poor bioavailability.[1] As progesterone is virtually unabsorbed orally, the vaginal route has become the most established way to deliver natural progesterone because it is easily administered, avoids liver first-pass metabolism, and has no systemic side-effects. Absorption through the vagina produces higher uterine levels and is called the 'uterine first-pass effect'. A study by Levine[2] suggests the area under the curve is about 38 times less with oral administration as with progesterone vaginal gel (Crinone). Thus fewer systemic effects are noted with oral administration.

With the use of progesterone in breastfeeding mothers, two principles are of paramount interest. What effect does it have on milk production and the components of milk? Does it transfer into milk in high enough levels to affect the infant directly? In general, there is significant confusion in the literature as to the effect of progestins on milk composition, but the compositional changes do not appear major, volume is normal or higher, and some authors report minor changes in lipid and protein content.[3-5] However, the majority of the studies are with other progestins (e.g. medroxyprogesterone). Shaaban studied the effect of an intravaginal progesterone ring (10 mg/day) in 120 women and found no changes in growth and development of the infant or breastfeeding performance of the study participants.[6] The author suggests the ring adds a measure of safety because the amount of steroid present in milk would not be effectively absorbed from the infant's gut. Another new study also suggests no impact on breastfeeding from the intravaginal progesterone ring.[7] The effect of progestins on milk production is poorly studied. Early postpartum, while progestin receptors are still present in the breast, administering progestins may actually suppress milk production just as it does in the pregnant women. This has been seen occasionally in patients early postpartum. Several days to a week later, most progestin receptors disappear from the lactocyte and breast tissues become relatively immune to the effects of progestins. Thus it is advisable to wait as long as possible postpartum prior to instituting therapy with progesterone to avoid reducing the milk supply.

The direct effect of progesterone therapy on the nursing infant is generally unknown, but it is believed minimal to none as natural progesterone is poorly bioavailable to the infant via milk. Several cases of gynecomastia in infants have been reported but are extremely rare.

Pregnancy Risk	B	Lactation Risk	L3
T ½	= 13–18 hours	M/P	=
Vd	=	PB	= 99%
Tmax	= 6 hours	Oral	= Low
MW	= 314	pKa	=

Adult Concerns: Bloating, cramps, pain, dizziness, headache, nausea, breast pain, constipation, diarrhea, nausea, somnolence, breast enlargement.

Pediatric Concerns: None reported, not bioavailable.

Drug Interactions: May increase estrogen levels when coadministered with estrogen-containing tablets. Increased doxorubicin-induced neutropenia when coadministered. Ketoconazole may increase levels of progesterone.

Relative Infant Dose:

Adult Dose: 90 mg daily.

Alternatives:

References:
1. Levy T, Gurevitch S, Bar-Hava I, Ashkenazi J, Magazanik A, Homburg R, Orvieto R, Ben Rafael Z. Pharmacokinetics of natural progesterone administered in the form of a vaginal tablet. Hum Reprod 1999; 14(3): 606–610.
2. Naqvi HM, Baseer A. Milk composition changes--a simple and non-invasive method of detecting ovulation in lactating women. J Pak Med Assoc 2001; 51(3): 112–115.
3. Rodriguez-Palmero M, Koletzko B, Kunz C, Jensen R. Nutritional and biochemical properties of human milk: II. Lipids, micronutrients, and bioactive factors. Clin Perinatol 1999; 26(2): 335–359.
4. Costa TH, Dorea JG. Concentration of fat, protein, lactose and energy in milk of mothers using hormonal contraceptives. Ann Trop Paediatr 1992; 12(2): 203–209.
5. Sas M, Gellen JJ, Dusitsin N, Tunkeyoon M, Chalapati S, Crawford MA, Drury PJ, Lenihan T, Ayeni O, Pinol A. An investigation on the influence of steroidal contraceptives on milk lipid and fatty acids in Hungary and Thailand. WHO Special Programme of Research, Development and Research Training in Human Reproduction. Task Force on oral contraceptives. Contracep 1986; 33(2): 159–178.
6. Shaaban MM. Contraception with progestogens and progesterone during lactation. J Steroid Biochem Mol Biol 1991; 40(4–6): 705–710.
7. Massai R, Quinteros E, Reyes MV, Caviedes R, Zepeda A, Montero JC, et al. Extended use of a progesterone-releasing vaginal ring in nursing women: a phase II clinical trial. Contracep 2005 Nov; 72(5): 352–7.

PROGUANIL   L3

Trade:

Other Trades:

Category: Antimalarials

Proguanil is a prophylactic antimalarial drug.[1] It is often used in combination with atovaquone to treat and prevent malaria. Only trace quantities of proguanil were found in human milk. Concentrations achieved in human milk are too low to be therapeutically protective in an infant.[2] Therefore, a nursing infant should also receive appropriate prophylactic measures for prevention of malaria. Proguanil is currently being used in infants and children for malaria prevention.

Pregnancy Risk	Probably Safe	Lactation Risk	L3
T ½	= 20 hours	M/P	=
Vd	= 23.1–35.7 l/kg	PB	= 75%
Tmax	= 2–4 hours	Oral	= 60%
MW	= 254	pKa	=

Adult Concerns: Diarrhea, hypersensitivity, aphthous ulceration.

Pediatric Concerns:

Drug Interactions: Concomitant use with anti-coagulants such as warfarin, heparin may cause major bleeding complications.

Relative Infant Dose:

Adult Dose: 200 mg/day.

Alternatives:

References:
1. Pharmaceutical manufacturer prescribing information, 2002.
2. Product Information: Paludrine (R), proguanil. Zeneca GmbH, Plankstadt, 1995.

PROMETHAZINE   L2

Trade: Phenergan, Promethegan
Other Trades: Avomine, Histanil, Phenergan, PMS Promethazine
Category: Phenothiazine used as antihistamine

Promethazine is a phenothiazine that is primarily used for nausea, vomiting, and motion sickness. It has been used safely for many years in adult and pediatric patients for vomiting, particularly associated with pregnancy. No data are available on the transfer of promethazine into milk, but small amounts probably do transfer. However, this product has been safely used in many pediatric conditions, and it is unlikely to produce untoward effects in older infants and children. Observe for sedation and apnea, particularly in younger infants. There are numerous suggestions that this product may increase the risk of SIDS. Do not use in infants subject to apnea. Long term follow-up (6 years) has found no untoward effects on development.[1]

Pregnancy Risk	C	Lactation Risk	L2
T ½	= 9–16 hours	M/P	=
Vd	= 13.9 l/kg	PB	= 93%
Tmax	= 4.5 hours	Oral	= 25%
MW	= 284	pKa	= 9.1

Adult Concerns: Sedation, apnea, extrapyramidal symptoms.

Pediatric Concerns: None reported via breastmilk, but promethazine has been implicated in SIDS. Some caution is recommended.

Drug Interactions: Epinephrine may cause significant decrease in blood pressure.

Relative Infant Dose:

Adult Dose: 12.5–25 mg every 4–6 hours.

Alternatives:

References:
1. Kris EB. Children born to mothers maintained on pharmacotherapy during pregnancy and postpartum. Recent Adv Biol Psychiatry 1961; 4: 180–187.

PROPAFENONE   L2

Trade: Rythmol

Other Trades: Arythmol

Category: Antiarrhythmic agent

Propafenone is a class 1C antiarrhythmic agent with structural similarities to propranolol. In a mother receiving 300 mg three times daily and at 3 days postpartum, maternal serum levels of propafenone and 5–OH-propafenone (active metabolite) were 219 µg/L and 86 µg/L respectively. The breastmilk level of propafenone and 5–OH-propafenone was 32 µg/L and 47 µg/L respectively.[1] The milk/plasma ratios for drug and metabolite were 0.15 and 0.54 respectively. The authors estimate that the daily intake of drug and active metabolite in the infant (3.3 kg) would have been 16 µg and 24 µg per day respectively.

Pregnancy Risk	C	Lactation Risk	L2
T ½	= 2–10 hours, 10–32 hours (poor metabolizer)	M/P	= 0.15
Vd	= 3.6 l/kg	PB	= 85–97%
Tmax	= 2–3 hours	Oral	= 5–50%
MW	= 341	pKa	= 16.34

Adult Concerns: Adverse effects include dizziness, unusual taste, first degree AV block, intraventricular conduction delay, nausea and/or vomiting, and constipation. In addition, dyspnea, CHF and proarrhythmia has been reported. Less frequently, hepatotoxicity, agranulocytosis, leukopenia, and positive ANA have been reported. Other side effects include sexual dysfunction.

Pediatric Concerns: None reported via milk. Levels are quite low.

Drug Interactions: Increased levels with cimetidine, beta blockers, quinidine, warfarin, cyclosporin and other drugs metabolized by this enzyme. Rifampin may reduce levels of propafenone.

Relative Infant Dose: 0.09%

Adult Dose: 150–225 mg three times daily.

Alternatives:

References:
1. Libardoni M, Piovan D, Busato E, Padrini R. Transfer of propafenone and 5–OH-propafenone to foetal plasma and maternal milk. Br J Clin Pharmacol 1991; 32(4): 527–528.

PROPOFOL   L2

Trade: Diprivan
Other Trades: Diprivan
Category: Preanesthetic sedative

Propofol is an IV sedative hypnotic agent for induction and maintenance of anesthesia. It is particularly popular in various pediatric procedures. Although the terminal half-life is long, it is rapidly distributed out of the plasma compartment to other peripheral compartments (adipose) so that anesthesia is short (3–10 minutes). Propofol is incredibly lipid soluble. However, only very low concentrations of propofol have been found in breastmilk.

In one study of 4 women who received propofol 2.5 mg/kg IV followed by a continuous infusion, the breastmilk levels at 4 hours ranged from 0.04 to 0.24 mg/L during the induction phase only.[1] Following continued infusion of propofol in some patients at 5 mg/kg/h, milk samples at 4 hours ranged from 0.04 to 0.74 mg/L. The second breastmilk level, obtained 24 hours after delivery, contained only 6% of the 4-hour sample. Similar levels (0.12–0.97 mg/L) were noted by Schmitt in colostrum samples obtained 4–8 hours after induction with propofol.[2] From these data it is apparent that only minimal amounts of propofol are transferred to human milk. No data are available on the oral absorption of propofol. Propofol is rapidly cleared from the neonatal circulation.[1]

Pregnancy Risk	B	Lactation Risk	L2
T ½	= 1–3 days	M/P	=
Vd	= 60 l/kg	PB	= 99%
Tmax	= Instant (IV)	Oral	=
MW	= 178	pKa	= 11.0

Adult Concerns: Sedation, apnea.

Pediatric Concerns: None reported in several studies.

Drug Interactions: Anaphylactoid reactions when used with atracurium. May potentiate the neuromuscular blockade of vecuronium. May be additive with other CNS depressants. Theophylline may antagonize the effect of propofol.

Relative Infant Dose: 4.4%

Adult Dose: 6–12 mg/kg/hour

Alternatives: Midazolam

References:
1. Dailland P, Cockshott ID, Lirzin JD, Jacquinot P, Jorrot JC, Devery J, Harmey JL, Conseiller C. Intravenous propofol during cesarean section: placental transfer, concentrations in breast milk, and neonatal effects. A preliminary study. Anesthesiology 1989; 71(6): 827–834.
2. Schmitt JP, Schwoerer D, Diemunsch P, Gauthier-Lafaye J. [Passage of propofol in the colostrum. Preliminary data]. Ann Fr Anesth Reanim 1987; 6(4): 267–268.

PROPOXYPHENE   L2

Trade: Darvocet N, Propacet, Darvon

Other Trades: Dextropropoxyphene, Capadex, Paradex, Di-Gesic, Darvon-N, Novo-Propoxyn, Doloxene

Category: Mild narcotic analgesic

Propoxyphene is a mild narcotic analgesic similar in efficacy to aspirin. The amount secreted into milk is extremely low and is generally too low to produce effects in infant (<1 mg/day).[1] Maternal plasma levels peak at 2 hours. Propoxyphene is metabolized to norpropoxyphene (which has weaker CNS effects). Adult half-life= 6–12 hours (propoxyphene), 30–36 hours (norpropoxyphene). The milk to plasma ratio averages 0.417 for propoxyphene, and 0.382 for norpropoxyphene.[2] Thus far, no reports of untoward effects in infants have been reported.

Pregnancy Risk	C	Lactation Risk	L2
T ½	= 6–12 hours (propoxyphene)	M/P	= 0.41
Vd	= 12–26 l/kg	PB	= 78%
Tmax	= 2 hours	Oral	= Complete
MW	= 339	pKa	= 6.3

Adult Concerns: Nausea, respiratory depression, sedation, agitation, seizures, anemia, liver toxicity, withdrawal symptoms.

Pediatric Concerns: None reported but observe for sedation.

Drug Interactions: Additive sedation may occur when used with CNS depressants such as barbiturates. Carbamazepine levels may be increased. Use with cimetidine may produce CNS toxicity such as confusion, disorientation, apnea, seizures.

Relative Infant Dose:

Adult Dose: 65 mg every 4 hours as needed.

Alternatives: Ibuprofen, Acetaminophen

References:
1. Catz CS, Giacoia GP. Drugs and breast milk. Pediatr Clin North Am 1972; 19(1): 151–166.
2. Kunka RL, Venkataramanan R, Stern RM, Ladick CF. Excretion of propoxyphene and norpropoxyphene in breast milk. Clin Pharmacl Ther 1984; 35(5): 675–680.

PROPRANOLOL   L2

Trade: Inderal

Other Trades: Deralin, Detensol, Inderal, Novo-Pranol, Cardinol

Category: Beta-blocker, antihypertensive

Propranolol is a popular beta blocker used in treating hypertension, cardiac arrhythmias, migraine headache, and numerous other syndromes. In general, the maternal plasma levels are exceedingly low, hence the milk levels are low as well. Milk/plasma ratios are generally less than one. In one study of 3 patients, the average milk concentration was only 35.4 µg/L after multiple dosing intervals.

The milk/plasma ratio varied from 0.33 to 1.65.[1] Using this data, the authors suggest that an infant would receive only 70 µg/L of milk per day, which is <0.1% of the maternal dose. In another patient who was receiving 20 mg orally every 8 hours, levels of propranolol ranged from zero to 5 µg/L.[2] In another study of a patient receiving 20 mg twice daily, milk levels varied from 4 to 20 µg/L with an estimated average dose to infant of 3 µg/day.[3] In another patient receiving 40 mg four times daily, the peak concentration occurred at 3 hours after dosing.[4] Milk levels varied from zero to 9 µg/L. After a 30 day regimen of 240 mg/day propranolol, the pre-dose and post dose concentrations in breastmilk was 26 and 64 µg/L respectively.[4] No symptoms or signs of beta blockade were noted in this infant. The above amounts in milk would likely be clinically insignificant. Long term exposure has not been studied, and caution is urged. Of the beta blocker family, propranolol is probably preferred in lactating women. Use with great caution, if at all, in mothers or infants with asthma.

Pregnancy Risk	C	Lactation Risk	L2
T ½	= 3–5 hours	M/P	= 0.5
Vd	= 3–5 l/kg	PB	= 90%
Tmax	= 60–90 minutes	Oral	= 30%
MW	= 259	pKa	= 9.5

Adult Concerns: Bradycardia, asthmatic symptoms, hypotension, sedation, weakness, hypoglycemia. Do not use in asthmatics.

Pediatric Concerns: None reported via breastmilk in numerous studies. Do not use in mothers breastfeeding infants subject to reactive airway disease (asthma).

Drug Interactions: Decreased effect when used with aluminum salts, barbiturates, calcium salts, cholestyramine, NSAIDs, ampicillin, rifampin, and salicylates. Beta blockers may reduce the effect of oral sulfonylureas (hypoglycemic agents). Increased toxicity/effect when used with other antihypertensives, contraceptives, monoamine oxidase inhibitors, cimetidine, and numerous other products. See drug interactions reference for complete listing.

Relative Infant Dose: 0.3%–0.5%

Adult Dose: 160–240 mg daily.

Alternatives: Metoprolol

References:
1. Smith MT, Livingstone I, Hooper WD, Eadie MJ, Triggs EJ. Propranolol, propranolol glucuronide, and naphthoxylactic acid in breast milk and plasma. Ther Drug Monit 1983; 5(1): 87–93.
2. Lewis AM, Patel L, Johnston A, Turner P. Mexiletine in human blood and breast milk. Postgrad Med J. 1981 Sep; 57(671): 546–7.
3. Taylor EA, Turner P. Anti-hypertensive therapy with propranolol during pregnancy and lactation. Postgrad Med J 1981; 57(669): 427–430.
4. Bauer JH, Pape B, Zajicek J, Groshong T. Propranolol in human plasma and breast milk. Am J Cardiol 1979; 43(4): 860–862.

PROPYLHEXEDRINE   L5

Trade: Benzedrex
Other Trades:
Category: Decongestant

Propylhexedrine is a stimulant with similar structure to methamphetamine. Propylhexedrine is used as a nasal decongestant but can also be used as a drug of abuse when taken orally or IV. There are no adequate and well-controlled studies or case reports in breast feeding women. Systemic effects include headache, hypertension, nervousness, and tachycardia. There have been fatalities due to myocardial infarction, pulmonary hypertension, and psychosis.

Pregnancy Risk	C	Lactation Risk	L5
T ½	=	M/P	=
Vd	=	PB	=
Tmax	=	Oral	=
MW	= 155.3	pKa	=

Adult Concerns: Sneezing, stinging, burning, rebound congestion. Systemic side-effects are hypertension, headache, tachycardia, nervousness.

Pediatric Concerns:

Drug Interactions:

Relative Infant Dose:

Adult Dose: 2 inhalations per nostril every 2 hours.

Alternatives: Oxymetazoline

References:

PROPYLTHIOURACIL   L2

Trade: PTU
Other Trades: Propyl-Thyracil
Category: Antithyroid

Propylthiouracil (PTU) reduces the production and secretion of thyroxine by the thyroid gland. Only small amounts are secreted into breastmilk. Reports thus far suggest that levels absorbed by infant are too low to produce side effects.[1] In one study of nine patients given 400 mg doses, mean serum and milk levels were 7.7 mg/L and 0.7 mg/L respectively.[2] No changes in infant thyroid have been reported. PTU is the best of antithyroid medications for use in lactating mothers. Monitor infant thyroid function (T4, TSH) carefully during therapy.

Pregnancy Risk	D	Lactation Risk	L2
T ½	= 1.5–5 hours	M/P	= 0.1
Vd	= 0.87 l/kg	PB	= 80–95%
Tmax	= 1 hour	Oral	= 50–95%
MW	= 170	pKa	= 12.89

Adult Concerns: Hypothyroidism, liver toxicity, aplastic anemia, anemia.

Pediatric Concerns: None reported, but observed closely for thyroid function.

Drug Interactions: Activity of oral anticoagulants may be potentiated by propylthiouracil associated anti-vitamin K activity.

Relative Infant Dose: 1.8%

Adult Dose: 100 mg three times daily.

Alternatives:

References:
1. Cooper DS. Antithyroid drugs: to breast-feed or not to breast-feed. Am J Obstet Gynecol 1987; 157(2): 234–235.
2. Kampmann JP, Johansen K, Hansen JM, Helweg J. Propylthiouracil in human milk. Revision of a dogma. Lancet 1980; 1(8171): 736–737.

PSEUDOEPHEDRINE   L3

Trade: Sudafed, Dimetapp Decongestant, Simply Stuffy, Cenafed, Biofed, Contac 12–Hour, 12 Hour Cold Maximum Strength

Other Trades:

Category: Decongestant

Pseudoephedrine is an adrenergic compound primarily used as a nasal decongestant. It is secreted into breast milk but in low levels. In a study of 3 lactating mothers who received 60 mg of pseudoephedrine, the milk/plasma ratio was as high as 2.6–3.9.[1] The average pseudoephedrine milk level over 24 hours was 264 µg/L. The calculated dose that would be absorbed by the infant was still very low (0.4 to 0.6% of the maternal dose). In a study of eight lactating women who received a single 60 mg dose of pseudoephedrine, the 24 hour milk production was reduced by 24% from 784 mL/day in the placebo period to 623 mL/day in the pseudoephedrine period.[2] While this study was done with a single 60 mg dose, if the normal dosing rate of 60 mg four times daily was used, the estimated infant dose of pseudoephedrine would have been 4.3% of the weight-adjusted maternal dose. While these results are preliminary, it is apparent that mothers in late-stage lactation may be more sensitive to pseudoephedrine and have greater loss in milk production. Therefore, breastfeeding mothers with poor or marginal milk production should be exceedingly cautious in using pseudoephedrine. While there are anecdotal reports of its use in mothers with engorgement, we do not know if it is effective, or recommend its use for this purpose at this time.

Pregnancy Risk	C	Lactation Risk	L3
T ½	= 9–16 hours	M/P	= 2.6–3.3
Vd	=	PB	=
Tmax	= 1–3 hours	Oral	= 90%
MW	= 165	pKa	= 9.7

Adult Concerns: Irritability, agitation, anorexia, stimulation, insomnia, hypertension, tachycardia.

Pediatric Concerns: One case of irritability via milk. Reduced milk production has been reported in late stage lactation. Mothers with marginal production should avoid this medication.

Drug Interactions: May have increased toxicity when used with monoamine oxidase inhibitors.

Relative Infant Dose: 4.7%

Adult Dose: 60 mg every 4–6 hours.

Alternatives: Oxymetazoline

References:
1. Findlay JW, Butz RF, Sailstad JM, Warren JT, Welch RM. Pseudoephedrine and triprolidine in plasma and breast milk of nursing mothers. Br J Clin Pharmacol 1984; 18(6): 901–906.
2. Aljazaf K, Hale TW, Ilett KF, Hartmann PE, Mitoulas LR, Kristensen JH, Hackett LP. Pseudoephedrine: effects on milk production in women and estimation of infant exposure via breastmilk. Br J Clin Pharmacol 2003; 56(1): 18–24.

PYRANTEL L3

Trade: Ascarel, Pamix, Pin-X, Pinworm

Other Trades: Early Bird

Category: Anthelmintic

Pyrantel is an anthelmintic used to treat pinworm, hookworm, and round worm infestations.[1] It is only minimally absorbed orally, with the majority being eliminated in feces. Peak plasma levels are generally less than 0.05 to 0.13 µg/mL and occur prior to 3 hours. Reported side effects are few and minimal. No data on transfer of pyrantel in human milk are available, but due to minimal oral absorption, and low plasma levels, it is unlikely that breastmilk levels would be clinically relevant. Generally it is administered as a single dose.

Pregnancy Risk	C	Lactation Risk	L3
T ½	=	M/P	=
Vd	=	PB	=
Tmax	= <3 hours	Oral	= <50%
MW	= 206	pKa	=

Adult Concerns: Side effects are generally minimal and include headache, dizziness, somnolence, insomnia, nausea, vomiting, abdominal cramps, diarrhea and pain. Only moderate changes in liver enzymes have been noted, without serious hepatotoxicity.

Pediatric Concerns: None reported via milk.

Drug Interactions: Pyrantel and piperazine should not be mixed because they are antagonistic. Pyrantel increases theophylline plasma levels.

Relative Infant Dose:

Adult Dose: 11 mg/kg X 2 over two weeks

Alternatives:

References:
1. Pharmaceutical manufacturer Prescribing Information, 2008.

PYRAZINAMIDE   L3

Trade: Pyrazinamide, D-50, MK-56

Other Trades: Zinamide, PMS-pyrazinamide, Tebrazid

Category: Antitubercular antibiotic

Pyrazinamide is a typical antituberculosis antibiotic used as first-line therapy in tuberculosis infections. In one patient three hours following an oral dose of 1000 mg, peak milk levels were 1.5 mg/L of milk.[1] Peak maternal plasma levels at 2 hours were 42 µg/mL. This amounts to a relative infant dose of 1.5%. This is probably too low to be clinically relevant in the breastfed infant.

Pregnancy Risk	C	Lactation Risk	L3
T ½	= 9–10 hours	M/P	=
Vd	= 0.75–1.65 l/kg	PB	= 5–10%
Tmax	= 2 hours	Oral	= Complete
MW	= 123	pKa	=

Adult Concerns: The most common side effect is hepatotoxicity, nausea and vomiting. Transient increases in liver enzymes, including fever, anorexia, malaise, jaundice, and liver tenderness have been reported. Hyperuricemia including gout has been reported. Maculopapular rashes, arthralgia, acne and numerous other side effects have been noted.

Pediatric Concerns: None reported via milk.

Drug Interactions:

Relative Infant Dose: 1.5%

Adult Dose: 15–30 mg/kg daily.

Alternatives:

References:
1. Holdiness MR. Antituberculosis drugs and breast-feeding. Arch Intern Med 1984; 144(9): 1888.

PYRETHRUM EXTRACT + PIPERONYL BUTOXIDE   L3

Trade: Licide, Rid, Tisit, Lice-X, A200 Maximum Strength, A200 Time-Tested Formula, Medi-Lice Maximum Strength, Pronto Maximum Strength, Pronto Plus

Other Trades:

Category: Lice treatment

This is a shampoo which contains Pyrethrum extract (equivalent to 0.33% pyrethrins) and Piperonyl butoxide (4%) used for the treatment of head and body lice.[1] Pyrethrins are natural insecticides derived from Chrysanthemum plants. They have minimal systemic toxicity. Topical absorption through the skin is negligible, so levels in milk are likely nil. However, there are no adequate and well-controlled studies or case reports in breastfeeding women.

Pregnancy Risk	C	Lactation Risk	L3
T ½	=	M/P	=
Vd	=	PB	=
Tmax	=	Oral	= Poor topically
MW	= 316	pKa	=

Adult Concerns: Dermatitis, allergies in children. Oral toxicity is significant in children.

Pediatric Concerns:

Drug Interactions:

Relative Infant Dose:

Adult Dose:

Alternatives:

References:
1. Pharmaceutical manufacturer prescribing information, 2011.

PYRIDOSTIGMINE   L2

Trade: Mestinon, Regonol

Other Trades: Mestinon, Regonol

Category: Anticholinesterase muscle stimulant

Pyridostigmine is a potent cholinesterase inhibitor used in myasthenia gravis to stimulate muscle strength. In a group of 2 mothers receiving from 120–300 mg/day, breastmilk concentrations varied from 5 to 25 µg/L.[1] The calculated milk/plasma ratios varied from 0.36 to 1.13. No cholinergic side effects were noted in the infants and no pyridostigmine was found in the infants' plasma. Because the oral bioavailability is so poor (10–20%), the actual dose received by the breastfed infant would be significantly less than the above concentrations. Please note the dosage is highly variable and may be as high as 600 mg/day in divided doses. The authors estimated total daily intake at 0.1% or less of the maternal dose.

Pregnancy Risk	C	Lactation Risk	L2
T ½	= 3.3 hours	M/P	= 0.36–1.13
Vd	= 0.53–1.76 l/kg	PB	=
Tmax	= 1–2 hours	Oral	= 10–20%
MW	= 261	pKa	=

Adult Concerns: Nausea, vomiting, salivation, sweating, weakness, asthmatic symptoms, muscle cramps, fasciculations, constricted pupils.

Pediatric Concerns: None reported in one study of two infants.

Drug Interactions: Increased effect of neuromuscular blockers such as succinylcholine. Increased toxicity with edrophonium.

Relative Infant Dose: 0.09%

Adult Dose: 60–180 mg 2–4 times daily.

Alternatives:

References:
1. Hardell LI, Lindstrom B, Lonnerholm G, Osterman PO. Pyridostigmine in human breast milk. Br J Clin Pharmacol 1982; 14(4): 565–567.

PYRIDOXINE   L2

Trade: Vitamin B$_6$, Hexa-Betalin
Other Trades: Pyroxin, Hexa-Betalin, Comploment continus
Category: Vitamin B$_6$

Pyridoxine is vitamin B$_6$. The recommended daily allowance for non-pregnant women is 1.6 mg/day. Pyridoxine is secreted in milk in direct proportion to the maternal intake and concentrations in milk vary from 123 to 314 ng/mL depending on the study. Pyridoxine is required in slight excess during pregnancy and lactation and most prenatal vitamin supplements contain from 12–25 mg/day. Very high doses (600 mg/day) were reported to suppress prolactin secretion and therefore production of breastmilk.[1,2] However, this data has been refuted in two studies where high doses of pyridoxine failed to suppress prolactin levels or lactation.[3,4]

It is not advisable to use in excess of 100 mg/day. One study clearly indicates that pyridoxine readily transfers into breastmilk and that B$_6$ levels in milk correlate closely with maternal intake, thus the reason for not using excessive doses.[5] Breastfeeding mothers who are deficient in pyridoxine should be supplemented with modest amounts (≤40 mg/day).

Pregnancy Risk	A	Lactation Risk	L2/L4 in high doses
T ½	= 15–20 days	M/P	=
Vd	=	PB	=
Tmax	= 1–2 hours	Oral	= Complete
MW	= 205	pKa	=

Adult Concerns: Reduced milk production, sensory neuropathy, gastrointestinal distress, sedation. Seizures at high doses (>360 mg/day).

Pediatric Concerns: Excessive oral doses have been reported to produce sedation, hypotonia and respiratory distress in infants, although none have been reported via breastmilk.

Drug Interactions: Decreased serum levels with levodopa, phenobarbital, and phenytoin.

Relative Infant Dose:

Adult Dose: 40 mg/day or less.

Alternatives:

References:
1. Marcus RG. Suppression of lactation with high doses of pyridoxine. S Afr Med J 1975; 49(52): 2155–2156.
2. Foukas MD. An antilactogenic effect of pyridoxine. J Obstet Gynaecol Br Commonw 1973; 80(8): 718–720.
3. de Waal JM, Steyn AF, Harms JH, Slabber CF, Pannall PR. Failure of pyridoxine to suppress raised serum prolactin levels. S Afr Med J 1978; 53(8): 293–294.
4. Canales ES, Soria J, Zarate A, Mason M, Molina M. The influence of pyridoxine on prolactin secretion and milk production in women. Br J Obstet Gynaecol 1976; 83(5): 387–388.
5. Kang-Yoon SA, Kirksey A, Giacoia G, West K. Vitamin B-6 status of breast-fed neonates: influence of pyridoxine supplementation on mothers and neonates. Am J Clin Nutr 1992; 56(3): 548–558.

PYRILAMINE — L3

Trade: Corzall, Dextrophenylpril, Polyhist, Atac, Ban-Tuss

Other Trades:

Category: Anti-histamine

Pyrilamine is an antihistamine which blocks the H_1 receptor.[1] It is used in many over-the-counter products. Antihistamines in this class may cause excitement in children, or sleeplessness. Pyrilamine also has anticholinergic (drying) effects as well. Use of these older antihistamines in pregnant and breastfeeding mothers should be avoided. Use the newer non-sedating antihistamines, such as loratadine or cetirizine.

Pregnancy Risk	C		Lactation Risk	L3
T ½	=		M/P	=
Vd	=		PB	=
Tmax	=		Oral	= Complete
MW	= 401		pKa	=

Adult Concerns: Sedation, incoordination, anticholinergic effects, excitement in children, CNS depression.

Pediatric Concerns:

Drug Interactions: Antihistamines may enhance the effect of tricyclic antidepressants, barbiturates, alcohol, and other CNS depressants. Monoamine oxidase inhibitors prolong and intensify the anticholinergic effects of antihistamines.

Relative Infant Dose:

Adult Dose: 75–200 mg per day in 4 divided doses.

Alternatives: Cetirizine, loratadine

References:
1. Pharmaceutical manufacturer prescribing information, 2011.

PYRIMETHAMINE   L3

Trade: Daraprim

Other Trades: Fansidar, Maloprim, Daraprim

Category: Antimalarial, folic acid antagonist

Pyrimethamine is a folic acid antagonist that has been used for prophylaxis of malaria. Maternal peak plasma levels occur 2–6 hours post-dose.[1] Pyrimethamine is secreted into human milk. In a group of mothers receiving 25, 50, and 75 mg/day of pyrimethamine for 10 days, milk levels ranged from 0.125 to 0.155 µg/L twenty four hours following the dose. The peak concentration was 3.3 mg/L.[2] An infant would receive an estimated dose of 3–4 mg in a 48 hour period (following 75 mg maternal dose). In another study, three women received a dose of 12.5 mg orally 2–5 days postpartum. The infants were reported to receive about 0.14, 0.21, and 0.34 mg pyrimethamine over 5 days.[3] The authors estimate the relative infant dose to be 46% of the maternal dose. No adverse effects were reported in any of the infants. Pyrimethamine is used in pediatric patients for the treatment and prophylaxis of malaria.

Pregnancy Risk	C		Lactation Risk	L3
T ½	= 96 hours		M/P	= 0.2–0.43
Vd	=		PB	= 87%
Tmax	= 2–6 hours		Oral	= Complete
MW	= 249		pKa	=

Adult Concerns: Anemia, blood dyscrasias, folate deficiency states, carcinogenesis, insomnia, headache, anorexia, vomiting, megaloblastic anemia, leukopenia.

Pediatric Concerns: None reported, but possible carcinogenesis may preclude its use in breastfed infants.

Drug Interactions: Use of pyrimethamine with other antifolate drugs (methotrexate, sulfonamides, TMP-SMZ) may increase the risk of bone marrow suppression and folate deficiency states.

Relative Infant Dose: 45.8%

Adult Dose: 25 mg every week.

Alternatives:

References:
1. Pharmaceutical manufacturer prescribing information, 1996.
2. Clyde DF, Press J, Shute GT. Transfer of pyrimethamine in human milk. J Trop Med Hyg 1956; 59(12): 277–284.
3. Edstein MD, Veenendaal JR, Newman K et al. Excretion of chloroquine, dapsone and pyrimethamine in human milk. Br J Clin Pharmacol. 1986; 22: 733–5.

PYRITHIONE ZINC   L3

Trade:

Other Trades:

Category: Dandruff and seborrheal dermatitis treatment

Pyrithione zinc is an antibacterial and anti-fungal agent that is used in dandruff treatment. Animal studies suggested that systemic absorption from topical administration of pyrithione zinc is low, in the order of 1–2%.[1] Because of minimal systemic absorption from topical administration, pyrithione zinc is unlikely to be present in milk. There are no adequate and well-controlled studies or case reports in breastfeeding women.

Pregnancy Risk	Probably Safe	Lactation Risk	L3
T ½	=	M/P	=
Vd	=	PB	=
Tmax	=	Oral	=
MW	= 318	pKa	=

Adult Concerns: Peripheral neuritis. Can cause irritation to mucous membranes with contact. If accidentally ingested, can cause hypernatremia, tachycardia, hypotension, nausea, vomiting, and diarrhea.

Pediatric Concerns:

Drug Interactions:

Relative Infant Dose:

Adult Dose:

Alternatives:

References:
1. Zinc pyrithione. In: REPROTOX Æ Database [Internet database]. Greenwood Village, Colo: Thomson Reuters (Healthcare) Inc. Updated periodically. Accessed 7/1/2011.

QUAZEPAM   L2

Trade: Doral, Dormalin
Other Trades:
Category: Sedative, hypnotic

Quazepam is a long half-life benzodiazepine medication used as a sedative and hypnotic. It is selectively metabolized to several metabolites that have even longer half-lives. In a study of four breastfeeding mothers who received a single 15 mg dose of quazepam, the average milk/plasma ratio (AUC) was 4.18.[1] The C_{max} of quazepam in milk occurred at 3 hours and was 95.8 µg/L and over the 48 hours, only 11.59 µg quazepam was recovered. The average concentration (AUC) of quazepam equivalents over 48 hours was 19.6 µg/L. However, including metabolites, the authors suggest that 17.1 µg of quazepam equivalents or 0.11% of the administered dose was recovered in milk. The authors estimated that 28.7 µg quazepam equivalents, or 0.19% of the quazepam dose would be excreted in breast milk every 24 hours. These estimates were not weight-adjusted. Observe for sedation in the breastfed infant.

Pregnancy Risk	X		Lactation Risk	L2
T ½	= 39 hours		M/P	= 4.18
Vd	= 5–8.6 l/kg		PB	= >95%
Tmax	= 2 hours		Oral	= Complete
MW	= 387		pKa	=

Adult Concerns: Drowsiness, sedation.

Pediatric Concerns: None reported via breastmilk. Observe for sedation.

Drug Interactions: May increase sedation when used with CNS depressants such as alcohol, barbiturates, opioids. Cimetidine may decrease metabolism and clearance of benzodiazepines. Valproic acid may displace benzodiazepines from binding sites, thus increasing sedative effects. SSRIs (fluoxetine, sertraline, paroxetine) can dramatically increase benzodiazepine levels by altering clearance, thus leading to sedation .

Relative Infant Dose: 1.4%

Adult Dose: 15 mg daily.

Alternatives: Lorazepam, alprazolam

References:
1. Hilbert JM, Gural RP, Symchowicz S, Zampaglione N. Excretion of quazepam into human breast milk. J Clin Pharmacol 1984; 24(10): 457–462.

QUETIAPINE   L2

Trade: Seroquel, Seroquel XR
Other Trades:
Category: Antipsychotic drug

Quetiapine is indicated for the treatment of psychotic disorders.[1] It has some affinity for histamine receptors, which may account for its sedative properties. It has been shown to increase the incidence of seizures, prolactin levels, and to lower thyroid levels in adults. In a patient (92 kg) receiving 200 mg/day of quetiapine throughout pregnancy, samples were expressed just before dosing, and at 1,2,4, and 6 hours post dose.[2] The average milk concentration of quetiapine over the 6 hours was 13 µg/L, with a maximum concentration of 62 µg/L at 1 hour. Levels of quetiapine rapidly fell to almost predose levels by 2 hours. The authors report that an exclusively breastfed infant would ingest only 0.09% of the weight-adjusted maternal dose. At maximum, the infant would ingest 0.43% of the weight-adjusted maternal dose. Although only one patient was studied, the data suggests levels in milk are minimal at this maternal dose. One study of 6 mothers taking a combination of quetiapine, paroxetine, clonazepam, trazodone, and/or venlafaxine showed that no medication was detectable in 3 of the mothers' milk. In two of the other cases, quetiapine levels were below 0.01 mg/kg/day infant dose, while the final mother expressed an infant dose of less than 0.10 mg/kg/day. The mothers' doses of quetiapine ranged from 25–400 mg. The authors reported that no correlation was noted between drug exposure and developmental outcomes.[3] In another study of one mother receiving 400 mg quetiapine per day 3 months postpartum, expressed milk contained with an average drug concentration of 41 µg/L, and a milk-to-plasma ratio of 0.29. The relative infant dose reported was 0.09% of the mother's dose. The infant's plasma concentration was 1.4 µg/L, or 6% of the mother's plasma concentration. No adverse effects were reported in the infant, but the authors suggest monitoring the infant's progress and quetiapine serum concentrations.[4]

Pregnancy Risk	C	Lactation Risk	L2
T ½	= 6 hours	M/P	= 0.29
Vd	= 10 l/kg	PB	= 83%
Tmax	= 1.5 hours	Oral	= 100%
MW	= 883	pKa	=

Adult Concerns: The side effects of quetiapine are similar to other antipsychotic drugs and include sedation, tardive dyskinesia, seizures, priapism, hypothermia, dysphagia, hyperprolactinemia, orthostatic hypotension, cataracts, and hypothyroidism.

Pediatric Concerns: None reported via milk in one small study.

Drug Interactions: Phenytoin increases clearance of quetiapine significantly (5X). Other drugs which increase clearance include: cimetidine, thioridazine, and other

P450 3a inhibitors. Lorazepam levels may be reduced by 20% when used with quetiapine.

Relative Infant Dose: 0.07%–0.1%

Adult Dose: 300–400 mg daily.

Alternatives: Risperidone, olanzapine

References:
1. Pharmaceutical manufacturer prescribing information, 1999.
2. Lee A, Giesbrecht B, Dunn E, Ito S. Excretion of Quetiapine in Breast Milk. Am J Psychiatry 2004; 161(9): 1715–6.
3. Misri S, Corral M, Wardrop AA, Kendrick K. Quetiapine Augmentation in Lactation: A Series of Case Reports. J Clin Psychopharmacol 2006; 26(5): 508–511.
4. Rampono J, Kristensen JH, Ilett KF, Hackett P, Kohan R. Quetiapine and Breast Feeding. Ann Pharmacother 2007; 41: 711–714.

QUINACRINE   L4

Trade: Atabrine

Other Trades:

Category: Antimalarial, giardiasis

Quinacrine was once used for malaria but has been replaced by other preparations. It is primarily used for giardiasis.[1,2] Small to trace amounts are secreted into milk. No known harmful effects except in infants with G6PD deficiencies. However, quinacrine is eliminated from the body very slowly, requiring up to 2 months for complete elimination. Quinacrine levels in liver are extremely high. Accumulation in infant is likely due to slow rate of excretion. Caution is urged.

Pregnancy Risk	C	Lactation Risk	L4
T ½	= >5 days	M/P	=
Vd	=	PB	= High
Tmax	= 1–3 hours	Oral	= Complete
MW	= 400	pKa	=

Adult Concerns: Gastrointestinal distress, liver toxicity, seizures, aplastic anemia, retinopathy.

Pediatric Concerns: None reported via milk, but accumulation may occur after prolonged exposure. Use with caution.

Drug Interactions: Primaquine toxicity is increased by quinacrine. Concomitant use is contraindicated.

Relative Infant Dose:

Adult Dose: 100 mg three times daily.

Alternatives:

References:
1. Drug Facts and Comparisons 1994 ed. ed. St. Louis: 1994.
2. McEvoy GE. (ed): AFHS Drug Information. 1992.

QUINAPRIL   L2/L4

Trade: Accupril, Accuretic
Other Trades: Accupril, Asig, Accupril, Accupro
Category: ACE inhibitor, antihypertensive

Quinapril is an angiotensin converting enzyme inhibitor (ACE) used as an antihypertensive. Once in the plasma compartment, quinapril is rapidly converted to quinaprilat, the active metabolite. In a study of 6 women who received 20 mg/day, the milk/plasma ratio for quinapril was 0.12.[1] Quinapril was not detected in milk after 4 hours. No quinaprilat (metabolite) was detected in any of the milk samples. The estimated 'dose' of quinapril that would be received by the infant was 1.6% of the maternal dose, adjusted for respective weights. The authors suggest that quinapril appears to be 'safe' during breastfeeding although, as always, the risk:benefit ratio should be considered when it is to be given to a nursing mother. ACE inhibitors are generally contraindicated during pregnancy due to increased fetal morbidity. The drug should not be used early postpartum in preterm infants.

Pregnancy Risk	C/D in 2nd and 3rd trimester	Lactation Risk	L2/L4 in preterm infants
T ½	= 2 hours	M/P	= 0.12
Vd	=	PB	= 97%
Tmax	= 2 hour	Oral	= Complete
MW	= 474	pKa	=

Adult Concerns: Cough, hypotension, nausea, vomiting.

Pediatric Concerns: None reported in one study. Levels are so low this agent is probably quite safe in most instances.

Drug Interactions: Probenecid increases plasma levels of ACE inhibitors. ACE inhibitors and diuretics have additive hypotensive effects. Antacids reduce bioavailability of ACE inhibitors. NSAIDS reduce hypotension of ACE inhibitors. Phenothiazines increase effects of ACE inhibitors. ACE inhibitors increase digoxin and lithium plasma levels. May elevate potassium levels when potassium supplementation is added.

Relative Infant Dose: 1.6%

Adult Dose: 20–80 mg daily.

Alternatives: Captopril, enalapril

References:
1. Begg EJ, Robson RA, Gardiner SJ, Hudson LJ, Reece PA, Olson SC, Posvar EL, Sedman AJ. Quinapril and its metabolite quinaprilat in human milk. Br J Clin Pharmacol 2001; 51(5): 478–481.

QUINIDINE   L2

Trade: Quinaglute, Quinidex

Other Trades: Kinidin Durules, Apo-Quinidine, Cardioquin, Novo-Quinidin, Kiditard

Category: Antiarrhythmic agent

Quinidine is used to treat cardiac arrhythmias. Three hours following a dose of 600 mg, the level of quinidine in the maternal serum was 9.0 mg/L and the concentration in her breast milk was 6.4 mg/L.[1] Subsequently, a level of 8.2 mg/L was noted in breastmilk. Quinidine is selectively stored in the liver. Long-term use could expose an infant to liver toxicity. Monitor liver enzymes.

Pregnancy Risk	C	Lactation Risk	L2
T ½	= 6–8 hours	M/P	= 0.71
Vd	= 1.8–3.0 l/kg	PB	= 87%
Tmax	= 1–2 hours	Oral	= 80%
MW	= 324	pKa	= 4.2, 8.3

Adult Concerns: Blood dyscrasias, hypotension, thrombocytopenia, depression, fever.

Pediatric Concerns: None reported, but observe for changes in liver function.

Drug Interactions: Quinidine levels may be elevated with amiodarone, certain antacids, cimetidine, verapamil. Digoxin plasma levels may be increased with quinidine. Quinidine may increase anticoagulant levels when used with warfarin. Quinidine levels or effects may be reduced when used with barbiturates, nifedipine, rifampin, sucralfate, or phenytoin. Effects of procainamide may be dangerously increased when used with quinidine. Clearance of tricyclic antidepressants may be decreased by quinidine.

Relative Infant Dose: 14.4%

Adult Dose: 200–400 mg 3–4 times daily.

Alternatives:

References:
1. Hill LM, Malkasian GD, Jr. The use of quinidine sulfate throughout pregnancy. Obstet Gynecol 1979; 54(3): 366–368.

QUININE   L2

Trade: Quinamm

Other Trades: Biquinate, Myoquin, Quinbisul, Quinate, Novo-Quinine

Category: Antimalarial

Quinine is a cinchona alkaloid primarily used in malaria prophylaxis and treatment. Small to trace amounts are secreted into milk. No reported harmful effects have been reported except in infants with G6PD deficiencies. In a study of 6 women receiving 600–1300 mg/day, the concentration of quinine in breastmilk ranged from 0.4 to 1.6 mg/L at 1.5 to 6 hours post-dose.[1] The authors suggest these levels are clinically insignificant. In another study, with maternal plasma concentrations of 0.5 to 8 mg/L, the milk/plasma ratio ranged from 0.11 to 0.53.[2] The total daily consumption by a breastfed infant was estimated to be 1–3 mg/day.

Pregnancy Risk	D	Lactation Risk	L2
T ½	= 11 hours	M/P	= 0.11–0.53
Vd	= 1.8–3.0 l/kg	PB	= 93%
Tmax	= 1–3 hours	Oral	= 76%
MW	= 324	pKa	= 4.3, 8.4

Adult Concerns: Blood dyscrasias, thrombocytopenia, retinal toxicity, tongue discoloration, kidney damage.

Pediatric Concerns: None reported via breastmilk in several studies.

Drug Interactions: Aluminum containing antacids may delay or decrease absorption. Quinine may depress vitamin K dependent clotting factors thereby increasing warfarin effects. Cimetidine may reduce quinine clearance. Digoxin serum levels may be increased. Do not use with mefloquine.

Relative Infant Dose: 0.7%–1.3%

Adult Dose: 650 mg every 8 hours.

Alternatives:

References:
1. Terwillinger WG, Hatcher RA. The elimination of morphine and quinine in human milk. Surg Gynecol Obstet 1934; 58: 823.
2. Phillips RE, Looareesuwan S, White NJ, Silamut K, Kietinun S, Warrell DA. Quinine pharmacokinetics and toxicity in pregnant and lactating women with falciparum malaria. Br J Clin Pharmacol 1986; 21(6): 677–683.

RABEPRAZOLE   L3

Trade: Aciphex

Other Trades:

Category: Antisecretory, antacid

Rabeprazole is an antisecretory proton pump inhibitor similar to omeprazole. Rodent studies suggest a high milk/plasma ratio, but as we know, these do not correlate well with humans. No data are available in humans. Further, rabeprazole is only 52% bioavailable in adults even when enteric coated due to its instability in gastric acids.[1] When presented in milk, it would be virtually destroyed in the infant's stomach prior to absorption.

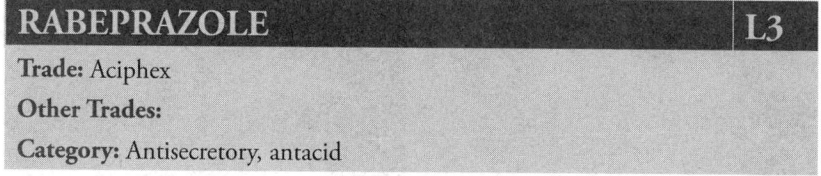

Pregnancy Risk	B	Lactation Risk	L3
T ½	= 1–2 hours	M/P	=
Vd	=	PB	= 96.3
Tmax	= 2–5 hours	Oral	= 52% (enteric)
MW	= 381	pKa	=

Adult Concerns: Asthenia, fever, allergies, malaise, chest pain, photosensitivity. Myalgia, arthritis, leg cramps and bone pain have been reported.

Pediatric Concerns: None reported via milk.

Drug Interactions: None are reported.

Relative Infant Dose:

Adult Dose: 20 mg daily.

Alternatives: Omeprazole

References:
1. Pharmaceutical manufacturer prescribing information, 2002.

RABIES INFECTION   L3

Trade: Rabies Infection
Other Trades:
Category: Viral infection

Rabies is an acute rapidly progressing illness caused by an RNA-containing virus that is usually fatal. Infection occurs via exposure to infected saliva, usually following animal bites. Incubation is prolonged and can be up to 4–6 weeks.[1] The virus multiplies locally, passes into local neurons and progressively ascends to the central nervous system. The virus is seldom found in the plasma compartment. The issue of breastfeeding following exposure to an animal bite is contentious and somewhat obscure. Person to person transmission has not been documented, nor has there been documentation of transmission of the rabies virus into human milk.[2,3] If a breastfeeding woman is exposed to the rabies virus, she should receive the human rabies immune globulin and begin the vaccination series.[4] Most sources agree that once immunization has begun, the mother can continue breastfeeding. For a thorough review, see reference 4.

Pregnancy Risk	Possibly Hazardous		Lactation Risk	L3
T½	=		M/P	=
Vd	=		PB	=
Tmax	=		Oral	=
MW	=		pKa	=

Adult Concerns:

Pediatric Concerns:

Drug Interactions:

Relative Infant Dose:

Adult Dose:

Alternatives:

References:
1. American Academy of Pediatrics. In: Pickering LK, ed. 2000 Red Book: Report of the Committee on Infectious Diseases. 25th ed. ed. Elk Grove Village, IL: 2000.

2. Lawrence RA. Breastfeeding: A guide for the medical profession. St. Louis: Mosby Publishers, 1994.
3. Hall TG. Diseases Transmitted from Animal to Man. Springfield, IL: Thomas, 1963.
4. Meerwood A, Philipp B. Breastfeeding: Conditions and Diseases. 1st ed. Amarillo, TX: Pharmasoft Publishing L.P., 2001.

RABIES VACCINE   L3

Trade: Imovax Rabies Vaccine, RabAvert

Other Trades:

Category: Vaccination for rabies.

Rabies vaccine is prepared from inactivated rabies virus. No data are available on transmission to breastmilk. Even if transferred to breastmilk, it is unlikely to produce untoward effects.[1]

Pregnancy Risk	C	Lactation Risk	L3
T ½	=	M/P	=
Vd	=	PB	=
Tmax	= 30–60 days	Oral	=
MW	=	pKa	=

Adult Concerns: Rash, anaphylactoid reactions, nausea, vomiting, diarrhea, etc.

Pediatric Concerns: No untoward effect reported.

Drug Interactions: Radiation therapy, antimalarials, corticosteroids, other immunosuppressive agents and immunosuppressive illnesses can interfere with the development of active immunity after vaccination, and may diminish the protective efficacy of the vaccine.

Relative Infant Dose:

Adult Dose: 1 mL X 3 over 21–28 days.

Alternatives:

References:
1. Pharmaceutical manufacturer prescribing information, 1995.

RALOXIFENE   L3

Trade: Evista

Other Trades: Evista

Category: Selective estrogen receptor modulator

Raloxifene hydrochloride is a selective estrogen receptor modulator (SERM) that has estrogenic actions on bone and anti-estrogenic actions on the uterus and breast. It blocks such estrogen effects as those that lead to breast cancer and uterine cancer. In addition, it also prevents bone loss and improved lipid profiles. It is used to prevent osteoporosis in postmenopausal women.[1] It is poorly absorbed orally (2%). While we do not have data on its transfer into human milk, levels are probably quite low. That present in milk would not be orally absorbed to any degree in infants. While the manufacturer suggests it is contraindicated in breastfeeding women, short-term exposure may not be overtly hazardous. Long-term exposure should be avoided, short-term exposure is probably of minimal risk.

Pregnancy Risk	X	Lactation Risk	L3
T ½	= 27–32 hours	M/P	=
Vd	= 2348 l/kg	PB	= >95%
Tmax	=	Oral	= 2%
MW	= 510	pKa	=

Adult Concerns: Adverse reactions include hot flashes, arthralgia, flu syndrome, infection, and headache.

Pediatric Concerns: No data are available.

Drug Interactions: Cholestyramine may decrease the absorption of raloxifene, and raloxifene may decrease levothyroxine absorption.

Relative Infant Dose:

Adult Dose: 60 mg/day.

Alternatives:

References:
1. Pharmaceutical manufacturer prescribing information, 2010.

RAMELTEON   L3

Trade: Rozerem
Other Trades:
Category: Nonbenzodiazepine hypnotic

Used for insomnia, ramelteon is a melatonin receptor agonist, and assists in the synchronization of the circadian rhythm and induces sleep.[1] Unlike the benzodiazepines, ramelteon does not bind to the GABA receptors. There have been no studies of levels of ramelteon in human milk. However, probable small amount in milk would only be 1.8% bioavailable. It is unlikely to sedate an infant.

Pregnancy Risk	C	Lactation Risk	L3
T ½	= 1–2.6 hours	M/P	=
Vd	= 1.06 l/kg	PB	= 82%
Tmax	= 0.5–1.5 hours	Oral	= 1.8%
MW	= 259	pKa	=

Adult Concerns: Adverse reactions include headache, fatigue, somnolence, dizziness, and nausea.

Pediatric Concerns: No data are available.

Drug Interactions: CNS depressants may have an additive effect on the depressant effect of ramelteon. CYP1A2 inhibitors will increase concentrations of ramelteon, as will fluconazole, fluvoxamine, and ketoconazole. Rifampin will decrease serum concentrations of ramelteon. Do not take with fluvoxamine or if you have liver problems.

Relative Infant Dose:

Adult Dose: 8 mg nightly.

Alternatives:

References:
1. Pharmaceutical manufacturer prescribing information, 2006.

RAMIPRIL   L3

Trade: Altace
Other Trades: Ramace, Tritace, Altace
Category: ACE inhibitor, antihypertensive

Ramipril is rapidly metabolized to ramiprilat which is a potent ACE inhibitor with a long half-life. It is used in hypertension. ACE inhibitors can cause increased fetal and neonatal morbidity and should not be used in pregnant women. Ingestion of a single 10 mg oral dose produced an undetectable level in breastmilk.[1,2] However, animal studies have indicated that ramiprilat is transferred into milk in concentrations about one-third of those found in serum, but animal studies (lactation) are always high and do not at all correlate with humans. Only 0.25% of the total dose is estimated to penetrate into milk.

Pregnancy Risk	C/D in 2nd and 3rd trimester	Lactation Risk	L3
T ½	= 13–17 hours	M/P	=
Vd	=	PB	= 56%
Tmax	= 2–4 hours	Oral	= 60%
MW	= 417	pKa	=

Adult Concerns: Hypotension, cough, nausea, vomiting, dizziness.

Pediatric Concerns: None reported via milk. Observe for hypotension.

Drug Interactions: Probenecid increases plasma levels of ACE inhibitors. ACE inhibitors and diuretics have additive hypotensive effects. Antacids reduce bioavailability of ACE inhibitors. NSAIDS reduce hypotension of ACE inhibitors. Phenothiazines increase effects of ACE inhibitors. ACE inhibitors increase digoxin and lithium plasma levels. May elevate potassium levels when potassium supplementation is added.

Relative Infant Dose: 0.3%

Adult Dose: 2.5–20 mg daily.

Alternatives: Captopril, enalapril

References:
1. Pharmaceutical manufacturer prescribing information, 1996.
2. Ball SG, Robertson JI. Clinical pharmacology of ramipril. Am J Cardiol 1987; 59(10): 23D-27D.

RANIBIZUMAB   L3

Trade: Lucentis
Other Trades:
Category: Angiogenesis inhibitor

Ranibizumab binds to and inhibits human vascular endothelial growth factor A, inhibiting it from binding to its receptor and suppressing neovascularization and slowing vision loss.[1] It is used in the treatment of macular degeneration. No data are available on the transfer of ranibizumab into the milk compartment, however, due to the large molecular weight, it is unlikely that this drug would pose a threat to a breastfeeding infant after the first week postpartum.

Pregnancy Risk	C	Lactation Risk	L3
T ½	= 9 days	M/P	=
Vd	=	PB	=
Tmax	=	Oral	= Nil
MW	= 48,000	pKa	=

Adult Concerns: Adverse reactions include headache, arthralgia, conjunctival hemorrhage, eye pain, increased intraocular pressure, nasopharyngitis and upper respiratory tract infection.

Pediatric Concerns: No data are available.

Drug Interactions: Drug interaction studies have not been conducted with ranibizumab.

Relative Infant Dose:

Adult Dose: 0.5 mg every month.

Alternatives: Pegaptanib

References:
1. Pharmaceutical manufacturer prescribing information, 2007.

RANITIDINE   L2

Trade: Zantac, Taladine, FusePaq Deprizine
Other Trades:
Category: Reduces gastric acid secretion

Ranitidine is a prototypic histamine-2 blocker used to reduce acid secretion in the stomach. It has been widely used in pediatrics without significant side effects primarily for gastroesophageal reflux (GER). Following a dose of 150 mg for four doses, concentrations in breastmilk were 0.72, 2.6, and 1.5 mg/L at 1.5, 5.5 and 12 hours respectively.[1] The milk/serum ratios varied from 6.81, 8.44 to 23.77 at 1.5, 5.5 and 12 hours respectively. Although the milk/plasma ratios are quite high, using this data, an infant would ingest at most 0.4 mg/kg/day. This amount is quite small considering the pediatric dose currently recommended is 2–4 mg/kg/24 hours. Consider nizatidine or famotidine as alternatives.

Pregnancy Risk	B	Lactation Risk	L2
T ½	= 2–3 hours	M/P	= 1.9–6.7
Vd	= 1.6–2.4 l/kg	PB	= 15%
Tmax	= 1–3 hours	Oral	= 50%
MW	= 314	pKa	= 2.3, 8.2

Adult Concerns: Side effects are generally minimal and include headache, gastrointestinal distress, dizziness.

Pediatric Concerns: None reported via milk. Although ranitidine is concentrated in milk, the overall dose is less than therapeutic.

Drug Interactions: Ranitidine may decrease the renal clearance of procainamide. May decrease oral absorption of diazepam. Ranitidine may increase the hypoglycemic effect of glipizide or glyburide. Ranitidine may reduce warfarin clearance, thus increasing anticoagulation.

Relative Infant Dose: 1.3%–4.6%

Adult Dose: 150 mg twice daily.

Alternatives: Famotidine, nizatidine

References:
1. Kearns GL, McConnell RF, Jr., Trang JM, Kluza RB. Appearance of ranitidine in breast milk following multiple dosing. Clin Pharm 1985; 4(3): 322–324.

REGADENOSON   L4

Trade: Lexiscan

Other Trades:

Category: Radiopharmaceutical Imaging Agent

Regadenoson is a pharmacologic stress agent that is used for myocardial perfusion imaging in patients unable to undergo stress from exercise. It is most often administered in a dose of 5 mL by rapid intravenous injection. This dose is quickly followed by a saline flush and radiopharmaceutical agent.[1] It is currently unknown if regadenoson is excreted into human milk. Due to the potential for serious adverse effects in infants, the necessity of the drug to the mother must be evaluated to determine if the interruption of nursing or the cessation of regadenoson is the appropriate choice. Based on the pharmacokinetics of regadenoson, it should be cleared after ten hours. It is recommended that nursing women wait ten hours before resuming breastfeeding.[1]

Pregnancy Risk	C	Lactation Risk	L4
T ½	= Initial phase: 2–4 minutes, Intermediate phase: 30 minutes, Terminal phase: 2 hours	M/P	=
Vd	= 1.04 l/kg	PB	= 27–33%
Tmax	= 1–4 minutes	Oral	=
MW	= 408.37	pKa	=

Adult Concerns: Dyspnea, headache, flushing, chest discomfort, angina pectoris, ST segment depression, dizziness, chest pain, nausea, abdominal discomfort, dysgeusia, feeling hot, heart block, asystole, marked hypertension, symptomatic hypertension, seizure, syncope, arrhythmias.

Pediatric Concerns:

Drug Interactions: Methylxanthines (caffeine, theophylline) may interfere with the vasodilatory effects of regadenoson. Avoid consumption of products containing methylxanthines for twelve hours after regadenoson administration.[1] Dipyridamole–May change the effects of regadenoson. Withhold dipyridamole for at least two days before regadenoson administration.[1]

Relative Infant Dose:

Adult Dose: 5 mL by rapid IV injection.

Alternatives:

References:
1. Pharmaceutical manufacturer prescribing information, 2011.

REMIFENTANIL   L3

Trade: Ultiva

Other Trades: Ultiva

Category: Opioid analgesic

Remifentanil is a new opioid analgesic similar in potency and use as fentanyl. It is primarily metabolized by plasma and tissue esterases (in adults and neonates) and has an incredibly short elimination half-life of only 10–20 minutes, with an effective biological half-life of only 3 to 10 minutes.[1] Unlike other fentanyl analogs, the half-life of remifentanil does not increase with prolonged administration. Although remifentanil has been found in rodent milk, no data are available on its transfer into human milk. It is cleared for use in children >2 years of age. As an analog of fentanyl, breastmilk levels should be similar and probably exceedingly low. In addition, remifentanil metabolism is not dependent on liver function and should be exceedingly short even in neonates. Due to its kinetics and brief half-life and its poor oral bioavailability, it is unlikely this product will produce clinically relevant levels in human breastmilk.

Pregnancy Risk	C	Lactation Risk	L3
T ½	= 10–20 minutes	M/P	=
Vd	= 0.1 l/kg	PB	= 70%
Tmax	=	Oral	= Poor
MW	= 412	pKa	= 7.07

Adult Concerns: Nausea, hypotension, sedation, vomiting, bradycardia.

Pediatric Concerns: None reported via milk. Not orally bioavailable.

Drug Interactions: May potentiate the effects of other opioids.

Relative Infant Dose:

Adult Dose: 0.25–0.4 µg/kg/minute

Alternatives:

References:
1. Pharmaceutical manufacturer prescribing information, 1997.

REPAGLINIDE   L4

Trade: Prandin

Other Trades: Gluconorm, Novonorm

Category: Antidiabetic agent

Repaglinide is a non-sulfonylurea hypoglycemic agent that lowers blood glucose levels in type 2 non-insulin dependent diabetics by stimulating the release of insulin from functional beta cells.[1] No data are available on its transfer to human milk, but rodent studies suggest that it may transfer into milk and induce hypoglycemic and skeletal changes in young animals via milk.[2] Unfortunately, no dosing regimens were mentioned in these studies, so it is not known if normal therapeutic doses would produce such changes in humans. Dosing of repaglinide is rather unique, with doses taken prior to each meal due to its short half-life and according to the need of each patient. At this point, we do not know if it is safe for use in breastfeeding patients. But if it is used, the infant should be closely monitored for hypoglycemia and should not be breastfed until at least several hours after the dose to reduce exposure.

Pregnancy Risk	C	Lactation Risk	L4
T ½	= 1 hour	M/P	=
Vd	= 31 l/kg	PB	= 98%
Tmax	= 1 hour	Oral	= 56%
MW	=	pKa	=

Adult Concerns: In adults, hypoglycemia and headache were the most common side effects.

Pediatric Concerns: Hypoglycemia in animal studies via milk, but doses were not mentioned.

Drug Interactions: Metabolism and increased effect may occur when used with azole antifungals such as ketoconazole, itraconazole and other drugs which inhibit liver enzymes such as erythromycin. Decreased effect may result following use of rifampin, troglitazone, barbiturates and carbamazepine. Reduced protein binding and increased effect may result when repaglinide is used with NSAIDs, salicylates, sulfonamides, etc. Numerous other drugs may interfere with the hypoglycemic effect. Check a drug interaction reference for a complete listing. Use with gemfibrozil may cause a significant reduction in blood glucose levels.

Relative Infant Dose:

Adult Dose: 0.5–4 mg 2–4 times daily.

Alternatives:

References:
1. Pharmaceutical manufacturer prescribing information, 1999.
2. Drug Facts and Comparisons 1999 ed. ed. St. Louis: 1999.

RESERPINE   L4

Trade: Raudixin, Serpasil

Other Trades: Adelphane, Serpasil, Abicol

Category: Antihypertensive

Reserpine is an old and seldom used antihypertensive. Reserpine is known to be secreted into human milk although the levels are unreported.[1,2,3] Increased respiratory tract secretions, severe nasal congestion, cyanosis, and loss of appetite can occur. Some reports suggest no observable effect but should use with extreme caution if at all. Because safer, more effective products are available, reserpine should be avoided in lactating patients.

Pregnancy Risk	C	Lactation Risk	L4
T ½	= 50–100 hours	M/P	=
Vd	=	PB	= 96%
Tmax	= 2 hours	Oral	= 40%
MW	= 609	pKa	=

Adult Concerns: Hypotonia, sedation, hypotension, nasal congestion, diarrhea, nausea, vomiting.

Pediatric Concerns: None reported via milk, but observe for nasal stuffiness, sedation, hypotonia. Use with caution.

Drug Interactions: Reserpine may decrease the effect of other sympathomimetics. May increase the effect of monoamine oxidase inhibitors and tricyclic antidepressants.

Relative Infant Dose:

Adult Dose: 125–250 µg 1–2 times daily.

Alternatives:

References:
1. O'Brien TE. Excretion of drugs in human milk. Am J Hosp Pharm 1974; 31(9): 844–854.
2. Vorherr H. Drug excretion in breast milk. Postgrad Med 1974; 56(4): 97–104.
3. Anderson PO. Drugs and breast feeding. Semin Perinatol 1979; 3(3): 271–278.

RESORCINOL   L3

Trade: Resinol, R A Acne

Other Trades:

Category: Analgesic, topical

Resorcinol is a topical agent used to treat a wide variety of dermatologic disorders, including acne, seborrheic dermatitis, eczema, and psoriasis. It is a benzene alcohol that is fully absorbed by the oral route, but has only limited bioavailability when absorbed through intact skin. Approximately 1.64% of a topical dose reaches the systemic circulation.[1] Information regarding excretion into breast milk is limited, though studies in rats have shown no untoward effects in either the lactating mother or the offspring. Decreases in weight were noted at a dose of 3000 mg/L of drinking water, but lower doses did not carry the same effect.[2] Exposure is likely minimal due to low topical absorption.

Pregnancy Risk	Probably Safe	Lactation Risk	L3
T ½	= 8–10 hours	M/P	=
Vd	=	PB	=
Tmax	= 15 minutes	Oral	= 100%
MW	= 110.1	pKa	=

Adult Concerns: Skin irritation, diarrhea, nausea, stomach pain, vomiting, dizziness, drowsiness, headache, nervousness, troubled breathing, sweating, weakness. All adverse effects other than skin irritation are associated with resorcinol poisoning, which is unlikely unless dosed with extremely high amounts.

Pediatric Concerns:

Drug Interactions: There are currently no known drug interactions.

Relative Infant Dose:

Adult Dose: Apply to affected area no more than 3–4 times daily.

Alternatives:

References:
1. Yeung, D., Kantor, S., Nacht, S., and Gans, E. H. (1983). Percutaneous absorption, blood levels, and urinary excretion of resorcinol applied topically in humans. Int. J. Dermatol. 22, 321–324.
2. F. Welsch, M. D. Nemec and W. B. Lawrence. Two-Generation Reproductive Toxicity Study of Resorcinol Administered Via Drinking Water to Crl: CD(SD) Rats. International Journal of Toxicology. January, 2008. vol. 27 no. 1 43–57.

RETAPAMULIN   L3

Trade: Altabax
Other Trades:
Category: Antibacterial

Retapamulin is a topical antibacterial used to treat impetigo caused by S. aureus (not MRSA) in both children and adults. It is only minimally absorbed systemically when applied topically.[1] No data are available on the transfer of retapamulin into human milk, however since systemic absorption is quite low, and this medication is used in children, retapamulin would probably be safe for use in breastfeeding mothers.

Pregnancy Risk	B	Lactation Risk	L3
T ½	=	M/P	=
Vd	=	PB	= 94%
Tmax	=	Oral	=
MW	= 517.8	pKa	=

Adult Concerns: Adverse reactions include headache, application site irritation, and nasopharyngitis.

Pediatric Concerns: Adverse effects seen in pediatric patients over 9 months of age include itching, eczema, and diarrhea. No data on transfer into milk.

Drug Interactions: Ketoconazole increases retapamulin concentrations.

Relative Infant Dose:

Adult Dose: Apply to affected area twice daily.

Alternatives: Mupirocin

References:
1. Pharmaceutical manufacturer prescribing information, 2007.

rhBMP-2   L3

Trade: Infuse bone graft

Other Trades:

Category: Bone Morphogenetic Protein

Recombinant human bone morphogenetic protein-2 (rhBMP-2) is a growth factor used to stimulate bone and cartilage growth. Implantable bone graft kits may contain rhBMP-2 soaked collagen sponge that is designed to disappear after a certain amount of time. RhBMP-2 is a very large molecule (26 kDa) and unlikely to be absorbed and secreted in breastmilk. In one case study, rhBMP-2 was not detected in breastmilk (minimum detection level of 62.5 pg/mL) after implantation of the Infuse bone graft kit which contains rhBMP-2.[1]

Pregnancy Risk	Possibly Hazardous	Lactation Risk	L3
T ½	=	M/P	=
Vd	=	PB	=
Tmax	=	Oral	=
MW	= 26 kDa	pKa	=

Adult Concerns: Ectopic bone formation, hematoma, swelling, dysphagia

Pediatric Concerns:

Drug Interactions:

Relative Infant Dose:

Adult Dose:

Alternatives:

References:
1. Tzeng ST, Liao JC, Murray SS, Brochmann EJ, Carlson GD, Wang JC. Absence of bone morphogenetic protein-2 in human breast milk after spinal surgery. Spine J. 2010 Jun; 10(6): e17–20.

RHO (D) IMMUNE GLOBULIN   L2

Trade: Rhogam, Gamulin RH, Hyprho-D, Mini-Gamulin RH

Other Trades:

Category: Immune globulin

Rho(D) immune globulin is an immune globulin prepared from human plasma containing high concentrations of Rh antibodies. Only trace amounts of anti-Rh are present in colostrum and none in mature milk in women receiving large doses of Rh immune globulin. No untoward effects have been reported. Most immunoglobulins are destroyed in the gastric acidity of the newborn infant. Rh immune globulins are not contraindicated in breastfeeding mothers.[1]

Pregnancy Risk	C	Lactation Risk	L2
T ½	= 24 days	M/P	=
Vd	=	PB	=
Tmax	=	Oral	= Nil
MW	=	pKa	=

Adult Concerns: Infrequent allergies, discomfort at injection site.

Pediatric Concerns: None reported via milk.

Drug Interactions:

Relative Infant Dose:

Adult Dose: 300 µg X 1–2

Alternatives:

References:
1. Lawrence RA. Breastfeeding: A guide for the medical profession. St. Louis: Mosby Publishers, 1994.

RIBAVIRIN   L4

Trade: Virazole, Rebetol, Copegus

Other Trades: Virazide, Virazole

Category: Antiviral agent.

Ribavirin is a synthetic nucleoside used as an antiviral agent and is effective in a wide variety of viral infections.[1] It has heretofore been used acutely in respiratory syncytial virus (RSV) infections in infants without major complications. However, its current use in breastfeeding patients for treatment of hepatitis C infections when combined with interferon-alfa (Rebetron) for periods up to one year may be more problematic as high concentrations of ribavirin could accumulate in the breastfed infant. No data are available on its transfer to human milk, but it is probably low and its oral bioavailability is low as well. However, ribavirin concentrates in peripheral tissues and in the red blood cells in high concentrations over time (Vd= 802).[2] Its elimination half-life at steady state averages 298 hours, which reflects slow elimination from non-plasma compartments. Red cell concentrations on average are 60 fold higher than plasma levels and may account for the occasional hemolytic anemia. It is likely the acute exposure of a breastfed infant would produce minimal side effects. However, chronic exposure over 6–12 months may be more risky, so caution is recommended.

Pregnancy Risk	X	Lactation Risk	L4
T ½	= 298 hours (SS)	M/P	=
Vd	= 2859 L l/kg	PB	= None
Tmax	= 1.5 hours	Oral	= 64%
MW	= 244	pKa	=

Adult Concerns: Rash, conjunctivitis, hemolytic anemia, congestive heart failure, seizures, asthenia, hypotension, bradycardia, reticulocytosis, bronchospasm, pulmonary edema, etc. Ribavirin may be a potent teratogen. Nursing personnel exposed to inhaled ribavirin should avoid environmental exposure.

Pediatric Concerns: None yet reported via breast milk.

Drug Interactions:

Relative Infant Dose:

Adult Dose: 12.5 L mist/min (190 µg/L) 12–18 hours daily.

Alternatives:

References:
1. Pharmaceutical manufacturer prescribing information, 1999.
2. Lertora JJ, Rege AB, Lacour JT, Ferencz N, George WJ, VanDyke RB, Agrawal KC, Hyslop NE, Jr. Pharmacokinetics and long-term tolerance to ribavirin in asymptomatic patients infected with human immunodeficiency virus. Clin Pharmacol Ther 1991; 50(4): 442–449.

RIBOFLAVIN   L1

Trade: Vitamin B$_2$
Other Trades: Abdec
Category: Vitamin B$_2$

Riboflavin is a B complex vitamin, also called Vitamin B$_2$. Riboflavin is absorbed by the small intestine by a well established transport mechanism. It is easily saturable, so excessive levels are not absorbed. Riboflavin is transported into human milk in concentrations proportional to dietary intake but generally averaged 400 ng/mL.[1] Maternal supplementation is permitted if dose is not excessive. No untoward effects have been reported.

Pregnancy Risk	A	Lactation Risk	L1
T ½	= 14 hours	M/P	=
Vd	=	PB	=
Tmax	= Rapid	Oral	= Complete
MW	= 376	pKa	=

Adult Concerns: Yellow colored urine.

Pediatric Concerns: None reported via milk.

Drug Interactions:

Relative Infant Dose:

Adult Dose: 1–4 mg daily.

Alternatives:

References:

1. Deodhar AD, Hajalakshmi R, Ramakrishnan CV. Studies on human lactation. III. Effect of dietary vitamin supplementation on vitamin contents of breastfmilk. Acta Paediatr 1964; 53: 42–48.

RIFAMPIN   L2

Trade: Rifadin, Rimactane

Other Trades: Rifampicin, Rimycin, Rifadin, Rimactane, Rofact

Category: Antitubercular drug

Rifampin is a broad-spectrum antibiotic with particular activity against tuberculosis. It is secreted into breastmilk in very small levels. One report indicates that following a single 450 mg oral dose, maternal plasma levels averaged 21.3 mg/L and milk levels averaged 3.4–4.9 mg/L.[1] Vorherr reported that after a 600 mg dose of rifampin, peak plasma levels were 50 mg/L while milk levels were 10–30 mg/L.[2] These studies suggest a milk dose 0.45–0.75 mg/kg/day, far lower than the generally recommended clinical doses (10–20 mg/kg/day). Therefore, the amounts of rifampin ingested through breastmilk are most likely not clinically relevant. No adverse effects in breastfed infants have been reported. Observe for diarrhea in the infant.

Pregnancy Risk	C	Lactation Risk	L2
T ½	= 3.5 hours	M/P	= 0.16–0.23
Vd	=	PB	= 80%
Tmax	= 2–4 hours	Oral	= 90–95%
MW	= 823	pKa	=

Adult Concerns: Hepatitis, anemia, headache, diarrhea, pseudomembranous colitis.

Pediatric Concerns: None reported via milk.

Drug Interactions: Rifampin is known to reduce the plasma level of a large number of drugs including: acetaminophen, anticoagulants, barbiturates, benzodiazepines, beta blockers, contraceptives, corticosteroids, cyclosporine, digitoxin, phenytoin, methadone, quinidine, sulfonylureas, theophylline, verapamil, and a large number of others.

Relative Infant Dose: 5.3%–11.5%

Adult Dose: 600 mg daily.

Alternatives:

References:
1. Lenzi E, Santuari S. Preliminary observations on the use of a new semi-synthetic rifamycin derivative in gynecology and obstetrics. Atti Accad Lancisiana Roma 1969; 13(suppl 1): 87–94.
2. Vorherr H. Drug excretion in breast milk. Postgrad Med 1974; 56(4): 97–104.

RIFAXIMIN L3

Trade: Xifaxan

Other Trades:

Category: Non-systemic antibiotic for diarrhea.

Rifaximin is a new antibiotic used for the treatment of traveler's diarrhea. It is poorly absorbed orally (<0.4%) and plasma levels are extremely low.[1] While we do not have data in breastfeeding mothers, it is unlikely enough would enter the maternal plasma compartment to produce clinically relevant levels in milk.

Pregnancy Risk	C	Lactation Risk	L3
T ½	= 5.85 hours	M/P	=
Vd	=	PB	=
Tmax	= 1.25 hours	Oral	= <0.4%
MW	= 785	pKa	=

Adult Concerns: Flatulence, headache, nausea, increased sweating, abdominal pain have been reported in adults.

Pediatric Concerns: Maternal plasma levels are extremely low. It is unlikely enough would enter the plasma compartment to produce clinically relevant levels in milk.

Drug Interactions: An *in vitro* study suggests that rifaximin is a substrate of P-glycoprotein. In the presence of P-glycoprotein inhibitor verapamil, the efflux ratio of rifaximin was reduced greater than 50% *in vitro*. The effect of P-glycoprotein inhibition on rifaximin was not evaluated *in vivo*.

Relative Infant Dose:

Adult Dose: 200 mg three times daily for 3 days.

Alternatives:

References:
1. Pharmaceutical manufacturer prescribing information, 2005.

RIMANTADINE   L3

Trade: Flumadine

Other Trades:

Category: Antiviral, anti-influenza A

Rimantadine hydrochloride is an antiviral agent primarily used for influenza A infections. It is concentrated in rodent milk.[1] Levels in animal milk 2–3 hours after administration were approximately twice those of the maternal serum, suggesting a milk/plasma ratio of about 2. The manufacturer alludes to toxic side effects but fails to state them. No side effects yet reported in breastfeeding infants. Rimantadine is, however, indicated for prophylaxis of influenza A in pediatric patients >1 year of age.

Pregnancy Risk	C	Lactation Risk	L3
T ½	= 25.4 hours	M/P	= 2
Vd	=	PB	= 40%
Tmax	= 6 hours	Oral	= 92%
MW	= 179	pKa	=

Adult Concerns: Gastrointestinal distress, nervousness, fatigue, and sleep disturbances.

Pediatric Concerns: None reported via milk.

Drug Interactions: The use of acetaminophen significantly reduces rimantadine plasma levels by 11%. Peak plasma levels of rimantadine were reduce by 10% by aspirin. Rimantadine clearance was reduced by 16% when used with cimetidine.

Relative Infant Dose:

Adult Dose: 100 mg twice daily.

Alternatives:

References:
1.   Pharmaceutical manufacturer prescribing information, 1996.

RISEDRONATE   L3

Trade: Actonel

Other Trades: Actonel

Category: Prevents bone resorption

Risedronate is a bisphosphonate that slows the dissolution of hydroxyapatite crystals in the bone, thus reducing bone calcium loss in certain syndromes such as Paget's syndrome.[1] Its penetration into milk is possible due to its small molecular weight, but it has not yet been reported except in rats. However, due to the presence of fat and calcium in milk, its oral bioavailability in infants would be exceedingly low. However, the presence of this product in an infant's growing bones is concerning, and due caution is recommended.

Pregnancy Risk	C	Lactation Risk	L3
T ½	= 480 hours	M/P	=
Vd	= 6.3 l/kg	PB	= 24%
Tmax	= 1 hour	Oral	= 0.63%
MW	= 305	pKa	=

Adult Concerns: Nausea, diarrhea, flatulence, gastritis, arthralgia have been reported.

Pediatric Concerns: None via milk.

Drug Interactions: Oral products containing calcium or magnesium will significantly reduce oral bioavailability. Take on empty stomach.

Relative Infant Dose:

Adult Dose: 30 mg/day for 2 months.

Alternatives:

References:
1. Pharmaceutical manufacturer prescribing information, 2002.

RISPERIDONE   L3

Trade: Risperdal

Other Trades: Risperdal

Category: Antipsychotic

Risperidone is a potent antipsychotic agent belonging to a new chemical class and is a dopamine and serotonin antagonist. Risperidone is metabolized to an active metabolite, 9-hydroxyrisperidone. In a study of one patient receiving 6 mg/day of risperidone at steady state, the peak plasma level of approximately 130 µg/L occurred 4 hours after an oral dose.[1] Peak milk levels of risperidone and 9-hydroxyrisperidone were approximately 12 µg/L and 40 µg/L respectively. The estimated daily dose of risperidone and metabolite (risperidone equivalents) was 4.3% of the weight-adjusted maternal dose. The milk/plasma ratios calculated from areas under the curve over 24 hours were 0.42 and 0.24 respectively for risperidone and 6-hydroxyrisperidone. In another study, the transfer of risperidone and 9-hydroxyrisperidone into milk was studied in 2 breastfeeding women and one woman with risperidone-induced galactorrhea.[2] In case two (risperidone dose= 42.1 µg/kg/day), the average concentration of risperidone and 9-hydroxyrisperidone in milk (Cav) was 2.1 and 6 µg/L respectively. The relative infant dose was 2.8% of the maternal dose. In case 3 (risperidone dose= 23.1 µg/kg/day), the average concentration of risperidone and 9-hydroxyrisperidone in milk (Cav) was 0.39 and 7.06 µg/L respectively. The milk/plasma ratio determined in 2 women was <0.5 for both risperidone compounds. The relative infant doses were 2.3%, 2.8%, and 4.7% (as risperidone equivalents) of the maternal weight-adjusted doses in these three cases. Risperidone and 9-hydroxyrisperidone were not detected in the plasma of the 2 breastfed infants studied, and no adverse effects were noted.

Pregnancy Risk	C	Lactation Risk	L3
T ½	= 3–20 hours	M/P	= 0.42
Vd	=	PB	= 90%
Tmax	= 3–17 hours	Oral	= 70–94%
MW	= 410	pKa	=

Adult Concerns: Risks include neuroleptic malignant syndrome, tardive dyskinesia, myocardial arrhythmias, orthostatic hypotension, seizures, hyperprolactinemia, somnolence. Galactorrhea has been reported.

Pediatric Concerns: None reported via milk.

Drug Interactions: Do not use with alcohol. May enhance the hypotensive response of other antihypertensives. May antagonize the effect of levodopa. Carbamazepine or clozapine may increase clearance of risperidone.

Relative Infant Dose: 2.8%–9.1%

Adult Dose: 3 mg twice daily.

Alternatives: Quetiapine

References:
1. Hill RC, McIvor RJ, Wojnar-Horton RE, Hackett LP, Ilett KF. Risperidone distribution and excretion into human milk: case report and estimated infant exposure during breast-feeding. J Clin Psychopharmacol 2000; 20(2): 285–286.
2. Ilett KF, Hackett LP, Kristensen JH, Vaddadi KS, Gardiner SJ, Begg EJ. Transfer of risperidone and 9-hydroxyrisperidone into human milk. Ann Pharmacother 2004; 38(2): 273–276.

RITODRINE   L3

Trade: Pre-Par, Yutopar
Other Trades: Yutopar
Category: Adrenergic agent

Ritodrine is primarily used to reduce uterine contractions in premature labor due to its beta-2 adrenergic effect on uterine receptors.[1] No data are available on its transfer to human milk. Its pharmacokinetic parameters suggest that transfer into milk is likely, but low oral bioavailability suggests that little would be absorbed in the infant's gut. Nevertheless, caution is advised with its use. Use only if potential benefit to mother outweighs potential risk to breastfed infant.

Pregnancy Risk	B	Lactation Risk	L3
T ½	= 15 hours	M/P	=
Vd	= 0.7 l/kg	PB	= 32%
Tmax	= 40–60 minutes	Oral	= 30%
MW	= 287	pKa	= 9

Adult Concerns: Fetal and maternal tachycardia, hypertension, lethargy, sleepiness, ketoacidosis, pulmonary edema.

Pediatric Concerns: None reported via milk.

Drug Interactions: Use cautiously with steroids due to pulmonary edema. Acebutolol and other beta blockers would block efficacy of ritodrine. Use with atropine may lead to systemic exaggerated hypertension. Use with bupivacaine has led to extreme hypotension. Numerous other interactions are listed, please refer a drug interactions reference for a complete listing.

Relative Infant Dose:

Adult Dose: 10–20 mg every 4–6 hours.

Alternatives:

References:
1. Gandar R, de Zoeten LW, van der Schoot JB. Serum level of ritodrine in man. Eur J Clin Pharmacol 1980; 17(2): 117–122.

RITONAVIR   L3

Trade: Norvir

Other Trades:

Category: Antiretroviral agent used in HIV infections

Ritonavir is an antiretroviral agent used in the treatment of HIV infection. There are no adequate and well-controlled studies or case reports in breastfeeding women. Breastfeeding is not recommended in mothers who have HIV.[1,2] No data are available on its transfer into human milk.

Pregnancy Risk	B	Lactation Risk	L3
T ½	= 3–5 hours	M/P	=
Vd	= 0.16–0.56 l/kg	PB	= 98–99%
Tmax	= 2–4 hours	Oral	= 80%
MW	= 720.95	pKa	=

Adult Concerns: The most common side effects are diarrhea, nausea, abdominal pain, asthenia, vomiting, headache, and dyspepsia

Pediatric Concerns:

Drug Interactions: Ritonavir may interact with many medications, resulting in potentially serious and/or life-threatening adverse events. Use with caution in patients taking strong CYP3A4 inhibitors, moderate or strong CYP3A4 inducers and major CYP3A4 substrates; consider alternative agents that avoid or lessen the potential for CYP-mediated interactions. Not recommended for use with fluticasone, salmeterol or high-dose or long-term use of meperidine.

Relative Infant Dose:

Adult Dose: 600 mg twice a day.

Alternatives:

References:
1. World Health Organization: Global Programme on AIDS. Consensus statement from the WHO/UNICEF consultation on HIV transmission and breast-feeding. Geneva: WHO, 1992.
2. Latham MC, Greiner T: Breastfeeding versus formula feeding in HIV infection. Lancet 352: 737, 1998.

RITUXIMAB   L4

Trade: Rituxan

Other Trades:

Category: Antineoplastic agent, monoclonal antibody

Rituximab, an IgG antibody, binds to the CD20 antigen found on the surface of B lymphocytes.[1] It is used in the treatment of non-Hodgkin's lymphoma, rheumatoid arthritis, and lymphoid leukemia. There are no reported levels in human milk, but due to its large molecular weight, it is unlikely to enter milk in clinically relevant concentrations. In addition, the low oral bioavailability of this protein suggests little absorption in the infant's gut. Mothers who are less than two weeks postpartum should not breastfeed. Because of numerous risks and the prolonged half-life of this product, mothers should probably not breastfeed following the use of this product.

Pregnancy Risk	C	Lactation Risk	L4
T ½	= 206 hours	M/P	=
Vd	= 4.3 l/kg	PB	=
Tmax	=	Oral	= Nil
MW	= 145,000	pKa	=

Adult Concerns: Common adverse effects include fever and chills, nausea, pruritus, angioedema, asthenia, hypotension, headache, bronchospasm.

Pediatric Concerns: No data are available. Due to its large molecular weight, it is unlikely to enter milk in clinically relevant concentrations.

Drug Interactions: Rituximab interacts with live vaccines, increasing the risk of infection by the vaccines. Cisplatin used concurrently increases the risk of renal failure.

Relative Infant Dose:

Adult Dose: 375 mg/square meter IV

Alternatives:

References:
1. Pharmaceutical manufacturer prescribing information, 2007.

RIVAROXABAN   L4

Trade: Xarelto

Other Trades:

Category: Anticoagulant, Factor Xa inhibitor

Rivaroxaban is a Factor Xa inhibitor. It selectively binds and inactivates endogenous Factor Xa, which plays a crucial role in the blood coagulation cascade. Rivaroxaban, therefore is used as an anti-coagulant agent in the prevention of postoperative deep vein thrombosis and in the prevention of strokes in those with nonvalvular atrial fibrillation.[1] Currently there are no data available on the transfer of this drug into breastmilk. Due to the risk of hemorrhagic complications in the breastfeeding infant, especially in the premature, it is advised that the use of this drug during lactation be based on a relative assessment of the potential benefits to the mother versus the potential risks to the infant.

Pregnancy Risk	C	Lactation Risk	L4
T ½	= 5–9 hours	M/P	=
Vd	= 50 L l/kg	PB	= 92–95%
Tmax	= 2–4 hours	Oral	= 66–100%
MW	= 435.89	pKa	=

Adult Concerns: Hemorrhage, hypersensitivity reactions. Cessation of rivaroxaban use in those with nonvalvular atrial fibrillation puts the patient at an increased risk for strokes. Patients receiving spinal anesthesia while on rivaroxaban therapy are at increased risk for spinal/epidural hematomas, which could result in neurological impairment and paralysis. Exercise caution in those with impaired liver or kidney function.

Pediatric Concerns:

Drug Interactions: Concomitant use of NSAIDs, platelet inhibitors such as aspirin or clopidogrel, or other anticoagulants such as warfarin and enoxaparin increases risk of hemorrhage. Concomitant use with the following drugs decreases efficacy of rivaroxaban: carbamazepine, phenytoin, rifampin, St. John's wort. Concomitant use with the following drugs increases plasma levels of rivaroxaban: ketoconazole, itraconazole, clarithromycin, lopinavir/ritonavir, ritonavir, indinavir/ritonavir, and conivaptan.

Relative Infant Dose:

Adult Dose: 10–20 mg once daily orally.

Alternatives:

References:
1. Pharmaceutical manufacturer prescribing information, 2011.

RIZATRIPTAN   L3

Trade: Maxalt
Other Trades: Maxalt
Category: Antimigraine

Rizatriptan is a selective serotonin receptor agonist, similar in effect to sumatriptan.[1] It is primarily indicated for acute migraine headache treatment. No data are available on its transfer into human milk, but it is concentrated in rodent milk (M/P=5). Until we have clear data on breastmilk levels, the kinetics of this drug may predispose to higher milk levels and sumatriptan should be preferred. Wait 4 hours after dose, then may breastfeed.

Pregnancy Risk	C	Lactation Risk	L3
T ½	= 2–3 hours	M/P	=
Vd	= 2 l/kg	PB	= 14%
Tmax	= 1–1.5 hours	Oral	= 45%
MW	= 269	pKa	=

Adult Concerns: Do not use in patients with ischemic heart disease, coronary artery vasospasm, or significant underlying cardiac disease. Rizatriptan should not be used within 24 hours of an ergot alkaloid, dihydroergotamine, or methysergide. Side effects include chest pain, paresthesia, dry mouth, nausea, dizziness, and somnolence.

Pediatric Concerns: None reported via milk, but caution is recommended.

Drug Interactions: Plasma levels may be increased when used with a monoamine oxidase inhibitor, or shortly thereafter. Concurrent use of propranolol produced a 70% increase in plasma levels of rizatriptan. No interactions were noted with nadolol or metoprolol.

Relative Infant Dose:

Adult Dose: 5–10 mg orally, repeat only after 2 hours.

Alternatives: Sumatriptan

References:
1. Pharmaceutical manufacturer prescribing information, 1999.

ROFECOXIB   L2

Trade: Vioxx
Other Trades: Vioxx
Category: NSAID analgesic

Rofecoxib is one of the newer cyclooxigenase-2 (COX-2) inhibitors. It was recently removed from the market in this country for increasing the risk of cardiovascular events following long-term use. In a new study of six breastfeeding mothers at steady state who received 25 mg/day, the absolute infant dose in milk was about 0.008 mg/kg per day.[1] The relative infant dose ranged from 1.8 to 3.2% of the maternal dose. The time to achieve peak concentrations for milk ranged from 1 to 4 hours. The authors suggest that rofecoxib is compatible with breastfeeding.

Pregnancy Risk	C	Lactation Risk	L2
T ½	= 17 hours	M/P	= 0.16–0.32
Vd	= 1.3 l/kg	PB	= 87%
Tmax	= 2–3 hours	Oral	= 93%
MW	= 314	pKa	=

Adult Concerns: Abdominal pain, fatigue, dizziness, diarrhea, headache

Pediatric Concerns: None reported via milk but observe for gastrointestinal cramping, distress, diarrhea. Probably quite safe for breastfeeding infants.

Drug Interactions: May reduce efficacy of ACE inhibitors with elevation of blood pressure. Increased plasma concentrations of rofecoxib result when coadministered with cimetidine. May increase lithium levels, and reduce the efficacy of diuretics. May increase plasma concentrations of methotrexate by 23%. Rifampin may increase rofecoxib plasma levels by 50%. When added to warfarin therapy, may increase INR by 8%.

Relative Infant Dose: 0%

Adult Dose: 12.5 to 25 mg once daily.

Alternatives: Ibuprofen, celecoxib

References:
1. Gardiner SJ, Begg EJ, Zhang M, Hughes RC. Transfer of rofecoxib into human milk. Eur J Clin Pharmacol 2005; 61: 405–408.

ROPINIROLE   L4

Trade: Requip

Other Trades:

Category: Dopamine stimulating agent used for Restless Legs and Parkinson's s

Ropinirole is a non-ergoline dopamine agonist. It is used to treat Parkinson's and Restless leg syndromes.[1] While it has not been studied in breastfeeding mothers, it should not be used. Ropinirole is known to reduce prolactin levels, even in men, and would likely reduce milk production in breastfeeding mothers.

Pregnancy Risk	C	Lactation Risk	L4
T ½	= 6 hours	M/P	=
Vd	= 7.5 l/kg	PB	= 40%
Tmax	= 1–2 hours	Oral	= 55%
MW	= 297	pKa	=

Adult Concerns: Ropinirole may potentiate the dopaminergic side effects of L-dopa and may cause and/or exacerbate pre-existing dyskinesia in patients treated with L-dopa. Cases of retroperitoneal fibrosis, pulmonary infiltrates, pleural effusion, pleural thickening, pericarditis, and cardiac valvulopathy have been reported. Patients should be advised that they may develop postural (orthostatic) hypotension with or without symptoms such as dizziness, nausea, fainting, and sometimes sweating. Daytime sleepiness or episodes of falling asleep have been reported and are of some concern for active individuals.

Pediatric Concerns: None reported, but a reduction of prolactin could severely reduce milk supply.

Drug Interactions: Co-administration of ciprofloxacin with ropinirole increased ropinirole AUC by 84% on average and C_{max} by 60% in 12 patients. Estrogens may reduce the oral clearance of ropinirole by 36%. Dopamine antagonists (metoclopramide, domperidone, etc.) may diminish the effectiveness of ropinirole.

Relative Infant Dose:

Adult Dose: 0.25–1.0 mg three times daily.

Alternatives:

References:
1. Pharmaceutical manufacturer prescribing information, 2005.

ROPIVACAINE   L2

Trade: Naropin

Other Trades: Naropin

Category: Local anesthetic

Ropivacaine is a newer local anesthetic commonly used as a regional anesthetic and for epidural infusions.[1] It is believed to produce less hypotension when compared to bupivacaine. No data are available on its transfer into human milk, but the manufacture suggests it is probably much lower than the infant receives in utero. This agent is commonly used in obstetrics and probably poses few if any problems to a breastfeeding infant.

Pregnancy Risk	B	Lactation Risk	L2
T ½	= 4.2 hours (epidural)	M/P	=
Vd	= 0.58 l/kg	PB	= 94%
Tmax	= 43 minutes (epidural)	Oral	=
MW	= 328	pKa	= 8.07

Adult Concerns: Adverse effects following epidural administration include hypotension, tachycardia, shivering, urinary retention, vomiting, nausea, headache, and back pain.

Pediatric Concerns: None reported in breastmilk. This agent is commonly used in obstetrics and is unlikely to affect the infant via milk.

Drug Interactions: Fluvoxamine and other CYP1A2 inhibitors may reduce plasma clearance of ropivacaine metabolites by 70%. CYP2A4 inhibitors such as ketoconazole may reduce clearance of ropivacaine as well.

Relative Infant Dose:

Adult Dose: Epidural = 75–150 mg.

Alternatives: Bupivacaine

References:
1. Pharmaceutical manufacturer prescribing information, 2003.

ROSIGLITAZONE   L3

Trade: Avandia
Other Trades:
Category: Oral antidiabetic agent

Rosiglitazone is an oral antidiabetic agent which acts primarily by increasing insulin sensitivity. In essence, the insulin receptor is activated reducing insulin resistance. It also decreases hepatic gluconeogenesis and increases insulin-dependent muscle glucose uptake. It does not increase the release of or secretion of insulin. No data are available on its entry into human milk. The maximum plasma concentration following a 2 mg dose is only 156 nG/mL.[1] Assuming a dose of 2 mg every 12 hours and a theoretical milk/plasma ratio of 1.0 (which is probably high), an infant would likely ingest about 23.4 µg/kg/day via milk. In a 5 kg infant, this would be approximately 2.8% of the maternal dose; too low to be clinically relevant in an infant. But these data are only theoretical.

Pregnancy Risk	C	Lactation Risk	L3
T ½	= 3–4 hours	M/P	=
Vd	= 0.25 l/kg	PB	= 99.8%
Tmax	= 1 hour	Oral	= 99%
MW	= 357	pKa	= 6.8

Adult Concerns: Elevated liver enzymes in small percentage of patients. Hypoglycemia, increased body weight gain, edema, anemia.

Pediatric Concerns: None via milk, but it has not been studied.

Drug Interactions: Metformin may enhance hypoglycemic effect. Rosiglitazone may reduce effectiveness of oral contraceptives containing estrogen and progestins by reducing plasma levels of these hormones. These changes could result in loss of contraception. Consider a higher dose contraceptive. Rosiglitazone may reduce cyclosporine levels.

Relative Infant Dose:

Adult Dose: 2–8 mg daily.

Alternatives:

References:
1. Pharmaceutical manufacturer prescribing information, 2011.

ROSUVASTATIN CALCIUM   L3

Trade: Crestor
Other Trades: Crestor
Category: HMG-CoA reductase inhibitor

Rosuvastatin, like other statins, is used to reduce cholesterol synthesis in patients with hypercholesterolemia. It works by blocking HMG-CoA reductase, the rate limiting enzyme in cholesterol synthesis.[1] No data are available on the excretion of this product into human milk, however due to the large molecular weight and high protein binding, it would be unlikely that a therapeutic concentration would be passed to a breastfeeding infant. Nevertheless, atherosclerosis is a chronic process and the discontinuation of lipid-lowering medications while breastfeeding would have little to no effect on the overall treatment of hypercholesterolemia. Therefore, since cholesterol and other products of cholesterol biosynthesis are so vital to proper infant development, the potential harm to an infant would outweigh the benefit a mother would receive from continued therapy. The use of anti-hyperlipidemia medications would not be advisable under most circumstances in breastfeeding mothers.

Pregnancy Risk	X	Lactation Risk	L3
T ½	= 19 hours	M/P	=
Vd	= 1.9 l/kg	PB	= 90%
Tmax	= 3–5 hours	Oral	= 20%
MW	= 1001	pKa	=

Adult Concerns: Adverse reactions include chest pain, hypertension, headache, anxiety, depression, rash, pharyngitis, bruising, myalgia, and cough.

Pediatric Concerns: No data are available.

Drug Interactions: Antacids and cholestyramine reduce plasma concentrations of rosuvastatin. Niacin, clofibrate, and colchicine can increase the risk of myopathy. Cyclosporine and gemfibrozil can increase serum concentrations of rosuvastatin. Rosuvastatin may increase serum plasma concentrations of ethinyl estradiol and norgestrel.

Relative Infant Dose:

Adult Dose: 5–40 mg/day.

Alternatives:

References:
1. Pharmaceutical manufacturer prescribing information, 2007.

ROTIGOTINE   L4

Trade: Neupro
Other Trades:
Category: Dopamine agonist

Rotigotine is a dopamine agonist used to treat the signs and symptoms of Parkinson's disease. It is thought to stimulate postsynaptic dopamine D_2-type auto receptors in the brain, leading to improved dopaminergic transmission in the motor areas of the basal ganglia.[1] No data are available on the transfer of rotigotine into human milk. According to the manufacturer, rotigotine stimulates dopamine and thus reduces prolactin secretion from the pituitary. It is possible that this medication could significantly decrease prolactin release and in turn, decrease milk production. Therefore, milk production should be monitored carefully if this medication is used in a lactating mother.

Pregnancy Risk	C	Lactation Risk	L4
T ½	= 5–7 hours	M/P	=
Vd	= 84 l/kg	PB	= 90%
Tmax	= 15–18 hours	Oral	=
MW	= 315.48	pKa	=

Adult Concerns: Adverse reactions include somnolence, dizziness, headache, nausea, vomiting, and application site reactions.

Pediatric Concerns: No data are available.

Drug Interactions: Typical antipsychotics and metoclopramide may decrease the efficacy of rotigotine, while CNS depressants may enhance the adverse effects.

Relative Infant Dose:

Adult Dose: 1–2 mg/24 hour patch daily.

Alternatives:

References:
1. Pharmaceutical manufacturer prescribing information, 2004.

RUBELLA VIRUS VACCINE, LIVE   L2

Trade: Meruvax, Rubella Vaccine

Other Trades:

Category: Live attenuated (measles) vaccine

Rubella virus vaccine contains a live attenuated virus. The American College of Obstetricians and Gynecologists (ACOG) and the CDC currently recommends the early postpartum immunization of women who show no or low antibody titers to rubella. At least four studies have found rubella virus to be transferred via milk although presence of clinical symptoms was not evident.[1-3] Rubella virus has been cultured from the throat of one infant while another infant was clinically ill with minor symptoms and serologic evidence of rubella infection.[4] In general, the use of rubella virus vaccine in breastfeeding mothers of full-term, normal infants has not been associated with untoward effects and is generally recommended.[5]

Pregnancy Risk	X	Lactation Risk	L2
T ½	=	M/P	=
Vd	=	PB	=
Tmax	=	Oral	=
MW	=	pKa	=

Adult Concerns: Burning, stinging, lymphadenopathy, rash, malaise, sore throat, etc.

Pediatric Concerns: One case report of rash, vomiting, and mild rubella infection.

Drug Interactions: Immunosuppressants and immune globulins may reduce immunogenicity. Concurrent use of interferon may reduce antibody response.

Relative Infant Dose:

Adult Dose: 0.5 mL X 1

Alternatives:

References:

1. Buimovici-Klein E, Hite RL, Byrne T, Cooper LZ. Isolation of rubella virus in milk after postpartum immunization. J Pediatr 1977; 91(6): 939–941.
2. Losonsky GA, Fishaut JM, Strussenberg J, Ogra PL. Effect of immunization against rubella on lactation products. I. Development and characterization of specific immunologic reactivity in breast milk. J Infect Dis 1982; 145(5): 654–660.
3. Losonsky GA, Fishaut JM, Strussenberg J, Ogra PL. Effect of immunization against rubella on lactation products. II. Maternal-neonatal interactions. J Infect Dis 1982; 145(5): 661–666.
4. Landes RD, Bass JW, Millunchick EW, Oetgen WJ. Neonatal rubella following postpartum maternal immunization. J Pediatr 1980; 97(3): 465–467.
5. Lawrence RA. Breastfeeding: A guide for the medical profession. St. Louis: Mosby Publishers, 1994.

S-ADENOSYL-L-METHIONINE   L3

Trade:

Other Trades:

Category: Herbal supplement

S-adenosyl-l-methionine (Sam-e) is derived from adenosine triphosphate and the amino acid, l-methionine. S-adenosyl-l-methionine is a naturally occurring substance in most body tissues and fluids. Sam-e appears to increase the central processing of dopamine and serotonin.[1] Sam-e has been used to treat depression, fibromyalgia, liver disease, osteoarthritis, migraine headaches, and sleep disturbances. Parenteral use of s-adenosyl-l-mehtionine improved symptoms of depression by 7 days and further improvement by 14 days with no serious side effects.[2] There have been no reports of Sam-e use in breastfeeding women.

Pregnancy Risk	Probably Safe	Lactation Risk	L3
T ½	= 80 minutes	M/P	=
Vd	= 0.4 l/kg	PB	=
Tmax	=	Oral	= 80–90%
MW	= 398.4	pKa	=

Adult Concerns: Headache, nausea, vomiting, flatulence, constipation, diarrhea, xerostomia, anxiety.

Pediatric Concerns:

Drug Interactions:

Relative Infant Dose:

Adult Dose: 200–1600 mg daily.

Alternatives:

References:

1. Shippy RA, Mendez D, Jones K, Cergnul I, Karpiak SE. S-adenosylmethionine (SAM-e) for the treatment of depression in people living with HIV/AIDS. BMC Psychiatry. 2004 Nov 11; 4: 38.
2. Fava M, Giannelli A, Rapisarda V, Patralia A, Guaraldi GP. Rapidity of onset of the antidepressant effect of parenteral S-adenosyl-L-methionine. Psychiatry Res. 1995 Apr 28; 56(3): 295–7.

SACCHARIN   L3

Trade:

Other Trades:

Category: Sweetener

Saccharin is a common sweetener. In one group of 6 women who received 126 mg (per 12 oz drink) every 6 hours for 9 doses, milk levels varied greatly from <200 µg/L after one dose to 1.765 mg/L after 9 doses.[1] Under these dosing conditions, saccharin levels appear to accumulate over time. Half-life in serum and milk were 4.84 hours and 17.9 hours respectively after 3 days. Even after such doses, these milk levels are considered minimal. Moderate intake should be compatible with nursing.

Pregnancy Risk	C	Lactation Risk	L3
T ½	= 4.84 hours	M/P	=
Vd	=	PB	=
Tmax	=	Oral	= Complete
MW	= 183	pKa	=

Adult Concerns: Rare side effects include allergic reactions and photosensitivity. There was a case report regarding elevated liver enzymes.

Pediatric Concerns: None reported via milk.

Drug Interactions:

Relative Infant Dose: 3.6%

Adult Dose:

Alternatives:

References:

1. Egan PC, Marx CM. et.al. Saccharin excretion in mature human milk. Drug Intell Clin Pharm 1984; 18: 511.

SAGE   L4

Trade: Sage, Dalmatian, Sage, Spanish

Other Trades:

Category: Herbal product

Salvia officinalis L. (Dalmatian sage) and Salvia lavandulaefolia Vahl (Spanish sage) are most common of the species. Extracts and teas have been used to treat digestive disorders (antispasmodic), as an antiseptic and astringent, for treating diarrhea, gastritis, sore throat, and other maladies.[1] The dried and smoked leaves have been used for treating asthma symptoms. These uses are largely unsubstantiated in the literature. Sage extracts have been found to be strong antioxidants and with some antimicrobial properties (staph. aureus) due to the phenolic acid salvin content. Sage oil has antispasmodic effects in animals and this may account for its moderating effects on the gastrointestinal tract. For the most part, sage is relatively nontoxic and nonirritating. Ingestion of significant quantities may lead to cheilitis, stomatitis, dry mouth, or local irritation.[2] Due to drying properties and pediatric hypersensitivity to anticholinergics, sage should be used with some caution in breastfeeding mothers.

Pregnancy Risk	Possibly Hazardous	Lactation Risk	L4
T ½	=	M/P	=
Vd	=	PB	=
Tmax	=	Oral	=
MW	=	pKa	=

Adult Concerns: Observe for typical anticholinergic effects such as cheilitis, stomatitis, dry mouth or local irritation.

Pediatric Concerns: None reported but observe for dry mouth, stomatitis, cheilitis.

Drug Interactions:

Relative Infant Dose:

Adult Dose:

Alternatives:

References:
1. Leung AY. Encyclopedia of Common Natural Ingredients used in Food, Drugs and Cosmetics. J Wiley and Sons, 1980.
2. Bissett NG. In: Herbal Drugs and Phytopharmaceuticals. Medpharm Scientific Publishers, CRC Press, Boca Raton, 1994.

SALICYLAMIDE   L3

Trade:

Other Trades:

Category: Analgesic

Salicylamide is not hydrolyzed to salicylate. It is well absorbed; however, its bioavailability is very low due to first pass metabolism. Only 1 µg/mL is in the plasma after ingesting a 650 mg dose.[1] Its purported use is as an analgesic and antipyretic. There are no data on transfer of salicylamide into breastmilk. Aspirin has been implicated in Reye syndrome. Since salicylamide is similar to aspirin, it may have similar issues as aspirin. Avoid the use of salicylamide if the infant has a viral syndrome.

Pregnancy Risk	Probably Safe	Lactation Risk	L3
T ½	=	M/P	=
Vd	=	PB	= 40–55%
Tmax	= 1.5–2 hours	Oral	= Good
MW	= 137	pKa	= 15.45

Adult Concerns: Heartburn, nausea, vomiting, diarrhea, dizziness, dry mouth, rash.

Pediatric Concerns:

Drug Interactions:

Relative Infant Dose:

Adult Dose: 325–650 mg 3–4 times daily.

Alternatives:

References:
1. Salicylamide. Available in: Lexi-Comp OnlineTM ,AHFS-DI, Hudson, Ohio: Lexi-Comp, Inc.; 2011; Updated May 26, 2011.

SALICYLIC ACID, TOPICAL   L3

Trade: Compound W, Duofilm, Mediplast, Occlusal-HP, Sal-Plant Gel, Trans-Ver-Sal, Stri-Dex, Avosil

Other Trades:

Category: Keratolytic, Antiacne

Salicylic acid,[1] is often used in anti-acne preparations, as well as in many wart and corn removal products. It produces desquamation of hyperkeratotic epithelium by dissolving the intercellular cement, thus leading to softening, maceration of the tissue, and ultimately desquamation. Concentrations vary, ranging from 0.5% to 60%, in gels, shampoos, ointments and creams. Salicylic acid acts as a keratolytic at concentrations of 3–6%, and above 6% becomes destructive. Systemic absorption depends on the concentration of the product used, the amount applied, the surface area treated, and duration of use. Absorption increases with the duration of use. The systemic absorption relative to the dose has been found to range from 9.3 to 25.1%. Due to systemic absorption, topical salicylic acid should probably not be used while breastfeeding. It is known that salicylates are excreted in mothers' milk, and have been attributed to cause certain conditions such as Reye's syndrome in children. Avoid its use in lactating mother if the infant has a viral illness.

Pregnancy Risk	Possibly Hazardous	Lactation Risk	L3
T ½	= 2–3 hours	M/P	=
Vd	= 0.17 l/kg	PB	= 50–80%
Tmax	=	Oral	= Complete
MW	= 138.12	pKa	=

Adult Concerns: Adverse reactions include burning and stinging, as well as redness around the application area.

Pediatric Concerns: No data are available in breastfeeding women.

Drug Interactions: May exacerbate anticoagulant effect of low molecular weight heparins. Concurrent with Tamarind, glyburide, and Tan-Shen may increase salicylate serum levels.

Relative Infant Dose:

Adult Dose: Topical

Alternatives: Azelaic acid

References:
1.   Pharmaceutical manufacturer prescribing information, 2003.

SALINE LAXATIVES   L2

Trade: Phillips Milk of Magnesia, Fleet, Visicol, Tridate, X-Prep
Other Trades:
Category: Laxative

Saline laxatives work by retaining water content in the gastrointestinal tract.[1] Saline laxatives come in two forms, magnesium salts and phosphate-containing salt forms. Neither are substantially absorbed in normal individuals, but instead most is retained in the gut. Magnesium and phosphate salts absorbed systemically would be rapidly eliminated by the kidneys in normal individuals. Caution is recommended in individuals with cardiovascular or renal anomalies. Magnesium Forms (Milk of Magnesia, Citrate of Magnesia, Phillips Milk of Magnesia, etc.): magnesium citrate, magnesium hydroxide, and magnesium sulfate compose the usual forms of magnesium laxatives. Only 15–30% of magnesium salts may be absorbed from the gastrointestinal tract, the remaining is retained in the intestinal lumen and keeps water in the intestinal lumen thus producing a laxative effect. Phosphate Forms (Fleet, Visicol): Sodium phosphate solutions containing both dibasic sodium phosphate and monobasic sodium phosphate are used to empty the bowel prior to colonoscopy and other procedures. Approximately 1–20% of the sodium and phosphate in such preparations is absorbed. It is very unlikely that the use of these saline laxatives would increase maternal plasma levels high enough to induce changes in electrolyte content of human milk. While we do not have specific data on the use of higher doses of oral magnesium salts or of the phosphates, the lactocyte controls the microelectrolyte concentrations of milk closely. Minute changes in maternal levels which could potentially occur following the use of these laxatives, would not likely alter milk content of these electrolytes. Caution is recommended in individuals with cardiovascular or renal anomalies.

Pregnancy Risk	Probably Safe	Lactation Risk	L2
T ½	=	M/P	=
Vd	=	PB	=
Tmax	=	Oral	= 33%
MW	=	pKa	=

Adult Concerns: Diarrhea, gut cramping, hyperphosphatemia and serious electrolyte disturbances have been reported in some patients at increased risk for electrolyte disturbances. With magnesium salts, especially in renally impaired patients, hypotension, cardiac arrhythmias or arrest, loss of deep tendon reflexes, and confusion may occur.

Pediatric Concerns: None reported via milk.

Drug Interactions: May reduce oral bioavailability of many drugs.

Relative Infant Dose:

Adult Dose: Highly variable.

Alternatives:

References:
1.   AHFS Drug Information. Bethesda, Md; American Society of Health System Pharmacists, 2003.

SALMETEROL XINAFOATE   L2

Trade: Serevent

Other Trades: Serevent

Category: Long acting beta adrenergic bronchodilator

Salmeterol is a long acting beta-2 adrenergic stimulant used as a bronchodilator in asthmatics. Maternal plasma levels of salmeterol after inhaled administration are very low (85–200 pg/mL), or undetectable.[1] Studies in animals have shown that plasma and breastmilk levels are very similar. Oral absorption of both salmeterol and the xinafoate moiety are good. The terminal half-life of salmeterol is 5.5 hours, xinafoate is 11 days. No reports of use in lactating women are available.

Pregnancy Risk	C	Lactation Risk	L2
T ½	= 5.5 hours	M/P	= 1.0
Vd	=	PB	= 98%
Tmax	= 10–45 minutes	Oral	= Complete
MW	=	pKa	=

Adult Concerns: Tremor, dizziness, hypertension.

Pediatric Concerns: None reported via milk, but studies are limited.

Drug Interactions: Use with monoamine oxidase inhibitors may result in severe hypertension, severe headache, and hypertensive crisis. Tricyclic antidepressants may potentiate the pressure response. The pressor response of salmeterol may be reduced by lithium.

Relative Infant Dose:

Adult Dose: 50 µg twice daily.

Alternatives:

References:
1. Pharmaceutical manufacturer prescribing information, 1996.

SALSALATE   L4

Trade: Amigesic
Other Trades: Amigesic, Salflex, Disalcid
Category: NSAID

Salsalate is a non-steroidal anti-inflammatory drug used to treat minor pain or fever and arthritis. Salsalate is a dimer of salicylic acid, that when ingested releases pure salicylic acid.[1] Absorption of salicylic acid (SA) is complete. SA inhibits prostaglandin synthesis and acts on the hypothalamus heat-regulating center to reduce fever. Salicylic acid is excreted in breast milk (see aspirin) and chronic use of salicylates should be avoided. Therefore, salsalate should not be used while breastfeeding. Avoid its use in a lactating mother if the infant has a viral illness.

Pregnancy Risk	C/D in 3rd trimester	Lactation Risk	L4
T ½	= 7–8 hours	M/P	=
Vd	=	PB	= 80–90%
Tmax	=	Oral	= Complete
MW	= 258	pKa	=

Adult Concerns: Adverse effects include nausea, heartburn, stomach pain, and dyspepsia.

Pediatric Concerns: Avoid use in breastfeeding mothers due to the risk of Reye Syndrome in infants. One case of neonatal metabolic acidosis has been reported in a mother consuming aspirin.[2]

Drug Interactions: A decreased effect is seen with urinary alkalinizer, antacids, and corticosteroids. Salsalate can decrease the effect of uricosurics and spironolactone. Also, ACE inhibitor effects may be decreased with NSAID use.

Relative Infant Dose:

Adult Dose: 3000 mg/day in 2–3 divided doses

Alternatives: Acetaminophen, ibuprofen

References:
1. Pharmaceutical manufacturer prescribing information, 1997.
2. Clark JH, Wilson WG. A 16-day-old breast-fed infant with metabolic acidosis caused by salicylate. Clin Pediatr. 1981; 20: 53–4.

SAQUINAVIR   L3

Trade: Fortovase, Invirase

Other Trades:

Category: Antiretroviral agent for HIV infections.

Saquinavir is an antiretroviral agent used for HIV infections. Due to its kinetics, milk levels will probably be low. Oral bioavailability is only 4%. There are no adequate and well-controlled studies or case reports in breastfeeding women. Breastfeeding is not recommended in mothers who have HIV.[1,2]

Pregnancy Risk	B	Lactation Risk	L3
T ½	= 9–15 hours	M/P	=
Vd	= 700 L l/kg	PB	= 97%
Tmax	= 3 hours	Oral	= 4%
MW	= 670.86	pKa	=

Adult Concerns: Nausea, vomiting, diarrhea, abdominal pain, and pneumonia. Blood disorders such as anemia, hemolytic anemia, leukopenia, lymphadenopathy, neutropenia, pancytopenia, thrombocytopenia.

Pediatric Concerns: None yet reported.

Drug Interactions: Avoid the concomitant administration of the following drugs: alfuzosin, amiodarone, dofetilide, flecainide, lidocaine, propafenone, quinidine, trazodone, rifampin, Ergot containing medicines, statins, sildenafil, triazolam, and midazolam. Refer a drug interactions reference for a complete listing.

Relative Infant Dose:

Adult Dose: 1000 mg twice daily but is highly variable.

Alternatives:

References:
1. World Health Organization: Global Programme on AIDS. Consensus statement from the WHO/UNICEF consultation on HIV transmission and breast-feeding. Geneva: WHO, 1992.
2. Latham MC, Greiner T: Breastfeeding versus formula feeding in HIV infection. Lancet 352: 737, 1998.

SCOPOLAMINE   L3

Trade: Transderm Scope

Other Trades: Benacine, Transderm-V, Buscopan, Scopoderm TTS

Category: Anticholinergic

Scopolamine is a typical anticholinergic used primarily for motion sickness and pre-operatively to produce amnesia and decrease salivation.[1-3] Scopolamine is structurally similar to atropine but is known for its prominent CNS effects, including reducing motion sickness. There are no reports on its transfer into human milk, but due to its poor oral bioavailability it is generally believed to be minimal.

However, following prolonged exposure in a newborn, some anticholinergic symptoms could appear, and include drying, constipation, and urinary retention.

Pregnancy Risk	C	Lactation Risk	L3
T ½	= 2.9 hours	M/P	=
Vd	= 1.4 l/kg	PB	=
Tmax	= 1 hour	Oral	= 27%
MW	= 303	pKa	= 7.55

Adult Concerns: Blurred vision, dry mouth, drowsiness, constipation, confusion, drowsiness, bradycardia, hypotension, dermatitis.

Pediatric Concerns: None via milk. Observe for anticholinergic symptoms such as drowsiness, dry mouth.

Drug Interactions: Decreased effect of acetaminophen, levodopa, ketoconazole, digoxin. Gastrointestinal absorption of the following drugs may be altered: ketoconazole, digoxin, potassium supplements, acetaminophen, levodopa.

Relative Infant Dose:

Adult Dose: 0.3–0.6 mg once.

Alternatives:

References:
1. Lacy C. Drug information handbook. Lexi-Comp Inc. Cleveland, OH, 1996.
2. Drug Facts and Comparisons 1996 ed. ed. St. Louis: 1996.
3. Pharmaceutical manufacturer prescribing information, 1997.

SECOBARBITAL   L3

Trade: Seconal

Other Trades: Novo-Secobarb, Seconal

Category: Short acting barbiturate sedative

Secobarbital is a sedative, hypnotic barbiturate. It is probably secreted into breastmilk, although levels are unknown, and may be detectable in milk for 24 hours or longer.[1,2,3] Recommend mothers to delay breastfeeding for 3-4 hours to reduce possible transfer to infant if exposure to this barbiturate is required.

Pregnancy Risk	D	Lactation Risk	L3
T ½	= 15–40 hours	M/P	=
Vd	= 1.6–1.9 l/kg	PB	= 30–45%
Tmax	= 2–4 hours	Oral	= 90%
MW	= 260	pKa	= 7.9

Adult Concerns: Respiratory depression, sedation, addiction.

Pediatric Concerns: None reported via milk, but observe for sedation.

Drug Interactions: Anticoagulants: Phenobarbital lowers the plasma levels of dicumarol and causes a decrease in anticoagulant activity as measured by the prothrombin time. Corticosteroids: Barbiturates appear to enhance the metabolism of exogenous corticosteroids, probably through the induction of hepatic microsomal enzymes. Griseofulvin: Phenobarbital appears to interfere with the absorption of orally administered griseofulvin, thus decreasing its blood level. Doxycycline: Phenobarbital has been shown to shorten the half-life of doxycycline for as long as 2 weeks after barbiturate therapy is discontinued. Phenytoin, Sodium Valproate, Valproic Acid: The effect of barbiturates on the metabolism of phenytoin appears to be variable. Some investigators report an accelerating effect, whereas others report no effect. Monoamine Oxidase Inhibitors (MAOIs): MAOIs prolong the effects of barbiturates, probably because metabolism of the barbiturate is inhibited. Estradiol, Estrone, Progesterone, and Other Steroidal Hormone: Pretreatment with or concurrent administration of phenobarbital may decrease the effect of estradiol by increasing its metabolism.

Relative Infant Dose:

Adult Dose: 100 mg daily.

Alternatives:

References:
1. Tyson RM, Shrader EA, Perlman HH. Drugs transmitted through breast milk. II Barbiturates. J Pediatr 1938; 14: 86–90.
2. Kaneko S, Sato T, Suzuki K. The levels of anticonvulsants in breast milk. Br J Clin Pharmacol 1979; 7(6): 624–627.
3. Wilson JT, Brown RD, Cherek DR, Dailey JW, Hilman B, Jobe PC, Manno BR, Manno JE, Redetzki HM, Stewart JJ. Drug excretion in human breast milk: principles, pharmacokinetics and projected consequences. Clin Pharmacokinet 1980; 5(1): 1–66.

SELEGILINE   L4

Trade: Eldepryl, Emsam, Zelapar

Other Trades:

Category: Monoamine Oxidase Inhibitor

Selegiline is a selective irreversible inhibitor of monoamine oxidase, which in turn increases dopaminergic activity.[1] It is used to treat parkinsonian patients, major depressive disorder, and ADHD. It is available in a capsule form, an orally disintegrating tablet, as well as a transdermal system. The transdermal application has a half-life of 18–25 hours, and an absorption of 25–30% over 24 hours. The orally disintegrating tablet concentration peaks at 10–15 minutes, and has a half-life of 10 hours. No data are available on the transfer of selegiline into human milk. However, monoamine oxidase inhibitors require extraordinarily careful use and have many food-drug and drug-drug interactions that could be dangerous. These products should not be used in breastfeeding mothers.

Pregnancy Risk	C	Lactation Risk	L4
T ½	= 10 hours	M/P	=
Vd	=	PB	= 99.5%
Tmax	=	Oral	= 5.5%
MW	= 187	pKa	=

Adult Concerns: Adverse effects include headache, insomnia, nausea, and dizziness. As with most antidepressant therapies, caution should be taken toward suicidal ideations.

Pediatric Concerns: Do not use in breastfeeding mothers.

Drug Interactions: There are many drug interactions, particularly with amphetamines, anorexiants, atomoxetine, barbiturates, and SSRIs. See product information for a complete list of drug interactions.

Relative Infant Dose:

Adult Dose: 10 mg daily (capsule).

Alternatives:

References:
1. Pharmaceutical manufacturer prescribing information, 2007.

SELENIUM   L3

Trade: Selenicaps, Selenimin, SE-Aspartate, Se-100
Other Trades:
Category: Minerals

Selenium is an essential trace element which is needed for antioxidant enzymes. Recommended dietary allowance of selenium for breastfeeding women is 70 µg/day.[1] Foods that are rich is selenium includes tuna, brazil nuts, beef, cod, chicken, turkey, egg, cheese, rice, oatmeal, bread, and walnut.

Pregnancy Risk	C		Lactation Risk	L3
T ½	=		M/P	=
Vd	=		PB	=
Tmax	=		Oral	=
MW	= 79		pKa	=

Adult Concerns: Abdominal pain, fatigue, tremor, excessive sweating.

Pediatric Concerns:

Drug Interactions:

Relative Infant Dose:

Adult Dose: 20–40 µg/day.

Alternatives:

References:
1. Selenium. Dietary Supplement Fact Sheet. Office of Dietary Supplements. National Institute of Health. November 12 2009.

SELENIUM SULFIDE   L3

Trade: Dandrex, Selsun Blue Medicated Treatment, Selseb, Selenos, Tersi Foam
Other Trades:
Category: Topical antimicrobial

Selenium sulfide is an anti-infective compound with mild antibacterial and antifungal activity. It is commonly used for tinea versicolor and seborrheic dermatitis such as dandruff. Selenium is not apparently absorbed significantly through intact skin but is absorbed by damaged skin or open lesions.[1] There are no data on its transfer into human milk. If used properly on undamaged skin, it is very unlikely that enough would be absorbed systemically to produce untoward effects in a breastfed infant. Do not apply directly to nipple as enhanced absorption by the infant could occur.

Pregnancy Risk	C		Lactation Risk	L3
T ½	=		M/P	=
Vd	=		PB	=
Tmax	=		Oral	=
MW	=		pKa	=

Adult Concerns: Changes in hair color and loss of hair have been reported. Extensive washing of hair reduces the incidence of these problems. Extensive systemic absorption can occur with application to broken skin. Nausea, vomiting, diarrhea.

Pediatric Concerns: None reported via milk. Do not apply directly to nipple.

Drug Interactions:

Relative Infant Dose:

Adult Dose: Apply topic twice weekly.

Alternatives: Topical clotrimazole, itraconazole

References:
1.   McEvoy GE. (ed): AFHS Drug Information. New York, NY: 2003.

SENNA LAXATIVES   L3

Trade: Sennosides A, Sennosides B, Senokot
Other Trades:
Category: Laxative

Senna is a potent, proven laxative. Anthraquinones, its key ingredient, are believed to increase bowel activity due to secretion of anthraquinones into the colon. Side effects such as abdominal cramping and colic are unpredictable with homemade varieties of this plant. Most sources recommend taking a standardized formulation commonly available. This product is only recommended for short use, such as 10 days. Do not use for intestinal obstruction, or appendicitis, or abdominal pain of unknown origin. Senna laxatives are occasionally used in postpartum women to alleviate constipation. In one study of 23 women who received Senokot (100 mg containing 8.602 mg of Sennosides A and B), no sennoside A or B was detectable in their milk.[1] Of 15 mothers reporting loose stools, two infants had loose stools.

Pregnancy Risk	C	Lactation Risk	L3
T ½	=	M/P	=
Vd	=	PB	=
Tmax	=	Oral	=
MW	=	pKa	=

Adult Concerns: Diarrhea, abdominal cramps, dark colored urine, chronic diarrhea, fluid loss.

Pediatric Concerns: Several infants had loose stools although no drug was detected in milk.

Drug Interactions:

Relative Infant Dose:

Adult Dose: 100 mg daily.

Alternatives:

References:
1. Werthmann MW, Jr., Krees SV. Quantitative excretion of Senokot in human breast milk. Med Ann Dist Columbia 1973; 42(1): 4–5.

SERTRALINE   L2

Trade: Zoloft

Other Trades: Zoloft, Lustral

Category: Antidepressant

Sertraline is a typical serotonin reuptake inhibitor similar to fluoxetine and paroxetine, but unlike fluoxetine, the longer half-life metabolite of sertraline is only marginally active. In one study of a single patient taking 100 mg of sertraline daily for 3 weeks postpartum, the concentration of sertraline in milk was 24, 43, 40, and 19 µg/L of milk at 1, 5, 9, and 23 hours respectively following the dose.[1] The maternal plasma levels of sertraline after 12 hours was 48 ng/mL. Sertraline plasma levels in the infant at three weeks were below the limit of detection (<0.5 ng/mL) at 12 hours post-dose. Routine pediatric evaluation after 3 months revealed a neonate of normal weight who had achieved the appropriate developmental milestones.

In another study of 3 breastfeeding patients who received 50–100 mg sertraline daily, the maternal plasma levels ranged from 18.4 to 95.8 ng/mL, whereas the plasma levels of sertraline and its metabolite, desmethylsertraline, in the 3 breastfed infants was below the limit of detection (<2 ng/mL).[2] Milk levels were not measured. Desmethylsertraline is poorly active, less than 10% of the parent sertraline.

Another recent publication reviewed the changes in platelet serotonin levels in breastfeeding mothers and their infants who received up to 100 mg of sertraline daily.[3] Mothers treated with sertraline had significant decreases in their platelet serotonin levels, which is expected. However, there was no change in platelet serotonin levels in breastfed infants of mothers consuming sertraline, suggesting that only minimal amounts of sertraline are actually transferred to the infant. This confirms other studies.

Studies by Stowe of 11 mother/infant pairs (maternal dose= 25–150 mg/day) further suggest minimal transfer of sertraline into human milk.[4] From this superb study, the concentration of sertraline peaked in the milk at 7–8 hours and the metabolite (desmethylsertraline) at 5–11 hours. The reported concentrations of sertraline and desmethylsertraline in breastmilk were 17–173 µg/L and 22–294 µg/L respectively. The reported dose of sertraline to the infant via milk varied from undetectable (5 of 11) to 0.124 mg/day in one infant. The infant's serum concentration of sertraline varied from undetectable to 3.0 ng/mL but was undetectable in 7 of 11 patients. No developmental abnormalities were noted in any of the infants studied.

In a study of 8 women taking sertraline (1.05 mg/kg/day) the mean milk/plasma ratio was 1.93 and 1.64 for sertraline and N-desmethylsertraline.[5] Infant exposure estimated from actual milk produced was 0.2% and 0.3% of the weight-adjusted maternal dose for sertraline and N-desmethylsertraline (sertraline equivalents) respectively. Assuming a 150 mL/kg/day intake, infant exposure was significantly greater at 0.90% and 1.32% for sertraline and N-desmethylsertraline respectively. Neither sertraline nor its N-desmethyl metabolite could be detected in plasma samples from the four infants tested. No adverse effects were observed in any of the eight infants and all had achieved normal developmental milestones.

Sertraline is a potent inhibitor of 5–HT transporter function both in the CNS and platelets. One recent study assessed the effect of sertraline on platelet 5–HT transporter function in 14 breastfeeding mothers (dose= 25–200 mg/day) and their infants to determine if even low levels of sertraline exposure could perhaps lead to changes in the infant's blood platelet 5–HT levels and, therefore, CNS serotonin levels.[6] While a significant reduction in platelet levels of 5–HT were noted in the mothers, no changes in 5–HT levels were noted in the 14 infants. Thus, it appears that at typical clinical doses, maternal sertraline has a minimal effect on platelet 5–HT transport in breastfeeding infants.

These studies generally confirm that the transfer of sertraline and its metabolite to the infant is minimal, and that attaining clinically relevant plasma levels in infants is remote at maternal doses less than 150 mg/day. Thorough reviews of antidepressant use in breastfeeding mothers are available.[7–9]

Pregnancy Risk	C	Lactation Risk	L2
T ½	= 26 hours	M/P	= 0.89
Vd	= 20 l/kg	PB	= 98%
Tmax	= 7–8 hours	Oral	= Complete
MW	= 306	pKa	=

Adult Concerns: Diarrhea, nausea, tremor, and increased sweating.

Pediatric Concerns: Of the cases reported in the literature, only one infant developed benign neonatal sleep at age 4 months which spontaneous resolved at 6 months. Its relationship, if any, to sertraline is unknown.

Drug Interactions: All SSRIs inhibit cytochrome P450 enzymes and may inhibit metabolism of desipramine, dextromethorphan, encainide, haloperidol, metoprolol, etc. May induce serotonergic hyperstimulation when added too soon after MAO inhibitors, tricyclic antidepressants, and lithium. May displace warfarin from binding sites increasing anticoagulation. Two recent cases of serotonin-like reactions (agitation, dysarthria, diaphoresis and extrapyramidal movement disorder) have been reported when metoclopramide was used in patients receiving sertraline or venlafaxine.[7]

Relative Infant Dose: 0.4%–2.2%

Adult Dose: 50–200 mg daily.

Alternatives: Escitalopram, paroxetine, fluoxetine

References:

1. Altshuler LL, Burt VK, McMullen M, Hendrick V. Breastfeeding and sertraline: a 24-hour analysis. J Clin Psychiatry 1995; 56(6): 243–245.
2. Mammen OK, Perel JM, Rudolph G, Foglia JP, Wheeler SB. Sertraline and norsertraline levels in three breastfed infants. J Clin Psychiatry 1997; 58(3): 100–103.
3. Epperson CN. et.al. Sertraine and Breastfeeding. NEJM 1997; 336(16): 1189–1190.
4. Stowe ZN, Owens MJ, Landry JC, Kilts CD, Ely T, Llewellyn A, Nemeroff CB. Sertraline and desmethylsertraline in human breast milk and nursing infants. Am J Psychiatry 1997; 154(9): 1255–1260.
5. Kristensen JH, Ilett KF, Dusci LJ, Hackett LP, Yapp P, Wojnar-Horton RE, Roberts MJ, Paech M. Distribution and excretion of sertraline and N-desmethylsertraline in human milk. Br J Clin Pharmacol 1998; 45(5): 453–457.
6. Epperson N, Czarkowski KA, Ward-O'Brien D, Weiss E, Gueorguieva R, Jatlow P, Anderson GM. Maternal sertraline treatment and serotonin transport in breast-feeding mother-infant pairs. Am J Psychiatry 2001; 158(10): 1631–1637.
7. Wisner KL, Perel JM, Findling RL. Antidepressant treatment during breast-feeding. Am J Psychiatry 1996; 153(9): 1132–1137.
8. Stowe ZN, Hostetter AL, Owens MJ, Ritchie JC, Sternberg K, Cohen LS, Nemeroff CB. The pharmacokinetics of sertraline excretion into human brest milk: determinants of infant serum concentrations. J Clin Psychiatry 2003; 64(1): 73–80.
9. Weissman AM, Levy BT, Hartz AJ, et.al. Pooled Analysis of Antidepressant Levels in Lactating Mothers, Breast Milk, and Nursing Infants. Am J Psychiatry 2004 June; 161(6): 1066–1078.

SEVELAMER HYDROCHLORIDE   L3

Trade: Renagel

Other Trades:

Category: Phosphate Binder

Sevelamer is a chelating resin that is used to treat elevated plasma phosphate levels in patients with chronic kidney disease who are on dialysis. Sevelamer hydrochloride is not systemically absorbed and is retained in the gastrointestinal tract.[1] Hence, it would not readily enter milk at all.

Pregnancy Risk	C		Lactation Risk	L3
T ½	=		M/P	=
Vd	=		PB	=
Tmax	=		Oral	= Nil
MW	= High		pKa	=

Adult Concerns: Most common side effects are dyspepsia, peritonitis, diarrhea, nausea, constipation, and pruritus

Pediatric Concerns: This product unabsorbed from the gastrointestinal tract and would not pose a hazard to a breastfeeding infant.

Drug Interactions: Ciprofloxacin, digoxin, warfarin, enalapril, metoprolol, and iron.

Relative Infant Dose:

Adult Dose: 800–1600 mg three times a day with meals.

Alternatives:

References:
1.   Pharmaceutical manufacturer prescribing information, 2010.

SEVOFLURANE   L3

Trade: Ultane
Other Trades:
Category: Anesthetic gas

Sevoflurane is a gaseous halogenated general anesthetic drug that is particularly popular because of its rapid wash-out. Average patient time to emergence is approximately 8.2 minutes. It is commonly used in adult and pediatric patients, and is used in cesarean sections. The manufacturer states that while the concentration of sevoflurane have not been measured in breastmilk, they are probably of no clinical importance 24 hours after anesthesia. Because of its rapid wash-out, sevoflurane concentrations in milk are predicted to be below those found with many other volatile anaesthetics.[1] Sevoflurane follows a three term exponential decay with half-lives of 11 min (18% of the dose in plasma compartment), 1.8 hours (15% from muscle compartment), and 20 hours (6% from fat compartment).[2] Small (3%) amounts of sevoflurane are metabolized and result in plasma levels that average 36 µM/L. Levels reported are temporary and completely dissipate by 6 days. The fluoride ion released is not high enough to be a contraindication to breastfeeding. Further, the oral absorption of fluoride in infants is believed poor as it is chelated with calcium ions orally in milk.

While no data on levels of sevoflurane in breast milk are available, this product, due to its rapid clearance from the body (100-fold drop in 120 minutes), should not pose a problem for continued breastfeeding soon after exposure.

Pregnancy Risk	B		Lactation Risk	L3
T ½	= 1.8–3.8 hours		M/P	=
Vd	= 0.5 l/kg		PB	=
Tmax	=		Oral	=
MW	= 200		pKa	=

Adult Concerns: Malignant hyperthermia, bradycardia, agitation, laryngospasm, shivering, hypotension, etc. Check anesthesia text for more.

Pediatric Concerns: None reported via milk. Milk levels are likely insignificant, and oral bioavailability is unlikely.

Drug Interactions: Sevoflurane increases intensity and duration of neuromuscular blockade by nondepolarizing muscle relaxants.

Relative Infant Dose:

Adult Dose: Variable.

Alternatives:

References:
1. Pharmaceutical manufacturer prescribing information, 2003.
2. Holaday DA, Smith FR. Clinical characteristics and biotransformation of sevoflurane in healthy volunteers. Anesthesiology 1981; 54: 100–106.

SILDENAFIL   L3

Trade: Viagra, Revatio

Other Trades: Viagra

Category: For erectile dysfunction and pulmonary hypertension

Sildenafil is a phosphodiesterase type 5 (PDE-5) inhibitor. It has vasodilating and smooth muscle relaxing properties. It is used in the treatment of pulmonary hypertension and in erectile dysfunction in men.[1] No data are available on the transfer of sildenafil into human milk, but due to its pharmacokinetic parameters, it is unlikely that significant transfer will occur. However, caution is recommended in breastfeeding mothers. Oral sildenafil has been used successfully in infants for the management of pulmonary hypertension.[2,3] No untoward effects were reported in these infants.

Pregnancy Risk	B		Lactation Risk	L3
T ½	= 4 hours		M/P	=
Vd	= 1.5 l/kg		PB	= 96%
Tmax	= 60 minutes		Oral	= 40%
MW	= 666		pKa	=

Adult Concerns: Changes in visual color perception is common. Other side effects include headache, flushing, dyspepsia, nasal congestion, and hypotension.

Pediatric Concerns: None reported via milk.

Drug Interactions: Do not admix with any form of nitrates, including nitroglycerine. Because it is metabolized by cytochrome P450 CYP3A4 and 2C9, increased plasma levels may result when admixed with azole antifungals, erythromycins, cimetidine and other such enzyme inhibitors. Serious prolonged erections have been reported with the coadministration of dihydrocodeine.

Relative Infant Dose:

Adult Dose: Pulmonary hypertension: 20 mg three times daily; 10 mg IV three times daily.

Alternatives:

References:

1. Pharmaceutical manufacturer prescribing information, 1999.
2. Palma G, Giordano R, Russolillo V, Cioffi S, Palumbo S, Mucerino M, Poli V, Vosa C. Sildenafil therapy for pulmonary hypertension before and after pediatric congenital heart surgery. Tex Heart Inst J. 2011; 38(3): 238–42.]
3. Humpl T, Reyes JT, Erickson S, Armano R, Holtby H, Adatia I. Sildenafiltherapy for neonatal and childhood pulmonary hypertensive vascular disease.Cardiol Young.

SILICONE BREAST IMPLANTS   L3

Trade:

Other Trades:

Category: Silicone mammoplasty

Augmentation mammoplasty with silicone implants has only recently been available in the USA. Millions of women have silicone implants for various esthetic reasons. In general, placement of the implant behind the breast seldom produces interruption of vital ducts, nerve supply, or blood supply. Peri areolar incisions should be avoided, as they might interrupt nerves vital to prolactin production. Most women have been able to breastfeed. Breast reduction surgery, on the other hand, has been found to produce significant interruption of the nervous supply (particularly the ductile tissue), leading to a reduced ability to lactate. Other reports suggesting autoimmune diseases such as scleroderma with esophageal dysfunction in breastfed infants[1,2] have failed to be confirmed.

Silicone transfer to breastmilk has been studied in one group of 15 lactating mothers with bilateral silicone breast implants.[3] Silicon levels were measured in breastmilk, whole blood, cow's milk, and 26 brands of infant formula. Comparing implanted women to controls, mean silicon levels were not significantly different in breastmilk (55.45 ± 35 and 51.05 ± 31 ng/mL respectively) or in blood (79.29 ± 87 and 103.76 ± 112 ng/mL respectively). Mean silicon level measured in store-bought cow's milk was 708.94 ng/mL and that for 26 brands of commercially available infant formula was 4402.5 ng/mL (ng/mL= parts per billion). The authors concluded that lactating women with silicone implants are similar to control women with respect to levels of silicon in their breastmilk and blood. From these studies, silicon levels are 10 times higher in cow's milk and even higher in infant formulas. It is not known for certain if ingestion of leaking silicone by a nursing infant is dangerous. Although one article has been published showing esophageal strictures, it has subsequently been recalled by the author. Silicone by nature is extremely inert and is unlikely to be absorbed in the gastrointestinal tract by a nursing infant although good studies are lacking. Silicone is a ubiquitous substance, found in all foods, liquids, etc.

Pregnancy Risk	Probably Safe	Lactation Risk	L3
T ½	=	M/P	=
Vd	=	PB	=
Tmax	=	Oral	=
MW	=	pKa	=

Adult Concerns:

Pediatric Concerns: None reported via milk.

Drug Interactions:

Relative Infant Dose:

Adult Dose: N/A

Alternatives:

References:

1. Spiera RF, Gibofsky A, Spiera H. Scleroderma in women with silicone breast implants: comment on the article by Sanchez-Guerrero et al. Arthritis Rheum. May 1995; 38(5): 719, 721.
2. Spiera H, Kerr LD. Scleroderma following silicone implantation: a cumulative experience of 11 cases. J Rheumatol. Jun 1993; 20(6): 958–961.
3. Semple JL, Lugowski SJ, Baines CJ, Smith DC, McHugh A. Breast milk contamination and silicone implants: preliminary results using silicon as a proxy measurement for silicone. Plast Reconstr Surg 1998; 102(2): 528–533.

SILODOSIN   L3

Trade: Rapaflo

Other Trades:

Category: Alpha-1 adrenergic receptor antagonist

Silodosin is an alpha-1 adrenergic receptor antagonist used for the treatment of benign prostatic hyperplasia. Silodosin relaxes the smooth muscles of the bladder neck and prostate. The drug is not indicated for the treatment of hypertension. Side effects include postural hypotension, dizziness, diarrhea, headache, nasopharyngitis, and nasal congestion. In one animal study, administration of silodosin 300 mg/kg/day did not suggest physical and development abnormalities in offsprings of rats.[1] There are no studies on the transfer of silodosin into human milk. Due to the pharmacokinetic properties, little of the drug is expected to transfer into milk. Observe baby for nasal congestion and hypotension.

Pregnancy Risk	B	Lactation Risk	L3
T ½	= 13 hours	M/P	=
Vd	= 49.5 L l/kg	PB	= 97%
Tmax	= 2.6 hours	Oral	= 32%
MW	= 495.5	pKa	=

Adult Concerns: Dizziness, diarrhea, orthostatic hypotension, headache, nasopharyngitis, and nasal congestion

Pediatric Concerns: Observe baby for nasal congestion and hypotension.

Drug Interactions: Concurrent use with strong CYP3A4 inhibitors (such as, clarithromycin, itraconazole, ketoconazole, ritonavir).

Relative Infant Dose:

Adult Dose: 8 mg once daily.

Alternatives:

References:
1. Physicians Total Care, Inc. manufacturer product information, 11/2009.

SILVER   L4

Trade: Silver pellet, Silver nitrate liquid

Other Trades:

Category: Antiseptic

There are many different forms of silver such as colloidal silver, silver nitrate, and silver sulfadiazine. Colloidal silver solution is normally labeled by silver content in parts per million. Silver ions are present in humans at low concentrations (2.3 µg/L) from environmental exposure (inhaled, food and drinking water contamination, etc).[1] One study suggests that less than 4% of topical silver nitrate administration is absorbed transcutaneously.[1] Another *in vitro* study suggests that nanoparticulate silver absorption is very low, in the order of 0.46 ng/cm^2 for intact skin and 2.32 ng/cm^2 for damaged skin. The oral bioavailability of silver is estimated to be less than 10%.

Silver toxicity occurs when excessive exposure over a long period of time exceeds the capacity of liver or kidney excretion. The NOAEL(Human No Observable Adverse Effect Level) for silver is 10 gm of lifetime intake. Silver is not acutely toxic; however, accumulation of silver can cause adverse effects such as argyria, argyrosis, leukopenia, and anemia. In one case, ingestion of 30 mg/day of silver nitrate for an extended period with total intake of 6.4 gm caused generalized argyria. Argyria is a greenish discoloration of the skin that is irreversible. There have been reported cases of argyria with total silver exposure of 3.8–6 grams. Another study of 30 healthy volunteers did not suggest significant adverse effects after ingesting 50 mg/day of silver leaf for 20 days (total dose of 1 g).[2] There is one case of argyria (limited to finger nails) after ingesting 550 mg of silver colloidal over two years.[3]

There are no studies regarding silver transfer into breastmilk, however the long term use of this drug should be avoided in all humans, particularly breastfeeding mothers.

Pregnancy Risk	Possibly Hazardous	Lactation Risk	L4
T ½	= 52 days	M/P	=
Vd	=	PB	=
Tmax	=	Oral	= Poor
MW	= 108	pKa	=

Adult Concerns: Silver toxicity: Argyria, argyrosis, leukopenia, and anemia.

Pediatric Concerns:

Drug Interactions:

Relative Infant Dose:

Adult Dose:

Alternatives:

References:
1. Lansdown AB. A pharmacological and toxicological profile of silver as an antimicrobial agent in medical devices. Adv Pharmacol Sci. 2010; 2010: 910686. Epub 2010 Aug 24.
2. Sharma DC, Sharma P, Sharma S. Effect of silver leaf on circulating lipids and cardiac and hepatic enzymes. Indian J Physiol Pharmacol. 1997 Jul; 41(3): 285–8. Abstract.
3. McKenna JK, Hull CM, Zone JJ. Argyria associated with colloidal silver supplementation. Int J Dermatol. 2003 Jul; 42(7): 549.

SILVER SULFADIAZINE   L3

Trade: Silvadene, SSD Cream, Thermazene

Other Trades: Silvazine, Flamazine, Dermazin, SSD,

Category: Topical antimicrobial cream

Silver sulfadiazine is a topical antimicrobial cream primarily used for reducing sepsis in burn patients. The silver component is not absorbed from the skin.[1] Sulfadiazine is partially absorbed. After prolonged therapy of large areas, sulfadiazine levels in plasma may approach therapeutic levels. Although sulfonamides such as sulfadiazine, are known to be secreted into human milk, they are not particularly problematic except in the newborn period when they may produce kernicterus. The WHO considers silver sulfadiazine as compatible with breastfeeding.[2]

Pregnancy Risk	B/X in third trimester	Lactation Risk	L3
T ½	= 10 hours (sulfa)	M/P	=
Vd	=	PB	=
Tmax	=	Oral	= Complete
MW	=	pKa	=

Adult Concerns: Allergic rash, renal failure, crystalluria.

Pediatric Concerns: None reported, but studies are limited. Observe caution during the neonatal period.

Drug Interactions:

Relative Infant Dose:

Adult Dose:

Alternatives:

References:
1. McEvoy GE. (ed): AFHS Drug Information. New York, NY: 2003.
2. Anon: Breastfeeding and Maternal Medication. World Health Organization, Geneva, Switzerland, 2002.

SIMETHICONE   L3

Trade: Mylicon, Gas-X, Maalox Anti-Gas, Mylanta Gas, Genasyme, Mytab Gas, Phazyme, Alka-Seltzer Anti-Gas

Other Trades:

Category: Antiflatulent

Simethicone is an anti-flatulent, used to relieve upper gastrointestinal gas and also used as an adjunct in ultrasonography. Because the drug is not absorbed, the risk to a nursing infant from maternal use of simethicone is thought to be negligible.[1] There was no evidence of medication-related adverse effects in the neonate with simethicone exposure.[2] Simethicone is not systemically absorbed, so none would enter milk.

Pregnancy Risk	Probably Safe	Lactation Risk	L3
T ½	=	M/P	=
Vd	=	PB	=
Tmax	=	Oral	= Unabsorbed orally
MW	=	pKa	=

Adult Concerns: Rash, diarrhea, nausea, vomiting, pharyngitis.

Pediatric Concerns: None reported. Commonly used in pediatric patients.

Drug Interactions: Concurrent use of simethicone with levothyroxine may result in decreased absorption of levothyroxine.

Relative Infant Dose:

Adult Dose: 40–360 mg daily.

Alternatives:

References:
1. Briggs GG, Freeman RK, Yaffe SJ. Drugs in Pregnancy and Lactation: A reference Guide to Fetal and Neonatal Risk. Philadelphia: Lippincott Williams and Wilkins, 2008.
2. Hodgkinson R et al: Comparison of cimetidine (Tagamet) with antacid for safety and effectiveness in reducing gastric acidity before elective cesarean section. Anesthesiology 59: 86–90, 1983.

SIMVASTATIN   L3

Trade: Zocor

Other Trades: Lipex, Zocor

Category: Reduces cholesterol

Simvastatin is an HMG-CoA reductase inhibitor that reduces the production of cholesterol in the liver. Like lovastatin, simvastatin reduces blood cholesterol levels. Others in this family are known to be secreted into human and rodent milk, but no data are available on simvastatin.[1] It is likely that milk levels will be low because less than 5% of simvastatin reaches the plasma, most being removed by first-pass by the liver. Atherosclerosis is a chronic process and discontinuation of lipid-lowering drugs during pregnancy and lactation should have little to no impact on the outcome of long-term therapy of primary hypercholesterolemia. Cholesterol and other products of cholesterol biosynthesis are essential components for fetal and neonatal development, and the use of cholesterol-lowering drugs would not be advisable.

Pregnancy Risk	X		Lactation Risk	L3
T ½	= Long		M/P	=
Vd	=		PB	= 95%
Tmax	= 1.3–2.4 hours		Oral	= Poor
MW	= 419		pKa	=

Adult Concerns: Gastrointestinal distress, headache, hypotension, elevated liver enzymes.

Pediatric Concerns: None reported.

Drug Interactions: Increased toxicity when added to gemfibrozil (myopathy, myalgia, etc), clofibrate, niacin (myopathy), erythromycin, cyclosporine, oral anticoagulants (elevated bleeding time).

Relative Infant Dose:

Adult Dose: 5–10 mg daily.

Alternatives:

References:
1. Facts and Comparisons. St. Louis: 2010..

SINCALIDE   L3

Trade: Kinevac

Other Trades:

Category: Diagnostic agent for cholecystography

Sincalide is a synthetically prepared, C-terminal octapeptide fragment of cholecystokinin (CCK).[1] When injected intravenously, it produces a substantial contracture of the gall bladder. Sincalide is therefore used for diagnostic purposes to assess biliary and gall bladder function. A reduction in radiographic gall bladder size of up to 40% is considered satisfactory contraction.[2,3] The half-life of Sincalide was found to be approximately 1.3 minutes, with a high molecular weight of 1143. Data from a study conducted in rats reveal that sincalide has a large volume of distribution and tends to concentrate in the liver, pancreas, upper digestive tract and in the thyroid. It does not penetrate the blood brain barrier. No data are available on the transfer of this peptide into human milk, but due to its high molecular weight, brief plasma half-life and extensive volume of distribution, it is extremely unlikely significant quantities would reach the milk compartment. Therefore, sincalide may be considered compatible with breastfeeding. A brief interruption of breastfeeding (1–2 hours) would preclude any possible side effects.

Pregnancy Risk	B	Lactation Risk	L3
T ½	= 1.3 minutes	M/P	=
Vd	= Widely distributed l/kg	PB	=
Tmax	= 5–15 min	Oral	= Nil
MW	= 1143	pKa	=

Adult Concerns: Adverse effects include gastrointestinal and abdominal pain, nausea, the urge to defecate, flushing, dizziness, and cramping. Contraindicated in those hypersensitive to sincalide.

Pediatric Concerns: None reported via milk. While it is unlikely to enter milk, a brief interruption of breastfeeding (1–2 hours) would preclude any possible side effects.

Drug Interactions:

Relative Infant Dose:

Adult Dose: 0.02 µg/kg over 30 seconds.

Alternatives:

References:
1. Pharmaceutical manufacturer Package Insert, 2003.
2. Sturdevant RAL, Stern DH, Resin H, et al: Effect of graded doses of octapeptide of cholecystokinin on gallbladder size in man. Gastroenterology 1973; 64: 452–456.3
3. Sargent EN, Meyers HI, and Hubsher J: Cholecystokinetic cholecystography: efficacy and tolerance study of sincalide. Am J Roentgenol 1976; 127: 267–271.

SIROLIMUS   L4

Trade: Rapamune, Rapamycin, NSC-226080

Other Trades: Rapamune

Category: Immunosuppressant

Sirolimus is an immunosuppressant sometimes used in combination with cyclosporin in renal transplants. No data are available on its transfer to human milk. Average plasma levels are quite low (264 ng x hr/mL) and the drug is strongly attached to cellular components and plasma levels are low. It is not likely it will penetrate milk in levels that are significant. However, it is a potent inhibitor of the enzyme 70 K S6 kinase, which is stimulated in breast tissue by prolactin. This agent, in rodent mammary tissue, strongly inhibits milk component production.[1]

It could potentially suppress milk production in lactating mothers and caution is recommended.

Pregnancy Risk	C	Lactation Risk	L4
T ½	= 57–63 hours	M/P	=
Vd	= 12 l/kg	PB	=
Tmax	= 1–3 hours	Oral	= 15%
MW	= 914	pKa	=

Adult Concerns: Anemia, thrombocytopenia, leukopenia, hypertension, headache, hyperlipidemia, hypophosphatemia, urinary tract infection, interstitial pneumonitis.

Pediatric Concerns: None via milk, but reduced milk production could occur.

Drug Interactions: Drugs which inhibit cytochrome P450 3A4 may significantly increase levels of sirolimus. These include: bromocriptine, carbamazepine, cimetidine, cisapride, clarithromycin, clotrimazole, danazol, diltiazem, erythromycin, fluconazole, fosphenytoin, metoclopramide, etc. Co-administration with cyclosporine may increase levels of sirolimus. Numerous other drug-drug contraindications may exist, consult drug interaction reference.

Relative Infant Dose:

Adult Dose: 2 mg/day.

Alternatives:

References:
1. Hang J, Rillema JA. Effect of rapamycin on prolactin-stimulated S6 kinase activity and milk product formation in mouse mammary explants. Biochim Biophys Acta 1997; 1358(2): 209–214.

SITAGLIPTIN PHOSPHATE   L3

Trade: Januvia

Other Trades:

Category: Antidiabetic agent in Type 2 diabetics

Sitagliptin phosphate is a dipeptidyl peptidase IV inhibitor resulting in prolonged active incretin levels, thus increasing insulin release from pancreatic beta cells in type 2 diabetics and decreasing glucagon secretion from pancreatic alpha cells, and ultimately decreasing blood glucose levels.[1] It does not lower blood glucose or cause hypoglycemia in healthy subjects. There are no data available on the transfer of sitagliptin into human milk. Levels will probably be quite low due to its size and kinetics. Some caution is recommended until we have data.

Pregnancy Risk	B	Lactation Risk	L3
T ½	= 12 hours	M/P	=
Vd	= 2.8 l/kg	PB	= 38%
Tmax	= 1–4 hours	Oral	= 87%
MW	= 523	pKa	=

Adult Concerns: Adverse reactions include headache, diarrhea, upper respiratory tract infection, and nasopharyngitis.

Pediatric Concerns: No data are available.

Drug Interactions: Sitagliptin is a minor substrate of CYP2C8 and CYP3A4, but has not shown any significant drug interactions.

Relative Infant Dose:

Adult Dose: 100 mg once daily.

Alternatives: Metformin

References:
1. Pharmaceutical manufacturer prescribing information, 2008.

SMALLPOX VACCINE   L4

Trade: Smallpox Vaccine, Dryvax, ACAM2000
Other Trades:
Category: Vaccine for vaccinia virus

Smallpox is a viral syndrome caused by infection with the vaccinia virus. The smallpox vaccine contains a live but attenuated (weakened) preparation of vaccinia virus. The reconstituted vaccine contains approximately 100 million infectious vaccinia viruses per mL. Introduction of potent smallpox vaccine into the superficial layers of the skin results in viral multiplication, immunity, and cellular hypersensitivity. With the primary vaccination, a papule appears at the site of vaccination on the 2nd to 5th day. It then becomes a pustule surrounded by erythema and induration. The erythema and swelling then subside after about 10 days and the crust forms. Secretions from the lesions are capable of inoculating other individuals and care should be exercised around pregnant women, infants, and particularly premature infants.

No data are available suggesting the degree of transmission into human milk, but it is likely to enter milk to some degree. Infants are at increased risk from vaccinia infections and the use of smallpox vaccine in infants is contraindicated unless it is an emergency situation. Although the use of the smallpox vaccine in children is not recommended in non-emergent situations, it was safely used in the past. The product information suggests that pregnant and breastfeeding mothers should not receive the vaccination under non-emergent conditions. However, there are no absolute contraindications regarding vaccination of a person with a high-risk exposure to smallpox. In breastfeeding mothers who are not at high risk, the use of smallpox vaccinations is not justified (Centers of Disease Control).

Pregnancy Risk	C		Lactation Risk	L4
T ½	=		M/P	=
Vd	=		PB	=
Tmax	=		Oral	=
MW	=		pKa	=

Adult Concerns: Adverse effects include fever, lymphedema, urticaria, secondary pyogenic infections, vesicular rash.

Pediatric Concerns: No data are available on its use in breastfeeding mothers or its transfer into human milk. However, vaccinia virus is likely transmitted via milk and is probably infectious. Its use in breastfeeding mothers is not recommended in non-emergent situations.

Drug Interactions:

Relative Infant Dose:

Adult Dose:

Alternatives:

References:
1. Pharmaceutical manufacturer prescribing information, 2003.

SODIUM OXYBATE   L4

Trade: Xyrem

Other Trades: Xyrem

Category: CNS depressant

Sodium oxybate is a central nervous system depressant used to treat excessive daytime sleepiness and cataplexy in patients with narcolepsy. Its mechanism of action is unknown, but it may work by inhibiting GABA receptors.[1] No data are available on the transfer of oxybate into human breastmilk, but due to the low molecular weight and low protein binding, it is likely this medication will be secreted in human milk and be passed to a breastfeeding infant. Due to the sedative properties of this drug, this product should be used very cautiously in breastfeeding mothers, if at all. Mothers consuming this product, might pump and discard milk at night, and continue breastfeeding during the day. This product has a very brief half-life.

Pregnancy Risk	B	Lactation Risk	L4
T ½	= 0.5–1 hour	M/P	=
Vd	= 0.19–0.384 l/kg	PB	= <1%
Tmax	= 0.5–1.25 hours	Oral	= 25%
MW	= 126	pKa	=

Adult Concerns: Adverse reactions include dizziness, headache, nausea, vomiting, confusion, hyperglycemia, hypernatremia, and pain. CNS side effects include: confusion, hallucinations, psychosis, vertigo, and nightmares.

Pediatric Concerns: No data are available but caution recommended.

Drug Interactions: Use with other central nervous system depressants is contraindicated.

Relative Infant Dose:

Adult Dose: < 6–9 gm/day.

Alternatives:

References:
1. Pharmaceutical manufacturer prescribing information, 2005.

SODIUM TETRADECYL SULFATE   L3

Trade: Sotradecol

Other Trades:

Category: Sclerosing Agent

Sodium tetradecyl sulfate (STS) is a sclerosing agent used to treat varicose veins.[1] This agent, when injected into the affected vein, acts as an anionic surfactant and causes local inflammation, and thrombus formation, thereby occluding and eventually obliterating the affected vein. Severe reactions such as anaphylactic shocks, precipitation of asthma and pulmonary embolism have been reported with its use, although rare. There are no data available on its transfer into human milk. There are no studies done in nursing women. This product could be hazardous if introduced in the infant through breastmilk. Therefore, extreme caution is recommended with its use in a lactating mother. Use only if the potential benefit to mother outweighs the potential risks to the infant.

Pregnancy Risk	C		Lactation Risk	L3
T ½	=		M/P	=
Vd	=		PB	=
Tmax	=		Oral	=
MW	= 316		pKa	=

Adult Concerns: Local injection site reactions, pain, urticaria, ulceration, permanent discoloration, necrosis, allergic reactions.

Pediatric Concerns: None reported

Drug Interactions: Caution while administering in patients on oral contraceptives.

Relative Infant Dose:

Adult Dose: 0.5–1 mL IV.

Alternatives: Glycerin, polidocanol

References:
1. Pharmaceutical manufacturer prescribing information, 2009.

SOLIFENACIN SUCCINATE   L4

Trade: VESIcare

Other Trades:

Category: Muscarinic agonist for bladder hyperactivity

Solifenacin is a muscarinic agonist drug that reduces the symptoms of overactive bladder disorder (OAB) and has a high affinity for the M3 muscarinic receptor.[1] OAB is a medical condition that causes the bladder muscle (known as the detrusor muscle) to contract while the bladder is filling with urine, rather than when the bladder is full. Patients with OAB feel the urge to urinate more often (urgency), without advance warning, and when the bladder isn't completely full.

Solifenacin is an unusual anticholinergic, structurally different but similar in effect to atropine. We do not have data on its use in breastfeeding mothers. However, the potency of this product, its effect on numerous important organs, the sensitivity of infants to anticholinergic agents, and its long-half life make this product problematic for breastfeeding infants. While I predict that milk levels will ultimately be low (due to its structure), we do not have that data at present, and caution is recommended. The manufacturer reports some side effects (reduced body weight, etc.) in lactating mice at doses 3.6 times the normal dose. The relevance of rodent studies to humans is usually minimal. This product should be used with significant caution in breastfeeding mothers, if at all. Infants should be closely watched for urinary retention, dry mouth, constipation, UTI, and other antimuscarinic symptoms.

Pregnancy Risk	C	Lactation Risk	L4
T ½	= 45–68 hours	M/P	=
Vd	= 8.57 l/kg	PB	= 98%
Tmax	= 3–8 hours	Oral	= 90%
MW	= 480	pKa	=

Adult Concerns: Dry mouth, constipation, nausea, dyspepsia, blurred vision, tachycardia, and drowsiness. Do not use in patients with glaucoma.

Pediatric Concerns: None reported but caution is recommended due to the anticholinergic effects and long half-life of this product.

Drug Interactions: Do not exceed doses of 5 mg/day when used with ketoconazole or other azole antifungals.

Relative Infant Dose:

Adult Dose: 5–10 mg daily.

Alternatives: Tolterodine

References:
1. Pharmaceutical manufacturer prescribing information, 2005.

SOMATREM, SOMATROPIN   L3

Trade: Human Growth Hormone, Nutropin, Humatrope, Growth Hormone, Saizen, Norditropin, Serostim, Zorbtive, Omnitrope

Other Trades: Genotropin, Norditropin, Somatropin, Protropin, Humatrope, Tev-Tropin

Category: Human growth hormone

Somatrem and somatropin are purified anterior pituitary hormones of recombinant DNA origin. It is a large protein. They are structurally similar or identical to the human growth hormone (hGH). One study in 16 women indicates that hGH treatment for 7 days stimulated breastmilk production by 18.5% (verses 11.6%

in controls) in a group of normal lactating women.[1] No adverse effects were noted. Leukemia has occurred in a small number of children receiving hGH, but the relationship is uncertain. Because it is a peptide of 191 amino acids and its molecular weight is so large, its transfer into milk is very unlikely. Further, its oral absorption would be minimal to nil.

Pregnancy Risk	C		Lactation Risk	L3
T ½	=		M/P	=
Vd	=		PB	=
Tmax	= 7.5 hours		Oral	= Poor
MW	= 22,124		pKa	=

Adult Concerns: Some fatalities have been reported in pediatric patients with Prader-Willi syndrome. Hypothyroidism and hypoglycemia have been reported.

Pediatric Concerns: None reported via milk. Absorption is very unlikely.

Drug Interactions: Caution while coadministering with the following agents: corticosteroids, sex steroids, anticonvulsants, cyclosporine. Dosages of the following may need to be adjusted during concomitant use: insulin, oral hypoglycemic agents, oral estrogen.

Relative Infant Dose:

Adult Dose: 0.1–0.3 mg/kg every week.

Alternatives:

References:
1. Milsom SR, Breier BH, Gallaher BW, Cox VA, Gunn AJ, Gluckman PD. Growth hormone stimulates galactopoiesis in healthy lactating women. Acta Endocrinol (Copenh) 1992; 127(4): 337–343.

SOTALOL   L3

Trade: Betapace

Other Trades: Cardol, Sotacor, Apo-Sotalol, Rylosol

Category: Antihypertensive, beta-blocker

Sotalol is a typical beta blocker antihypertensive with low lipid solubility. It is secreted into milk in high levels. Sotalol concentrations in milk ranged from 4.8 to 20.2 mg/L (mean= 10.5 mg/L) in 5 mothers.[1] The mean maternal dose was 433 mg/day. Although these milk levels appear high, no evidence of toxicity was noted in 12 infants. Another study of a 22-year-old mother taking 120 to 240 mg daily reported an infant dose of 20–23% of the weight adjusted maternal dose in milk. This would relate to an infant dose of 0.41 to 0.58 mg/kg. However, there were no untoward effects noted in the infant.[2] It is suggested that if a mother decides to breastfeed while taking sotalol, the baby should receive close monitoring for side effects. Observe for sedation, bradycardia, hypotension, weakness, poor suckling in the breastfed infant.

Pregnancy Risk	B		Lactation Risk	L3
T ½	= 12 hours		M/P	= 5.4
Vd	= 1.6–2.4 l/kg		PB	=
Tmax	= 2.5–4 hours		Oral	= 90–100%
MW	= 272		pKa	= 8.3, 9.8

Adult Concerns: Bradycardia, hypotension, sedation.

Pediatric Concerns: None reported via milk, but observe for sedation, bradycardia, hypotension, weakness, poor suckling.

Drug Interactions: Decreased effect when used with aluminum salts, barbiturates, calcium salts, cholestyramine, NSAIDs, ampicillin, rifampin, and salicylates. Beta blockers may reduce the effect of oral sulfonylureas (hypoglycemic agents). Increased toxicity/effect when used with other antihypertensives, contraceptives, monoamine oxidase inhibitors, cimetidine, and numerous other products. See drug interaction reference for complete listing.

Relative Infant Dose: 25.5%

Adult Dose: 80–160 mg twice daily.

Alternatives: Propranolol, metoprolol

References:
1. O'Hare MF, Murnaghan GA, Russell CJ, Leahey WJ, Varma MP, McDevitt DG. Sotalol as a hypotensive agent in pregnancy. Br J Obstet Gynaecol 1980; 87(9): 814–820.
2. Hackett LP, Wojnar-Horton RE, Dusci LJ, Ilett KF, Roberts MJ. Excretion of sotalol in breast milk. Br J Clin Pharmac 1990; 29: 277–279.

SPINOSAD   L3

Trade: ParaPro Natroba Topical Suspension, Natroba

Other Trades:

Category: Pediculicide

Spinosad is an insecticide used in the treatment of pediculosis capitis (head lice). Spinosad causes neuronal excitation in lice followed by paralysis and death. Spinosad topical suspension is a mixture of spinosyn A and spinosyn D in a 5:1 ratio. Spinosad is approved for children older than 4 years. The drug should not be used in infants, especially preterm infants as it contains benzoyl alcohol. One study of 14 pediatric patients using one application to the scalp of 1.8% topical suspension of spinosad for 10 minutes revealed no drug detected in the plasma of the patients. No studies have been located on the use of spinosad during lactation.[1] Spinosad is not absorbed systemically when used in topical preparations. The benzyl alcohol in spinosad formulations may be absorbed and mothers may wish to pump and discard for 8 hours to avoid any benzyl alcohol exposure to the child.[1]

Pregnancy Risk	B		Lactation Risk	L3
T ½	=		M/P	=
Vd	=		PB	=
Tmax	=		Oral	=
MW	=		pKa	=

Adult Concerns: Skin erythema, skin irritation, ocular erythema, ocular irritation, ocular hyperemia.

Pediatric Concerns:

Drug Interactions:

Relative Infant Dose:

Adult Dose: Apply on scalp and hair, leave on for 10 min.

Alternatives:

References:
1. Pharmaceutical manufacturer prescribing information, 2011.

SPIRONOLACTONE   L2

Trade: Aldactone

Other Trades: Spiractin, Aldactone, Novospiroton

Category: Potassium sparing diuretic/aldosterone receptor antagonist

Spironolactone is an aldosterone receptor antagonist used as a diuretic in various edematous conditions, as well as in the treatment of hypertension, hypokalemia and primary aldosteronism. Spironolactone is metabolized to canrenone, which is known to be secreted into breastmilk. In one mother receiving 25 mg of spironolactone, at 2 hours post-dose the maternal serum and milk concentrations of canrenone were 144 and 104 µg/L respectively.[1] At 14.5 hours, the corresponding values for serum and milk were 92 and 47 µg/L respectively. Milk/plasma ratios varied from 0.51 at 14.5 hours, to 0.72 at 2 hours. Based on these values, the calculated relative infant dose is 2–4%. The amounts ingested by the infant through breastmilk are probably too low to be clinically significant.

Pregnancy Risk	C (D if used in gestational hypertension)		Lactation Risk	L2
T ½	= 10–35 hours		M/P	= 0.51–0.72
Vd	=		PB	= >90%
Tmax	= 1–2 hours		Oral	= 70%
MW	= 417		pKa	=

Adult Concerns: Nausea, vomiting, elevated serum potassium, hepatitis.

Pediatric Concerns: None reported via milk, but suppression of milk supply is possible but unlikely.

Drug Interactions: Use with anticoagulants may reduce the anticoagulant effect. Use with potassium preparations may increase potassium levels in plasma. Use with ACE inhibitors may elevate serum potassium levels. The diuretic effect of spironolactone may be decreased by use with salicylates.

Relative Infant Dose: 2%–4.3%

Adult Dose: 50–100 mg daily.

Alternatives:

References:
1. Phelps DL, Karim Z. Spironolactone: relationship between concentrations of dethioacetylated metabolite in human serum and milk. J Pharm Sci 1977; 66(8): 1203.

ST. JOHN'S WORT   L2

Trade: Hypericum perforatum, Tipton's weed, Chase-devil, Klamath weed
Other Trades:
Category: Antidepressant

St. John's Wort (hypericum perforatum L.) consists of the whole fresh or dried plant or its components containing not less than 0.04% naphthodianthrones of the hypericin group. Hypericum contains many biologically active compounds and most researchers consider its effect due to a combination of constituents rather than any single component.[1] However, the naphthodianthrones hypericin and pseudohypericin and numerous flavonoids have stimulated the most interest as antidepressants and antivirals.

Following doses of (3 x 300 mg/day), peak steady state concentrations of hypericin and pseudohypericin were 8.5 ng/mL and 5.8 ng/mL respectively.[2] Concentrations in brain appear to be the least of all compartments. Hypericum has become increasingly popular for the treatment of depression following results from numerous studies showing efficacy and good data suggesting that it is associated with fewer and less severe side effects. Many studies have been flawed due to the use of poor extracts or questionable preparations. However the German extract WS5570 has grown in popularity and is now often used as the standard preparation for clinical studies.

Two recent studies using this St. John's Wort (SJW) extract WS5570 showed this preparation to be very effective in treating depression,[3,4] and just as effective as the SSRI paroxetine.[4] The latter study was double blinded and well done. These newer studies suggest that SJW may indeed be an active and clinically effective product for treating depression when good preparations are used.

Several other studies show that St. John's Wort may significantly stimulate cytochrome P450 3A4, which is a major drug metabolizing enzyme in the liver.[5–9] Following such induction, major reductions (50% or more) in plasma levels of a number of important drugs have been reported and include: cyclosporin, midazolam, indinavir, and possibly numerous other drugs. Patients taking anticonvulsants and other critically important drugs should be advised about the possible interaction with these medications leading to major reductions in plasma levels. Patients should always inform their physicians of their use of St. John's Wort.

In a recent prospective, observational, cohort study of the safety of SJW in 33 breastfeeding mothers, along with matched controls, no significant differences were found in maternal or infant demographics or maternal adverse effects following treatment with SJW.[10] In another study of a single patient receiving 3 daily doses of Jarsin 300, hypericin levels in milk were undetectable (<0.2 ng/mL).[11] Hyperforin levels in milk ranged from 0.58 to 18.2 ng/mL. Maternal plasma levels of hypericin and hyperforin were 10.71 and 154 ng/mL respectively. Both components were undetectable in the plasma of the infant. No side effects of any kind were noted in the infant and the Denver Developmental Screen was normal.

Please be aware that many products produced and sold in the USA and Canada may be of poor quality and contain little or no SJW. Users should only purchase standardized or assayed products from reputable sources.

Pregnancy Risk	C	Lactation Risk	L2
T ½	= 26.5 hours	M/P	=
Vd	=	PB	=
Tmax	= 5.9 hours	Oral	=
MW	= 504	pKa	=

Adult Concerns: Caution, because of uterotonic effects, hypericum should not be used in pregnant patients. Dry mouth, dizziness, constipation, and confusion have been infrequently reported. Overt toxicity is generally considered quite low. Photosensitization in fair-skinned people has been noted. No teratogenic effects has been documented.

Pediatric Concerns: None reported in two studies. Probably safe.

Drug Interactions: May prolong narcotic-induced sedation and sleeping times. May reduce barbiturate-induced sleeping times. A recent report in Lancet suggests St. John's wort may induce the cytochrome P-450 enzyme system. The data indicates a major interaction between St. John's wort and the HIV-1 protease inhibitor, Indinavir, where indinavir AUC was reduced by a mean of 57%. In addition, trough concentrations of indinavir at 8 hours were reduced by 81%. Another report indicates acute rejection episodes in two heart transplant patients who had initiated St. John's wort for depression. Although each patient recovered after the St. John's wort was discontinued, this again implicates P-450 induction activity of St. John's wort. SJW may decrease digoxin plasma levels (AUC) by 25%, and theophylline levels significantly.

Relative Infant Dose:

Adult Dose: 300 mg three times daily, dry-powdered (0.3% hypericin).

Alternatives: Sertraline, paroxetine

References:

1. Upton R. St. John's Wort. American Herbal Pharmacopoeia and Therapeutic Compendium 1997.
2. Stock S, Holzl J. Pharmacokinetic tests of (14C)-labeled hypericin and pseudohypericin from Hypericum perforatum and serum kinetics of hyperich in man. Planta Medica 1991; 57(suppl 2): A61.

3. Lecrubier Y, Clerc G, Didi R, Kieser M. Efficacy of St. John's wort extract WS 5570 in major depression: a double-blind, placebo-controlled trial. Am J Psychiatry 2002 Aug; 159(8): 1361–6.
4. Szegedi A, Kohnen R, Dienel A, Kieser M. Acute treatment of moderate to severe depression with hypericum extract WS 5570 (St John's wort): randomised controlled double blind non-inferiority trial versus paroxetine. BMJ 2005 Mar 5; 330(7490): 503.
5. Durr D, Stieger B, Kullak-Ublick GA, Rentsch KM, Steinert HC, Meier PJ, Fattinger K. St John's Wort induces intestinal P-glycoprotein/MDR1 and intestinal and hepatic CYP3A4. Clin Pharmacol Ther 2000; 68(6): 598–604.
6. Barone GW, Gurley BJ, Ketel BL, Lightfoot ML, Abul-Ezz SR. Drug interaction between St. John's wort and cyclosporine. Ann Pharmacother 2000; 34(9): 1013–1016.
7. Obach RS. Inhibition of human cytochrome P450 enzymes by constituents of St. John's Wort, an herbal preparation used in the treatment of depression. J Pharmacol Exp Ther 2000; 294(1): 88–95.
8. Roby CA, Anderson GD, Kantor E, Dryer DA, Burstein AH. St John's Wort: effect on CYP3A4 activity. Clin Pharmacol Ther 2000; 67(5): 451–457.
9. De Smet PA, Touw DJ. Safety of St John's wort (Hypericum perforatum). Lancet 2000; 355(9203): 575–576.
10. Lee A, Minhas R, Matsuda N et al. The safety of St. John's wort (Hypericum perforatum) during breastfeeding. J Clin Psychiatry. 2003; 64: 966–968.
11. Klier CM, Schafer MR, Schmid-Siegel B et al. St. John's wort (Hypericum perforatum)--is it safe during breastfeeding? Pharmacopsychiatry 2002; 35: 29–30.

STAVUDINE   L4

Trade: Zerit

Other Trades:

Category: Antiretroviral agent used in HIV infections.

Stavudine is an antiretroviral agent used in HIV infections. There are no adequate and well-controlled studies or case reports in breastfeeding women. Breastfeeding is not recommended in mothers who have HIV.[1,2] Fatal lactic acidosis has occurred in patients treated with stavudine in combination with other antiretroviral agents. Caution is recommended.

Pregnancy Risk	C	Lactation Risk	L4
T ½	= 2.3 hours	M/P	=
Vd	= 0.73 l/kg	PB	= Low
Tmax	=	Oral	= 86%
MW	= 224	pKa	=

Adult Concerns: Headache, diarrhea, peripheral neurologic symptoms/neuropathy, rash, nausea and vomiting.

Pediatric Concerns: Adverse reactions and serious laboratory abnormalities in pediatric patients from birth through adolescence were similar in type and frequency to those seen in adult patients.

Drug Interactions: Zidovudine in combination with stavudine should be avoided.

Relative Infant Dose:

Adult Dose: 40 mg twice daily.

Alternatives:

References:
1. World Health Organization: Global Programme on AIDS. Consensus statement from the WHO/UNICEF consultation on HIV transmission and breast-feeding. Geneva: WHO, 1992.
2. Latham MC, Greiner T: Breastfeeding versus formula feeding in HIV infection. Lancet 352: 737, 1998.

STEVIA   L3

Trade: Stevia, Only Sweet, PureVia, Reb-A, Rebiana, SweetLeaf, Truvia, Rebaudioside A, Candy leaf

Other Trades: Sweet herb of Paraguay, Sweet honey leaf, Sugar leaf

Category: Sweetener

Stevia[1] is the genus name for over 240 species of herbs that belong to the sunflower family. They have become popular as natural sweeteners with minimal effects on blood glucose levels. Since we do not know what is contained in each of these herbs, its use in breastfeeding is not indicated and caution should be advised in women who are breastfeeding and taking this drug. The highly refined, purified component of stevia is Rebaudioside A,[2] which has been approved by the FDA to be used in the following food products: Sweet Green Fields, Blue California, McNeil Nutritionals, Cargill, and Whole Earth Sweetener/Merisant. There are no studies of the use of Rebaudioside A in pregnant or lactating women and so is not recommended for use.

Pregnancy Risk	Probably Safe	Lactation Risk	L3
T ½	=	M/P	=
Vd	=	PB	=
Tmax	=	Oral	=
MW	=	pKa	=

Adult Concerns: Headache, nausea, myalgias, muscle weakness, dizziness, hypersensitivity to daisy family such as ragweed, chrysanthemum, marigold and many other herbs. High doses can affect renal perfusion.

Pediatric Concerns:

Drug Interactions:

Relative Infant Dose:

Adult Dose:

Alternatives:

References:
1. Chatsudthipong V, Muanprasat C. Stevioside and related compounds: therapeutic benefits beyond sweetness. Pharmacol Ther. Jan 2009; 121(1): 41–54.
2. FDA. Rebaudioside A which is a component of Stevia has been approved for use in food products. Available at: www.fda.gov/AboutFDA/Basics/ucm214865.htm. Accessed 8/4/2010.

STREPTOMYCIN   L3

Trade:

Other Trades: Streptobretin, Streptotriad

Category: Antibiotic

Streptomycin is an aminoglycoside antibiotic from the same family as gentamicin. It is primarily administered IM or IV although it is seldom used today with exception of the treatment of tuberculosis. One report suggests that following a 1 gm dose (IM), levels in breastmilk were 0.3 to 0.6 mg/L (2–3% of plasma level).[1] Another report suggests that only 0.5% of a 1 gm IM dose is excreted in breastmilk within 24 hours.[2] Because the oral absorption of streptomycin is very poor, absorption by infant is probably minimal (unless premature or early neonate).

Pregnancy Risk	D	Lactation Risk	L3
T ½	= 2.6 hours	M/P	= 0.12–1.0
Vd	=	PB	= 34%
Tmax	= 1–2 hours (IM)	Oral	= Poor
MW	= 582	pKa	=

Adult Concerns: Deafness, anemia, kidney toxicity.

Pediatric Concerns: None reported via milk, but observe for changes in gastrointestinal flora.

Drug Interactions: Increased toxicity when used with certain penicillins, cephalosporins, amphotericin B, loop diuretics, and neuromuscular blocking agents.

Relative Infant Dose: 0.3%–0.6%

Adult Dose: 1–2 gm daily.

Alternatives:

References:
1. Wilson J. Drugs in Breast Milk. New York: ADIS Press 1981.
2. Snider DE, Jr., Powell KE. Should women taking antituberculosis drugs breast-feed? Arch Intern Med 1984; 144(3): 589–590.

STRONTIUM-89 CHLORIDE   L5

Trade: Metastron

Other Trades:

Category: Radioactive product for bone pain

Strontium-89 chloride behaves similarly to calcium. It is rapidly cleared from plasma and sequestered into bone where its radioactive emissions relieve metastatic bone pain.[1] Radioactive half-life is 50.5 days. Transfer into milk is unreported but likely. This radioactive product is too dangerous to use in lactating mothers.

Pregnancy Risk	D		Lactation Risk	L5	
T ½	= 50.5 days		M/P	=	
Vd	=		PB	=	
Tmax	= Immediate (IV)		Oral	=	
MW	= 159		pKa	=	

Adult Concerns: Severe bone marrow suppression, septicemia.

Pediatric Concerns: None reported via milk. But this product is probably too dangerous to use with breastfed infants.

Drug Interactions:

Relative Infant Dose:

Adult Dose: 4 mCi every 90 days.

Alternatives:

References:
1. Facts and Comparisons. St. Louis: 2010..

SUCCIMER   L3

Trade: Chemet

Other Trades:

Category: Lead Chelator for lead poisoning

Succimer is a chelating agent containing dimercaptosuccinic acid. It is commonly used to chelate and increase the urinary excretion of lead.[1] While removing lead is important, some chelators (EDTA) are noted for increasing the plasma levels of lead and promoting its migration to neural and other tissues. In the instance of a breastfeeding woman, this could theoretically increase milk lead levels. However, succimer as studied in rodents has been found to increase the urinary elimination of lead without redistribution of lead to other compartments (this would theoretically include milk).[2] While we do not have studies of succimer transfer into human milk, due to its low pKa of succimer, it is unlikely that lead, chelated to succimer, would transfer into human milk. But this is not known for sure. Clinical studies in succimer-treated patients indicate that lead levels reach their lowest point after 4–5 days of therapy with succimer.[3] If breastfeeding patients were to pump and discard milk for 5 days while under therapy with succimer, it would significantly remove the risk of lead transfer into milk (if this occurs). However, more data are required before breastfeeding can be recommended following the use of succimer.

Pregnancy Risk	C		Lactation Risk	L3	
T ½	= 2–48 hours		M/P	=	
Vd	=		PB	=	
Tmax	= 1–2 hours		Oral	= Complete	
MW	= 182		pKa	= 3.0	

Adult Concerns: Nausea, vomiting, diarrhea, appetite loss, thrombocytosis, intermittent eosinophilia, arrhythmias, neutropenia, drowsiness, dizziness, neuropathies, headache, rash, and paresthesias.

Pediatric Concerns: None reported.

Drug Interactions:

Relative Infant Dose:

Adult Dose: 30 mg/kg/day for 5 days.

Alternatives:

References:
1. Pharmaceutical manufacturer prescribing information, 2001.
2. Graziano JH, Lolacono NJ, Moulton T, Mitchell ME, Slavkovich V, Zarate C. Controlled study of meso-2,3-dimercaptosuccinic acid for the management of childhood lead intoxication. J Pediatr 1992; 120(1): 133–139.
3. Graziano JH, Lolacono NJ, Meyer P. Dose-response study of oral 2,3-dimercaptosuccinic acid in children with elevated blood lead concentrations. J Pediatr 1988; 113(4): 751–757.

SUCRALFATE   L2

Trade: Carafate

Other Trades: Carafate, SCF, Ulcyte, Sulcrate, Novo-Sucralfate, Nu-Sucralfate, Antepsin

Category: For peptic ulcers

Sucralfate is a sucrose aluminum complex used for stomach ulcers. When administered orally, sucralfate forms a complex that physically covers stomach ulcers.[1] Less than 5% is absorbed orally. At these plasma levels it is very unlikely to penetrate into breastmilk.

Pregnancy Risk	B	Lactation Risk	L2
T ½	=	M/P	=
Vd	=	PB	=
Tmax	=	Oral	= <5%
MW	= 2087	pKa	=

Adult Concerns: Constipation.

Pediatric Concerns: None reported via milk. Absorption is very unlikely.

Drug Interactions: The use of aluminum containing antacids and sucralfate may increase the total body burden of aluminum. Sucralfate may reduce the anticoagulant effect of warfarin. Serum digoxin levels may be reduced. Phenytoin absorption may be decreased. Ketoconazole bioavailability may be decreased. Serum quinidine levels may be reduced. Bioavailability of the fluoroquinolone family may be decreased.

Relative Infant Dose:

Adult Dose: 1 gm four times daily.

Alternatives:

References:
1. Facts and Comparisons. St. Louis: 2010..

SUCRALOSE   L2

Trade: Splenda
Other Trades:
Category: Sweetener

Sucralose is a non-caloric artificial sweetener that is 600 times sweeter than sucrose. There are no adequate or well-controlled case reports in breastfeeding women. Sucralose is not fully absorbed, and is excreted unchanged in the urine; no toxicity or carcinogenic activity has been noted in animal studies. FDA deems sucralose is safe for consumption in pregnant and lactating women.

Pregnancy Risk	Probably Safe	Lactation Risk	L2
T ½	=	M/P	=
Vd	=	PB	=
Tmax	=	Oral	=
MW	= 398	pKa	=

Adult Concerns: No evidence of side effects.

Pediatric Concerns:

Drug Interactions:

Relative Infant Dose:

Adult Dose:

Alternatives:

References:
1. ACOG Practice Bulletin # 60. Available at: www.acog.org/from_home/publications/green_journal/PBListOfTitles.pdf. Accessed July 21, 2010.
2. NCI. Artificial Sweeteners. U.S. Institute of Health. Aug. 5, 2009. Available at: http://www.cancer.gov/cancertopics/factsheet/Risk/artificial-sweeteners. Accessed July 22, 2010.
3. WedMD. Artificial Sweeteners. June 18, 2009. Available at: www.MedicineNet.com/artificial-sweeteners/page10.htm. Accessed July 22, 2010.

SULBACTAM   L1

Trade:
Other Trades:
Category: Extended spectrum

Sulbactam is a beta-lactamase inhibitor used in combination with penicillin or cephalosporin antibiotics. Its structure is similar to penicillin. Its absorption from gastrointestinal tract is poor.[1] After a dose of 0.5 to 1 gram, sulbactam is secreted into milk at an average concentration of 0.52 µg/mL. This would lead to a maximal dose of 0.7 mg/kg/day in a breastfeeding infant, which equates to less than 1% of the maternal dose. Therefore, untoward effects are unlikely in a breastfeeding infant.[2]

Pregnancy Risk	Safer	Lactation Risk	L1
T ½	=	M/P	=
Vd	=	PB	=
Tmax	=	Oral	=
MW	= 233	pKa	=

Adult Concerns: Most common side effects: rash and diarrhea. Less common side effects: nausea, urticaria, vomiting, abdominal distention, itching, malaise, chills, edema and epistaxis.

Pediatric Concerns:

Drug Interactions:

Relative Infant Dose:

Adult Dose:

Alternatives:

References:
1. Sweetman S (Ed), Martindale: The complete drug reference. London: Pharmaceutical Press. Electronic version. 2010.
2. Foulds G, Miller RD, Knirsch AK, Thrupp LD. Sulbactam kinetics and excretion into breast milk in postpartum women. Clin Pharmacol Ther 1985; 38(6): 692–696.

SULCONAZOLE NITRATE   L3

Trade: Exelderm

Other Trades: Exelderm

Category: Antifungal cream

Sulconazole nitrate is a broad-spectrum antifungal topical cream.[1] Although no data exist on transfer into human milk, it is unlikely that the degree of transdermal absorption would be high enough to produce significant milk levels. Only 8.7% of the topically administered dose is transcutaneously absorbed.

Pregnancy Risk	C	Lactation Risk	L3
T ½	=	M/P	=
Vd	=	PB	=
Tmax	=	Oral	=
MW	=	pKa	=

Adult Concerns: Rash, skin irritation, burning, stinging.

Pediatric Concerns: None reported via milk.

Drug Interactions:

Relative Infant Dose:

Adult Dose: Topical

Alternatives:

References:
1. Pharmaceutical manufacturer prescribing information, 1996.

SULFACETAMIDE SODIUM OPHTHALMIC DROPS   L2

Trade: Bleph-10, Isopto Cetamide, Sulf-10

Other Trades:

Category: Sulfonamide antibiotic

Sulfacetamide is one of the N-acetyl derivatives of sulfanilamide.[1] Sodium sulfacetamide is a bacteriostatic medication that inhibits the bacterial enzyme system. It provides coverage for many gram positive organisms but does not provide coverage for Neisseria species, Serratia marcescens or Pseudomonas aeruginosa. Sulfanilamide, when given orally, has been found to be excreted into breast milk in large quantities but because sodium sulfacetamide is instilled topically, the amount of the drug excreted in milk would be expected to be minimal. Because sulfonamides, as a drug class, may increase the risk of kernicterus in the first few weeks of life, sodium sulfacetamide should not be used during the neonatal period. Avoid in premature infants and in neonates.

Pregnancy Risk	C	Lactation Risk	L2
T ½	= 7–13 hours	M/P	=
Vd	=	PB	=
Tmax	=	Oral	=
MW	= 214.2	pKa	=

Adult Concerns: May cause burning and stinging.

Pediatric Concerns:

Drug Interactions:

Relative Infant Dose:

Adult Dose: 1–2 drops every 3 hours for 7 to 10 days.

Alternatives:

References:
1. Pharmaceutical manufacturer prescribing information, 2010.

SULFAMETHOXAZOLE   L3

Trade: Gantanol

Other Trades: Bactrim, Resprim, Septrin, Gantanol

Category: Sulfonamide antibiotic

Sulfamethoxazole is a common and popular sulfonamide antimicrobial. It is secreted in breastmilk in small amounts.[1] It has a longer half-life than other sulfonamides. Use with caution in weakened infants and premature infants or neonates with hyperbilirubinemia. Sulfisoxazole (Gantrisin) is considered the best choice of sulfonamides due to reduced transfer to infant. Compatible but exercise caution. Pediatric half-life = 14.7–36.5 hours (neonate), 8–9 hours (older infants).

Pregnancy Risk	C/D in 3rd trimester	Lactation Risk	L3
T ½	= 10.1 hours	M/P	= 0.06
Vd	=	PB	= 62%
Tmax	= 1–4 hours	Oral	= Complete
MW	= 253	pKa	=

Adult Concerns: Anemia, blood dyscrasias, allergies.

Pediatric Concerns: None reported via milk, but use with caution in hyperbilirubinemic neonates and in infants with G6PD.

Drug Interactions: Decreased effect with para-aminobenzoic acid (PABA) metabolites of drugs such as procaine and tetracaine. Increased effect of oral anticoagulants, oral hypoglycemic agents, and methotrexate.

Relative Infant Dose:

Adult Dose: 1–2 gm 1–2 times daily.

Alternatives:

References:
1. Rasmussen F. Mammary excretion of sulphonamides. Acta Pharmacol Toxicol 1958; 15: 138–148.

SULFAMETHOXAZOLE + TRIMETHOPRIM | L3

Trade: Bactrim, Septra, Sulfatrim, Cotrim, Duclor

Other Trades: Resprim-Forte, Apo-Sulfatrim, Novo-Trimel, Novo-Trimox, Nu-Cotrimox

Category: Antibiotic

Sulfamethoxazole and Trimethoprim is a combined drug product. It is used as an antibiotic in conditions such as acute otitis media, pneumocystis pneumonia, traveller's diarrhea, shigellosis and urinary tract infections.

Sulfamethoxazole is secreted in breastmilk in small amounts.[1] It has a longer half-life than other sulfonamides. Use with caution in mothers with weakened infants, premature infants, or neonates with hyperbilirubinemia, or in mothers with newborn infants (first 22 days). Compatible but exercise caution. Pediatric half-life = 14.7–36.5 hours (neonate), 8–9 hours (older infants).

In one study of 50 patients, average milk levels of trimethoprim were 2.0 mg/L.[2] Milk/plasma ratio was 1.25. In another group of mothers receiving 160 mg 2–4 times daily, concentrations of 1.2 to 5.5 mg/L were reported in milk. Because it may interfere with folate metabolism, its long-term use should be avoided in breastfeeding mothers, or the infant should be supplemented with folic acid. However, trimethoprim apparently poses few problems in full term or older infants where it is commonly used clinically.[3] The relative infant dose is 4–9%.

Pregnancy Risk	C	Lactation Risk	L3
T ½	= Sulfamethoxazole/trimethoprim: 10.1 hours/8–10 hours	M/P	= Sulfamethoxazole/trimethoprim: 0.06/1.25
Vd	= Sulfamethoxazole/trimethoprim: l/kg	PB	= Sulfamethoxazole/trimethoprim: 62%/44%
Tmax	= Sulfamethoxazole/trimethoprim: 1–4 hours/1–4 hours	Oral	= Sulfamethoxazole/trimethoprim: Complete/complete
MW	= Sulfamethoxazole/trimethoprim: 253/290	pKa	= Sulfamethoxazole/trimethoprim:/6.6

Adult Concerns: Nausea, vomiting, rash, urticaria, loss of appetite, Steven-Johnson syndrome, erythema, diarrhea, anaphylaxis, hematologic disorder.

Pediatric Concerns: May increase the risk of hyperbilirubinemia in newborns. Caution recommended first 30 days postpartum.

Drug Interactions: Increased risk of thrombocytopenia with purpura when used in the elderly on diuretics, especially thiazides. Increased risk of bleeding when used in those on warfarin. May potentiate the effect of phenytoin. May decrease the clearance of digoxin and cause increased plasma digoxin levels. May decrease the efficacy of tricyclic antidepressants. Potentiates the effect of oral hypoglycemics.

Relative Infant Dose:

Adult Dose: Sulfamethoxazole/trimethoprim: 400–800 mg/80–160 mg twice daily.

Alternatives:

References:
1. Rasmussen F. Mammary excretion of sulphonamides. Acta Pharmacol Toxicol 1958; 15: 138–148.
2. Miller RD, Salter AJ. The passage of trimethoprim/sulphamethoxazole into breast milk and its significance. In Daikos GK, ed. Progress in Chemotherapy, Proceedings of the Eight International Congress of Chemotherapy, Athens, 1973. Athens: Hellenic Society for Chemotherapy, 1974.
3. Pagliaro, Levin. Problems in Pediatric Drug Therapy. Hamilton, IL: Drug Intelligence Publications, 1979.

SULFASALAZINE   L3

Trade: Azulfidine

Other Trades: PMS Sulfasalazine, Salazopyrin, SAS-500

Category: Anti-inflammatory for ulcerative colitis

Sulfasalazine is a conjugate of sulfapyridine and 5-aminosalicylic acid (5–ASA) and is used as an anti-inflammatory for ulcerative colitis. Only one-third of the dose is absorbed by the mother. Most stays in the gastrointestinal tract. Secretion of 5–ASA (active compound) and its inactive metabolite (acetyl -5–ASA) into human milk is very low.

In one study of 12 women receiving 1 to 2 gm/day of sulfasalazine, the amount of sulfasalazine in milk in patients receiving 1 gm/day was far less than 1 mg/L and approximately 0.5 to 2 mg/L in those receiving 2 gm/day.[1] In this study, small milk levels were found in only 2 women. It was estimated by the authors that breastfed infants would receive approximately 0.3 mg/kg/day of sulfapyridine. This very small amount may be regarded as negligible in considering kernicterus because sulfapyridine and sulfadiazine are known to have a poor bilirubin-displacing capacity. Berlin reported a single case treated with salicylazosulfapyridine (Azulfidine).[2] No 5–ASA was found in milk. The sulfapyridine levels were approximately 3 to 6 mg/L.

The study by Jarnerot suggests that while sulfasalazine levels in milk were negligible, sulfapyridine levels were approximately 45% of the maternal serum levels and the infant was likely to receive about 3–4 mg/kg of body weight.[1] In a study of a patient receiving 1 gm of 5–ASA three times daily, the milk levels for 5–ASA and acetyl-5–ASA were 0.1 µg/mL and 12.3 µg/mL respectively at 5 days postpartum. These results suggest that even with high doses (3 gm/day) the amount of 5–ASA transferred is minimal.[3]

In another study of 3 mothers receiving a dose of 0.5 gm four times per day, the average maternal serum concentration of sulfasalazine and 5–ASA was 8.8 and 0.6 µg/mL, respectively. The milk concentrations were 2.7 and 0.8 µg/mL, respectively. The authors reported sulfasalazine levels in breastmilk are approximately 30% of maternal serum levels. No adverse reactions were noted in any infant.[4]

Few if any adverse effects have been observed in most nursing infants. However, one reported case of toxicity which may have been an idiosyncratic allergic response.[5] Use with caution.

Pregnancy Risk	B/D in third trimester	Lactation Risk	L3
T ½	= 7.6 hours	M/P	= 0.09–0.17
Vd	=	PB	=
Tmax	=	Oral	= Poor
MW	= 398	pKa	=

Adult Concerns: Watery diarrhea, gastrointestinal distress, nausea, vomiting, rapid breathing.

Pediatric Concerns: Only one reported case of hypersensitivity. Most studies show minimal effects via milk. Observe for diarrhea, gastrointestinal discomfort.

Drug Interactions: Decreased effect when used with iron, digoxin, and para-aminobenzoic acid containing drugs. Decreased effect of oral anticoagulants, methotrexate, and oral hypoglycemic agents.

Relative Infant Dose: 0.3%–1.1%

Adult Dose: 500 mg every 6 hours.

Alternatives:

References:
1. Jarnerot G, Into-Malmberg MB. Sulphasalazine treatment during breast feeding. Scand J Gastroenterol 1979; 14(7): 869–871.
2. Berlin CM, Jr., Yaffe SJ. Disposition of salicylazosulfapyridine (Azulfidine) and metabolites in human breast milk. Dev Pharmacol Ther 1980; 1(1): 31–39.
3. Klotz U, Harings-Kaim A. Negligible excretion of 5-aminosalicylic acid in breast milk. Lancet 1993; 342(8871): 618–619.
4. Khan AK, Truelove SC. Placental and mammary transfer of sulphasalazine. Br Med J 1979; 2(6204): 1553.
5. Branski D, Kerem E, Gross-Kieselstein E, Hurvitz H, Litt R, Abrahamov A. Bloody diarrhea--a possible complication of sulfasalazine transferred through human breast milk. J Pediatr Gastroenterol Nutr 1986; 5(2): 316–317.

SULFISOXAZOLE   L2

Trade: Gantrisin, AZO-Gantrisin

Other Trades: Novo-Soxazole, Sulfizole

Category: Sulfonamide antibiotic

Sulfisoxazole is a popular, sulfonamide antimicrobial. It is secreted in breastmilk in small amounts although the actual levels are somewhat controversial.[1] Kauffman (1980) reports the total amount of sulfisoxazole recovered over 48 hours following a dose of 1 gm every 6 hours (total=4 gm) was 0.45% of the total dose.[2] The milk/plasma ratio was quite low for sulfisoxazole, only 0.06, and for n-acetyl sulfisoxazole, 0.22. The infant secreted 1,104 µg total sulfisoxazole in his urine over 24 hours, compared to the 1,142 µg secreted in milk. Less than 1% of the maternal dose is secreted into human milk. This is probably insufficient to produce problems in a normal newborn. Sulfisoxazole appears to be best choice with lowest milk/plasma ratio. Use with caution in weakened infants or those with hyperbilirubinemia.

Pregnancy Risk	C	Lactation Risk	L2
T ½	= 4.6–7.8 hours	M/P	= 0.06
Vd	=	PB	= 91%
Tmax	= 2–4 hours	Oral	= 100%
MW	= 267	pKa	=

Adult Concerns: Elevated bilirubin, rash.

Pediatric Concerns: None reported via milk. Use with caution in hyperbilirubinemia neonates and in infants with G6PD.

Drug Interactions: The anesthetic effects of thiopental may be enhanced with sulfisoxazole. Cyclosporine concentrations may be decreased by sulfonamides. Serum phenytoin levels may be increased. The risk of methotrexate induced bone marrow suppression may be enhanced. Increased sulfonylurea half-lives and hypoglycemia when used with sulfonamides.

Relative Infant Dose: 0.3%

Adult Dose: 1–4 gm every 4–6 hours.

Alternatives:

References:

1. Rasmussen F. Mammary excretion of sulphonamides. Acta Pharmacol Toxicol 1958; 15: 138–148.
2. Kauffman RE, O'Brien C, Gilford P. Sulfisoxazole secretion into human milk. J Pediatr 1980; 97(5): 839–841.

SULPIRIDE   L2

Trade:

Other Trades: Dolmatil, Sulparex, Sulpitil

Category: Antidepressant, antipsychotic

Sulpiride is a selective dopamine antagonist used as an antidepressant and antipsychotic. Sulpiride is a strong neuroleptic antipsychotic drug; however, several studies using smaller doses have found it to significantly increase prolactin levels and breastmilk production in smaller doses that do not produce overt neuroleptic effects on the mother.[1] In a study with 14 women who received sulpiride (50 mg three times daily), and in a subsequent study with 36 breastfeeding women, Ylikorkala found major increases in prolactin levels and significant but only moderate increases in breastmilk production.[2,3] In a group of 20 women who received 50 mg twice daily, breastmilk samples were drawn 2 hours after the dose.[4] The concentration of sulpiride in breastmilk ranged from 0.26 to 1.97 mg/L. No effects on breastfed infants were noted. The authors concluded that sulpiride, when administered early in the postpartum period, is useful in promoting initiation of lactation. In a study by McMurdo, sulpiride was found to be a potent stimulant of maternal plasma prolactin levels.[5] Interestingly, it appears that the prolactin response to sulpiride is not dose-related and reached a maximum at 3–10 mg and thereafter, further increased doses did not further increase prolactin levels. Sulpiride is not available in the USA.

Pregnancy Risk	Possibly Hazardous	Lactation Risk	L2
T ½ = 6–8 hours		M/P =	
Vd = 2.7 l/kg		PB =	
Tmax = 2–6 hours		Oral = 27–34%	
MW = 341		pKa =	

Adult Concerns: Tardive dyskinesia, extrapyramidal symptoms, sedation, neuroleptic malignant syndrome, cholestatic jaundice.

Pediatric Concerns: None reported via milk.

Drug Interactions: Antacids and sucralfate may reduce absorption of sulpiride. Increased risk of seizures from use of tramadol or zotepine with sulpiride.

Relative Infant Dose: 2.7%–20.7%

Adult Dose: 50 mg twice daily.

Alternatives: Metoclopramide, domperidone

References:

1. Wiesel FA, Alfredsson G, Ehrnebo M, Sedvall G. The pharmacokinetics of intravenous and oral sulpiride in healthy human subjects. Eur J Clin Pharmacol 1980; 17(5): 385–391.
2. Ylikorkala O, Kauppila A, Kivinen S, Viinikka L. Sulpiride improves inadequate lactation. Br Med J (Clin Res Ed) 1982; 285(6337): 249–251.
3. Ylikorkala O, Kauppila A, Kivinen S, Viinikka L. Treatment of inadequate lactation with oral sulpiride and buccal oxytocin. Obstet Gynecol 1984; 63(1): 57–60.
4. Aono T, Shioji T, Aki T, Hirota K, Nomura A, Kurachi K. Augmentation of puerperal lactation by oral administration of sulpiride. J Clin Endocrinol Metab 1979; 48(3): 478–482.
5. McMurdo ME, Howie PW, Lewis M, Marnie M, McEwen J, McNeilly AS. Prolactin response to low dose sulpiride. Br J Clin Pharmacol 1987; 24(2): 133–137.

SUMATRIPTAN SUCCINATE   L3

Trade: Imitrex, Alsuma, Sumavel DosePro

Other Trades: Imitrex, Imigran

Category: Anti-migraine medication

Sumatriptan is a 5–HT (Serotonin) receptor agonist and a highly effective new drug for the treatment of migraine headache. It is not an analgesic, rather, it produces a rapid vasoconstriction in various regions of the brain, thus temporarily reducing the cause of migraines. In one study using 5 lactating women, each were given 6 mg subcutaneous injections and samples drawn for analysis over 8 hours.[1] The highest breastmilk levels were 87.2 µg/L at 2.6 hours post-dose and rapidly disappeared over the next 6 hours. The mean total recovery of sumatriptan in milk over the 8 hour duration was only 14.4 µg. On a weight-adjusted basis, this concentration in milk corresponded to a mean infant exposure of only 3.5% of the maternal dose. Further, assuming an oral bioavailability of only 14%, the weight-adjusted dose an infant would absorb would be approximately 0.49% of the maternal dose. The authors suggest that continued breastfeeding following sumatriptan use would not pose a significant risk to the suckling infant. The maternal plasma half-life is 1.3 hours; the milk half-life is 2.2 hours. Although the milk/plasma ratio was 4.9 (indicating significant concentrating mechanisms in milk), the absolute maternal plasma levels were small; hence, the absolute milk concentrations were low.

Pregnancy Risk	C	Lactation Risk	L3
T ½	= 1.3 hours	M/P	= 4.9
Vd	=	PB	= 14–21%
Tmax	= 12 minutes (IM)	Oral	= 10–15%
MW	= 413	pKa	=

Adult Concerns: Flushing, hot tingling sensations.

Pediatric Concerns: None reported via milk.

Drug Interactions: Monoamine oxidase inhibitors can markedly increase sumatriptan systemic effect and elimination including elevated sumatriptan plasma levels. Ergot containing drugs have caused prolonged vasospastic reactions. There have been rare reports of weakness, hyperreflexia, and incoordination with combined use with SSRIs such as fluoxetine, paroxetine, sertraline and fluvoxamine.

Relative Infant Dose: 3.5%–15.3%

Adult Dose: 25–100 mg two-three times daily.

Alternatives: Zolmitriptan

References:

1. Wojnar-Horton RE, Hackett LP, Yapp P, Dusci LJ, Paech M, Ilett KF. Distribution and excretion of sumatriptan in human milk. Br J Clin Pharmacol 1996; 41(3): 217–221.

SYNEPHRINE   L4

Trade: Bitter Orange, Advantra, Oxedrine

Other Trades:

Category: Weight-loss agent

Synephrine (or oxedrine) is commonly used as an ephedrine-free weight loss agent. There is little to no data on its use during lactation. Its effectiveness as a weight-loss agent is highly speculative and debated. It is likely transferred into breast milk due to its small molecular weight and chemical structure. This product should be used with caution as little is known about its pharmacology.

Pregnancy Risk	Possibly Hazardous	Lactation Risk	L4
T ½	= 2–3 hours	M/P	=
Vd	= 16347L l/kg	PB	=
Tmax	= 90 min	Oral	= 22%
MW	= 167	pKa	= 9.3

Adult Concerns: Cardiovascular toxicity, myocardial infarction, arrhythmia, excitement.

Pediatric Concerns:

Drug Interactions: Do not take with monoamine oxidase inhibitors and midazolam. Moderate drug interaction with caffeine, QT-prolonging agents.

Relative Infant Dose:

Adult Dose:

Alternatives:

References:

SYPHILIS   L2

Trade: Treponema pallidum

Other Trades:

Category: Infectious disease

Syphilis is a sexually transmitted disease that is caused by a bacterium called Treponema pallidum, which belongs to the family of spirochetes. Syphilis is caused due to sexual contact to infected lesions. Primary syphilis is characterized by the appearance of painless skin ulcers or chancres in the genital area. These chancres are infectious and disappear spontaneously without treatment within a few weeks. This is followed by secondary syphilis characterized by the appearance of a generalized rash that involves the palms and soles, and also the appearance of warts in the genital area called condyloma lata. This stage also resolves spontaneously to cause latent syphilis years later, characterized by neurological and cardiac manifestations.

The treatment of syphilis is with parenteral Penicillin G. When a lactating mother has been diagnosed with syphilis, treatment should be instituted immediately. Mother and infant should be separated for 24 hours following initiation of therapy, and breastfeeding is avoided during this period. The mother may resume breastfeeding within 24 hours of initiation of therapy. Any wet sores on the body may be infectious and should be adequately covered during breastfeeding to avoid contact with the infant. If there are wet sores on one breast, breastfeeding should be avoided from that breast and the infant may breastfeed from the opposite breast. Breastfeeding should be avoided from the affected breast until the skin sores completely heal.

Pregnancy Risk	Hazardous	Lactation Risk	L2
T ½	=	M/P	=
Vd	=	PB	=
Tmax	=	Oral	=
MW	=	pKa	=

Adult Concerns: Primary syphilis is characterized by the appearance of painless skin ulcers or chancres in the genital area. These chancres are infectious and disappear spontaneously without treatment within a few weeks. This is followed by secondary syphilis characterized by the appearance of a generalized rash that involves the palms and soles, and also the appearance of warts in the genital area called condyloma lata. This stage also resolves spontaneously to cause latent syphilis years later, characterized by neurological and cardiac manifestations.

Pediatric Concerns:

Drug Interactions:

Relative Infant Dose:

Adult Dose:

Alternatives:

References:

TACROLIMUS   L3

Trade: Prograf, Protopic
Other Trades: Protopic
Category: Immunosuppressant

Tacrolimus is an immunosuppressant formerly known as SK506. It is used to reduce rejection of transplanted organs including liver and kidney.[1] In one report of 21 mothers who received tacrolimus while pregnant, milk concentrations in colostrum averaged 0.79 ng/mL and varied from 0.3 to 1.9 ng/mL.[2] Maternal doses

(PO) ranged from 9.8 to 10.3 mg/day. Milk/blood ratio averaged 0.54. Using this data and an average daily milk intake of 150 mL/kg/day, the average dose to the infant per day via milk would be <0.1 µg/kg/day. Because the oral bioavailability is poor (<32%), an infant would likely ingest less than 100 ng/kg/day. The usual pediatric dose (PO) for preventing rejection varies from 0.15 to 0.2 mg/kg/day (equivalent to 150,000–200,000 ng/kg/day).

In a 32-year-old woman who had taken tacrolimus 0.1 mg/kg/day throughout pregnancy, samples were manually expressed at 0(trough), 1,6, 9, 11, and 12 hours after the morning dose.[3] The C_{max} occurred at 1 hour and was 0.57 µg/L. Using AUC data, the mean milk concentration was calculated to be 0.429 ng/mL. From these measurements, the exclusively breast-fed infant would ingest, on average, 0.06 µg/kg/day, which corresponds to 0.06% of the mother's weight-normalized dose. Given the low oral bioavailability of tacrolimus, the maximum amount the baby would receive is 0.02% of the mother's weight-adjusted dose. The milk/blood ratios of tacrolimus at pre-dosing and 1-hour post-dosing concentrations were calculated to be 0.08 and 0.09, respectively. At 2.5 months of age, the infant was developing well both physically and neurologically. The authors suggest that maternal therapy with tacrolimus for liver transplant may be compatible with breastfeeding.

In a more recent study, a 29-year-old woman with a 3-month-old breastfed infant, was receiving 2 mg tacrolimus twice daily, azathioprine 100 mg, prednisone 5 mg, diltiazem 180 mg, atenolol 100 mg, and furosemide 20 mg daily.[4] The milk-to-blood ratio was 0.23, and the average tacrolimus concentration in milk was 1.8 µg/L. The authors estimated the daily intake in the infant to be 0.5% of the maternal weight-adjusted dose (RID) or 0.27 µg/kg/day. This is less than 0.2% of the recommended pediatric dose for renal or liver transplant. The concentration-time profile of tacrolimus in milk was essentially flat. The highest concentration of tacrolimus in milk was at 4 and 8.5 hours post dose.

Recently the FDA has approved a topical form of tacrolimus (Protopic) for use in moderate to severe eczema, in those for whom standard eczema therapies are deemed inadvisable because of potential risks, or who are not adequately treated by, or who are intolerant to standard eczema therapies. Absorption via skin is minimal. In a study of 46 adult patients after multiple doses, plasma levels ranged from undetectable to 20 ng/mL, with 45 of the patients having peak blood concentrations less than 5 ng/mL.[1] In another study, the peak blood levels averaged 1.6 ng/mL, which is significantly less than the therapeutic range in kidney transplantation (7–20 ng/mL). While the absolute transcutaneous bioavailability is unknown, it is apparently very low. Combined with the poor oral bioavailability of this product, it is not likely a breastfed infant will receive enough following topical use (maternal) to produce adverse effects.

Pregnancy Risk	C	Lactation Risk	L3
T ½	= 34.2 hours	M/P	= 0.54
Vd	= 2.6 l/kg	PB	= 99%
Tmax	= 1.6 hours	Oral	= 14–32%
MW	= 822	pKa	=

Adult Concerns: Edema, renal shutdown. The US FDA has issued a warning concerning elevated risks of skin cancers and lymphomas in patients exposed to this product. This warning is highly controversial and is not supported by many dermatologic organizations.

Pediatric Concerns: None reported. The US FDA has issued a warning concerning elevated risks of skin cancers and lymphomas in patients exposed to this product. This warning is highly controversial and is not supported by many dermatologic organizations.

Drug Interactions: Drugs that may increase tacrolimus levels include: calcium channel blockers, azole antifungals, macrolide antibiotics (erythromycin, clarithromycin), cisapride, metoclopramide, bromocriptine, cimetidine, cyclosporine, danazol, methylprednisolone, protease inhibitors. Drugs that may decrease tacrolimus blood levels include: carbamazepine, phenobarbital, phenytoin, rifabutin, rifampin.

Relative Infant Dose: 0.1%–0.5%

Adult Dose: 0.15–0.3 mg/kg daily.

Alternatives:

References:
1. Pharmaceutical manufacturer prescribing information, 2001.
2. Jain A, Venkataramanan R, Fung JJ, Gartner JC, Lever J, Balan V, Warty V, Starzl TE. Pregnancy after liver transplantation under tacrolimus. Transplantation 1997; 64(4): 559–565.
3. French AE, Soldin SJ, Soldin OP, Koren G. Milk transfer and neonatal safety of tacrolimus. Ann Pharmacother 2003; 37(6): 815–818.
4. Gardiner SJ, Begg EJ. Breastfeeding during tacrolimus therapy. Obstet Gynecol 2006; 107: 453–5.

TAMOXIFEN   L5

Trade: Nolvadex

Other Trades: Tamoxen, Genox, Apo-Tamox, Nolvadex, Tamofen, Tamone, Eblon, Noltam

Category: Anti-estrogen, anticancer

Tamoxifen is a nonsteroidal antiestrogen. It attaches to the estrogen receptor and produces only minimal stimulation, thus it prevents estrogen from stimulating the receptor. Aside from this, it also produces a number of other effects within the cytoplasm of the cell and some of its anticancer effects may be mediated by its effects at sites other than the estrogen receptor. Tamoxifen is metabolized by the liver and has an elimination half-life of greater than 7 days (range 3–21 days).[1] It is well absorbed orally, and the highest tissue concentrations are in the liver (60 fold). It is 99% protein bound and normally reduces plasma prolactin levels significantly (66% after 3 months).

At present, there are no data on its transfer into breastmilk; however, it has been shown to inhibit lactation early postpartum in several studies. In one study, doses of 10–30 mg twice daily early postpartum, completely inhibited postpartum engorgement and lactation.[2] In a second study, tamoxifen doses of 10 mg four times daily significantly reduced serum prolactin and inhibited milk production as well.[3] We do not know the effect of tamoxifen on established milk production. It has a pKa of 8.85 which may suggest some trapping in milk compared to the maternal plasma levels. This product has a very long half-life, and the active metabolite is concentrated in the plasma (2 fold). This drug has all the characteristics that would suggest a concentrating mechanism in breastfed infants over time. Its prominent effect on reducing prolactin levels will inhibit early lactation and may ultimately inhibit established lactation. In this instance, the significant risks to the infant from exposure to tamoxifen probably outweigh the benefits of breastfeeding. Mothers receiving tamoxifen should not breastfeed until we know more about the levels transferred into milk and the plasma/tissue levels found in breastfed infants.

Pregnancy Risk	D	Lactation Risk	L5
T ½	= 3–21 days	M/P	=
Vd	=	PB	= 99%
Tmax	= 2–3 hours	Oral	= Complete
MW	= 371	pKa	= 8.85

Adult Concerns: Hot flashes, nausea, vomiting, vaginal bleeding/discharge, menstrual irregularities, amenorrhea.

Pediatric Concerns: None reported but caution is urged.

Drug Interactions: Avoid SSRI or SNRI antidepressants such as paroxetine, fluoxetine, bupropion, and duloxetine; substitute venlafaxine, desvenlafaxine, reboxetine, escitalopram, or mirtazapine. Avoid antipsychotics thioridazine, perphenazine, and pimozide; substitute thiothixene, clozapine, risperidone, olanzapine, ziprasidone, or quetiapine. Avoid cardiac drugs quinidine and ticlopidine, but diltiazem is acceptable. Avoid terfenadine and quinidine to treat infectious disease; substitute indinavir, saquinavir, nelfinavir, delavirdine, nevirapine, or efavirenz. Cinacalcet should be avoided, whereas gabapentin has little CYP2D6 inhibition. If possible, avoid prescription and over-the-counter antihistamines that are intermediate inhibitors of CYP2D6; preferable alternatives with little inhibition include chlorpheniramine, cetirizine, and loratadine. If possible, avoid the histamine H_2-blocker cimetidine, which is an intermediate inhibitor of CYP2D6; substitute ranitidine, which has little inhibition. Increased anticoagulant effect when used with coumarin-type anticoagulants. Tamoxifen is a potent inhibitor of drug metabolizing enzymes in the liver, observe for elevated levels of many drugs.

Relative Infant Dose:

Adult Dose: 10–20 mg twice daily.

Alternatives:

References:
1. Pharmaceutical manufacturer prescribing information, 1997.
2. Shaaban MM. Suppression of lactation by an antiestrogen, tamoxifen. Eur J Obstet Gynecol Reprod Biol 1975; 4(5): 167–169.
3. Masala A, Delitala G, Lo DG, Stoppelli I, Alagna S, Devilla L. Inhibition of lactation and inhibition of prolactin release after mechanical breast stimulation in puerperal women given tamoxifen or placebo. Br J Obstet Gynaecol 1978; 85(2): 134–137.

TAMSULOSIN HYDROCHLORIDE   L3

Trade: Flomax

Other Trades: Flomax, Flomax CR

Category: Alpha1 adrenergic antagonist

Tamsulosin is used in men for benign prostatic hyperplasia[1] and in women for problems in voiding, and in all patients to facilitate kidney stone passage.[2,3] It works by blocking the alpha-1A adrenoreceptors, thus reducing ureter contractility. Due to its high protein binding, and larger molecular weight, it is unlikely that tamsulosin would be excreted in human milk in clinically relevant amounts, but no breastfeeding data are presently available.

Pregnancy Risk	B	Lactation Risk	L3
T ½	= 13 hours	M/P	=
Vd	= 0.23 l/kg	PB	= 94–99%
Tmax	= 4–7 hours	Oral	= 90%
MW	= 445	pKa	=

Adult Concerns: Adverse reactions include orthostatic hypotension, headache, dizziness, rhinitis, and infection.

Pediatric Concerns: No data are available.

Drug Interactions: Calcuim channel blockers and beta blockers may both increase the risk of hypotension when used with tamulosin. Cimetidine decreases tamsulosin clearance. CYP3A4 and CYP2D6 inhibitors may increase the levels of tamulosin.

Relative Infant Dose:

Adult Dose: 0.4 mg once daily.

Alternatives:

References:
1. Pharmaceutical manufacturer prescribing information, 2008.
2. Singh SK, Pawar DS, Griwan MS, Indora JM, Sharma S. Role of tamsulosin in clearance of upper ureteral calculi after extracorporeal shock wave lithotripsy: a randomized controlled trial. Urol J. 2011 Winter; 8(1): 14–20.
3. Vincendeau S, Bellissant E, Houlgatte A, Doré B, Bruyère F, Renault A, Mouchel C, Bensalah K, Guillé F; Tamsulosin Study Group. Tamsulosin hydrochloride vs placebo for management of distal ureteral stones: a multicentric, randomized, double-blind trial. Arch Intern Med. 2010 Dec 13; 170(22): 2021–7.

TAPENTADOL   L3

Trade: Nucynta

Other Trades:

Category: Opiate analgesic

Tapentadol is an opiate analgesic and norepinephrine reuptake inhibitor.[1] There have been no studies done on the effects of tapentadol in breastfeeding mothers. However, from a pharmacokinetic standpoint, we believe it is likely that tapentadol is secreted into breast milk. Tapentadol has a relatively small molecular weight of 258 daltons, it is only 20% protein bound, and has a large volume of distribution; all of these factors facilitate the transfer of the drug into breast milk. Since the pka of the drug is quite basic, ion trapping may occur which leads to concentration of the drug within the milk. Also, the oil: water partition coefficient log P value is 2.87, which is very lipophilic; this means tapentadol can cross easily into milk. However, tapentadol undergoes extensive first pass metabolism and has a short half life. Thus, this may limit the effects of tapentadol on mother's milk. Nonetheless, caution is advised.

Pregnancy Risk	C		Lactation Risk	L3
T ½	= 6 hours		M/P	=
Vd	= 540 ± 98 L l/kg		PB	= 20%
Tmax	= 1.25 hours		Oral	= 32%
MW	= 257.80		pKa	= 9.34 and 10.45

Adult Concerns: Nausea, vomiting, dizziness, somnolence.

Pediatric Concerns:

Drug Interactions: Concurrent use with monoamine oxidase inhibitors is contraindicated. Avoid concurrent use with the following drugs due to enhanced risk of respiratory depression: barbiturates, benzodiazepines, other opioids, alcohol. Co-administration with the following increases risk of serotonin syndrome: tricyclic antidepressants, venlafaxine, desvenlafaxine, sumatriptan. For a complete list, refer a drug interactions text.

Relative Infant Dose:

Adult Dose: 50–150 mg four times daily.

Alternatives:

References:
1. Pharmaceutical manufacturer prescribing information, 2010.

TAZAROTENE — L3

Trade: Tazorac

Other Trades: Zorac

Category: Anti-psoriatic

Tazarotene is a specialized retinoid for topical use and is used for the topical treatment of stable plaque psoriasis and acne. Following topical application, tazarotene is converted to an active metabolite; transcutaneous absorption is minimal (<1%).[1] Applied daily, it is indicated for treatment of stable plaque psoriasis of up to 20% of the body surface area. Only 2–3% of the topically applied drug is absorbed transcutaneously. Tazarotene is metabolized to the active ingredient, tazarotenic acid. Little compound could be detected in the plasma. At steady state, plasma levels were only 0.09 ng/mL although this value is largely a function of surface area treated. When applied to large surface areas, systemic absorption is increased. Data on transmission to breastmilk are not available. The manufacturer reports some is transferred to rodent milk, but it has not been tested in humans.

Pregnancy Risk	X	Lactation Risk	L3
T ½	= 18 hours (met)	M/P	=
Vd	=	PB	= 99%
Tmax	= 8 hours	Oral	= Complete
MW	= 351	pKa	= 1.5

Adult Concerns: Hypertriglyceridemia, peripheral edema, pruritus, erythema, burning, contact dermatitis have been reported. This drug is potentially a significant teratogen and should not ever be used in pregnant patients or those not protected with a suitable birth-control measure.

Pediatric Concerns: None via milk. Some caution is recommended if used over large surface areas (20–30%).

Drug Interactions: Do not use concomitantly with drying agents.

Relative Infant Dose:

Adult Dose: Apply daily.

Alternatives:

References:
1. Pharmaceutical manufacturer prescribing information, 2002.

TAZOBACTAM   L2

Trade:

Other Trades:

Category: Antibiotic beta lactamase inhibitor

Tazobactam is a penicillin-like inhibitor of the enzyme beta lactamase and has few clinical effects. It is usually available in combination with piperacillin. Tazobactam concentrations in human milk have not been studied. Studies in women suggest that this medication poses minimal risk to the infant when used during breastfeeding. Its poor oral absorption would limit its absorption.[1] There has been one report that this medication turned the milk blue.

Pregnancy Risk	Safer	Lactation Risk	L2
T ½	= 0.69–0.78 hours	M/P	=
Vd	=	PB	=
Tmax	=	Oral	=
MW	= 322	pKa	= 2.1

Adult Concerns: Adverse effects for piperacillin/tazobactam: Diarrhea, nausea, vomiting, headache, insomnia, rash, itching, fever, moniliasis.

Pediatric Concerns:

Drug Interactions:

Relative Infant Dose:

Adult Dose:

Alternatives:

References:

1.   Chaplin S, Sanders GL, Smith JM. Drug excretion in human breast milk. Adv Drug React Ac Pois Rev 1982; 1: 255–287.

TEA TREE OIL   L3

Trade: Melaleuca oil

Other Trades:

Category: Antibacterial, antifungal

Tee tree oil (TTO), as derived from Melaleuca alternifolia, has recently gained popularity for its antiseptic properties. The essential oil, derived by steam distillation of the leaves, contains terpin-4-ol in concentrations of 40% or more.[1] TTO is primarily noted for its antimicrobial effects without irritating sensitive tissues. It is an antimicrobial when tested against Candida albicans, E. coli, S. Aureus, Staph. epidermidis, and pseudomonas aeruginosa. In several reports it is suggested to have antifungal properties equivalent to tolnaftate and clotrimazole. Although the use of TTO in adults is mostly nontoxic, the safe use in infants is unknown. Use directly on the nipple is not recommended. In one case, ingestion of about 10 mL of tea tree oil caused ataxia and fussiness in a 17-month-old baby.[2]

Pregnancy Risk	Possibly Hazardous	Lactation Risk	L3
T ½	=	M/P	=
Vd	=	PB	=
Tmax	=	Oral	=
MW	=	pKa	=

Adult Concerns: Toxic effects include allergic eczema. Petechial body rash and leukocytosis in one individual who ingested ½ teaspoonful orally. Ataxia and drowsiness following oral ingestion of < 10 cc by a 17-month-old infant.

Pediatric Concerns: None reported via milk.

Drug Interactions:

Relative Infant Dose:

Adult Dose:

Alternatives:

References:

1.   Review of Natural Products Ed: Facts and Comparisons 1997.
2.   Tea tree oil. In: AltMedDex Æ Evaluations Database [Internet database]. Greenwood Village, Colo: Thomson Reuters (Healthcare) Inc. Updated periodically. Accessed 7–18–2011.

TECHNETIUM[99m]   L4

Trade: [99m]Technetium

Other Trades:

Category: Radioactive imaging

Radioactive [99m]Technetium (^{99m}Tc) is present in milk for at least 15 hours to 3 days, and significant quantities have been reported in the thyroid and gastric mucosa of infants ingesting milk from treated mothers. Technetium is one of the halide elements and is handled, biologically, much like iodine. Like iodine, it concentrates in thyroid tissues, the stomach, and breastmilk of nursing mothers. It has a radioactive half-life of 6.02 hours. Following a dose of 15 mCi of ^{99m}Tc for a brain scan, the concentration of ^{99m}Tc in breastmilk at 4, 8.5, 20, and 60 hours was 0.5 µCi, 0.1 µCi, 0.02 µCi, and 0.006 µCi respectively.[1] In another study, following a dose of 10 mCi of NaTcO4, breastmilk levels were 5.7, 1.5, 0.015 µCi/mL at 3.25, 7.5, and 24 hours respectively.[2] The estimated dose to infant was 1,036, 284, and 2.7 µCi/180 mL milk. These authors recommended pumping and discarding of milk for 48 hours. [99m]Technetium is used in many salt and chemical forms, but the radioactivity and decay are the same although the concentrations in milk may be influenced by the salt form. In another study using [99m]Technetium MAG3 in two mothers receiving 150 MBq of radioactivity, the total percent of ingested radioactivity ranged from 0.7 to 1.6% of the total.[3] These authors suggested that the DTPA salt of [99m]Technetium would produce the least breastmilk levels and would be preferred in breastfeeding mothers. The NRC table suggests duration of interruption of breastfeeding of 12 to 24 hours for 12 and 30 mCi respectively, but this depends on the salt form used. See close contact and breastfeeding restriction table and appendix and for numerous other preparations and recommendations. The American Academy of Pediatrics (AAP) recommends temparry cessation of breastfeeding following administration of this agent.[4]

International Commission of Radiological Protection (ICRP) recommends 4 hours breastfeeding interruption for [99m]Technetium DISIDA, DMSA, DTPA, ECD, MDP, gluconate, glucoheptonate, HM-PAO, sulfur colloid, MAG3, MIBI, PYP, Technegas, and Tetrofosmin.[5] ICRP recommends 12 hours interruption for [99m]Technetium MAA, HAM, pertechnetate, RBC, and WBC.[5]

Close contact restrictions (6 feet separation from infant):

[99m]Tc (Static renal scan): 30 or less mCi dose: Limit close contact to 35 min/hour with maximum 9 hours/day.[6]

[99m]Tc (Dynamic renal scan, thyroid scan, liver scan, brain scan): 10 or less mCi dose: Limit close contact to 35 min/hour with maximum 9 hours/day.[6]

[99m]Tc (Dynamic renal scan, thyroid scan, liver scan, brain scan): 10–22.9 mCi dose: Avoid contact for first 4 hours. Limit close contact to 35 min every 3 hours.[6]

[99m]Tc (Bone scan, lung V/Q scan, bile scan): 16 or less mCi dose: Limit close contact to 35 min/hour with maximum 9 hours/day.[6]

[99m]Tc (Bone scan, lung V/Q scan, bile scan): 16–30 mCi dose: Avoid contact for first 4 hours. Limit close contact to 35 min every 3 hours.[6]

^{99m}Tc (Marrow scan): 8 or less mCi dose: Limit close contact to 35 min/hour with maximum 9 hours/day.[6]

^{99m}Tc (Marrow scan): 8–16 mCi dose: Avoid contact for first 4 hours. Limit close contact to 35 min every 3 hours.[6]

Note: These recommendations still permit a minimal amount of <1 mSv of radiation transfer to the infant. Exposure of 1 mSv has a cancer incidence risk of 1 in 10,000 people. This amount of exposure is less than the amount an average American is exposed to from the natural environment (6.2 mSv/year). The only way to avoid all radiation exposure is to wait for 5-10 half-lives, until all of the radioisotope decays (1–3 days).

Pregnancy Risk	C	Lactation Risk	L4
T ½	= <6 hours	M/P	=
Vd	=	PB	=
Tmax	=	Oral	= Complete
MW	=	pKa	=

Adult Concerns: Hypersensitivity, edema, nausea, vomiting, arthralgia, rash, malaise, hypotension, headache.

Pediatric Concerns: None reported, but may be transferred to infant thyroid. Pump and dump for a minimum of 48 hours.

Drug Interactions:

Relative Infant Dose:

Adult Dose: 15–20 mCi X 1

Alternatives:

References:
1. Rumble WF, Aamodt RL, Jones AE, Henkin RI, Johnston GS. Accidental ingestion of Tc-^{99m} in breast milk by a 10-week-old child. J Nucl Med 1978; 19(8): 913–915.
2. Maisels MJ, Gilcher RO. Excretion of technetium in human milk. Pediatrics 1983; 71(5): 841–842.
3. Evans JL, Mountford AN, Herring AN, Richardson MA. Secretion of radioactivity in breast milk following administration of 99Tcm-MAG3. Nuc Med Comm 1993; 14: 108–111.
4. American Academy of Pediatrics, Committee on Drugs. Transfer of drugs and other chemicals into human milk. Pediatrics 2001; 108(3): 776–89.
5. ICRP, 2008. Radiation Dose to Patients from Radiopharmaceuticals–Addendum 3 to ICRP Publication 53. ICRP Publication 106. Ann. ICRP 38 (1–2).
6. Mountford PJ, O'Doherty MJ, Forge NI, Jeffries A, Coakley AJ. Radiation dose rates from adult patients undergoing nuclear medicine investigations. Nucl Med Commun. 1991 Sep; 12(9): 767–77.

TECHNETIUM^{99m} SESTAMIBI   L4

Trade: Cardiolite, Sestamibi

Other Trades:

Category: Imaging agent

Technetium^{99m} sestamibi is a myocardial imaging agent that is also sometimes used as an oncologic imaging agent. The radioactive Technetium^{99m} ion is chelated to the sestamibi molecule. It is used as an alternative to Thallium-201 imaging.[1] Sestamibi is largely distributed to the myocardium and is a function of myocardial viability.[2] Technetium^{99m} is a weak gamma emitter with a radioactive half-life of only 6.02 hours. The biological half-life of this product is approximately 6 hours, but the effective half-life (both biological and radioactive) is only about 3 hours. Transfer of significant amounts of sestamibi into human milk is yet unreported but is rather unlikely as sestamibi binds irreversible to myocardial tissue and does not redistribute to other tissues to a significant degree. Other forms of Technetium^{99m} have been reported to enter milk, but entry would be largely determined by the chemical form, not the radioactive agent.[3]

Pregnancy Risk	C	Lactation Risk	L4
T ½	= 6 hours	M/P	=
Vd	=	PB	= <1%
Tmax	=	Oral	= Complete
MW	=	pKa	=

Adult Concerns: Dysgeusia, headache, flushing, angina, hypersensitivity, and hypertension.

Pediatric Concerns: It is not known if the sestamibi chelate is transferred into human milk. But Technetium salts in general do transfer. Pump and discard for 24–30 hours or pump and hold the milk for approximately 24–30 hours prior to feeding.

Drug Interactions:

Relative Infant Dose:

Adult Dose: 10–30 mCi X 1

Alternatives:

References:
1. Berman DS. Introduction--Technetium-^{99m} myocardial perfusion imaging agents and their relation to thallium-201. Am J Cardiol 1990; 66(13): 1E-4E.
2. Berman DS, Kiat H, Maddahi J. The new Tc-^{99m} myocardial perfusion imaging agents: Tc-^{99m} sestamibi and Tc-^{99m} teboroxime. Circulation 1991; 84((suppl)): 7–21.
3. Maisels MJ, Gilcher RO. Excretion of technetium in human milk. Pediatrics 1983; 71(5): 841–842.

TEGASEROD MALEATE   L3

Trade: Zelnorm

Other Trades: Zelnorm

Category: Treatment of irritable bowel syndrome

Tegaserod is a serotonin agonist (stimulant) used to treat the symptoms of irritable bowel syndrome. Oral absorption is only 10% (fasting) and is reduced to 40–65% by food. In patients receiving oral doses of 2, 6, and 12 mg, mean peak plasma concentrations were 0.9, 2.9, and 6.3 µg/L respectively.[1] Studies in rats suggest it transfers with a higher milk/plasma ratio, but this is common for rodent studies and the dose was 320 times that given in humans.[2] No data are available on its transfer to human milk. Tegaserod is a lipophilic drug which would assist its transfer into human milk, however, its low plasma levels, poor oral bioavailability (particularly with food), and large volume of distribution suggests that the actual amount transferred into human milk is probably quite low. Recently this drug was restricted for use by the FDA due to reported higher chances of heart attack, stroke and unstable angina.

Pregnancy Risk	B	Lactation Risk	L3
T ½	= 11 hours	M/P	=
Vd	= 368 l/kg	PB	= 98%
Tmax	= 1 hour	Oral	= 10%
MW	= 417	pKa	= 5.83

Adult Concerns: Adverse events may include abdominal pain, diarrhea, nausea, flatulence, headache, pain, flushing, hypotension, and vertigo. Use of tegaserod was previously restricted at the request of FDA in 2007 following a safety analysis that found a higher chance of heart attack, stroke, and unstable angina (heart/chest pain) in patients treated with tegaserod compared with those treated with an inactive substance (placebo).

Pediatric Concerns: None reported via milk, but rat milk levels have been detected. Note new warnings on this drug.

Drug Interactions: None reported.

Relative Infant Dose:

Adult Dose: 6 mg twice daily.

Alternatives:

References:
1. Pharmaceutical manufacturer prescribing information, 2003.
2. Appel-Dingemanse S. Clinical pharmacokinetics of tegaserod, a serotonin 5–HT(4) receptor partial agonist with promotile activity. Clin Pharmacokinet 2002; 41(13): 1021–1042.

TELBIVUDINE   L4

Trade: Tyzeka
Other Trades:
Category: Hepatitis B antiviral

Telbivudine is a thymidine nucleoside analog that inhibits reverse transcriptase and DNA polymerase in hepatitis B virus infections. It does not inhibit human cellular polymerase. Telbivudine is used in adults with chronic hepatitis B that have evidence of either increased liver function tests or an active infection.[1] It is considered safe in pregnancy, but is very lipid soluble, therefore its transfer into milk may be likely, but probably not clinically relevant. However, this product is intended for chronic use, and exposing an infant to a potential hepatotoxin such as this over a prolonged period is not justified.

Pregnancy Risk	B		Lactation Risk	L4
T ½	= 40–49 hours		M/P	=
Vd	=		PB	= 3.3%
Tmax	= 1–4 hours		Oral	=
MW	= 242		pKa	= 9.61

Adult Concerns: Adverse reactions include fatigue, muscle pain, headache, lactic acidosis, hepatomegaly, steatosis and abdominal pain.

Pediatric Concerns: No data are available.

Drug Interactions: Telbivudine is renally excreted, therefore medications that altar renal function may alter plasma concentrations.

Relative Infant Dose:

Adult Dose: 600 mg daily.

Alternatives:

References:
1. Pharmaceutical manufacturer prescribing information, 2006.

TELITHROMYCIN   L3

Trade: Ketek
Other Trades:
Category: Erythromycin-like antibiotic

Telithromycin is an erythromycin-like antibiotic.[1] No data are available on its transfer into human milk. Due to its large molecular weight, the amount in milk is likely low. About 1–2% of the maternal dose of erythromycin passes into milk. Please be advised that telithromycin is an erythromycin-like antibiotic and perhaps hundreds of drug-drug interactions are possible.

Pregnancy Risk	C		Lactation Risk	L3
T ½	= 9.8 hours		M/P	=
Vd	= 2.9 l/kg		PB	= 60–70%
Tmax	= 1 hour		Oral	= 57%
MW	= 812		pKa	= 2.4, 5.1, 8.7

Adult Concerns: Side effects include: diarrhea (10.8%), nausea (7.9%), headache (5.5%), dizziness, vomiting, loose stools, visual disturbances have been reported. May produce changes in QTc prolongation. Do not use in patients with myasthenia gravis.

Pediatric Concerns: No data are available on the transfer of telithromycin into human milk. Probably similar to azithromycin.

Drug Interactions: Numerous drug-drug interactions exist, including the azole antifungals. Please check other authoritative sources or your pharmacist.

Relative Infant Dose:

Adult Dose: 800 mg every 24 hours.

Alternatives: Azithromycin, clarithromycin

References:
1.   Pharmaceutical manufacturer prescribing information, 2005.

TELMISARTAN   L4

Trade: Micardis, Micardis HCT, Twynsta
Other Trades: Micardis
Category: Angiotensin II receptor antagonist

Telmisartan is a potent antihypertensive that blocks the angiotensin II receptor site.[1] It is also available in combination with hydrochlorothiazide. This agent should never be used in pregnant patients, as fetal demise has been reported with similar agents in this class. No data are available on its use in lactating mothers. However, its use early postpartum in lactating mothers should be approached with caution, particularly in mothers with premature infants.

Pregnancy Risk	C/D in 2nd and 3rd trimester	Lactation Risk	L4
T ½	= 24 hours	M/P	=
Vd	= 7.14 l/kg	PB	= 99.5%
Tmax	= 1 hour	Oral	= 42–58%
MW	= 514	pKa	= 3.83

Adult Concerns: UTI infection, back pain, sinusitis and diarrhea have been reported. Flu-like symptoms, myalgia, coughing, hypotension have been reported.

Pediatric Concerns: None reported, but use caution early postpartum.

Drug Interactions: When coadministered with digoxin, a 50% increase in digoxin peak plasma levels occurred, and a 13–20% increase in trough levels.

Relative Infant Dose:

Adult Dose: 40 mg daily.

Alternatives:

References:
1.   Pharmaceutical manufacturer prescribing information, 2002.

TEMAZEPAM   L3

Trade: Restoril

Other Trades: Euhypnos, Noctume, Temaze, Temtabs, Restoril, PMS-Temazepam, Normison

Category: Short acting benzodiazepine (Valium-like) hypnotic

Temazepam is a short acting benzodiazepine primarily used as a nighttime sedative. In a study of ten breastfeeding mothers (<15 days postpartum) who received doses of 10–20 mg at bedtime for two days prior to the study, the milk/plasma ratio varied from <0.09 to <0.63 (mean= 0.18).[1] Levels of temazepam were undetectable (<5 µg/L) in 9 out of 10 subjects. The tenth mother had plasma levels of temazepam of 234 µg/L and milk levels that ranged from 26–28 µg/L. Temazepam is relatively water soluble and therefore partitions poorly into breastmilk. Levels of temazepam were undetectable in the infants studied although these studies were carried out 15 hours post-dose. Although the study shows low neonatal exposure to temazepam via breastmilk, the infant should be monitored carefully for sleepiness and poor feeding.

Pregnancy Risk	X	Lactation Risk	L3
T ½	= 9.5–12.4 hours	M/P	= 0.18
Vd	= 0.8–1.0 l/kg	PB	= 96%
Tmax	= 2–4 hours	Oral	= 90%
MW	= 301	pKa	= 1.6

Adult Concerns: Sedation.

Pediatric Concerns: None reported via milk, but observe for sedation, poor feeding.

Drug Interactions: Increased effect when used with other CNS depressants.

Relative Infant Dose:

Adult Dose: 7.5–30 mg daily.

Alternatives: Lorazepam, alprazolam

References:
1. Lebedevs TH, Wojnar-Horton RE, Yapp P, Roberts MJ, Dusci LJ, Hackett LP, Ilett KF. Excretion of temazepam in breast milk. Br J Clin Pharmacol 1992; 33(2): 204–206.

TEMOZOLOMIDE   L5

Trade: Temodar, Temodal

Other Trades:

Category: Anticancer drug

Temozolomide is an alkylating agent used to treat refractory anaplastic astrocytoma and newly-diagnosed glioblastoma multiforme. Temozolomide is converted to a metabolite MTIC spontaneously under physiologic conditions.[1] No studies have been performed regarding the transmission of the drug into milk, however, it is highly likely that temozolomide would transfer into the milk compartment, due to the low volume of distribution, low protein binding, and low molecular weight. Temozolomide would be orally bioavailable to an infant and thus should not be used in a nursing mother. In male infants, it could be genotoxic or cause damage to DNA. Temozolomide is an extremely toxic agent, and infants should be withdrawn from the breast for a prolonged period of at least seven days.

Pregnancy Risk	D	Lactation Risk	L5
T ½	= 1.8 hours (parent drug)	M/P	=
Vd	= 0.1 l/kg	PB	= 15%
Tmax	= 1–2.25 hours	Oral	=
MW	= 194	pKa	= 15.29

Adult Concerns: Alopecia, fatigue, nausea, vomiting, headache, constipation, anorexia, convulsions, rash, hemiparesis, diarrhea, asthenia, fever, dizziness, coordination abnormal, viral infection, amnesia, and insomnia

Pediatric Concerns: Potentially very toxic.

Drug Interactions: Valproic Acid may increase the serum concentration of temozolomide.

Relative Infant Dose:

Adult Dose: Highly variable.

Alternatives:

References:
1.   Pharmaceutical manufacturer prescribing information, 2005.

TENIPOSIDE   L4

Trade: Vumon, Vehem
Other Trades: Vumon
Category: Anticancer drug

Teniposide is a semisynthetic derivative of podophyllotoxin. It is similar to etoposide chemically. Teniposide has a broad spectrum of *in vivo* antitumor activity against murine tumors, including hematologic malignancies and various solid tumors. Plasma drug levels declined biexponentially following intravenous infusion (155 mg/m^2 over 1 to 2.5 hours) of teniposide given to eight children (4–11 years old) with newly diagnosed acute lymphoblastic leukemia (ALL).[1] The terminal elimination half-life was 5.4 hours. Mean steady-state volumes of distribution range from 8 to 44 L/m^2 for adults and 3 to 11 L/m^2 for children. Teniposide is highly (99%) protein bound and does not readily enter the CNS. These kinetics alone would suggest milk levels are probably exceedingly low. However, no data are yet available on the transfer of this product into human milk. Withhold breastfeeding for a minimum of 36–48 hours.

Pregnancy Risk	D		Lactation Risk	L4
T ½	= 5.4 hours		M/P	=
Vd	= 8–44 L/m²		PB	= 99.4
Tmax	=		Oral	=
MW	= 656.7		pKa	= 9.95

Adult Concerns: Risk of infection, anemia, mouth irritation, nausea or vomiting, diarrhea, and hair loss

Pediatric Concerns: Hazardous. Wait 36–48 hours following exposure to breastmilk.

Drug Interactions: Caution should be used in administering teniposide to patients receiving tolbutamide, sodium salicylate, and sulfamethizole due to possible drug toxicity. An increase in intracellular levels of methotrexate was observed *in vitro* in the presence of teniposide.

Relative Infant Dose:

Adult Dose: Varies according to cancer type/treatment.

Alternatives:

References:
1. Pharmaceutical manufacturer prescribing information, 2005.

TENOFOVIR DISOPROXIL FUMARATE   L3

Trade: Viread
Other Trades: Viread
Category: Antiretroviral agent

Tenofovir is used in the management of HIV and hepatitis B infections. It interferes with the viral RNA-dependent DNA polymerase, inhibiting viral replication.[1] In a recent study in two Rhesus macaques monkeys, and following a subcutaneous dose of 30 mg/kg tenofovir, peak plasma levels were reported to be 18.3 and 30.3 µg/mL.[2] Peak levels in milk were reported to be 0.808 and 0.610 µg/mL. The AUC levels were 68.9 and 12.8 µg.h/mL for plasma and milk in one animal and 56.2 and 12.1 µg.h/mL for plasma and milk in the second animal. Using this peak data, the relative infant dose would only be 0.4% of the maternal dose. In addition, the oral bioavailability of tenofovir (non salt form) is negligible (5%). Thus the overall risk to a breastfeeding infant would probably be low.

Pregnancy Risk	B		Lactation Risk	L3
T ½	= 17 hours		M/P	=
Vd	= 1.2–1.3 l/kg		PB	= 7%
Tmax	= 36–144 minutes		Oral	= 25–40%
MW	= 636		pKa	= 3.75

Adult Concerns: Adverse reactions include pain, nausea, diarrhea, and weakness.

Pediatric Concerns: Data on humans is not available, but milk levels in monkeys are quite low.

Drug Interactions: Antiviral agents may increase the serum concentrations of tenofovir. Concurrent use of didanosine will increase serum concentrations of didanosine. Nephrotoxic agents will decrease the elimination of tenofovir. Tenofovir will decrease the serum concentrations of protease inhibitors.

Relative Infant Dose: 0.4%

Adult Dose: 300 mg daily.

Alternatives:

References:
1. Pharmaceutical manufacturer prescribing information, 2005.
2. K. Van Rompay, M. Hamilton, B. Kearney and N. Bischofberger, Pharmacokinetics of tenofovir in breast milk of lactating rhesus macaques. Antimicrob Agents Chemother 49, 2093–2094 (2005).

TERAZOSIN HCL   L4

Trade: Hytrin

Other Trades: Hytrin

Category: Antihypertensive

Terazosin is an antihypertensive that belongs to the alpha-1 blocking family. This family is generally very powerful, produces significant orthostatic hypotension and other side effects.[1] Terazosin has rather powerful effects on the prostate and testes producing testicular atrophy in some animal studies (particularly newborn) and is therefore not preferred in pregnant or in lactating women. No data are available on transfer into human milk.

Pregnancy Risk	C	Lactation Risk	L4
T ½	= 9–12 hours	M/P	=
Vd	=	PB	= 94%
Tmax	= 1–2 hours	Oral	= 90%
MW	= 423	pKa	= 7.1

Adult Concerns: Hypotension, bradycardia, sedation.

Pediatric Concerns: None reported, but extreme caution is recommended.

Drug Interactions: Decreased antihypertensive effect when used with NSAIDs. Increased hypotensive effects when used with diuretics and other antihypertensive beta blockers.

Relative Infant Dose:

Adult Dose: 1–10 mg daily.

Alternatives:

References:
1. Pharmaceutical manufacturer prescribing information, 1995.

TERBINAFINE   L2

Trade: Lamisil, Terbinex
Other Trades:
Category: Antifungal

Terbinafine is an antifungal agent primarily used for tinea species such as athletes foot and ringworm. Systemic absorption following topical therapy is minimal.[1] Following an oral dose of 500 mg in two volunteers, the total dose of terbinafine secreted in breastmilk during the 72 hour post-dosing period was 0.65 mg in one mother and 0.15 mg in another.[2] The total excretion of terbinafine in breastmilk ranged from 0.13% to 0.03% of the total maternal dose respectively. Topical absorption through the skin is minimal.[3]

Pregnancy Risk	B	Lactation Risk	L2
T ½	= 26 hours	M/P	=
Vd	= >28 l/kg	PB	= 99%
Tmax	= 1–2 hours	Oral	= 80%
MW	= 291	pKa	= 7.1

Adult Concerns: Topical: burning, pruritus. Oral: fatigue, headache, gastrointestinal distress, elevated liver enzymes, alopecia.

Pediatric Concerns: None reported via milk.

Drug Interactions: Terbinafine clearance is decreased 33% by cimetidine, and 16% by terfenadine. Terbinafine increases clearance of cyclosporin(15%). Rifampin increases terbinafine clearance by 100%.

Relative Infant Dose:

Adult Dose: 250 mg daily.

Alternatives: Fluconazole

References:
1. Pharmaceutical manufacturer prescribing Information, 1996.
2. Drug Facts and Comparisons 1996 ed. St. Louis: 1996.
3. Birnbaum JE. Pharmacology of the allylamines. J Am Acad Dermatol 1990; 23(4 Pt 2): 782–785.

TERBUTALINE   L2

Trade: Bricanyl, Brethine
Other Trades: Bricanyl
Category: Bronchodilator for asthma

Terbutaline is a popular beta-2 adrenergic receptor agonist used for bronchodilation in asthmatics. It is secreted into breastmilk but in low quantities. Following doses of 7.5 to 15 mg/day of terbutaline, milk levels averaged 3.37 µg/L.[1] Assuming a daily milk intake of 165 m, these levels would suggest a daily intake of less than 0.5 µg/kg/day which corresponds to 0.2 to 0.7% of maternal dose. In another study of a patient receiving 5 mg three times daily, the mean milk concentrations ranged from 3.2 to 3.7 µg/L.[2] The author calculated the daily dose to infant at 0.4–0.5 µg/kg body weight. Terbutaline was not detectable in the infant's serum. No untoward effects have been reported in breastfeeding infants.

Pregnancy Risk	B	Lactation Risk	L2
T ½	= 14 hours	M/P	= <2.9
Vd	= 1–2 l/kg	PB	= 20%
Tmax	= 5–30 minutes	Oral	= 33–50%
MW	= 225	pKa	= 10.1

Adult Concerns: Tremors, nervousness, tachycardia.

Pediatric Concerns: None reported via milk.

Drug Interactions: Decreased effect when used with beta blockers. May increase toxicity when used with monoamine oxidase inhibitors and tricyclic antidepressants.

Relative Infant Dose: 0.2%–0.3%

Adult Dose: 5 mg three times daily.

Alternatives:

References:
1. Lindberg C, Boreus LO, De Chateau P, Lindstrom B, Lonnerholm G, Nyberg L. Transfer of terbutaline into breast milk. Eur J Respir Dis Suppl 1984; 134: 87–91.
2. Lonnerholm G, Lindstrom B. Terbutaline excretion into breast milk. Br J Clin Pharmacol 1982; 13(5): 729–730.

TERCONAZOLE   L3

Trade: Terazol 3, Terazol 7

Other Trades: Terazol

Category: Antifungal, vaginal.

Terconazole is an antifungal primarily used for vaginal candidiasis. It is similar to fluconazole and itraconazole. When administered intravaginally, only a limited amount (5–16%) is absorbed systemically (mean peak plasma level=6 ng/mL).[1,2] It is well absorbed orally. Even at high doses, the drug is not mutagenic, nor fetotoxic. At high doses, terconazole is known to enter breastmilk in rodents although no data are available on human milk. The milk levels are probably too small to be clinically relevant.

Pregnancy Risk	C	Lactation Risk	L3
T ½	= 4–11.3 hours	M/P	=
Vd	=	PB	=
Tmax	=	Oral	= Complete
MW	= 532	pKa	= 7.23

Adult Concerns: Vaginal burning, itching, flu-like symptoms.

Pediatric Concerns: None reported due to minimal studies.

Drug Interactions:

Relative Infant Dose:

Adult Dose: 5 gm daily.

Alternatives: Fluconazole

References:
1. Pharmaceutical manufacturer prescribing information, 1996.
2. McEvoy GE. (ed): AFHS Drug Information. New York, NY: 2003.

TERIPARATIDE   L3

Trade: Forteo

Other Trades:

Category: Human parathyroid hormone

Teriparatide is the identical peptide hormone secreted by the parathyroid gland in humans. This leads to an increase in skeletal mass, markers of bone formation and resorption, and bone strength. Teriparatide is used to treat osteoporosis.[1] No studies are available on the levels in breast milk, however, due to the high molecular weight and poor oral bioavailablility, it is unlikely that teriparatide will cross into the milk or be absorbed by an infant.

Pregnancy Risk	C		Lactation Risk	L3
T ½	= 1 hour		M/P	=
Vd	= 0.12 l/kg		PB	=
Tmax	=		Oral	= Nil
MW	= 4118		pKa	=

Adult Concerns: Adverse reactions include dizziness, nausea, dyspepsia, arthralgia, weakness, rhinitis, and pharyngitis.

Pediatric Concerns: No data are available, but this is the normal human parathyroid hormone.

Drug Interactions: Hypercalcemia may increase the risk of digitalis toxicity.

Relative Infant Dose:

Adult Dose: 20 µg subcutaneous daily.

Alternatives:

References:
1. Pharmaceutical manufacturer prescribing information, 2004.

TETANUS TOXOID VACCINE   L2

Trade: TE Anatoxal Berna

Other Trades:

Category: Vaccine Tetanus, Tdap

Tetanus toxoid contains a large molecular weight protein. Tetanus vaccine is made from inactivated tetanus toxoid by formaldehyde.[1] Tetanus vaccine is part of Tdap, DT, Td, DTaP, Pediarix, Pentacel and DTP vaccines. Because tetanus vaccine is an inactivated bacterial product, there is no specific contraindication in breastfeeding following injection with this vaccine. It is extremely unlikely proteins of this size would be secreted in breastmilk.

While the USA has removed mercury from virtually all pediatric immunizations, other countries have not. In infants receiving three doses of hepatitis B vaccine and three DTP vaccines during the first 6 months of life, the exposure to ethylmercury was 25 µg Hg for each vaccine. Infant hair-Hg increased 446% during these six months, while maternal hair-Hg decreased 57%. This provides evidence that the extra mercury exposure is due to the vaccinations rather than maternal milk.[2]

Pregnancy Risk	C		Lactation Risk	L2
T ½	=		M/P	=
Vd	=		PB	=
Tmax	=		Oral	=
MW	=		pKa	=

Adult Concerns: Local injection site reactions, fever, pain, hypotension. Rare cases: Peripheral neuropathy, Guillain-Barre syndrome.

Pediatric Concerns:

Drug Interactions:

Relative Infant Dose:

Adult Dose:

Alternatives:

References:
1. Atkinson W, Wolfe S, Hamborsky J, eds. 2011. Tetanus. "Centers for Disease Control and Prevention. Epidemiology and Prevention of Vaccine-Preventable Diseases". 12th ed. Washington DC: Public Health Foundation.
2. Marques, RC, Dorea JG, Fonseca MF, Bastos WR, Malm O. Hair mercury in breast-fed infants exposed to thimerosal-preserved vaccines. Eur J Pediatr 2007; [Epub ahead of print].

TETRACYCLINE   L2

Trade: Achromycin, Sumycin, Terramycin
Other Trades: Mysteclin, Tetrex, Achromycin, Aureomycin, Tetracyn, Tetrachel
Category: Antibiotic

Tetracycline is a broad-spectrum antibiotic with significant side effects in pediatric patients, including dental staining and reduced bone growth. It is secreted into breastmilk in extremely small levels. Because tetracyclines bind to milk calcium they would have reduced oral absorption in the infant. Posner reports that in a patient receiving 500 mg four times daily, the average concentration of tetracycline in milk was 1.14 mg/L.[1] The maternal plasma level was 1.92 mg/L and the milk/plasma ratio was 0.59. The absolute dose to the infant ranged from 0.17

to 0.39 mg/kg/day. None was detected in the plasma compartment of the infant (limit of detection 0.05 mg/L). In a mother receiving 275 mg/day, milk levels averaged 1.25 mg/L with a maximum of 2.51 mg/L.[2] None was detected in the infant's plasma. In another study of 2–3 patients receiving a single 150 mg/day dose, milk levels ranged from 0.3 to 1.2 mg/L at 4 hours (C_{max}). The maximum reported milk level was 1.2 mg/L.[3] A milk/plasma ratio of 0.58 was reported. From the above studies, the relative infant dose is 0.6%, 4.77% and 8.44%. Thus a high degree of variability exists in these studies. Invariably, mixture of tetracyclines in milk would greatly limit their oral bioavailability.

The short-term exposure of infants to tetracyclines (via milk) is not contraindicated (<3 weeks). However, the long-term exposure of breastfeeding infants to tetracyclines, such as when used daily for acne, could cause problems. The absorption of even small amounts over a prolonged period could result in dental staining.

Pregnancy Risk	D		Lactation Risk	L2
T ½	= 6–12 hours		M/P	= 0.58–1.28
Vd	=		PB	= 25%
Tmax	= 1.5–4 hours		Oral	= 75%
MW	= 444		pKa	= 3.3, 7.68, 9.69

Adult Concerns: Pediatric: dental staining, decreased bone growth, altered gastrointestinal flora.

Pediatric Concerns: None reported via milk. Poor oral absorption of tetracyclines generally limits effects. Avoid long-term exposure.

Drug Interactions: Absorption may be reduced or delayed when used with dairy products, calcium, magnesium, or aluminum containing antacids, oral contraceptives, iron, zinc, sodium bicarbonate, penicillins, cimetidine. Increased toxicity may result when used with methoxyflurane anesthesia. Use with warfarin anticoagulants may increase anticoagulation.

Relative Infant Dose: 0.6%

Adult Dose: 500 mg four times daily.

Alternatives:

References:
1. Posner AC, Prigot A, Konicoff NG. Further observations on the use of tetracycline hydrochloride in prophylaxis and treatment of obstetric infections. New York: Antibiotics Annual 1954–1955. In: Medical Encyclopedia, 1955.
2. Graf von H, Riemann S. Untersuchungen uber die konzentration von pyrrolidino-methyl-tetracyclin in der muttermilch. Dtsch med wochenschr 1959; 84: 1694–1696.
3. Matsuda S. Transfer of antibiotics into maternal milk. Biol Res Pregnancy Perinatol 1984; 5(2): 57–60.

TETRAHYDROZOLINE   L3

Trade: Visine, Altazine, Eye-Zine, Geneye, Opti-Clear, Optigene 3, Medidrops Eye Drops, Steri-Optics Redness Reliever

Other Trades:

Category: Decongestion

Tetrahydrozoline is present in ophthalmic drops and in nasal decongestant sprays for the treatment of conjunctivitis and rhinitis.[1] Over the counter products have low tetrahydrozoline concentration (0.05–0.1%) such that systemic absorption is probably low especially from ophthalmic preparations. There are no adequate or well-controlled studies in breastfeeding women; however, the risk of side effects to a breastfed infant is probably minimal. Tetrahydrozoline should only be given only if the potential benefit justifies the potential risk to the infant.

Pregnancy Risk	C	Lactation Risk	L3
T ½	=	M/P	=
Vd	=	PB	=
Tmax	=	Oral	=
MW	= 200	pKa	=

Adult Concerns: Local irritation, blurred vision, headache, sneezing, tremor.

Pediatric Concerns:

Drug Interactions: Combination with monoamine oxidase inhibitors may increase hypertensive effect.

Relative Infant Dose:

Adult Dose: 1–2 drop per eye 2–4 times/day (0.05%), 3–4 spray per nostril every 3–4 hours (0.1%).

Alternatives: Saline nasal spray, oxymetazoline nasal spray, naphazoline eye solution.

References:
1. Pharmaceutical manufacturer prescribing information, 2011.

THALIDOMIDE   L5

Trade: Thalomid

Other Trades:

Category: Antineoplastic agent

Thalidomide is used in the treatment of multiple myeloma and also for the treatment of skin manifestations in leprosy patients.[1] There is no data on the transfer of thalidomide into human milk. Because many drugs are transferred into human milk and because of the potential for serious adverse reactions in nursing infants, the manufacturer recommends a decision to be made whether or not to discontinue nursing or to discontinue the drug taking into account the importance of the drug to the nursing woman.

Pregnancy Risk	X	Lactation Risk	L5
T ½	= 5–7 hours	M/P	=
Vd	= 120 L l/kg	PB	= 55–66%
Tmax	= 2–6 hours	Oral	= 90%
MW	= 258.2	pKa	= 16.74

Adult Concerns: Fatigue, edema, sensory neuropathy, hypocalcemia, dyspnea, thrombosis, rash, nausea, constipation, leukopenia, anemia, increase in liver enzymes levels, weakness, diaphoresis, somnolence.

Pediatric Concerns:

Drug Interactions: Enhanced sedation when used concomitantly with sedative/hypnotics such as barbiturates, benzodiazepines such as carbamazepine, alcohol and reserpine. concomitant use with midazolam and cyclosporine caused their decreased efficacy. Increased risk of toxic epidermal necrolysis when used with dexamethasone. Avoid use with other drugs that cause peripheral neuropathy such as phenytoin, some anti-cancer drugs such as vincristine, antiretroviral drugs, isoniazid, dapsone, fluoroquinolones, amiodarone, hydralazine.

Relative Infant Dose:

Adult Dose: 100–300 mg daily.

Alternatives:

References:
1. Pharmaceutical manufacturer prescribing information, 2011.

THALLIUM-[201]   L3

Trade: Thallium-[201], Thallous chloride Tl [201]

Other Trades:

Category: Radioactive tracer

Thallium-[201] in the form of thallous chloride is used extensively for myocardial perfusion imaging to delineate ischemic myocardium. Following infusion, almost 85% of the administered dose is extracted into the heart on the first pass. Less than 5% of the dose remains free in the plasma in as little as 5 minutes after administration. Whereas Thallium-[201] has a radioactive half-life of only 73 hours, the terminal elimination half-life of the Thallium ion from the body is about 10 days. Most all radiation will be decayed in 5–6 half-lives (15 days). In a study of one breastfeeding patient who received 111MBq (3 mCi) for a brain scan, the amount of Thallium-[201] in breastmilk at 4 hours was 326 Bq/mL and subsequently dropped to 87 Bq/mL after 72 hours.[1] Even without interrupting breastfeeding, the infant would have received less than the NCRP radiation safety guideline dose for infrequent exposure for a 1-year-old infant. However, a brief interruption of breastfeeding was nevertheless recommended. The length of interrupted breastfeeding is dependent on age of infant and dose of Thallium. With an interruption time varying from 2, 24, 48, to 96 hours, the respective Thallium dose to the infant would be 0.442, 0.283, 0.197, and 0.101 MBq compared to the maternal dose of 111 MBq. In another study of a breastfeeding mother who received 111 MBq (3 mCi), the calculated dose an infant (without any interruption of breastfeeding and assuming the consumption of 1000 mL of milk daily) would receive is approximately 0.81 MBq, which is presently less than the maximal allowed radiation dose (NCRP) for an infant.[2] The authors therefore recommend that breastfeeding be discontinued for at least 24–48 hours following the administration of 111 MBq of Thallium-201. The amount of infant exposure from close contact with the mother was also measured and found to be very small in comparison to the orally ingested dose via milk.

Thus the interruption of breastfeeding largely depends on the dose and the volume of milk consumed by the infant. Most authors recommend interruption for 24 up to 96 hours[1,2,3], although the Nuclear Regulatory commission (NRC) recommends interruption for 2 weeks.[4] International Commission of Radiological Protection (ICRP) recommends interruptions of breastfeeding for 48 hours.[5] Estimated radiation exposure from breastmilk is 0.63 mSv after administration of 3 mCi with 48 hours interruption.[1]

Breastfeeding restrictions:

201Tl-chloride (Brain scan): 3 mCi dose: 48 hours interruption.[1,5]

201Tl-chloride (Cardiac perfusion and stress test): 2.5–3.5 mCi: 2 weeks interruption.[4]

Close contact restrictions (6 feet separation from infant) for 201–Tl-chloride at a dose of 3 mCi or less: Avoid close contact for the first 4 hours. Limit close contact to 35 min every 2–3 hours.[1]

Note: These recommendations still permit a minimal amount of <1 mSv of radiation transfer to the infant. Exposure of 1 mSv has a cancer incidence risk of 1 in 10,000 people. This amount of exposure is less than the amount an average American is exposed to from the natural environment (6.2 mSv/year). The only way to avoid all radiation exposure is to wait for 5–10 half-lives, until all of the radioisotope decays (15–30 days).

Pregnancy Risk	C	Lactation Risk		L3 with interruption
T ½	= 73 hours	M/P	=	
Vd	=	PB	=	
Tmax	= <60 minutes	Oral	=	
MW	=	pKa	=	

Adult Concerns: Anaphylaxis, flushing, hypotension, rash, nausea, vomiting, fever, chills, blurred vision, shortness of breath.

Pediatric Concerns: None reported in one case, but a brief interruption for 24–48 hours (depending on dose) is advised.

Drug Interactions:

Relative Infant Dose:

Adult Dose:

Alternatives:

References:
1. Johnston RE, Mukherji SK, Perry RJ, Stabin MG. Radiation dose from breastfeeding following administration of thallium-201. J Nucl Med 1996; 37(12): 2079–2082.
2. Murphy PH, Beasley CW, Moore WH, Stabin MG. Thallium-201 in human milk: observations and radiological consequences. Health Phys 1989; 56(4): 539–541.
3. Stabin MG, Breitz HB. Breast milk excretion of radiopharmaceuticals: mechanisms, findings, and radiation dosimetry. J Nucl Med 2000 May; 41(5): 863–73.
4. Activities of Radiopharmaceuticals from the Nuclear Regulatory Commission.
5. ICRP, 2008. Radiation Dose to Patients from Radiopharmaceuticals–Addendum 3 to ICRP Publication 53. ICRP Publication 106. Ann. ICRP 38 (1–2).

THEOPHYLLINE   L3

Trade: Aminophylline, Quibron, Theo-Dur

Other Trades: Austyn, Nuelin, Theo-Dur, Pulmophylline, Quibron-T/SR

Category: Bronchodilator

Theophylline is a methylxanthine bronchodilator. It has a prolonged half-life in neonates which may cause retention. Milk concentrations are approximately equal to the maternal plasma levels. If a mother is maintained at 10–20 μg/mL, the milk concentrations are closely equivalent. Estimates generally indicate that less than 1% of dose is absorbed by infant. Assuming maternal plasma levels of 10–20 μg/mL, the theophylline levels in a neonate would range from 0.9 to 3.6 μg/mL.[1] In another study of 12 patients receiving 300 mg theophylline, followed 5 hours later by 200 mg, the reported milk concentration was 2.8 mg/L and the milk/plasma ratio ranged from 0.6 to 0.89.[2] The reported maximum concentration was 6.0 mg/L. The relative infant dose would be approximately 5.8% of the weight normalized maternal dose. One reported case of irritability and fretful sleeping was reported in an infant exposed to breastmilk only on days when the mother reported taking theophylline. The average milk concentration of theophylline in this case was 0.7 mg/L.[3]

Pregnancy Risk	C	Lactation Risk	L3
T ½	= 3–12.8 hours	M/P	= 0.67
Vd	= 0.3–0.7 l/kg	PB	= 56%
Tmax	= 1–2 hours (oral)	Oral	= 76%
MW	= 180	pKa	= 8.6

Adult Concerns: Irritability, nausea, vomiting, tachycardia, seizures.

Pediatric Concerns: None reported via milk. One case of irritability and fretful sleeping.

Drug Interactions: Numerous drug interactions exist. Agents that decrease theophylline levels include barbiturates, phenytoin, ketoconazole, rifampin, cigarette smoking, carbamazepine, isoniazid, loop diuretics, and others. Agents that increase theophylline levels include allopurinol, beta blockers, calcium channel blockers, cimetidine, oral contraceptives, corticosteroids, disulfiram, ephedrine, influenza virus vaccine, interferon, macrolides, mexiletine, quinolones, thiabendazole, thyroid hormones, carbamazepine, isoniazid, and loop diuretics.

Relative Infant Dose: 5.9%

Adult Dose: 3 mg/kg every 8 hours.

Alternatives:

References:

1. Stec GP, Greenberger P, Ruo TI, Henthorn T, Morita Y, Atkinson AJ, Jr., Patterson R. Kinetics of theophylline transfer to breast milk. Clin Pharmacol Ther 1980; 28(3): 404–408.
2. Reinhardt D, Richter O, Brandenburg G. [Pharmacokinetics of drugs from the breast-feeding mother passing into the body of the infant, using theophylline as an example]. Monatsschr Kinderheilkd 1983; 131(2): 66–70.
3. Yurchak AM, Jusko WJ. Theophylline secretion into breast milk. Pediatrics 1976; 57(4): 518–520.

THIABENDAZOLE   L3

Trade: Mintezol

Other Trades: Mintezol

Category: Anthelmintic, antiparasitic

Thiabendazole is an antiparasitic agent for the treatment of roundworm, pinworm, hookworm, whipworm, and other parasitic infections.[1] After absorption, it is completely eliminated from the plasma by 48 hours although most is excreted by 24 hours. Can be used in children. Although it is effective in pinworms, other agents with less side effects are preferred. No reports on its transfer to breastmilk have been found.

Pregnancy Risk	C	Lactation Risk	L3
T ½	=	M/P	=
Vd	=	PB	=
Tmax	= 1–2 hours	Oral	= Complete
MW	= 201	pKa	= 4.7

Adult Concerns: Hypotension, nausea, vomiting, psychotic reactions (seizures, hallucinations, delirium), rash, pruritus, intrahepatic cholestasis.

Pediatric Concerns: None reported.

Drug Interactions: May increase theophylline and other xanthines levels by 50%.

Relative Infant Dose:

Adult Dose: 1.5 gm twice daily.

Alternatives: Pyrantel

References:

1. Pharmaceutical manufacturer prescribing information, 2007.

THIAMINE   L1

Trade: Vitamin B₁

Other Trades: Betaxin

Category: Vitamin

Thiamine, also known as Vitamin B_1, is used to treat thiamine deficiency. It is an essential coenzyme in carbohydrate metabolism, combining with adenosine triphosphate to form thiamine pyrophosphate. Thiamine has been shown to cross into human milk, with average concentrations in milk of 200 µg/L under normal circumstances.[1] Thiamine deficiency causes beriberi, which presents with weight loss, mental changes, muscle weakness, or cardiovascular effects. The recommended daily allowance for infants 0 to 12 months is 0.03 mg/kg/day. The recommended daily intake for pregnant and lactating females is 1.2 mg/day. The concentration of thiamine in human milk increases with the progression of lactation, with an average milk level of 200 µg/L.[2] We do not know what milk levels would be following the use of extraordinarily large oral doses, although it appears that it would be a linear increase in milk levels. Supra-therapeutic doses should be avoided in breastfeeding mothers. Long term high doses (3 gm/day) have been associated with adult toxicity.

Pregnancy Risk	A		Lactation Risk	L1	
T ½	=		M/P	=	
Vd	=		PB	=	
Tmax	=		Oral	= Adequate	
MW	= 265		pKa	= 19.26	

Adult Concerns: Adverse reactions include cyanosis, restlessness, nausea, edema, and weakness.

Pediatric Concerns: No data are available.

Drug Interactions:

Relative Infant Dose:

Adult Dose: 1.4 mg daily.

Alternatives:

References:
1. Dietary Reference Intakes for Thiamin, Riboflavin, Niacin, Vitamin B₆, Folate, Vitamin B₁₂, Pantothenic Acid, Biotin, and Choline. Food and Nutrition Board. Institude of Medicine. Washington DC: National Academy Press; 1998.
2. Picciano MF. Handbook of milk composition. Jensen RG, ed. San Diego: Academic Press; 1995.

THIOPENTAL SODIUM   L3

Trade: Pentothal

Other Trades: Pentothal, Intraval

Category: Barbiturate anesthetic agent

Thiopental is an ultra short-acting, barbiturate sedative. Used in the induction phase of anesthesia, it rapidly redistributes from the brain to adipose and muscle tissue; hence, the plasma levels are small, and the sedative effects are virtually gone in 20 minutes. Thiopental sodium is secreted into milk in low levels. In a study of two groups of 8 women who received from 5.0 to 5.4 mg/kg thiopental sodium, the maximum concentration in breastmilk was 0.9 mg/L in mature milk and in colostrum was 0.34 mg/L.[1] The milk/plasma ratio was 0.3 for colostrum and 0.4 for mature milk. The maximum daily dose to infant would be 0.135 mg/kg or approximately 2.5% of the adult dose.

Pregnancy Risk	C	Lactation Risk	L3
T ½	= 3–8 hours	M/P	= 0.3–0.4
Vd	= 1.4 l/kg	PB	= 60–96%
Tmax	= 1–2 minutes	Oral	= Variable
MW	= 264	pKa	= 7.6

Adult Concerns: Hemolytic anemia has been reported. Respiratory depression, renal failure, delirium, nausea, vomiting, pruritus.

Pediatric Concerns: None reported in a study of 16 women receiving induction doses.

Drug Interactions: Increased depression when used with CNS depressants (especially opiates and phenothiazines), and with salicylates or sulfisoxazole.

Relative Infant Dose: 2.6%

Adult Dose: 50–100 mg X 2.

Alternatives:

References:
1. Andersen LW, Qvist T, Hertz J, Mogensen F. Concentrations of thiopentone in mature breast milk and colostrum following an induction dose. Acta Anaesthesiol Scand 1987; 31(1): 30–32.

THIORIDAZINE   L4

Trade: Mellaril
Other Trades: Aldazine, Apo-Thioridazine, Mellaril, Novo-Ridazine
Category: Antipsychotic

Thioridazine is a potent phenothiazine tranquilizer. It has a high volume of distribution and long half-life. No data are available on its secretion into human milk, but it should be expected.[1] Pediatric indications (2–12 years of age) are available although neonatal apnea is associated with this family of drugs.

Pregnancy Risk	C	Lactation Risk	L4
T ½	= 21–24 hours	M/P	=
Vd	= 18 l/kg	PB	=
Tmax	=	Oral	= Complete
MW	= 371	pKa	= 9.5

Adult Concerns: Blood dyscrasias, arrhythmias, sedation, gynecomastia, nausea, vomiting, constipation, dry mouth, retinopathy.

Pediatric Concerns: None reported due to limited studies. Neonatal apnea is common in this family of drugs.

Drug Interactions: Thioridazine is a phenothiazine. Alcohol may enhance CNS depression. Aluminum salts may reduce gastrointestinal absorption. Other anticholinergics may reduce the therapeutic actions of phenothiazines. Barbiturates may reduce phenothiazine plasma levels. Bromocriptine effectiveness may be inhibited by phenothiazines. Propranolol and phenothiazines may result in increased plasma levels of both drugs. Tricyclic antidepressant serum concentrations may be increased with phenothiazines. Valproic acid clearance may be decreased.

Relative Infant Dose:

Adult Dose: 100–400 mg daily.

Alternatives:

References:
1.   O'Brien TE. Excretion of drugs in human milk. Am J Hosp Pharm 1974; 31(9): 844–854.

THIOTHIXENE   L4

Trade: Navane

Other Trades: Navane

Category: Antipsychotic agent

Thiothixene is an antipsychotic agent similar in action to the phenothiazines, butyrophenones, and chlorprothixene. There are no data on its transfer into human milk. Of this family, thiothixene has a rather higher risk of extrapyramidal symptoms and lowered seizure threshold.[1,2] Only two agents in these families have been studied with respect to milk levels: haloperidol and chlorpromazine. Both produced rather low milk levels. However these agents generally have long half-lives and some concern exists for long-term exposure. Observe infant for sedation, seizures, or jerks.

Pregnancy Risk	C	Lactation Risk	L4
T ½	= 34 hours	M/P	=
Vd	=	PB	=
Tmax	= 1–2 hours	Oral	= Complete
MW	= 443	pKa	=

Adult Concerns: Decreases seizure threshold. Sedation, lethargy, extrapyramidal jerking motion.

Pediatric Concerns: None via milk.

Drug Interactions: Thiothixene may be additive when coadministered with other sedative drugs, alcohol, anticholinergics, and hypotensive agents. Aluminum salts may reduce oral absorption of phenothiazines. Anticholinergics may reduce efficacy of thiothixene. Thiothixene may increase tricyclic antidepressant plasma levels.

Relative Infant Dose:

Adult Dose: 5–15 mg three to four times daily.

Alternatives: Haloperidol

References:
1. Drug Facts and Comparisons 1999 ed. ed. St. Louis: 1999.
2. McEvoy GE. (ed): AFHS Drug Information. New York, NY: 2003.

THYROID SCAN   L5

Trade: Thyroid Scan

Other Trades:

Category: Radiographic scan of thyroid gland

Thyroid scanning with ^{131}Iodine or ^{99m}Technetium is useful in delineating structural abnormalities of the thyroid, e.g., to distinguish Grave's disease from multinodular goiter and a single toxic adenoma or to determine the functional state of a single nodule ("hot" vs. "cold"). In one procedure, the radiologist uses radioactive ^{99m}Technetium pertechnetate, which has a short half-life of 6.02 hours. At least 97% of the radioactivity would be decayed in 5 half-lives (30.1 hours), after which it would be presumably safe to breastfeed. In the second procedure (an uptake scan) radioactive ^{131}Iodine is used. The radioactive half-life of ^{131}Iodine is 8.1 days. Five half-lives in this situation is 40.5 days. Although the biologic half-life of iodine would be less than the 40.5 days, it is not known with certainty how long is required before breastmilk samples are at background levels. For safety in this case, breast milk samples should be counted by a gamma counter prior to reinstituting breastfeeding. ^{131}Iodine is sequestered in high concentrations in breastmilk, and breastmilk levels could be exceedingly high. Excessive exposure of the infant's thyroid to ^{131}Iodine is exceedingly dangerous.[1-6]

Pregnancy Risk	Hazardous	Lactation Risk	L5
T ½	= 8 days (radioactive)	M/P	=
Vd	=	PB	=
Tmax	=	Oral	= Complete
MW	= 131	pKa	=

Adult Concerns: High radioactive exposure to the patients thyroid gland. High radioactive exposure to the breasts of breastfeeding mothers if Iodine-131 is used.

Pediatric Concerns: Possible thyroid suppression is possible if high levels of ^{131}I are used. Count breastmilk samples to determine radiation levels.

Drug Interactions:

Relative Infant Dose:

Adult Dose:

Alternatives:

References:
1. American Academy of Pediatrics, Committee on Drugs. Transfer of drugs and other chemicals into human milk. Pediatrics 2001; 108(3): 776–89.

2.   Palmer KE. Excretion of 125I in breast milk following administration of labelled fibrinogen. Br J Radiol 1979; 52(620): 672–673.

3.   Karjalainen P, Penttila IM, Pystynen P. The amount and form of radioactivity in human milk after lung scanning, renography and placental localization by 131 I labelled tracers. Acta Obstet Gynecol Scand 1971; 50(4): 357–361.

4.   Hedrick WR, Di Simone RN, Keen RL. Radiation dosimetry from breast milk excretion of radioiodine and pertechnetate. J Nucl Med 1986; 27(10): 1569–1571.

5.   Romney B, Nickoloff EL, Esser PD. Excretion of radioiodine in breast milk. J Nucl Med 1989; 30(1): 124–126.

6.   Robinson PS, Barker P, Campbell A, Henson P, Surveyor I, Young PR. Iodine-131 in breast milk following therapy for thyroid carcinoma. J Nucl Med 1994; 35(11): 1797–1801.

THYROTROPIN   L1

Trade: Thyrotropin, TSH, Thyrogen

Other Trades: Thytropar

Category: Thyroid-stimulating hormone

Thyrotropin (TSH) is known to be secreted into breastmilk, but in low levels. Virtually none of it would be orally bioavailable or transferred into human milk. Because TSH is significantly elevated in hypothyroid mothers, if present in milk at high levels, it could theoretically cause a hyperthyroid condition in the breastfeeding infant. In a 34-year-old breastfeeding mother with severe hypothyroidism, maternal plasma levels of TSH were measured at 110 mU/L. Milk levels of TSH were 1.4 mU/L.[1] The author suggests that breastmilk TSH was too low to affect thyroid function in a breastfeeding infant, even with milk from a mother with extremely elevated TSH.

Thyrotropin is most often used to detect malignant thyroid nodules. In this situation, it is often used with radioactive Iodine-131. Radioactive Iodine is absolutely contraindicated in breastfeeding women. Be sure that radioactive Iodine-131 is NOT being concomitantly used in this therapy, and if it is, you must stop breastfeeding completely.

Pregnancy Risk	C		Lactation Risk	L1	
T ½	=		M/P	=	
Vd	=		PB	=	
Tmax	=		Oral	= Poor	
MW	= 359		pKa	=	

Adult Concerns: Elevated thyroxine levels in breastfeeding infant.

Pediatric Concerns: None reported via milk. Breastfeeding by hypothyroid mother is permissible.

Drug Interactions:

Relative Infant Dose:

Adult Dose: 10 units daily.

Alternatives:

References:
1.   Robinson P, Hoad K. Thyrotropin in human breast milk. Aust N Z J Med 1994; 24(1): 68.

TIAGABINE   L3

Trade: Gabitril
Other Trades: Gabitril
Category: Anticonvulsant

Tiagabine is a GABA inhibitor useful for the treatment of partial epilepsy. It works by enhancing the activity of gamma aminobutyric acid (GABA), the major inhibitory neurotransmitter in the central nervous system.[1] No data are available on its transfer to human milk. It has been used in pediatric patients 3–10 years of age. Use in women who are breastfeeding only if the benefits clearly outweigh the risks.

Pregnancy Risk	C	Lactation Risk	L3
T ½	= 7–9 hours	M/P	=
Vd	=	PB	= 96%
Tmax	= 45 minutes	Oral	= 90%
MW	= 412	pKa	= 9.4, 13.3

Adult Concerns: Asthenia, sedation, dizziness, headache, mild memory impairment, and abdominal pain and nausea have been reported.

Pediatric Concerns: None reported via milk. Observe for somnolence.

Drug Interactions: Enhanced clearance of tiagabine has been reported when coadministered with carbamazepine, fosphenytoin, phenytoin, primidone, and phenobarbital. Clearance was 60% or more greater when admixed with other enzyme-inducing anti-epileptic drugs (phenobarbital, phenytoin, etc). Valproic acid produces a 10% drop in tiagabine plasma levels but with a significant drop in plasma protein binding (may enhance the effect).

Relative Infant Dose:

Adult Dose: 32–56 mg daily.

Alternatives: Gabapentin, lamotrigine

References:
1. Pharmaceutical manufacturer prescribing information, 2005.

TICAGRELOR   L4

Trade: Brilinta
Other Trades:
Category: Anticoagulant, antiplatelet

Ticagrelor is an anticoagulant similar to clopidogrel and prasugrel. Unlike these other agents, ticagrelor exerts a reversible effect and is not a direct ADP antagonist, but rather prevents ADP from binding to the platelet through allosteric action. There are currently no studies of this drug in breastfeeding women, though it is known to be excreted in the milk of lactating rats. In animal studies, radioactive ticagrelor was found to be in greater concentrations in milk than in the maternal plasma. The majority of the radiation was from unchanged drug, while small amounts were from several different metabolites, of which one, AR-C124910XX, is pharmacologically active. Ticagrelor and its active metabolites are highly protein bound and do not exhibit extensive oral bioavailability.[1,2]

Pregnancy Risk	C	Lactation Risk	L4
T ½	= 6.2–6.9 hours	M/P	=
Vd	=	PB	= 99.7%
Tmax	= 1.5–3 hours	Oral	= 39%
MW	= 522.27	pKa	= 4.12

Adult Concerns: Bleeding, atrial fibrillation, arrhythmia, chest pain, hyper/hypotension, syncope, diarrhea, nausea, vomiting, backache, dizziness, headache, cough.

Pediatric Concerns:

Drug Interactions: Aspirin: Recent studies suggest that high doses of aspirin may decrease the effect of this medication. CYP3A4 Inhibitors: These agents may decrease the metabolism of ticagrelor. NSAIDS: These agents may increase the toxic effects of ticagrelor. Thrombolytic Agents: These agents may increase the risk of bleeding associated with ticagrelor.

Relative Infant Dose:

Adult Dose: 180 mg loading dose, followed by 90 mg twice daily each day afterwards.

Alternatives:

References:
1. Li Y, Landqvist C, Scott GW. Disposition and Metabolism of Ticagrelor, a Novel P2Y12 Receptor Antagonist, in Mice, Rats, and Marmosets. Drug Metab Dispos. 2011 Jun 13.
2. Product Information: BRILINTA(TM) oral tablets, ticagrelor oral tablets. AstraZeneca LP (per manufacturer), Wilmington, DE, 2011.

TICARCILLIN   L1

Trade: Ticar, Timentin

Other Trades: Tarcil, Ticillin, Ticar

Category: Penicillin antibiotic

Ticarcillin is an extended-spectrum penicillin, used only IM or IV, and is not appreciably absorbed via oral ingestion.[1,2] In a study of 2–3 patients who received 1000 mg IV, only trace amounts were detected in milk and were too low to measure.[3] In a study of 10 patients who received 5 gm three times daily IV, the amount of ticarcillin in milk ranged from 2– 2.5 mg/L.[4] Twelve hours after discontinuing ticarcillin, it was undetectable in milk. As with many penicillins, only minimal levels are secreted into milk. Poor oral absorption would limit exposure of breastfeeding infant. May cause changes in gastrointestinal flora and possibly fungal overgrowth. Timentin is ticarcillin with clavulanate added.

Pregnancy Risk	B	Lactation Risk	L1
T ½	= 0.9–1.3 hours	M/P	=
Vd	=	PB	= 54%
Tmax	= 0.5–1.25 hours (IM)	Oral	= Poor
MW	= 384	pKa	= 4.12

Adult Concerns: Neutropenia, anemia, kidney toxicity. Changes in gastrointestinal flora, diarrhea, candida overgrowth.

Pediatric Concerns: None reported via milk. Observe for changes in gastrointestinal flora, diarrhea.

Drug Interactions: Probenecid may increase penicillin levels. Tetracyclines may decrease penicillin effectiveness.

Relative Infant Dose: 0.2%

Adult Dose: 150–300 mg daily.

Alternatives:

References:
1. Facts and Comparisons. St. Louis: 2010..
2. Pharmaceutical manufacturer prescribing information, 1995.
3. Matsuda S. Transfer of antibiotics into maternal milk. Biol Res Pregnancy Perinatol 1984; 5(2): 57–60.
4. von Kobyletzki D, Dalhoff A, Lindemeyer H, Primavesi CA. Ticarcillin serum and tissue concentrations in gynecology and obstetrics. Infection 1983; 11(3): 144–149.

TICLOPIDINE   L4

Trade: Ticlid

Other Trades: Tilodene, Ticlid, Apo-Ticlopidine

Category: Inhibits platelet aggregation

Ticlopidine is useful in preventing thromboembolic disorders, increased cardiovascular mortality, stroke, infarcts, and other clotting disorders. Ticlopidine is reported to be excreted into rodent milk.[1] No data are available on penetration into human breastmilk. However it is highly protein bound, and the levels of ticlopidine in plasma are quite low.

Pregnancy Risk	B	Lactation Risk	L4
T ½	= 12.6 hours	M/P	=
Vd	=	PB	= 98%
Tmax	= 2 hours	Oral	= 80%
MW	= 264	pKa	=

Adult Concerns: Bleeding, neutropenia, maculopapular rash.

Pediatric Concerns: None reported via milk, but caution is recommended.

Drug Interactions: Antacids may reduce absorption of ticlopidine. Chronic cimetidine administration has reduced the clearance of ticlopidine by 50%. Use of aspirin may alter platelet aggregation. Digoxin plasma levels may be slightly decreased by 15%. Theophylline elimination half-life was significantly increased from 8–10 hours.

Relative Infant Dose:

Adult Dose: 250 mg twice daily.

Alternatives:

References:
1. Pharmaceutical manufacturer prescribing information, 1996.

TIGECYCLINE   L3

Trade: Tygacil
Other Trades:
Category: Antibiotic

Tigecycline is a glycylcycline antibiotic similar to related tetracyclines. Tigecycline is not affected by the major mechanisms of resistance, and thus is effective against a broad-spectrum of bacterial pathogens.[1] Tigecycline may cause fetal harm when administered to a pregnant woman, as well as tooth discoloration when used during tooth development. There have been no studies performed on the transmission of tigecycline into a mother's breastmilk, however, due to the limited oral bioavailability, it would be unlikely that the infant would absorb clinically relevant levels over a brief exposure. However, prolonged exposure (>3 weeks) is not recommended.

Pregnancy Risk	D	Lactation Risk	L3
T ½	= 27–42 hours	M/P	=
Vd	= 7–9 l/kg	PB	= 71–89%
Tmax	=	Oral	= Nil
MW	= 586	pKa	= 4.37

Adult Concerns: Adverse effects include nausea, vomiting, diarrhea, fever, and abdominal pain.

Pediatric Concerns: Use of tigecycline during tooth development (fetus-age 8) has resulted in tooth discoloration.

Drug Interactions: Decreased effectiveness of oral contraceptives, increased warfarin exposure, and increased risk of pseudotumor cerebri with retinoic acid derivatives have been observed with concurrent use of tygecycline.

Relative Infant Dose:

Adult Dose: 50 mg IV every 12 hours for 5–14 days.

Alternatives:

References:
1. Pharmaceutical manufacturer prescribing information, 2007.

TIMOLOL   L2

Trade: Blocadren

Other Trades: Tenopt, Timpilo, Apo-Timol, Blocadren, Timoptic, Novo-Timol, Betimolol, Betim, Timoptol

Category: Beta blocker for hypertension and glaucoma

Timolol is a beta blocker used for treating hypertension and glaucoma. It is secreted into milk. Following a dose of 5 mg three times daily, milk levels averaged 15.9 µg/L.[1] Both oral and ophthalmic drops produce modest levels in milk. Breastmilk levels following ophthalmic use of 0.5% timolol drops was 5.6 µg/L at 1.5 hours after the dose.[2] Untoward effects on infant have not been reported. These levels are probably too small to be clinically relevant.

Pregnancy Risk	C		Lactation Risk	L2
T ½	= 4 hours		M/P	= 0.8
Vd	= 1–3 l/kg		PB	= 10%
Tmax	= 1–2 hours		Oral	= 50%
MW	= 316		pKa	= 9.21

Adult Concerns: Hypotension, bradycardia, depression, sedation.

Pediatric Concerns: None reported via milk, but observe for hypotension, weakness, hypoglycemia, sedation, depression.

Drug Interactions: Decreased effect when used with aluminum salts, barbiturates, calcium salts, cholestyramine, NSAIDs, ampicillin, rifampin, and salicylates. Beta blockers may reduce the effect of oral sulfonylureas (hypoglycemic agents). Increased toxicity/effect when used with other antihypertensives, contraceptives, monoamine oxidase inhibitors, cimetidine, and numerous other products. See drug interaction reference for complete listing.

Relative Infant Dose: 1.1%

Adult Dose: 10–20 mg twice daily.

Alternatives: Propranolol, metoprolol

References:
1. Fidler J, Smith V, De Swiet M. Excretion of oxprenolol and timolol in breast milk. Br J Obstet Gynaecol 1983; 90(10): 961–965.
2. Lustgarten JS, Podos SM. Topical timolol and the nursing mother. Arch Ophthalmol 1983; 101(9): 1381–1382.

TINIDAZOLE   L3

Trade: Tindamax

Other Trades: Fasigyn

Category: Antimicrobial agent for protozoal and anaerobic bacterial infections.

Tinidazole is an antimicrobial agent that is sometimes used for the treatment of anaerobic infections and protozoal infections such as intestinal amebiasis, giardiasis and trichomoniasis. It is similar to metronidazole. Tinidazole is highly lipophilic and passes membranes easily attaining high concentrations in virtually all body tissues. Concentrations in saliva and bile are equivalent to that of the plasma compartment.

In a study of 24 women, who received a single IV infusion immediately postpartum of 500 mg, aliquots of milk and serum were collected at 12, 24, 48, 72, and 96 hours after the injection.[1] At 48 and 72 hours, fore and hind milk samples were also taken, whereas at 12 and 24 hours only mixed milk samples were collected. Milk levels at 12 and 24 hours were 5.8 and 3.5 mg/L respectively. Serum levels at 12 and 24 hours averaged 6.1 and 3.7 mg/L respectively. The milk/serum ratios at 12 and 24 hours were 0.94 and 0.95 respectively, further suggesting the high lipid solubility of this product. At 48 and 72 hours, the fore milk levels were 1.28 and 0.32 mg/L respectively. Hind milk levels at these same times were 1.2 and 0.3 respectively. At 96 hours only trace amounts were present in milk and none in serum. As this study was done early postpartum, when milk levels are low and lipid content is low, as well, it should be presumed that milk levels in mature, more lipid rich milk, might actually be higher than reported in this study. The maximum relative infant dose (12 hours) would be 12.1%, but this is assuming milk intake of 150 mL/kg/day.

One other study of 5 women taking a dose of 1600 mg IV reported milk-to-plasma ratios of between 0.62 and 1.39. After 72 hours, the majority of the milk samples were below 0.5 μg/mL. The authors therefore concluded that breastfeeding should be withheld for 72 hours after a 1600 mg IV dose of tinidazole.[2]

Following the oral use of a 2 gram dose, maternal levels at 30 hours are exceedingly low. With this dosage regimen, recommend withholding breastfeeding for 30 hours.

Pregnancy Risk	C		Lactation Risk	L3	
T ½	= 11–14.7 hours		M/P	= 1.28	
Vd	= 0.8 l/kg		PB	= 12%	
Tmax	= 2 hours		Oral	= 100%	
MW	=		pKa	= 4.7	

Adult Concerns: Headaches, confusion, dizziness, fatigue, malaise and weakness occur in 2% or less of patients. Agitation, tingling, numbness, and drowsiness have been reported. Dark-colored urine is common. A metallic or bitter taste has been reported, as well as nausea and anorexia. A disulfiram-like reaction when taken with alcohol.

Pediatric Concerns: Levels in milk were low in 24 women studied, no untoward effects were reported in breastfed infants.

Drug Interactions: None reported.

Relative Infant Dose: 12.2%

Adult Dose: 2 grams daily for 1 to 3 days.

Alternatives: Metronidazole

References:

1. Mannisto PT, Karhunen M, Koskela O et al. Concentrations of tinidazole in breast milk. Acta Pharmacol Toxicol (Copenh) 1983; 53: 254–256.
2. Evaldson GR, Lindgren S, Nord CE, Rane AT. Tinidazole milk excretion and pharmacokinetics in lactating women. Br J Clin Pharmac 1985; 19: 503–507.

TINZAPARIN SODIUM   L3

Trade: Innohep

Other Trades: Logiparin, Innohep

Category: Anticoagulant low molecular weight heparin

Tinzaparin is a depolymerized heparin (low molecular weight heparin)[1] similar to several others such as dalteparin, enoxaparin, nadroparin or parnaparin. The average molecular weight range of tinzaparin is approximately one-half that of regular (unfractionated) heparin (5500–7500 vs 12,000 daltons). No data are available on the transfer of this anticoagulant into human milk but it is likely low. In studies with dalteparin none was found in milk in one study, and only small amounts in another (see dalteparin). In studies with enoxaparin, no changes in anti-Xa activity were noted in breastfed infants. It is very unlikely any would be orally bioavailable.

Other typical low molecular weight heparins: Dalteparin (Fragmin), enoxaparin (Lovenox), nadroparin (Fraxiparin), parnaparin (Fluxum).

Pregnancy Risk	B	Lactation Risk	L3
T ½	= 3–4 hours	M/P	=
Vd	= 3.1–5.0 l/kg	PB	=
Tmax	= 4–5 hours (SC)	Oral	= Nil
MW	= <7500	pKa	=

Adult Concerns: Hemorrhage, thrombocytopenia, hematoma at site of injection, allergic reaction, and vaginal bleeding.

Pediatric Concerns: None reported via milk. Milk levels in other LMWHs are reportedly low, it is likely similar for tinzaparin as well.

Drug Interactions: Do not use with other anticoagulants which includes many NSAIDs, aspirin, herbal remedies, and other agents which inhibit thrombus formation. Check other sources for complete lists.

Relative Infant Dose:

Adult Dose: 175 IU/kg/day (highly variable).

Alternatives: Dalteparin, enoxaparin

References:

1. Pharmaceutical manufacturer prescribing information, 2002.

TIOCONAZOLE   L3

Trade: Monistat 1, Tioconazole 1, Vagistat-1
Other Trades:
Category: Antifungal

Tioconazole is an anti-fungal agent used in the treatment of candida vulvovaginitis.[1] There are no adequate and well-controlled studies or case reports in breast feeding women. Oral bioavailability following topical or vaginal application is minimal to nil. Therefore, it is unlikely that any exposure through breastmilk would be clinically significant in the infant.

Pregnancy Risk	C	Lactation Risk	L3
T ½	=	M/P	=
Vd	=	PB	=
Tmax	=	Oral	= 2.9% (topical), negligible (vaginal)
MW	= 387.7	pKa	= 6.42

Adult Concerns: Burning, Itching, rash, erythema.

Pediatric Concerns:

Drug Interactions:

Relative Infant Dose:

Adult Dose:

Alternatives:

References:
1. Pharmaceutical manufacturer prescribing information, 2011.

TIOPRONIN   L4

Trade: Thiola
Other Trades:
Category: Nephrolithiasis prevention for cystinuria

Tiopronin is a reducing agent used in the treatment of cystinuria. It has similar structure with penicillamine such that it may have similar adverse reactions.[1] Tiopronin has been approved for children aged 9 years or older. Tiopronin is excreted in urine, up to 48% after 4 hours and 78% after 72 hours. There are no data on its transfer to breastmilk; however, manufacturer does not suggest breastfeeding while taking tiopronin. Recommend discontinuing lactation if this drug is mandatory.

Pregnancy Risk	C	Lactation Risk	L4
T ½	= 53 hours	M/P	=
Vd	= 6.5 l/kg	PB	=

Tmax	= 3–6 hours	Oral	= 63%
MW	= 163	pKa	=

Adult Concerns: Fatigue, fever, rash, pruritus, anemia, leukopenia, jaundice, Goodspasture's syndrome, hematuria, loss of smell, bronchiolitis, dyspnea.

Pediatric Concerns:

Drug Interactions:

Relative Infant Dose:

Adult Dose: 1000 mg/day in 3 divided dose.

Alternatives:

References:
1. Thiola. Full prescribing information, Mission Pharmacal Company, San Antonio, TX.

TIZANIDINE   L4

Trade: Zanaflex

Other Trades:

Category: Muscle relaxant

Tizanidine is a centrally acting muscle relaxant. It has demonstrated efficacy in the treatment of tension headache and spasticity associated with multiple sclerosis. It is not known if it is transferred into human milk although the manufacturer states that due to its lipid solubility, it likely penetrates milk.[1] This product has a long half-life, high lipid solubility, and significant CNS penetration, all factors that would increase milk penetration. While the half-life of the conventional formulation is only 4–8 hours, the half-life of the sustained release formulation is 13–22 hours.[2] Further, 48% of patients complain of sedation. Use caution if used in a breastfeeding mother.

Pregnancy Risk	C	Lactation Risk	L4
T ½	= 13–22 hours	M/P	=
Vd	= 2.4 l/kg	PB	= 30%
Tmax	= 1.5 hours	Oral	= 40%
MW	=	pKa	= 7.47

Adult Concerns: Hypotension (49%), sedation (48%), dry mouth, asthenia, dizziness, and other symptoms have been reported. Nausea and vomiting have been reported. A high risk of elevated liver enzymes (5%).

Pediatric Concerns: None reported via milk, but caution is recommended.

Drug Interactions: Alcohol may increase plasma levels of tizanidine by 20%. Oral contraceptives may significantly (50%) reduce clearance of tizanidine.

Relative Infant Dose:

Adult Dose: 8 mg every 6 hours PRN.

Alternatives:

References:
1. Pharmaceutical manufacturer prescribing information, 1999.
2. Wagstaff AJ, Bryson HM. Tizanidine. A review of its pharmacology, clinical efficacy and tolerability in the management of spasticity associated with cerebral and spinal disorders. Drugs 1997; 53(3): 435–452.

TOBRAMYCIN   L3

Trade: Nebcin, Tobrex, Tobi

Other Trades: Tobi, Nebcin, Tobrex, Tobralex

Category: Antibiotic

Tobramycin is an aminoglycoside antibiotic similar to gentamicin.[1] Although small levels of tobramycin are known to transfer into milk, they probably pose few problems. In one study of 5 patients, following an 80 mg IM dose, tobramycin levels in milk ranged from undetectable to 0.5 mg/L in only one patient.[2] In a case report of a mother receiving 150 mg three times daily for 14 days (IV), milk concentrations were determined on day four, before administration, and 60, 120, 180, 240, and 300 minutes after dosing. Tobramycin was undetectable in all samples. The limit of detection was >0.18 mg/L. No untoward effects were noted in the infant.[3] In another study of one mother who received 80 mg every 8 hours (IM), milk levels ranged from 0.6 mg/L at 1 hour to 0.58 mg/L at 8 hours post dose.[4] Levels in milk are generally low, but could produce minor changes in gut flora. As oral tobramycin is not absorbed orally, systemic levels in infant would be unexpected.

Pregnancy Risk	D		Lactation Risk	L3
T ½	= 2–3 hours		M/P	=
Vd	= 0.22–0.31 l/kg		PB	= <5%
Tmax	= 30–90 minutes (IM)		Oral	= Nil
MW	= 468		pKa	= 13.13

Adult Concerns: Changes in gastrointestinal flora.

Pediatric Concerns: Observe for changes in gastrointestinal flora.

Drug Interactions: Increased toxicity when used with certain penicillins, cephalosporins, amphotericin B, loop diuretics, and neuromuscular blocking agents.

Relative Infant Dose: 2.6%

Adult Dose: 1 mg/kg every 8 hours.

Alternatives:

References:
1. Pharmaceutical manufacturer prescribing information, 1996.
2. Takase Z. Laboratory and clinical studies on tobramycin in the field of obstetrics and gynecology. Chemotherapy (Tokyo) 1975; 23: 1402.

3. Festini F, Ciuti R, Taccetti G, Repetto T, Campana S, Martino M. Breast feeding in a woman with cystic fibrosis undergoing antibiotic intravenous treatment. J Matern Fetal Neonatal Med 2006; 19(6): 375–376.
4. Uwaydah M, Bibi S. and Salman S, Therapeutic efficacy of tobramycin--a clinical and laboratory evaluation. J Antimicrob Chemother 1975; 1: 429–437.

TOCAINIDE   L4

Trade: Tonocard

Other Trades: Xylotocan

Category: Antiarrhythmic

Tocainide is an antiarrhythmic reserved for the treatment of ventricular arrhythmias. It is an oral analogue of and similar in structure and pharmacology to lidocaine. In a study of a single patient who received 400 mg every 8 hours, milk and serum levels were drawn 0.5 hours before administration and 2 hours after administration of a 400 mg dose.[1] The reported level in plasma and milk were 5.6 and 12 µg/mL respectively, 0.5 hours before the dose. Levels at 2 hours following the dose were 9.2 and 28 µg/mL respectively. The relative infant dose via milk would then be approximately 24.5% of the weight-normalized maternal dose. Caution is recommended as these levels are quite high and this product is well absorbed.

Pregnancy Risk	C	Lactation Risk	L4
T ½	= 11–22 hours	M/P	= 1.6–2.3
Vd	= 1.4–32 l/kg	PB	= 22%
Tmax	= 0.5–2 hours	Oral	= 100%
MW	= 192	pKa	= 7.7

Adult Concerns: Prolonged QRS complex. Severe vomiting followed by nodal bradycardia. Heart failure, hypotension, pericarditis has been reported.

Pediatric Concerns: None reported via milk.

Drug Interactions: Cimetidine, rifampin, and rifapentine may reduce its effectiveness. Coadministration of lidocaine may increase their combined toxicity.

Relative Infant Dose: 24.5%

Adult Dose: 400 mg three times daily.

Alternatives: Lidocaine

References:
1. Wilson JH. Breast milk tocainide levels. J Cardiovasc Pharmacol 1988 Oct; 12(4): 497.

TOCILIZUMAB   L3

Trade: Actemra

Other Trades:

Category: Interleukin 6 receptor inhibitor

Tocilizumab is an interleukin 6 (IL-6) receptor inhibitor used in the treatment of rheumatoid arthritis (RA). Tocilizumab is used in severe cases of RA or in cases where the RA had a subclinical response to TNF antagonists.[1] The dose starts at 4 mg/kg and is increased to 8 mg/kg depending on clinical response. There are no studies on the passage of tocilizumab into human milk. Tocilizumab has a large molecular weight of 148 kilodaltons and is unlikely to pass into breast milk. The studies on a similar medication, infliximab have shown no passage into milk.

Pregnancy Risk	C	Lactation Risk	L3
T ½	= 6.3 days (single dose); 11–13 days (multiple doses)	M/P	=
Vd	=	PB	=
Tmax	=	Oral	=
MW	= 148 kilodaltons	pKa	=

Adult Concerns: Infections, increased liver enzymes (AST, ALT), neutropenia, local infusion site reactions, dizziness, headache, nasopharyngitis, bronchitis, rash, abdominal pain, diarrhea.

Pediatric Concerns:

Drug Interactions:

Relative Infant Dose:

Adult Dose: 4–8 mg/kg every 4 weeks.

Alternatives: Infliximab

References:
1. Pharmaceutical manufacturer prescribing information, 2011.

TOLBUTAMIDE   L3

Trade: Oramide, Orinase

Other Trades: Apo-Tolbutamide, Mobenol, Novo-Butamide, Orinase, Glyconon, Rastinon

Category: Antidiabetic

Tolbutamide is a short-acting sulfonylurea used to stimulate insulin secretion in type II diabetics. Only low levels are secreted into breastmilk. Following a dose of 500 mg twice daily, milk levels in two patients were 3 and 18 µg/L respectively.[1] Maternal serum levels averaged 35 and 45 µg/L. Observe infant closely for jaundice and hypoglycemia.

Pregnancy Risk	C	Lactation Risk	L3
T ½	= 4.5–6.5 hours	M/P	= 0.09–0.4
Vd	= 0.10–0.15 l/kg	PB	= 93%
Tmax	= 3.5 hours	Oral	= Complete
MW	= 270	pKa	= 5.3

Adult Concerns: Hypoglycemia, nausea, dyspepsia.

Pediatric Concerns: None reported via milk.

Drug Interactions: The hypoglycemic effect may be enhanced by anticoagulants, chloramphenicol, clofibrate, fenfluramine, fluconazole, H_2 antagonists, magnesium salts, methyldopa, monoamine oxidase inhibitors, probenecid, salicylates, tricyclic antidepressants, sulfonamides. The hypoglycemic effect may be reduced by beta blockers, cholestyramine, diazoxide, phenytoin, rifampin, thiazide diuretics.

Relative Infant Dose: 0.004%–0.02%

Adult Dose: 250–2000 mg daily.

Alternatives:

References:
1.   Moiel RH, Ryan JR. Tolbutamide orinase in human breast milk. Clin Pediatr (Phila) 1967; 6(8): 480.

TOLMETIN SODIUM   L3

Trade: Tolectin

Other Trades: Tolectin

Category: Non-steroidal analgesic, used for arthritis, etc.

Tolmetin is a standard non-steroidal analgesic. Tolmetin is known to be distributed into milk but in small amounts. In one patient given 400 mg, the milk level at 0.67 hours was 0.18 mg/L.[1] The estimate of dose per day an infant would receive is 115 µg in 1 L of milk. Tolmetin is sometimes used in pediatric rheumatoid patients (>2 years).

Pregnancy Risk	C/D in 3rd trimester	Lactation Risk	L3
T ½	= 1–1.5 hours	M/P	= 0.0055
Vd	=	PB	= 99%
Tmax	= 0.5–1 hour	Oral	= Complete
MW	= 257	pKa	= 3.5

Adult Concerns: Gastrointestinal distress, bleeding, vomiting, nausea, edema.

Pediatric Concerns: None reported via milk.

Drug Interactions: Tolmetin is an NSAID. May prolong prothrombin time when used with warfarin. Antihypertensive effects of ACE inhibitors may be blunted or completely abolished by NSAIDs. Some NSAIDs may block antihypertensive effect of beta blockers, diuretics. Used with cyclosporin, may dramatically increase renal toxicity. May increase digoxin, phenytoin, lithium levels. May increase toxicity of methotrexate. May increase bioavailability of penicillamine. Probenecid may increase NSAID levels.

Relative Infant Dose: 0.5%

Adult Dose: 200–600 mg three times daily.

Alternatives: Ibuprofen

References:
1. Sagraves R, Waller ES, Goe hours HR. Tolmetin in breast milk. Drug Intell Clin Pharm 1985; 19(1): 55–56.

TOLNAFTATE   L3

Trade: Tinactin, Aftate, Blis-To-Sol, Dermasept Antifungal, Fungi-Guard, Podactin, Q-Naftate, Absorbine Jr. Antifungal

Other Trades:

Category: OTC antifungal

Tolnaftate is a topical antifungal agent that is used in over-the-counter products. There are no adequate and well-controlled studies of tolnaftate use in breastfeeding women. In an *in vitro* study, dermal absorption of 1% tolnaftate from topical application is 0.92 µg/cm^2.[1] It is not recommended for use on the nipple or areas that may be in direct contact with the infant. Water-based creams, liquid, and gels are preferred compared to ointment bases because of possible infant ingestion of mineral paraffins.[2]

Pregnancy Risk	C	Lactation Risk	L3
T ½	=	M/P	=
Vd	=	PB	=
Tmax	=	Oral	=
MW	= 307	pKa	=

Adult Concerns: Local irritation, contact dermatitis, pruritus.

Pediatric Concerns:

Drug Interactions:

Relative Infant Dose:

Adult Dose: 1–3 drop or small amount of cream twice a day.

Alternatives:

References:
1. Kezutyte T, Kornysova O, Maruska A, Briedis V. Assay of tolnaftate in human skin samples after in vitro penetration studies using high performance liquid chromatography. Acta Pol Pharm. 2010 Jul-Aug; 67(4): 327–34.
2. Noti A, Grob K, Biedermann M et al. Exposure of babies to C(15)-C(45) mineral paraffins from human milk and breast salves. Regul Toxicol Pharmacol. 2003; 38: 317–25.

TOLTERODINE   L3

Trade: Detrol

Other Trades: Detrol, Detrusitol

Category: Urinary incontinence

Tolterodine is a muscarinic anticholinergic agent similar in effect to atropine but is more selective for the urinary bladder.[1] Tolterodine levels in milk have been reported in mice, where offsprings exposed to extremely high levels had slightly reduced body weight gain, but no other untoward effects. While it is more selective for the urinary bladder, preclinical trials still showed adverse effects including blurred vision, constipation, and dry mouth in adults. While we have no data on human milk, it is unlikely concentrations will be high enough to produce untoward effects in infants. However, the infant should be monitored for classic anticholinergic symptoms including dry mouth, constipation, poor tearing, etc.

Pregnancy Risk	C	Lactation Risk	L3
T ½	= 1.9–3.7 hours	M/P	=
Vd	= 1.6 l/kg	PB	= 96%
Tmax	= 1–2 hours	Oral	= 77%
MW	=	pKa	= 9.87

Adult Concerns: Blurred vision, constipation, and dry mouth in adults.

Pediatric Concerns: None by milk, but observe for anticholinergic symptoms such as dry mouth, constipation, poor tearing, poor urinary output.

Drug Interactions: Fluoxetine reduces metabolism of tolterodine significantly and may increase plasma levels by 4.8 fold.

Relative Infant Dose:

Adult Dose: 2 mg twice daily.

Alternatives:

References:
1. Pharmaceutical manufacturer prescribing information, 2011.

TOPIRAMATE   L3

Trade: Topamax

Other Trades: Topamax

Category: Anticonvulsant

Topiramate is an anticonvulsant used in controlling refractory partial seizures. In a group of 2 women receiving topiramate (150–200 mg/day) at three weeks postpartum the mean milk/plasma ratio was 0.86 (range=0.67–1.1).[1] The concentration of topiramate in milk averaged 7.9 µM (range=1.6 to 13.7). The weight normalized relative infant dose (RID), assuming a milk intake of 150 mg/kg/day, was 3–23% of the maternal dose/day. The absolute infant dose was 0.1 to 0.7 mg/kg/day. The plasma concentrations of topiramate in two infants were 1.4 and 1.6 µM, respectively. The plasma level in another infant was undetectable. The plasma concentrations in the two infants were 10–20% of the maternal plasma level. At 4 weeks, the milk/plasma ratio had dropped to 0.69 and plasma levels in the infant were <0.9 µM and 2.1 µM, respectively. Topiramate has become increasingly popular due to its fewer adverse side effects.[2-5] Due to the fact that the plasma levels found in breastfeeding infants were significantly less than in maternal plasma, the risk of using this product in breastfeeding mothers is probably acceptable. Close observation for sedation is advised.

Pregnancy Risk	D	Lactation Risk	L3
T ½	= 18–24 hours	M/P	= 0.86
Vd	= 0.7 l/kg	PB	= 15%
Tmax	= 1.5–4 hours	Oral	= 75%
MW	= 339	pKa	= 8.7

Adult Concerns: Topiramate induces a significant cognitive dysfunction, particularly in older patients. Paresthesias, sedation, weight loss(7%), diarrhea.

Pediatric Concerns: None reported in two cases. Milk levels were moderate and infant plasma levels were 10–20% of maternal levels.

Drug Interactions: A 40% decrease in topiramate concentration has been reported when carbamazepine was added to topiramate therapy. Do not use topiramate with dichlorphenamide due to increased risk of nephrolithiasis. Serum digoxin levels (AUC) are decreased by 12% in patients receiving digoxin and topiramate. Efficacy of combination birth control pills may be reduced when adding topiramate. A 25% decrease in phenytoin levels have been reported when topiramate was added. Phenobarbital may reduce half-life of topiramate by 11%.

Relative Infant Dose: 24.5%

Adult Dose: 200 mg twice daily.

Alternatives:

References:
1. Ohman I, Vitols S, Luef G, Soderfeldt B, Tomson T. Topiramate kinetics during delivery, lactation, and in the neonate: preliminary observations. Epilepsia 2002; 43(10): 1157–1160.
2. Patsalos PN, Sander JW. Newer antiepileptic drugs. Towards an improved risk-benefit ratio. Drug Saf 1994; 11(1): 37–67.
3. Bialer M. Comparative pharmacokinetics of the newer antiepileptic drugs. Clin Pharmacokinet 1993; 24(6): 441–452.
4. Britton JW, So EL. New antiepileptic drugs: prospects for the future. J Epilepsy 1995; 8: 267–281.
5. Pharmacokinetics of topiramate in pregnancy and lactation-transplacental transfer and excretion in breast-milk. Fifth Eilat Conference on Antiepileptic Drugs, Eilat, Israel. 00 Jun; 2000.

TOREMIFENE   L4

Trade: Fareston
Other Trades: Fareston
Category: Anticancer drug

Toremifene is a nonsteroidal agent that binds to estrogen receptors without producing an estrogenic response, hence blocking estrogenic activity. It is well absorbed orally (100%).[1] The plasma concentration time profile of toremifene declines biexponentially after absorption, with a mean distribution half-life of about four hours and an elimination half-life of about five days. Toremifene has an apparent volume of distribution of 580 L and binds extensively (>99.5%) to serum proteins, mainly to albumin. No data are available on its transfer to milk, but its molecular weight of 580 and high protein binding will probably reduce its entry into milk. However, the potential for severe interruption of estrogen levels in breastfed infants would largely suggest this agent should not be used in breastfeeding mothers. Breastfeeding mothers should withhold breastfeeding for a minimum of 25–30 days.

Pregnancy Risk	D		Lactation Risk	L4
T ½	= 5 days		M/P	=
Vd	= 580 L/m²		PB	= 99.5%
Tmax	= 3–6 hours		Oral	= Complete
MW	= 598.1		pKa	= 8.0

Adult Concerns: Nausea, sudden sweating and feeling of warmth, blurred vision, change in vaginal discharge, changes in vision, confusion, increased urination, loss of appetite, pain or feeling of pressure in pelvis, tiredness, vaginal bleeding.

Pediatric Concerns:

Drug Interactions: Drugs such as thiazide diuretics, may increase the risk of hypercalcemia in patients receiving toremifene. There is a known interaction with coumarin-type anticoagulants (such as, warfarin) which can lead to an increased prothrombin time.

Relative Infant Dose:

Adult Dose: 60 mg once daily.

Alternatives:

References:
1. Pharmaceutical manufacturer prescribing information, 2005.

TORSEMIDE   L3

Trade: Demadex
Other Trades: Demadex, Torem
Category: Potent Loop diuretic

Torsemide is a potent loop diuretic generally used in congestive heart failure and other conditions which require a strong diuretic.[1] There are no reports of its transfer into human milk. Its extraordinarily high protein binding would likely limit its transfer into human milk. As with many diuretics, reduction of plasma volume and hypotension may adversely reduce milk production although this is rare.

Pregnancy Risk	B	Lactation Risk	L3
T ½	= 3.5 hours	M/P	=
Vd	= 0.21 l/kg	PB	= >99%
Tmax	= 1 hour	Oral	= 80%
MW	= 348	pKa	= 16.74

Adult Concerns: Hypotension, hypokalemia, volume depletion, headache, excessive urination, dizziness.

Pediatric Concerns: None reported. Renal calcification has been reported with other loop diuretics in premature infants, but not via milk supply.

Drug Interactions: When used with salicylates, elevated plasma salicylate levels may occur. Co-administration with other NSAIDS may increase the risk of renal dysfunction. Cholestyramine administration reduces bioavailability of torsemide. Use caution in using with lithium.

Relative Infant Dose:

Adult Dose: 5–10 mg daily.

Alternatives: Furosemide

References:
1. Pharmaceutical manufacturer prescribing information, 1997.

TOXOPLASMA GONDII   L3

Trade: Toxoplasmosis
Other Trades:
Category: Infectious disease

Toxoplasmosis is an infection caused by the parasite *Toxoplasma gondii* commonly spread by eating undercooked meat of infected animals, by contact with the feces of infected cats, or through contact with infected soil or insects in the soil. The infection can get into the blood causing a parasitemia that can get into the placenta and cause fetal infection. Although the disease seems to be self-limited in healthy adults, it can affect the infants of affected mothers. Some of the clinical signs of infection in infants include hearing loss, mental retardation, rash, and seizures. According to the CDC, there are no studies documenting breast milk transmission of toxoplasmosis in humans. Even though the breastfeeding infant was probably exposed to this parasite long before the diagnosis was made, it still may be advisable to withhold breastfeeding until treatment has been initiated.

Pregnancy Risk	Hazardous		Lactation Risk	L3
T ½	=		M/P	=
Vd	=		PB	=
Tmax	=		Oral	=
MW	=		pKa	=

Adult Concerns: Symptoms in adults include cervical lymphadenopathy, fever, night sweats, myalgias, and hepatosplenomegaly.

Pediatric Concerns:

Drug Interactions:

Relative Infant Dose:

Adult Dose:

Alternatives:

References:

TRAMADOL   L2

Trade: Ultram, Ultram ER, Ryzolt, Rybix ODT, FusePaq Synapryn, ConZip
Other Trades: Tramal, Nycodol, Tramake, Zydol, Zamadol, Dromadol
Category: Analgesic

Tramadol is a new class analgesic that most closely resembles the opiates although it is not a controlled substance and appears to have reduced addictive potential. It appears to be slightly more potent than codeine. After oral use, its onset of analgesia is within 1 hour and reaches a peak in 2–3 hours. Following a single IV 100 mg dose of tramadol, the cumulative excretion in breastmilk within 16 hours was 100 µg of tramadol (1.05% of the maternal dose) and 27 µg of the M1 metabolite.[1]

In a recent study of 75 mothers who received 100 mg every 6 hours after cesarean section, milk samples were taken on days 2–4 postpartum in transitional milk.[2] At steady state, the milk/plasma ratio averaged 2.4 for rac-tramadol and 2.8 for rac-O-desmethyltramadol. The estimated absolute and relative infant doses were 112 µg/kg/day and 30 µg/kg/day for rac-tramadol and its desmethyl metabolite. The relative infant dose was 2.24% and 0.64% for rac-tramadol and its desmethyl metabolite, respectively. No significant neurobehavioral adverse effects were noted between controls and exposed infants.

Based on these studies, it may be concluded that tramadol is compatible with breastfeeding.

Pregnancy Risk	C	Lactation Risk	L2
T ½	= 7 hours	M/P	= 2.4
Vd	=	PB	= 20%
Tmax	= 2 hours	Oral	= 60%
MW	= 263	pKa	= 9.4

Adult Concerns: Sedation, respiratory depression, nausea, vomiting, constipation.

Pediatric Concerns: None reported via milk. Observe for sedation. Safety and efficacy for use in those under 16–18 years of age has not been studied.

Drug Interactions: Use with carbamazepine dramatically increases tramadol metabolism and reduces plasma levels. Use with monoamine oxidase inhibitors may increase toxicity.

Relative Infant Dose: 1.1%–2.9%

Adult Dose: 50–100 mg every 4–6 hours PRN.

Alternatives: Hydrocodone

References:
1. Pharmaceutical manufacturer prescribing information, 1996.
2. Ilett KF, Paech MJ, Page-Sharp M, et.al. Use of a sparse sampling study design to assess transfer of tramadol and its O-desmethyl metabolite into transitional breast milk. Br J Clin Pharmacol 65(5): 661–666, 2008.

TRANEXAMIC ACID   L3

Trade: Cyklokapron, Lysteda

Other Trades: Cyklokapron, Tranexamic Acid Injection BP

Category: Antifibrinolytic Agent; Antihemophilic Agent; Hemostatic Agent

Tranexamic acid is used to reduce or prevent hemorrhage (excessive bleeding) in hemophilia and in other bleeding disorders. This is accomplished by inhibiting the conversion of plasminogen to plasmin.[1] From unpublished data from the manufacturer, tranexamic acid is excreted into human milk and is present in the mother's milk at a concentration of about one-hundredth of the corresponding serum concentrations.[1] In one unpublished study, it was determined that after a 2 day treatment of tranexamic acid in lactating women, the milk concentration was approximately 1% of the peak serum concentration. The effects on an infant receiving a small amount of tranexamic acid is not known.

Pregnancy Risk	B	Lactation Risk	L3
T ½	= 2–11 hours	M/P	=
Vd	= 0.39 l/kg	PB	= 3%, primarily to plasminogen
Tmax	= 3 hours	Oral	= 45%
MW	= 157.2	pKa	= 4.77

Adult Concerns: Adverse reactions can include nausea, vomiting, diarrhea, allergic skin reactions, and dizziness

Pediatric Concerns:

Drug Interactions: No drug-drug interaction studies were conducted with tranexamic acid. Because tranexamic acid is antifibrinolytic, the use of a hormonal contraceptive may further exacerbate the increased thrombotic risk associated with combination hormonal contraceptives. Factor IX Complex Concentrates or Anti-inhibitor Coagulant Concentrates -Tranexamic acid is not recommended in patients taking either Factor IX complex concentrates or anti-inhibitor coagulant concentrates because the risk of thrombosis may be increased. Tissue Plasminogen Activators–Concomitant therapy with tissue plasminogen activators may decrease the efficacy of both tranexamic acid and tissue plasminogen activators.

Relative Infant Dose: 1%

Adult Dose: Oral: 1300 mg 3 times daily (3900 mg/day) for up to 5 days during monthly menstruation (for heavy menstrual bleeding).

Alternatives:

References:
1. Pharmaceutical manufacturer prescribing information, 2010.

TRASTUZUMAB   L4

Trade: Herceptin
Other Trades: Herceptin
Category: Anticancer antibody

Trastuzumab is a therapy for women with metastatic breast cancer, whose tumors have too much HER2 protein. For patients with this disease, herceptin is approved for first-line use in combination with paclitaxel. Trastuzumab is a recombinant DNA-derived monoclonal antibody that selectively binds to the extracellular receptor domain of the human epidermal growth factor protein (HER2). The antibody is an IgG1 kappa antibody that binds to HER2 receptor. The manufacturer reports conducting a study in lactating cynomolgus monkeys at doses 25 times the weekly human maintenance dose of 2 mg/kg trastuzumab, which demonstrated that trastuzumab is secreted in their milk (no levels reported).[1] The presence of trastuzumab in the serum of infant monkeys was not associated with any adverse effects on their growth or development from birth to three months of age. It is not known whether trastuzumab is secreted in human milk. IgG levels in colostrum are much higher, but IgG is normally present in mature human milk only at low levels, only 4 mg/dL. After a dose of 2 mg/kg trastuzumab, only 1 in approximately every 432 molecules of IgG would be this drug, thus the dose to infant daily would be infinitesimally small. It is unlikely that levels in mature, human milk will be high enough to produce untoward symptoms in human infants, but this has not yet been demonstrated. Caution is nevertheless recommended.

The risk is low, but unknown at this time. Mothers should probably not breastfeed while taking this medication.

Pregnancy Risk	D	Lactation Risk	L4
T ½	= 5.8 days	M/P	=
Vd	= 44 ml/kg	PB	=
Tmax	=	Oral	= Nil
MW	= 185,000	pKa	=

Adult Concerns: Adverse events include pain, asthenia, fever, chills, back and abdominal pain, headache, nausea, diarrhea, vomiting, insomnia, cough, dyspnea, rhinitis, and rash.

Pediatric Concerns:

Drug Interactions: Increased risk of cardiac toxicity when admixed with anthracyclines, and cyclophosphamide. Paclitaxel may increase the plasma levels of trastuzumab by 1.5 times.

Relative Infant Dose:

Adult Dose: 2 mg/kg/week.

Alternatives:

References:
1. Pharmaceutical manufacturer prescribing information, 2005.

TRAVOPROST   L3

Trade: Travatan, Travatan Z

Other Trades:

Category: Prostaglandin for glaucoma (ophthalmic solution)

Travoprost is a prostaglandin analog that is used to treat intraocular hypertension and open angle glaucoma. Travoprost is undetectable in plasma one hour after eye drops are instilled. The drug appears in rat milk after oral administration but there were no studies located on the use of travoprost and human lactation.[1] Due to its use as an ophthalmic agent, it is unlikely to be absorbed systemically and thus unlikely to enter milk.

Pregnancy Risk	C	Lactation Risk	L3
T ½	= 45 minutes	M/P	=
Vd	=	PB	=
Tmax	= 0.5 hours	Oral	=
MW	= 500.5	pKa	= 14.62

Adult Concerns: May cause increased pigmentation of iris and eyelid along with increased growth and pigmentation of eyelashes. Has caused macular edema. Don't use with contact lenses. Plasma levels undetectable within 1 hour of application to the eye.

Pediatric Concerns:

Drug Interactions:

Relative Infant Dose:

Adult Dose: One drop in affected eye once daily.

Alternatives:

References:
1. Pharmaceutical manufacturer prescribing information, 2006.

TRAZODONE   L2

Trade: Desyrel, Oleptro

Other Trades: Desyrel, Trazorel, Apo-Trazodone, Novo-Trazodone, Molipaxin

Category: Antidepressant, serotonin reuptake inhibitor

Trazodone is an antidepressant whose structure is dissimilar to the tricyclics and to the other antidepressants. In six mothers who received a single 50 mg dose, the milk/plasma ratio averaged 0.14.[1] Peak milk concentrations occurred at 2 hours and were approximately 110 µg/L (taken from graph) and declined rapidly thereafter. On a weight basis, an adult would receive 0.77 mg/kg whereas a breastfeeding infant, using this data, would consume only 0.005 mg/kg. The authors estimate that about 0.6% of the maternal dose was ingested by the infant over 24 hours. Milk levels are probably low to be clinically relevant in the breastfed infant.

Pregnancy Risk	C		Lactation Risk	L2
T ½	= 4–9 hours		M/P	= 0.142
Vd	= 0.9–1.5 l/kg		PB	= 85–95%
Tmax	= 1–2 hours		Oral	= 65%
MW	= 372		pKa	= 6.74

Adult Concerns: Dry mouth, sedation, hypotension, blurred vision.

Pediatric Concerns: None reported via milk.

Drug Interactions: May enhance the CNS depressant effect of alcohol, barbiturates, and other CNS depressants. Digoxin serum levels may be increased. Use caution when administering with monoamine oxidase inhibitors. Phenytoin serum levels may be increased. Use with warfarin may increase anticoagulant effect.

Relative Infant Dose: 2.8%

Adult Dose: 150–400 mg daily.

Alternatives:

References:
1. Verbeeck RK, Ross SG, McKenna EA. Excretion of trazodone in breast milk. Br J Clin Pharmacol 1986; 22(3): 367–370.

TRETINOIN   L4/L3

Trade: Retin-A, Renova
Other Trades: Vesanoid, Retin-A, Stieva-A, Vitamin A, Acid, Renova
Category: Treatment of acne

Tretinoin is a retinoid derivative similar to Vitamin A. It is primarily used topically for acne and wrinkling and sometimes administered orally for leukemias and psoriasis. Used topically, tretinoin stimulates epithelial turnover and reduces cell cohesiveness.[1] Blood concentrations measured 2–48 hours following application are essentially zero. Absorption of Retin-A via topical sources is reported to be minimal, and breastmilk would likely be minimal to none.[2] However, if it is used orally, transfer into milk is likely and should be used with great caution in a breastfeeding mother.

Pregnancy Risk	D oral/C topical	Lactation Risk	L4 orally/L3 topically
T ½	= 2 hours	M/P	=
Vd	= 0.44 l/kg	PB	=
Tmax	=	Oral	= 70%
MW	= 300	pKa	= 4.79

Adult Concerns: Leukocytosis, dry skin, skin irritation, blistering, scaling, pigmentary changes, nausea, vomiting. Side effects of oral use are similar to hypervitaminosis A, and include headache, increased CSF pressure, anorexia, nausea, scaling of skin, fatigue, hepatosplenomegaly.

Pediatric Concerns: None reported via milk. Do not breastfeed if used orally.

Drug Interactions: Use other topical medications such as sulfur, resorcinol, benzoyl peroxide or salicylic acid with caution due to accelerated skin irritation.

Relative Infant Dose:

Adult Dose: Variable.

Alternatives:

References:
1. Zbinden G. Investigation on the toxicity of tretinoin administered systemically to animals. Acta Derm Verereol Suppl(Stockh) 1975; 74: 36–40.
2. Lucek RW, Colburn WA. Clinical pharmacokinetics of the retinoids. Clin Pharmacokinet 1985; 10(1): 38–62.

TRIAMCINOLONE ACETONIDE | L3

Trade: Nasacort, Azmacort, Tri-Nasal, Cinolar, Triesence, Trianex, Triamcot, Oralone

Other Trades: Aristocort, Kenalone, Aristocort, Azmacort, Kenalog, Triaderm, Nasacort, Adcortyl

Category: Corticosteroid

Triamcinolone is a typical corticosteroid that is available for topical, intranasal, injection, inhalation, and oral use. When administered intranasally to the nose or by inhalation to the lungs, only minimal doses are used and plasma levels are exceedingly low to undetectable.[1] When applied topically, absorption varies between 1–36% depending on amount used and surface area covered on application.[2] Absorption after topical application is promoted with use of higher doses, increased dosing frequency and use of occlusive dressings.[3,4] Derendorf,[5] found that absorption was complete within two to three weeks after intra-articular injection and low systemic levels of corticosteroid were attained. Although no data are available on triamcinolone secretion into human milk, it is likely that the milk levels would be exceedingly low and not clinically relevant when administered via inhalation or intranasally. There is virtually no risk to the infant following use of the intranasal or aerosol products in breastfeeding mothers. With topical application, limit the dose and frequency of use. For intra-articular and intramuscular injections, mothers should pump and discard for a minimum of 12 hours after injection.

Pregnancy Risk	C		Lactation Risk	L3
T ½	= Intranasal/inhalation/oral: 88 minutes; IM/joint: 18–36 hours		M/P	=
Vd	= IM: 99.5 L l/kg		PB	= IM: 68%
Tmax	= IM: 8 to 10 hours		Oral	= Complete
MW	= 434		pKa	= 13.4

Adult Concerns: Intranasal and inhaled: nasal irritation, dry mucous membranes, sneezing, throat irritation, hoarseness, candida overgrowth.

Pediatric Concerns: None reported via milk. Observe growth rate.

Drug Interactions: Concurrent use of triamcinolone and rotavirus vaccine is contraindicated. Concurrent use of triamcinolone and quetiapine may result in decreased serum quetiapine concentrations. Concurrent use of triamcinolone and fluoroquinolones may result in increased risk of tendon rupture.

Relative Infant Dose:

Adult Dose: 220 µg/day (intranasal), 200 µg 3–4 times daily (inhaled), 4–48 mg/day(oral), 2.5–15 mg (intra-articular), 40–80 mg (IM).

Alternatives:

References:

1. Pharmaceutical manufacturer prescribing information, 1996.
2. Kelly R and Keipert JA: Selecting a topical corticosteroid. Curr Ther 1979; 20: 89,90,93–95.
3. Pellanda C, Strub C, Figueiredo V, Rufli T, Imanidis G, Surber C. Topicalbioavailability of triamcinolone acetonide: effect of occlusion. Skin PharmacolPhysiol. 2007; 20(1): 50–6.
4. Pellanda C, Ottiker E, Strub C, Figueiredo V, Rufli T, Imanidis G, Surber C.Topical bioavailability of triamcinolone acetonide: effect of dose andapplication frequency. Arch Dermatol Res. 2006 Oct; 298(5): 221–30.
5. Derendorf H, Möllmann H, Grüner A, Haack D, Gyselby G. Pharmacokinetics and pharmacodynamics of glucocorticoid suspensions after intra-articular administration. Clin Pharmacol Ther. 1986 Mar; 39(3): 313–7.

TRIAMTERENE   L3

Trade: Dyrenium

Other Trades: Dyazide, Hydrene, Dyrenium

Category: Diuretic

Triamterene is a potassium-sparing diuretic, commonly used in combination with thiazide diuretics such as hydrochlorothiazide. Plasma levels average 26–30 ng/mL.[1] No data are available on the transfer of triamterene into human milk, but it is known to transfer into animal milk. Because of the availability of other less dangerous diuretics, triamterene should be used as a last resort in breastfeeding mothers.

Pregnancy Risk	C		Lactation Risk	L3
T ½	= 1.5–2.5 hours		M/P	=
Vd	=		PB	= 55%
Tmax	= 1.5–3 hours		Oral	= 30–70%
MW	= 253		pKa	= 6.2

Adult Concerns: Leukopenia, hyperkalemia, diarrhea, nausea, vomiting, hepatitis.

Pediatric Concerns: None reported via milk.

Drug Interactions: Hyperkalemia when administered with potassium supplements. Triamterene may reduce clearance of amantadine. May increase plasma potassium levels when administered with amiloride, or ACE inhibitors, cyclosporine. May reduce clearance of lithium. Enhanced bone marrow suppression when administered with methotrexate. Use with spironolactone may result in hyperkalemia.

Relative Infant Dose:

Adult Dose: 25–100 mg daily.

Alternatives: Hydrochlorothiazide

References:
1. Mutschler E, Gilfrich HJ, Knauf H, Mohrke W, Volger KD. Pharmacokinetics of triamterene. Clin Exp Hypertens A 1983; 5(2): 249–269.

TRIAZOLAM   L3

Trade: Halcion

Other Trades: Apo-Triazo, Halcion, Novo-Triolam

Category: Benzodiazepine (Valium-like) hypnotic

Triazolam is a typical benzodiazepine used as a nighttime sedative. Animal studies indicate that triazolam is secreted into milk although levels in human milk have not been reported.[1] As with all the benzodiazepines, some penetration into breastmilk is likely. Observe for sedation in the breastfed infant.

Pregnancy Risk	X		Lactation Risk	L3
T ½	= 1.5–5.5 hours		M/P	=
Vd	= 1.1–2.7 l/kg		PB	= 89%
Tmax	= 0.5–2 hours		Oral	= 85%
MW	= 343		pKa	= 1.5

Adult Concerns: Sedation, addiction.

Pediatric Concerns: None reported for triazolam, but side effects for benzodiazepines include sedation, depression.

Drug Interactions: Additive CNS depressant effects when used with other benzodiazepines, barbiturates, anticonvulsants, anesthetics, antihistamines, opiates or alcohol. Use with itraconazole, ketoconazole and nefazodone is contra-indicated. Use with isoniazid, oral contraceptives, ranitidine and grapefruit juice increases the plasma levels and efficacy of triazolam. Caution while coadministering with the following: ergotamine, cyclosporine, amiodarone, nicardipine, and nifedipine

Relative Infant Dose:

Adult Dose: 0.125–0.25 mg daily.

Alternatives: Lorazepam, alprazolam

References:
1.   Facts and Comparisons. St. Louis: 2010.

TRICLOSAN   L3

Trade:

Other Trades:

Category: Antibacterial

Triclosan is a chlorinated phenol compound used in antiseptic hygiene products. In a study including 36 mothers, investigators reported a low level of triclosan up to 0.95 ng/g of breastmilk from the use of triclosan-containing products (toothpaste, soap, and etc).[1] The authors extrapolate 11–570 ng/day of triclosan ingested by breastfed infant per day. Women who used triclosan containing toothpaste have a higher plasma level of triclosan. In another study, milk samples from 62 mothers had up to 35.8 ng of triclosan per 1 gm of breastmilk.[2] The authors calculated a maximum of 7.4 µg/kg/day of triclosan may be ingested by breastfed infant. Based on no observed adverse effect level (NOAEL) of 50 mg/kg/day for triclosan, infant exposure to it is very small. Two studies have shown decreased serum thyroxine levels or impaired thyroid homeostasis in rats and fetal toxicity in offspring.[34] Triclosan absorbed through skin have been indicated to be 6.3% in one study.[5] Greater than 80% of absorbed triclosan is metabolized to triclosan glucuronide and triclosan sulfate by the skin.

Pregnancy Risk	Probably Safe	Lactation Risk	L3
T ½	= 21 hours	M/P	= 0.25
Vd	=	PB	= 99%
Tmax	= 1–3 hours	Oral	= Dermal absorption 6.7%
MW	= 289.5	pKa	= 7.9

Adult Concerns: Can cause hypersensitivity reactions such as skin redness, irritation, and rash

Pediatric Concerns:

Drug Interactions:

Relative Infant Dose: 0.06%

Adult Dose:

Alternatives:

References:

1. Allmyr M, Adolfsson-Erici M, McLachlan MS, Sandborgh-Englund G. Triclosan in plasma and milk from Swedish nursing mothers and their exposure via personal care products. Sci Total Environ. 2006 Dec 15; 372(1): 87–93. Epub 2006 Sep 26.
2. Dayan AD. Risk assessment of triclosan [Irgasan] in human breast milk. Food Chem Toxicol. 2007 Jan; 45(1): 125–9. Epub 2006 Aug 30.
3. Rodriguez PE, Sanchez MS. Maternal exposure to triclosan impairs thyroid homeostasis and female pubertal development in Wistar rat offspring. J Toxicol Environ Health A. 2010; 73(24): 1678–88.
4. Paul KB, Hedge JM, Devito MJ, Crofton KM. Developmental triclosan exposure decreases maternal and neonatal thyroxine in rats. Environ Toxicol Chem. 2010 Dec; 29(12): 2840–4. doi: 10.1002/etc.339. Epub 2010 Oct 15.
5. Moss T, Howes D, Williams FM. Percutaneous penetration and dermal metabolism of triclosan (2,4, 4-trichloro-2-hydroxydiphenyl ether). Food Chem Toxicol. 2000 Apr; 38(4): 361–70.

TRIFLUOPERAZINE   L3

Trade:

Other Trades: Apo-Trifluoperazine, Novo-Trifluzine, PMS-Trifluoperazine, Terfluzine

Category: Antipsychotic, phenothiazine

Trifluoperazine is an antipsychotic drug used for the treatment of schizophrenia and anxiety. Though there is limited information regarding the matter, it appears that doses of this drug up to 10 mg each day do not have adverse effects in breastfed infants. Limited long-term follow-up data indicates that adverse effects do not develop in children who are administered other drugs of this class. Combination therapies should be avoided due to the possibility of negative effects from breastfeeding. Reports from two mothers indicate that use of trifluoperazine at doses of 5 and 10 mg did not result in measurable levels in milk. It has also been observed that concentrations of this drug were undetectable(<2 µg/L) in infant urine during maternal therapy while breastfeeding.[1] Trifluoperazine does enter the infant's blood stream, as evidenced by one report wherein an infant showed plasma levels of 1 µg/L following the use of 10 mg/day by the mother. This concentration may have occurred due to the use of trifluoperazine during pregnancy.[2] No adverse effects have been reported in infants who were exposed to trifluoperazine in breastmilk.[1,2,3] Another study that involved twelve mothers observed the effects of haloperidol, chlorpromazine, and trifluoperazine on breastfeeding. It was found that up to 3% per kilogram of body weight of the administered maternal dose was transferred to the infant through breastmilk. Small levels of drug were present in both infant plasma and urine. Those infants who were exposed to combination therapy containing haloperidol and chlorpromazine showed a decline in developmental scores, while those who were exposed to single drug regimens did not show adverse effects. Caution may be needed when the mother is prescribed one or two antipsychotics at near maximum doses.[1] It should be noted that trifluoperazine and other drugs in its class can cause galactorrhea due to increasing prolactin levels.[4–8] The hyperprolactinemia is likely due to dopamine-blocking action in the tuberoinfundibular pathway of the pituitary.[9]

Pregnancy Risk	Probably Safe	Lactation Risk	L3
T ½	= 24 hours	M/P	=
Vd	=	PB	= 90–99%
Tmax	= 2–4 hours	Oral	=
MW	= 480.4	pKa	=

Adult Concerns: Cardiac arrest, hypotension, orthostatic hypotension, extrapyramidal symptoms, headache, dizziness, photosensitivity, discoloration of skin, breast pain, galactorrhea, hyperglycemia, hypoglycemia, constipation, nausea, vomiting, dry mouth, sexual dysfunction.

Pediatric Concerns:

Drug Interactions: CYP1A2 Inhibitors–These agents may decrease the metabolism of trifluoperazine. Droperidol–Trifluoperazine may enhance the depressant effect of this drug. Methotrimeprazine–Trifluoperazine may enhance the depressant effect of this drug. Metoclopramide–This drug may enhance the toxic effects of antipsychotics.

Relative Infant Dose:

Adult Dose: 1–2 mg twice daily, up to 15–20 mg twice daily.

Alternatives:

References:
1. Yoshida K, Smith B, Craggs M et al. Neuroleptic drugs in breast-milk: a study of pharmacokinetics and of possible adverse effects in breast-fed infants. Psychol Med. 1998; 28: 81–91.
2. Birnbaum CS, Cohen LS, Bailey JW et al. Serum concentrations of antidepressants and benzodiazepines in nursing infants: a case series. Pediatrics. 1999; 104: e11.

3. Goldstein DJ, Corbin LA, Fung MC. Olanzapine-exposed pregnancies and lactation: early experience. J Clin Psychopharmacol. 2000; 20: 399–403.
4. Polishuk WZ, Kulcsar S. Effects of chlorpromazine on pituitary function. J Clin Endocrinol Metab. 1956; 16: 292–3.
5. Hooper JH Jr, Welch VC, Shackelford RT. Abnormal lactation associated with tranquilizing drug therapy. JAMA. 1961; 178: 506–7.
6. Turkington RW. Prolactin secretion in patients treated with various drugs: phenothiazines, tricyclic antidepressants, reserpine, and methyldopa. Arch Intern Med. 1972; 130: 349–54.
7. Turkington RW. Serum prolactin levels in patients with gynecomastia. J Clin Endocrinol Metab. 1972; 34: 62–6.
8. Meltzer HY, Fang VS. The effect of neuroleptics on serum prolactin in schizophrenic patients. Arch Gen Psychiatry. 1976; 33: 279–86.
9. Maguire GA. Prolactin elevation with antipsychotic medications: mechanisms of action and clinical consequences. J Clin Psychiatry. 2002; 63(suppl 4): 56–62.

TRIFLURIDINE OPHTHALMIC DROPS | L3

Trade: Viroptic

Other Trades:

Category: Antiviral agent

Trifluridine, also known as trifluorothymidine, is a fluorinated pyrimidine nucleoside used in the treatment of both epithelial keratitis and keratoconjunctivitis of the eye which is caused by herpes simplex viruses 1 and 2. The drug interferes with DNA synthesis in cultured mammalian cells, but the actual mechanism of action is unknown. The major metabolite is 5-carboxy-2'-deoxyuridine. If the corneal epithelium is not intact, there is a two fold increase in penetration of the drug into the eye. Trifluridine is not effective against infections of the cornea by chlamydia, bacteria, or fungi. Trifluridine should not be used longer than 21 days. Systemic absorption of trifluridine ophthalmic preparation following therapeutic dosing appears to be negligible. No detectable concentrations of trifluridine or 5-carboxy-2'-deoxyuridine were found in the sera of adult healthy normal subjects who had trifluridine instilled into their eyes seven times daily for 14 consecutive days. Trifluridine ophthalmic drops are unlikely to be excreted in human milk after ophthalmic instillation because of the relatively small dosage (<5 mg/day), its dilution in body fluids and its extremely short half-life (approximately 12 minutes). The drug should not be prescribed for nursing mothers unless the potential benefits outweigh the potential risks.[1]

Pregnancy Risk	C	Lactation Risk	L3
T ½	= 12 minutes	M/P	=
Vd	=	PB	=
Tmax	=	Oral	=
MW	= 296.2	pKa	= 13.91

Adult Concerns: Most common side effects: transient burning or stinging and palpebral edema. Less common side effects: contact dermatitis, impaired stomal wound healing and increased ocular pressure.

Pediatric Concerns:

Drug Interactions:

Relative Infant Dose:

Adult Dose: 1 drop every 2 hours, total 9 drops/day until corneal ulcer is healed; followed by 1 drop every 4 hours, total 5 drops/day for 7 days. Treatment should not exceed 21 days.

Alternatives:

References:
1. NLM. Daily Med. U.S. Dept of Health and Human Services. June 1, 2010. Available at: daily. nlm.nih.gov/dailymed/about.cfm. Accessed March 30, 2011.
2. Carmine AA, Brogden RN, Heel RC, Speight TM, Avery GS. Trifluridine: a review of its antiviral activity and therapeutic use in the topical treatment of viral eye infections. Drugs. 1982 May; 23(5): 329–53.

TRIMEBUTINE MALEATE   L3

Trade: Timotor, Debridat, Recutin, Polybutin

Other Trades: Apo-Trimebutine, Modulon

Category: 5HT3 receptor antagonist

Trimebutine is a spasmolytic agent with some opioid agonistic action. It is used to treat irritable bowel syndrome and to accelerate intestinal transit following abdominal surgery.[1] Trimebutine maleate is not available in the U.S. No data are available on the use of this product in breastfeeding mothers. However, a review of its pharmacokinetic properties suggests that transfer into breastmilk is likely. Therefore, use of this drug during lactation is best avoided and should be used only if the potential benefits to the mother outweigh the potential risks to the infant.

Pregnancy Risk	Possibly Hazardous	Lactation Risk	L3
T ½	= 10–12 hours	M/P	= 78–82
Vd	=	PB	= <5%
Tmax	= 1 hour	Oral	=
MW	= 387	pKa	= 6.71

Adult Concerns: Adverse reactions include dry mouth, diarrhea, foul taste, epigastric pain, nausea, drowsiness, and headache.

Pediatric Concerns: Not recommended for patients under 12 years of age.

Drug Interactions: Neuromuscular blocking agents may have prolonged effects.

Relative Infant Dose: 0%

Adult Dose: 20 mg three times daily.

Alternatives:

References:
1. Pharmaceutical manufacturer prescribing information, 2002.

TRIMEPRAZINE   L3

Trade: Temaril, Alimemazine, Levoprome
Other Trades: Panectyl, Vallergan
Category: Antihistamine, antipruritic.

Trimeprazine is an antihistamine from the phenothiazine family used for itching, common cold and as an anti-emetic in motion sickness.[1] It has also been used to induce sedation in young children.[2] Its use in infants is limited due to the increased risk of apnea and sudden infant death syndrome (SIDS). It is secreted into human milk but in very low levels.[3] Exact data is not available. The use of this drug in lactating women is best avoided.

Pregnancy Risk	C	Lactation Risk	L3
T ½	= 5–8 hours	M/P	=
Vd	=	PB	=
Tmax	= 3.5–4.5 hours	Oral	= 70%
MW	= 298	pKa	= 9.1

Adult Concerns: Sedation, hypotension, bradycardia.

Pediatric Concerns: None reported, but as with other antihistamines, observe for sedation.

Drug Interactions: Do not use concomitantly with other CNS depressants such as barbiturates, benzodiazepines, anticonvulsants, anesthetics, opioid narcotics, antihistamines and alcohol. Use with monoamine oxidase inhibitors increases the plasma levels of trimeprazine. Trimeprazine decreases the effect of heparin and other anti-coagulants.

Relative Infant Dose:
Adult Dose: 5 mg twice daily.
Alternatives:

References:
1. Levoprome, Flexyx on-line drug info.
2. Vallergan product information, pages 1–6, date of TGA approval 2 Feb 2011.
3. O'Brien TE. Excretion of drugs in human milk. Am J Hosp Pharm 1974; 31(9): 844–854.

TRIMETHADIONE   L4

Trade: Tridione
Other Trades:
Category: Anticonvulsant

Trimethadione is an oxazolidinedione compound used as an anticonvulsant.[1] There are no adequate and well-controlled studies or case reports in breastfeeding women. Due to its numerous side effects and toxicities, including significant risks of blood dyscrasias, this is not a preferred anticonvulsant for breastfeeding mothers.

Pregnancy Risk	D	Lactation Risk	L4
T ½	=	M/P	=
Vd	=	PB	= 90%
Tmax	= 0.5 to 2 hours	Oral	= Complete
MW	= 143	pKa	=

Adult Concerns: Nausea, vomiting, abdominal pain, anorexia, weight loss, gastric distress. Observe for blood dyscrasias including aplastic anemia, neutropenia, agranulocytosis, and bleeding disorders. Hepatitis and jaundice have been reported.

Pediatric Concerns:

Drug Interactions: Caution while administering with other CNS depressants such as barbiturates, benzodiazepines, other anticonvulsants, anti-histamines, opioid narcotics and alcohol.

Relative Infant Dose:

Adult Dose: 900 mg/day in 3–4 divided doses.

Alternatives:

References:
1.   Trimethadione package insert.

TRIMETHOBENZAMIDE   L4

Trade: Tigan, Trimazide, Tebamide, T-Gen, Arrestin, Ticon
Other Trades:
Category: Antiemetic, antivertigo

Trimethobenzamide is an older generation antiemetic whose use has been supplanted by newer more effective agents.[1] It is most commonly used in suppository form in adults and rarely in infants. Maternal plasma levels following a 500 mg oral dose are 1–2 µg/mL. No data are available on breastmilk levels. But if one were to assume a milk/plasma ratio of 1.0 (which is probably high), then the theoretical infant dose would only be about 0.3 mg/kg/day, which is far less than the oral dose of 300–400 mg/day used in 15 kg infants. It is unlikely the amount of trimethobenzamide present in breastmilk would produce a clinical effect in an infant.

Pregnancy Risk	C	Lactation Risk	L4
T ½	= Short	M/P	=
Vd	=	PB	=
Tmax	=	Oral	= Good
MW	=	pKa	= 8.27

Adult Concerns: Extrapyramidal symptoms, drowsiness, depression, dizziness, headache, vertigo, blood dyscrasias have been reported following higher oral/IM/rectal doses.

Pediatric Concerns: None reported via milk.

Drug Interactions: Concomitant use with metoclopramide is contra-indicated due to increased risk of extrapyramidal symptoms.

Relative Infant Dose:

Adult Dose: 250 mg three to four times daily.

Alternatives: Ondansetron

References:
1. Drug Facts and Comparisons 1999 ed. ed. St. Louis: 1999.

TRIMETHOPRIM   L2

Trade: Proloprim, Trimpex
Other Trades: Alprim, Triprim, Proloprim, Ipral, Monotrim Monotrim, Tiempe
Category: Antibiotic

Trimethoprim is an inhibitor of folic acid production in bacteria. In one study of 50 patients, average milk levels were 2.0 mg/L.[1] Milk/plasma ratio was 1.25. In another group of mothers receiving 160 mg 2–4 times daily, concentrations of 1.2 to 5.5 mg/L were reported in milk. Because it may interfere with folate metabolism, its long-term use should be avoided in breastfeeding mothers, or the infant should be supplemented with folic acid. However, trimethoprim apparently poses few problems in full term or older infants where it is commonly used clinically.[2]

Pregnancy Risk	C	Lactation Risk	L2
T ½	= 8–10 hours	M/P	= 1.25
Vd	=	PB	= 44%
Tmax	= 1–4 hours	Oral	= Complete
MW	= 290	pKa	= 6.6

Adult Concerns: Rash, pruritus nausea, vomiting, anorexia, altered taste sensation.

Pediatric Concerns: None reported via milk.

Drug Interactions: May increase phenytoin plasma levels.

Relative Infant Dose: 3.9%–9%

Adult Dose: 80 mg twice daily, 160 mg twice daily, 200 mg daily.

Alternatives:

References:
1. Miller RD, Salter AJ. The passage of trimethoprim/sulphamethoxazole into breast milk and its significance. In Daikos GK, ed. Progress in Chemotherapy, Proceedings of the Eight International Congress of Chemotherapy, Athens, 1973. Athens: Hellenic Society for Chemotherapy, 1974.
2. Pagliaro, Levin. Problems in Pediatric Drug Therapy. Hamilton, IL: Drug Intelligence Publications, 1979.
3. Arnauld R. Etude du passage de la trimethoprime dans le lait maternel.Ouest Med. 1972; 25: 959.
4. American Academy of Pediatrics, Committee on Drugs. Transfer of drugs and other chemicals into human milk. Pediatrics 2001; 108(3): 776–89.

TRIPELENNAMINE   L4

Trade: Pyribenzamine
Other Trades:
Category: Antihistamine

Tripelennamine is an older class of antihistamine. This product is generally not recommended in pediatric patients, particularly neonates due to increased sleep apnea.[1] The drug has been shown to be secreted into milk of animals.[2] No human data exist.

Pregnancy Risk	B		Lactation Risk	L4
T ½	= 2–3 hours		M/P	=
Vd	= 9–12 l/kg		PB	=
Tmax	= 2–3 hours		Oral	= Complete
MW	= 255		pKa	= 4.2, 8.7

Adult Concerns: Sleep apnea in children, peptic ulcer, sedation, dry mouth, gastrointestinal distress.

Pediatric Concerns: None reported, but observe for sedation, sleep apnea.

Drug Interactions: Increased sedation when used with CNS depressants, other antihistamines, alcohol, monoamine oxidase inhibitors.

Relative Infant Dose:

Adult Dose: 25–50 mg every 4–6 hours.

Alternatives:

References:
1. O'Brien TE. Excretion of drugs in human milk. Am J Hosp Pharm 1974; 31(9): 844–854.
2. Pharmaceutical manufacturer prescribing information, 1996.

TRIPROLIDINE   L1

Trade: Zymine, Tripohist
Other Trades:
Category: Antihistamine

Triprolidine is an antihistamine. It is secreted into milk but in very small levels and is marketed with pseudoephedrine as Actifed. In a study of three patients who received 2.5 mg triprolidine, the average concentration in milk ranged from 1.2 to 4.4 µg/L over 24 hours.[1] The relative infant dose is less than 1.8% of the weight-normalized maternal dose. This dose is far too low to be clinically relevant. The drug combination of triprolidine and pseudoephedrine should be avoided by breastfeeding mothers since pseudoephedrine is known to decrease milk supply.

Pregnancy Risk	C	Lactation Risk	L1
T ½	= 5 hours	M/P	= 0.5–1.2
Vd	=	PB	=
Tmax	= 2 hours	Oral	= Complete
MW	= 278	pKa	= 6.5

Adult Concerns: Sedation, dry mouth, anticholinergic side effects.

Pediatric Concerns: None reported. Observe for sedation.

Drug Interactions: Increased sedation when used with CNS depressants, other antihistamines, alcohol, monoamine oxidase inhibitors.

Relative Infant Dose: 1.8%

Adult Dose: 2.5 mg every 4–6 hours.

Alternatives:

References:
1. Findlay JW, Butz RF, Sailstad JM, Warren JT, Welch RM. Pseudoephedrine and triprolidine in plasma and breast milk of nursing mothers. Br J Clin Pharmacol 1984; 18(6): 901–906.

TRIPTORELIN PAMOATE   L3

Trade: Trelstar LA, Trelstar Depo, Trelstar

Other Trades:

Category: Analog of luteinizing hormone releasing hormone

Triptorelin is an analog of endogenous luteinizing hormone releasing hormone (LHRH). It is a potent inhibitor of gonadotropin secretion when given continuously. After chronic administration, a sustained decrease of luteinizing hormone (LH) and follicle stimulating hormone (FSH) secretion and marked reduction of testicular and ovarian steroidogenesis occurs. Continuous use in breastfeeding mothers would ultimately lead to reduced levels of ovulation and sex steroids. In a study in males, prolactin levels were actually increased.[1] Thus it is difficult to discern what, if any, effect this agent would have on milk production in breastfeeding mothers. Some caution is recommended until more is known about its effect on milk production. It is extremely unlikely this agent would penetrate milk due to its high molecular weight. Also, it is not orally bioavailable, so it is very unlikely to harm a breastfeeding infant.

Pregnancy Risk	X	Lactation Risk	L3
T ½	= 3 hour IV	M/P	=
Vd	= 33 l/kg	PB	=
Tmax	= 1 week	Oral	= Nil
MW	= 1699	pKa	=

Adult Concerns: Side effects include vaginal dryness, hot flashes, leg pain, headache, breakthrough bleeding, skeletal pain, edema in legs, decreased libido, and dizziness.

Pediatric Concerns: None reported. Unlikely to penetrate milk, or be orally bioavailable.

Drug Interactions: Avoid use with anti-dopaminergics such as anti-psychotics, metoclopramide, domperidone, cisapride due to additive hyperprolactinemia.

Relative Infant Dose:

Adult Dose: 11.25 mg every 84 days IM.

Alternatives:

References:
1. Stoffel-Wagner B, Sommer L, Bidlingmaier F, Klingmuller D. Effects of the gonadotropin-releasing-hormone agonist, D-Trp-6–GnRH, on prolactin secretion in healthy young men. Horm Res 1995; 43: 266–272.

TROLAMINE   L3

Trade: Myoflex, Mobisyl, Joint-Ritis, FlexPower, Arthricream, Asper-Flex

Other Trades:

Category: Topical Analgesic

Trolamine is the salt formed by combining salicylic acid and triethanolamine.[1] It is used in sunscreens and analgesic topical balms, and cosmetics. As a topical salicylate it has not been formally assigned a pregnancy risk category by the FDA. Because trolamine is used topically for a local effect, it is unlikely to be absorbed systemically or produce problems for a breastfeeding mother or her infant. Topical absorption is estimated to be <10%. There are no adequate and well-controlled studies or case reports in breastfeeding women.

Pregnancy Risk	Possibly Hazardous	Lactation Risk	L3
T ½	= 1–2 hours	M/P	=
Vd	=	PB	= 50% to 90%
Tmax	=	Oral	= Significant
MW	= 287	pKa	= 7.8

Adult Concerns: Allergic reaction, rash, hives, nausea, vomiting.

Pediatric Concerns:

Drug Interactions: May exacerbate anticoagulant effect of low molecular weight heparins. Concurrent with tamarind, glyburide, and Tan-Shen may increase salicylate serum levels.

Relative Infant Dose:

Adult Dose: Apply topically 3–4 times a day.

Alternatives: Ibuprofen, acetaminophen

References:
1. Pharmaceutical manufacturer prescribing information, 2011.

TROPICAMIDE   L3

Trade: Mydral, Mydriacyl, Tropicacyl
Other Trades: Diotrope, Mydriacyl
Category: Mydriatic ophthalmic agent

Tropicamide is used as a short-acting pupil dilator used in diagnostic procedures. It is an antimuscarinic agent which produces competitive antagonism of the actions of acetylcholine, thus preventing the sphincter muscle of the iris and the muscle of the ciliary body from responding to cholinergic stimulation.[1] It is unlikely that systemic levels in adults will be sufficient to produce clinically relevant levels in milk. Infants, however should be observed for anticholinergic effects (dry mouth, mydriasis, sedation, tachycardia). A brief waiting period of 3–4 hours would eliminate most risks.

Pregnancy Risk	C	Lactation Risk	L3
T ½	=	M/P	=
Vd	=	PB	= 45%
Tmax	=	Oral	=
MW	= 284	pKa	= 5.2

Adult Concerns: Adverse reactions include cardiorespiratory collapse, tachycardia, sedation, dry mouth, blurred vision, corneal irritation, and increased intraocular pressure.

Pediatric Concerns: Pediatric patients may require smaller doses to avoid systemic effects. Levels in milk are probably too low to affect an infant.

Drug Interactions: Cisapride may lose effectiveness when administered with tropicamide.

Relative Infant Dose:

Adult Dose: 1–2 drops 15–20 minutes before exam.

Alternatives:

References:
1. Pharmaceutical manufacturer prescribing information, 2000.

TROPISETRON   L3

Trade:
Other Trades: Navoban
Category: Antiemetic for chemotherapy

Tropisetron is a serotonergic (5–HT3) receptor antagonist with antiemetic activity similar to ondansetron and many others.[1] No data are available on its transfer to human milk. Consider ondansetron as alternative in USA.

Pregnancy Risk	B		Lactation Risk	L3
T ½	= 5.6–8.6		M/P	=
Vd	= 7.14 l/kg		PB	= 71%
Tmax	= 2 hours		Oral	= 60%
MW	=		pKa	=

Adult Concerns: Adverse effects include occasional extrapyramidal reactions, headache, rash, fever, constipation, fatigue, sedation, dizziness, diarrhea, and hypotension or hypertension.

Pediatric Concerns: None reported via milk.

Drug Interactions: None reported.

Relative Infant Dose:

Adult Dose: 5 mg orally every 6–24 hours.

Alternatives: Ondansetron

References:
1. Pharmaceutical manufacturer prescribing information, 2003.

TROVAFLOXACIN MESYLATE   L4

Trade: Trovan, Alatrofloxacin
Other Trades:
Category: Antibiotic

Trovafloxacin mesylate is a synthetic broad-spectrum fluoroquinolone antibiotic for oral use. Its IV form is called alatrofloxacin mesylate which is metabolized to trovafloxacin *in vivo*. Trovafloxacin was found in measurable but low concentrations in breastmilk of three breastfeeding mothers.[1] Following an IV dose of 300 mg trovafloxacin equivalent and repeated oral 200 mg doses of trovafloxacin mg daily, breastmilk levels averaged 0.8 mg/L and ranged from 0.3 to 2.1 mg/L of milk. This would average less than 4% of the weight-normalized maternal dose. New data on this antibiotic documents a higher risk of hepatotoxicity and its use is restricted. This agent has been withdrawn from the US market due to risk of acute liver failure.

Pregnancy Risk	C		Lactation Risk	L4
T ½	= 12.2 hours		M/P	=
Vd	= 1.3 l/kg		PB	= 76%
Tmax	= 1.2 hours		Oral	= 88%
MW	= 512		pKa	= 8.09

Adult Concerns: Dizziness, nausea, headache, vomiting, diarrhea have been reported.

Pediatric Concerns: None reported via milk. Only small amounts are secreted in milk.

Drug Interactions: Antacids, morphine, sucralfate, and iron significantly reduce oral absorption.

Relative Infant Dose: 4.2%

Adult Dose: 200–300 mg daily.

Alternatives: Norfloxacin, ofloxacin

References:
1. Pharmaceutical manufacturer prescribing information, 2006.

TUBERCULIN PURIFIED PROTEIN DERIVATIVE	L2

Trade: Tubersol, Aplisol, Sclavo, PPD, Mantoux
Other Trades:
Category: Tuberculin skin test

Tuberculin (also called Mantoux, PPD, Tine test) is a skin-test using antigen derived from the concentrated, sterile, soluble products of growth of M. tuberculosis or M. bovis. Small amounts of this purified product when placed intradermally, produce a hypersensitivity reaction at the site of injection in those individuals with antibodies to M. tuberculosis.[1,2] Preliminary studies also indicate that breast-fed infants may passively acquire sensitivity to mycobacterial antigens from mothers who are sensitized. There are no contraindications to using PPD tests in breastfeeding mothers as the proteins are sterilized and unlikely to penetrate milk.

Pregnancy Risk	C		Lactation Risk	L2
T ½	=		M/P	=
Vd	=		PB	=
Tmax	=		Oral	=
MW	=		pKa	=

Adult Concerns: Local vesiculation, irritation, bruising, and rarely hypersensitivity.

Pediatric Concerns: None via milk.

Drug Interactions:

Relative Infant Dose:

Adult Dose: 5 units X 1

Alternatives:

References:
1. Drug Facts and Comparisons 1999 ed. ed. St. Louis: 1999.
2. McEvoy GE. (ed): AFHS Drug Information. New York, NY: 2003.

TURMERIC   L3

Trade: Curcumin, Diferuloylmethane, Indian saffron, Zingiberaceae ginger, Curcuma longa, Curcum, Haridra

Other Trades:

Category: Herbal Anti-Oxidant

The active compound in turmeric is curcumin (diferuloylmethane), a polyphenol from the Zingiberaceae ginger family. In a study by Ganiger et al, during lactation, using oral doses of 250–320 mg/kg body weight or below of curcumin, the rat pups gained weight. In doses higher than 320 mg/kg body weight, the rat pups had slightly less weight gain prior to weaning.[1] In a study by Singh, et al, curcumin increased the liver enzymes of both the mother mice and their suckling pups.[2] Incidentally, human clinical trials are under-way on curcumin use in the treatment of various types of cancers such as multiple myeloma, pancreatic cancer, and colon cancer. Also, curcumin can either potentiate or decrease the action of certain medications and therefore, caution should be used when taking prescription medications and using curcumin. Curcumin does appear to have anti-oxidant, anti-inflammatory, and cytotoxic properties along with inhibiting platelet aggregation (can cause bleeding). These properties have been seen in lab tests but because curcumin is poorly soluble in water and poorly bioavailable to tissues, the effect following human consumption may not be the same.

Probably safe during breastfeeding, but due to possible interaction with metabolism of prescription drugs, minimize use if mother or infant are on other medications concurrently.

Pregnancy Risk	Possibly Hazardous	Lactation Risk	L3
T ½	=	M/P	=
Vd	=	PB	=
Tmax	=	Oral	=
MW	=	pKa	= 9.12

Adult Concerns: Diarrhea, nausea, contact dermatitis (topical use).

Pediatric Concerns:

Drug Interactions: Patients should be monitored when turmeric is taken with P-gp substrate drugs

Relative Infant Dose:

Adult Dose:

Alternatives:

References:
1. Ganiger S, Malleshappa HN, Krishnappa H, Rajashekhar G, Ramakrishna Rao V,Sullivan F. A two generation reproductive toxicity study with curcumin, turmeric yellow, in Wistar rats. Food Chem Toxicol. 2007 Jan; 45(1): 64–9
2. Singh A, Singh SP, Bamezai R. Postnatal modulation of hepatic biotransformation system enzymes via translactational exposure of F1 mouse pups to turmeric and curcumin. Cancer Lett. 1995 Sep 4; 96(1): 87–93.

TYPHOID VACCINE   L3

Trade: Vivotif Berna, Typhim Vi

Other Trades: Vivotif Berna

Category: Vaccination

Typhoid vaccine promotes active immunity against typhoid fever. It is available in an oral form (Ty21a) which is a live attenuated vaccine for oral administration.[1] The parenteral (injectable) form is derived from acetone-treated killed and dried bacteria, phenol-inactive bacteria, or a special capsular polysaccharide vaccine extracted from killed S. typhi Ty21a strains. Due to a limited lipopolysaccharide coating, the Ty21a strains are limited in their ability to produce infection. No data are available on its transfer into human milk. If immunization is required, the injectable form would be preferred, as infection of the neonate would be unlikely.

Pregnancy Risk	C		Lactation Risk	L3 (injectable)
T ½	=		M/P	=
Vd	=		PB	=
Tmax	=		Oral	=
MW	=		pKa	=

Adult Concerns: Following oral administration, nausea, abdominal cramps, vomiting, urticaria. IM preparations may produce soreness at injection site, tenderness, malaise, headache, myalgia, fever.

Pediatric Concerns: None reported, but injectable killed vaccine suggested.

Drug Interactions: Use cautiously in patients receiving anticoagulants. Do not coadminister with plague vaccine. Do not administer the live-attenuated varieties to immunocompromised patients. Phenytoin may reduce antibody response to this product. Do not use with sulfonamides.

Relative Infant Dose:

Adult Dose: 0.5 mL X 2 over 4 weeks.

Alternatives:

References:
1. Pharmaceutical manufacturer prescribing information, 2008.

TYROPANOATE   L3

Trade: Bilopaque

Other Trades:

Category: Radiological Contrast Agent

Tyropanoate is an oral contrast agent used for examining the gallbladder, when gallstones are suspected. It contains 57.4% bound iodine and is only used in adults.[1] Safety in pediatrics has not been established. There have been no studies done on the transfer of tyropanoate into human milk. It is possible that minimal drug would transfer into the milk compartment; however, levels are unknown.

Pregnancy Risk	D	Lactation Risk	L3
T ½	= 45% gone in 24 hours	M/P	=
Vd	=	PB	= Moderate
Tmax	=	Oral	= Well absorbed
MW	= 641	pKa	=

Adult Concerns: Hypotension, tachycardia, fever, chills, perspiration, nausea, vomiting, diarrhea, pain, and cramping of extremities. Rarely allergic reactions occur including rash, urticaria, pruritus, dysphagia, syncope, shock and chest pain, conjunctivitis.

Pediatric Concerns:

Drug Interactions:

Relative Infant Dose:

Adult Dose:

Alternatives:

References:
1. Pharmaceutical manufacturer prescribing information, 1997.

ULIPRISTAL ACETATE   L2

Trade: Ella

Other Trades:

Category: Progesterone agonist/antagonist

Ulipristal acetate is a selective progesterone receptor modulator used for emergency contraception within 120 hours of unprotected sex. No data are available on its use in breastfeeding mothers. However, as it is a steroid, levels in milk are probably low. Ulipristal has been shown to be excreted in the milk of lactating rats.[1]

Pregnancy Risk	X	Lactation Risk	L2
T ½	= 32 hours	M/P	=
Vd	=	PB	= 96.7 to 99.5%
Tmax	= 1 hour	Oral	= 100%
MW	= 475.6	pKa	=

Adult Concerns: Headache, nausea, abdominal pain, delayed menses.

Pediatric Concerns:

Drug Interactions: Concomitant use of the following drugs may decrease the plasma drug levels of ulipristal: barbiturates, bosentan, carbamazepine, felbamate, griseofulvin, oxcarbazepine, phenytoin, rifampin, St. John's Wort, topiramate. Concomitant use with itraconazole and ketoconazole may decrease plasma drug levels of ulipristal.

Relative Infant Dose:

Adult Dose: 30 mg within 120 hours of intercourse.

Alternatives:

References:
1. Pharmaceutical manufacturer prescribing information, 2010.

UNDECYLENIC ACID   L3

Trade: Desenex, Trifungol, Cruex
Other Trades:
Category: Antifungal for tinea pedis

Undecylenic acid and its derivatives are fatty acids that are used topically in the treatment of fungal infections, most often in tinea pedis, tinea cruris, and ringworm. This medication exerts a fungistatic action, though fungicidal properties have been observed at extremely high doses. Undecylenic acid is found naturally in human sweat, and is absorbed orally.[1] Presently, there are no data regarding the use of undecylenic acid or its derivatives in breastfeeding women. As a topical agent it is unlikely that undecylenic acid will be absorbed systemically in a high enough concentration to have an adverse effect on breastfeeding infants.

Pregnancy Risk	Probably Safe	Lactation Risk	L3
T ½	=	M/P	=
Vd	=	PB	=
Tmax	=	Oral	=
MW	= 184.27	pKa	=

Adult Concerns: Rash, skin irritation, stinging, sensitization.

Pediatric Concerns:

Drug Interactions: There are no known drug interactions with undecylenic acid.

Relative Infant Dose:

Adult Dose: Apply as needed twice daily for 2–4 weeks

Alternatives:

References:
1. Gomez I: [The teratogenic effect of unsaturated short-chain fatty acids in Rhodnium prolixus]. Mem Inst Oswaldo Cruz 80: 375–85, 1985.

UREA   L3

Trade:
Other Trades:
Category: Humectant

Urea is a chemical that is formed from protein breakdown. It is a large source of nitrogen in urine. It acts as a humectant in creams to improve hydration of the skin. Urea is naturally found in human milk[1]. Urea comprises approximately 15%

of milk nitrogen, and some of this urea may be used by gut bacteria as a nitrogen source.[1,2]

Pregnancy Risk	C		Lactation Risk	L3
T ½	=		M/P	=
Vd	=		PB	=
Tmax	=		Oral	= Rapid
MW	= 60.06		pKa	= 0.18

Adult Concerns: Local irritation, stinging.

Pediatric Concerns:

Drug Interactions:

Relative Infant Dose:

Adult Dose: Apply 1–3 times/day (topical).

Alternatives:

References:
1. Harzer G, Franzke V, Bindels JG. Human milk nonprotein nitrogen components: changing patterns of free amino acids and urea in the course of early lactation. Am J Clin Nutr. 1984 Aug; 40(2): 303–9.
2. Jackson AA. Urea as a nutrient: bioavailability and role in nitrogen economy. Arch Dis Child. 1994 Jan; 70(1): 3–4.

URSODIOL　　L3

Trade: Actigall, Ursodeoxycholic acid
Other Trades: Urso, Combidol, Destolit, Lithofalk, Urdox, Ursogal
Category: Bile acid for dissolving gall stones

Ursodiol (ursodeoxycholic acid) is a bile salt found in small amounts in humans that is used to dissolve cholesterol gallstones. It is almost completely absorbed orally via the portal circulation and is extracted almost completely by the liver. Ursodiol suppresses hepatic synthesis and excretion of cholesterol. Following extraction by the liver, it is conjugated with glycine or taurine and is re-secreted into the hepatic bile duct. Only trace amounts are found in the plasma and it is not likely significant amounts would be present in milk.[1] While no breastfeeding data are available, only small amounts of bile salts are known to be present in milk.[2] It is not likely with the low levels of ursodiol in the maternal plasma, that clinically relevant amounts would enter milk.

Pregnancy Risk	B		Lactation Risk	L3
T ½	=		M/P	=
Vd	=		PB	=
Tmax	=		Oral	= 90%
MW	= 392		pKa	= 4.76

Adult Concerns: Insomnia, headache, abdominal pain, flatulence, cholecystitis, constipation, diarrhea (rare), nausea, vomiting.

Pediatric Concerns: None via breast milk.

Drug Interactions: Cholestyramine, antacids, charcoal and colestipol may interfere with gastrointestinal absorption.

Relative Infant Dose:

Adult Dose: 8–10 mg/kg/day in 3 divided doses.

Alternatives:

References:
1. Bachrach WH, Hofmann AF. Ursodeoxycholic acid in the treatment of cholesterol cholelithiasis. part I. Dig Dis Sci 1982; 27(8): 737–761.
2. Forsyth JS, Ross PE, Bouchier IA. Bile salts in breast milk. Eur J Pediatr 1983; 140(2): 126–127.

USTEKINUMAB   L3

Trade: Stelara

Other Trades:

Category: Antirheumatic /Antipsoritic antibody

Ustekinumab is a human IgG1 monoclonal antibody against the p40 subunit of the IL-12 and IL-23 cytokines. It is comprised of 1326 amino acids and has an estimated molecular mass that ranges from 148,079 to 149,690 daltons.[1] It is used in the treatment of severe plaque psoriasis who are candidates for phototherapy or systemic therapy. The drug has also been used in treating rheumatoid arthritis. According to the manufacturer, ustekinumab is excreted in the milk of lactating monkeys. While some IgG is excreted into human milk, levels of ustekinumab are probably exceedingly low. It is not known if ustekinumab is absorbed systemically after ingestion; however, published data suggest that antibodies in breast milk do not enter the neonatal and infant circulation in substantial amounts.

Pregnancy Risk	B	Lactation Risk	L3
T ½	= 14.9–45.6 days	M/P	=
Vd	= 161 ml/kg	PB	=
Tmax	= 13.5 days	Oral	= Nil
MW	= 148,079 daltons	pKa	=

Adult Concerns: Infections, headache, seizures, confusion, vision problems

Pediatric Concerns: No studies available. Observe infant for infection, diarrhea.

Drug Interactions: Do not administer live vaccines with ustekinumab. Use caution in using with other immunosuppressants.

Relative Infant Dose:

Adult Dose: 45–90 mg every 12 weeks.

Alternatives: Etanercept, infliximab

References:
1. Pharmaceutical manufacturer prescribing information, 2010.

VALACYCLOVIR   L1

Trade: Valtrex
Other Trades: Valaciclovir, Valtrex
Category: Antiviral, for herpes simplex

Valacyclovir is a prodrug that is rapidly metabolized in the plasma to acyclovir. In a study of 5 women who received 500 mg twice daily for 7 days after delivery, the median peak acyclovir concentration in breast milk was 4.2 mg/L at 4 hours while the average concentration (AUC) was 2.24 mg/L if 12 hour dosing intervals were used.[1] Thus the relative infant dose would be 4.7% of the weight-normalized maternal dose. The milk/serum ratio was highest 4 hours after the initial dose at 3.4 and reached steady state ratio at 1.85. Valacyclovir is rapidly converted to acyclovir which transfers into breast milk. However, the amount of acyclovir in breast milk after valacyclovir administration is considerably less than that used in therapeutic dosing of neonates.

Pregnancy Risk	B	Lactation Risk	L1
T ½	= 2.5–3 hours	M/P	= 0.6–4.1
Vd	=	PB	= 9–33%
Tmax	= 1.5 hours	Oral	= 54%
MW	=	pKa	=

Adult Concerns: Nausea, vomiting, diarrhea, sore throat, edema, and skin rashes.

Pediatric Concerns: None reported via milk.

Drug Interactions:

Relative Infant Dose: 4.7%

Adult Dose: 500–1000 mg 2–3 times daily.

Alternatives: Acyclovir

References:
1. Sheffield JS, Fish DN, Hollier LM, Cadematori S, Nobles BJ, Wendel GD, Jr. Acyclovir concentrations in human breast milk after valaciclovir administration. Am J Obstet Gynecol 2002; 186(1): 100–102.

VALDECOXIB   L3

Trade: Bextra
Other Trades:
Category: Analgesic for pain.

Valdecoxib is a selective cyclo-oxygenase-2 (COX-2) inhibitor, used for the relief of pain associated with osteoarthritis, rheumatoid arthritis and primary dysmenorrhea.[1] It is no longer approved in the United States. Valdecoxib is an active metabolite of parecoxib. There are currently no studies on transfer of valdecoxib into breastmilk, however, valdecoxib is a metabolite of parecoxib. In one study, 40 women were administered 40 mg IV parecoxib within 41 hours following birth for the relief of post-cesarean pain.[2] Breastmilk samples and plasma samples were obtained from these women over the subsequent 24 hours. In the study, the authors reported a median milk/plasma ratio of valdecoxib alone as 0.14, with a median absolute infant dose (AID) of 1.82 µg/kg/day and a median relative infant dose (RID) of 0.47%. The half-life of valdecoxib in milk was reported to be 8.5 hours. No untoward effects were noted in the infants. The authors of this study conclude that the RID for valdecoxib is low and is probably compatible with breastfeeding.

Therefore, although valdecoxib transfers into breastmilk, it does so in minimal quantities. Nonetheless, since this drug has a sulfonamide group in its chemical structure, some caution is advised in the newborn and premature infants due to the increased risk of hemorrhage and kernicterus.

Pregnancy Risk	C	Lactation Risk	L3
T ½	= 8–11 hours	M/P	= 0.14
Vd	= 83 L l/kg	PB	= 98%
Tmax	= 3 hours	Oral	= 83%
MW	= 314.36	pKa	=

Adult Concerns: Peripheral edema, skin rash, abdominal pain, nausea, vomiting, upper respiratory infection Some of the serious but rare side-effects include anaphylactic reactions, hepatitis, life-threatening skin reactions such as Stevens-Johnson syndrome, toxic epidermal necrolysis, myocardial infarction, strokes, deep vein thrombosis, pulmonary embolism. This drug is contra-indicated in those with known hypersensitivity to other sulfonamides, aspirin, NSAIDs. Contra-indicated for the relief of post-operative pain following coronary artery bypass graft (CABG).

Pediatric Concerns:

Drug Interactions: Concomitant use with fluconazole and itraconazole causes increased plasma levels of valdecoxib. Co-administration with phenytoin decreases the plasma levels of valdecoxib. Concomitant use increases the plasma levels of the following drugs: warfarin, diazepam, glyburide, norethindrone, ethinyl estradiol, probably other oral contraceptives, omeprazole, dextromethorphan. Co-administration with ACE-inhibitors, furosemide, and lithium decreases their plasma concentrations and efficacy. Do not co-administer with aspirin due to increased risk of gastrointestinal ulceration.

Relative Infant Dose: 0.3%

Adult Dose: 10–20 mg once daily.

Alternatives: Acetaminophen, ketorolac, ibuprofen.

References:

1. Pharmaceutical manufacturer prescribing information, 2006.
2. Paech MJ, Salman S, Ilett KF, O'Halloran SJ, Muchatuta NA. Transfer ofParecoxib and Its Primary Active Metabolite Valdecoxib via TransitionalBreastmilk Following Intravenous Parecoxib Use After Cesarean Delivery: AComparison of Naive Pooled Data Analysis and Nonlinear Mixed-Effects Modeling.Anesth Analg. 2012 Feb 17.

VALERIAN OFFICINALIS   L3

Trade: Garden valerian, Garden heliotrope, All-heal
Other Trades:
Category: Herbal sedative

Valerian root is most commonly used as a sedative/hypnotic. Of the numerous chemicals present in the root, the most important chemical group appears to be the valepotriates. This family consists of at least a dozen or more related compounds and is believed responsible for the sedative potential of this plant although it is controversial. The combination of numerous components may inevitability account for the sedative response. Controlled studies in man have indicated a sedative/hypnotic effect with fewer night awakenings and significant somnolence.[1-3] The toxicity of valerian root appears to be low, with only minor side effects reported. However, the valepotriates have been found to be cytotoxic, with alkylating activity similar to other nitrogen mustard-like anticancer agents. Should this prove to be so *in vivo*, it may preclude the use of this product in humans. No data are available on the transfer of valerian root compounds into human milk. However, the use of sedatives in breastfeeding mothers is generally discouraged, due to a possible increased risk of sudden infant death syndrome (SIDS).

Pregnancy Risk	Probably Safe	Lactation Risk	L3
T ½	=	M/P	=
Vd	=	PB	=
Tmax	=	Oral	=
MW	=	pKa	= 4.8

Adult Concerns: Ataxia, hypothermia, muscle relaxation. Headaches, excitability, cardiac disturbances.

Pediatric Concerns: None reported via human milk.

Drug Interactions:

Relative Infant Dose:

Adult Dose:

Alternatives:

References:
1. Leathwood PD, Chauffard F, Heck E, Munoz-Box R. Aqueous extract of valerian root (Valeriana officinalis L.) improves sleep quality in man. Pharmacol Biochem Behav 1982; 17(1): 65–71.
2. von Eickstedt KW, Rahman S. [Psychopharmacologic effect of valepotriates]. Arzneimittelforschung 1969; 19(3): 316–319.
3. Leathwood PD, Chauffard F. Aqueous extract of valerian reduces latency to fall asleep in man. Planta Med 1985; 51(2): 144–148.

VALGANCICLOVIR   L3

Trade: Valcyte, Cytovene
Other Trades: Valcyte
Category: Antiviral

Valganciclovir is a prodrug that is rapidly metabolized to the active antiviral drug ganciclovir.[1] It is used for cytomegalovirus infections particularly in HIV infected patients. The oral bioavailability of valganciclovir is 60% while only 6% with its active metabolite ganciclovir. Further it is very water soluble and lipophobic, which would suggest milk levels will be low. No data are available on its use in breastfeeding mothers but its oral absorption in the infant is likely low.

Pregnancy Risk	C	Lactation Risk	L3
T ½	= 4 hours	M/P	=
Vd	= 0.7 l/kg	PB	= 1–2%
Tmax	= 1–3 hours	Oral	= 61%
MW	= 390	pKa	= 14.6

Adult Concerns: Adverse events include diarrhea, neutropenia, nausea, headache, insomnia, abdominal pain, anemia, and catheter-related infections.

Pediatric Concerns: None reported via milk. No studies thus far. Due to its use in HIV infected patients, it is unlikely this agent will be used in breastfeeding mothers. Poor oral bioavailability would limit absorption in an infant.

Drug Interactions: The plasma levels of zidovudine and didanosine may be increased when used concomitantly with valganciclovir. The plasma levels of valganciclovir are increased when used concomitantly with probenecid.

Relative Infant Dose:

Adult Dose: 450–900 mg daily.

Alternatives:

References:
1. Pharmaceutical manufacturer package insert, 2000.

VALPROIC ACID   L3

Trade: Depakene, Depakote, Stavzor, Depacon
Other Trades: Epilim, Valpro, Depakene, Novo-Valproic, Deproic, Convulex
Category: Anticonvulsant

Valproic acid is a popular anticonvulsant used in grand mal, petit mal, myoclonic, temporal lobe seizures, and the treatment of mania. In a study of 16 patients receiving 300–2400 mg/day, valproic acid concentrations ranged from 0.4 to 3.9 mg/L (mean=1.9 mg/L).[1] The milk/plasma ratio averaged 0.05. In a study of one patient receiving 250 mg twice daily, milk levels ranged from 0.18 to 0.47 mg/L. The milk/plasma ratio ranged from 0.01 to 0.02.[2] Alexander reports milk levels of 5.1 mg/L following a larger dose of up to 1600 mg/day.[3] In a study of 6 women receiving 9.5 to 31 mg/kg/day valproic acid, milk levels averaged 1.4 mg/L while serum levels averaged 45.1 mg/L.[4] The average milk/serum ratio was 0.027. Most authors agree that the amount of valproic acid transferring to the infant via milk is low. Breastfeeding would appear safe. However, the infant may need monitoring for liver and platelet changes. Prior studies have shown that cognitive delay can occur in infants exposed to valproic acid during pregnancy. We do not know that this would occur during breastfeeding, but some concern is justified.

Pregnancy Risk	D	Lactation Risk	L3
T ½	= 14 hours	M/P	= 0.42
Vd	= 0.1–0.4 l/kg	PB	= 94%
Tmax	= 1–4 hours	Oral	= Complete
MW	= 144	pKa	= 4.8

Adult Concerns: Sedation, thrombocytopenia, tremor, nausea, diarrhea, liver toxicity.

Pediatric Concerns: None reported via milk. Observe infant for changes in liver enzymes, clinical status, and platelet levels.

Drug Interactions: Valproic acid levels may be reduced by charcoal, rifampin, carbamazepine, clonazepam, lamotrigine, phenytoin. Valproic acid levels may be increased when used with chlorpromazine, cimetidine, felbamate, salicylates, alcohol. Valproic acid use may increase levels or the effect of barbiturates, warfarin, benzodiazepines, clozapine.

Relative Infant Dose: 1.4%–1.7%

Adult Dose: 10–30 mg/kg daily.

Alternatives:

References:
1. von Unruh GE, Froescher W, Hoffmann F, Niesen M. Valproic acid in breast milk: how much is really there? Ther Drug Monit 1984; 6(3): 272–276.
2. Dickinson RG, Harland RC, Lynn RK, Smith WB, Gerber N. Transmission of valproic acid (Depakene) across the placenta: half-life of the drug in mother and baby. J Pediatr 1979; 94(5): 832–835.
3. Alexander FW. Sodium valproate and pregnancy. Arch Dis Child 1979; 54(3): 240.
4. Nau H, Rating D, Koch S, Hauser I, Helge H. Valproic acid and its metabolites: placental transfer, neonatal pharmacokinetics, transfer via mother's milk and clinical status in neonates of epileptic mothers. J Pharmacol Exp Ther 1981; 219(3): 768–777.

VALSARTAN   L3

Trade: Diovan, Valturna

Other Trades: Diovan

Category: Antihypertensive

Valsartan is a new angiotensin-II receptor antagonist used to treat hypertension. While it is believed to enter the milk of rodents, no human data are available.[1,2] Use with caution in breastfeeding mothers.

Pregnancy Risk	C/D in 2nd and 3rd trimester		Lactation Risk	L3	
T ½	= 9 hours		M/P	=	
Vd	= 0.24 l/kg		PB	= 97%	
Tmax	= 2–4 hours		Oral	= 23%	
MW	=		pKa	= 8.15	

Adult Concerns: Occasional increase in liver enzymes. Small decreases in hemoglobin have been reported. Significant increases (>20%) in serum potassium levels have been reported. Dizziness, insomnia, viral infection, cough, diarrhea, etc. have been reported.

Pediatric Concerns: None via milk, but caution is recommended.

Drug Interactions: May significantly increase digoxin levels by 49%.

Relative Infant Dose:

Adult Dose: 80–320 mg daily.

Alternatives:

References:
1. Pharmaceutical manufacturer prescribing information, 1999.
2. McEvoy GE. (ed): AFHS Drug Information. New York, NY: 2003.

VANCOMYCIN   L1

Trade: Vancocin

Other Trades: Vancoled, Vancocin

Category: Antibiotic

Vancomycin is an antimicrobial agent. Only low levels are secreted into human milk. Milk levels were 12.7 mg/L four hours after infusion in one woman receiving 1 gm every 12 hours for 7 days.[1] Its poor absorption from the infant's gastrointestinal tract would limit its systemic absorption. Low levels in infant could provide alterations of gastrointestinal flora.

Pregnancy Risk	C		Lactation Risk	L1	
T ½	= 5.6 hours		M/P	=	
Vd	= 0.3–0.7 l/kg		PB	= 10–30%	
Tmax	=		Oral	= Minimal	
MW	= 1449		pKa	= 8.78	

Adult Concerns: Alteration of gastrointestinal flora, neutropenia, hypotension, kidney and hearing damage.

Pediatric Concerns: None reported via milk.

Drug Interactions: When used with aminoglycosides, risk of nephrotoxicity may be increased. Use with anesthetics may produce erythema and histamine-like flushing in children. May increase risk of neuromuscular blockade when used with neuromuscular blocking agents.

Relative Infant Dose: 6.7%

Adult Dose: 125–500 mg every 6 hours.

Alternatives:

References:
1.   Reyes MP, Ostrea EM, Jr., Cabinian AE, Schmitt C, Rintelmann W. Vancomycin during pregnancy: does it cause hearing loss or nephrotoxicity in the infant? Am J Obstet Gynecol 1989; 161(4): 977–981.

VARENICLINE   L4

Trade: Chantix

Other Trades: Champix

Category: Smoking cessation

Varenicline is used to assist smoking cessation. It is a partial alpha-4-beta-2-nicotinic receptor partial agonist that binds to nicotine receptors in the brain, thus preventing nicotine stimulation. It stimulates dopamine activity, but to a lesser extent than does nicotine, thus reducing craving and withdrawal symptoms.[1] There have been no studies performed on the transfer of varenicline into human milk, but it is nearly identical in structure and would probably transfer into human milk easily. Caution should be used in breastfeeding mothers.

Pregnancy Risk	C	Lactation Risk	L4
T ½	= 24 hours	M/P	=
Vd	=	PB	= 20%
Tmax	= 3–4 hours	Oral	= High
MW	= 361	pKa	= 9.2

Adult Concerns: Adverse effects include nausea, sleep disturbance, neuropsychiatric changes, constipation, flatulence, and vomiting. Dose adjustments must be made in severe renal failure.

Pediatric Concerns: No data are available on levels in milk, but due to long half-life and kinetics, some caution should be exercised in using this in breastfeeding mothers.

Drug Interactions: Cimetidine increases varenicline concentrations by as much as 29% due to decreased varenicline clearance. Co-administration of transdermal nicotine with varenicline increases incidence of dyspepsia, nausea, vomiting, headache, dizziness, and fatigue.

Relative Infant Dose:

Adult Dose: 1mg twice daily.

Alternatives:

References:
1.   Pharmaceutical manufacturer prescribing information, 2006.

VARICELLA VACCINE   L2

Trade: Varivax

Other Trades:

Category: Vaccination for Varicella (Chickenpox)

A live attenuated varicella vaccine (Varivax–Merck) was recently approved for marketing by the US Food and Drug Administration. Although effective, it does not apparently provide the immunity attained from infection with the parent virus and may not provide life-long immunity. The Oka/Merck strain used in the vaccine is attenuated by passage in human and embryonic guinea pig cell cultures. It is not known if the vaccine-acquired VZV is secreted in human milk, nor its infectiousness to infants. Interestingly, in two women with varicella-zoster infections, the virus was not culturable from milk. The antibody from the varicella zoster vaccine has been isolated in breast milk along with the DNA.[2] Mothers of immunodeficient infants should not breastfeed following use of this vaccine. Recommendations for Use: Varicella vaccine is only recommended for children >1 year of age up to 12 years of age with no history of varicella infection. Both the AAP[3] and the Centers for Disease Control approve the use of varicella-zoster vaccines in breastfeeding mothers, if the risk of infection is high.

Pregnancy Risk	C	Lactation Risk	L2
T ½	=	M/P	=
Vd	=	PB	=
Tmax	=	Oral	=
MW	=	pKa	=

Adult Concerns: Tenderness and erythema at the injection site in about 25% of vaccinees and a sparse generalized maculopapular rash occurring within one month after immunization in about 5%. Spread of the vaccine virus to others has been reported. Susceptible, immunodeficient individuals should be protected from exposure.

Pediatric Concerns: None reported via milk, but no studies are available. Immunocompromised infants should not be exposed to this product.

Drug Interactions:

Relative Infant Dose: 0%

Adult Dose: 0.5 mL X 2 over 4–8 weeks.

Alternatives:

References:
1. Frederick IB, White RJ, Braddock SW. Excretion of varicella-herpes zoster virus in breast milk. Am J Obstet Gynecol 1986; 154(5): 1116–1117.
2. Yoshida M, Yamagami N, Tezuka T, Hondo R. Case report: detection of varicella-zoster virus DNA in maternal breast milk. J Med Virol. 1992Oct; 38(2): 108–10.
3. American Academy of Pediatrics. Committee on Infectious Diseases. Red Book. 1997.

VARICELLA-ZOSTER VIRUS   L4

Trade: Chickenpox
Other Trades:
Category: Chickenpox

The Varicella- Zoster Virus (VZV) belongs to the family of herpes viruses. Mode of transmission includes direct contact, aerosol droplet transmission, contact with the infected vesicular rash and transplacental passage.[1] The incubation period is generally 14–16 days after exposure. In the unimmunized or in those exposed for the first time, VZV establishes a primary infection, otherwise known as Chickenpox. It is characterized by a generalized rash and mild flu-like symptoms. Following the primary infection, VZV tends to remain latent in the dorsal root ganglia and may become re-activated later in life causing herpes zoster infection, popularly known as 'shingles'.

Chickenpox virus has been reported to be transferred via breastmilk in one 27-year-old mother who developed chickenpox postpartum.[2] Her 2-month-old son also developed the disease 16 days after the mother. Chickenpox virus was detected in the mother's milk and may suggest that transmission can occur via breastmilk. However, in a study of 2 breastfeeding patients who developed varicella-herpes zoster infections, in neither case was the virus isolated and cultured from their milk.[3] According to the American Academy of Pediatrics, neonates born to mothers with active varicella should be placed in isolation at birth and, if still hospitalized, until 21 or 28 days of age, depending on whether they received VZIG (Varicella Zoster Immune Globulin).[4] Candidates for VZIG include: immunocompromised children, pregnant women, and a newborn infant whose mother has onset of VZV within 5 days before or 48 hours after delivery. For an excellent review of VZV and breastfeeding see Merewood and Philipp.[5]

Pregnancy Risk	Hazardous	Lactation Risk	L4
T ½	=	M/P	=
Vd	=	PB	=
Tmax	=	Oral	=
MW	=	pKa	=

Adult Concerns:

Pediatric Concerns: Varicella-zoster virus transfers into human milk. Infants should not breastfeed unless protected with VZIG.

Drug Interactions:

Relative Infant Dose:

Adult Dose:

Alternatives:

References:

1. AAP CoID: Varicella-Zoster Infections. In: Red Book: 2009 Report of the Committe on Infectious Diseases. Edited by Pickering LK BC, Kimberlin DW, Long SS, 28 edn; 2009: 714–727.

2. Yoshida M, Yamagami N, Tezuka T, Hondo R. Case report: detection of varicella-zoster virus DNA in maternal breast milk. J Med Virol 1992; 38(2): 108–110.
3. Frederick IB, White RJ, Braddock SW. Excretion of varicella-herpes zoster virus in breast milk. Am J Obstet Gynecol 1986; 154(5): 1116–1117.
4. Report of the committee on Infectious Diseases. American Academy of Pediatrics. 1994.
5. Meerwood A, Philipp B. Breastfeeding: Conditions and Diseases. 1st ed. ed. Amarillo, TX: Pharmasoft Publishing L.P., 2001.

VASOPRESSIN   L3

Trade: Pitressin

Other Trades: Pitresin, Pitressin, Pressyn

Category: Antidiuretic hormone

Vasopressin, also know as the antidiuretic hormone, is a small peptide (8 amino acids) that is normally secreted by the posterior pituitary.[1] It reduces urine production by the kidney. Although it probably passes to some degree into human milk, it is rapidly destroyed in the gastrointestinal tract by trypsin and must be administered by injection or intranasally. Hence, oral absorption by a nursing infant is very unlikely. Desmopressin is virtually identical and milk levels have been reported to be very low.

Pregnancy Risk	C	Lactation Risk	L3
T ½	= 10–20 minutes	M/P	=
Vd	=	PB	=
Tmax	= 1 hour	Oral	= Nil
MW	=	pKa	= 8.0

Adult Concerns: Increased blood pressure, water retention and edema, sweating, tremor, and bradycardia.

Pediatric Concerns: None reported via milk.

Drug Interactions: Caution while coadministering with the following drugs: Tricyclic antidepressants, selective serotonin re-uptake inhibitors, chlorpromazine, opiate analgesics, NSAIDs, lamotrigine and carbamazepine.

Relative Infant Dose:

Adult Dose: 5–10 units daily.

Alternatives:

References:
1. McEvoy GE. (ed): AFHS Drug Information. New York, NY: 2003.

VENLAFAXINE   L3

Trade: Effexor

Other Trades: Efexor

Category: Antidepressant

Venlafaxine is a new serotonin reuptake inhibitor antidepressant. It inhibits both serotonin reuptake and norepinephrine reuptake. It is somewhat similar in mechanism to other antidepressants such as fluoxetine, but has fewer anticholinergic side-effects. In an excellent study of three mothers (mean age = 34.5 years, 84.5 kg) receiving venlafaxine (225–300 mg/day), the mean milk/plasma ratios for venlafaxine (V) and O-desmethylvenlafaxine (ODV) were 2.5 and 2.7 respectively.[1] The mean maximum concentrations of V and ODV in milk were 1.16 mg/L and 0.796 mg/L. The peak concentrations in milk occurred at 2.25 hours. The mean infant exposure was 3.2% for V and 3.2% for ODV of the weight-adjusted maternal dose. Venlafaxine was detected in the plasma of one of the seven infants while ODV was detected in four of the seven infants. The infants were healthy and showed no acute adverse effects.

In a study of 11 women consuming an average of 194.3 mg/day of venlafaxine, the theoretical infant dose of venlafaxine and desvenlafaxine was 0.208 mg/kg/day, or a relative infant dose of 8.1% of the maternal dose. The maximum level in milk occurred at 8 hours after maternal ingestion. Infant plasma levels for V + D were 37.1% of maternal levels. No adverse effects were noted in any of the infants.[2] However, recent data (MedWatch, FDA) has suggested that infants exposed in utero to various serotonin reuptake inhibitors such as venlafaxine, may have profound adverse effects immediately upon delivery. These include: respiratory distress, cyanosis, apnea, seizures, temperature instability, etc. It is not known if these adverse events are due to a direct toxic effect of venlafaxine on the fetus, or due to a discontinuation (withdrawal) syndrome. Studies have shown that these adverse effects may be partially relieved with venlafaxine received through breast milk.[3]

Pregnancy Risk	C		Lactation Risk	L3
T ½	= 5 hours (venlafaxine).		M/P	= 2.75
Vd	= 4–12 l/kg		PB	= 27%
Tmax	= 2.25		Oral	= 92%
MW	= 313		pKa	= 9.4

Adult Concerns: Nausea/vomiting, somnolence, dry mouth, dizziness, headache, weakness.

Pediatric Concerns: None reported via milk, but no studies are available. Recent data has suggested that infants exposed during pregnancy to venlafaxine and other SNRIs have developed complications requiring prolonged hospitalization, respiratory support, and tube feeding. Such complications arise immediately upon delivery. The implication for breastfeeding is not known.

Drug Interactions: Serious, sometimes fatal reactions when used with monoamine oxidase inhibitors, or if used within 7–14 days of their use. Serious organic psychosis has been reported with the coadministration of propafenone. Two recent cases of serotonin-like reactions (agitation, dysarthria, diaphoresis and extrapyramidal movement disorder) have been reported when metoclopramide was used in patients receiving sertraline or venlafaxine.[2]

Relative Infant Dose: 6.8%–8.1%

Adult Dose: 75 mg three times daily.

Alternatives: Sertraline, fluoxetine

References:

1. Ilett KF, Kristensen JH, Hackett LP, Paech M, Kohan R, Rampono J. Distribution of venlafaxine and its O-desmethyl metabolite in human milk and their effects in breastfed infants. Br J Clin Pharmacol 2002; 53(1): 17–22.
2. Newport DJ, Ritchie JC, Knight BT, Glover BA, Zach EB, Stowe ZN. Venlafaxine in human breast milk and nursing infant plasma: determination of exposure. J Clin Psychiatry. Sep 2009; 70(9): 1304–1310.
3. Koren G, Moretti, Kapur B. Can Venlafaxine in Breast Milk Attenuate the Norepinephrine and Serotonin Reuptake Neonatal Withdrawal Syndrome? JOGC 2006 April; 28(4): 299–302.

VERAPAMIL   L2

Trade: Calan, Isoptin, Covera-HS

Other Trades: Anpec, Coridlox, Veracaps SR, Apo-Verap, Isoptin, Novo-Veramil, Berkatens, Univer

Category: Calcium channel blocker for hypertension

Verapamil is a typical calcium channel blocker used as an antihypertensive. It is secreted into milk but in very low levels, which are highly controversial. Anderson reports that in one patient receiving 80 mg three times daily, the average steady-state concentrations of verapamil and norverapamil in milk were 25.8 and 8.8 µg/L respectively.[1] The respective maternal plasma level was 42.9 µg/L. The milk/plasma ratio for verapamil was 0.60. No verapamil was detected in the infant's plasma. Inoue reports that in one patient receiving 80 mg four times daily, the milk level peaked at 300 µg/L at approximately 14 hours.[2] These levels are considerably higher than the aforementioned. In another study of a mother receiving 240 mg daily, the concentrations in milk were never higher than 40 µg/L.[3]

From these three studies, the relative infant doses were 0.15%, 0.98%, and 0.18% respectively. Regardless of the variability, the relative amount transferred to the infant is still quite small.

Pregnancy Risk	C	Lactation Risk	L2
T ½	= 3–7 hours	M/P	= 0.94
Vd	= 2.5–6.5 l/kg	PB	= 83–92%
Tmax	= 1–2.2	Oral	= 90%
MW	= 455	pKa	= 8.8

Adult Concerns: Hypotension, bradycardia, peripheral edema.

Pediatric Concerns: None reported via milk. Observe for hypotension, bradycardia, weakness.

Drug Interactions: Verapamil is a calcium channel blocker (CCB). Barbiturates may reduce bioavailability of CCBs. Calcium salts may reduce hypotensive effect. Dantrolene may increase risk of hyperkalemia and myocardial depression. H_2 blockers may increase bioavailability of certain CCBs. Hydantoins may reduce plasma levels. Quinidine increases risk of hypotension, bradycardia, tachycardia. Rifampin may reduce effects of CCBs. Vitamin D may reduce efficacy of CCBs. CCBs may increase carbamazepine, cyclosporin, encainide, prazosin levels.

Relative Infant Dose: 0.2%

Adult Dose: 80–100 mg three times daily.

Alternatives: Bepridil, nifedipine, nimodipine

References:

1. Anderson P, Bondesson U, Mattiasson I, Johansson BW. Verapamil and norverapamil in plasma and breast milk during breast feeding. Eur J Clin Pharmacol 1987; 31(5): 625–627.
2. Inoue H, Unno N, Ou MC, Iwama Y, Sugimoto T. Level of verapamil in human milk. Eur J Clin Pharmacol 1984; 26(5): 657–658.
3. Andersen HJ. Excretion of verapamil in human milk. Eur J Clin Pharmacol 1983; 25(2): 279–280.

VERTEPORFIN   L3

Trade: Visudyne

Other Trades: Visudyne

Category: Photosensitizing agent to treat macular degeneration

Verteporfin is a photosensitizing agent used in the treatment of neovascularization associated with macular degeneration. When administered, verteporfin is transported to the neovascular endothelium, where it needs to be activated by nonthermal red light, resulting in local damage to the endothelium. This leads to temporary choroidal vessel occlusion.[1] The manufacturer reports verteporfin and its metabolites have been found in the breast milk of one women after a 6 mg/m^2 infusion.[1] Milk levels were up to 66% of the corresponding plasma levels. Verteporfin was undetectable after 12 hours but its metabolites were present for up to 48 hours. A waiting period of 24 hours is recommended.

Pregnancy Risk	C		Lactation Risk	L3
T ½	= 5–6 hours		M/P	=
Vd	=		PB	=
Tmax	=		Oral	= Nil
MW	= 718		pKa	= 14.94

Adult Concerns: Adverse reactions include headache, blurred vision, decreased visual acuity, and visual disturbances.

Pediatric Concerns: Milk levels are significant but brief. Breastfeeding should be interrupted for 24 hours.

Drug Interactions: Calcium channel blockers, polymyxin B, and radiation therapy could enhance the rate of uptake of verteporfin. Drugs that decrease clotting, beta-carotene, dimethyl sulfoxide, ethanol, formate, mannitol, or other drugs that decrease oxygen radicals can decrease the efficacy of verteporfin. Also, increased photosensitivity is seen when taken with drugs such as griseofulvin, sulfonamides, sulfonylureas, tetracyclines, or thiazide diuretics.

Relative Infant Dose:

Adult Dose: 6 mg/m^2.

Alternatives:

References:
1. Pharmaceutical manufacturer prescribing information, 2005.

VIGABATRIN   L3

Trade: Sabril
Other Trades:
Category: Anticonvulsant

Vigabatrin is a newer anticonvulsant. It is a mixture consisting of 50% active S-enantiomer and 50% inactive R-enantiomer. This drug acts by inhibiting the metabolism of the inhibitory neurotransmitter GABA, thereby raising its levels in the human brain.[1] It is an effective adjunctive anticonvulsant for the treatment of multi-drug resistant complex partial seizures. It has also shown efficacy in controlling seizures and spasm in infants 3 months and older.

Milk levels of vigabatrin were estimated in two mothers who had been on 2000 mg/day vigabatrin therapy during pregnancy.[2] Case 1 had been on therapy since third trimester and case 2 had taken vigabatrin throughout her pregnancy. The milk levels of both enantiomers were assessed in this study. Milk samples were collected from case 1 and case 2 on the 7th and 8th day postpartum respectively, at pre-dose and then at 3 and 6 hours post-dose. Assuming that the infants consumed 0.15 / day of breastmilk, it was found that the doses received by the infants through milk of the active S-enantiomer were 108 µg/kg/day and 160 µg/kg/day respectively for case 1 and 2. Likewise, the absolute infant doses for the inactive R-enantiomer for case 1 and 2 were 333 µg/kg/day and 601 µg/kg/day respectively. The relative infant doses for the active S-enantiomer were <0.06% and 0.96% for case 1 and 2 respectively. The relative infant doses for the inactive R-enantiomer for case 1 and 2 were <2% and 3.6% respectively. The milk/plasma ratio at all times throughout the study were always <1. The authors suggest that the maximum relative infant dose for vigabatrin (R- + S-enantiomer) will barely exceed 4%. The total relative infant dose of the active S-enantiomer in this study barely exceeded 1%.

Vigabatrin enters milk in small amounts and is not likely to be clinically relevant in the breastfed infant. However, since this drug acts by raising the levels of inhibitory GABA in the brain,[1] the effect of this property on neonatal brains is not known. Some caution is recommended. Observe for CNS depressant effects in the infant such as excessive sleepiness, sedation and poor suckling. As with all CNS depressants, the risk of apnea also exists, especially in the premature and newborn infants.

Pregnancy Risk	C	Lactation Risk	L3
T ½	= 7 hours	M/P	= <1
Vd	= 0.8 l/kg	PB	=
Tmax	= 0.5–2 hours	Oral	= 50%
MW	= 129	pKa	=

Adult Concerns: Changes in visual field defects have been noted. Drowsiness, fatigue, and acute psychosis (7%) have been described particularly in patients with a history of psychiatric disorders. Psychosis and an increased frequency of seizures have been reported upon abrupt withdrawal of vigabatrin therapy.

Pediatric Concerns: None reported via milk.

Drug Interactions: May decrease phenytoin levels by 30%. Few other interactions are noted which is a plus for this drug.

Relative Infant Dose: 1.5%–2.7%

Adult Dose: 1 - 4 gm daily.

Alternatives:

References:
1. Dichter MA, Brodie MJ. New antiepileptic drugs. N Engl J Med 1996; 334(24): 1583–1590.
2. Tran A, O'Mahoney T, Rey E, Mai J, Mumford JP, Olive G. Vigabatrin: placental transfer in vivo and excretion into breast milk of the enantiomers. Br J ClinPharmacol. 1998 Apr; 45(4): 409–11.

VILAZODONE   L3

Trade: Viibryd
Other Trades:
Category: SSRI, 5–HT1a receptor agonist

Vilazodone is a selective serotonin re-uptake inhibitor as well as a 5–HT1 alpha receptor agonist. It is indicated for the treatment of depression. At present there are no data on its transfer into human milk. It is currently not known if vilazodone is excreted into breastmilk, though it is known to be excreted into the milk of lactating rats.[1]

Pregnancy Risk	C	Lactation Risk	L3
T ½	= 25 hours	M/P	=
Vd	= Large l/kg	PB	= 96–99%
Tmax	= 4–5 hours	Oral	= 72%
MW	= 477.99	pKa	=

Adult Concerns: Palpitations, night sweats, decreased appetite, diarrhea, flatulence, gastroenteritis, indigestion, increased appetite, nausea, vomiting, xerostomia, arthralgia, dizziness, insomnia, migraine, paresthesia, somnolence, tremor, serotonin syndrome, dry eye, sexual dysfunction, suicidal ideation, mania, restlessness.

Pediatric Concerns:

Drug Interactions: Do not use with monoamine oxidase inhibitors or methylene blue. May increase anticoagulation when used with warfarin. Do not use concomitantly with tramadol, or the triptans.

Relative Infant Dose:

Adult Dose: 10 mg daily for 1 week, then 20 mg daily for 1 week, then 40 mg daily.

Alternatives: Sertraline, paroxetine.

References:
1. Product Information: VIIBRYD(R) oral tablets, vilazodone HCl oral tablets. Trovis Pharmaceuticals, LLC, New Haven, CT, 2011.

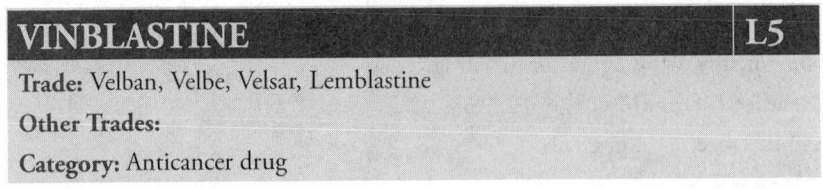

VINBLASTINE   L5

Trade: Velban, Velbe, Velsar, Lemblastine

Other Trades:

Category: Anticancer drug

Vinblastine is an antineoplastic agent derived from the Catharanthus alkaloids family. It is commonly used in numerous cancers including breast cancer, Kaposi's sarcoma, Hodgkin's choriocarcinoma, and many others. Vinblastine has a triphasic elimination with half-lives of 3.7 minutes, 1.6 hours, and 24.8 hours respectively.[1] No data are available on its transfer into human milk, but its levels are probably low due to a relatively higher molecular weight of 909 daltons. However, mothers should be advised to withhold breastfeeding for a minimum of 10 days following treatment.

Pregnancy Risk	D	Lactation Risk	L5
T ½	= 24.8 hours	M/P	=
Vd	= 18.9–27.3 (dose dependent). l/kg	PB	= 99%
Tmax	=	Oral	=
MW	= 909.07	pKa	= 5.4, 7.4

Adult Concerns: Cough or hoarseness, fever or chills, lower back or side pain, painful or difficult urination, nausea, and vomiting.

Pediatric Concerns:

Drug Interactions: The simultaneous oral or intravenous administration of phenytoin and antineoplastic chemotherapy combinations that included vinblastine sulfate has been reported to have reduced blood levels of the anticonvulsant and to have increased seizure activity.

Relative Infant Dose:

Adult Dose: Given once weekly for duration of treatment; dosage amounts vary according to body surface area and duration of treatment.

Alternatives:

References:
1. Grochow LB, Ames MM. A clinician's guide to chemotherapy pharmacokinetics and pharmacodynamics. 1st ed. Baltimore, MD: Williams and Wilkins; 1998.

VINCRISTINE   L5

Trade: Vincasar PFS, Oncovin, Citomid, Farmistin, Ifavin, Norcristine, Vincizina

Other Trades: Vincristine

Category: Anticancer drug

Vincristine is an antineoplastic agent derived from the Catharanthus alkaloids family. It is commonly used in numerous cancers including breast cancer, Kaposi's sarcoma, non-Hodgkin's, lymphoma, and many others. Vincristine has a molecular weight of 923 Da. The kinetic studies thus far are highly variable and exact data is lacking. Vincristine exhibits a large and variable volume of distribution and ranges from 8.4 to 10.8 .[1] Studies in patients suggest it has a triphasic elimination pattern with initial, middle, and terminal half-lives of five minutes, 2.3 hours, and 85 hours respectively. However, the terminal elimination half-live sometimes ranges from 19–155 hours depending on the individual patient. No data are available on its transfer into human milk, but its levels are probably low due to a relatively higher molecular weight of 923 daltons. However, mothers should be advised to withhold breastfeeding for a minimum of 35 days following treatment, as this product is slowly eliminated from the body.[2] Withhold breastfeeding for a minimum of 35 days.

Pregnancy Risk	D	Lactation Risk	L5
T ½	= (gamma) 19–55 hours	M/P	=
Vd	= 8.4–10.8 l/kg	PB	=
Tmax	=	Oral	=
MW	= 923	pKa	= 5.0, 7.4

Adult Concerns: Common side effects: Impaired walking (may last several months), constipation and alopecia. Less common side effects: Convulsions, often with hypertension, abdominal pain and urinary disturbances.

Pediatric Concerns:

Drug Interactions: The simultaneous oral or intravenous administration of phenytoin and antineoplastic chemotherapy combinations that included vincristine sulfate has been reported to reduce blood levels of the anticonvulsant and to increase seizure activity.

Relative Infant Dose:

Adult Dose: A maximum of 2 mg/dose; amount of medication varies according to treatment plan.

Alternatives:

References:
1. Grochow LB, Ames MM. A clinician's guide to chemotherapy pharmacokinetics and pharmacodynamics. 1st ed. Baltimore, MD: Williams and Wilkins; 1998.
2. Pharmaceutical manufacturer prescribing information, 2005.

VINORELBINE   L5

Trade: Navelbine, Biovelbin

Other Trades:

Category: Anticancer drug

Vinorelbine is a close congener of vincristine. It is used for the treatment of advanced breast cancer, non-small cell lung cancer, non-Hodgkin's lymphoma, Hodgkin's disease, and ovarian carcinoma.[1] In a number of studies, the terminal elimination half-life ranged from 31.2 to 80 hours. The volume of distribution in these studies ranged from 25 to 75.6 .[2] No data are available on the transfer of this agent into human milk. Mothers should abstain from breastfeeding for a minimum of 30 days.

Pregnancy Risk	D		Lactation Risk	L5
T ½	= (gamma) 31.2–80 hours		M/P	=
Vd	= 25–75.6 l/kg		PB	= 80%-91%
Tmax	=		Oral	=
MW	= 1079.1		pKa	= 5.4, 7.4

Adult Concerns: Cough or hoarseness, fever or chills, lower back or side pain, painful or difficult urination, redness, increased warmth, pain, or discoloration of vein at injection site, sore throat, nausea, and vomiting.

Pediatric Concerns:

Drug Interactions: Acute pulmonary reactions have been reported with vinorelbine when used in conjunction with mitomycin. Patients who receive vinorelbine and paclitaxel, either concomitantly or sequentially, should be monitored for signs and symptoms of neuropathy. Administration of vinorelbine to patients with prior or concomitant radiation therapy may result in radiosensitizing effects.

Relative Infant Dose:

Adult Dose: 30 mg/m²/weekly.

Alternatives:

References:
1. Grochow LB, Ames MM. A clinician's guide to chemotherapy pharmacokinetics and pharmacodynamics. 1st ed. Baltimore, MD: Williams and Wilkins; 1998.
2. Pharmaceutical manufacturer prescribing information, 2005.

VITAMIN A   L3

Trade: A-25, A-Natural, A-Natural-25, Aquasol A

Other Trades:

Category: Vitamin supplement

Vitamin A (retinol) is a typical retinoid. It is a fat soluble vitamin that is secreted into human milk and primarily sequestered in high concentrations in the liver (90%).[1] Retinol is absorbed in the small intestine by a selective carrier-mediated uptake process. Levels in infants are generally unknown. The overdose of Vitamin A is extremely dangerous and is characterized by nausea, vomiting, headache, vertigo, and muscular incoordination. Acute toxicity generally occurs at doses of 25,000 IU/kg. Chronic exposure to levels of 4,000 IU/kg daily for 6 or more months is hazardous. Liver damage can occur at doses as low as 15,000 IU per day. In infants, a bulging fontanel is also indicative of Vitamin A toxicity. The suggested adult female dose is listed at 700 µg or 2300 IU. Upper limit is normally 3000 µg or 10,000 IU. Adults should never exceed 5000 units/day unless under the direct supervision of a physician and for specific diseases. Use normal doses in breastfeeding mothers if at all possible. Mature human milk is rich in retinol and contains 750 µg/L (2800 units). At this point we do not know if vitamin A levels in milk correlate with maternal plasma levels, but they probably do. Caution is recommended in supratherapeutic dosing in breastfeeding mothers.

Pregnancy Risk	A		Lactation Risk	L3
T ½	=		M/P	=
Vd	=		PB	=
Tmax	=		Oral	= Complete
MW	= 286		pKa	=

Adult Concerns: Liver toxicity in overdose. Numerous other symptoms are possible including drying of mucous membranes, alopecia, fever, fatigue, weight loss, etc.

Pediatric Concerns: None reported via milk, but do not use vitamin A in excess of 5000 IU/day.

Drug Interactions:

Relative Infant Dose:

Adult Dose: <5000 IU daily.

Alternatives:

References:
1. McEvoy GE. (ed): AFHS Drug Information. New York, NY: 2005.

VITAMIN B-12 | L1

Trade: Cyanocobalamin

Other Trades: Rubramin, Anacobin, Cytacon

Category: Vitamin supplement

Vitamin B_{12} is also called cyanocobalamin and is used for the treatment of pernicious anemia. It is an essential vitamin that is secreted in human milk at concentrations of 0.1 µg/100 mL. B_{12} deficiency is very dangerous (severe brain damage) to an infant. Vegan mothers and certain other vegetarians should be supplemented during pregnancy. Milk levels vary in proportion to maternal serum levels.[1] Vegetarian mothers may have low levels unless supplemented. Supplementation of nursing mothers is generally recommended. Following the maternal administration of radiolabeled cyanocobalamin during a Schilling test, peak concentrations occur at 24 hours post-dose. However, the amount absorbed by an infant is less than the current regulatory limit at any time. Therefore, discarding the first feed at four hours after administration (as advised by the Administration of Radioactive Substances Advisory Committee) is not warranted.[2] B_{12} is now available in many forms, including injections, oral tablets, and intranasal gels, all of which are safe in breastfeeding mothers and infants.

Pregnancy Risk	C		Lactation Risk	L1
T ½	=		M/P	=
Vd	=		PB	=
Tmax	= 2 hours		Oral	= Variable
MW	= 1355		pKa	=

Adult Concerns: Itching, skin rash, mild diarrhea, megaloblastic anemia in vegetarian mothers.

Pediatric Concerns: None reported with exception of B_{12} deficiency states.

Drug Interactions:

Relative Infant Dose:

Adult Dose: 25 µg daily.

Alternatives:

References:
1. Lawrence RA. Breastfeeding: A guide for the medical profession. St. Louis: Mosby Publishers, 1994.
2. Pomeroy KM, Sawyer LJ, Evans MJ. Estimated radiation dose to breast feeding infant following maternal administration of 57Co labelled to vitamin B_{12}. Nucl Med Commun 2005 Sept; 26(9): 839–41.

VITAMIN D   L2

Trade: Calciferol, Cholecalciferol, Ergocalciferol, Bio-D-Mulsion, D3–50, Ddrops, Delta, Enfamil D-Vi-Sol

Other Trades: D-Vi-Sol

Category: Vitamin D supplement

Vitamin D is secreted into milk in limited concentrations and is somewhat proportional to maternal serum levels.[1] Excessive doses can produce elevated calcium levels in the infant[2]; therefore, doses lower than 10,000 IU/day are suggested in undernourished mothers. There has been some concern that mothers deficient in vitamin D may not provide sufficient vitamin D to the infant and hence impede bone mineralization in their infants. In a study by Greer[3], breastfed infants who received oral vitamin D supplementation had greater bone mineralization than those who were not supplemented. However, a more recent study of Korean women in winter who were not supplemented with vitamin D, and whose infants were either fed with human milk or artificial cow's formula (with vitamin D added), suggested that even though the breastfed groups plasma 25-hydroxyvitamin D concentration was lower, bone mineralization was equivalent in both breastfed and formula-fed infants.[4] The authors speculated that adequate bone mineralization occurs during the breastfeeding period from a predominantly vitamin D independent passive transport mechanism.

Human milk is known to have rather minimal concentrations of vitamin D. On average, breast milk contains approximately 26 IU/L (range= 5–136). Supplementing a mother with even moderate doses of vitamin D does not substantially increase milk levels.

In 2003, the Academy of Pediatrics, responding to the increased reports of rickets in breastfeeding infants, published a recommendation that all US infants should consume at least 200 IU of vitamin D per day by supplementation if needed. These recommendations are somewhat controversial for at least two reasons. One, we do not know with certainty the minimal but adequate dose of vitamin D required by breastfed infants, and two, they suggest that a mother's milk may in some cases be nutritionally inadequate. Regardless of these concerns, mothers who have limited vitamin D intake due to poor nutrition, or whose bodies have limited exposure to sunlight, probably need supplementation as their milk is likely deficient in vitamin D. In addition, infants of these mothers (who have limited or no exposure to sunlight or inadequate intake) may need supplementation, as these infants (particularly dark skinned) are most at risk for developing rickets. The most recent study to evaluate the use of higher maternal doses of vitamin D and its transmission into human milk suggests that relatively higher maternal doses may actually increase milk levels of vitamin D significantly.

In two groups of exclusively lactating women (n= 18) who were consuming 1600 IU vitamin D_2 and 400 IU vitamin D_3 (prenatal vitamin), or 3600 IU vitamin D_2 and 400 IU vitamin D_3, supplementation at these higher levels increased circulating 25-hydroxyvitamin D 25(OH)D] concentrations for both groups.[5] The vitamin D activity of milk from mothers receiving 2000 IU/day vitamin D increased by 34.2 IU/L, on average, whereas the activity in the 4000 IU/day group increased by 94.2 IU/L. Infants of mothers receiving 4000 IU/day exhibited increases in circulating 25(OH)D_3 and 25(OH)D_2 concentrations from 12.7 to 18.8 ng/mL and from 0.8 to 12.0 ng/mL, respectively. Total circulating 25(OH)D concentrations increased from 13.4 to 30.8 ng/mL. This latter study clearly shows that increasing the maternal intake of vitamin D significantly increases milk vitamin D content. Further using the typical 400 IU dose (RDA) in adults is all but worthless in increasing maternal or the infants plasma 25(OH)D concentrations. Maternal doses of 4000 IU/day may be required to facilitate increased transfer of 25(OH)D to the infant. For a review of this issue read Greer.[6]

In summary, human milk is known to have rather minimal concentrations of vitamin D. Supplementing a mother with even moderate doses of vitamin D does not substantially increase milk levels. Using the typical 400 IU dose (RDA) in adults is all but worthless in increasing maternal or the infant's plasma 25(OH)D concentrations. Maternal doses of 4000 IU/day may be required to facilitate increased transfer of 25(OH)D to the infant. Excessive doses can produce elevated calcium levels in the infant[2]; therefore, doses lower than 10,000 IU/day are suggested in undernourished mothers. Mothers who have limited vitamin D intake due to poor nutrition, or whose bodies have limited exposure to sunlight, probably need supplementation as their milk is likely deficient in vitamin D. In addition, infants of these mothers (who have limited or no exposure to sunlight or inadequate intake) may need supplementation as well, as these infants (particularly dark skinned) are most at risk for developing rickets.

Pregnancy Risk	C	Lactation Risk	L2
T ½	=	M/P	=
Vd	=	PB	=
Tmax	=	Oral	= Variable
MW	= 396	pKa	=

Adult Concerns: Elevated calcium levels in the plasma following chronic high doses (>10,000 IU/day).

Pediatric Concerns: None reported via milk. The AAP recommends an infant dose of 200 IU/day.

Drug Interactions:

Relative Infant Dose:

Adult Dose: RDA = 400 IU/day.

Alternatives:

References:
1. Rothberg AD, Pettifor JM, Cohen DF, Sonnendecker EW, Ross FP. Maternal-infant vitamin D relationships during breast-feeding. J Pediatr 1982; 101(4): 500–503.
2. Goldberg LD. Transmission of a vitamin-D metabolite in breast milk. Lancet 1972; 2(7789): 1258–1259.
3. Greer FR, Searcy JE, Levin RS, Steichen JJ, Asch PS, Tsang RC. Bone mineral content and serum 25-hydroxyvitamin D concentration in breast-fed infants with and without supplemental vitamin D. J Pediatr 1981; 98(5): 696–701.
4. Park MJ, Namgung R, Kim DH, Tsang RC. Bone mineral content is not reduced despite low vitamin D status in breast milk-fed infants versus cow's milk based formula-fed infants. J Pediatr 1998; 132(4): 641–645.
5. Hollis BW, Wagner CL. Vitamin D requirements during lactation: high-dose maternal supplementation as therapy to prevent hypovitaminosis D for both the mother and the nursing infant. Am J Clin Nutr 2004 Dec; 80(6 Suppl): 1752S-8S.
6. Greer FR. Issues in establishing vitamin D recommendations for infants and children. Am J Clin Nutr 2004 Dec; 80(6 Suppl): 1759S-62S.

VITAMIN E   L2

Trade: Alpha Tocopherol, Aquasol E
Other Trades: Aquasol E, Bio E
Category: Vitamin E supplement

Vitamin E (alpha tocopherol) is secreted in milk in higher concentrations than in the maternal serum. Vitamin E is particularly important biologically to infants and premature infants may require supplementation with oral vitamin E as they are relatively deficient at birth, and the amount in milk may not be sufficient due to their more rapid growth rate, and their poor absorption via the gut. Vitamin E has been repeatedly found to reduce the risk of intraventricular hemorrhage and retinopathy of prematurity to slight degrees. Following topical administration to nipples (400 IU/feeding), Vitamin E plasma levels in breastfeeding infants were

40% higher than controls in just 6 days.[1] In numerous studies, the concentration of alpha tocopherol varies enormously from as little as 0.1 mg/dL to as much as 0.86 mg/dL.[2,3] Further, vitamin E levels also change with stage of lactation. In one study, the mean value for vitamin E at 2 weeks postpartum was 0.67 mg/dL and subsequently dropped to 0.4, 0.37, and 0.37 at 6, 12, and 16 weeks postpartum.[4] The effect of maternal supplementation with vitamin E is obscure. In one study, supplementing with as little as 50 mg/day did not increase vitamin E content in human milk.[4] However a later study suggests that supplementing with large quantities may indeed increase milk levels to a minimal degree. In a study of a mother who supplemented with an average of 1090 mg/day, milk levels averaged 1.1 mg/dL.[5]

Do not overdose. Do not apply concentrated products to nipples unless concentrations are low (<50–100 IU) and then, only infrequently. The application of pure vitamin E oil (1000 IU/gm) to nipples could be hazardous to the infant. For an excellent review see Jensen.[6]

Pregnancy Risk	A	Lactation Risk	L2
T ½	= 282 hours (IV)	M/P	=
Vd	=	PB	=
Tmax	=	Oral	= Variable
MW	= 431	pKa	= 11.4

Adult Concerns: Thrombophlebitis, pulmonary embolism, contact dermatitis (topical), eczematous lesions (topical).

Pediatric Concerns: None reported via milk, but caution is recommended. Do not use highly concentrated vitamin E oils directly on nipple.

Drug Interactions:

Relative Infant Dose:

Adult Dose: 16–18 IU (1 mg d-Alpha-tocopherol) daily.

Alternatives:

References:

1. Marx CM, Izquierdo A, Driscoll JW, Murray MA, Epstein MF. Vitamin E concentrations in serum of newborn infants after topical use of vitamin E by nursing mothers. Am J Obstet Gynecol 1985; 152(6 Pt 1): 668–670.
2. Kobayashi H, Kanno C, Yamauchi K, Tsugo T. Identification of alpha-, beta-, gamma-, and delta-tocopherols and their contents in human milk. Biochim Biophys Acta 1975 Feb 20; 380(2): 282–90.
3. Haug M, Laubach C, Burke M, Harzer G. Vitamin E in human milk from mothers of preterm and term infants. J Pediatr Gastroenterol Nutr 1987 Jul; 6(4): 605–9.
4. Lammi-Keefe CJ. Tocopherols in human milk: analytical method using high-performance liquid chromatography. J Pediatr Gastroenterol Nutr 1986 Nov; 5(6): 934–7.
5. Anderson DM, Pittard WB, III. Vitamin E and C concentrations in human milk with maternal megadosing: a case report. J Am Diet Assoc 1985 Jun; 85(6): 715–7.
6. Lammi-Keefe, CJ. Vitamins D and E in Human Milk. In: Handbook of milk composition. San Diego: Academic Press; 1995.

WARFARIN   L2

Trade: Coumadin, Panwarfin
Other Trades: Marevan, Coumadin, Warfilone
Category: Anticoagulant

Warfarin is a potent anticoagulant. Warfarin is highly protein bound in the maternal circulation and therefore very little is secreted into human milk. Very small and insignificant amounts are secreted into milk but it depends to some degree on the dose administered. In one study of two patients who were anticoagulated with warfarin, no warfarin was detected in the infant's serum, nor were changes in coagulation detectable.[1] In another study of 13 mothers, less than 0.08 μmol/L (25 ng/mL) was detected in milk, and no warfarin was detected in the infants' plasma.[2] According to these authors, maternal warfarin apparently poses little risk to a nursing infant and thus far has not produced bleeding anomalies in breastfed infants. Other anticoagulants, such as phenindione, should be avoided. Observe infant for bleeding such as excessive bruising or reddish petechia (spots). While the risks in breastfeeding premature infants (which are more susceptible to intracranial bleeding) is still low, oral supplementation with vitamin K_1 will preclude any chance of hemorrhage. Even modest doses of Vitamin K_1 counteract high doses of warfarin.

Pregnancy Risk	X	Lactation Risk	L2
T ½	= 1–2.5 days	M/P	=
Vd	= 0.1–0.2 l/kg	PB	= 99%
Tmax	= 0.5–3 days	Oral	= Complete
MW	= 308	pKa	= 4.5

Adult Concerns: Bleeding, bruising.

Pediatric Concerns: None reported via milk, but observe for bleeding, bruising.

Drug Interactions: The drug interactions of warfarin are numerous. Agents that may increase the anticoagulant effect and the risk of bleeding include: acetaminophen, androgens, beta blockers, clofibrate, corticosteroids, disulfiram, erythromycin, fluconazole, hydantoins, ketoconazole, miconazole, sulfonamides, thyroid hormones, and numerous others. Agents that may decrease the anticoagulant effect of warfarin include: ascorbic acid, dicloxacillin, ethanol, griseofulvin, nafcillin, sucralfate, trazodone, amino glutethimide, barbiturates, carbamazepine, etretinate, rifampin. Due to numerous drug interactions, please consult additional references.

Relative Infant Dose:

Adult Dose: 2–10 mg daily.

Alternatives:

References:
1. McKenna R, Cole ER, Vasan U. Is warfarin sodium contraindicated in the lactating mother? J Pediatr 1983; 103(2): 325–327.
2. Orme ML, Lewis PJ, De Swiet M, Serlin MJ, Sibeon R, Baty JD, Breckenridge AM. May mothers given warfarin breast-feed their infants? Br Med J 1977; 1(6076): 1564–1565.

WEST NILE FEVER   L4

Trade:

Other Trades:

Category: Viral febrile infection

West Nile Virus (WNV), which belongs to the flaviviridae family, is transmitted to humans from infected birds via the bite of culex mosquito. Although prevalent in many parts of the world, there have been increasing reports of WNV infection in the United States since 1999. Several modes of transmission have been reported which includes air-borne, blood-borne, trans-placental, organ transplantation and also possible transmission through breast milk. Mosquitoes, largely bird-feeding species, are the principal vectors of West Nile virus. The virus has been isolated from 43 mosquito species, predominantly of the genus Culex.[1,2,3] West Nile fever in humans usually is a febrile, influenza-like illness characterized by an abrupt onset (incubation period is 3 to 6 days) of moderate to high fever (3 to 5 days, infrequently biphasic, sometimes with chills), headache (often frontal), sore throat, backache, myalgia, arthralgia, fatigue, conjunctivitis, retrobulbar pain, maculopapular or roseolar rash, lymphadenopathy, anorexia, nausea, abdominal pain, diarrhea, and respiratory symptoms.

Only one established case of transmission of WNV in breast milk occurred in Michigan, 2002 when a mother was transfused with WNV-contaminated blood one day after delivering a healthy infant. The mother started breastfeeding her baby on the day of delivery. Twelve days after delivery, the mother developed WNV illness and her serum tested positive for WNV-specific IgM antibody. Sixteen days after delivery her breast milk sample tested positive for WNV–RNA as well as for WNV specific IgM antibodies. Although the infant's serum also tested positive for IgM antibodies, the infant did not develop WNV illness and remained healthy.[4] In 2003, 6 infants known to have breastfed from WNV infected mothers were studied.[5] Of the 6, 5 remained healthy without any serological evidence of WNV infection. One infant did develop a rash, but breast milk transmission could not be established since neither infant serum nor breast milk samples were collected. Therefore, although WNV transmission by breast milk could be a possibility, it is rare.[5] The American Academy of Pediatrics states, "Because the benefits of breastfeeding seem to outweigh the risk of any WNV illness in breastfeeding infants, mothers should be encouraged to breastfeed even in areas of ongoing WNV transmission."

For answers to questions about West Nile virus, please see the CDC web site http://www.cdc.gov/ncidod/dvbid/westnile/qanda.htm

Pregnancy Risk	Probably Safe	Lactation Risk	L4
T ½	=	M/P	=
Vd	=	PB	=
Tmax	=	Oral	=
MW	=	pKa	=

Adult Concerns: Febrile influenza-like illness, characterized by an abrupt onset of moderate to high fever, headache (often frontal), sore throat, backache, myalgia, arthralgia, fatigue, conjunctivitis, retrobulbar pain, maculopapular or roseolar rash, lymphadenopathy, anorexia, nausea, abdominal pain, diarrhea, and respiratory symptoms.

Pediatric Concerns: No transmission reported via milk but it has not been studied.

Drug Interactions:

Relative Infant Dose:

Adult Dose:

Alternatives:

References:

1. Hayes C. West Nile Fever. In: Monath TP (ed). The arboviruses: epidemiology and ecology, Vol 5. Boca Raton, FL: CRC Press, 1989.
2. Shope RE. Other Flavivirus Infections. In: Guerrant RL, Walker DH, and Weller PF (eds). Tropical Infectious Diseases: Principals, Pathogens, and Practice. Philadelphia, PA: Churchill Livingstone, 2004.
3. Hubalek Z, Halouzka J. West Nile fever--a reemerging mosquito-borne viral disease in Europe. Emerg Infect Dis 1999; 5(5): 643–650.
4. Centers for Disease Control and Prevention (CDC). Possible West Nile virustransmission to an infant through breast-feeding--Michigan, 2002. MMWR MorbMortal Wkly Rep. 2002 Oct 4; 51(39): 877–8.
5. Hinckley AF, O'Leary DR, Hayes EB. Transmission of West Nile virus throughhuman breast milk seems to be rare. Pediatrics. 2007 Mar; 119(3): e666–71.
6. AAP CoID: West Nile Virus. In: Red Book: 2009 Report of the Committe on Infectious Diseases. Edited by Pickering LK BC, Kimberlin DW, Long SS, 28 edn; 2009: 730–732.

XENON-[133]   L3

Trade: Xenon-[133]

Other Trades:

Category: Evaluation of pulmonary obstruction

Xenon-[133] (T½ = 5.3 days) and Xenon-[127] (T½=36.4 days) are noble gases.[1] As such they are chemically inert and are used often for ventilation and for cerebral blood flow studies. The patient is asked to inhale a gas mixed with either of these isotopes, followed by a brief 5 min wash out period. Obstructions in the lung appear as hot spots. Because these gases are inert, they would not be stored for any length of time in the human and would be rapidly exhaled within minutes. This is a typical case were the biological half-life (time stored in body, minutes in this case) is incredibly short compared to the radioactive half-life (5.3 days). Xenon-[133] would not likely be hazardous to a breastfeeding infant as long as a brief wash out period of an hour or more is used. International Commission of Radiological Protection recommends no interruption for breastfeeding.[2] The Nuclear Regulatory Commission (NRC) recommends 1 hour interruption of breastfeeding for a dosage of 10–30 mCi of Xenon-[133].[3]

Pregnancy Risk	C	Lactation Risk	L3
T ½	= 5.3 days	M/P	=
Vd	=	PB	=
Tmax	=	Oral	= Nil
MW	=	pKa	=

Adult Concerns: None.

Pediatric Concerns: None, if brief wash out period is used.

Drug Interactions:

Relative Infant Dose:

Adult Dose:

Alternatives:

References:

1. Gopal B, Saha. Fundamentals of Nuclear Pharmacy. 3rd ed. ed. Springer-Verlag Publishers, 1992.
2. ICRP, 2008. Radiation Dose to Patients from Radiopharmaceuticals–Addendum 3 to ICRP Publication 53. ICRP Publication 106. Ann. ICRP 38 (1–2).
3. Activities of Radiopharmaceuticals from the Nuclear Regulatory Commission.

XYLOMETAZOLINE   L3

Trade:

Other Trades:

Category: Decongestant

Xylometazolione is a vasocontrictive agent used both nasally and ophthalmically. No reports are available regarding the use of xylometazoline during lactation and effects on the infant with exposure of the drug in human milk are unknown. Generally, use of topical agents possess less risk than systemically absorbed agents. However, xylometazoline may be absorbed systemically when used nasally. Caution is warranted when contemplating use of xylometazoline while breastfeeding.[1]

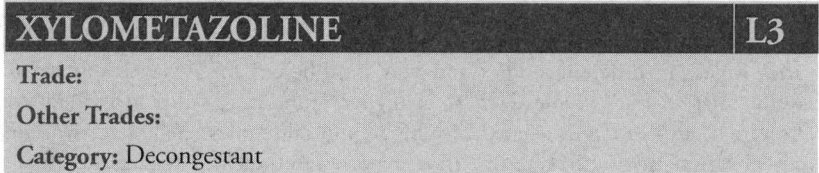

Pregnancy Risk	C	Lactation Risk	L3
T ½	=	M/P	=
Vd	=	PB	=
Tmax	=	Oral	= Good (nasal)
MW	= 244	pKa	=

Adult Concerns: Minimal increase in blood pressure, but only in hypertensive individuals. With excessive use or dose, hypertension and arrhythmias are possible. Headache, insomnia, and dizziness have been reported.

Pediatric Concerns:

Drug Interactions:

Relative Infant Dose:

Adult Dose: 2–3 drops of a 0.1% solution every 12 hours.

Alternatives: Oxymetazoline, pseudoephedrine.

References:

1. Xylometazoline. In: DRUGDEX Æ System [Internet database]. Greenwood Village, Colo: Thomson Reuters (Healthcare) Inc. Updated periodically.

YELLOW FEVER VACCINE   L4

Trade: YF-Vax

Other Trades: Arilvax, Stamaril

Category: Vaccine

Yellow fever is an acute viral illness caused by a mosquito-borne flavivirus. The clinical spectrum of yellow fever is highly variable, from subclinical infection to overwhelming pansystemic disease. Yellow fever has an abrupt onset after an incubation period of 3 to 6 days, and usually includes fever, prostration, headache, photophobia, lumbosacral pain, extremity pain (especially the knee joints), epigastric pain, anorexia, and vomiting. The illness may progress to liver and renal failure, and hemorrhagic symptoms and signs caused by thrombocytopenia and abnormal clotting and coagulation may occur. The case-fatality rate of yellow fever varies widely in different studies and may be different for Africa compared to South America, but is typically 20% or higher. Jaundice or other gross evidence of severe liver disease is associated with higher mortality rates.[1] Yellow fever occurs only in Africa and South America. Those reported in the United States are usually imported cases.[2] The World Health Organization (WHO) estimates that a total of 200,000 cases of yellow fever occur each year worldwide.

Yellow fever vaccine is a live, attenuated virus preparation made from the 17D yellow fever virus strain.[1] Historically, the 17D vaccine has been considered to be one of the safest and most effective live virus vaccines ever developed. The virus is grown in chick embryos. Being a live attenuated vaccine, there is significant risk to the infant following breastmilk exposure to this vaccine. A report of possible yellow fever virus transmission in breast milk occurred in Brazil 2009 when a 23-day old breast-fed infant developed fever and seizures 8 days after the mother received the yellow fever vaccine. The infant's CSF tested positive for yellow fever vaccine virus (17D). A case of yellow fever viral meningoencephalitis was established.[3,4] The Canadian Medical Association Journal recently published a report of a five–week old breastfed infant who developed yellow fever encephalitis 30 days after his mother received the 17D yellow fever vaccine. The infant presented with fever, focal seizures, irritability and vomiting. The infant's serum tested positive for yellow fever–specific IgM antibody, and more importantly the cerebrospinal fluid (CSF) of the infant demonstrated the presence of yellow fever antigen.[5] Although in both cases breast milk samples were not available for investigation, all evidence points to breast milk being the possible route of infection to the infant. In both cases, the infants recovered fully and were devoid of any neurological sequelae at five and six month follow-ups respectively.[3–5]

According to CDC recommendations, all persons aged >9 months, traveling to, or living in areas of high yellow fever transmission should be vaccinated. For infants between 6–8 months of age, travel should preferably be avoided or postponed. But if travel is unavoidable, then a risk vs benefit assessment has to be made and the infant be vaccinated accordingly. Yellow fever vaccine is absolutely contra-indicated in infants 1–5 months of age.[6] According to CDC, immunization of lactating mothers with infants <9 months of age, should preferably be avoided. However, if travel of a lactating mother to an endemic area cannot be avoided or postponed, or in situations where exposure to the yellow fever virus is high, then the potential benefits of the vaccine out weigh the potential risks, and immunization in such a situation should be considered.[6]

Studies have found that in up to 80–100% of cases, the 17D vaccine virus is no longer present in maternal serum 10–13 days following vaccination.[6,7] This would suggest that breastfeeding poses little risk to an infant 10–13 days after immunization.

Pregnancy Risk	C		Lactation Risk	L4
T ½	=		M/P	=
Vd	=		PB	=
Tmax	=		Oral	=
MW	=		pKa	=

Adult Concerns: Adverse effects are numerous and include: mild headaches, myalgia, low-grade fevers. Local reactions include edema, hypersensitivity, and pain at the injection site.

Pediatric Concerns: One reported case of severe seizures and vaccine encephalitis in an infant who's mother received yellow fever vaccination eight days prior. While not adequately documented that the infection was via milk, the CDC strongly suggests that this infant probably received the virus via its mother's breastmilk. Risks in infants and children can be severe and include vaccine-induced encephalitis, most of which have occurred in infants <4 months of age (n=14), and in children >3 years (n=7).

Drug Interactions:

Relative Infant Dose: 0%

Adult Dose:

Alternatives:

References:
1. Pharmaceutical manufacturer prescribing information, 2005.
2. AAP CoID. In: Red Book: 2009 Report of the Committee on Infectious Diseases. Edited by Pickering LK BC, Kimberlin DW, Long SS, 29 edn; 2009.
3. Chen LH, Zeind C, Mackell S, LaPointe T, Mutsch M, Wilson ME: Yellow fever virus transmission via breastfeeding: follow-up to the paper on breastfeeding travelers. J Travel Med 2010, 17(4): 286–287.
4. Couto AM SM: Transmission of Yellow Fever Vaccine Virus Through Breast-Feeding–Brazil, 2009. MMWR Morbidity and Mortality Weekly Report 2010, 59.
5. Kuhn S, Twele-Montecinos L, MacDonald J, Webster P, Law B: Case report: probable transmission of vaccine strain of yellow fever virus to an infant via breast milk. Cmaj 2011, 183(4): E243–245.

6. Staples JE, Gershman M, Fischer M: Yellow fever vaccine: recommendations of the Advisory Committee on Immunization Practices (ACIP). MMWR Recomm Rep 2010, 59(RR-7): 1–27.
7. Reinhardt B, Jaspert R, Niedrig M, Kostner C, L'Age-Stehr J. Development of viremia and humoral and cellular parameters of immune activation after vaccination with yellow fever virus strain 17D: a model of human flavivirus infection. J Med Virol. Oct 1998; 56(2): 159–167.

ZAFIRLUKAST   L3

Trade: Accolate

Other Trades: Accolate

Category: Leukotriene inhibitor for asthma

Zafirlukast is a new competitive receptor antagonist of leukotriene D_4, which is a mediator of bronchoconstriction in asthmatic patients. Zafirlukast is not a bronchodilator and should not be used for acute asthma attacks. Zafirlukast is excreted into milk in low concentrations. Following repeated 40 mg doses twice daily (please note: average adult dose is 20 mg twice daily), the average steady-state concentration in breastmilk was 50 µg/L compared to 255 ng/mL in maternal plasma.[1] Zafirlukast is poorly absorbed when administered with food. It is likely the oral absorption via ingestion of breastmilk would be low. The manufacturer recommends against using in breastfeeding mothers.

Pregnancy Risk	B	Lactation Risk	L3
T ½	= 10–13 hours	M/P	= 0.15
Vd	=	PB	= >99%
Tmax	= 3 hours	Oral	= Poor
MW	= 575	pKa	= 4.01

Adult Concerns: Pharyngitis, aggravation reaction, headache, nausea, diarrhea have been reported.

Pediatric Concerns: None reported.

Drug Interactions: Erythromycin reduces oral bioavailability of zafirlukast by 40%. Aspirin increases zafirlukast plasma levels by 45%. Theophylline reduces zafirlukast plasma levels by 30%. Zafirlukast increases warfarin anticoagulation by 35%. Terfenadine reduces zafirlukast plasma levels by 54%.

Relative Infant Dose: 0.7%

Adult Dose: 20 mg twice daily.

Alternatives:

References:
1. Pharmaceutical manufacturer prescribing information, 1997.

ZALEPLON   L2

Trade: Sonata

Other Trades: Starnoc, Sonata

Category: Hypnotic agent used for insomnia.

Zaleplon is a nonbenzodiazepine hypnotic sedative that interacts at the GABA receptor. In a study of 5 lactating mothers who received doses of 10 mg orally, the peak milk level occurred at 1.2 hours and averaged 14 µg/L.[1] Milk levels decreased rapidly following a peak at 1.2 hours to less than 3 µg/L four hours following administration. The authors suggest that these levels would be subclinical to the infant.

Pregnancy Risk	C		Lactation Risk	L2
T ½	= 1.2 hours		M/P	= 0.5
Vd	=		PB	=
Tmax	= 1.2 hours		Oral	= Complete
MW	= 305		pKa	= -1.47

Adult Concerns: Headache, drowsiness, peripheral edema, dizziness have been reported. Avoid alcohol and other depressants.

Pediatric Concerns: None reported via milk. Milk levels were reported to be subclinical.

Drug Interactions: Zaleplon potentiates the CNS effects of alcohol, imipramine, thioridazine. Rifampin decreases the plasma levels of zaleplon. Cimetidine produces a significant increase in plasma levels of zaleplon.

Relative Infant Dose: 1.5%

Adult Dose: 10 mg nightly.

Alternatives:

References:
1. Darwish M, Martin PT, Cevallos WH, Tse S, Wheeler S, Troy SM. Rapid disappearance of zaleplon from breast milk after oral administration to lactating women. J Clin Pharmacol 1999; 39(7): 670–674.

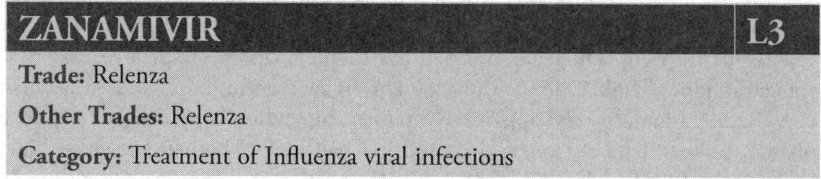

ZANAMIVIR   L3

Trade: Relenza

Other Trades: Relenza

Category: Treatment of Influenza viral infections

Zanamivir is a viral neuraminidase inhibitor that blocks or prevents viral seeding or release from infected cells and prevents viral aggregation.[1] It is only moderately effective and is believed to reduce symptoms by only 30% or several days, and only if treatment is instituted within 2 days of infection. It is administered via inhalation using a diskhaler device. Only 4–17% of the inhaled drug is systemically absorbed. Peak plasma concentrations are only 17–142 ng/mL within 2 hours of administration and then rapidly decline. The manufacturer reports that it is present in the milk of rodents although no human data are available. Due to the poor oral or inhaled absorption and the incredibly low plasma levels, it is unlikely to produce untoward effects in breastfed infants. However, due to its limited efficacy (reduces length of illness by 1 to 1.5 days), its use in breastfeeding mothers is probably not warranted, unless in high-risk patients with other severe medical conditions.

Pregnancy Risk	C	Lactation Risk	L3
T ½	= 2.5–5.1 hours	M/P	=
Vd	=	PB	= <10%
Tmax	= 1–2 hours	Oral	= 4–17%
MW	= 332	pKa	= 11.3

Adult Concerns: Bronchospasm may occur in patients with asthma or obstructive pulmonary disease.

Pediatric Concerns: None reported via milk but no studies exist.

Drug Interactions: None yet reported.

Relative Infant Dose:

Adult Dose: 10 mg twice daily.

Alternatives:

References:
1. Drug Facts and Comparisons 1999 ed. ed. St. Louis: 1999.

ZIDOVUDINE   L3

Trade: Retrovir, Combivir

Other Trades: Combivir, Novo-Azt

Category: Antiretroviral agent used in HIV

Zidovudine in an antiretroviral agent used in the treatment of HIV. In a study of 18 women receiving 300 mg twice daily at steady state, median zidovudine levels at 5.4 hours post dose in maternal serum, breast milk, and infant serum were 58 ng/mL, 207 ng/mL and 123 ng/mL, respectively.[1] The milk/serum ratio was 3.21. The median infant serum concentration of zidovudine (123 ng/mL) was at least 25 times the 50% inhibitory concentration for HIV. Infant serum concentrations of zidovudine were a median of 2.5 times higher than the respective maternal concentration of zidovudine. The elevated infant serum levels are somewhat inexplicable. In adults, and apparently infants, zidovudine has a delayed terminal phase half-life (4.8 hours) longer than its initial half-life (<3 hours). The rather high serum levels in infant is worrisome and some caution is recommended although no untoward effects were reported in this study of 18 patients. Close monitoring of the infant for changes in CBC (granulocytopenia, anemia, leukopenia), liver function, CNS symptoms (i.e. headache, seizures), drug-induced myopathy, and numerous other symptoms, is recommended.

Pregnancy Risk	C	Lactation Risk	L3
T ½	= <3 hours	M/P	= 3.21
Vd	= 1.6 l/kg	PB	= <38%
Tmax	= 1.5 hours	Oral	= 61%
MW	= 267	pKa	= 9.96

Adult Concerns: Side effects include cardiomyopathy, congestive heart failure, skin and nail discoloration, gynecomastia, lactic acidosis, anorexia, nausea, vomiting, esophageal ulcer, dyspnea, cough, headache. Many other side effects have been reported. Consult the prescribing information.

Pediatric Concerns: None reported but milk levels are moderately high, and serum levels in infants are 3.2 times higher than maternal serum levels.

Drug Interactions: Drug interactions are numerous. Nelfinavir, trimethoprim/sulfa, atovaquone, fluconazole, methadone, probenecid, ritonavir, valproic acid are a few that have been reported to alter the plasma levels of zidovudine. Consult other texts for full list of drug-drug interactions.

Relative Infant Dose: 0.4%

Adult Dose: 300 mg twice daily.

Alternatives: Nevirapine, lamivudine

References:
1. Shapiro RL, Holland DT, Capparelli E, Lockman S, Thior I, Wester C, et al. Antiretroviral concentrations in breast-feeding infants of women in Botswana receiving antiretroviral treatment. J Infect Dis 2005 Sep 1; 192(5): 720–7.

ZILEUTON   L3

Trade: Zyflo

Other Trades:

Category: Lipoxygenase inhibitor

Zileuton is used for chronic treatment of asthma. It inhibits leukotriene formation, which in turn inhibits neutrophil and eosinophil migration, neutrophil and monocyte aggregation, and leukocyte adhesion, minimizing inflammation and bronchoconstriction in the airways.[1] No data are available on its transfer into human milk. It is not significantly toxic nor does it have severe side effects.

Pregnancy Risk	C	Lactation Risk	L3
T ½	= 2.5 hours	M/P	=
Vd	= 1.2 l/kg	PB	= 93%
Tmax	= 1.7 hours	Oral	=
MW	= 236	pKa	= 9.96

Adult Concerns: Adverse reactions include headache, pain, dyspepsia, nausea, asthenia, and abdominal pain.

Pediatric Concerns: No data are available.

Drug Interactions: Zileuton may increase the levels of aminophylline, fluvoxamine, mexiletine, mirtazapine, ropinirole, theophylline, propranolol and trifluoperazine. Concomitant use with warfarin can increase prothrombin time.

Relative Infant Dose:

Adult Dose: 600 mg four times daily.

Alternatives:

References:
1. Pharmaceutical manufacturer prescribing information, 2005.

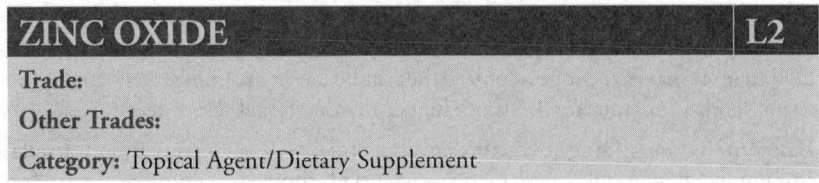

ZINC OXIDE			**L2**
Trade:			
Other Trades:			
Category: Topical Agent/Dietary Supplement			

Zinc oxide is a metal compound found in a number of topical preparations and dietary supplements. Studies in rats show that the administration of dietary zinc oxide or other organic zinc salts at levels not exceeding 38 mg per day had no effect on breastfeeding pups.[1] A sign of zinc toxicity, metal fume fever, which can be identified by fever, chills, myalgias, vomiting, and malaise, may decrease milk production.[2] Dermal absorption of zinc oxide is minimal.[3] No statistically significant increases in zinc levels occurred in the serum following administration of 40% zinc oxide ointment.[4]

Pregnancy Risk	C	Lactation Risk	L2
T ½	=	M/P	=
Vd	=	PB	=
Tmax	=	Oral	= 41%
MW	=	pKa	=

Adult Concerns: Dermal preparations of zinc may result in irritation and skin sensitivity. Gastrointestinal upset and gastritis may result from oral intake.

Pediatric Concerns:

Drug Interactions: Zinc may reduce absorption of ciprofloxacin, tetracyclines, norfloxacin, ofloxacin. Iron salts may reduce absorption of zinc. Foods containing high concentrations of phosphorus, calcium (diary foods), or phytates (bran, brown bread) may reduce oral zinc absorption. Coffee reduces zinc absorption by 50%.

Relative Infant Dose:

Adult Dose: Dermal: Apply to affected area several times each day; Oral: 25–50 mg/day.

Alternatives:

References:
1. Thompson PK, Marsh M, and Drinker KR: The effect of zinc administration upon reproduction and growth in the albino rat, together with a demonstration of the constant concentration of zinc in a given species, regardless of age. Am J Physiol 1927; 80: 65–74.
2. HSDB: Hazardous Substances Data Bank. National Library of Medicine. Bethesda, MD (Internet Version). Edition expires 2001; provided by Thomson Healthcare Inc., Greenwood Village, CO.

3. TERIS: Teratogen Information System database. CD-ROM Version. 28. University of Washington. Seattle, WA (Internet Version). Edition expires 4/30/1996; provided by Thomson Healthcare Inc., Greenwood Village, CO.
4. Derry JE, McLean WM, and Freeman JB: A study of percutaneous absorption from topically applied zinc oxide ointment. J Parent Enteral Nutr 1983; 7: 131–135.

ZINC SALTS   L2

Trade:

Other Trades:

Category: Zinc supplements

Zinc is an essential element that is required for enzymatic function within the cell. Zinc deficiencies have been documented in newborns and premature infants with symptoms such as anorexia nervosa, arthritis, diarrheas, eczema, recurrent infections, and recalcitrant skin problems. The Recommended Daily Allowance (RDA) for adults is 12–15 mg/day. The average oral dose of supplements is 25–50 mg/day; higher doses may lead to gastritis. Doses used for treatment of cold symptoms averaged 13.3 mg (lozenges) every 2 hours while awake for the duration of cold symptoms. The acetate or gluconate salts are preferred due to reduced gastric irritation and higher absorption. Zinc sulfate should not be used.

Excessive intake is detrimental. Eleven healthy males who ingested 150 mg twice daily for 6 weeks showed significant impairment of lymphocyte and polymorphonuclear leukocyte function and a significant reduction of HDL cholesterol. Intranasal zinc salts should not be used as their use was recently implicated in damage to the olfactory cells, leading the complete loss of smell.

Interestingly, absorption of dietary zinc is nearly twice as high during lactation as before conception. In 13 women studied, zinc absorption at preconception averaged 14% and during lactation, 25%.[1] There was no difference in serum zinc values between women who took iron supplements and those who did not although iron supplementation may reduce oral zinc absorption. Zinc absorption by the infant from human milk is high, averaging 41%, which is significantly higher than from soy or cow formulas (14% and 31% respectively). Minimum daily requirements of zinc in full term infants vary from 0.3 to 0.5 mg/kg/day.[2] Daily ingestion of zinc from breastmilk has been estimated to be 0.35 mg/kg/day and declines over the first 17 weeks of life as older neonates require less zinc due to slower growth rate.

Supplementation with 25–50 mg/day is probably safe, but excessive doses are discouraged. Another author has shown that zinc levels in breastmilk are independent of maternal plasma zinc concentrations or dietary zinc intake.[3] Other body pools of zinc (i.e., liver and bone) are perhaps the source of zinc in breastmilk. Therefore, higher levels of oral zinc intake probably have minimal effect on zinc concentrations in milk but excessive doses are not recommended.

Pregnancy Risk	A	Lactation Risk	L2
T ½	=	M/P	=
Vd	=	PB	=
Tmax	=	Oral	= 41%
MW	=	pKa	=

Adult Concerns: Oral zinc salts may cause gastritis, gastrointestinal upset. Gluconate salts, and lower doses are preferred.

Pediatric Concerns: None reported via milk.

Drug Interactions: Zinc may reduce absorption of ciprofloxacin, tetracyclines, norfloxacin, ofloxacin. Iron salts may reduce absorption of zinc. Foods containing high concentrations of phosphorus, calcium (dairy foods), or phytates (bran, brown bread) may reduce oral zinc absorption. Coffee reduces zinc absorption by 50%.

Relative Infant Dose:

Adult Dose: 15 mg daily.

Alternatives:

References:
1. Fung EB, Ritchie LD, Woodhouse LR, Roehl R, King JC. Zinc absorption in women during pregnancy and lactation: a longitudinal study. Am J Clin Nutr 1997; 66(1): 80–88.
2. Drug Facts and Comparisons 1997 ed. ed. St. Louis: 1997.
3. Krebs NF, Reidinger CJ, Hartley S, Robertson AD, Hambidge KM. Zinc supplementation during lactation: effects on maternal status and milk zinc concentrations. Am J Clin Nutr 1995; 61(5): 1030–1036.

ZIPRASIDONE   L2

Trade: Geodon

Other Trades:

Category: Antipsychotic

Ziprasidone is an atypical antipsychotic agent chemically unrelated to phenothiazines or butyrophenones.[1] In a brief case report of 1 patient receiving a dose of 160 mg/day with a plasma level of 177 ng/mL, milk levels were undetectable until day 10 of therapy which was 11 ng/mL and 170 ng in maternal plasma.[2] Milk/plasma ratio was 0.06. The authors estimated the relative infant dose to be 1.2% of the weight-normalized maternal dose. No untoward effects were noted in the infant. In another case report of an infant exposed throughout pregnancy and subsequently breastfed for 6 months, the infant (2.64 kg) was delivered at 39 weeks, and did not exhibit withdrawal symptoms or any other drug-related symptoms.[3] While milk levels were not determined, no symptoms of ziprasidone were noted. The infant developed normally over the following 6 months.

Pregnancy Risk	C	Lactation Risk	L2
T ½	= 7 hours	M/P	= 0.06
Vd	= 1.5 l/kg	PB	= 99%
Tmax	= 4–5 hours	Oral	= 60%
MW	= 419	pKa	= 14.89

Adult Concerns: Side effects include somnolence, prolonged QT/QTc intervals, nausea, dyspepsia, headache, skin rash, elevated liver enzymes. Relative incidence of extrapyramidal symptoms is low. Elevation of serum prolactin levels is common with this family and should be expected, although it appears minimal with this agent. Prolonged QT intervals are potentially quite hazardous so should be used with caution in individuals with bradycardia, hypokalemia, and/or hypomagnesemia.

Pediatric Concerns: None reported in one case report.

Drug Interactions: Too numerous to list. The manufacturer states that concomitant use of ziprasidone and Class III antiarrhythmic agents is contraindicated. An increased risk of cardiotoxicity is reported for many drugs (QT prolongation, torsades de pointes, cardiac arrest).

Relative Infant Dose: 0.07%–1.2%

Adult Dose: 20–80 mg twice daily.

Alternatives: Risperidone, olanzapine

References:
1. Pharmaceutical manufacturer prescribing information, 2003.
2. Schlotterbeck P, Saur R, Hiemke C, et al. Low concentration of ziprasidone in human milk: a case report. Int J Neuropsychopharmacol. Apr 2009; 12(3): 437–438.
3. Werremeyer A. Ziprasidone and citalopram use in pregnancy and lactation in a woman with psychotic depression. Am J Psychiatry. Nov 2009; 166(11): 1298.

ZOLMITRIPTAN   L3

Trade: Zomig, Zomig-ZMT, AscoTop, Zomigoro, Zomigon

Other Trades: Zomig, Rapimelt

Category: Migraine analgesic

Zolmitriptan is a selective serotonin-1D receptor antagonist that is specifically indicated for treating acute migraine headaches. Peak plasma levels of zolmitriptan during migraine attacks are generally 8–14 ng/mL and occur before 4 hours.[1,2] Zolmitriptan is structurally similar to sumatriptan but has better oral bioavailability, higher penetration into the CNS, and may have dual mechanisms of action. No data are available on its penetration into human milk, but transfer is likely. Consider sumatriptan as a preferred alternative.

Pregnancy Risk	C	Lactation Risk	L3
T ½	= 3 hours	M/P	=
Vd	=	PB	= 25%
Tmax	= 2–4 hours	Oral	= 48%
MW	= 287	pKa	= 9.64

Adult Concerns: Asthenia, dizziness, paresthesias, drowsiness, nausea, throat tightness, tight chest. Tachycardia and palpitations have been reported.

Pediatric Concerns: None reported via milk. Consider sumatriptan as alternative.

Drug Interactions: Slight increase in zolmitriptan levels when used with propranolol. Half-life doubled when used with cimetidine.

Relative Infant Dose:

Adult Dose: 2.5 mg every 2 hours PRN.

Alternatives: Sumatriptan

References:
1. Seaber E, On N, Dixon RM, Gibbens M, Leavens WJ, Liptrot J, Chittick G, Posner J, Rolan PE, Pack RW. The absolute bioavailability and metabolic disposition of the novel antimigraine compound zolmitriptan (311C90). Br J Clin Pharmacol 1997; 43(6): 579–587.
2. Palmer KJ, Spencer CM. Zolmitriptan (Adis new drug profile). CNS Drugs Jun 1997; 7(6): 468–478.

ZOLPIDEM TARTRATE   L3

Trade: Ambien, Ambien CR, Edluar

Other Trades:

Category: Sedative, sleep aid

Zolpidem, although not a benzodiazepine, interacts with the same GABA-BZ receptor site and shares some of the same pharmacologic effects of the benzodiazepine family.[1] It is used for the treatment of insomnia and difficulty falling asleep after middle of the night awakening. In a study of 5 lactating mothers receiving 20 mg daily, the maximum plasma concentration occurred between 1.75 and 3.75 hours and ranged from 90 to 364 µg/L.[2] The authors suggest that the amount of zolpidem recovered in breastmilk 3 hours after administration ranged between 0.76 and 3.88 µg or 0.004 to 0.019% of the total dose administered. Breastmilk clearance of zolpidem is very rapid and none was detectable (below 0.5 ng/mL) by 4–5 hours post dose.

One case of infant sedation and poor appetite related to zolpidem use has been reported following the nightly use of sertraline (100 mg) and 10 mg zolpidem.[3] Upon discontinuation of zolpidem, the infant regained appetite and became more alert.

Pregnancy Risk	C	Lactation Risk	L3
T ½	= 2.5–5 hours	M/P	= 0.13–0.18
Vd	=	PB	= 92.5%
Tmax	= 1.6 hours	Oral	= 70%
MW	= 307	pKa	=

Adult Concerns: Sedation, anxiety, fatigue, irritability. Sweating, tachycardia, tachypnea, tremors, and severe anxiety have been reported upon discontinuation of zolpidem.

Pediatric Concerns: One case of infant drowsiness and poor feeding. Discontinuation symptoms are known in adults and may be present in infants following long exposure.

Drug Interactions: Use with food may significantly decrease plasma levels by 25%.

Relative Infant Dose: 4.7%–19.1%

Adult Dose: 5–10 mg daily.

Alternatives: Zopiclone, eszopiclone

References:

1. Pharmaceutical manufacturer prescribing information, 1996.
2. Pons G, Francoual C, Guillet P, Moran C, Hermann P, Bianchetti G, Thiercelin JF, Thenot JP, Olive G. Zolpidem excretion in breast milk. Eur J Clin Pharmacol 1989; 37(3): 245–248.
3. A.K. Personnal communication, 1999.

ZONISAMIDE   L4

Trade: Zonegran

Other Trades:

Category: Anticonvulsant

Zonisamide is a broad-spectrum anticonvulsant medication chemically classified as a sulfonamide. It is especially effective in partial seizures and in patients whose seizures are drug resistant. It has a long half-life and high pKa which from the data below leads to high maternal milk and plasma concentrations. In pregnant patients, it readily (92%) transfers through the placenta to the fetus.

In a study of one patient receiving 100 mg three times daily of zonisamide on postpartum days 0, 3, 6, 14, and 30, the reported milk levels were drawn at 1.5 to 2.5 hours following administration of the medication.[1] The reported milk levels ranged from 8.25 to 10.5 mg/L (mean= 9.5) while the maternal plasma levels ranged from 9.52 to 10.6 mg/L (mean=10.13). The milk/plasma ratio averaged 0.93. Using the highest reported milk level, the average relative infant dose would be about 33% of the maternal dose.

In another study in a patient receiving 400 mg zonisamide during and after pregnancy, the plasma levels of zonisamide at delivery were 15.7 µg/mL in the mother and 14.4 µg/mL in the infant at birth.[2] Thus the placental transfer was 92%. Levels in maternal plasma and maternal milk were similar, 10.7–13.3 µg/mL. The authors suggested the rate of breast milk transfer was 41–57%. The breastfed infant plasma level of zonisamide at day 24 was 3.9 µg/mL. While significantly less than the cord blood level of 14.4 µg/mL at birth, these levels are still quite high and are equal to that of an adult receiving 300 mg/day doses (C_{max}= 3.479 µg/mL).[3] Significant caution is recommended with this medication as a number of pediatric adverse effects have been noted in older children.

Pregnancy Risk	C	Lactation Risk	L4
T ½	= 63 hours	M/P	= 0.93
Vd	= 1.45 l/kg	PB	= 40%
Tmax	= 2–6 hours	Oral	=
MW	= 212	pKa	= 10.2

Adult Concerns: Adverse reactions include somnolence, dizziness, headache, nausea, anorexia, agitation, irritability, speech abnormalities, diplopia, chest pain, paresthesias, psychosis, leukopenia, weight loss, Steven-Johnson syndrome, oligohydrosis and hyperthermia in pediatric patients. Seizures on withdrawal have been reported. Nephrolithiasis is reported in 4% of patients.

Pediatric Concerns: None via breastmilk, but levels are extremely high.

Drug Interactions: Carbamazepine may increase the plasma clearance of zonisamide. Do not use with Evening primrose oil or Ginko as seizure thresholds may be lowered. Phenobarbital reduces plasma half-life of zonisamide significantly.

Relative Infant Dose: 28.9%–36.8%

Adult Dose: 100–200 mg/day.

Alternatives:

References:
1. Shimoyama R, Ohkubo T, Sugawara K. Monitoring of zonisamide in human breast milk and maternal plasma by solid-phase extraction HPLC method. Biomed Chromatogr 1999; 13(5): 370–372.
2. Kawada K, Itoh S, Kusaka T, Isobe K, Ishii M. Pharmacokinetics of zonisamide in perinatal period. Brain Dev. 2002 Mar; 24(2): 95–7.
3. Maanen R, Bentley D. Bioequivalence of zonisamide orally dispersible tablet and immediate-release capsule formulations: results from two open-label, randomized-sequence, single-dose, two-period, two-treatment crossover studies in healthy male volunteers. Clin Ther. 2009 Jun; 31(6): 1244–55.

ZOPICLONE   L2

Trade:

Other Trades: Imovane, Apo-Zopiclone, Dom-Zopiclone, PMS-Zopiclone, Rhovan, Alti-Zopiclone, Ratio-Zopiclone, Zileze, Zimmovane

Category: Hypnotic sedative

Zopiclone is a sedative/hypnotic which, although structurally dissimilar to the benzodiazepines, shares their pharmacologic profile.[1] In a group of 12 women who received 7.5 mg of zopiclone, the average peak milk concentration at 2.4 hours was 34 µg/L[2], but the average milk concentration was 10.92 µg/L. The milk half-life was 5.3 hours compared to the maternal plasma half-life of 4.9 hours. The milk/plasma AUC ratio was 0.51 and ranged from 0.4 to 0.7. The authors report that the average infant dose of zopiclone via milk would be 1.4% of the weight adjusted dose ingested by the mother.

Pregnancy Risk	C	Lactation Risk	L2
T ½	= 4–5 hours	M/P	= 0.51
Vd	= 1.51 l/kg	PB	= 45%
Tmax	= 1.6 hours	Oral	= 75%
MW	= 388	pKa	= 6.7

Adult Concerns: Sedation.

Pediatric Concerns: None reported via milk.

Drug Interactions:

Relative Infant Dose: 1.5%

Adult Dose: 7.5 mg orally.

Alternatives:

References:

1. Gaillot J, Heusse D, Hougton GW, Marc AJ, Dreyfus JF. Pharmacokinetics and metabolism of zopiclone. Pharmacology 1983; 27 Suppl 2: 76–91.
2. Matheson I, Sande HA, Gaillot J. The excretion of zopiclone into breast milk. Br J Clin Pharmacol 1990; 30(2): 267–271.

ZOSTER VACCINE, LIVE   L3

Trade: Zostavax

Other Trades:

Category: Vaccine

The varicella zoster virus (VZV) belongs to the family of herpes viruses. Primary VZV infection is commonly called chickenpox and occurs usually in childhood. After the primary illness subsides, this virus remains latent in the ganglia and may get re-activated decades later to cause herpes zoster, or shingles. The infectivity of shingles to other susceptible individuals is 15%. Transmission can be reduced by covering the lesions of shingles, until they dry up and form crusts.

The zoster vaccine is prepared from a live, attenuated VZV strain. This vaccine is routinely recommended for all those more than 60 years of age. There is currently no established evidence of transmission of the zoster virus vaccine in breastmilk. This vaccine is not contra-indicated in breastfeeding.[1,2]

Pregnancy Risk	Hazardous	Lactation Risk	L3
T ½	=	M/P	=
Vd	=	PB	=
Tmax	=	Oral	=
MW	=	pKa	=

Adult Concerns: Redness, pain, tenderness, swelling at the site of injection, varicella-like rash, hypersensitivity reactions. This vaccine is contra-indicated in those with neomycin allergy. Avoid in those with an ongoing viral illness, and those with immunodeficiency disorders.

Pediatric Concerns:

Drug Interactions: Avoid administration in those with an ongoing viral illness, on cancer therapy, on immunosupressants, on corticosteroids.

Relative Infant Dose:

Adult Dose: 0.65 mL, subcutaneous, in the deltoid.

Alternatives:

References:
1. Anon: Resource materials: general recommendations on immunization. Am J Prev Med 1994; 10(suppl): 60–82.
2. Schaefer CSchaefer C: Drugs During Pregnancy and Lactation, Elsevier Science B.V., Amsterdam, The Netherlands, 2001.

ZUCLOPENTHIXOL   L3

Trade:

Other Trades: Clopixol-Acuphase, Clopixol Depot, Clopixol

Category: Antipsychotic agent

Zuclopenthixol is a typical antipsychotic agent used in the management of schizophrenia. It is not available in the USA. It works by blocking the postsynaptic dopaminergic receptors.[1] In a study of a single patient who initially received 24 mg zuclopenthixol for 4 days and then 14 mg/day thereafter, levels in milk averaged 20 µg/L following the 24 mg dose, and 5 µg/L at the 14 mg dose. Based on these concentrations, the authors estimated the absolute infant dose at 0.8 to 3.0 µg/kg and the relative infant dose at 0.3 to 0.8% of the maternal dose.[2] In a group of six patients ranging from 3 days to 10 months postpartum, the dose ranged from 4 mg/day to 72 mg/2 weeks (IM).[3] In all instances, milk levels were much lower than plasma. Zuclopenthixol levels in milk averaged 29% of the maternal plasma levels. The daily dose to an infant was estimated to be approximately 0.5–5 µg/day which roughly corresponds to a relative infant dose of 0.03 to 0.38% of the weight-adjusted maternal dose.

The plasma levels of zuclopenthixol in infants were low in both studies. No untoward effects were noted in the infants although some caution is recommended with prolonged exposure to this medication.

Pregnancy Risk	C		Lactation Risk	L3
T ½	= 20 hours		M/P	= 0.29
Vd	= 15–20 l/kg		PB	= 98
Tmax	= 4 hours		Oral	= 49%
MW	= 443–555		pKa	= 3.3, 7.6

Adult Concerns: Adverse reactions include drowsiness, anxiety, insomnia, xerostomia, hypertonia, tremor, and weakness.

Pediatric Concerns: No untoward effects were noted in 7 infants studied thus far.

Drug Interactions: Zuclopenthixol is a major substrate of CYP2D6, and thus drug interactions are numerous. Some reported are aluminum salts, anticholinergics, antihypertensives, bromocriptine, CNS depressants, epinephrine, levodopa, lithium, phenytoin, propranolol, tricyclic antidepressants, trazodone, and valproic acid. Consult other texts for a full list of drug-drug interactions.

Relative Infant Dose: 0.4%–0.9%

Adult Dose: Oral=10–150 mg/day: IM=50–150 mg every 48–72 hours.

Alternatives: Risperidone, olanzapine.

References:
1. Pharmaceutical manufacturer prescribing information, 2006.
2. Matheson I, Skjaeraasen J. Milk concentrations of flupenthixol, nortriptyline and zuclopenthixol and between-breast differences in two patients. Eur J Clin Pharmacol 1988; 35(2): 217–220.
3. Aaes-Jorgensen T, Bjorndal F, Bartels U. Zuclopenthixol levels in serum and breast milk. Psychopharmacology (Berl) 1986; 90(3): 417–418.

APPENDIX A

USING RADIOPHARMACEUTICAL PRODUCTS IN BREASTFEEDING MOTHERS

The use of radioactive products in breastfeeding mothers must be approached with great care. Invariably, the administration of a radiopharmaceutical to a lactating mother will result in some transfer of radioactivity into her milk. The relative dose received by the infant is dependent on a number of factors, but most importantly by the radioactive dose administered, the absorption and distribution of the radioisotope, the biological and radioactive half-life of the product, and the amount that enters milk. The following table presents data from some of the best sources in the world and provides their recommendations on interrupting breastfeeding to allow for the decay and/or clearance of the radiopharmaceutical. Most of their decisions were based on the probable radioactive 'dose' transferred to the infant, and whether or not it was considered hazardous. Please note that some of their recommendations conflict. Ultimately the mother and her radiologist will have to assess the relevancy of this data in their own situation.

- When evaluating radiopharmaceuticals, it is important to understand that all of these products have "two" half-lives. One is the radioactive half-life of the isotope. This half-life is set and invariable. While we prefer shorter half-life products like ^{99m}Technetium (6.02 h), many other isotopes have important uses in medicine. The second half-life is the 'biological' or 'effective' half-life of the specific product. Many of these products are rapidly eliminated from the body via the kidney, some within minutes to hours. Thus the 'biological or effective' half-life is critical and sometimes is so fast that the radiopharmaceutical is gone from body long before its isotope is decayed (see ^{111}In-Octreotide). However, some isotopes such as the radioactive iodides (^{131}I, ^{125}I) may be retained in the body for long periods and present extraordinary hazards to the breastfeeding infant. Lastly, two units of radioactivity are commonly used by differing sources. Just remember that one mCi (millicurie) is equal to 37 MBq (megabecquerel). Regardless of the unit you are given, you can now convert them easily.

1 MILLICURIE = 37 MEGABECQUEREL

Some important points to remember about evaluating these products in breastfeeding mothers are:

- Use the shortest half-life product permitted such as ^{99m}Technetium. It's half-life is so short, and its radioactive emissions are so weak, that it poses little risk (but this depends on dose). While the table that follows often does not even require interrupting breastfeeding, I still suggest that waiting even 12-24 hours before breastfeeding would virtually eliminate all possible risks associated with this isotope.

- Regardless of the isotope used, if the dose is extremely high, then withholding breastfeeding for a minimum of five to as many as ten radioactive half-lives is probably advisable.

- Measuring the radioactivity present in milk is the most accurate way to determine risk. This often requires sophisticated equipment not available in most hospitals, but it is the "final" determinant of risk to the infant. If the isotope present in milk approaches 'background' levels, there is no risk to the infant.

- Use great caution before returning to breastfeeding if the radioactive Iodides are used. Iodine is selectively concentrated in the thyroid gland, the lactating breast (27% of dose), and breastmilk, and high doses could potentially lead to thyroid cancer in the infant. ^{131}I and ^{125}I are potentially of high risk due to their long radioactive half-lives and their affinity for thyroid tissues. ^{123}I has a much shorter half-life, and brief interruptions may eliminate most risks. In mothers who have had their thyroid removed, the return to breastfeeding will be much quicker. Further even close contact can produce high radiation exposure to an individual in close contact with the individual. Thus we have added a close contact restriction table.

- Because radioactivity decays at a set rate, milk can be stored in the freezer for at least eight to ten half-lives and then fed to the infant without problem. All of the radioactivity will be gone.

TYPICAL RADIOACTIVE HALF-LIVES

RADIOACTIVE ELEMENT	HALF-LIFE
^{99}Mo	2.75 Days
^{201}Tl	3.05 Days
^{201}Tl	73.1 Hours
^{67}Ga	3.26 Days
^{67}Ga	78.3 Hours
^{131}I	8.02 Days
^{133}Xe	5.24 Days
^{111}In	2.80 Days
^{51}Cr	27.7 Days
^{125}I	60.1 Days
^{89}Sr	50.5 Days
^{99m}Tc	6.02 Hours
^{123}I	13.2 Hours
^{153}Sm	47.0 Hours

ACTIVITIES OF RADIOPHARMACEUTICALS THAT REQUIRE INSTRUCTIONS AND RECORDS WHEN ADMINISTERED TO PATIENTS WHO ARE BREAST-FEEDING AN INFANT OR CHILD.*

RADIOPHARMACEUTICAL	COLUMN 1 ACTIVITY ABOVE WHICH INSTRUCTIONS ARE REQUIRED		COLUMN 3 EXAMPLES OF RECOMMENDED DURATION OF INTERRUPTION OF BREAST-FEEDING*
	MBq	mCi	
^{131}I NaI	0.01	0.0004	Complete cessation (for this infant or child)
^{123}I NaI	20	0.5	
^{123}I OIH	100	4	
^{123}I mIBG	70	2	24 hr for 370 MBq (10 mCi) 12 hr for 150 MBq (4 mCi)
^{125}I OIH	3	0.08	
^{131}I OIH	10	0.30	
^{99m}Tc DTPA	1,000	30	
^{99m}Tc MAA	50	1.3	12.6 hr for 150 Mbq (4 mCi)
^{99m}Tc Pertechnetate	100	3	24 hr for 1,100 Mbq (30 mCi) 12 hr for 440 Mbq (12 mCi)
^{99m}Tc DISIDA	1,000	30	
^{99m}Tc Glucoheptonate	1,000	30	
^{99m}Tc HAM	400	10	
^{99m}Tc MIBI	1,000	30	
^{99m}Tc MDP	1,000	30	
^{99m}Tc PYP	900	25	
^{99m}Tc Red Blood Cell In Vivo Labeling	400	10	6 hr for 740 Mbq (20 mCi)
^{99m}Tc Red Blood Cell In Vitro Labeling	1,000	30	
^{99m}Tc Sulphur Colloid	300	7	6 hr for 440 Mbq (12 mCi)
^{99m}Tc DTPA Aerosol	1,000	30	
^{99m}Tc MAG3	1,000	30	
^{99m}Tc White Blood Cells	100	4	24 hr for 1,100 Mbq (5 mCi) 12 hr for 440 Mbq (2 mCi)

ACTIVITIES OF RADIOPHARMACEUTICALS THAT REQUIRE INSTRUCTIONS AND RECORDS WHEN ADMINISTERED TO PATIENTS WHO ARE BREAST-FEEDING AN INFANT OR CHILD.*		
RADIOPHARMACEUTICAL	COLUMN 1 ACTIVITY ABOVE WHICH INSTRUCTIONS ARE REQUIRED		COLUMN 3 EXAMPLES OF RECOMMENDED DURATION OF INTERRUPTION OF BREAST-FEEDING*
^{67}Ga Citrate	1	0.04	1 month for 150 Mbq (4 mCi) two weeks for 50 Mbq (1.3 mCi) 1 week for 7 Mbq (0.2 mCi)
^{51}Cr EDTA	60	1.6	
^{111}In White Blood Cells	10	0.2	1 week for 20 Mbq (0.5 mCi)
^{201}T1 Chloride	40	1	two weeks for 110 Mbq (3 mCi)

*   The duration of interruption of breast-feeding is selected to reduce the maximum dose to a newborn infant to less than 1 millisievert (0.1 rem), although the regulatory limit is 5 millisieverts (0.5 rem). The actual doses that would be received by most infants would be far below 1 millisievert (0.1 rem). Of course, the physician may use discretion in the recommendation, increasing or decreasing the duration of the interruption.

If there is no recommendation in Column 3 of this table, the maximum activity normally administered is below the activities that require instructions on interruption or discontinuation of breast-feeding.

*   Source: Nuclear Regulatory Commission. For a more complete table see: http://neonatal.ttuhsc.edu/lact/

Breastfeeding Interruption Recommendations

Diagnostic Procedure	Radiopharmaceuticals	T½ Hours	Dose Range (mCi)	Breastfeeding Restrictions to limit exposure to <1 mSv*	Breastfeeding Restrictions to limit exposure to zero mSv** (5 half-lives)
Brain Serotonin Level	^{11}C-Way 100635	0.34	14.2	100 minutes interruption	1.7 hours
	^{11}C-Raclopride	0.34	10.3	100 minutes interruption[8]	1.7 hours
WBC Scan	^{99m}Tc-WBC	6	10-15	12-24 hours interruption for 2-5 mCi or more	30 hours
	^{99m}Tc-Ceretec	6	10-24		30 hours
	^{111}In-WBC	67.2	0.5	11 week interruption for 0.5 mCi[1]	14 days
Cystogram (Voiding)	^{99m}Tc-SC, ^{99m}Tc-O$_4$	6	0.5-1	6 hours interruption for 12 mCi[1]	30 hours
Liver/spleen scan	^{99m}Tc-SC (sulfur colloid)	6	2-4	6 hours interruption for 12 mCi[1]	30 hours
Bone marrow scan	^{99m}Tc-SC	6	<20	6 hours interruption for 12 mCi[1]	30 hours
Lymphoscintigraphy	^{99m}Tc-SC	6	0.1-0.8	No interruption[1]	30 hours
Liver SPECT (hemangioma)	^{99m}Tc-pyp-RBCs	6	20-30	13 hour interruption for 25-30 mCi[14]	30 hours
Myocardial (MI) scan	^{99m}Tc-pyp	6	20-30	12 hour interruption for 25-30 mCi[14]	30 hours
Meckel's diverticulum	^{99m}Tc-O$_4$	6	10-15	24 hours for 30 mCi[1]	30 hours
		6		12 hours for 12 mCi[1]	30 hours
Testicular scan	^{99m}Tc-O$_4$	6	0-25	24 hours for 30 mCi[1]	30 hours
		6		12 hours for 12 mCi[1]	30 hours
Thyroid scan	^{99m}Tc-O$_4$	6	1-2	24 hours for 30 mCi[1]	30 hours
		6		12 hours for 12 mCi[1]	30 hours
Bone scan	^{99m}Tc-MDP,-HDP	6	<30	No interruption for 30 mCi or less[1]	30 hours

BREASTFEEDING INTERRUPTION RECOMMENDATIONS

Diagnostic Procedure	Radiopharmaceuticals	T½ Hours	Dose Range (mCi)	Breastfeeding Restrictions to limit exposure to <1 mSv*	Breastfeeding Restrictions to limit exposure to zero mSv** (5 half-lives)
MUGA scan	99mTc-labeled-RBCs	6	20-30	6 hour interruption of breastfeeding for 20 mCi[1]	30 hours
Lung ventilation imaging	99mTc-DTPA (labeled aerosol)	6	30	No interruption for 30 mCi or less[1]	30 hours
Renal scan	99mTc-DTPA	6	10-15	No interruption for 30 mCi or less[1]	30 hours
Renal scan	99mTc-DMSA	6	3-10	No interruption for 2-5 mCi or less[1]	30 hours
Brain scan	99mTc-D₄-, DTPA-GH	6	<20-30	No interruption for 30 mCi or less[1]	30 hours
HIDA (cholescintigraphy)	99mTc-Choletec; Hepatolite'	6	3-5	No interruption for 4 mCi or less[2]	30 hours
Brain scan-SPECT	99mTc-Choletec; Neurolite'	6	20-30	24 hours for 30 mCi[1]	30 hours
Brain scan-SPECT	99mTc-Cardiolite	6	16-30	No interruption for	30 hours
Parathyroid scan Subtraction:	201Tl	73	2-3	<30 mCi[3]; two week interruption for 3 mCi[1]	15 days
	99mTc-D₄	6	5-12		30 hours
Scintimammo-graphy	99mTc-Cardiolite	6	20	No interruption for 30 mCi or less[3]	30 hours
CEA-ScanR	99mTc-arcitumomab	6	20-30	24 hour interruption for 30 mCi[3]	30 hours
Cardiac Studies	99mTc-Cardiolite or Myoview	6	7-30	No interruption for <30 mCi[3]	30 hours

Breastfeeding Interruption Recommendations

Diagnostic Procedure	Radiopharmaceuticals	T½ Hours	Dose Range (mCi)	Breastfeeding Restrictions to limit exposure to <1 mSv[*]	Breastfeeding Restrictions to limit exposure to zero mSv[**] (5 half-lives)
Infections – labeled with HMPAO	99mTc WBC	6	3–10	24 hours for 5 mCi[1]	30 hours
Gastroesophageal emptying time-liquids		6	1	12 hours for 2 mCi[1]	30 hours
		6	0.5	6 hours for 12 mCi[1]	30 hours
Gastroesophageal emptying time-solids	99mTc-SC (sulfur colloid)	6	5	6 hours for 12 mCi[1]	30 hours
		6		6 hours for 12 mCi[1]	30 hours
SPECT Analysis – Liver		6	2	No interruption period[2]	30 hours
Perfusion study –cardiac	99mTc Sestamibi Teboroxime	6	25	No interruption for <30 mCi[3]	30 hours
Adenoma-parathyroid		6	20		30 hours
MUGA Scan for cardiac-gated ventriculo-graphy	99mTc RBC	6	20	6-12 hours of interruption of breastfeeding[1]	30 hours
Bleeding Scan of GI tract					
Liver Scan for Hemangioma		6		6-12 hours of interruption of breastfeeding[2]	30 hours
Myocardial Infarct	99mTc Pyrophosphate	6	15	No interruption reqiered[1,2,4]	30 hours
		6	20		30 hours
	99mTc Plasmin	6	0.5		30 hours

Breastfeeding Interruption Recommendations

Diagnostic Procedure	Radiopharmaceuticals	T½ Hours	Dose Range (mCi)	Breastfeeding Restrictions to limit exposure to <1 mSv*	Breastfeeding Restrictions to limit exposure to zero mSv** (5 half-lives)
Meckel's Scan of GI tract	99mTc Pertechnetate	6	21	47 hour interruption[2]	47 hours
	99mTc Microspheres	6	2	25 hour interruption[2]	30 hours
	99mTc Microspheres	6	2.7	17 hour interruption[2]	30 hours
	99mTc MIBI	6	27	No interruption[2]	30 hours
Bone-osteomyelitis	99mTc MDP	6	20	No interruption for 30 mCi or less[1]	30 hours
	99mTc Leukoscan	6	20.3	10 hour interruption[9]	30 hours
		6	10	No interruption for 30 mCi or less[1]	30 hours
Renal Blood Flow Clearance	99mTc MAG3	6	11	Interruption for 5 hours[2]	30 hours
		6	2.7	No interruption[2]	30 hours
Perfusion studies of Lung	99mTc-MAA (microaggregated albumin)	6		12.6 hours for 4 mCi[1,4]	30 hours
Biliary Atresia—Cholecystitis-HIDA	99mTc IDA derivative	6	5	No interruption required[1]	30 hours
SPECT Analysis of Brain Perfusion	99mTc HMPAO	6	20	No interruption required[1,2]	30 hours
		6	13.5		30 hours
	99mTc Glucoheptonate	6	22	No interruption[2]	30 hours
	99mTc HAM	6	8	No interruption[4]	30 hours
	99mTc-SC (sulfur colloid)	6	12	No interruption[4]	30 hours
	99mTc Ferrous hydroxide MA	6		Interruption with measurement[2]	30 hours

Breastfeeding Interruption Recommendations

Diagnostic Procedure	Radiopharmaceuticals	T½ Hours	Dose Range (mCi)	Breastfeeding Restrictions to limit exposure to <1 mSv	Breastfeeding Restrictions to limit exposure to zero mSv** (5 half-lives)
	99mTc Erythrocytes	6	22	17 hours interruption[2]	30 hours
	99mTc EDTA	6	10	No interruption[2]	30 hours
CNS Perfusion	99mTc DTPA	6	30	No interruption for 30 mCi or less[1]	30 hours
Renal perfusion/filtration	99mTc DTPA	6	10 or 20	No interruption[2]	30 hours
		6	22		30 hours
	99mTc-DMSA	6	2.2	No interruption[2]	30 hours
		6	5		30 hours
Kidney parenchyma imaging kidney DTPA + DMSA	99mTc-DMSA Glucoheptonate		10	No interruption[1,2,4]	
		6	2.2		30 hours
Unspecific uses	99mTc DISIDA	6	4-8	No interruption[2,4]	30 hours
	99mTc Diphosphonate	6	16.2	No interruption[2]	30 hours
	75Se Methionine	120 days	0.3	450 hours interruption or complete cessation[2]	600 days
Infections Tumors imaging	67Ga Citrate	78.2	4	1 month interruption for 4 mCi[1]	30 days
		78.2	1.3	two weeks interruption for 1.3 mCi[1]	16 days
		78.2		1 weeks interruption for 0.2 mCi[1]	16 days
		78.2	4	20 days interruption[2]	30 days
Gallium scan (tumor)	67Ga	78.2	5-10	1 month interruption for 4 mCi[1]	30 days
Gallium scan for infections	67Ga	78.2	5-10	1 month interruption for 4 mCi[1]	30 days

BREASTFEEDING INTERRUPTION RECOMMENDATIONS

Diagnostic Procedure	Radiopharmaceuticals	T½ Hours	Dose Range (mCi)	Breastfeeding Restrictions to limit exposure to <1 mSv*	Breastfeeding Restrictions to limit exposure to zero mSv** (5 half-lives)
Schilling	57Co-B$_{12}$	271.8 days	0.3-0.5	Avoid feeding at 24 hour peak if possible[5] Exposure at 72 hours is virtually nil.	1359 days
Unspecified	51Cr EDTA	27.7 days	0.1	No interruption[2,4]	138.5 days
	32P Na phosphate	14.3 days	Any	Complete cessation of breastfeeding[2]	Complete cessation of breastfeeding[2]
Cardiac perfusion and stress test	201Tl Chloride	73	3	two weeks interruption for 3 mCi[1]	15 days
		73	2.2	No interruption[2]	15 days
Glucose Metabolism	18F-FDG	1.83		Interruption for first 4 hours[14]	9 hours
Tumor Imaging		1.83	1.35-4.32	Risk from proximity to breast not milk itself[10]	9 hours
Lung ventilation	133Xe Gas	127.2	10-30	1 hour interruption for washout[1]	26.5 days
Lung ventilation imaging	133Xe Gas	127.2	10-15	1 hour interruption for washout[1]	26.5 days
Renogram	131I-OIH	192.5	0.15-0.3	No interruption[1]	40.5 days
MIBG (adrenal medulla)	131I-MIBG	192.5	0.5	25 days interruption[3]	40.5 days
Adrenocortical Scan	131I-Iodomethyinorcholesterol	192.5	2	Complete cessation of breastfeeding or until count are baseline[3]	40.5 days
Thyroid hyperthyroid therapy	131I-Sodium diffuse nodular	192.5	1-10	Complete cessation of breastfeeding or until count are baseline[1]	Complete cessation of breastfeeding or until count are baseline[1]
		192.5	<30		
Thyroid ablation		192.5	30-300		
		192.5	108		

BREASTFEEDING INTERRUPTION RECOMMENDATIONS

Diagnostic Procedure	Radiopharmaceuticals	T½ Hours	Dose Range (mCi)	Breastfeeding Restrictions to limit exposure to <1 mSv*	Breastfeeding Restrictions to limit exposure to zero mSv** (5 half-lives)
Thyroid diagnostic imaging-post thyroidectomy	131I-Sodium	192.5	5	Complete cessation of breastfeeding or until count are baseline[1]	Complete cessation of breastfeeding or until count are baseline[1]
Tumor Imaging	131I-MIBG	192.5	1.5	Complete cessation of breastfeeding or until count are baseline[3]	Complete cessation of breastfeeding or until count are baseline[3]
	131I-HAS	192.5		Complete cessation of breastfeeding or until count are baseline[2]	Complete cessation of breastfeeding or until count are baseline[2]
Renal Blood flow and clearance	131I-Hippuran	192.5	0.25	34 hours interruption[2]	40.5 days
		192.5	0.05		40.5 days
Thyroid scan (substernal)	131I	192.5	< 0.1	Complete cessation of breastfeeding or until count are baseline[1]	Complete cessation of breastfeeding or until count are baseline[1]
Whole-body 131I carcinoma work-up	131I	192.5	1-5	Complete cessation of breastfeeding or until count are baseline[1]	Complete cessation of breastfeeding or until count are baseline[1]
	125I HAS	60.2 days	0.2	277 hour interruption or complete cessation[2]	301 days
	125I-Hippuran	60.2 days	0.05	23 hours cessation[2]	301 days
	125I-Fibrinogen	60.2 days	0.1	620 hour interruption of breastfeeding or until counts are baseline[3]	301 days

BREASTFEEDING INTERRUPTION RECOMMENDATIONS

Diagnostic Procedure	Radiopharmaceuticals	T½ Hours	Dose Range (mCi)	Breastfeeding Restrictions to limit exposure to <1 mSv	Breastfeeding Restrictions to limit exposure to zero mSv.** (5 half-lives)
Pheochromo-cytoma scan	[123]I	13.2	< 0.35	No interruption[1]	2.75 days
	[123]I Sodium	13.2	0.4	Complete cessation of breastfeeding or until counts are baseline[1]	Complete cessation of breastfeeding or until counts are baseline[1]
Thyroid Imaging Scans	[123]I Hippuran	13.2	0.5	27 hours interruption[2]	2.75 days
	[123]I MIBG	13.2	0.5	11 hours interruption[2]	2.75 days
		13.2	11	21 hours interruption[2]	2.75 days
OncoScint	^{111}In-satumomab pendetide	67.2	4-6	14 days interruption[3]	14 days
OctreoScan	^{111}In-pentetriotide	67.2	6	72 hours interruption[3]	14 days
Cisternogram	[111]Indium-DTPA	67.2	0.5-1.5	14 days interruption[3]	14 days
ProstaScint	^{111}In-CYT-356	67.2	5-17	14 days interruption[3]	14 days
Infections	^{111}In-WBC	67.2	0.5	1 week interruption for 0.5 mCi[1]	14 days
CSF-imaging neuroendocrie tumors	^{111}In-Octreotide	67.2	5.3	<10 day interruption (see monograph)	14 days
CSF-cternogram/ shunt patency	^{111}In-DTPA	67.2	0.5	1 week interruption for 0.5 mCi[1]	14 days
	^{111}In-Leucocytes	67.2	0.5	No interruption[2]	1 days

*   IMPORTANT: The recommendations in the table above were derived by calculating the dose and time required to limit the ingested effective dose to the infant below 1 mSv. Please be advised, these recommendations still permit a minimal amount of radiation transfer to the infant that is considered safe by the authorities. Average American radiation exposure is 6.2 mSv per year. The only way to totally avoid any radiation is to wait for all of it to decay (5-10 half-lives).

**   To avoid all radiation exposure to the breastfed infant, breastfeeding must be interrupted for at least 5 half-lives.

Recommendations by the following sources:

1. Activities of Radiopharmaceuticals from the Nuclear Regulatory Commission

2. Montford PJ. Textbook of Radiopharmacy. Third Edition. Gordon and Breach Publishers 1999.

3. T.W. Hale Ph.D.

4. Stabin MG, Breitz HB. Breast milk excretion of radiopharmaceuticals: mechanisms, findings, and radiation dosimetry. J Nucl Med 2000 41(5): 863-73.

5. Pomeroy KM, Sawyer LJ, Evans MJ. Estimated radiation dose to breastfeeding infant following maternal administration of 57Co labelled to vitamin B12. Nucl Med Commun 2005 Sep; 26(9): 839-41.

6. Robinson PS, Barker P, Campbell A, Henson P, Surveyor I, Young PR. Iodine-131 in breast milk following therapy for thyroid carcinoma. J Nucl Med 1994 Nov; 35(11): 1797-801.

7. Johnson RE, Mukherji SK, Perry RJ, Stabin MG. Radiation dose from breastfeeding following administration of thallium-201. J. Nucl Med 1996 Dec; 37(12): 2079-82.

8. Moses-Kolko EL, Meltzer CC, Helsel JC, Sheetz M, Mathis C, Ruszkiewicz J et al. No interruption of lactation is needed after (11) C-WAY 100635 or (11) C-raclopride PET. J Nucl Med 2005 Oct; 46(10): 1765.

9. Prince JR, Rose MR. Measurement of radioactivity in breast milk following 99mTc-Leukoscan injection.Nucl Med Commun 2004 Sep; 25(9): 963-6."

10. Hicks RJ, Binns D, Stabin MG. Pattern of uptake and excretion of (18)F-FDG in the lactating breast. J Nucl Med 2001 Aug; 42(8): 1238-42."

11. Mountford PJ, O'Doherty MJ, Forge NI, Jeffries A, Coakley AJ. Radiation dose rates from adult patients undergoing nuclear medicine investigations. Nucl Med Commun. 1991 Sep; 12(9): 767-77.

12. Mountford PJ. Estimation of close contact doses to young infants from surface dose rates on radioactive adults. Nucl Med Commun. 1987 Nov;8(11): 857-63.

13. Rose MR, Prescott MC, Herman KJ. Excretion of iodine-123-hippuran, technetium-99m-red blood cells, and technetium-99m-macroaggregated albumin into breast milk. J Nucl Med. 1990 Jun;31(6):978-84.

14. Leide-Svegborn S. Radiation exposure of patients and personnel from a PET/CT procedure with 18F-FDG. Radiat Prot Dosimetry. 2010 Apr-May;139(1-3):208-13.

Radioactive [131]Iodine Close Contact Restrictions

Treatment of Hyperthyroidism (assuming 50% uptake)*,**				
RADIATION DOSE	10 mCi	15 mCi	20mCi	30mCi
Sleeping restriction (6 feet separation sleeping arrangement) for adult.	3 nights	6 nights	8 nights	11 nights
Sleeping restriction (6 feet separation of sleeping arrangement) for infant children and pregnant women.	15 nights	18 nights	20 nights	23 nights
Close contact restriction (6 feet separation) from children and pregnant women.	1 day	1 day	2 days	5 days

Treatment of Thyroid cancer remnant ablation (assuming 2% uptake) (No thyroid)*,**				
RADIATION DOSE	50 mCi	100 mCi	150mCi	200mCi
Sleeping restriction (6 feet separation sleeping arrangement) for adult.	1 night	1 night	2 nights	4 nights
Sleeping restriction (6 feet separation of sleeping arrangement) for infant children and pregnant women.	6 nights	13 nights	18 nights	21 nights
Close contact restriction (6 feet separation) from children and pregnant women.	1 day	1 day	1 day	1 day

Adapted from American Thyroid Association Taskforce On Radioiodine Safety, Sisson JC, Freitas J, McDougall IR, Dauer LT, Hurley JR, Brierley JD, Edinboro CH, Rosenthal D, Thomas MJ, Wexler JA, Asamoah E, Avram AM, Milas M, Greenlee C. Radiation safety in the treatment of patients with thyroid diseases by radioiodine [131]I: practice recommendations of the American Thyroid Association. Thyroid. 2011 Apr;21(4):335-46. Epub 2011 Mar 18.

* IMPORTANT: The recommendations in the table above were derived by calculating the dose and time required to limit the effective dose to the infant below 1 mSv. Please be advised, these recommendations still permit a minimal amount of radiation transfer to the infant that is considered safe by the authorities. An average adult American is exposed to 6.2 mSv/year according to the Nuclear Regulatory Commission. The only way to totally avoid any radiation is to wait for all of it to decay (5-10 half-lives). Exposure of 1 mSv slightly increases the incidence of cancer to 1 in10,000 people.

** The half-life of 131I is around 8 days. To avoid all radiation exposure to the breastfed infant, close contact must be avoided for at least 5 half-lives, ie. 40 days.

RECOMMENDATIONS FOR CLOSE CONTACT EXPOSURE

PROCEDURE	ISOTOPE	HALF-LIFE (HOURS)	DOSE (mCI)	CLOSE CONTACT RECOMMENDATIONS TO LIMIT EXPOSURE TO <1 mSv***	CLOSE CONTACT RECOMMENDATIONS TO LIMIT EXPOSURE TO ZERO mSv**** (5 HALF-LIVES)
Static Renal Scan	^{99m}Tc	6	30 or less	Limit close contact to 35 min per hour with maximum 9 hours per day.[5,*] Estimated exposure = 0.429 mSv. Estimated dose for 1 mSv is 70 mCi[5]	30 hours
Dynamic Renal Scan	^{99m}Tc	6	10 or less	Limit close contact to 35 min per hour with maximum 9 hours per day.[5,*] Estimated exposure = 0.433 mSv. Estimated dose for 1 mSv is 22.9 mCi[5]	30 hours
			10 –22.9	Avoid contact for the first 4 hours. Limit close contact to 35 min every 3 hours. Estimated exposure is < 1 mSv[5,**]	
Bone	^{99m}Tc	6	16 or less	Limit close contact to 35 min per hour with maximum 9 hours per day.[5,*] Estimated exposure = 0.462 mSv. Estimated dose for 1 mSv is 35 mCi[5]	30 hours
			16–30	Avoid contact for the first 4 hours. Limit close contact to 35 min every 3 hours. Estimated exposure is < 1 mSv[5,**]	
Lung V/Q	^{99m}Tc	6	16 or less	Limit close contact to 35 min per hour with maximum 9 hours per day.[5,*] Estimated exposure = 0.462 mSv. Estimated dose for 1 mSv is 35 mCi[5]	30 hours
			16–30	Avoid contact for the first 4 hours. Limit close contact to 35 min every 3 hours. Estimated exposure is < 1 mSv[5,**]	
Thyroid	^{99m}Tc	6	10 or less	Limit close contact to 35 min per hour with maximum 9 hours per day.[5,*] Estimated exposure = 0.433 mSv. Estimated dose for 1 mSv is 22.9 mCi[5]	30 hours
			10–22.9	Avoid contact for the first 4 hours. Limit close contact to 35 min every 3 hours. Estimated exposure is < 1 mSv[5,**]	
Liver	^{99m}Tc	6	10 or less	Limit close contact to 35 min per hour with maximum 9 hours per day.[5,*] Estimated exposure = 0.433 mSv. Estimated dose for 1 mSv is 22.9 mCi[5]	30 hours
			10–22.9	Avoid contact for the first 4 hours. Limit close contact to 35 min every 3 hours. Estimated exposure is < 1 mSv[5,**]	

RECOMMENDATIONS FOR CLOSE CONTACT EXPOSURE

Procedure	Isotope	Half-Life (Hours)	Dose (mCi)	Close Contact Recommendations to Limit Exposure to <1 mSv***	Close Contact Recommendations to Limit Exposure to Zero mSv**** (5 half-lives)
Marrow	99mTc	6	8 or less	Limit close contact to 35 min per hour with maximum 9 hours per day.[5,*] Estimated exposure = 0.462 mSv. Estimated dose for 1 mSv is 16 mCi)5	30 hours
			8–16	Avoid contact for the first 4 hours. Limit close contact to 35 min every 3 hours. Estimated exposure is < 1 mSv[5,**]	
Brain	99mTc	6	10 or less	Limit close contact to 35 min per hour with maximum 9 hours per day.[5,*] Estimated exposure = 0.433 mSv. Estimated dose for 1 mSv is 22.9 mCi[5]	30 hours
			10–22.9	Avoid contact for first 4 hours. Limit close contact to 35 min every 3 hours. Estimated exposure is < 1 mSv[5,**]	
Bile	99mTc	6	16 or less	Limit close contact to 35 min per hour with maximum 9 hours per day.[5,*] Estimated exposure = 0.462 mSv. Estimated dose for 1 mSv is 35 mCi[5]	30 hours
			16–30	Avoid contact for the first 4 hours. Limit close contact to 35 min every 3 hours. Estimated exposure is < 1 mSv[5,**]	
PET Scan	18F-FDG	1.83	8 or less	Avoid contact for the first 4 hours[7]. Limit close contact for 10 hours. Leide-Svegborn suggests to avoid close contact for few hours[1]. Estimated exposure is < 1mSv.	9.15 hours
Cardiac	201Tl-Chloride	73	3 or less	Avoid close contact for the first 4 hours. Limit close contact to 35 minutes every 2-3 hours. Estimated exposure is 0.32 mSv[2]	15.2 days
Leucocytes	111In- Leuko-cytes	67.2	0.21 or less	Avoid close contact for the first 4 hours. Limit close contact to 35 min per hour with maximum 9 hours per day.[5,*] Estimated exposure = 0.460 mSv. Estimated dose for 1 mSv is 0.46 mCi[5]; Restricting close contact to 35 min every 4 hours for 3 days reduce dose by 30%[5]	14 days

RECOMMENDATIONS FOR CLOSE CONTACT EXPOSURE

PROCEDURE	ISOTOPE	HALF-LIFE (HOURS)	DOSE (MCI)	CLOSE CONTACT RECOMMENDATIONS TO LIMIT EXPOSURE TO <1 mSv***	CLOSE CONTACT RECOMMENDATIONS TO LIMIT EXPOSURE TO ZERO mSv**** (5 HALF-LIVES)
	^{67}Ga-Citrate	78.2	2.5 or less	Limit close contact to 35 min per hour with maximum 9 hours per day.[5,*] Estimated exposure = 0.483 mSv. Estimated dose for 1mSv is 5.1 mCi[5]	16.3 days
			2.5–5.1	Avoid contact for the first 4 hours. Limit close contact to 35 min every 3 hours. Estimated exposure is < 1 mSv[5]	

References:

1. Leide-Svegborn S. Radiation exposure of patients and personnel from a PET/CT procedure with 18F-FDG. Radiat Prot Dosimetry. 2010 Apr-May;139(1-3):208-13. Epub 2010 Feb 18.

2. Johnston RE, Mukherji SK, Perry RJ, Stabin MG. Radiation dose from breastfeeding following administration of thallium-201. J Nucl Med. 1996 Dec;37(12):2079-82.

3. Stabin MG, Breitz HB. Breast milk excretion of radiopharmaceuticals: mechanisms, findings, and radiation dosimetry. J Nucl Med 2000 41(5):863-73.

4. Mountford PJ, Coakley AJ. Body surface dosimetry following re-injection of 111In-leucocytes. Nucl Med Commun. 1989 Jul;10(7):497-501. Abstract.

5. Mountford PJ, O'Doherty MJ, Forge NI, Jeffries A, Coakley AJ. Radiation dose rates from adult patients undergoing nuclear medicine investigations. Nucl Med Commun. 1991 Sep;12(9):767-77.

6. Mountford PJ. Estimation of close contact doses to young infants from surface dose rates on radioactive adults. Nucl Med Commun. 1987 Nov;8(11):857-63.

7. Hicks RJ, Binns D, Stabin MG. Pattern of uptake and excretion of (18)F-FDG in the lactating breast. J Nucl Med. 2001 Aug;42(8):1238-42.

* Assuming close contact of 9 hours/day; 35 min each hour for the first 8 h, 35 min each hour 4 h for 12 h, 35 min each hour for 4 h, in each 24 h period

** Limiting close contact for 20 min every 4 hours for the 1st day will reduce radiation exposure by 67%.

*** The recommendations in the table above were derived by calculating the dose and time required to limit the effective dose to the infant below 1 mSv. Please be advised, these recommendations still permit a minimal amount of radiation transfer to the infant that is considered safe by the authorities. An average American is exposed to 6.2 mSv/year according to the Nuclear Regulatory Commission. The only way to totally avoid any radiation is to wait for all of it to decay (5-10 half-lives). Exposure of 1 mSv increases risk of cancer incidence to 1 out of 10,000 people.

**** To avoid all radiation exposure to the breastfed infant, close contact has to be avoided for at least 5 half-lives.

APPENDIX B

Glossary

adipose	the fat tissue in the body
analgesic	drugs used to treat pain
androgen	drug that mimics the action of the male hormone testosterone
antiangina	drug used to treat the pain associated with reduced coronary flow in the heart
antidepressant	drugs that elevate or treat mental depression
antiemetic	compound used to treat nausea and vomiting
antihypertensive	drug used to treat high blood pressure
antimetabolite	drug generally used to inhibit the immune response, such as in arthritis or cancer
antineoplastic	drug used to treat neoplasms or cancers
antivertigo	compound used to treat dizziness, bradycardia, slow heart rate
anxiolytic	reduces anxiety, sedative drug
arthropathy	painful inflammation of joints
bronchodilator	drug that dilates the bronchi in the lungs
CCB	calcium channel blocker
candidiasis	fungal infection, candida, yeast, thrush
cholinergic	nerve transmitter, acetylcholine
d	day
diuretic	drug that induces excretion of water by kidneys
dL	deciliter, 100ml
DNA	deoxyribonucleic acid, chromosome, genetic components of human cells
estrogen	drugs that mimic the action of estrogens or female hormones
flora	bacteria normally residing within the intestine
GI	gastrointestinal
half-life	the time required for the concentration of a drug to diminish by one-half in the specified compartment (blood)
hepatoxic	drug that produces liver damage
hyperglycemia	elevated blood sugar (dextrose)
hypoglycemia	low blood sugar (dextrose)
hypotension	low blood pressure
immune	antibody system which fights infection, foreign protein, etc.
immunosuppressive	drugs that diminish or reduce the immune (antibody)response
L	liter, 1000 ml, 1000 cc, approximately 1 quart
lipid	fat
maternal	mother
mg	milligram, one thousandth of a gram
mg/L	milligram per Liter
milk-plasma ratio	ratio of drug in milk to plasma. Higher ratios indicate more drug penetration into milk. A ratio of 1 means that the amount of drug in milk is identical to that in plasma.
ng	nanogram, 1×10^{-9} gm

Glossary

NICU	Neonatal intensive care unit
NSAID	Nonsteroidal anti-inflammatory
perineal	area between the anus and scrotum
progestational	drug that mimics the action of progesterone, a female hormone
prolactin	hormone that promotes breast milk production
pseudomembranous	severe, sometimes bloody diarrhea caused colitis by overgrowth of offending colonic bacteria
RNA	ribonucleic acid, genetic component of human cell
tachycardia	rapid heart rate
teratogenic	drugs or conditions that produce birth defects in pregnant women
µg	microgram, one millionth of a gram
µg/L	microgram per liter

Recommended immunization schedule for ages 0 through 6 years

FIGURE 1: Recommended immunization schedule for persons aged 0 through 6 years—United States, 2012 (for those who fall behind or start late, see the catch-up schedule [Figure 3])

Vaccine ▼ / Age ▶	Birth	1 month	2 months	4 months	6 months	9 months	12 months	15 months	18 months	19–23 months	2–3 years	4–6 years
Hepatitis B[1]	Hep B	HepB			HepB							
Rotavirus[2]			RV	RV	RV[2]							
Diphtheria, tetanus, pertussis[3]			DTaP	DTaP	DTaP		see footnote[3]	DTaP				DTaP
Haemophilus influenzae type b[4]			Hib	Hib	Hib[4]		Hib					
Pneumococcal[5]			PCV	PCV	PCV		PCV				PPSV	
Inactivated poliovirus[6]			IPV	IPV		IPV						IPV
Influenza[7]							Influenza (Yearly)					
Measles, mumps, rubella[8]							MMR		see footnote[8]			MMR
Varicella[9]							Varicella		see footnote[9]			Varicella
Hepatitis A[10]							Dose 1[10]				HepA Series	
Meningococcal[11]							MCV4 — see footnote[11]					

Range of recommended ages for all children

Range of recommended ages for certain high-risk groups

Range of recommended ages for all children and certain high-risk groups

This schedule includes recommendations in effect as of December 23, 2011. Any dose not administered at the recommended age should be administered at a subsequent visit, when indicated and feasible. The use of a combination vaccine generally is preferred over separate injections of its equivalent component vaccines. Vaccination providers should consult the relevant Advisory Committee on Immunization Practices (ACIP) statement for detailed recommendations, available online at http://www.cdc.gov/vaccines/pubs/acip-list.htm. Clinically significant adverse events that follow vaccination should be reported to the Vaccine Adverse Event Reporting System (VAERS) online (http://www.vaers.hhs.gov) or by telephone (800-822-7967).

1. **Hepatitis B (HepB) vaccine. (Minimum age: birth)**
   At birth:
   - Administer monovalent HepB vaccine to all newborns before hospital discharge.
   - For infants born to hepatitis B surface antigen (HBsAg)–positive mothers, administer HepB vaccine and 0.5 mL of hepatitis B immune globulin (HBIG) within 12 hours of birth. These infants should be tested for HBsAg and antibody to HBsAg (anti-HBs) 1 to 2 months after completion of at least 3 doses of the HepB series, at age 9 through 18 months (generally at the next well-child visit).
   - If mother's HBsAg status is unknown, within 12 hours of birth administer HepB vaccine for infants weighing ≥2,000 grams, and HepB vaccine plus HBIG for infants weighing <2,000 grams. Determine mother's HBsAg status as soon as possible and, if she is HBsAg-positive, administer HBIG for infants weighing ≥2,000 grams (no later than age 1 week).

7. **Influenza vaccines. (Minimum age: 6 months for trivalent inactivated influenza vaccine [TIV]; 2 years for live, attenuated influenza vaccine [LAIV])**
   - For most healthy children aged 2 years and older, either LAIV or TIV may be used. However, LAIV should not be administered to some children, including 1) children with asthma, 2) children 2 through 4 years who had wheezing in the past 12 months, or 3) children who have any other underlying medical conditions that predispose them to influenza complications. For all other contraindications to use of LAIV, see MMWR 2010;59(No. RR-8), available at http://www.cdc.gov/mmwr/pdf/rr/rr5908.pdf.
   - For children aged 6 months through 8 years:
     — For the 2011–12 season, administer 2 doses (separated by at least 4 weeks) to those who did not receive at least 1 dose of the 2010–11 vaccine. Those who received at least 1 dose of the 2010–11 vaccine

Doses after the birth dose:

- The second dose should be administered at age 1 to 2 months. Monovalent HepB vaccine should be used for doses administered before age 6 weeks.
- Administration of a total of 4 doses of HepB vaccine is permissible when a combination vaccine containing HepB is administered after the birth dose.
- Infants who did not receive a birth dose should receive 3 doses of a HepB-containing vaccine starting as soon as feasible (Figure 3).
- The minimum interval between dose 1 and dose 2 is 4 weeks, and between dose 2 and 3 is 8 weeks. The final (third or fourth) dose in the HepB vaccine series should be administered no earlier than age 24 weeks and at least 16 weeks after the first dose.

2. **Rotavirus (RV) vaccines.** (Minimum age: 6 weeks for both RV-1 [Rotarix] and RV-5 [Rota Teq])
   - The maximum age for the first dose in the series is 14 weeks, 6 days; and 8 months, 0 days for the final dose in the series. Vaccination should not be initiated for infants aged 15 weeks, 0 days or older.
   - If RV-1 (Rotarix) is administered at ages 2 and 4 months, a dose at 6 months is not indicated.

3. **Diphtheria and tetanus toxoids and acellular pertussis (DTaP) vaccine.** (Minimum age: 6 weeks)
   - The fourth dose may be administered as early as age 12 months, provided at least 6 months have elapsed since the third dose.

4. **Haemophilus influenzae type b (Hib) conjugate vaccine.** (Minimum age: 6 weeks)
   - If PRP-OMP (PedvaxHIB or Comvax [HepB-Hib]) is administered at ages 2 and 4 months, a dose at age 6 months is not indicated.
   - Hiberix should only be used for the booster (final) dose in children aged 12 months through 4 years.

5. **Pneumococcal vaccines.** (Minimum age: 6 weeks for pneumococcal conjugate vaccine [PCV]; 2 years for pneumococcal polysaccharide vaccine [PPSV])
   - Administer 1 dose of PCV to all healthy children aged 24 through 59 months who are not completely vaccinated for their age.
   - For children who have received an age-appropriate series of 7-valent PCV (PCV7), a single supplemental dose of 13-valent PCV (PCV13) is recommended for:
     — All children aged 14 through 59 months
     — Children aged 60 through 71 months with underlying medical conditions.
   - Administer PPSV at least 8 weeks after last dose of PCV to children aged 2 years or older with certain underlying medical conditions, including a cochlear implant. See MMWR 2010:59(No. RR-11), available at http://www.cdc.gov/mmwr/pdf/rr/rr5911.pdf.

6. **Inactivated poliovirus vaccine (IPV).** (Minimum age: 6 weeks)
   - If 4 or more doses are administered before age 4 years, an additional dose should be administered at age 4 through 6 years.
   - The final dose in the series should be administered on or after the fourth birthday and at least 6 months after the previous dose.

require 1 dose for the 2011–12 season.
— For the 2012–13 season, follow dosing guidelines in the 2012 ACIP influenza vaccine recommendations.

8. **Measles, mumps, and rubella (MMR) vaccine.** (Minimum age: 12 months)
   - The second dose may be administered before age 4 years, provided at least 4 weeks have elapsed since the first dose.
   - Administer MMR vaccine to infants aged 6 through 11 months who are traveling internationally. These children should be revaccinated with 2 doses of MMR vaccine, the first at ages 12 through 15 months and at least 4 weeks after the previous dose, and the second at ages 4 through 6 years.

9. **Varicella (VAR) vaccine.** (Minimum age: 12 months)
   - The second dose may be administered before age 4 years, provided at least 3 months have elapsed since the first dose.
   - For children aged 12 months through 12 years, the recommended minimum interval between doses is 3 months. However, if the second dose was administered at least 4 weeks after the first dose, it can be accepted as valid.

10. **Hepatitis A (HepA) vaccine.** (Minimum age: 12 months)
    - Administer the second (final) dose 6 to 18 months after the first.
    - Unvaccinated children 24 months and older at high risk should be vaccinated. See MMWR 2006;55(No. RR-7), available at http://www.cdc.gov/mmwr/pdf/rr/rr5507.pdf.
    - A 2-dose HepA vaccine series is recommended for anyone aged 24 months and older, previously unvaccinated, for whom immunity against hepatitis A virus infection is desired.

11. **Meningococcal conjugate vaccines, quadrivalent (MCV4).** (Minimum age: 9 months for Menactra [MCV4-D], 2 years for Menveo [MCV4-CRM])
    - For children aged 9 through 23 months 1) with persistent complement component deficiency; 2) who are residents of or travelers to countries with hyperendemic or epidemic disease; or 3) who are present during outbreaks caused by a vaccine serogroup, administer 2 primary doses of MCV4-D, ideally at ages 9 months and 12 months or at least 8 weeks apart.
    - For children aged 24 months and older with 1) persistent complement component deficiency who have not been previously vaccinated; or 2) anatomic/functional asplenia, administer 2 primary doses of either MCV4 at least 8 weeks apart.
    - For children with anatomic/functional asplenia, if MCV4-D (Menactra) is used, administer at a minimum age of 2 years and at least 4 weeks after completion of all PCV doses.
    - See MMWR 2011;60:72–6, available at http://www.cdc.gov/mmwr/pdf/wk/mm6003.pdf, and Vaccines for Children Program resolution No. 6/11-1, available at http://www.cdc.gov/vaccines/programs/vfc/downloads/resolutions/06-11mening-mcv.pdf, and MMWR 2011;60:1391–2, available at http://www.cdc.gov/mmwr/pdf/wk/mm6040.pdf, for further guidance, including revaccination guidelines.

Recommended immunization schedule for ages 7 through 18 years

FIGURE 2: Recommended immunization schedule for persons aged 7 through 18 years—United States, 2012 (for those who fall behind or start late, see the schedule below and the catch-up schedule [Figure 3])

Vaccine ▼　　Age ▶	7–10 years	11–12 years	13–18 years
Tetanus, diphtheria, pertussis[1]	1 dose (if indicated)	1 dose	1 dose (if indicated)
Human papillomavirus[2]	see footnote[2]	3 doses	Complete 3-dose series
Meningococcal[3]	See footnote[3]	Dose 1	Booster at 16 years old
Influenza[4]		Influenza (yearly)	
Pneumococcal[5]		See footnote[5]	
Hepatitis A[6]		Complete 2-dose series	
Hepatitis B[7]		Complete 3-dose series	
Inactivated poliovirus[8]		Complete 3-dose series	
Measles, mumps, rubella[9]		Complete 2-dose series	
Varicella[10]		Complete 2-dose series	

Range of recommended ages for all children

Range of recommended ages for catch-up immunization

Range of recommended ages for certain high-risk groups

This schedule includes recommendations in effect as of December 23, 2011. Any dose not administered at the recommended age should be administered at a subsequent visit, when indicated and feasible. The use of a combination vaccine generally is preferred over separate injections of its equivalent component vaccines. Vaccination providers should consult the relevant Advisory Committee on Immunization Practices (ACIP) statement for detailed recommendations, available online at http://www.cdc.gov/vaccines/pubs/acip-list.htm. Clinically significant adverse events that follow vaccination should be reported to the Vaccine Adverse Event Reporting System (VAERS) online (http://www.vaers.hhs.gov) or by telephone (800-822-7967).

1. **Tetanus and diphtheria toxoids and acellular pertussis (Tdap) vaccine.** (Minimum age: 10 years for Boostrix and 11 years for Adacel).
   - Persons aged 11 through 18 years who have not received Tdap vaccine should receive a dose followed by tetanus and diphtheria toxoids (Td) booster doses every 10 years thereafter.
   - Tdap vaccine should be substituted for a single dose of Td in the catch-up series for children aged 7 through 10 years. Refer to the catch-up schedule if additional doses of tetanus and diphtheria toxoid–containing vaccine are needed.
   - Tdap vaccine can be administered regardless of the interval since the last tetanus and diphtheria toxoid–containing vaccine.

   - For children aged 6 months through 8 years:
     — For the 2011–12 season, administer 2 doses (separated by at least 4 weeks) to those who did not receive at least 1 dose of the 2010–11 vaccine. Those who received at least 1 dose of the 2010–11 vaccine require 1 dose for the 2011–12 season.
     — For the 2012–13 season, follow dosing guidelines in the 2012 ACIP influenza vaccine recommendations.

5. **Pneumococcal vaccines (pneumococcal conjugate vaccine [PCV] and pneumococcal polysaccharide vaccine [PPSV]).**
   - A single dose of PCV may be administered to children aged 6 through 18 years who have anatomic/functional asplenia, HIV infection or other

2. **Human papillomavirus (HPV) vaccines (HPV4 [Gardasil] and HPV2 [Cervarix]). (Minimum age: 9 years)**
- Either HPV4 or HPV2 is recommended in a 3-dose series for females aged 11 or 12 years. HPV4 is recommended in a 3-dose series for males aged 11 or 12 years.
- The vaccine series can be started beginning at age 9 years.
- Administer the second dose 1 to 2 months after the first dose and the third dose 6 months after the first dose (at least 24 weeks after the first dose).
- See MMWR 2010;59:626–32, available at http://www.cdc.gov/mmwr/pdf/wk/mm5920.pdf.

3. **Meningococcal conjugate vaccines, quadrivalent (MCV4).**
- Administer MCV4 at age 11 through 12 years with a booster dose at age 16 years.
- Administer MCV4 at age 13 through 18 years if patient is not previously vaccinated.
- If the first dose is administered at age 13 through 15 years, a booster dose should be administered at age 16 through 18 years with a minimum interval of at least 8 weeks after the preceding dose.
- If the first dose is administered at age 16 years or older, a booster dose is not needed.
- Administer 2 primary doses at least 8 weeks apart to previously unvaccinated persons with persistent complement component deficiency or anatomic/functional asplenia, and 1 dose every 5 years thereafter.
- Adolescents aged 11 through 18 years with human immunodeficiency virus (HIV) infection should receive a 2-dose primary series of MCV4, at least 8 weeks apart.
- See MMWR 2011;60:72–76, available at http://www.cdc.gov/mmwr/pdf/wk/mm6003.pdf, and Vaccines for Children Program resolution No. 6/11-1, available at http://www.cdc.gov/vaccines/programs/vfc/downloads/resolutions/06-11mening-mcv.pdf, for further guidelines.

4. **Influenza vaccines (trivalent inactivated influenza vaccine [TIV] and live, attenuated influenza vaccine [LAIV]).**
- For most healthy, nonpregnant persons, either LAIV or TIV may be used, except LAIV should not be used for some persons, including those with asthma or any other underlying medical conditions that predispose them to influenza complications. For all other contraindications to use of LAIV, see MMWR 2010;59(No.RR-8), available at http://www.cdc.gov/mmwr/pdf/rr/rr5908.pdf.
- Administer 1 dose to persons aged 9 years and older.

immunocompromising condition, cochlear implant, or cerebral spinal fluid leak. See MMWR 2010;59(No. RR-11), available at http://www.cdc.gov/mmwr/pdf/rr/rr5911.pdf.
- Administer PPSV at least 8 weeks after the last dose of PCV to children aged 2 years or older with certain underlying medical conditions, including a cochlear implant. A single revaccination should be administered after 5 years to children with anatomic/functional asplenia or an immunocompromising condition.

6. **Hepatitis A (HepA) vaccine.**
- HepA vaccine is recommended for children older than 23 months who live in areas where vaccination programs target older children, who are at increased risk for infection, or for whom immunity against hepatitis A virus infection is desired. See MMWR 2006;55(No. RR-7), available at http://www.cdc.gov/mmwr/pdf/rr/rr5507.pdf.
- Administer 2 doses at least 6 months apart to unvaccinated persons.

7. **Hepatitis B (HepB) vaccine.**
- Administer the 3-dose series to those not previously vaccinated.
- For those with incomplete vaccination, follow the catch-up recommendations (Figure 3).
- A 2-dose series (doses separated by at least 4 months) of adult formulation Recombivax HB is licensed for use in children aged 11 through 15 years.

8. **Inactivated poliovirus vaccine (IPV).**
- The final dose in the series should be administered at least 6 months after the previous dose.
- If both OPV and IPV were administered as part of a series, a total of 4 doses should be administered, regardless of the child's current age.
- IPV is not routinely recommended for U.S. residents aged18 years or older.

9. **Measles, mumps, and rubella (MMR) vaccine.**
- The minimum interval between the 2 doses of MMR vaccine is 4 weeks.

10. **Varicella (VAR) vaccine.**
- For persons without evidence of immunity (see MMWR 2007;56[No. RR-4], available at http://www.cdc.gov/mmwr/pdf/rr/rr5604.pdf), administer 2 doses if not previously vaccinated or the second dose if only 1 dose has been administered.
- For persons aged 7 through 12 years, the recommended minimum interval between doses is 3 months. However, if the second dose was administered at least 4 weeks after the first dose, it can be accepted as valid.
- For persons aged 13 years and older, the minimum interval between doses is 4 weeks.

Catch-up immunization

Persons aged 4 months through 6 years

Vaccine	Minimum Age for Dose 1	Minimum Interval Between Doses			
		Dose 1 to dose 2	Dose 2 to dose 3	Dose 3 to dose 4	Dose 4 to dose 5
Hepatitis B	Birth	4 weeks	8 weeks and at least 16 weeks after first dose; minimum age for the final dose is 24 weeks		
Rotavirus[1]	6 weeks	4 weeks	4 weeks[1]		
Diphtheria, tetanus, pertussis[2]	6 weeks	4 weeks	4 weeks	6 months	6 months[2]
Haemophilus influenzae type b[3]	6 weeks	4 weeks if first dose administered at younger than age 12 months 8 weeks (as final dose) if first dose administered at age 12–14 months No further doses needed if first dose administered at age 15 months or older	4 weeks[3] if current age is younger than 12 months 8 weeks (as final dose)[3] if current age is 12 months or older and first dose administered at younger than age 12 months and second dose administered at younger than 15 months No further doses needed if previous dose administered at age 15 months or older	8 weeks (as final dose) This dose only necessary for children aged 12 months through 59 months who received 3 doses before age 12 months	
Pneumococcal[4]	6 weeks	4 weeks if first dose administered at younger than age 12 months 8 weeks (as final dose for healthy children) if first dose administered at age 12 months or older or current age 24 through 59 months No further doses needed for healthy children if first dose administered at age 24 months or older	4 weeks if current age is younger than 12 months 8 weeks (as final dose for healthy children) if current age is 12 months or older No further doses needed for healthy children if previous dose administered at age 24 months or older	8 weeks (as final dose) This dose only necessary for children aged 12 months through 59 months who received 3 doses before age 12 months or for children at high risk who received 3 doses at any age	
Inactivated poliovirus[5]	6 weeks	4 weeks	4 weeks	6 months[5] minimum age 4 years for final dose	
Meningococcal[6]	9 months	8 weeks[6]			
Measles, mumps, rubella[7]	12 months	4 weeks			
Varicella[8]	12 months	3 months			
Hepatitis A	12 months	6 months			

	Persons aged 7 through 18 years			
Tetanus, diphtheria/tetanus, diphtheria, pertussis[9]	7 years[9]	4 weeks	4 weeks if first dose administered at younger than age 12 months / 6 months if first dose administered at 12 months or older	6 months if first dose administered at younger than age 12 months
Human papillomavirus[10]	9 years	Routine dosing intervals are recommended[10]		
Hepatitis A	12 months	6 months		
Hepatitis B	Birth	4 weeks	8 weeks (and at least 16 weeks after first dose)	
Inactivated poliovirus[5]	6 weeks	4 weeks	4 weeks[5]	6 months[5]
Meningococcal[6]	9 months	8 weeks[6]		
Measles, mumps, rubella[7]	12 months	4 weeks		
Varicella[8]	12 months	3 months if person is younger than age 13 years / 4 weeks if person is aged 13 years or older		

1. **Rotavirus (RV) vaccines (RV-1 [Rotarix] and RV-5 [Rota Teq]).**
   - The maximum age for the first dose in the series is 14 weeks, 6 days; and 8 months, 0 days for the final dose in the series. Vaccination should not be initiated for infants aged 15 weeks, 0 days or older.
   - If RV-1 was administered for the first and second doses, a third dose is not indicated.

2. **Diphtheria and tetanus toxoids and acellular pertussis (DTaP) vaccine.**
   - The fifth dose is not necessary if the fourth dose was administered at age 4 years or older.

3. **Haemophilus influenzae type b (Hib) conjugate vaccine.**
   - Hib vaccine should be considered for unvaccinated persons aged 5 years or older who have sickle cell disease, leukemia, human immunodeficiency virus (HIV) infection, or anatomic/functional asplenia.
   - If the first 2 doses were PRP–OMP (PedvaxHIB or Comvax) and were administered at age 11 months or younger, the third (and final) dose should be administered at age 12 through 15 months and at least 8 weeks after the second dose.
   - If the first dose was administered at age 7 through 11 months, administer the second dose at least 4 weeks later and a final dose at age 12 through 15 months.

4. **Pneumococcal vaccines.** (Minimum age: 6 weeks for pneumococcal conjugate vaccine [PCV]; 2 years for pneumococcal polysaccharide vaccine [PPSV])
   - For children aged 24 through 71 months with underlying medical conditions, administer 1 dose of PCV if 3 doses of PCV were received previously, or administer 2 doses of PCV at least 8 weeks apart if fewer than 3 doses of PCV were received previously.
   - A single dose of PCV may be administered to certain children aged 6 through 18 years with underlying medical conditions. See age-specific schedules for details.
   - Administer PPSV to children aged 2 years or older with certain underlying medical conditions. See *MMWR* 2010;59(No. RR-11), available at http://www.cdc.gov/mmwr/pdf/rr/rr5911.pdf.

5. **Inactivated poliovirus vaccine (IPV).**
   - A fourth dose is not necessary if the third dose was administered at age 4 years or older and at least 6 months after the previous dose.
   - In the first 6 months of life, minimum age and minimum intervals are only recommended if the person is at risk for imminent exposure to circulating poliovirus (i.e., travel to a polio-endemic region or during an outbreak).
   - IPV is not routinely recommended for U.S. residents aged 18 years or older.

6. **Meningococcal conjugate vaccines, quadrivalent (MCV4).** (Minimum age: 9 months for Menactra [MCV4-D]; 2 years for Menveo [MCV4-CRM])
   - See Figure 1 ("Recommended immunization schedule for persons aged 0 through 6 years") and Figure 2 ("Recommended immunization schedule for persons aged 7 through 18 years") for further guidance.

7. **Measles, mumps, and rubella (MMR) vaccine.**
   - Administer the second dose routinely at age 4 through 6 years.

8. **Varicella (VAR) vaccine.**
   - Administer the second dose routinely at age 4 through 6 years. If the second dose was administered at least 4 weeks after the first dose, it can be accepted as valid.

9. **Tetanus and diphtheria toxoids (Td) and tetanus and diphtheria toxoids and acellular pertussis (Tdap) vaccines.**
   - For children aged 7 through 10 years who are not fully immunized with the childhood DTaP vaccine series, Tdap vaccine should be substituted for a single dose of Td vaccine in the catch-up series; if additional doses are needed, use Td vaccine. For these children, an adolescent Tdap vaccine dose should not be given.
   - An inadvertent dose of DTaP vaccine administered to children aged 7 through 10 years can count as part of the catch-up series. This dose can count as the adolescent Tdap dose, or the child can later receive a Tdap booster dose at age 11–12 years.

10. **Human papillomavirus (HPV) vaccines (HPV4 [Gardasil] and HPV2 [Cervarix]).**
    - Administer the vaccine series to females (either HPV2 or HPV4) and males (HPV4) at age 13 through 18 years if patient is not previously vaccinated.
    - Use recommended routine dosing intervals for vaccine series catch-up; see Figure 2 ("Recommended immunization schedule for persons aged 7 through 18 years").

Contraception Methods

Trade name	Type	Estrogen	Progestin	Formulation	Comment
Alesse, Aviane, Lessina, Levlite, Lutera, Sronyx	Monophasic	Ethinyl estradiol 20 mcg	Levonorgestrel 0.1 mg	Oral	Avoid
Angeliq	Monophasic	Estradiol 1 mg	Drospirenone 0.5 mg	Oral	Avoid
Approved in Europe with US FDA approval expected early 2012.	Monophasic	17 p-estradiol 1.5 mg	Nomegestrol acetate 2.5 mg	Oral	Avoid
Apri, Desogen, Emoquette, Ortho-Cept, Reclipsen, Solia	Monophasic	Ethinyl estradiol 30 mcg	Desogestrel 0.15 mg	Oral	Avoid
Aranelle, Leena, Tri-Norinyl	Triphasic	Ethinyl estradiol 35 mcg	Norethindrone 0.5 mg (days 1-7), 1 mg (days 8-16), 0.5 mg (days 17-21)	Oral	Avoid
Azurette, Kariva, Mircette	Biphasic	Ethinyl estradiol 20 mcg (days 1-21), 10 mcg (days 24-28)	Desogestrel 0.15 mg	Oral	Avoid
Balziva-28, Briellyn 28, Ovcon-35, Zenchent	Monophasic	Ethinyl estradiol 35 mcg	Norethindrone 0.4 mg	Oral	Avoid
Beyaz, Gianvi, Loryna, Yaz	Monophasic + levomefolate calcium 0.451 mg	Ethinyl estradiol 20 mcg (days 1-24)	Drospirenone 3 mg (days 1-24)	Oral	Avoid
Brevicon, Modicon, Necon 0.5/35, Norrel 0.5/35	Monophasic	Ethinyl estradiol 35 mcg	Norethindrone 0.5 mg	Oral	Avoid
Camila, Errin, Jolivette, Micronor, Nora-BE, Norethindrone, Nor-QD, Ortho-Micronor	Progestin only		Norethindrone 0.35 mg	Oral	Acceptable

Contraception Methods

Trade name	Type	Estrogen	Progestin	Formulation	Comment
Caziant, Cesia, Cyclessa, Velivet	Triphasic	Ethinyl estradiol 25 mcg	Desogestrel 0.1 mg (days 1-7), 0.125 (days 8-14), 0.15 mg (days 15-21)	Oral	Avoid
Cryselle, Lo/Ovral, Low-Ogestrel	Monophasic	Ethinyl estradiol 30 mcg	Norgestrel 0.3 mg	Oral	Avoid
Demulen 1/35, Kelnor, Zovia 1/35	Monophasic	Ethinyl estradiol 35 mcg	Ethynodiol diacetate 1 mg	Oral	Avoid
Depo-Provera	Progestin only		Medroxyprogesterone 150 mg every 3 months	IM Injection	Acceptable
Depo-SubQ Provera	Progestin only		Medroxyprogesterone 104 mg every 3 months	SQ Injection	Acceptable
Enpresse, Levonest, Trivora	Triphasic	Ethinyl estradiol 30 mcg (days 1-6), 40 mcg (days 7-11), 30 mcg (days 12-21)	Levonorgestrel 0.05 mg (days 1-6), 0.075 mg (days 8-14), 0.15 mg (days 15-21)	Oral	Avoid
Estrostep 21, Tilia	Triphasic	Ethinyl estradiol 20 mcg (days 1-5), 30 mcg (days 6-12), 35 mcg (days 13-21)	Norethindrone 1 mg	Oral	Avoid
Estrostep Fe, Tilia Fe, Tri-Legest Fe	Triphasic/ iron days 22-28	Ethinyl estradiol 20 mcg (days 1-5), 30 mcg (days 6-12), 35 mcg (days 13-21)	Norethindrone 1mg	Oral	Avoid
Femcon Fe	Monophasic/ iron days 22-28	Ethinyl estradiol 35 mcg	Norethindrone 0.4 mg	Oral	Avoid
Gildess Fe, Junel FE 1/20, Loestrin 24 FE 1/20, Microgestin Fe 1/20	Monophasic/ iron days 25-28	Ethinyl estradiol 20 mcg (days 1-24)	Norethindrone acetate 1 mg (days 1-24)	Oral	Avoid

Contraception Methods

Trade name	Type	Estrogen	Progestin	Formulation	Comment
Gildess Fe 1.5/30, Gildess Fe 1.5/30, Junel Fe 1.5/30, Loestrin Fe 1.5/30, Microgestin Fe 1.5/30	Monophasic/ iron days 22-28	Ethinyl estradiol 30 mcg	Norethindrone acetate 1.5 mg	Oral	Avoid
Implanon	Progestin only		Etonogestrel 60-70 mcg/day (year 1), 35-45 mcg/day (year 2), 30-40 mcg/day (year 3)	Subdermal Implant	Acceptable
Introvale, Jolessa, Quasense, Seasonale	Continuous cycle regimen	Ethinyl estradiol 30 mcg (days 1-84)	Levonorgestrel 0.15 mg (days 1-84)	Oral	Avoid
Junel-21 1/20, Loestrin 21 1/20, Microgestin 1/20	Monophasic	Ethinyl estradiol 20 mcg	Norethindrone acetate 1 mg	Oral	Avoid
Junel-21 1.5/30, Loestrin-21 1.5/30, Microgestin 1.5/30	Monophasic	Ethinyl estradiol 30 mcg	Norethindrone acetate 1.5 mg	Oral	Avoid
Levlen, Levora, Nordette, Portia	Monophasic	Ethinyl estradiol 30 mcg	Levonorgestrel 0.15 mg	Oral	Avoid
Lo Loestrin Fe	Monophasic/ iron days 26-28	Ethinyl estradiol 10 mcg (days 1-26)	Norethindrone acetate 1 mg (days 1-24)	Oral	Avoid
LoSeasonique	Continuous cycle regimen	Ethinyl estradiol 20 mcg (days 1-84), 10 mcg (days 85-91)	Levonorgestrel 0.1 mg (days 1-84)	Oral	Avoid
Lybrel	Continuous	Ethinyl estradiol 20 mcg	Levonorgestrel 90 mcg	Oral	Avoid
Mirena	Progestin only		Levonorgestrel 20 mcg/day for 5 years	Intrauterine Device (IUD)	Acceptable
MonoNessa, Ortho-Cyclen, Previfem, Sprintec	Monophasic	Ethinyl estradiol 35 mcg	Norgestimate 0.25 mg	Oral	Avoid

Contraception Methods

Trade Name	Type	Estrogen	Progestin	Formulation	Comment
Natazia	Quadrephasic	Estradiol valerate 3 mg (days 1-2), 2 mg (days 3-24), 1 mg (25-26)	Dienogest none (days 1-2), 2 mg (days 3-7), 3 mg (days 8-24), none (days 25-28)	Oral	Avoid
Necon 1/35, Norinyl 1+35, Nortrel 1/35, Ortho-Novum 1/35	Monophasic	Ethinyl estradiol 35 mcg	Norethindrone 1 mg	Oral	Avoid
Necon 1/50, Norinyl 1+50, Ortho-Novum 1/50	Monophasic	Mestranol 50 mcg	Norethindrone 1 mg	Oral	Avoid
Necon 7/7/7, Nortrel 7/7/7, Ortho-Novum 7/7/7	Triphasic	Ethinyl estradiol 35 mcg	Norethindrone 0.5 mg (days 1-7), 0.75 mg (days 8-14), 1 mg (days 15-21)	Oral	Avoid
Necon 10/11, Ortho-Novum 10/11,	Biphasic	Ethinyl estradiol 35 mcg	Norethindrone 0.5 mg (days 1-10), 1 mg (days 11-21)	Oral	Avoid
Next Choice, Next Step, Plan B	Emergency Contraception		Levonorgestrel 0.75 mg	Oral	Acceptable
NuvaRing	Combination	Ethinyl estradiol 0.015 mg/day	Etonogestrel 0.12 mg/day	Vaginal ring	Avoid
Ocella, Syeda, Yasmin	Monophasic	Ethinyl estradiol 30 mcg	Drospirenone 3 mg	Oral	Avoid
Ogestrel 0.5/50	Monophasic	Ethinyl estradiol 50 mcg	Norgestrel 0.5 mg	Oral	Avoid
Ortho Evra	Combination	Ethinyl estradiol 20 mcg/day	Norelgestromin 150 mcg/day	Transdermal Patch	Avoid
Ortho-Tri-Cyclen, TriNessa, Tri-Previfem, Tri-Sprintec,	Triphasic	Ethinyl estradiol 35 mcg	Norgestimate 0.18 mg (days 1-7), 0.215 mg (days 8-14), 0.25 mg (days 15-21)	Oral	Avoid

Contraception Methods

Trade Name	Type	Estrogen	Progestin	Formulation	Comment
Ortho-Tri-Cyclen Lo, Tri-Lo-Sprintec	Triphasic	Ethinyl estradiol 25 mcg	Norgestimate 0.18 mg (days 1-7), 0.215 mg (days 8-14), 0.25 mg (days 15-21)	Oral	Avoid
Ovcon-50	Monophasic	Ethinyl estradiol 50 mcg	Norethindrone 1 mg	Oral	Avoid
Ovrette	Progestin only		Norgestrel 0.075 mg	Oral	Acceptable
ParaGard	Non-hormonal (copper)			Intrauterine Device (IUD)	Acceptable
Plan B One Step	Emergency contraception		Levonorgestrel 1.5 mg	Oral	Acceptable
Prefest	Multiphasic	Ethinyl estradiol 1mg (days 1-6)	Norgestimate 0.09 mg (days 4-6)	Oral	Avoid
Preven	Emergency contraception	Ethinyl estradiol 50 mcg	Levonorgestrel 0.25 mg	Oral	Avoid
Safyral	Monophasic + levomefolate calcium 0.451 mg days 22-28	Ethinyl estradiol 30 mcg	Drospirenone 3 mg	Oral	Avoid
Seasonique	Continuous cycle regimen	Ethinyl estradiol 30 mcg (days 1-84), 10 mcg (days 85-91)	Levonorgestrel 0.15 mg (days 1-84)	Oral	Avoid
Tri-Norinyl	Triphasic	Ethinyl estradiol 35 mcg	Norethindrone 0.5 mg (days 1-7), 1 mg (days 8-16), 0.5 mg (days 17-21)	Oral	Avoid
Zovia 1/50	Monophasic	Ethinyl estradiol 50 mcg	Ethynodiol diacetate 1 mg	Oral	Avoid

Normal Growth During Development

Boys Growth Chart

Age	Weight (lb.)	Length (in.)
Birth	7.5	19.7
3 months	14.1	24.0
6 months	17.6	26.8
9 months	19.8	28.3
12 months	21.1	29.9
15 months	22.9	31.1
18 months	24.2	32.3
24 months	26.8	34.6

Close approximate values taken from WHO growth charts for breastfed infants, 2010.

Normal Growth During Development

Girls Growth Chart

Age	Weight (lb.)	Length (in.)
Birth	7.0	19.3
3 months	12.8	23.6
6 months	15.8	26.0
9 months	18.0	27.6
12 months	19.9	29.1
15 months	21.1	30.7
18 months	22.4	31.9
24 months	25.1	33.9

Close approximate values taken from WHO growth charts for breastfed infants, 2010.

Thyroid Function Tests

Test	Time	Normal Range
T4(thyroxine)	1-7 days 8-14 days 1 month-1year >1 year	10.1-20.9 µg/dL 9.8-16.6 µg/dL 5.5-16 µg/dL 4-12 µg/dL
FTI	1-3 days 1-4 weeks 1-4 months 4-12 months 1-6 years >6 years	9.3-26.6 7.6-20.8 7.4-17.9 5.1-14.5 5.7-13.3 4.8-14
T3 by RIA	Newborns 1-5 years 5-10 years 10 years-adult	100-470 ng/dL 100-260 ng/dL 90-240 ng/dL 70-210 ng/dL
T3 uptake		35-45%
TSH	Cord 1-3 days 3-7 days >7 days	3-22 µIU/mL <40 µIU/mL <25 µIU/mL 0-10 µIU/mL

Therapeutic Drug Levels

REFERENCE (NORMAL) VALUES

DRUG		THERAPEUTIC RANGE
Acetaminophen		10-20 µg/ml
Theophylline		0-20 µg/ml
Carbamazepine		4-10 µg/ml
Ethosuximide		40-100 µg/ml
Phenobarbital		15-40 µg/ml
Phenytoin		
	Neonates	6-14 µg/ml
	Children, adults	10-20 µg/ml
Primidone		5-15 µg/ml
Valproic Acid		50-100 µg/m
Gentamicin		
	Peak	5-12 µg/ml
	Trough	<2.0 µg/ml
Vancomycin		
	Peak	20-40 µg/ml
	Trough	5-10 µg/ml
Digoxin		0.9-2.2 µg/ml
Lithium		0.3-1.3 mmol/L
Salicylates		20-25 mg/dL

From Therapeutic Drug Monitoring Guide, WE Evan, Editor, Abbott Laboratories, 1988.

Pediatric Laboratory Values

Test	Age	Range	Units
pH	< 1 mo	7.3-7.46	
pCO2	2-5d	4.1-6.3	kPa(mmHg)
pCO2	2-5d	5.6-7.7	kPa(mmHg)
Total CO2	<1 yr.	15-35	mmol/L
Albumin, Serum	< 1 yr.	3-4.9	gm/dL
Phenylalamine	Newborn	0.7-3.5	umol/L
Ammonia	<1 yr.	68	µmol/L
Total Bilirubin	< 2 w	< 11.7	µg/dL
	<10 yr.	<0.9	mg/dL
Calcium	< 1 yr.	7.8-11.2	mg/dL
Chloride	< 2 yr.	100-110	mmol/dL
Cholesteral Tota	< 1 yr.	93-260	mg/dL
Copper, Serum	1-5 yr.	80-150	µg/dL
Copper, Wiring	< 6 yr.	8-17	µg/dL
Creatine Kinose	1-3 yr.	50-305	IU/L
Creatine, Serum	< 10 yr.	0.2-1.02	mg/dL
Ferritin	1-4 yr.	6-24	µg/L
Fructosamine	5-17 yr.	1.4-2.2	mmol/L
Glucose	1-6 yr.	74-127	mg/dL
Hemoglobin A1C	2-12 yr.	5.1	%HbA1C
Cholesterol (HDL)	1-9 yr.	35-82	mg/dL
Iron	< 2 yr.	11-150	µg/dL
Magnesium	< 1 yr.	1.6-2.6	mg/dL
Osmolality	28d	274-305	mmol/dL
Phosphatose, alkaline	2-9 yr.	100-400	IU/L
Phosphorus, Serum	< 2 yr.	2.5-7.1	mg/dL
Potassium	< 2 mo.	3-7.0	mmol/dL
Prolactin	0-18 yr.	20 or less	ng/mL
Protein, Total	< 1 yr.	5-7.5	mg/dL
Protein, Urine	< 1 yr.	130-145	mmol/dL
Sodium, Urinary	1-6 mo.		
breast-fed		6.1	mmol/L
formula-fed		13.2	mmol/L

Drugs to Avoid in Lactation

GENERIC NAME	BRAND NAME
DOPAMINE AGONISTS	
Apomorphine	Apokyn
Bromocriptine	Parlodel
Cabergoline	Dostinex
Pramipexole	Mirapex
Ropinirole	Requip
Rotigotine	Neupro
Selegiline	Eldepryl, Emsam, Zelapar
Levodopa	Dopar, Larodopa, Sinemet

Drugs that are potentially
Hazardous in Breastfeeding Mothers

Generic Name	Trade Names	LRC
Acitretin	Soriatane	L5
Aminopterin		L5
Amiodarone	Aratac, Cordarone	L5
Anastrozole	Arimidex	L5
Anthrax (bacillus anthracis)	Anthrax Infection, Bacillus Anthracis	L5
Blue cohosh	Blue ginseng, Papoose root, Squaw root, Yellow ginseng	L5
Borage	Bee plant, Beebread, Borage, Borage oil, Burrage, Ox, Starflower	L5
Bromides		L5
Bromocriptine	Apo-Bromocriptine, Bromolactin, Kripton, Parlodel	L5
Busulfan	Busilvex, Myleran	L5
Cannabis	Marijuana, Tetrahydrocannabinol	L5
Capecitabine	Xeloda	L5
Carbetapentane	Exhall, Expectuss	L5
Carboplatin	Carboplat, Carbosin, Emorzim, Novoplat, Paraplatin, Paraplatin-AQ	L5
Carmustine	BCNU, Bicnu, Carmubris, Gliadel, Nitrumon	L5
Chlorambucil	Alti-Chlorambucil, Leukeran, Linfolysin	L5
Cisplatin	Abiplatin, Bioplatino, C-Platin, Cis-Gry, Cisplatin, Placis	L5
Cladribine	Leustat, Leustatin, Litak	L5
Clobetasol	Clobevate, Clobex, Cormax, Dermovate, Gen-Clobetasol, Novo-Clobetasol, Olux, Olux-E, Taro-Clobetasol, Temovate, Temovate E	L5
Cocaine	Crack	L5
Comfrey	Blackwort, Bruisewort, Knitbone, Russian comfrey, Slippery root	L5
Cyclophosphamide	Carloxan, Cycloblastin, Cytoxan, Endoxan, Endoxana, Neosar, Procytox	L5
Cytarabine	Alexan, Arabine, Cytarabine, Cytosar, Cytosar-U, Tarabine PFS	L5
Dactinomycin	Actinomycin D, Cosmegen	L5
Danazol	Azol, Cyclomen, Danocrine, Danol	L5
Daunorubicin	Cerubidin, Cerubidine, DaunoXome, Daunoblastin, Daunoblastina	L5
Dehydroepiandrosterone (DHEA)	DHEA	L5
Delavirdine	Rescriptor	L5

Drugs that are potentially Hazardous in Breastfeeding Mothers

Generic Name	Trade Names	LRC
Didanosine	Videx	L5
Diethylpropion	Dospan, Tenuate, Tepanil	L5
Diethylstilbestrol	Apstil, DES, Fosfestrol, Honvan, Honvol	L5
Disulfiram	Antabuse	L5
Docetaxel	Taxotere	L5
Doxepin	Adapin, Deptran, Novo-Doxepin, Silenor, Sinequan, Triadapin	L5
Doxorubicin	Adriamycin, Adriblastina, Caelyx	L5
Epirubicin	Ellence, Epi-Cell, Farmorubicina, Pharmarubicin, Rubina	L5
Etoposide	Abiposid, Celltop, Eposid, Eposin, Etopofos, Etopophos, Toposar, VP-16	L5
Etravirine	Intelence	L5
Etretinate	Tegison, Tigason	L5
Everolimus	Afinitor, Zortress	L5
Exemestane	Aromasin	L5
Gamma hydroxybutyric acid	GBH, GHB, Gamma-OH, Liquid Ecstasy, Oxybutyrate, Somsanit	L5
Gold compounds	Myochrysine, Myocrisin, Ridaura, Solganal	L5
Heroin	Heroin	L5
I-123	DaTscan, I-123, Iodine-123, Ioflupane I-123, Radioactive Iodine	L5
I-125	I-125, Iodine-125, Radioactive Iodine	L5
I-131	Hicon, I-131, Iodine-131, Iodotope, Radioactive Iodine	L5
Imatinib mesylate	Gleevec	L5
Isotretinoin	Accure, Accutane, Isotrex, Roaccutane	L5
Ixabepilone	Ixempra	L5
Kava-kava		L5
Kombucha tea		L5
Lead		L5
Leuprolide acetate	Eligard, Lupron, Prostap, Viadur	L5
Lysergic acid diethylamide (lsd)	LSD	L5
Melphalan	Alkeran	L5
Mercury	Mercury	L5

Drugs that are potentially Hazardous in Breastfeeding Mothers

Generic Name	Trade Names	LRC
Methamphetamine	Anadrex, Desoxyephedrine, Desoxyn, Methedrine, Pervitin	L5
Mitomycin	Mitomycin-C, Mutamycin	L5
Mitoxantrone	Formyxan, Genefadrone, Misostol, Mitoxl, Novantrone, Onkotrone, Pralifan	L5
Oxaliplatin	Eloxatin, Eloxatine, O-Plat, Oxalip	L5
Paclitaxel	Abitaxel, Abraxane, Anzatax, Biotax, Paxel, Paxene, Taxol	L5
Pazopanib	Votrient	L5
Pentostatin	Nipent	L5
Phencyclidine	Angel Dust, PCP	L5
Propylhexedrine	Benzedrex	L5
Strontium-89 chloride	Metastron	L5
Tamoxifen	Apo-Tamox, Eblon, Genox, Noltam, Nolvadex, Tamofen, Tamone, Tamoxen	L5
Temozolomide	Temodal, Temodar	L5
Thalidomide	Thalomid	L5
Thyroid scan	Thyroid Scan	L5
Vinblastine	Lemblastine, Velban, Velbe, Velsar	L5
Vincristine	Citomid, Farmistin, Ifavin, Norcristine, Oncovin, Vincasar PFS, Vincizina, Vincristine	L5
Vinorelbine	Biovelbin, Navelbine	L5

Drugs That Are Usually Contraindicated In Lactating Women*

DRUG	NATURE OF POSSIBLE INFANT RISK
Amiodarone	Relative infant dose 4-6% of maternal dose; may accumulate because of very long half-life; adverse cardiovascular and thyroid effects possible. However, short-term use is permissible.
Antineoplastic agents	Overtly toxic; avoid exposure; bone marrow suppression, damage to intestinal epithelial cells possible. Pump and discard for a suitable period following exposure.
Chloramphenicol	Relative infant dose 2% of maternal dose. Blood dyscrasias, aplastic anemia, etc. possible.
Ergotamine	Symptoms of ergotism (vomiting and diarrhea) reported; potential to inhibit prolactin secretion
Gold salts	Relative infant dose varies from 1-7%. Long half-life in adults suggests potential for accumulation. Possibility of diarrhea, dermatitis, nephrotoxicity and blood dyscrasia
Phenindione	Relative infant dose calculated at around 18% of maternal dose and abnormal blood coagulation in an infant has been reported
Radiopharmaceuticals	Temporary discontinuation of breastfeeding may be necessary. See Appendix A.
Retinoids	Secretion into milk is unknown, but is likely to be significant as these drugs are usually very lipid soluble (e.g. isotretinoin). Contraindicated because if the wide range of adverse effects in adults and mutagenic and carcinogenic actions in animals
Tetracyclines (Chronic)	While the short-term use of tetracyclines for up to three weeks is OK, chronic use over many months may lead to staining of immature teeth, or changes in epiphyseal bone growth
Pseudoephedrine	Data indicates that pseudoephedrine may inhibit milk production significantly, but primarily in late-stage lactation.

* Adapted from Hale TW, Ilett KF. Drug Therapy and Breastfeeding: From Theory to Clinical Practice, First Edition ed. London: Parthenon Publishing; 2002

Is It A Cold Or The Flu?

Symptoms	Cold	Flu
Fever	rare	characteristic, high (102-104F); lasts 3-4 days
Headache	rare	Prominent
General Aches, Pains	slight	usual; often severe
Fatigue, Weakness	quite mild	can last up to 2-3 weeks
Extreme Exhaustion	never	early and prominent
Stuffy Nose	common	Sometimes
Sneezing	usual	Sometimes
Sore Throat	common	Sometimes
Chest Discomfort, Cough	mild to moderate; hacking cough	common; can become severe

(Source: National Institute of Allergy and Infectious Diseases)
Publication No. (FDA) 99-1264 http://www.fda.gov/fdac/features/896_flu.html

Neuromuscular Blocking Agents

Agent (Brand Name)	Pharmacological Properties	Time of Onset (min.)	Clinical Duration (min.)	Half-Life (min.)
Atracurium (TRACRIUM)	intermediate duration	2 – 4	30 – 60	16 – 20 min
d-Tubocurarine	long duration	4 – 6	80 – 120	173 min
Doxacurium (NUROMAX)	long duration	4 – 6	90 – 120	120 min
Mivacurium (MIVACRON)	short duration	2 – 4	12 – 18	1.8 – 2 min
Pancuronium (PAVULON)	long duration	4 – 6	120 – 180	89 – 140 min
Pipecuronium (ARDUAN)	long duration	2 – 4	80 – 100	137 – 161 min
Rapacuronium (RAPLON)	intermediate duration	1 – 2	15 – 30	72 – 175 min
Rocuronium (ZEMURON)	intermediate duration	1 – 2	30 – 60	84 – 131 min
Succinylcholine (ANECTINE)	ultrashort duration	1 – 1.5	5 – 8	< 1 min
Vecuronium (NORCURON)	intermediate duration	2 – 4	60 – 90	80 min

Topical Corticosteroids

Potency	Topical corticosteroid (Brand name)	Preparation	Comment
Low potency	Alclometasone (Aclovate)	0.05% cream/ ointment	Probably safe if not used in large amounts on the nipple.
	Desonide (DesOwen, Tridesilon)	0.05% cream	
	Fluocinolone (Synalar solution, Derma Smoothe/FS)	0.01% cream/solution	
	Hydrocortisone (Anusol-HC, Cortaid, Cortizone, Dermarest, Hytone, ProctoCream)	0.25%; 0.5%; 1% & 2.5% in various dosage forms	
Intermediate potency	Betamethasone (Alphatrex, Betatrex)	0.025% cream/ gel/ lotion 0.05% lotion 0.1% cream	Probably safe if used in minimal amounts directly applied on the nipple. Some caution is recommended.
	Clocortolone (Cloderm)	0.1% cream	
	Desoximetasone (Topicort-LP)	0.05% cream	
	Fluocinolone (Synalar)	0.025% cream/ ointment	
	Flurandrenolide (Cordran)	0.05% cream/ ointment/ lotion/tape	
	Fluticasone (Cutivate)	0.005% ointment & 0.05% cream	
	Hydrocortisone butyrate or valerate (Locoid, Locoid Lipocream, Westcort)	0.1% ointment/ solution & 0.2% cream/ointment	
	Mometasone furoate (Elecon)	0.1% cream/ ointment/lotion	
	Prednicarbate (Dermatop)	0.1% cream/ointment	
	Triamcinolone acetonide (Aristocort, Kenalog, Triderm)	0.025% & 0.1% cream/ ointment/ lotion	

Topical Corticosteroids

Potency	Topical corticosteroid (Brand name)	Preparation	Comment
High potency	Amcinonide (Cyclocort)	0.1% cream/ ointment/lotion	Do not use on nipple. Some caution is recommended if used on large areas on the body.
	Betamethasone dipropionate or valerate (Alphatrex, Betatrex, Diprolene AF, Diprolene, Maxivate)	0.05% cream/ ointment & 0.1% ointment	
	Desoximetasone (Topicort)	0.05% gel & 0.25% cream/ ointment	
	Diflorasone diacetate (Maxiflor, Psorcon)	0.05% cream/ ointment	
	Fluocinonide (Lidex, Lidex-E)	0.05% cream/ ointment/gel	
	Halcinonide (Halog, Halog-E)	0.1% cream/ointment	
	Triamcinolone (Aristocort, Kenalog)	0.5% cream/ointment	
Very high potency	Clobetasol (Clobex, Cormax, Olux, Temovate)	0.05% cream/ ointment /lotion/foam	Never use on nipple. Caution is recommended if used on large areas on the body.
	Diflorasone diacetate (Maxiflor, Psorcon)	0.05% ointment	
	Halobetasol (Ultravate)	0.05% cream/ ointment	

Herbal Drugs To Avoid in Lactation*

Aloe

Blue Cohosh

Buckthorn Bark and Berry

Cascara Sagrada bark

Coltsfoot leaf

Comfrey

Extract of Senna leaf, peppermint and caraway oil

Germander

Ginseng

Goldenseal

Gordolobo yerba tea

Indian snakeroot

Jin Bu Huan

Kava Kava

Licorice

Male fern

Margosa Oil

Mate tea

Mistletoe

Pennyroyal oil

Petasites root

Podophyllum

Purging buckthorn

Rhubarb root

Sage

Senna leaf

Skullcap

Uva Uris

* Adapted in part from The Complete German Commission E Monographs. Ed. M. Blumenthal Amer Botanical Council 1998 and other literature.

Iodine Contents from Various Natural Sources

Iodine Sources	Descriptions	Quantity	Dose Form	Iodine Contents (MCG)	Percent of Daily Recommended Value
Bread[2]	White enriched	2 slice		45	30%
Cheese[2]	Cheddar	1 oz		12	8%
Cod[2]		3 oz		99	66%
Corn[2]	Creamy (canned)	1/2 cup		14	9%
Egg[2]		1 large		24	16%
Fish sticks[2]		3 oz		54	36%
Fruit cocktail[2]	Heavy syrup	1/2 cup		42	28%
Ice cream[2]	Chocolate	1/2 cup		30	20%
Macaroni[2]	Enriched	1 cup		27	18%
Milk[2]		1 cup		56	37%
Prunes[2]	Dried	5		13	9%
Iodized Salt[2]		3 g		142	94%
Sea weed[1]		1 g		16-8165	11-540%
Sea weed[1]	Arame	1 g		586 ± 56	391%
Sea weed[1]	Bladderwrack	1 g		276 ± 82	184%
Sea weed[1]	Dulse	1 g		72 ± 23	48%
Sea weed[1]	Fingered tangle	1 g		1997 ± 563	1331%
Sea weed[1]	Fingered tangle	1 g	Granules	8165 ± 373	5443%
Sea weed[1]	Hijiki	1 g		629 ± 153	419%
Sea weed[1]	Horsetail tangle	1 g		30 ± 1	20%
Sea weed[1]	Kelp	1 g	Capsule	1259 ± 200	839%
Sea weed[1]	Kelp	1 g		1513 ± 117	1009%
Sea weed[1]	Kelp (wild)	1 g	Capsule	1356 ± 665	904%
Sea weed[1]	Kelp Oarweed	1 g		746 ± 26	497%
Sea weed[1]	Knotted wrack	1 g		646 ± 153	431%
Sea weed[1]	Kombu	1 g		1350 ± 362	900%
Sea weed[1]	Mekabu	1 g	Tablet	22 ± 1	15%
Sea weed[1]	Mekabu	1 g	Powder	53 ± 3	35%
Sea weed[1]	Mitthsuishi-kombu	1 g	Powder	2353 ± 65	1569%
Sea weed[1]	Nori	1 g	Sheet	16 ± 2	11%
Sea weed[1]	Oarweed	1 g		1862 ± 520	1241%
Sea weed[1]	Paddle weed	1 g		2123 ± 352	1415%
Sea weed[1]	Sea palm	1 g		871 ± 231	581%
Sea weed[1]	Wakame	1 g		32-431	21-287%
Selenum[3]		1 tablet	Tablet	215	143%
Shrimp[2]		3 oz		35	23%

Iodine Contents from Various Natural Sources

Iodine Sources	Descriptions	Quantity	Dose Form	Iodine Contents (mcg)	Percent of Daily Recommended Value
Tuna[2]	Canned in oil	3 oz		17	11%
Yogurt[2]		1 cup		75	50%

References:

1. Teas J, Pino S, Critchley A, Braverman LE. Variability of iodine content in common commercially available edible seaweeds. Thyroid. 2004 Oct; 14(10): 836-41
2. Iodine: Dietary Supplement Fact Sheet. National Institutes of Health, Office of Dietary Supplements. Updated 4/18/2011. Accessed 5/27/2011
3. Arum SM, He X, Braverman LE. Excess iodine from an unexpected source. N Engl J Med. 2009 Jan 22; 360(4): 424-6

Environmental Pollutants And Toxins

Bisphenol A (Bpa)	**DESCRIPTION:** Bisphenol A is a chemical used in the manufacture of polycarbonate plastics. It is used in the production of water bottles, baby bottles, plastic wraps and food packaging. A significant amount of BPA was detected in liquid from canned vegetables that are exposed to high temperature during autoclaving and in saliva of dental patients fitted with restorative materials. The major source of exposure to humans is by oral route. Bisphenol A exposure is of concern due to its endocrine effects in humans.
	COMMENTS IN LACTATION: LRC – L3 Overall, even after high oral exposure to BPA, the serum levels of BPA are below levels of detection. Any BPA exposure is rapidly metabolized and cleared within 6 hours in the urine without any significant systemic accumulation. Therefore, negligible transfer into breastmilk and minimal lactational exposure to BPA is expected. However, since metabolic pathways are immature in babies, some concern does exist, especially in those 0-4 months of age. An infant would be exposed to more BPA from baby foods and baby formulas, than from breastmilk. Exclusive breastfeeding for at least first 4 months, without introduction of baby foods or formulas should minimize most exposure. The possible long-term endocrine and estrogenic effects associated with early BPA exposure while in utero or during lactation are not really known. However, due to some risk of behavioral and brain development, it is advised that use of BPA-containing plastic baby bottles and plastic products be avoided, and glass products be preferably used wherever possible.
Fragrant Musks	**DESCRIPTION:** Synthetic fragrant musks are found in many consumer products such as perfumes, deodorants, cosmetics, shampoos, soaps and detergents, to promote the fragrance of the product. Perfumes are widely used by women worldwide. The four most commonly used musk compounds are musk xylene, musk ketone, HHCB and AHTN. However, many different forms of musk compounds are present in commercial products. Musk compounds tend to accumulate in body fat as well as in milk fat.
	COMMENTS IN LACTATION: LRC – L1 Only a few studies have been conducted concerning the concentrations of musk compounds in breastmilk. In these studies, musk compounds have been detected in human milk in varying concentrations, with the mean concentrations of HHCB in breastmilk being the highest, as compared to the other musk compounds. While detectable, the daily dose of the musk compounds provided to the infant via breastmilk was found to be very low and probably insignificant clinically. Greater exposure to synthetic musks occurs by inhalational or dermal route. Exposure via breastmilk was found to be insignificant. The dose available to the infant via breastmilk was found to be 1-2 orders below the set tolerable daily intake values.

Environmental Pollutants And Toxins

JET FUELS

DESCRIPTION: Jet fuels contain a mixture of a large number of hydrocarbons. There are 2 types of jet fuels – kerosene-containing, and naphtha-containing fuels. The kerosene type is used more commonly for commercial aviation. The naphtha-type is used for extreme weather conditions because of its cold-weather endurance. The kerosene type jet fuels include Jet A, Jet A1, JP5 and JP8. The naphtha-type includes Jet B, JP4.

COMMENTS IN LACTATION: LRC – L3
Skin and oral exposure to jet fuels have been found to be of relatively low toxicity, but high inhalational exposure to jet fuels is expected. Although, reproductive, renal, neurological and immunological effects have been postulated with exposure to jet fuels, these effects have not been confirmed. Occupational exposure among aircraft personnel has also been found to be generally low. There are no studies currently of jet fuel exposure in lactating women. It is however prudent to wear all protective gear, including gloves and respirators to avoid exposure. Operations such as entering fuel tanks and repairing leaks are associated with high levels of exposure, and should preferably be avoided by breastfeeding women. The level of air pollution caused following combustion of jet fuels is no different from that found in highly urbanized areas.

Symptoms of acute exposure would include: CNS depression, headache, dizziness, respiratory irritation and cardiac palpitations or dysrhythmias. Mothers with these symptoms should pump and discard their milk for 24 hours.

Environmental Pollutants And Toxins

MOLD	**DESCRIPTION:** Molds are considered fungi. Molds can be found almost anywhere and they can grow on virtually any organic substance, as long as moisture and oxygen are present. Molds contaminate foods that have been stored in dark, unventilated humid conditions. When excessive moisture accumulates in buildings or on building materials, mold growth can occur. Molds release various mycotoxins and spores which cause health effects in humans on exposure. Humans are exposed to mycotoxins and mold spores by ingesting them in contaminated foods, or by inhalation or by skin contact with mold growing on building surfaces. Mytotoxins are carcinogenic and have been known to cause hepatocellular cancer (liver cancer) as well as renal failure and glomerulonephritis. Inhalational exposure to mycotoxins may cause significant complications such as respiratory allergies, lung inflammatory conditions, asthma, neurotoxicity. In infants, exposure to indoor molds may cause pulmonary hemorrhage. Due to the many toxic effects of mold exposure, and because mold causes pulmonary hemorrhage in infants, concerns have been raised of the effects of its exposure in breastmilk.
	COMMENTS IN LACTATION: LRC – L2 Although mycotoxins released from molds have been found in breastmilk, the exposure of infants to molds in breastmilk has not been associated with untoward effects in the breastfed infant. The effects of exposure to long-term, high doses of mycotoxins in breastmilk are yet to be determined. However, current data suggests that lactational exposure to molds does not warrant cessation of breastfeeding, nor does it warrant interruption of the breastfeeding period. In fact, early weaning could increase mycotoxin exposure due to introduction of various weaning foods, and therefore is not recommended. The presence of mycotoxins in breastmilk does not alter its nutritional value. Current data does not suggest any changes in the general breastfeeding recommendations. However, it is prudent to control indoor mold growth since inhalational exposure to mold causes pulmonary hemorrhage in infants. Repair any sources of moisture in the house such as leaks in the plumbing system or obstruction in the ventilation ducts. Maintain low indoor humidity and discard mold-contaminated furnishings.

Environmental Pollutants And Toxins

OXYBENZONE	**DESCRIPTION**: Oxybenzone is a chemical found in many sunscreens. This organic compound has been shown to penetrate into the skin where it acts as a photosensitizer. This results in an increased production of free radicals under illumination, possibly making this substance a photocarcinogen. Studies in human subjects have shown that even after 24 hours of exposure, the concentration of sunscreens found in human epidermis was found to be 5-fold lower than the dose known to cause toxicity in in-vitro studies. Although about 97% of Americans have the compound in their urine, current exposure limits are deemed safe.
	COMMENTS IN LACTATION: LRC – L1 The skin penetration of oxybenzone following topical application of sunscreens containing this chemical is found to be minimal. Therefore minimal transfer to milk is expected, if any.
PARABENS	**DESCRIPTION**: Parabens are synthetic preservatives commonly used in food and in cosmetics such as moisturizers, hair care and shaving products. Parabens belong to a group of chemicals called p-hydroxybenzoic acid esters and includes different parabens, but the most commonly used are methylparaben, ethylparaben, n-propylparaben and n-butylparaben. When administered either orally or applied topically, the parabens are metabolized to form p-hydroxybenzoic acid, which has weak estrogenic activity: and therefore, may produce endocrine effects in individuals exposed to high levels of these chemicals.
	COMMENTS IN LACTATION: LRC – L1 The margin of safety of parabens present in commercially available products is very high. Parabens are rapidly absorbed, metabolized and excreted in the urine. Parabens do not accumulate in the body. Several studies in animals have not confirmed mutagenicity and carcinogenicity of parabens. Potency of methyl, ethyl, propyl and butylparaben is 1000 times less than natural estradiol. Therefore, negligible exposure to parabens through breastmilk is expected. Even if exposure occurs, only limited endocrine activity in the infant would be expected.

Environmental Pollutants And Toxins

PERCHLORATE	**DESCRIPTION:** Ammonium perchlorate is a primary ingredient in rocket fuels. It is also an essential component of military explosives, bottle rockets, fireworks, highway flares, automobile airbags and old-fashioned black powder. Perchlorate is also present in bleach and fertilizers. Workers working at perchlorate production plants are exposed to high levels of perchlorate on a regular basis. Workplace exposure most commonly occurs by inhalational route and contact. Community exposure is mainly by ingestion in the diet. Perchlorate exposure has raised concerns due to its effects on thyroid function. High doses of perchlorate can block iodide uptake in the thyroid and could cause iodine deficiency and hypothyroidism. This especially raises concerns in exclusively breastfed infants who depend solely on breastmilk for their daily iodine requirement. Perchlorate exposure is highest in the younger age groups, because higher perchlorate consumption per kilogram body weight occurs in this population group.
	COMMENTS IN LACTATION: LRC – L3 Although perchlorate has been detected in several breastmilk samples, sometimes in high concentrations, there are no data to establish that lactational exposure to perchlorate causes thyroid disruption in the infant. Further, perchlorate is less likely to have untoward effects if the iodine content of breastmilk is adequate, which in turn depends on the iodine status of the mother. Therefore, consumption of foods rich in iodine, and modest iodine-supplementation is recommended in lactating women, particularly those exposed to perchlorates. Five to nine servings of fruits and vegetables is recommended by the CDC. This is especially important in mothers of premature and newborn infants. The risk declines as age advances. No perchlorate has been detected in bottled water and treatment by reverse osmosis removes 80% of perchlorate from drinking water. Therefore, although tap water has not been found to be a significant source of perchlorate, bottled water or water treated by reverse osmosis may be preferred in breastfeeding women. Women exposed to high levels of perchlorate at their workplace are likely to have high perchlorate levels in their milk. But perchlorate has a short half-life of 8 hours, it is unlikely that breastfeeding could pose a source of continuous exposure to the infant. In a study done on workers exposed to high perchlorate for 2-6 years, no thyroid function disruption was observed suggesting that long-term, intermittent high exposure to perchlorate does not have significant effects on thyroid function. However, to minimize exposure, workers are encouraged to avoid inhalation or contact with perchlorate by using protective garments, face masks, respirators and gloves.

Environmental Pollutants And Toxins

PERFLUORO-OCTANOIC ACID (PFOA)	**DESCRIPTION**: PFOA belongs to a group of chemicals called perfluorinated compounds (PFCs). PFOA is a component of Teflon nonstick coatings. This chemical is found in tap water, nonstick pots and pans. PFOA may cause hormonal disruption and reproductive abnormalities following excessive and repeated exposure. Exposure has been associated with hypercholesterolemia and hyperuricemia, and recently higher serum levels of PFOA were found to be associated with increased risk of chronic kidney disease.
	COMMENTS IN LACTATION: LRC – L3 Although overall PFCs have been detected in breastmilk, PFOA has only rarely been detected in milk. When detected, the levels have almost always been below recommended acceptable daily intake (ADI) levels. However, the occupation and geographical location of the breastfeeding mother also influences PFC levels in milk, with the highest levels occurring in chemical plant employees and surrounding subpopulations. Comparatively higher levels of PFCs and PFOA have been detected in breastmilk of Japanese women. But even in these women, the PFC and PFOA concentrations in breastmilk rarely exceeded ADI. While efforts are underway to curb the use of PFOA, avoiding heating empty Teflon cookware to high temperatures can help minimize some exposure.

Environmental Pollutants And Toxins

PERSISTENT ORGANIC POLLUTANTS (POPS)	**DESCRIPTION:** Polychlorinated biphenyls (PCBs), dioxins, polybrominated biphenyl ethers (PBDEs), furans and other organochlorines and organobromines are together grouped as persistent organic pollutants (POPs). These have become ubiquitous in our environment and have become a part of our food chain. Exposure to POPs is unavoidable. PCBs/dioxins have been known to cause endocrine disruption. PBDEs have been known to decrease fertility. When ingested by lactating women, POPs may accumulate in the milk fat, exposing infants to these potentially hazardous chemicals. Further, the gastrointestinal absorption of POPs in nursing infants is 95-100%.
	COMMENTS IN LACTATION: LRC – L3 Although POPs have been consistently detected in breastmilk, its effects on breastfed infants are not established. In fact, inspite of high PCB/dioxin exposure in breastmilk, breastfeeding has been found to be beneficial in the improvement of cognition and fluency of movements in breastfed infants. Based on currently published data, the ill-effects of exposure to POPs through breastmilk does not override the numerous benefits of breastfeeding, and therefore, no changes are made in the current breastfeeding recommendations. Since POPs mainly accumulate in milk fat, some authorities advise pumping and dumping of breastmilk during the early lactational period. However, these claims have also been refuted by a study that suggested that in spite of changes in concentration of milk fat over the period of lactation, no significant alterations were observed in the concentration of the POPs in breastmilk. Women exposed to these chemicals at work are advised to minimize exposure by using protective gear, including gloves and respirators. Community exposure is mostly by ingestion of meats and fatty fish. Since these chemicals accumulate in the fatty tissues, consumption of lean meats reduces exposure. A vegetarian diet is considered safer than a non-vegetarian diet. Lastly, it is important to understand, that most environmental pollutants, and particularly POPs transfer significantly during pregnancy, and far less during breastfeeding. So in breastfeeding mothers, the infant will receive the largest exposure during pregnancy, not breastfeeding.

BISPHENOL A (BPA)

1 A.V. Krishnan, P. Stathis, S.F. Permuth, L. Tokes, D. Feldman Bisphenol A: an estrogenic substance is released from polycarbonate flasks during autoclaving. Endocrinology, 132 (1993), pp. 2279–2286

2 N. Olea, R. Pulgar, P. Perez, F. Olea-Serrano, A. Novillo-Fertrell, V. Pedraza, A.M. Soto, C. Sonnenschein. Estrogenicity of resin-based composites and sealants used in dentistry. Environ. Health Perspect., 104 (1996), pp. 298–305

3 Kunz N, Camm EJ, Somm E, Lodygensky G, Darbre S, Aubert ML, Hüppi PS, Sizonenko SV, Gruetter R. Developmental and metabolic brain alterations in rats exposed to bisphenol A during gestation and lactation. Int J Dev Neurosci. 2011 Feb;29(1):37-43.

4 Tsutsumi O. Assessment of human contamination of estrogenic endocrine-disrupting chemicals and their risk for human reproduction. J Steroid Biochem Mol Biol. 2005 Feb;93(2-5):325-30.

5 Hanioka N, Naito T, Narimatsu S. Human UDP-glucuronosyltransferase isoforms involved in bisphenol A glucuronidation. Chemosphere. 2008 Dec;74(1):33-6.

6   Trdan Lušin T, Roškar R, Mrhar A. Evaluation of bisphenol A glucuronidation according to UGT1A1*28 polymorphism by a new LC-MS/MS assay. Toxicology. 2012 Feb 6;292(1):33-41.

7   Teeguarden JG, Calafat AM, Ye X, Doerge DR, Churchwell MI, Gunawan R, Graham MK. Twenty-four hour human urine and serum profiles of bisphenol a during high-dietary exposure. Toxicol Sci. 2011 Sep;123(1):48-57.

8   Völkel W, Colnot T, Csanády GA, Filser JG, Dekant W. Metabolism and kinetics of bisphenol a in humans at low doses following oral administration. Chem Res Toxicol. 2002 Oct;15(10):1281-7.

9   Pandelova M, Piccinelli R, Lopez WL, Henkelmann B, Molina-Molina JM, Arrebola JP, Olea N, Leclercq C, Schramm KW. Assessment of PCDD/F, PCB, OCP and BPA dietary exposure of non-breast-fed European infants. Food Addit Contam Part A Chem Anal Control Expo Risk Assess. 2011 Aug;28(8):1110-22.

FRAGRANT MUSKS

1   G.G. Rimkus, M. Wolf Polycyclic musk fragrances in human adipose tissue and human milk Chemosphere, 33 (1996), pp. 2033–2043

2   Zhang X, Liang G, Zeng X, Zhou J, Sheng G, Ful J. Levels of synthetic musk fragrances in human milk from three cities in the Yangtze River Delta in Eastern China. J Environ Sci (China). 2011;23(6):983-90.

3   Reiner JL, Wong CM, Arcaro KF, Kannan K. Synthetic musk fragrances in human milk from the United States. Environ Sci Technol. 2007 Jun 1;41(11):3815-20.

4   Yin J, Wang H, Zhang J, Zhou N, Gao F, Wu Y, Xiang J, Shao B. The occurrence of synthetic musks in human breast milk in Sichuan, China. Chemosphere. 2011 Dec 21.

JET FUELS

1   NRC. 2003. Toxicologic Assessment of Jet-Propulsion Fuel 8. National Research Council, National Academy of Sciences, Washington, DC.

2   L.R. Kaufman, G.K. Lemasters, D.M. Olsen, P. Succop Effects of concurrent noise and jet fuel exposure on hearing loss. J. Occup. Environ. Med., 47 (2005), pp. 212–218

3   Mattie DR, Sterner TR. Past, present and emerging toxicity issues for jet fuel. Toxicol Appl Pharmacol. 2011 Jul 15;254(2):127-32.

4   McDougal JN, Rogers JV. Local and systemic toxicity of JP-8 from cutaneous exposures. Toxicol Lett. 2004 Apr 1;149(1-3):301-8.

5   Peden-Adam MM, Eudaly J, Eudaly E, Dudley A, Zeigler J, Lee A, Robbs J, Gilkeson G, Keil DE. Evaluation of immunotoxicity induced by single or concurrent exposure to N,N-diethyl-m-toluamide (DEET), pyridostigmine bromide (PYR), and JP-8 jet fuel. Toxicol Ind Health. 2001 Jun;17(5-10):192-209.

6   Neely, W.B., 1994. Introduction to Chemical Exposure and Risk Assessment. CRC Press, Boca Raton, FL

7   Subcommittee on Jet-Propulsion 8 fuel of Committee on Toxicology, 2003. NRC Toxicologic Assessment of Jet-Propulsion Fuel, vol. 8. The National Academics Press, Washington, DC.

8   G.K. LeMasters, D.M. Olsen, J.H. Yiin, J.E. Lockey, R. Shukla, S.G. Selevan, S.M. Schrader, G.P. Toth, D.P. Evenson, G.B. Huszar. Male reproductive effects of solvent and fuel exposure during aircraft maintenance. Reprod. Toxicol., 13 (1999), pp. 155–166

9   Ritchie G, Still K, Rossi J 3rd, Bekkedal M, Bobb A, Arfsten D. Biological and health effects of exposure to kerosene-based jet fuels and performance additives. J Toxicol Environ Health B Crit Rev. 2003 Jul-Aug;6(4):357-451.

10   Smith KW, Proctor SP, Ozonoff AL, McClean MD. Urinary biomarkers of occupational jet fuel exposure among air force personnel. J Expo Sci Environ Epidemiol. 2012 Jan-Feb;22(1):35-45.

11   MacDonald RD, Thomas L, Rusk FC, Marques SD, McGuire D. Occupational health and safety assessment of exposure to jet fuel combustion products in air medical transport. Prehosp Emerg Care. 2010 Apr 6;14(2):202-8.

12   Reutman SR, LeMasters GK, Knecht EA, Shukla R, Lockey JE, Burroughs GE, Kesner JS. Evidence of reproductive endocrine effects in women with occupational fuel and solvent exposures. Environ Health Perspect. 2002 Aug;110(8):805-11.

13   Tesseraux I. Risk factors of jet fuel combustion products. Toxicol Lett. 2004 Apr 1;149(1-3):295-300.

MOLDS

1   Hifnawy MS, Mangoud AM, Eissa MH, Nor Edin E, Mostafa Y, Abouel-Magd Y, Sabee EI, Amin I, Ismail A, Morsy TA, Mahrous S, Afefy AF, el-Shorbagy E, el-Sa- dawy M, Ragab H, Hassan MI, el-

Hady G, Saber M (2004) The role of aflatoxin-contaminated food materials and HCV in developing hepatocellular carcinoma in Al-Sharkia Governorate, Egypt. J Egypt Soc Parasitol 34(Suppl 1):479–488

2   Hope JH, Hope BE. A review of the diagnosis and treatment of Ochratoxin A inhalational exposure associated with human illness and kidney disease including focal segmental glomerulosclerosis. J Environ Public Health. 2012;2012:835059.

3   Gürbay A, Girgin G, Sabuncuoğlu SA, Sahin G, Yurdakök M, Yigit S, Tekinalp G. Ochratoxin A: is it present in breast milk samples obtained from mothers from Ankara, Turkey? J Appl Toxicol. 2010 May;30(4):329-33.

4   Galvano F, Pietri A, Bertuzzi T, Gagliardi L, Ciotti S, Luisi S, Bognanno M, La Fauci L, Iacopino AM, Nigro F, Li Volti G, Vanella L, Giammanco G, Tina GL, Gazzolo D. Maternal dietary habits and mycotoxin occurrence in human mature milk. Mol Nutr Food Res. 2008 Apr;52(4):496-501.

5   Gürbay A, Sabuncuoğlu SA, Girgin G, Sahin G, Yiğit S, Yurdakök M, Tekinalp G. Exposure of newborns to aflatoxin M1 and B1 from mothers' breast milk in Ankara, Turkey. Food Chem Toxicol. 2010 Jan;48(1):314-9.

6   Keskin Y, Başkaya R, Karsli S, Yurdun T, Ozyaral O. Detection of aflatoxin M1 in human breast milk and raw cow's milk in Istanbul, Turkey. J Food Prot. 2009 Apr;72(4):885-9.

7   Polychronaki N, West RM, Turner PC, Amra H, Abdel-Wahhab M, Mykkänen H, El-Nezami H. A longitudinal assessment of aflatoxin M1 excretion in breast milk of selected Egyptian mothers. Food Chem Toxicol. 2007 Jul;45(7):1210-5.

8   Hassan AM, Sheashaa HA, Abdel Fatah MF, Ibrahim AZ, Gaber OA. Does aflatoxin as an environmental mycotoxin adversely affect the renal and hepatic functions of Egyptian lactating mothers and their infants? A preliminary report. Int Urol Nephrol. 2006;38(2):339-42.

9   Abdulrazzaq YM, Osman N, Yousif ZM, Al-Falahi S. Aflatoxin M1 in breast-milk of UAE women. Ann Trop Paediatr. 2003 Sep;23(3):173-9.

10   Zarba A, Wild CP, Hall AJ, Montesano R, Hudson GJ, Groopman JD. Aflatoxin M1in human breast milk from The Gambia, west Africa, quantified by combined monoclonal antibody immunoaffinity chromatography and HPLC. Carcinogenesis. 1992 May;13(5):891-4.

OYBENZONE

1   Hanson Kerry M.; Gratton Enrico; Bardeen Christopher J. (2006). "Sunscreen enhancement of UV-induced reactive oxygen species in the skin". Free Radical Biology and Medicine 41 (8): 1205–1212.

2   Xu C, Parsons PG. Cell cycle delay, mitochondrial stress and uptake of hydrophobic cations induced by sunscreens in cultured human cells. Photochem Photobiol. 1999 May;69(5):611-6.

3   Hayden, CG; Cross, SE; Anderson, C; Saunders, NA; Roberts, MS (20 May 2005). "Sunscreen penetration of human skin and related keratinocyte toxicity after topical application". Skin Pharmacol Physiol. Therapeutics Research Unit, University of Queensland, Southern Clinical School, University of Queensland, Princess Alexandra Hospital, Brisbane, Australia. Retrieved 16 May 2010.

4   Antonia M. Calafat, Lee-Yang Wong, Xiaoyun Ye, John A. Reidy, and Larry L. Needham (2008). "Concentrations of the Sunscreen Agent Benzophenone-3 in Residents of the United States: National Health and Nutrition Examination Survey 2003–2004" (in press). Environmental Health Perspectives 116 (7): 893–7.

PARABENS

1   S. Oishi Effects of butylparaben on the male reproductive system in rats Toxicol Ind Health, 17 (1) (2001), pp. 31–39

2   S. Oishi Effects of propyl paraben on the male reproductive system Food Chem Toxicol, 40 (12) (2002), pp. 1807-1813

3   Boberg J, Taxvig C, Christiansen S, Hass U. Possible endocrine disrupting effects of parabens and their metabolites. Reprod Toxicol. 2010 Sep;30(2):301-12.

4   Routledge EJ, Parker J, Odum J, Ashby J, Sumpter JP. Some alkyl hydroxy benzoate preservatives (parabens) are estrogenic. Toxicol Appl Pharmacol. 1998 Nov;153(1):12-9.

5   Final amended report on the safety assessment of Methylparaben, Ethylparaben, Propylparaben, Isopropylparaben, Butylparaben, Isobutylparaben, and Benzylparaben as used in cosmetic products. Int J Toxicol. 2008;27 Suppl 4:1-82.

6   Janjua NR, Mortensen GK, Andersson AM, Kongshoj B, Skakkebaek NE, Wulf HC. Systemic uptake of diethyl phthalate, dibutyl phthalate, and butyl paraben following whole-body topical application and reproductive and thyroid hormone levels in humans. Environ Sci Technol. 2007 Aug 1;41(15):5564-70.

PERCHLORATE

1   Greer, M. A.; Goodman, G.; Pleus, R. C.; Greer, S. E. Health effects assessment for environmental perchlorate contamination: The dose response for inhibition of thyroidal radioiodine uptake in humans. Environ. Health Perspect. 2002, 110, 927–37.

2   Valentín-Blasini L, Blount BC, Otero-Santos S, Cao Y, Bernbaum JC, Rogan WJ. Perchlorate exposure and dose estimates in infants. Environ Sci Technol. 2011 May1; 45(9): 4127-32. Epub 2011 Mar 30.

3   Dasgupta PK, Kirk AB, Dyke JV, Ohira S. Intake of iodine and perchlorate and excretion in human milk. Environ Sci Technol. 2008 Nov 1; 42(21): 8115-21.

4   Kirk AB, Dyke JV, Martin CF, Dasgupta PK. Temporal patterns in perchlorate, thiocyanate, and iodide excretion in human milk. Environ Health Perspect. 2007 Feb; 115(2): 182-6.

5   Pearce EN, Leung AM, Blount BC, Bazrafshan HR, He X, Pino S, Valentin-Blasini L, Braverman LE. Breast milk iodine and perchlorate concentrations in lactating Boston-area women. J Clin Endocrinol Metab. 2007 May; 92(5): 1673-7.

6   Baier-Anderson C, Blount BC, Lakind JS, Naiman DQ, Wilbur SB, Tan S. Estimates of exposures to perchlorate from consumption of human milk, dairy milk, and water, and comparison to current reference dose. J Toxicol Environ Health A. 2006 Feb; 69(3-4): 319-30.

7   Braverman LE, He X, Pino S, Cross M, Magnani B, Lamm SH, Kruse MB, Engel A, Crump KS, Gibbs JP. The effect of perchlorate, thiocyanate, and nitrate on thyroid function in workers exposed to perchlorate long-term. J Clin Endocrinol Metab. 2005 Feb; 90(2): 700-6.

PERFLUOROOCTANOIC ACID (PFOA)

1   Shankar, Anoop; Jie Xiao and Alan Ducatman (2011 Oct 15). "Perfluoroalkyl Chemicals and Chronic Kidney Disease in US Adults". American Journal of Epidemiology 174 (8): 893–900.

2   Kennedy GL, Butenhoff JL, Olsen GW, et al. (2004). "The toxicology of perfluorooctanoate". Crit. Rev. Toxicol. 34 (4): 351–84.

3   Bartell SM, Calafat AM, Lyu C, Kato K, Ryan PB, Steenland K (February 2010). "Rate of decline in serum PFOA concentrations after granular activated carbon filtration at two public water systems in Ohio and West Virginia". Environ. Health Perspect. 118 (2): 222–8.

4   Steenland K, Fletcher T, Savitz DA (2010). "Epidemiologic Evidence on the Health Effects of Perfluorooctanoic Acid (PFOA)". Environ. Health Perspect. 118 (8): 1100–8.

5   Brede E, Wilhelm M, Göen T, Müller J, Rauchfuss K, Kraft M, Hölzer J (June 2010). "Two-year follow-up biomonitoring pilot study of residents' and controls' PFC plasma levels after PFOA reduction in public water system in Arnsberg, Germany". Int J Hyg Environ Health 213 (3): 217–23.

6   Llorca M, Farré M, Picó Y, Teijón ML, Alvarez JG, Barceló D. Infant exposure of perfluorinated compounds: levels in breast milk and commercial baby food. Environ Int. 2010 Aug; 36(6): 584-92.

7   European Food Safety Authority (EFSA) Perfluorooctane sulfonate (PFOS), perfluorooctanoic acid (PFOA) and their salts J Eur Food Saf Auth, 653 (2008), pp. 1–31

8   Völkel W, Genzel-Boroviczény O, Demmelmair H, Gebauer C, Koletzko B, Twardella D, Raab U, Fromme H. Perfluorooctane sulphonate (PFOS) and perfluorooctanoic acid (PFOA) in human breast milk: results of a pilot study. Int J Hyg Environ Health. 2008 Jul; 211(3-4): 440-6.

9   Tao L, Kannan K, Wong CM, Arcaro KF, Butenhoff JL. Perfluorinated compounds in human milk from Massachusetts, U.S.A. Environ Sci Technol. 2008 Apr 15; 42(8): 3096-101.

10   Kärrman A, Ericson I, van Bavel B, Darnerud PO, Aune M, Glynn A, Lignell S,Lindström G. Exposure of perfluorinated chemicals through lactation: levels of matched human milk and serum and a temporal trend, 1996-2004, in Sweden. Environ Health Perspect. 2007 Feb; 115(2): 226-30

11   Kärrman A, Domingo JL, Llebaria X, Nadal M, Bigas E, van Bavel B, Lindström G. Biomonitoring perfluorinated compounds in Catalonia, Spain: concentrations and trends in human liver and milk samples. Environ Sci Pollut Res Int. 2010 Mar;17(3):750-8.

12   Tao L, Ma J, Kunisue T, Libelo EL, Tanabe S, Kannan K. Perfluorinated compounds in human breast milk from several Asian countries, and in infant formula and dairy milk from the United States. Environ Sci Technol. 2008 Nov 15; 42(22): 8597-602.

PERSISTENT ORGANIC POLLUTANTS

1   Longnecker MP, Rogan WJ, Lucier G. The human health effects of DDT (dichlorodiphenyltrichloroethane) and PCBs (polychlorinated biphenyls) and an overview of organochlorines in public health. Annual Review of Public Health. 1997; 18:211–244.

2   Seegal RF. Epidemiological and laboratory evidence of PCB-induced neurotoxicity. Critical Reviews in Toxicology. 1996; 26:709–737.

3   Hauser P, McMillin JM, Bhatara VS. Resistance to thyroid hormone: implications for neurodevelopmental research on the effects of thyroid hormone disruptors. Toxicology and Industrial Health. 1998; 14:85–101.

4   Hagmar L. Polychlorinated biphenyls and thyroid status in humans: a review. Thyroid. 2003;13:1021–1028.

5   Faroon OM, Keith S, Jones D, de Rosa C. Effects of polychlorinated biphenyls on development and reproduction. Toxicology and Industrial Health. 2001;17:63–93.

6   Harley, K.; Marks, A.; Chevrier, J.; Bradman, A.; Sjödin, A.; Eskenazi, B. (2010). "PBDE Concentrations in Women's Serum and Fecundability.". Environmental health perspectives 118 (5): 699–704.

7   Identifying PCB-Containing Capacitors. Australian and New Zealand Environment and Conservation Council (ANZECC). 1997. pp. 4–5. ISBN 0-642-54507-3. Retrieved 2007-07-07.

8   Uemura H, Arisawa K, Hiyoshi M, Satoh H, Sumiyoshi Y, Morinaga K, Kodama K, Suzuki T, Nagai M, Suzuki T. PCDDs/PCDFs and dioxin-like PCBs: recent body burden levels and their determinants among general inhabitants in Japan. Chemosphere. 2008 Aug; 73(1): 30-7.

9   Dahl P, Lindström G, Wiberg K, Rappe C. Absorption of polychlorinated biphenyls, dibenzo-p-dioxins and dibenzofurans by breast-fed infants. Chemosphere. 1995 Jun; 30(12): 2297-306.

10   Tsukimori K, Uchi H, Mitoma C, Yasukawa F, Fukushima K, Todaka T, Kajiwara J, Yoshimura T, Hirata T, Wake N, Furue M. Comparison of the concentrations of polychlorinated biphenyls and dioxins in mothers affected by the Yusho incident and their children. Chemosphere. 2011 Aug; 84(7): 928-35.

11   Tai PT, Nishijo M, Kido T, Nakagawa H, Maruzeni S, Naganuma R, Anh NT, Morikawa Y, Luong HV, Anh TH, Hung NN, Son le K, Tawara K, Nishijo H. Dioxin concentrations in breast milk of Vietnamese nursing mothers: a survey four decades after the herbicide spraying. Environ Sci Technol. 2011 Aug 1; 45(15): 6625-32.

12   Chovancová J, Čonka K, Kočan A, Sejáková ZS. PCDD, PCDF, PCB and PBDE concentrations in breast milk of mothers residing in selected areas of Slovakia. Chemosphere. 2011 May; 83(10): 1383-90.

13   Uemura H, Arisawa K, Hiyoshi M, Satoh H, Sumiyoshi Y, Morinaga K, Kodama K, Suzuki T, Nagai M, Suzuki T. PCDDs/PCDFs and dioxin-like PCBs: recent body burden levels and their determinants among general inhabitants in Japan. Chemosphere. 2008 Aug; 73(1): 30-7.

14   Yang J, Shin D, Park S, Chang Y, Kim D, Ikonomou MG. PCDDs, PCDFs, and PCBs concentrations in breast milk from two areas in Korea: body burden of mothers and implications for feeding infants. Chemosphere. 2002 Jan; 46(3): 419-28.

15   Tue NM, Sudaryanto A, Minh TB, Isobe T, Takahashi S, Viet PH, Tanabe S. Accumulation of polychlorinated biphenyls and brominated flame retardants in breast milk from women living in Vietnamese e-waste recycling sites. Sci Total Environ. 2010 Apr 1; 408(9): 2155-62.

16   Daniels JL, Pan IJ, Jones R, Anderson S, Patterson DG Jr, Needham LL, Sjödin A. Individual characteristics associated with PBDE levels in U.S. human milk samples. Environ Health Perspect. 2010 Jan; 118(1): 155-60.

17   Toms LM, Harden F, Paepke O, Hobson P, Ryan JJ, Mueller JF. Higher accumulation of polybrominated diphenyl ethers in infants than in adults. Environ Sci Technol. 2008 Oct 1; 42(19): 7510-5.

18   Schecter A, Pavuk M, Päpke O, Ryan JJ, Birnbaum L, Rosen R. Polybrominated diphenyl ethers (PBDEs) in U.S. mothers' milk. Environ Health Perspect. 2003 Nov; 111(14): 1723-9.

19   Toms LM, Hearn L, Kennedy K, Harden F, Bartkow M, Temme C, Mueller JF. Concentrations of polybrominated diphenyl ethers (PBDEs) in matched samples of human milk, dust and indoor air. Environ Int. 2009 Aug; 35(6): 864-9.

20   Pan IJ, Daniels JL, Herring AH, Rogan WJ, Siega-Riz AM, Goldman BD, Sjödin A. Lactational exposure to polychlorinated biphenyls, dichlorodiphenyltrichloroethane, and dichlorodiphenyldichloroethylene and infant growth: an analysis of the Pregnancy, Infection, and Nutrition Babies Study. Paediatr Perinat Epidemiol. 2010 May; 24(3): 262-71.

21   Pan IJ, Daniels JL, Goldman BD, Herring AH, Siega-Riz AM, Rogan WJ. Lactational exposure to polychlorinated biphenyls, dichlorodiphenyltrichloroethane, and dichlorodiphenyldichloroethylene and infant neurodevelopment: an analysis of the pregnancy, infection, and nutrition babies study. Environ Health Perspect. 2009 Mar; 117(3): 488-94.

22   Gladen BC, Ragan NB, Rogan WJ. Pubertal growth and development and prenatal and lactational exposure to polychlorinated biphenyls and dichlorodiphenyl dichloroethene. J Pediatr. 2000 Apr; 136(4): 490-6.

23   Lanting CI, Patandin S, Fidler V, Weisglas-Kuperus N, Sauer PJ, Boersma ER, Touwen BC. Neurological condition in 42-month-old children in relation to pre- and postnatal exposure to

polychlorinated biphenyls and dioxins. Early Hum Dev.1998 Feb 27; 50(3): 283-92.

24   Koopman-Esseboom C, Weisglas-Kuperus N, de Ridder MA, Van der Paauw CG, Tuinstra LG,
      Sauer PJ. Effects of polychlorinated biphenyl/dioxin exposure and feeding type on infants' mental
      and psychomotor development. Pediatrics. 1996 May; 97(5): 700-6.

25   Patandin S, Weisglas-Kuperus N, de Ridder MA, Koopman-Esseboom C, van Staveren WA, van
      der Paauw CG, Sauer PJ. Plasma polychlorinated biphenyl levels in Dutch preschool children either
      breast-fed or formula-fed during infancy. Am J Public Health. 1997 Oct; 87(10): 1711-4.

26   Kreuzer PE, Csanády GA, Baur C, et al. 2,3,7,8-Tetra- chlorodibenzo-p-dioxin (TCDD) and
      congeners in infants. A toxicokinetic model of human lifetime body burden by TCDD with special
      emphasis on its uptake by nutrition. Arch Toxicol 1997;71:383–400.

27   LaKind JS, Berlin CM, Park CN, et al. Methodology for characterizing distributions of incremental
      body burdens of 2,3,7,8-TCDD and DDE from breast milk in North American nursing infants. J
      Toxicol Environ Health A 2000;59:605–639.

28   Lorber M, Phillips L. Infant exposure to dioxin-like com- pounds in breast milk. Environ Health
      Perspect 2002;110: A325–A332.

29   Hsu JF, Guo YL, Liu CH, Hu SC, Wang JN, Liao PC. A comparison of PCDD/PCDFs exposure in
      infants via formula milk or breast milk feeding. Chemosphere. 2007 Jan; 66(2): 311-9.

30   Johnson-Restrepo B, Kannan K. An assessment of sources and pathways of human exposure to
      polybrominated diphenyl ethers in the United States. Chemosphere. 2009 Jul;76(4):542-8.

31   Weisglas-Kuperus N, Sas TC, Koopman-Esseboom C, van der Zwan CW, De Ridder MA,
      Beishuizen A, Hooijkaas H, Sauer PJ. Immunologic effects of background prenatal and
      postnatal exposure to dioxins and polychlorinated biphenyls in Dutch infants. Pediatr Res. 1995
      Sep;38(3):404-10.

32   Kaneko H, Matsui E, Shinoda S, Kawamoto N, Nakamura Y, Uehara R, Matsuura N, Morita M,
      Tada H, Kondo N. Effects of dioxins on the quantitative levels of immune components in infants.
      Toxicol Ind Health. 2006 Apr;22(3):131-6.

33   Giacomini SM, Hou L, Bertazzi PA, Baccarelli A. Dioxin effects on neonatal and infant thyroid
      function: routes of perinatal exposure, mechanisms of action and evidence from epidemiology
      studies. Int Arch Occup Environ Health. 2006 May;79(5):396-404.

34   Matsuura N, Uchiyama T, Tada H, Nakamura Y, Kondo N, Morita M, Fukushi M. Effects of
      dioxins and polychlorinated biphenyls (PCBs) on thyroid function in infants born in Japan--the
      second report from research on environmental health. Chemosphere. 2001 Dec;45(8):1167-71.

35   Boersma ER, Lanting CI. Environmental exposure to polychlorinated biphenyls (PCBs) and dioxins.
      Consequences for longterm neurological and cognitive development of the child lactation. Adv Exp
      Med Biol. 2000;478:271-87.

36   Huisman M, Koopman-Esseboom C, Lanting CI, van der Paauw CG, Tuinstra LG, Fidler V,
      Weisglas-Kuperus N, Sauer PJ, Boersma ER, Touwen BC. Neurological condition in 18-month-old
      children perinatally exposed to polychlorinated biphenyls and dioxins. Early Hum Dev. 1995 Oct
      2;43(2):165-76.

37   LaKind JS, Berlin CM, Mattison DR. The heart of the matter on breastmilk and environmental chemicals: essential points for healthcare providers and new parents. Breastfeed Med. 2008 Dec;3(4):251-9.

38   LaKind JS, Berlin CM Jr, Sjödin A, Turner W, Wang RY, Needham LL, Paul IM, Stokes JL, Naiman DQ, Patterson DG Jr. Do human milk concentrations of persistent organic chemicals really decline during lactation? Chemical concentrations during lactation and milk/serum partitioning. Environ Health Perspect. 2009 Oct;117(10):1625-31.

39   Hergenrather J, Hlady G, Wallace B, Savage E. Pollutants in breast milk of vegetarians. N Engl J Med. 1981 Mar 26;304(13):792.

Foul Tasting Drugs That Might Alter The Taste Of Milk

Common Foul Tasting Drugs	Trade Names
Acyclovir	Aciclover, Acyclo-V, Apo-Acyclovir, Aviraz, Lipsovir, Zovirax, Zyclir
Amlodipine	Istin, Norvasc
Azelastine	Astelin, Astepro, Azep, Optilast, Optivar, Rhinolast
Azithromycin	Zithromax
Captopril	Acenorm, Acepril, Apo-Capto, Capoten, Enzace, Novo-Captopril
Cetrizine	
Cholecalciferol	
Ciprofloxacin	Ciloxan, Cipro, Ciproxin
Clarithromycin	Biaxin, Klacid, Klaricid
Clindamycin	Cleocin Phosphate IV, Cleocin HCL
Clomipramine	Anafranil, Apo-Clomipramine, Placil
Cod Liver Oil	
Cromolyn Sodium	Cromese, Gastrocrom, Intal, Nalcrom, Nasalcrom, Opticrom, Rhynacrom, Rynacrom, Vistacrom
Desipramine	Norpramin, Novo-Desipramine, Pertofran, Pertofrane
Dextromethorphan	Babee Cof Syrup, Benylin Pediatric Formula, Creomulsion, Dexalone, Hold DM, Pediacare, Robitussin, Vicks 44 Cough Relief
Didanosine	Videx
Diethylpropion	Dospan, Tenuate, Tepanil
Diltiazem	Adizem, Apo-Diltiaz, Apo-Diltiazem, Britiazim, Cardcal, Cardizem, Cardizem CD, Cardizem SR, Cartia XT, Coras, Dilacor-XR, Dilzem, Tildiem
Disulfiram	Antabuse
Donepezil	Aricept
Doxepin	Adapin, Deptran, Novo-Doxepin, Silenor, Sinequan, Triadapin
Doxycycline	Apo-Doxy, Doryx, Doxychel, Doxycin, Doxylar, Doxylin, Periostat, Vibra-Tabs, Vibramycin
Efavirenz	Atripla, Sustiva
Emedastine	
Enalapril	Amprace, Innovace, Renitec, Vasotec
Enoxacin	Comprecin, Enoxin, Penetrex
Erythromycin	Ceplac, E-Mycin, E-mycin, EES, EMU-V, Ery-Tab, Eryc, Erycen, Erythrocin, Erythromide, Ilosone, Ilotyc, Novo-Rythro, PCE
Famotidine- some brands	Pepcid

Foul Tasting Drugs That Might Alter The Taste Of Milk

COMMON FOUL TASTING DRUGS	TRADE NAMES
Flecainide	Tambocor
Hydrochlorothiazide	Amizide, Apo-Hydro, Direma, Diuchlor H, Dyazide, Esidrex, Esidrix, Hydrodiuril, Modizide, Novo-Hydrazide, Oretic, Tekturna HCT
Imipramine	Apo-Imipramine, Impril, Janimine, Melipramine, Novo-Pramine, Tofranil
Indinavir	Crixivan
Labetolol	Labrocol, Normodyne, Presolol, Trandate
Lamivudine	3TC, Epivir-HBV
Metronidazole	Apo-Metronidazole, Flagyl, Metizol, Metrocream, Metrolotion, Metrozine, NeoMetric, Noritate, Novo-Nidazol, Protostat, Rozex, Trikacide
Mexiletene	Mexitil, Novo-Mexiletine
Nedocromil	Mireze, Tilade
Oxypentifylline	
Penicillins	
Phentermine	Adipex-P, Duromine, Fastin, Ionamin, Ponderax caps, Zantryl
Potassium chloride preparations – Koachlor, KayCiel	
Potassium Iodide	SSKI
Prednisolone powder	Desonate, Prednisolone, Prednisone
Procainamide	Apo-Procainamide, Procan, Procan SR, Pronestyl
Propafenone	Arythmol, Rythmol
Propranolol	Cardinol, Deralin, Detensol, Inderal, Novo-Pranol
Ritonavir	Norvir
Saquinanir	Fortovase, Invirase
Stavudine	Zerit
Sulfamethoxazole + Trimethoprim	Apo-Sulfatrim, Bactrim, Cotrim, Duclor, Novo-Trimel, Novo-Trimox, Nu-Cotrimox, Resprim-Forte, Septra, Sulfatrim
Tinidazole	Fasigyn, Tindamax
Valacyclovir	Valaciclovir, Valtrex
Zidovudine	Combivir, Novo-Azt, Retrovir

Foul smelling/tasting drugs when introduced to an infant in breastmilk, may cause alteration in the taste of breastmilk and could possibly cause a 'breastfeeding strike' in an infant. Of the antibiotics, clindamycin and macrolides such as erythromycin, azithromycin and clarithromycin are found to taste poorly by most individuals. Wherever possible, these maybe substituted for cephalosporins, which are known to be more palatable.

OTC NAME	DRUGS	LRC
4-Way Fast Acting Nasal Decogestant Spray	Phenylephrine	L3
4-Way Metholated Nasal Decongestant Spray	Phenylephrine	L3
4-Way Nasal Reg	Phenylephrine	L3
666 Cold Preparation Venom	Dextromethorphan	L1
	Acetaminophen	L1
	Phenylephrine	L3
666 Cough Syr	Dextromethorphan	L1
	Acetaminophen	L1
	Phenylephrine	L3
666 Cough Syr	Dextromethorphan	L1
	Acetaminophen	L1
	Phenylephrine	L3
A200	Pyrethrum	L3
A-200 Lice Contr Spray	Pyrethrum	L3
A200 Shampoo	Pyrethrum	L3
Abreva Cold Sore/Fever Blister Treatment	Docosanol	L3
Abreva Pump Cold Sore/Fever Blister Treatment	Docosanol	L3
Absorbine Arthritis Strength	Capsaicin	L3
	Menthol	L3
Absorbine Gel	Menthol	L3
Absorbine Jr Deep Pain Relief Patches	Menthol	L3
Absorbine Jr Orig Lin	Menthol	L3
Absorbine Jr X/S Lin	Menthol	L3
Absorbine Jrrlon	Menthol	L3
Ace Pain Relieving Patch Clear	Methyl Salicylate	L3 (L5 In Viral Syndromes)
	Menthol	L3
	Camphor	L3
Ace Pain Relieving Patch Hygel	Methyl Salicylate	L3 (L5 In Viral Syndromes)
	Menthol	L3
	Camphor	L3
Acephen	Acetaminophen	L1
Aceta Gesic 325/ 30Mg Tab	Acetaminophen	L1
Acetamin 120 Mg Sup	Acetaminophen	L1
Acetamin 325 Mg Tab	Acetaminophen	L1
Acetamin Af 100 Mg/Ml	Acetaminophen	L1
Acetaminophen	Acetaminophen	L1
Acetaminophen 650 Mg Sup	Acetaminophen	L1
Acetic Ac Ds Glacia Liq	Acetic Acid	L3
Acetic Acid 5 % Sol	Acetic Acid	L3
Aches Pains W/Arnica Chewable Tabt	Herbal Supplement/Teas	L4
Acidophillus Cap	Probiotics	L3
Acne 10 Lotion	Benzoyl Peroxide	L2
Acne Lot 5	Benzoyl Peroxide	L2

OTC NAME	DRUGS	LRC
Acne Medicat 10 % Gel	Benzoyl Peroxide	L2
Acnefree Kit Liq	Benzoyl Peroxide	L2
Acnomel	Resorcinol	L3
Acnomel Acne Crm	Resorcinol	L3
Acryline	Benzoyl Peroxide	L2
Act Cinnamon	Fluoride	L2
Actagen	Triprolidine	L1
	Pseudoephedrine	L3
Acticin(Permethrin) Cream	Permethrin	L2
Actidose Aqua 25 Gm Liq L	Charcoal Activated	L3
Actifed	Chlorpheniramine	L3
	Phenylephrine	L3
Actifed Cold & Allergy Tablets	Phenylephrine	L3
	Chlorpheniramine	L3
Actifed Cold & Sinus Caplets	Triprolidine	L1
	Pseudoephedrine	L3
	Acetaminophen	L1
Actron	Ketoprofen	L2
Actron 50Ct Caplets	Ketoprofen	L2
Acutrim Complete Caffeine Free	Phenylpropanolamine	L2
Acutrim Max Strength	Phenylpropanolamine	L2
A-D Ont	Vitamin A	L3
	Vitamin D	L2
Adult Low Strength Aspirin, 81 Mg	Aspirin	L3 (L5 In Viral Syndromes)
Advil	Ibuprofen	L1
Advil Allergy Sinus Caplets	Ibuprofen	L1
	Chlorpheniramine	L3
	Pseudoephedrine	L3
Advil Allergy Sinus Children's Liquid	Ibuprofen	L1
	Chlorpheniramine	L3
	Pseudoephedrine	L3
Advil Caplets Allergy Sinus	Ibuprofen	L1
	Chlorpheniramine	L3
	Pseudoephedrine	L3
Advil Cold & Sinus Caplets	Ibuprofen	L1
	Pseudoephedrine	L3
Advil Cold & Sinus Liqui-Gels	Ibuprofen	L1
	Pseudoephedrine	L3
Advil Cold & Sinus Tablets	Ibuprofen	L1
	Pseudoephedrine	L3
Advil Cold Sinus Caplets	Ibuprofen	L1
	Pseudoephedrine	L3

OTC NAME	DRUGS	LRC
Advil Cold Sinus Liqui-Gels	Ibuprofen	L1
	Pseudoephedrine	L3
Advil Congest Relief Cpl	Ibuprofen	L1
	Phenylephrine	L3
Advil Ez Open 200 Mg Lgl	Ibuprofen	L1
Advil Ibuprofen Tablets-50 50, 200Mg	Ibuprofen	L1
Advil Liqui-Gels 200 Mg	Ibuprofen	L1
Advil Migraine Capsules	Ibuprofen	L1
Advil Multi-Symptom Cold Caplets	Ibuprofen	L1
	Chlorpheniramine	L3
	Pseudoephedrine	L3
Advil Pm 200 Mg Cpl	Diphenhydramine	L2
	Ibuprofen	L1
Advil Pm 25% Bns 200 Mg Lgl	Diphenhydramine	L2
	Ibuprofen	L1
Advil Tablets	Ibuprofen	L1
Advil Tablets	Ibuprofen	L1
Advil Tablets Bns	Ibuprofen	L1
Advil Tablets Cold Sinus Whitehall-Robbins Heathcare	Pseudoephedrine	L3
	Ibuprofen	L1
Afrin	Oxymetazoline	L3
Afrin Severe	Oxymetazoline	L3
Afrin Sinus Nasal Spy	Oxymetazoline	L3
Aftate Antifungal Liquid Spray For Athelete's Foot	Tolnaftate	L3
After Bite Ant Chiggr Liq	Ammonia / Ammonium Salts	
Airborne	Zinc Salts	L2
	Vitamin E	L2
	Vitamin A	L3
	Selenium Sulfide	L3
	Magnesium Sulfate	L1
	Echinacea	L3
	Bicarbonate (Na/K)	L3
	Ascorbic Acid	L1
Airborne Berry Tab	Ginger	L3
	Echinacea	L3
	Lysine	L2
Airborne On T/Go Berry Pwd	Zinc Salts	L2
	Vitamin E	L2
	Vitamin A	L3
	Magnesium Sulfate	L1
	Ginger	L3
	Ascorbic Acid	L1
	Echinacea	L3

OTC NAME	DRUGS	LRC
Alahist Ir 2 Mg Tab	Dexbrompheniramine	L3
Alahist Pe 2/ 10 Mg Tab	Dexbrompheniramine	L3
	Phenylephrine	L3
Alavert 24-Hour Allergy Tablets	Loratadine	L1
Alavert D-12	Loratadine	L1
	Pseudoephedrine	L3
Alavert D-12 Allergy And Sinus Tablets	Loratadine	L1
	Pseudoephedrine	L3
Alberton's Allergy Capsules	Diphenhydramine	L2
Alcon Naphcon	Pheniramine	L3
Alcon Pantanol 0.1 Eye Drops	Olopatadine Ophthalmic	L2
Alcon Tobradex Eyedrops	Dexamethasone	L3
	Tobramycin	L3
Alconefrin	Phenylephrine	L3
Aleve	Naproxen	L3 For Acute Use/L4 For Chronic Use
Aleve Cold & Sinus Tablets	Naproxen	L3 For Acute Use/L4 For Chronic Use
	Pseudoephedrine	L3
Aleve D Sinus Head Ache Cpl	Naproxen	L3 For Acute Use/L4 For Chronic Use
	Pseudoephedrine	L3
Aleve Liquid Gels	Naproxen	L3 For Acute Use/L4 For Chronic Use
Aleve Sinus Headache	Naproxen	L3 For Acute Use/L4 For Chronic Use
	Pseudoephedrine	L3
Aleve Sinus Headache 12-Hr	Naproxen	L3 For Acute Use/L4 For Chronic Use
	Pseudoephedrine	L3
Aleve Tablets	Naproxen	L3 For Acute Use/L4 For Chronic Use
Align 28+7 Bns Pdq Cap	Probiotics	L3
Alka-Seltzer Blue Tab	Bicarbonate (Na/K)	L3
	Aspirin	L3 (L5 In Viral Syndromes)
	Citric Acid	L3
Alka-Seltzer Extra Strength Effervescent Tablets	Citric Acid	L3
	Aspirin	L3 (L5 In Viral Syndromes)
	Bicarbonate (Na/K)	L3
Alka-Seltzer Gold Tablets	Citric Acid	L3
	Bicarbonate (Na/K)	L3
Alka-Seltzer Heartburn Relief Tablets	Bicarbonate (Na/K)	L3
	Citric Acid	L3
Alka-Seltzer Lemn Lime Tab	Bicarbonate (Na/K)	L3
	Aspirin	L3 (L5 In Viral Syndromes)
	Citric Acid	L3

OTC NAME	DRUGS	LRC
Alka-Seltzer Morning Relief Effervescent Tablets	Aspirin	L3 (L5 In Viral Syndromes)
	Caffeine	L2
Alka-Seltzer Original	Bicarbonate (Na/K)	L3
	Aspirin	L3 (L5 In Viral Syndromes)
	Citric Acid	L3
Alka-Seltzer Original Effervescent Tablets	Bicarbonate (Na/K)	L3
	Aspirin	L3 (L5 In Viral Syndromes)
	Citric Acid	L3
Alka-Seltzer Plus Cherry Tab	Chlorpheniramine	L3
	Aspirin	L3 (L5 In Viral Syndromes)
	Phenylephrine	L3
Alka-Seltzer Plus Cldcgh Lgl	Phenylephrine	L3
	Dextromethorphan	L1
	Chlorpheniramine	L3
	Aspirin	L3 (L5 In Viral Syndromes)
Alka-Seltzer Plus Cold & Sinus Tablets	Acetaminophen	L1
	Phenylephrine	L3
Alka-Seltzer Plus Cold Cherry Burst Formula Effervescent Tablets	Chlorpheniramine	L3
	Acetaminophen	L1
	Phenylephrine	L3
Alka-Seltzer Plus Cold Effervescent Tablets	Chlorpheniramine	L3
	Acetaminophen	L1
	Phenylephrine	L3
Alka-Seltzer Plus Cold Pwd	Chlorpheniramine	L3
	Acetaminophen	L1
	Phenylephrine	L3
Alka-Seltzer Plus Cough & Cold Effervescent Tablets	Phenylephrine	L3
	Chlorpheniramine	L3
	Acetaminophen	L1
	Dextromethorphan	L1
Alka-Seltzer Plus Cough & Cold Liquid	Phenylephrine	L3
	Dextromethorphan	L1
	Chlorpheniramine	L3
	Acetaminophen	L1
Alka-Seltzer Plus Cough & Cold Liquid Gels	Phenylephrine	L3
	Chlorpheniramine	L3
	Acetaminophen	L1
	Dextromethorphan	L1
Alka-Seltzer Plus Day & Night Effervescent Tablets	Phenylephrine	L3
	Acetaminophen	L1
	Dextromethorphan	L1

OTC NAME	DRUGS	LRC
Alka-Seltzer Plus Day & Night Liquid Gels	Phenylephrine	L3
	Acetaminophen	L1
	Dextromethorphan	L1
Alka-Seltzer Plus Day Cold Liquid	Phenylephrine	L3
	Acetaminophen	L1
	Dextromethorphan	L1
Alka-Seltzer Plus Day Cold Liquid Gels	Phenylephrine	L3
	Acetaminophen	L1
	Dextromethorphan	L1
Alka-Seltzer Plus Day Nd Lgl	Dextromethorphan	L1
	Acetaminophen	L1
	Phenylephrine	L3
Alka-Seltzer Plus Effervescent Tablets	Phenylephrine	L3
	Doxylamine	L3
	Acetaminophen	L1
	Dextromethorphan	L1
Alka-Seltzer Plus Flu Effervescent Tablets	Dextromethorphan	L1
	Chlorpheniramine	L3
	Aspirin	L3 (L5 In Viral Syndromes)
Alka-Seltzer Plus Mucus & Congestion Effervescent Tablets	Dextromethorphan	L1
	Guaifenesin	L2
Alka-Seltzer Plus Mucus Lgl	Dextromethorphan	L1
	Guaifenesin	L2
Alka-Seltzer Plus Nghttm Tab	Doxylamine	L3
	Dextromethorphan	L1
	Aspirin	L3 (L5 In Viral Syndromes)
	Phenylephrine	L3
Alka-Seltzer Plus Night Cold Liquid	Phenylephrine	L3
	Doxylamine	L3
	Acetaminophen	L1
	Dextromethorphan	L1
Alka-Seltzer Plus Nighttime Cold Liquid-Gels	Dextromethorphan	L1
	Pseudoephedrine	L3
	Acetaminophen	L1
	Chlorpheniramine	L3
Alka-Seltzer Plus Nighttime Liquid Gels	Doxylamine	L3
	Acetaminophen	L1
	Dextromethorphan	L1
Alka-Seltzer Plus Orange Tab	Chlorpheniramine	L3
	Aspirin	L3 (L5 In Viral Syndromes)
	Phenylephrine	L3
Alka-Seltzer Plus Sinus Effervescent Tablets	Acetaminophen	L1
	Phenylephrine	L3

OTC NAME	DRUGS	LRC
Alka-Seltzer Plus Sinus Tab	Aspirin	L3 (L5 In Viral Syndromes)
	Phenylephrine	L3
Alka-Seltzer Pm	Aspirin	L3 (L5 In Viral Syndromes)
	Diphenhydramine	L2
Alka-Seltzer Pm Effervescent Tablets	Aspirin	L3 (L5 In Viral Syndromes)
	Diphenhydramine	L2
Alka-Seltzer Pm Lt/Frt Tab	Aspirin	L3 (L5 In Viral Syndromes)
	Diphenhydramine	L2
Alka-Seltzer Regular Seltzer Multi-Symptom Cold Relief Effervescent Tablets	Chlorpheniramine	L3
	Acetaminophen	L1
	Phenylephrine	L3
Alka-Seltzer Tablets, Extra Strength	Bicarbonate (Na/K)	L3
	Aspirin	L3 (L5 In Viral Syndromes)
	Citric Acid	L3
Alka-Seltzer Tablets, Original	Bicarbonate (Na/K)	L3
	Aspirin	L3 (L5 In Viral Syndromes)
	Citric Acid	L3
Allegra	Fexofenadine	L2
Allegra D	Fexofenadine	L2
	Pseudoephedrine	L3
Aller Chlor 4 Mg Tab	Chlorpheniramine	L3
Allerest	Chlorpheniramine	L3
	Pseudoephedrine	L3
Allerest No-Drowsiness Caplets	Acetaminophen	L1
	Pseudoephedrine	L3
Allerest Pe M/S Alg/Sn Tab	Chlorpheniramine	L3
	Phenylephrine	L3
Allerest Tablets	Chlorpheniramine	L3
	Phenylephrine	L3
Alpha Lipoic Acid 100 Mg Tab	Herbal Supplement/Teas	L4
Ambelesol	Benzocaine	L2
Americaine 20 % Aer	Benzocaine	L2
Amitone	Calcium Carbonate	L3
	Clavulanate	L3
Amphojel	Aluminum Hydroxide	L2
Anacin	Acetaminophen	L1
Anacin	Aspirin	L3 (L5 In Viral Syndromes)
Anacin Advanced Headache Tablets	Aspirin	L3 (L5 In Viral Syndromes)
	Acetaminophen	L1
	Caffeine	L2
Anacin Aspirin Free Extra Strength Tablets	Acetaminophen	L1
Anacin Coated Caplets-Unknown	Acetaminophen	L1
	Caffeine	L2

OTC NAME	DRUGS	LRC
Anacin Extra Strength Aspirin Free Tablets	Acetaminophen	L1
Anacin Max Strength Tablets	Aspirin	L3 (L5 In Viral Syndromes)
	Caffeine	L2
Anacin Tab	Acetaminophen	L1
	Caffeine	L2
Anbesol	Benzocaine	L2
Anbesol Baby Grape Gel	Benzocaine	L2
Anbesol C/MNT Reg Gel	Benzocaine	L2
Anbesol Cold Sore Therapy Ointment	Camphor	L3
	Benzocaine	L2
	Allantoin	L3
Anbesol Liq	Benzocaine	L2
Anbesol Maximum Strength Gel Core Sore Treatment	Benzocaine	L2
	Camphor	L3
Anbesol Mx/St Gel	Benzocaine	L2
Anti-Diarheal 2 Mg Cpl	Loperamide	L2
Anti-Diarrheal Caplets	Loperamide	L2
Antifungal 1 % Crm 15 Gm	Tolnaftate	L3
Antifungal Liquid	Undecylenic Acid	L3
Antifungal Spray Liquid Tolnaftate	Tolnaftate	L3
Anti-Gas (Simethicone 80Mg)	Simethicone	L3
Anusol Hc-1	Hydrocortisone Topical	L2
Anusol Hemorroidal Ointment	Pramoxine	L3
	Zinc Salts	L2
Apap 160 Mg/5Ml Elx	Acetaminophen	L1
Apap Pain/Fvr 500 Mg	Acetaminophen	L1
Apap Sup 325Mg 1943265	Acetaminophen	L1
Apap Sup 650Mg 2418788	Acetaminophen	L1
Apap X-Str Caplets	Acetaminophen	L1
Arnica Crm	Herbal Supplement/Teas	L4
Arnicare Gel	Herbal Supplement/Teas	L4
Arthricare Medicated Trial	Capsaicin	L3
	Menthol	L3
Arthricare Odor Free	Capsaicin	L3
	Menthol	L3
Arthricare Rub Dbl Ice	Camphor	L3
	Menthol	L3
Arthricare Women Extra Moisterizing	Capsaicin	L3
Arthri-Creme /Aloe	Trolamine	L3
	Aloe Vera	L3
Arthri-Flex Tab	Glucosamine	L3
	Chondroitin Sulfate	L3
	Hyaluronic Acid	L3

OTC NAME	DRUGS	LRC
Arthritis Hot Cream	Menthol	L3
Arthritis Pain Formula Release Caplets, 650Mg	Acetaminophen	L1
Arthritis Pain Relief Pump-A	Menthol	L3
	Camphor	L3
Arthx Glucosamine Tablets	Glucosamine	L3
	Chondroitin Sulfate	L3
Ascriptin	Magnesium Hydroxide	L1
	Aspirin	L3 (L5 In Viral Syndromes)
	Aluminum Hydroxide	L2
	Calcium Carbonate	L3
Ascriptin 500 Mg X/S Cpl	Magnesium Hydroxide	L1
	Aspirin	L3 (L5 In Viral Syndromes)
	Aluminum Hydroxide	L2
	Calcium Carbonate	L3
Ascriptin A/D Caplet	Magnesium Hydroxide	L1
	Aspirin	L3 (L5 In Viral Syndromes)
	Aluminum Hydroxide	L2
	Calcium Carbonate	L3
Ascriptin Regular Strength Tablets	Aluminum Hydroxide	L2
	Magnesium Hydroxide	L1
	Calcium Carbonate	L3
	Aspirin	L3 (L5 In Viral Syndromes)
Aspercreme	Trolamine	L3
Aspercreme Heat Gel	Menthol	L3
Aspercreme Ice	Trolamine	L3
Aspergum	Aspirin	L3 (L5 In Viral Syndromes)
Aspergum Cherry	Aspirin	L3 (L5 In Viral Syndromes)
Aspergum Chewable Tablets	Aspirin	L3 (L5 In Viral Syndromes)
Aspirin	Aspirin	L3 (L5 In Viral Syndromes)
Aspirin 325Mg	Aspirin	L3 (L5 In Viral Syndromes)
Aspirin 300 Mg	Aspirin	L3 (L5 In Viral Syndromes)
Asthmahaler	Epinephrine	L1
Astracaine	Articaine	L3
	Epinephrine	L1
Athlete's Foot Cream	Terbinafine	L2
Auro Ear 6.5 %	Carbamide Peroxide	L1
Aveeno 1% Hydrocortisone Anti-Itch Cream	Hydrocortisone Topical	L2
Aveeno Anti-Itch Concentrated Lotion	Pramoxine	L3
	Camphor	L3
Aveeno Anti-Itch Cream	Pramoxine	L3
	Camphor	L3
Aveeno Calamine Nd Pramoxine Hcl Anti-Itch Cream	Pramoxine	L3
Aveeno Clear Complexion Cleansing Bar	Salicylic Acid, Topical	L3

OTC NAME	DRUGS	LRC
Aveeno Clear Complexion Foaming Cleanser	Salicylic Acid, Topical	L3
Aveeno Correction Treatment Clear Complexion	Salicylic Acid, Topical	L3
Aveeno Hydrocortisone 1% Anti-Itch Cream	Hydrocortisone Topical	L2
Aveeno Skin Relief Moisturinzing Cream	Dimethicone	L3
Ayr Allergy Sins Mist	Benzalkonium Chloride	L3
Ayr Gel No Drip Sinus Spy	Sodium Chloride	L2
	Aloe Vera	L3
	Benzalkonium Chloride	L3
Azo Cranberry	Cranberry Extract	L3
Azo Itch Relief Maximum Strength Medicated Cream	Pramoxine	L3
Azo Itch Relief Medicated Wipes	Pramoxine	L3
Azo Standard	Phenazopyridine Hcl	L3
Azo-Gesic 95 Mg Tab	Phenazopyridine Hcl	L3
Bacid Cap	Probiotics	L3
Baciguent	Bacitracin	L2
Bacitr Zinc 500 Un/Gm Ont	Bacitracin	L2
	Zinc Salts	L2
Bacitr/Poly B Ont	Bacitracin	L2
	Polymyxin B Sulfate	L2
Bacitracin Ointment	Bacitracin	L2
Backaid Pills Tab	Acetaminophen	L1
	Pamabrom	L3
Bactimicina Pastilas	Acetaminophen	L1
Bactine Pain Relieving Protective Antibiotic	Polymyxin B Sulfate	L2
	Neomycin	L3/L5 On Nipple
	Bacitracin	L2
	Pramoxine	L3
Bactine Pain Relv Clnsng Spy	Benzalkonium Chloride	L3
	Lidocaine	L2
Banalg	Methyl Salicylate	L3 (L5 In Viral Syndromes)
	Menthol	L3
Band-Aid Corn Remover	Salicylic Acid, Topical	L3
Bayer Midol Mx St Teen Cp	Acetaminophen	L1
	Pamabrom	L3
Bayer Pm Relief Caplets	Aspirin	L3 (L5 In Viral Syndromes)
	Diphenhydramine	L2
Bayer Select	Acetaminophen	L1
Bc Allergy-Sinus-Headache Powders	Pseudoephedrine	L3
	Aspirin	L3 (L5 In Viral Syndromes)
	Chlorpheniramine	L3
Bc Allergy-Sinus-Cold	Phenylpropanolamine	L2
	Aspirin	L3 (L5 In Viral Syndromes)
	Chlorpheniramine	L3

OTC NAME	DRUGS	LRC
Bc Arthritis Strength Powders	Caffeine	L2
	Aspirin	L3 (L5 In Viral Syndromes)
Bc Fast Pain Relief Headache Powder	Aspirin	L3 (L5 In Viral Syndromes)
	Caffeine	L2
Bc Headache Powders	Aspirin	L3 (L5 In Viral Syndromes)
	Caffeine	L2
Bc Origonal Formula Powders	Aspirin	L3 (L5 In Viral Syndromes)
	Caffeine	L2
Beano Food Enzyme Dietary Supplement Drops	Alpha-Galactosidase Enzyme	L3
Bectracin Oint. 175-1858	Bacitracin	L2
Bee Pollen 500 Mg Tab	Herbal Supplement/Teas	L3
Beelith Tab	Magnesium Hydroxide	L1
	Pyridoxine	L2/L4 In High Doses
Benadryl	Diphenhydramine	L2
Benadryl Allergy & Cold Tablets	Diphenhydramine	L2
	Acetaminophen	L1
	Pseudoephedrine	L3
Benadryl Allergy & Sinus Headache Tablets	Diphenhydramine	L2
	Acetaminophen	L1
	Pseudoephedrine	L3
	Zinc Salts	L2
Benadryl Original Cream	Diphenhydramine	L2
	Zinc Salts	L2
Benadryl Redy Mst Reg Spy	Diphenhydramine	L2
	Zinc Salts	L2
Benadryl Severe Allergy & Sinus Headache Caplets	Diphenhydramine	L2
	Acetaminophen	L1
	Phenylephrine	L3
Benadryl Ultr 25 Mg Tab	Diphenhydramine	L2
Benadryl-D Allergy/Sinus Tablets	Diphenhydramine	L2
	Phenylephrine	L3
Bengay	Menthol	L3
	Camphor	L3
Benzaclin Topical Gel	Benzoyl Peroxide	L2
	Clindamycin	L2
Benzedrex	Propylhexedrine	L5
Benzedrex Inhaler	Propylhexedrine	L5
Benzocaine 20 % Spy	Benzocaine	L2
Benzodent Crm	Benzocaine	L2
Benzoin	Herbal Supplement/Teas	L4
Beta Carotene 10M Iu Cap	Beta-Carotene	L3
Beta Carotene 25M Iu Cap	Beta-Carotene	L3
Betadine Gel	Povidone Iodide	L4

OTC NAME	DRUGS	LRC
Betadine Md	Povidone Iodide	L4
Betadine Md Dch 1217306	Povidone Iodide	L4
Betadine Medicate Douc	Povidone Iodide	L4
Betadine Shampoo	Povidone Iodide	L4
Betadine Skin Cleanser	Povidone Iodide	L4
Betadine Solution	Povidone Iodide	L4
Betamide Lot	Povidone Iodide	L4
Betasept	Chlorhexidine	L4
Betdne Aero Spray	Povidone Iodide	L4
Betdne Med Douche	Povidone Iodide	L4
Biotin 1000 Mcg Tab	Biotin	L1
Bisacodyl	Bisacodyl	L2
Bisacodyl 10 Mg Sup	Bisacodyl	L2
Bisacodyl	Bisacodyl	L2
Bismatrol Liq	Bismuth Subsalicylate	L3
Bismatrol Tab	Bismuth Subsalicylate	L3
Black Cohosh	Black Cohosh	L4
Black Draught Laxatv Syr	Senna Laxatives	L3
	Magnesium Sulfate	L1
Black Draught Powder	Senna Laxatives	L3
	Magnesium Sulfate	L1
Black Elderberry Extract [Strength 1:2]	Herbal Supplement/Teas	L4
Blue Star Ointment	Camphor	L3
B-Natal Loz	Pyridoxine	L2/L4 In High Doses
Bonine	Meclizine	L3
Bonjela	Salicylic Acid, Topical	L3
Boric Acid	Boric Acid	L3
Bristol Myers Vagistat	Tioconazole	L3
Bromfed Syrup 339226	Dextromethorphan	L1
	Brompheniramine	L3
	Pseudoephedrine	L3
Bronkaid Cpl	Guaifenesin	L2
	Ephedrine	L4
Bufferin Extra Strength Tablets	Aspirin	L3 (L5 In Viral Syndromes)
	Calcium Carbonate	L3
Bufferin Tablets	Calcium Carbonate	L3
	Aspirin	L3 (L5 In Viral Syndromes)
	Magnesium Hydroxide	L1
C Lice Treatmnt Shmp	Pyrethrum	L3
Caladryl Clear Lotion	Zinc Salts	L2
	Pramoxine	L3
Caladryl Lotion	Pramoxine	L3
Caldecort	Hydrocortisone Topical	L2

OTC NAME	DRUGS	LRC
Caltrate	Calcium Carbonate	L3
Calvite P&D Tab	Calcium Carbonate	L3
	Vitamin D	L2
Campho Phn Liq	Camphor	L3
Cank-Aid Liq	Carbamide Peroxide	L1
Capaician Cream	Capsaicin	L3
Capsaicin	Capsaicin	L3
Carbamoxide Ed	Carbamide Peroxide	L1
Carmol 10 % Lot	Urea	L3
Carrington Antifungal 2% Topical Cream	Miconazole	L2
Carter's Laxative, Sodium Free Pills	Bisacodyl	L2
Cartilage Formula	Glucosamine	L3
Castiva Pain Rel Capscn Lot	Capsaicin	L3
Castor Oil	Castor Oil	L3
Cepacol	Benzocaine	L2
	Menthol	L3
Cepacol Cold Care Cherry	Benzocaine	L2
	Menthol	L3
Cepacol Cold Care Zinc Acetate Lozenges	Zinc Salts	L2
Cepacol Dual Chry Spy	Benzocaine	L2
Cepacol Max Spray Mint	Benzocaine	L2
Cepacol Max Strength Cherry Lozenges	Menthol	L3
	Benzocaine	L2
Cepacol Mint Mouthwash	Cetylpyridinium Chloride	L3
Cepacol Sore Throat Lozenges	Benzocaine	L2
Cepacol Sore Throat Spray	Benzocaine	L2
Cetaphil Retinol	Vitamin A	L3
Cetirizine 1 Mg/Ml Sol	Cetirizine	L2
Charcoal Hm Activ Pwd	Charcoal Activated	L3
Charcoal Capsules 260 Mg	Charcoal Activated	L3
Cheracol Cough Syrup	Dextromethorphan	L1
	Guaifenesin	L2
Cheracol D	Dextromethorphan	L1
	Guaifenesin	L2
Cherocol Pl	Phenylpropanolamine	L2
	Chlorpheniramine	L3
	Dextromethorphan	L1
Chlorasep S/T +Cgh Sf Chy Loz	Dextromethorphan	L1
	Benzocaine	L2
	Menthol	L3
Chloraseptic Cherry Sore Throat Spray	Phenol	L3
Chloraseptic Cherry Spy	Phenol	L3

OTC NAME	DRUGS	LRC
Chloraseptic Totl Cherry Loz	Dextromethorphan	L1
	Benzocaine	L2
	Menthol	L3
Chlorophyll 3 Mg Tab	Herbal Supplement/Teas	L4
Chlorpheniramine	Chlorpheniramine	L3
Chlorpherniramine Maleate Tablets	Chlorpheniramine	L3
Chlor-Trimetn 4 Hour Tab	Chlorpheniramine	L3
Chlor-Trimeton Allergy-D 12 Hour Tablets	Chlorpheniramine	L3
	Pseudoephedrine	L3
Cholesterol Care	Milk Thistle	L3
	Coenzyme Q10	L3
	Herbal Supplement/Teas	L4
Choline & Inositol [250 Mg Each]	Herbal Supplement/Teas	L4
Choline & Inositol 500 Mg	Herbal Supplement/Teas	L4
Chromium Pic 200 Mcg Cap	Chromium	L3
Citrate Of Magnesium Oral Cherry	Magnesium Salts	
Citric Ac Hm Grn	Citric Acid	L3
Citrocarbonat Antacd Grn	Citric Acid	L3
	Bicarbonate (Na/K)	L3
Citronella Hm Oil	Herbal Supplement/Teas	L4
Citrucel Caplets	Methylcellulose	L1
Citrucel Packets Orange	Methylcellulose	L1
Claritin	Loratadine	L1
Claritin-D 12 Hour Tablets	Loratadine	L1
	Pseudoephedrine	L3
Claritin-D 24 Hour Allergy & Congestion Tablets	Pseudoephedrine	L3
	Loratadine	L1
Clear Away Clear Wart Remover	Salicylic Acid, Topical	L3
Clearasil Acne Treatment Tinted Cream	Benzoyl Peroxide	L2
Clearasil Daily Acne Stay Clear Facial Scrub	Salicylic Acid, Topical	L3
Clearasil Stay Clear Deep Cleanse Acne Fighting Cleansing Wipes	Salicylic Acid, Topical	L3
Clearasil Stay Clear Skin Daily Pore Cleansing Pads	Salicylic Acid, Topical	L3
Clearasil Stay Clear Skin Perfecting Wash	Salicylic Acid, Topical	L3
Clearasil Total Acne Control	Benzoyl Peroxide	L2
Clearasil Ultra Acne Clearing Gel Wash	Salicylic Acid, Topical	L3
Clearasil Ultra Acne Scrub	Salicylic Acid, Topical	L3
Clearasil Ultra Acne Treatment Vanishing Cream	Benzoyl Peroxide	L2
Clearasil Ultra Daily Face Wash	Salicylic Acid, Topical	L3
Clearasil Ultra Deep Pore Cleansing Pads	Salicylic Acid, Topical	L3
Clotrimaz 2% Vag 3Dy Af Crm	Clotrimazole	L1
Clove Hm Oil	Herbal Supplement/Teas	L4

OTC NAME	DRUGS	LRC
Codal Dm Clr Cherry Syr	Pyrilamine	L3
	Phenylephrine	L3
	Dextromethorphan	L1
Co-Defense Mini-Tablets	Multivitamin	L3
Co-Defense Tablets	Multivitamin	L3
Codiclear	Guaifenesin	L2
	Hydrocodone	L3
Codimal	Pyrilamine	L3
	Phenylephrine	L3
Codimal Dm Liq	Phenylephrine	L3
	Dextromethorphan	L1
	Pyrilamine	L3
Codituss Dm Chry Punch Syr	Pyrilamine	L3
	Dextromethorphan	L1
Colace	Docusate	L2
Colace Glycer Adult Sup	Glycerin	L3
Colace Liquid	Docusate	L2
Coldec D Tablets	Carbinoxamine	L2
	Pseudoephedrine	L3
Cold-Fx 200 Mg Capsules	Ginseng	L3
Coldmist La Tablets	Guaifenesin	L2
	Pseudoephedrine	L3
Colon Cleanse Reg Pwd	Psyllium	L2
	Senna Laxatives	L3
Commit Stop Smoking 2Mg Lozenges	Nicotine	L2
Commit Stop Smoking 4Mg Lozenges	Nicotine	L2
Complete Allergy Medicine	Diphenhydramine	L2
Complete Allergy/Sinus Headache Tablets	Phenylephrine	L3
	Acetaminophen	L1
	Diphenhydramine	L2
Compound W	Salicylic Acid, Topical	L3
Compoz Nte Slp Aid	Diphenhydramine	L2
Comtres Acute Head Cold Maximum Strength	Brompheniramine	L3
	Acetaminophen	L1
	Pseudoephedrine	L3
Comtrex	Dextromethorphan	L1
	Chlorpheniramine	L3
	Acetaminophen	L1
	Phenylephrine	L3
Comtrex-Maximum Strength, Day Night Flu Therapy	Dextromethorphan	L1
	Chlorpheniramine	L3
	Acetaminophen	L1
	Phenylephrine	L3

OTC NAME	DRUGS	LRC
Comtrex Allergy-Sinus Treatment, Maximum Strength Tablets	Pseudoephedrine	L3
	Acetaminophen	L1
	Chlorpheniramine	L3
	Dextromethorphan	L1
Comtrex Caps	Dextromethorphan	L1
	Chlorpheniramine	L3
	Acetaminophen	L1
	Phenylephrine	L3
Comtrex Cold & Cough Tablets	Phenylephrine	L3
	Acetaminophen	L1
	Dextroamphetamine	L3 In Clinical Doses/L5 If Abused
Comtrex Cold Cough	Dextromethorphan	L1
	Acetaminophen	L1
	Phenylephrine	L3
Comtrex D/N Cold Cough Cpl	Dextromethorphan	L1
	Chlorpheniramine	L3
	Acetaminophen	L1
	Phenylephrine	L3
Comtrex D/Nt Flu Therpy Cpl	Dextromethorphan	L1
	Chlorpheniramine	L3
	Acetaminophen	L1
	Phenylephrine	L3
Comtrex Day & Night Severe Cold & Sinus Caplets	Chlorpheniramine	L3
	Acetaminophen	L1
	Phenylephrine	L3
Comtrex Deep Chest Cold	Acetaminophen	L1
	Guaifenesin	L2
Comtrex Deep Chest Cold Non-Drowsy	Acetaminophen	L1
	Guaifenesin	L2
Comtrex Deep Chest Congestion Relief Liquid	Guaifenesin	L2
	Acetaminophen	L1
Comtrex Flu And Fever	Chlorpheniramine	L3
	Acetaminophen	L1
	Pseudoephedrine	L3
Comtrex Nighttime Cold & Cough Caplets	Phenylephrine	L3
	Chlorpheniramine	L3
	Acetaminophen	L1
	Dextromethorphan	L1
Comtrex Non/D Cold Cough Cpl	Dextromethorphan	L1
	Acetaminophen	L1
	Pseudoephedrine	L3

OTC NAME	DRUGS	LRC
Comtrex Tabs	Dextromethorphan	L1
	Chlorpheniramine	L3
	Acetaminophen	L1
	Phenylephrine	L3
Congestac	Guaifenesin	L2
	Pseudoephedrine	L3
Congestac Cpl	Guaifenesin	L2
	Pseudoephedrine	L3
Contac	Diphenhydramine	L2
	Acetaminophen	L1
	Chlorpheniramine	L3
	Pseudoephedrine	L3
Contac 12 Hr. Capsules	Phenylpropanolamine	L2
Contac Allergy Tab	Clemastine	L4
Contac Cf M/S Pse Free Cpl	Chlorpheniramine	L3
	Acetaminophen	L1
	Phenylephrine	L3
Contac Cold & Flu Day & Night Caplets	Acetaminophen	L1
	Phenylephrine	L3
Contac Cold & Flu Maximum Strength Caplets	Chlorpheniramine	L3
	Acetaminophen	L1
	Phenylephrine	L3
Contac Cold & Flu Non-Drowsy Maximum Strength Caplets	Acetaminophen	L1
	Phenylephrine	L3
Contac Cold Continuous Action Medication 120Mg Caplet	Chlorpheniramine	L3
	Acetaminophen	L1
	Phenylephrine	L3
Contac Day/Nt C/F Pse Fr Cpl	Phenylephrine	L3
	Acetaminophen	L1
	Chlorpheniramine	L3
Contac-D Cold Decongestant Tablets	Phenylephrine	L3
Contact Trl	Pseudoephedrine	L3
Controlled Labs Blue Growth	Herbal Supplement/Teas	L4
Cool Mint Chlorasceptic Spray	Phenol	L3
Coricidin	Dextromethorphan	L1
	Acetaminophen	L1
	Chlorpheniramine	L3
	Pseudoephedrine	L3
Coricidin Cold & Flu Tablets	Acetaminophen	L1
	Chlorpheniramine	L3

OTC NAME	DRUGS	LRC
Coricidin Hbp	Guaifenesin	L2
	Dextromethorphan	L1
	Acetaminophen	L1
	Chlorpheniramine	L3
Coricidin Hbp Chest Congestion & Cough Softgels	Dextromethorphan	L1
	Guaifenesin	L2
Coricidin Hbp Cough & Cold Tablets	Dextromethorphan	L1
	Chlorpheniramine	L3
Coricidin Hbp Day/ Nt Tab	Guaifenesin	L2
	Dextromethorphan	L1
	Acetaminophen	L1
	Chlorpheniramine	L3
Coricidin Hbp Maximum Strength Flu Tablets	Chlorpheniramine	L3
	Acetaminophen	L1
	Dextromethorphan	L1
Coricidin Hbp Nt Cld Rl Liq	Doxylamine	L3
	Dextromethorphan	L1
	Acetaminophen	L1
Correctol Bis Lax Tab	Bisacodyl	L2
Correctol Stiik Softener Laxative Soft Gels	Docusate	L2
Correctol Stimulant Laxative Tablets For Women	Bisacodyl	L2
Cort Aid Cream Sensitive	Hydrocortisone Topical	L2
Cortaflex Ha Capsules For People	Glucosamine	L3
	Chondroitin Sulfate	L3
	Hyaluronic Acid	L3
Cortaid	Hydrocortisone Topical	L2
Cruex	Clotrimazole	L1
Cruex Medicated Spray Powder	Miconazole	L2
Dairy Digestive Caplets	Lactase	L3
Dairy Ease Caplets	Lactase	L3
Dakin's .125 % Sol	Boric Acid	L3
Daktacort 2% Topical Cream	Miconazole	L2
Daktar Mundgel Oral Gel/Jelly	Miconazole	L2
Daktarin	Miconazole	L2
Daktarin Topical Powder	Miconazole	L2
Dayquil +Vitc Cpl	Phenylephrine	L3
	Dextromethorphan	L1
	Acetaminophen	L1
	Ascorbic Acid	L1
Dayquil Allrgy Tab	Chlorpheniramine	L3
	Pseudoephedrine	L3

OTC NAME	DRUGS	LRC
Dayquil Bonus Cold Flu Lcp	Dextromethorphan	L1
	Acetaminophen	L1
	Phenylephrine	L3
Dayquil Bonus Liq	Dextromethorphan	L1
	Acetaminophen	L1
	Phenylephrine	L3
Dayquil Cold Flu Lcp	Dextromethorphan	L1
	Acetaminophen	L1
	Phenylephrine	L3
Dayquil Cough Liq	Dextromethorphan	L1
Dayquil Lcp	Dextromethorphan	L1
	Acetaminophen	L1
	Phenylephrine	L3
Dayquil Liquid	Dextromethorphan	L1
	Acetaminophen	L1
	Phenylephrine	L3
Dayquil Muc Cnt Ctr Bl Liq	Guaifenesin	L2
Dayquil Muc Cnt Dm Cb Liq	Guaifenesin	L2
	Dextromethorphan	L1
Dayquil Vit C Cap	Phenylephrine	L3
	Dextromethorphan	L1
	Acetaminophen	L1
	Ascorbic Acid	L1
Dayquil/Nyqui Cmbo Cough Liq	Phenylephrine	L3
	Dextromethorphan	L1
	Acetaminophen	L1
	Doxylamine	L3
Daytime Cold/Flu Relief	Dextromethorphan	L1
	Acetaminophen	L1
	Phenylephrine	L3
Daytime Liquigels	Phenylephrine	L3
	Acetaminophen	L1
	Dextromethorphan	L1
Debrox Drops Kit	Carbamide Peroxide	L1
Deconamine	Chlorpheniramine	L3
	Pseudoephedrine	L3
Deep Heat	Menthol	L3
	Methyl Salicylate	L3 (L5 In Viral Syndromes)
Deep Heating Rub Tub	Menthol	L3
	Methyl Salicylate	L3 (L5 In Viral Syndromes)
Delsym 12-Hour Cough Relief Liquid	Dextromethorphan	L1
Delsym Adt Nt C&C Cherry Liq	Doxylamine	L3
	Dextromethorphan	L1

OTC NAME	DRUGS	LRC
	Phenylephrine	L3
Delsym Adt Nt M/S Cherry Liq	Dextromethorphan	L1
	Doxylamine	L3
Denorex	Pyrithione Zinc	L3
Derifil 100Mg Tablet	Herbal Supplement/Teas	L4
Derma Gran Af Topical Ointment	Miconazole	L2
Dermacaine Cream	Lidocaine	L2
Dermafungal Topical Ointment	Miconazole	L2
Dermonistat Topical Cream	Miconazole	L2
Dermoplast A/B Spy	Benzocaine	L2
Dermoplast Pain Relvng	Menthol	L3
	Benzocaine	L2
Desenex	Miconazole	L2
Desenex Af 1% Value Crm	Clotrimazole	L1
Desenex Antifungal Powder	Miconazole	L2
Desenex Max	Terbinafine	L2
Desenex Prescription Strength Liquid Spray	Miconazole	L2
Desenex Topical Powder	Miconazole	L2
Desitin Ont	Zinc Oxide	L2
Dexatrim Caff Fr	Phenylpropanolamine	L2
Dexatrim Gelcaps	Phenylpropanolamine	L2
Dexatrim Grn Tea Naturl Cpl	Chromium	L3
	Herbal Supplement/Teas	L4
Diabet Aid Pain Tingln Lot	Capsaicin	L3
Diabetaid Antifungal Foot Bath Tablets	Miconazole	L2
Digestive Adv Cnstpd Cpl	Probiotics	L3
	Herbal Supplement/Teas	L4
Dimenhydrinate	Dimenhydrinate	L2
Dimetane Extentabs	Brompheniramine	L3
Dimetane-Dx Cough	Pseudoephedrine	L3
	Brompheniramine	L3
	Dextromethorphan	L1
Dimetapp	Phenylephrine	L3
	Brompheniramine	L3
Dimetapp Allergy	Brompheniramine	L3
	Phenylephrine	L3
Dimetapp Cold & Allergy Elixir	Brompheniramine	L3
	Pseudoephedrine	L3
Dimetapp Lond-Acting Cold Plus Cough Elixir	Dextromethorphan	L1
	Chlorpheniramine	L3
Dimtap Dm Elixir	Dextromethorphan	L1
	Brompheniramine	L3
	Phenylephrine	L3

OTC NAME	DRUGS	LRC
Dimtap Elixir	Brompheniramine	L3
	Phenylephrine	L3
Dimtap Extentabs	Phenylpropanolamine	L2
	Brompheniramine	L3
Doan's Caplets	Magnesium Salts	
Doans Extra Strength	Magnesium Salts	
Doan's Extra Strength Pm Caplets	Magnesium Salts	
	Diphenhydramine	L2
Doans Pm Cap	Magnesium Salts	
	Diphenhydramine	L2
Docusate	Docusate	L2
Domeboro Pkt Pwd	Aluminum Acetate	L3
Dormin Slp- Aid Cap	Diphenhydramine	L2
Doxidan Capsules	Bisacodyl	L2
Doxidan Liquigels	Bisacodyl	L2
Dr. Scholl's	Salicylic Acid, Topical	L3
Dramamine	Dimenhydrinate	L2
Dramamine 24H Less Drowsy	Meclizine	L3
Dristan	Pseudoephedrine	L3
	Chlorpheniramine	L3
	Acetaminophen	L1
	Phenylephrine	L3
	Ibuprofen	L1
Dristan 12 Hour Nasal Spray	Oxymetazoline	L3
Dristan Cold Multi-Symptom Tablets	Chlorpheniramine	L3
	Acetaminophen	L1
	Phenylephrine	L3
Dristan Juice Mixin Pk	Pseudoephedrine	L3
	Acetaminophen	L1
	Dextromethorphan	L1
Dristan Juice-Mix Trial-Trial	Pseudoephedrine	L3
	Acetaminophen	L1
	Dextromethorphan	L1
Drixoral	Pseudoephedrine	L3
	Acetaminophen	L1
	Dexbrompheniramine	L3
Drixoral Cold & Allergy Sustained Action Tablets	Dexbrompheniramine	L3
	Pseudoephedrine	L3
Drixoral Decongestant Nasal Punp	Oxymetazoline	L3
Drixoral Tablets	Dexbrompheniramine	L3
	Pseudoephedrine	L3
Dulcagen	Bisacodyl	L2
Dulcolax	Docusate	L2

OTC NAME	DRUGS	LRC
Dulcolax Suppository	Bisacodyl	L2
Dulcolax Tablets	Bisacodyl	L2
Duratuss	Pseudoephedrine	L3
	Guaifenesin	L2
	Hydrocodone	L3
Dura-Vent/Da Tablets	Phenylephrine	L3
	Chlorpheniramine	L3
	Methscopolamine	L3
Echinacea	Echinacea	L3
Ecotrin Low Strength Tablets	Aspirin	L3 (L5 In Viral Syndromes)
Efidac	Chlorpheniramine	L3
E-Lax Old Box	Senna Laxatives	L3
Emetrol Liquid	Phosphorated Carbohydrate Solution	L3
Endacon Syr	Phenylephrine	L3
	Guaifenesin	L2
	Dextromethorphan	L1
Endal	Guaifenesin	L2
	Pseudoephedrine	L3
Enema Complete Ready-To-Use Disposable	Sodium Phosphate Dibasic-Dibasic Anhydrous	L3
Enteric Omega 3 Sgt	Docosahexaenoic Acid (Dha)	L3
	Eicosapentaenoic Acid (Epa)	L3
Equate-Tolnaftate Cream Usp	Tolnaftate	L3
Equate Acid Reducer (Cimetidine)	Cimetidine	L1
Equate Acid Reducer (Ranitidine-Similar To Zantac)	Ranitidine	L2
Equate Advanced Healing Lotion	Dimethicone	L3
Equate Allergy Relief-25Mg	Diphenhydramine	L2
Equate Antacid Tablets	Calcium Carbonate	L3
Equate Chlortabs (Antihistamine (Chlorpheniramine Maleate))	Chlorpheniramine	L3
Equate Cimetidine Tablets 200Mg	Cimetidine	L1
Equate Cod Liver Oil Capsules (Walmart Brand)	Eicosapentaenoic Acid (Epa)	L3
	Vitamin D	L2
	Vitamin A	L3
	Docosahexaenoic Acid (Dha)	L3
Equate Complete Multivitamin	Multivitamin	L3
Equate Cough Drops	Menthol	L3
Equate Day Time Liquid Caps	Dextromethorphan	L1
	Acetaminophen	L1
	Phenylephrine	L3
Equate Enema Twin Pack	Sodium Phosphate Dibasic-Dibasic Anhydrous	L3
Equate Extra Strength Antacid	Calcium Carbonate	L3
Equate Extra Strength Non-Aspirin Pain Fever Relief (Acetaminophen 500 Mg)	Acetaminophen	L1

OTC NAME	DRUGS	LRC
Equate Headache Relief	Aspirin	L3 (L5 In Viral Syndromes)
	Acetaminophen	L1
	Caffeine	L2
Equate Hemorrhoidal Ointment	Phenylephrine	L3
Equate Ibuprofen Tablets 200Mg	Ibuprofen	L1
Equate Maximum Strenght/Non-Drowsy Sudephedrine (Expectorant Nasal Decongestant-Nondrying)	Pseudoephedrine	L3
Equate Multi-Purpose Solution	Phenylephrine	L3
	Chlorpheniramine	L3
	Acetaminophen	L1
	Dextromethorphan	L1
Equate Nicotine Gum	Nicotine	L2
Equate Nicotine Gun	Nicotine	L2
Equate Night Time Sleep Aid	Doxylamine	L3
Equate Nite Time Liquid Caps	Dextromethorphan	L1
	Acetaminophen	L1
	Doxylamine	L3
Equate Nite Time Multi-Symptom Cold/Flu Relief	Dextromethorphan	L1
	Acetaminophen	L1
	Doxylamine	L3
Equate Non-Drowsy Day Time Liquid Caps	Dextromethorphan	L1
	Acetaminophen	L1
	Phenylephrine	L3
Equate Severe Allergy Sinus Headache	Phenylephrine	L3
	Acetaminophen	L1
	Diphenhydramine	L2
Equate Stay Awake Caffeine Tablets 200Mg	Caffeine	L2
Equate Suphedrine 30Mg	Pseudoephedrine	L3
Equate Tussin Cold Congestion	Phenylephrine	L3
	Dextromethorphan	L1
	Acetaminophen	L1
	Guaifenesin	L2
Ergocalcifero Sol	Vitamin D	L2
Es Tums Smooth Dissolve Peppermint	Calcium Carbonate	L3
Esoterica Cream	Hydroquinone	L3
Estrin D	Herbal Supplement/Teas	L4
	Pyridoxine	L2/L4 In High Doses
Etrivine Spry 1 286252	Xylometazoline	L3
Evening Primrose	Herbal Supplement/Teas	L4
Ex St Phazyme	Simethicone	L3
Exact Acne Medication	Benzoyl Peroxide	L2

OTC NAME	DRUGS	LRC
Excederin Mig	Aspirin	L3 (L5 In Viral Syndromes)
	Acetaminophen	L1
	Caffeine	L2
Excederin Quicktabs	Acetaminophen	L1
	Caffeine	L2
Excedrin	Caffeine	L2
	Acetaminophen	L1
	Aspirin	L3 (L5 In Viral Syndromes)
Excedrin A/F Gel Tabs Xstrg	Aspirin	L3 (L5 In Viral Syndromes)
	Acetaminophen	L1
	Caffeine	L2
Excedrin Back & Body Caplets	Acetaminophen	L1
	Aspirin	L3 (L5 In Viral Syndromes)
Excedrin Caps	Aspirin	L3 (L5 In Viral Syndromes)
	Acetaminophen	L1
	Caffeine	L2
Excedrin Extra Strength Back Body	Acetaminophen	L1
	Aspirin	L3 (L5 In Viral Syndromes)
Excedrin Extra Strength Caplets	Aspirin	L3 (L5 In Viral Syndromes)
	Acetaminophen	L1
	Caffeine	L2
Excedrin Extra Strength Geltabs	Caffeine	L2
	Aspirin	L3 (L5 In Viral Syndromes)
	Acetaminophen	L1
Excedrin Extra Strength Tablets	Aspirin	L3 (L5 In Viral Syndromes)
	Acetaminophen	L1
	Caffeine	L2
Excedrin Geltabs	Aspirin	L3 (L5 In Viral Syndromes)
	Acetaminophen	L1
	Caffeine	L2
Excedrin Migraine Tablets	Aspirin	L3 (L5 In Viral Syndromes)
	Acetaminophen	L1
	Caffeine	L2
Excedrin Mnst Comp E/Gl Gcp	Aspirin	L3 (L5 In Viral Syndromes)
	Acetaminophen	L1
	Caffeine	L2
Excedrin Pm Tablets	Acetaminophen	L1
	Diphenhydramine	L2
Excedrin Quicktabs	Aspirin	L3 (L5 In Viral Syndromes)
	Acetaminophen	L1
	Caffeine	L2
Excedrin Sinus Headache Tablets	Acetaminophen	L1
	Phenylephrine	L3

OTC NAME	DRUGS	LRC
Excedrin Tabs	Aspirin	L3 (L5 In Viral Syndromes)
	Acetaminophen	L1
	Caffeine	L2
Excedrin Tension Headache Caplets	Acetaminophen	L1
	Caffeine	L2
Excedrin X/S Gtb	Aspirin	L3 (L5 In Viral Syndromes)
	Acetaminophen	L1
	Caffeine	L2
Excedrin X/S Migr Twin Gtb	Aspirin	L3 (L5 In Viral Syndromes)
	Acetaminophen	L1
	Caffeine	L2
Exlax	Senna Laxatives	L3
Ex-Lax Choc Tab	Senna Laxatives	L3
Ex-Lax Milk Of Magnesia Liquid	Magnesium Hydroxide	L1
Ex-Lax Stool Softener Tablets	Docusate	L2
Ex-Lax Tablets	Senna Laxatives	L3
Exlax Ultra Laxative Pills	Bisacodyl	L2
Eye Drops Tetrahydrozoline Hcl	Tetrahydrozoline	L3
Famotidine	Famotidine	L1
Femazole One	Metronidazole	L2
Femcare	Clotrimazole	L1
Femiron	Iron	L1
Femizol-M Vaginal Cream	Miconazole	L2
Femstat	Butoconazole	L3
Femstat 3	Econazole	L3
Feosol Cbl Ir 45Mg 30+10 Cpl	Iron	L1
Feosol Elixir	Iron	L1
Feosol Fs 65Mg 100+25 Tab	Iron	L1
Fer Iron Drp	Iron	L1
Ferate 27 Mg Tab	Iron	L1
Ferrous Sulfate	Iron	L1
Ff Cough Lozenge	Menthol	L3
Flax Seed Oil 1000 Mg Om3 Cap	Omega-3-Acid Ethyl Esters	L3
Flaxseed Bns 1000 Mg Sgc	Omega-3-Acid Ethyl Esters	L3
Flaxseed 1000 Mg Sgc	Omega-3-Acid Ethyl Esters	L3
Fleet	Sodium Phosphate Dibasic-Dibasic Anhydrous	L3
Fleet Bagenema	Sodium Phosphate Dibasic-Dibasic Anhydrous	L3
Fleet Bisacod 10Mg Enm	Bisacodyl	L2
Fleet Bisacod 5 Mg Tab	Bisacodyl	L2
Fleet Bisacodyl Suppositories	Bisacodyl	L2
Fleet Enema	Sodium Phosphate Dibasic-Dibasic Anhydrous	L3
Fleet Enema Adult Enm	Sodium Phosphate Dibasic-Dibasic Anhydrous	L3
Fleet Enema Min Oil Enm	Mineral Oil (Paraffin)	L3

OTC NAME	DRUGS	LRC
Fleet Enema	Sodium Phosphate Dibasic-Dibasic Anhydrous	L3
Fleet Extra Enm	Sodium Phosphate Dibasic-Dibasic Anhydrous	L3
Fleet Glycerine Suppostrs Adlt	Glycerin	L3
Fleet Glycern Adult Sup	Glycerin	L3
Fleet Lax	Bisacodyl	L2
Fleet Laxative	Bisacodyl	L2
Fleet Pain Relief Pre-Moistened Anorectal Pads	Pramoxine	L3
Fleet Phosphosoda Flavored	Sodium Phosphate Dibasic-Dibasic Anhydrous	L3
Fleet Phospho-Soda Oral Saline Laxative Flavored	Sodium Phosphate Dibasic-Dibasic Anhydrous	L3
Fleet Phosphosoda Unflavored	Sodium Phosphate Dibasic-Dibasic Anhydrous	L3
Folgard Tab	Folic Acid	L1
Folic Acid 400 Mcg Tab	Folic Acid	L1
Formaldehy Ds ⅗ % Usp Sol	Formaldehyde	L4
Fostex 10 Bpo Gel	Benzoyl Peroxide	L2
Fungi Nail Anti-Fungal Solution	Tolnaftate	L3
Gas-X Antigas Chewable Tablets	Simethicone	L3
Gaviscon Acid Breakthrough Chewable Tablets	Calcium Carbonate	L3
Gaviscon Extra Strength Liquid	Aluminum Hydroxide	L2
Gelusil Chewable Tablets	Magnesium Hydroxide	L1
	Aluminum Hydroxide	L2
	Simethicone	L3
Geritol Tab	Multivitamin	L3
Ginkgo Biloba	Ginkgo Biloba	L3
Ginseng Gold-Korean Ginseng Royal Jelly	Ginseng	L3
Gnp Acid Rdcr Bns 30+10 Tab	Famotidine	L1
Gyne Cure Vaginal Ovule	Tioconazole	L3
Gyne-Lotrimin 3-Day	Clotrimazole	L1
Gyno-Trosyd Vaginal Ointment	Tioconazole	L3
Hibclens	Chlorhexidine	L4
Hydrocort 0.5 % Ont	Hydrocortisone Topical	L2
Ibprofen Tablets	Ibuprofen	L1
Ichthammol 20 % Ont	Ichthammol	L3
Icy Hot	Menthol	L3
Icy Hot Balm Ont	Methyl Salicylate	L3 (L5 In Viral Syndromes)
	Menthol	L3
Imodium	Loperamide	L2
Iodine Hm 2% Mild Tnc	Iodine	L4
Iodine Mild 2 % Tnc	Iodine	L4
Ipecac Hm Usp Sol	Herbal Supplement/Teas	L4
Ipecac Syrup	Herbal Supplement/Teas	L4
Kaopectate Caplets	Bismuth Subsalicylate	L3
Kava Kava Extract 250Mg (30 Kavalactones)	Kava-Kava	L5
Kava Kava Root 337576	Kava-Kava	L5

OTC NAME	DRUGS	LRC
Kava Valerian	Kava-Kava	L5
	Valerian Officinalis	L3
Lac-Dose Tab	Lactase	L3
Lactaid	Lactase	L3
Lactaid Cpl	Mannitol	L3
Lactaid Fast Act Chw	Lactase	L3
Lactinex 1 Gm Grn	Probiotics	L3
Lamisil Af 1 % Crm	Terbinafine	L2
Lamisil At	Terbinafine	L2
Lamisil At 1 % Pwd	Terbinafine	L2
Lamisil At Antifungal Cream	Terbinafine	L2
Lanacane Maximum Strength	Benzocaine	L2
L-Carnitine 250 Mg Cap	Carnitine	L2
Loratadine 10 Mg Tab	Loratadine	L1
Lotrim Af Antifungal Aerosol Liquid Spray	Miconazole	L2
Lotrimin Cream	Clotrimazole	L1
Lotrimin Deo Pwdr Super Spy	Clotrimazole	L1
Lotrimin Spray	Miconazole	L2
Lotrimin Ultra Antifungal Cream	Butenafine	L3
Maalox	Magnesium Hydroxide	L1
	Aluminum Hydroxide	L2
	Simethicone	L3
Maalox Antacid-75 Tablets-Mint Creme Flavor	Calcium Carbonate	L3
Meclizine 12.5 Mg Tab	Meclizine	L3
Melatonin 1 Mg Tab	Melatonin	L3
Mentholatum Jar Ont	Camphor	L3
	Menthol	L3
Mercurochrome	Merbromin + Mercurochrome	Hazardous
Micatin	Miconazole	L2
Micatin Af Spray Powder	Miconazole	L2
Midol Cramp Formula	Ibuprofen	L1
Midol Extended Relief Caplets	Naproxen	L3 For Acute Use/L4 For Chronic Use
Midol M/S Gcp	Caffeine	L2
	Acetaminophen	L1
	Pyrilamine	L3
Milk Mag	Magnesium Hydroxide	L1
Milk Thistle	Herbal Supplement/Teas	L4
Milk Thistle 277339	Herbal Supplement/Teas	L4
Monistat 1 Vaginal Ointment	Tioconazole	L3
Monistat 1-Day	Miconazole	L2
Motrin Migraine	Ibuprofen	L1

OTC NAME	DRUGS	LRC
Motrin Pm Tab	Ibuprofen	L1
	Diphenhydramine	L2
Motrin Sinus Cold Flu	Ibuprofen	L1
	Pseudoephedrine	L3
Mucinex	Guaifenesin	L2
Mucinex D Extended Release Tablets	Pseudoephedrine	L3
	Guaifenesin	L2
Mucinex Dm Expectorant / Cough Suppressant, Extended Release Bi-Layer Tablets	Dextromethorphan	L1
	Guaifenesin	L2
Mucinex Exp 600 Mg Tab	Guaifenesin	L2
Mylanta	Calcium Carbonate	L3
	Magnesium Hydroxide	L1
Mylanta Ds Tablets Cherry	Simethicone	L3
Mylanta Gas Maximum Strength Softgels	Simethicone	L3
Mylanta Regular Strength Liquid	Magnesium Hydroxide	L1
	Aluminum Hydroxide	L2
	Simethicone	L3
Mylanta Supreme Antacid Liquid	Aluminum Hydroxide	L2
	Magnesium Hydroxide	L1
Mylanta Supreme Smooth Cherry Creme	Calcium Carbonate	L3
	Magnesium Hydroxide	L1
Mylanta Ultimate Strength Chewable Tablets	Calcium Carbonate	L3
	Magnesium Hydroxide	L1
Naproxen	Naproxen	L3 For Acute Use/L4 For Chronic Use
Neosporin	Neomycin	L3/L5 On Nipple
	Polymyxin B Sulfate	L2
Neosporin Af	Miconazole	L2
Neosporin Af Antifungal Cream	Miconazole	L2
Neosporin Ointment	Bacitracin	L2
	Polymyxin B Sulfate	L2
	Neomycin	L3/L5 On Nipple
Neosporin On The Go Spy	Polymyxin B Sulfate	L2
	Neomycin	L3/L5 On Nipple
	Pramoxine	L3
Neosporin Plus Crm	Polymyxin B Sulfate	L2
	Neomycin	L3/L5 On Nipple
	Pramoxine	L3
Neosporin Plus Ont	Polymyxin B Sulfate	L2
	Neomycin	L3/L5 On Nipple
	Pramoxine	L3

OTC NAME	DRUGS	LRC
Neosporin To Go Ointment	Polymyxin B Sulfate	L2
	Neomycin	L3/L5 On Nipple
	Bacitracin	L2
Neo-Synephrine 1/2 Spray Reg	Phenylephrine	L3
Neo-Synephrine 12 Hour Extra Decongestant Nasal Spray	Oxymetazoline	L3
Niacin 100 Mg Tab	Niacin	L3
Nicoderm Cq 21 Mg Pat	Nicotine	L2
Nicorette 2 Mg Gum	Nicotine	L2
Nix	Permethrin	L2
Nix Complete Lice Trmnt Kit	Permethrin	L2
Nupercainal	Dibucaine	L3
Nupercainal Ointment	Dibucaine	L3
Nuprin	Ibuprofen	L1
Nyquil Alc Fr Cold Flu Liq	Chlorpheniramine	L3
	Acetaminophen	L1
	Dextromethorphan	L1
Nyquil Bonus 20% Free Gcp	Doxylamine	L3
	Dextromethorphan	L1
	Acetaminophen	L1
Nyquil Bonus Orig Liq	Dextromethorphan	L1
	Acetaminophen	L1
	Doxylamine	L3
Nyquil Cherry Bonus Liq	Dextromethorphan	L1
	Acetaminophen	L1
	Doxylamine	L3
Nytol	Diphenhydramine	L2
Omeprazole Dr 20 Mg Tab	Omeprazole	L2
Ortivin Drops 737259	Xylometazoline	L3
Pamprin Max Tab	Aspirin	L3 (L5 In Viral Syndromes)
	Acetaminophen	L1
	Caffeine	L2
Pamprin Mcrf Cpl	Pamabrom	L3
	Acetaminophen	L1
	Pyrilamine	L3
Pamprin Multi Symp Cpl	Pamabrom	L3
	Acetaminophen	L1
	Pyrilamine	L3
Panadeine	Acetaminophen	L1
	Codeine	L3/L5 In Rapid Metabolizers
Panadol	Acetaminophen	L1
Pepcid Ac Chewable Tablets	Famotidine	L1

OTC NAME	DRUGS	LRC
Pepcid Complete Chewable Tablets	Famotidine	L1
	Calcium Carbonate	L3
	Magnesium Hydroxide	L1
Pepto-Bismol	Bismuth Subsalicylate	L3
Pepto-Bismol Liquid	Bismuth Subsalicylate	L3
Peri-Colace Tablets	Senna Laxatives	L3
	Docusate	L2
Permethrin Cream	Permethrin	L2
Pinworm Ds Medic Cpl	Pyrantel	L3
Pinworm Medic Sus	Pyrantel	L3
Pin-X 50 Mg/Ml Sol	Pyrantel	L3
Polysporin	Polymyxin B Sulfate	L2
	Bacitracin	L2
Prep H Suppos	Phenylephrine	L3
Preparation H Anti-Itch Cream	Hydrocortisone Topical	L2
Prevacid	Lansoprazole	L3
Prilosec Otc Tablets	Omeprazole	L2
Primatene	Epinephrine	L1
Pseudoephdrine	Pseudoephedrine	L3
Pyridoxine 50 Mg Tab	Pyridoxine	L2/L4 In High Doses
Ranitidine 150 Mg Tab	Ranitidine	L2
Robitussin	Dextromethorphan	L1
	Brompheniramine	L3
	Pseudoephedrine	L3
Robitussin Allergy & Cough Liquid	Pseudoephedrine	L3
	Brompheniramine	L3
	Dextromethorphan	L1
Robitussin Cf Liquid	Phenylephrine	L3
	Dextromethorphan	L1
	Guaifenesin	L2
Robitussin Cf Max Syr	Guaifenesin	L2
	Dextromethorphan	L1
	Phenylephrine	L3
Robitussin Cf To Go Syr	Phenylephrine	L3
	Guaifenesin	L2
	Dextromethorphan	L1
Robitussin Cold & Congestion Tablets	Chlorpheniramine	L3
	Acetaminophen	L1
	Phenylephrine	L3
Robitussin Cold & Cough Cf Liquid	Phenylephrine	L3
	Dextromethorphan	L1

OTC NAME	DRUGS	LRC
Robitussin Cold, Multisymptom Cold & Flu Softgels	Guaifenesin	L2
	Pseudoephedrine	L3
	Acetaminophen	L1
	Dextromethorphan	L1
Robitussin Cough & Cold Long-Acting Liquid	Chlorpheniramine	L3
	Dextromethorphan	L1
Robitussin Cough & Congestion Liquid	Dextromethorphan	L1
	Guaifenesin	L2
Robitussin Cough And Cold	Guaifenesin	L2
	Dextromethorphan	L1
	Phenylephrine	L3
Robitussin Cough Gels Liqui-Gels	Dextromethorphan	L1
Robitussin Cough Lgl	Dextromethorphan	L1
Robitussin Cough Long-Acting Liquid	Dextromethorphan	L1
Robitussin Cough Medicine	Dextromethorphan	L1
Robitussin Dm Cough Suppressant/Expectorant	Dextromethorphan	L1
	Guaifenesin	L2
Robitussin Dm Liquid	Dextromethorphan	L1
Rogaine	Minoxidil	L2 Topically/L3 Orally
Rolaids	Calcium Carbonate	L3
Selsun Bl	Selenium Sulfide	L3
Selsun Blue Dandruff Shampoo	Selenium Sulfide	L3
Senna Lax	Senna Laxatives	L3
Senokot Granls 2723377	Senna Laxatives	L3
Senokot Lax	Senna Laxatives	L3
Senokot Tab	Senna Laxatives	L3
Simethicone 80 Mg Tab	Simethicone	L3
Simethicone Chew 80 Mg Tab	Simethicone	L3
Sinutab	Guaifenesin	L2
	Acetaminophen	L1
	Pseudoephedrine	L3
	Chlorpheniramine	L3
Sinutab Coated Caplets	Acetaminophen	L1
	Phenylephrine	L3
Sinutab Max Wd Strngt Cpl	Acetaminophen	L1
	Phenylephrine	L3
Sleepeze	Diphenhydramine	L2
Sleepinal Cap	Diphenhydramine	L2
Solarcaine Aer	Lidocaine	L2
	Aloe Vera	L3
Sominex	Diphenhydramine	L2
St Johns Wort	St. John's Wort	L2
Stridex	Salicylic Acid, Topical	L3

OTC NAME	DRUGS	LRC
Sucrets	Menthol	L3
Sucrets Cgh Supp Cherry Loz	Dextromethorphan	L1
Sudafed	Pseudoephedrine	L3
Sudafed Cold & Cough Capsules	Pseudoephedrine	L3
	Dextromethorphan	L1
	Acetaminophen	L1
	Guaifenesin	L2
Sudafed Cold & Sinus Nondrowsy Liqui-Caps	Pseudoephedrine	L3
	Acetaminophen	L1
Sudafed Cold Cough Liquid Caps	Pseudoephedrine	L3
	Guaifenesin	L2
	Dextromethorphan	L1
	Acetaminophen	L1
Sudafed Pe Sinus Headache Caplets	Pseudoephedrine	L3
	Acetaminophen	L1
Sudafed Pe Tablets	Phenylephrine	L3
Sudafed Severe Cold Formula	Dextromethorphan	L1
	Acetaminophen	L1
	Pseudoephedrine	L3
Sudafed Sinus	Acetaminophen	L1
	Pseudoephedrine	L3
Sudafed Sinus & Allergy Tablets	Chlorpheniramine	L3
	Pseudoephedrine	L3
Sudafed Sinus & Cold Liquid Capsules	Acetaminophen	L1
	Pseudoephedrine	L3
Sudafed Sinus Caplets Bns	Acetaminophen	L1
	Pseudoephedrine	L3
Sudafed Sinus Nighttime Plus Pain Relief	Diphenhydramine	L2
	Acetaminophen	L1
	Pseudoephedrine	L3
Sudafed Sinus Nighttime Tablets	Triprolidine	L1
	Pseudoephedrine	L3
Sudafed Sinus Pe Nighttime Cold Caplets	Diphenhydramine	L2
	Acetaminophen	L1
	Phenylephrine	L3
Sudafed Sn/Pn 12Hr Pse Cpl	Pseudoephedrine	L3
	Acetaminophen	L1
	Diphenhydramine	L2
Surfak	Docusate	L2
Tagament Hb	Cimetidine	L1
Tavist Allergy/Sinus/Headache Tablets	Clemastine	L4
	Acetaminophen	L1
	Pseudoephedrine	L3

OTC NAME	DRUGS	LRC
Tavist Allrgy Tab	Clemastine	L4
Tavist D Allergy/Sinus/Headache	Pseudoephedrine	L3
	Clemastine	L4
	Acetaminophen	L1
Tavist-D Cld Rlf	Clemastine	L4
	Phenylpropanolamine	L2
Lidocaine	Lidocaine	L2
Terconazole	Terconazole	L3
Terbinafine	Terbinafine	L2
Tetrahydrozoline	Tetrahydrozoline	L3
Theraflu	Pheniramine	L3
	Dextromethorphan	L1
	Phenylephrine	L3
Theraflu Cold & Cough Hot Liquid	Acetaminophen	L1
	Phenylephrine	L3
	Dextromethorphan	L1
Theraflu Cold & Cough Nighttime Powder	Pseudoephedrine	L3
	Acetaminophen	L1
	Chlorpheniramine	L3
	Dextromethorphan	L1
Theraflu Cold & Sore Throat Hot Liquid	Phenylephrine	L3
	Pheniramine	L3
	Acetaminophen	L1
Theraflu Cold Cough Pwd	Pheniramine	L3
	Dextromethorphan	L1
	Phenylephrine	L3
Theraflu Cold Sore Throat Pwd	Pheniramine	L3
	Acetaminophen	L1
	Phenylephrine	L3
Theraflu Cold Warm Sinus Liq	Diphenhydramine	L2
	Acetaminophen	L1
	Phenylephrine	L3
Theraflu D/N Svr C&C Pk Pwd	Phenylephrine	L3
	Dextromethorphan	L1
	Acetaminophen	L1
	Diphenhydramine	L2
Theraflu Day Svr C&C Pwd	Phenylephrine	L3
	Dextromethorphan	L1
	Acetaminophen	L1
Theraflu Daytime Cold & Cough Liquid	Phenylephrine	L3
	Dextromethorphan	L1

OTC NAME	DRUGS	LRC
Theraflu Daytime Severe Cold Caplets	Phenylephrine	L3
	Acetaminophen	L1
	Dextromethorphan	L1
Theraflu Daytime Severe Cold Hot Liquid	Phenylephrine	L3
	Acetaminophen	L1
Theraflu Daytime Warming Relief Syrup	Phenylephrine	L3
	Acetaminophen	L1
	Dextroamphetamine	L3 In Clinical Doses/L5 If Abused
Theraflu Dt Ms Cold Cap	Dextromethorphan	L1
	Acetaminophen	L1
	Phenylephrine	L3
Theraflu Dynt Warm Combo Liq	Phenylephrine	L3
	Dextromethorphan	L1
	Acetaminophen	L1
	Diphenhydramine	L2
Theraflu Flu & Chest Liquid	Guaifenesin	L2
	Acetaminophen	L1
Theraflu Flu & Sore Throat Liquid	Pheniramine	L3
	Acetaminophen	L1
	Phenylephrine	L3
Theraflu Flu & Sore Throat Relief Syrup	Diphenhydramine	L2
	Acetaminophen	L1
	Phenylephrine	L3
Theraflu Flu, Cold & Cough And Sore Throat Maximum Strength Powder	Pseudoephedrine	L3
	Acetaminophen	L1
	Chlorpheniramine	L3
	Dextromethorphan	L1
Theraflu Flu/ Chst Congst Pwd	Acetaminophen	L1
	Guaifenesin	L2
Theraflu Flu/ Sore Throat Pwd	Pheniramine	L3
	Acetaminophen	L1
	Phenylephrine	L3
Theraflu Max Pse Severe Pwd	Guaifenesin	L2
	Dextromethorphan	L1
	Acetaminophen	L1
	Pseudoephedrine	L3
Theraflu Nght Svr C&C Pwd	Diphenhydramine	L2
	Acetaminophen	L1
	Phenylephrine	L3
Theraflu Nighttime Warning Relief Syrup	Diphenhydramine	L2
	Acetaminophen	L1
	Phenylephrine	L3

OTC NAME	DRUGS	LRC
Theraflu Nighttime Cold & Cough Thin Strips	Diphenhydramine	L2
	Phenylephrine	L3
Theraflu Nighttime Severe Cold Caplets	Phenylephrine	L3
	Chlorpheniramine	L3
	Acetaminophen	L1
	Dextromethorphan	L1
Theraflu Nighttime Severe Hot Liquid	Phenylephrine	L3
	Diphenhydramine	L2
	Acetaminophen	L1
Tinactin	Tolnaftate	L3
Titralac	Calcium Carbonate	L3
Titralac 420 Mg Tab	Calcium Carbonate	L3
Tolnaftate 1 % Anti Crm	Tolnaftate	L3
Triaminic	Acetaminophen	L1
Triaminic Cgh Rnny Nose Chw	Diphenhydramine	L2
Triaminic Chest & Nasal Liquid	Phenylephrine	L3
	Guaifenesin	L2
Triaminic Cng Ch/Nsl Liq	Guaifenesin	L2
	Phenylephrine	L3
Triaminic Cold & Allergy Liquid	Diphenhydramine	L2
Triaminic Cold With Stuffy Nose Thin Strips	Phenylephrine	L3
Triaminic Cough & Sore Throat Liquid	Acetaminophen	L1
	Dextromethorphan	L1
Triaminic D M/S Cold Liq	Dextromethorphan	L1
	Phenylephrine	L3
Triaminic Day Cold Cough Stp	Dextromethorphan	L1
	Phenylephrine	L3
Triaminic Daytime Cold & Cough Liquid	Phenylephrine	L3
	Dextromethorphan	L1
Triaminic Dt/ Nt Cc Pck Liq	Phenylephrine	L3
	Diphenhydramine	L2
	Dextromethorphan	L1
Triaminic Flu Cough & Fever Liquid	Chlorpheniramine	L3
	Acetaminophen	L1
	Dextromethorphan	L1
Triaminic Long Acting Cough Liquid	Dextromethorphan	L1
Triaminic Long Acting Cough Thin Strips	Dextromethorphan	L1
Triaminic Nighttime Cough & Cold Liquid	Diphenhydramine	L2
	Phenylephrine	L3
Triaminic Nighttime Cough & Cold Thin Strips	Diphenhydramine	L2
	Phenylephrine	L3
Triaminic Softchews Cough & Runny Nose	Chlorpheniramine	L3
	Dextromethorphan	L1

OTC NAME	DRUGS	LRC
Triaminic Softchews Cough & Sore Throat Daytime Liquid	Acetaminophen	L1
	Dextromethorphan	L1
Triaminic Sore Throat Grape Flavor	Acetaminophen	L1
	Dextromethorphan	L1
Triaminic Triaminicol (Cough Cold)	Phenylpropanolamine	L2
	Dextromethorphan	L1
	Chlorpheniramine	L3
Triaminicin	Chlorpheniramine	L3
	Acetaminophen	L1
	Pseudoephedrine	L3
Triple Antib 5M Un Ont	Bacitracin	L2
	Polymyxin B Sulfate	L2
	Neomycin	L3/L5 On Nipple
Triple Antib Foil Ont	Polymyxin B Sulfate	L2
	Neomycin	L3/L5 On Nipple
	Bacitracin	L2
Triple Antib Ont	Polymyxin B Sulfate	L2
	Neomycin	L3/L5 On Nipple
	Bacitracin	L2
Tylenol	Acetaminophen	L1
Tylenol 8-Hour	Acetaminophen	L1
Tylenol Allergy Complete Multi-Symptom Cool Burst Caplets	Chlorpheniramine	L3
	Acetaminophen	L1
	Phenylephrine	L3
Tylenol Allergy Complete Nighttime Cool Burst Caplets	Diphenhydramine	L2
	Acetaminophen	L1
	Phenylephrine	L3
Tylenol Allergy Multi-Symptom Caplets	Chlorpheniramine	L3
	Acetaminophen	L1
	Phenylephrine	L3
Tylenol Allergy Multi-Symptom Nighttime Caplets	Diphenhydramine	L2
	Acetaminophen	L1
	Phenylephrine	L3
Tylenol Allergy Sinus	Chlorpheniramine	L3
	Acetaminophen	L1
	Pseudoephedrine	L3
Tylenol Allergy Sinus, Maximum Strength Tablets, Gelcaps And Geltabs	Chlorpheniramine	L3
	Acetaminophen	L1
	Pseudoephedrine	L3
Tylenol Alrgy M/S Night Cpl	Diphenhydramine	L2
	Acetaminophen	L1
	Phenylephrine	L3

OTC NAME	DRUGS	LRC
Tylenol Alrgy M/S Severe Cpl	Acetaminophen	L1
	Diphenhydramine	L2
Tylenol Arth	Acetaminophen	L1
Tylenol Arthritis Caplets	Acetaminophen	L1
Tylenol C & C Day Clbrst Liq	Acetaminophen	L1
	Dextromethorphan	L1
Tylenol Cold Citr Ms Day Liq	Dextromethorphan	L1
	Acetaminophen	L1
	Phenylephrine	L3
Tylenol Cold Cng/ Pn Day Cpl	Dextromethorphan	L1
	Phenylephrine	L3
	Acetaminophen	L1
Tylenol Cold Complete Formula Tablets	Dextromethorphan	L1
	Acetaminophen	L1
	Chlorpheniramine	L3
	Pseudoephedrine	L3
Tylenol Cold Cool Ms Ngt Liq	Doxylamine	L3
	Dextromethorphan	L1
	Acetaminophen	L1
	Phenylephrine	L3
Tylenol Cold De Cngst Cpl	Dextromethorphan	L1
	Acetaminophen	L1
	Phenylephrine	L3
Tylenol Cold Extra Strength	Dextromethorphan	L1
	Acetaminophen	L1
	Phenylephrine	L3
Tylenol Cold Head Congestion Day/Night Pack	Phenylephrine	L3
	Acetaminophen	L1
	Dextromethorphan	L1
Tylenol Cold Head Congestion Daytime Caplets	Phenylephrine	L3
	Acetaminophen	L1
	Dextromethorphan	L1
Tylenol Cold Head Congestion Daytime Capsules	Phenylephrine	L3
	Acetaminophen	L1
	Dextromethorphan	L1
Tylenol Cold Head Congestion Nighttime Caplets	Phenylephrine	L3
	Chlorpheniramine	L3
	Acetaminophen	L1
	Dextromethorphan	L1
Tylenol Extra Strength Gelcaps	Acetaminophen	L1

OTC NAME	DRUGS	LRC
Tylenol Flu Day Night Convenience Pack	Phenylephrine	L3
	Dextromethorphan	L1
	Acetaminophen	L1
	Chlorpheniramine	L3
Tylenol Flu Daytime Gelcaps	Phenylephrine	L3
	Acetaminophen	L1
	Dextromethorphan	L1
Tylenol Pm Caplets	Acetaminophen	L1
	Diphenhydramine	L2
Tylenol Pm Caplets	Acetaminophen	L1
	Diphenhydramine	L2
Tylenol Sinus Congestion & Pain Daytime Caplets	Acetaminophen	L1
	Phenylephrine	L3
Tylenol Sinus Congestion & Pain Daytime Gelcaps	Acetaminophen	L1
	Phenylephrine	L3
Tylenol Sinus Congestion & Pain Daytime Rapid Release Gelcaps	Acetaminophen	L1
	Phenylephrine	L3
Tylenol Sinus Congestion & Pain Nighttime Caplets	Chlorpheniramine	L3
	Acetaminophen	L1
	Phenylephrine	L3
Tylenol Sinus Congestion & Severe Pain Caplets	Acetaminophen	L1
	Phenylephrine	L3
Tylenol Sinus Pain Day Cpl	Acetaminophen	L1
	Phenylephrine	L3
Tylenol Sinus Pain Nt Cpl	Phenylephrine	L3
	Acetaminophen	L1
	Chlorpheniramine	L3
Tylenol Sinus Severe Congestion	Guaifenesin	L2
	Acetaminophen	L1
	Pseudoephedrine	L3
Tylenol Sinus Severe Congestion Daytime Caplets	Pseudoephedrine	L3
	Acetaminophen	L1
	Guaifenesin	L2
Tylenol Sore Throat Nighttime Liquid	Acetaminophen	L1
	Diphenhydramine	L2
Tylenol Ultra	Acetaminophen	L1
	Caffeine	L2
Tylenol Women's Caplets	Acetaminophen	L1
	Pamabrom	L3
Tylenol Women's Mentral Relief	Acetaminophen	L1
	Pamabrom	L3
Tylenol X Strength Caplet Vial	Acetaminophen	L1

OTC NAME	DRUGS	LRC
Tylnl 50 S Flu Fs	Guaifenesin	L2
	Dextromethorphan	L1
	Acetaminophen	L1
	Phenylephrine	L3
Unisom	Diphenhydramine	L2
Unisom Pm Pain Cpl	Acetaminophen	L1
	Diphenhydramine	L2
Vaginex	Tripelennamine	L4
Vagisil Anti-Itch Creme	Lidocaine	L2
Vagisil Maximum Strength Anti-Itch Creme	Benzocaine	L2
Vagisil Orig Crm	Benzocaine	L2
Vagisil Wipe Wpe	Pramoxine	L3
Vagistat	Tioconazole	L3
Vagistat	Miconazole	L2
Vagnex Yeast Care	Zinc Oxide	L2
Valerian	Valerian Officinalis	L3
Vicks	Menthol	L3
	Camphor	L3
	Eucalyptus	L3
Vicks 44 C/C Cgh/ Cld Pm Liq	Dextromethorphan	L1
	Chlorpheniramine	L3
	Acetaminophen	L1
Vicks 44 C/C Chst Cgh Br Liq	Dextromethorphan	L1
	Guaifenesin	L2
Vicks 44 C/C Cngs Brry Liq	Dextromethorphan	L1
	Phenylephrine	L3
Vicks 44 C/C Dry Cgh Br Liq	Dextromethorphan	L1
Vicks 44 Cgh W/Vit C Drps	Dextromethorphan	L1
	Acetaminophen	L1
	Doxylamine	L3
Vicks 44 Liquid	Dextromethorphan	L1
Vicks 44 W/Free Drops	Menthol	L3
Vicks 44 W/Vit C Drops	Dextromethorphan	L1
	Acetaminophen	L1
	Phenylephrine	L3
Vicks 44D Cough & Congestion Relief Liquid	Phenylephrine	L3
	Dextromethorphan	L1
Vicks 44E Cough & Chest Congestion Relief	Dextromethorphan	L1
	Guaifenesin	L2
Vicks 44E Liquid	Dextromethorphan	L1
	Guaifenesin	L2

OTC NAME	DRUGS	LRC
Vicks 44M Liquid	Chlorpheniramine	L3
	Acetaminophen	L1
	Dextromethorphan	L1
Vicks Chloraseptic (Cool Mint Flavor)	Phenol	L3
Vicks Chloraseptic Phenol/Oral Anesthetic Sore Throat Spray-Menthol	Phenol	L3
Vicks Cough Drops Cherry Flavor	Menthol	L3
Vicks Dayquil	Pseudoephedrine	L3
	Acetaminophen	L1
	Dextromethorphan	L1
Vicks Dayquil Cough Liquid	Dextromethorphan	L1
Vicks Dayquil Liquicaps	Phenylephrine	L3
	Acetaminophen	L1
	Dextromethorphan	L1
Vicks Dayquil Liquid	Phenylephrine	L3
	Acetaminophen	L1
	Dextromethorphan	L1
Vicks Dayquil Multi-Symptom Cold/Flu Relief Non-Drowsy	Dextromethorphan	L1
	Acetaminophen	L1
	Phenylephrine	L3
Vicks Dayquil Sinus Liquicaps	Acetaminophen	L1
	Phenylephrine	L3
Vicks Formula 44E Ped Liq	Dextromethorphan	L1
	Guaifenesin	L2
Vicks Nyquil Original	Dextromethorphan	L1
	Doxylamine	L3
Vicks Nyquil Sinus Liquicaps	Doxylamine	L3
	Acetaminophen	L1
	Phenylephrine	L3
Vicks Sinex 12-Hour Nasal Spray	Phenylephrine	L3
Vicks Sinex Long Acting Nasal Spray For Sinus Relief	Oxymetazoline	L3
Vicks Sinex Nasal Spray	Phenylephrine	L3
Vivarin	Caffeine	L2
Zantac	Ranitidine	L2
Zyrtec	Cetirizine	L2
Zyrtec-D 12 Hour Tablets	Pseudoephedrine	L3
	Cetirizine	L2

*   Lactation Risk Category

Index

H

N

Ordering Information

Hale Publishing, L.P.
1712 N. Forest Street
Amarillo, Texas, USA 79106

8:00 am to 5:00 pm CST

Call » 806.376.9900
Sales » 800.378.1317
Fax » 806.376.9901

Online Web Orders
www.ibreastfeeding.com